BLACK'S MEDICAL DICTIONARY

BLACK'S
MEDICAL
DICTIONARY

WILLIAM A. R. THOMSON, M.D.

THIRTY-SECOND EDITION

WITH 2 COLOUR PLATES AND
455 OTHER ILLUSTRATIONS

LONDON
ADAM & CHARLES BLACK
1979

PUBLISHED BY A. AND C. BLACK (PUBLISHERS) LTD
35 BEDFORD ROW LONDON WC1R 4JH

FIRST EDITION (BY J. D. COMRIE, M.D.) 1906
SECOND EDITION 1906
THIRD EDITION 1907
FOURTH EDITION 1910
FIFTH EDITION 1914, REPRINTED 1916
SIXTH EDITION 1918, REPRINTED 1920
SEVENTH EDITION 1922, REPRINTED 1924
EIGHTH EDITION (ENTIRELY RESET) 1926
REPRINTED 1928 (TWICE)
NINTH EDITION 1930
TENTH EDITION 1931
ELEVENTH EDITION 1933
TWELFTH EDITION 1934
THIRTEENTH EDITION 1936
FOURTEENTH EDITION (COMPLETING 100,000) 1937
FIFTEENTH EDITION 1939
SIXTEENTH EDITION 1941
SEVENTEENTH EDITION 1942
REPRINTED 1943

REVISED BY H. A. CLEGG, F.R.C.P.:
EIGHTEENTH EDITION 1944
REPRINTED 1945
REPRINTED, WITH SLIGHT CHANGES, 1946
REPRINTED 1947

REVISED BY W. A. R. THOMSON, M.D.
NINETEENTH EDITION 1948
TWENTIETH EDITION (ENTIRELY RESET) 1951
TWENTY-FIRST EDITION 1953
TWENTY-SECOND EDITION 1955
TWENTY-THIRD EDITION 1958
TWENTY-FOURTH EDITION 1961
TWENTY-FIFTH EDITION 1963
TWENTY-SIXTH EDITION 1965
TWENTY-SEVENTH EDITION 1967
TWENTY-EIGHTH EDITION 1968
TWENTY-NINTH EDITION 1971
REPRINTED 1972
THIRTIETH EDITION (ENTIRELY RESET) 1974
THIRTY-FIRST EDITION 1976
REPRINTED 1978 AND 1979
THIRTY-SECOND EDITION 1979

ISBN 0 7136 1980 5

PRINTED IN GREAT BRITAIN
BY BUTLER AND TANNER LTD, FROME AND LONDON

PREFACE TO
THE THIRTY-SECOND EDITION

It was Thomas Carlyle who referred to 'the folly of that impossible precept, "Know thyself" till it be translated into this partially possible one, "Know what thou canst work at"'. Irritable and intolerant the 'wizard of Chelsea' may have been, but he was a shrewd observer of life. His aphorism is a typical example of his canny, down-to-earth approach to life, and it is one that is very applicable to matters of health.

The inner workings of the body are still sheathed in mystery, even for the medical practitioner. The searching mind in medicine is undoubtedly probing ever deeper into how the human body works, and the deeper it probes the more mysterious and wonderful does *homo sapiens* become. Its more dramatic discoveries, as well as its more sensational theories, are highlighted in the national press – as often as not with more enthusiasm than discrimination. The result is that that useful figment of the imagination – the man, or woman, in the street – becomes even more perplexed, worried or misled.

Hence the increasing necessity for a book such as this that attempts to provide the basic proven (or at least accepted) facts of healthy living so that its readers can 'know what they canst work at'. Healthy living is dependent upon knowledge of how the body works, which in turn is dependent upon an elementary knowledge of anatomy and physiology. This, of course, should be taught in our schools in the course on biology but, as every experienced family doctor knows, even the so-called 'top people' can be incredibly ignorant on such matters.

Equally important is it that the departures from normal that indicate the onset of disease should be appreciated – and for two major reasons. In the first place in order to be able to differentiate between the mild and the serious. In other words, to know when to treat oneself or one's family, and when to seek medical advice. Far too many people today are rushing off unnecessarily to their general practitioners and so cluttering up their surgeries that seriously ill patients are not receiving the attention they need and deserve. Many of the minor ills to which man is heir can be treated just as effectively at home as in the doctor's surgery.

The second major advantage of a modicum of self-knowledge is that it allows one to lead a reasonably healthy, yet still enjoyable, life. Literally, no two individuals are the same, and we must each of us learn our capabilities, mental and physical, and learn how to live within them. In addition, we must learn how to preserve them and how to make the most of them. There is far too much loose talk these days about 'stress and strain', and not enough about striving. Nature not only abhors a vacuum, it also abhors laziness and lack of activity. The muscle that is not regularly exercised to its optimal extent atrophies. So does the mind, the zest for life and every other part of the body. If we are to get the most out of life, and put the most into it, we must have an elementary knowledge of our capabilities and how to use them.

Such is, and always has been, the aim of this book. Over the years its contents have varied with the advances in knowledge but, so far as possible, it has avoided that waxing and waning inseparable from medical theorizing. Advances have been incorporated, not because they are recent, but because they seem to be real advances of practical significance. Superficially, medical research is advancing at a rapid, almost staggering, speed, but much of this is of theoretical interest and, to date, has little practical import. Most of the extravagant claims made by certain research workers, and all too eagerly picked up by Fleet Street, have been ignored, and attention devoted primarily to those problems of every-day life that worry the ordinary citizen, and to those advances that seem to be of practical value in helping him or her to live a healthier life.

This new edition includes around 150 new sections, covering subjects such as legionnaire's disease, thumb-sucking, nursing bottle mouth, burning mouth, budgerigar-fancier's lung, roughage, travel medicine, accident prevention in the home, immersion hypothermia, disabled persons and Remploy, as well as a selection of some of the more important, and apparently proven, new drugs introduced since the last edition. In addition, other sections, such as those on acne, acupuncture, adrenergic receptors, heredity and hypothermia, have been rewritten.

Respect for one's body and full utilization of its capabilities are two of the fundamental laws of healthy living. Both can be achieved with relative ease, and their fulfilment brings that joy of living and zest for life which are the ambition of us all. It is to assist in allowing as many as possible to make full and enjoyable use of their bodies that yet another edition of this book now goes forth.

LONDON, 1979   W.A.R.T.

EXCERPT FROM
PREFACE TO FIRST EDITION

In the preparation of this book the object sought has been to produce a work which would occupy a position somewhere between that of a technical Dictionary of Medicine and one intended merely for the domestic treatment of commoner ailments. An endeavour has accordingly been made to give information in simple language upon medical subjects of importance and general interest.

Definitions are given of most of the terms commonly used in medical science, though no attempt has been made to include all the compound and often hybrid words which have been lately introduced, especially into surgery. Brief notices upon anatomy and physiology precede the lists of diseases to which the various bodily organs are liable. They have been designed mainly with the object of making clear to the reader what are the normal functions and how these are affected by disease. With regard to such practically important matters as those in which unskilled persons can safely be trusted to render aid to the injured, and to increase the comfort of the sick, full details have been given. It is hoped, therefore, that these articles will be found useful to district nurses, ship captains, dwellers in remote districts, and others who may be called upon to treat the suffering in the absence of trained supervision. Those subjects, on the contrary, which are of a more theoretical and intricate nature are sketched only in outline. In this connection, too, it may be noted that almost no reference has been made to diagnosis, a highly technical matter, which lies entirely within the province of the trained medical man. Special attention has been given to subjects in which medical science has made recent advances, but care has been taken to avoid speculative and debatable views, and to keep as closely as possible to what are generally recognized as ascertained facts. In the case of surgical subjects, the principles upon which the measures of treatment are based have been explained, but the details of operations are quite foreign to the scope of this book. Proprietary medicines and food-stuffs are mentioned as seldom as possible.

J. D. C.

EDINBURGH, 1906

ABDOMEN is the lower part of the trunk. Above, and separated from it by the diaphragm or midriff, lies the thorax or chest, and below lies the pelvis, or basin, generally described as a separate cavity though directly continuous with that of the abdomen. Behind lie the spinal column and lower ribs which come within a few inches of the iliac or haunch bones; stomach, and of the various important movements of the organs associated with digestion. The shape of the abdomen varies; in children it may protrude considerably, though if this be too marked it may indicate disease; in healthy young adults it should be either very slightly prominent or slightly indrawn, and should show the outline of the muscular layer,

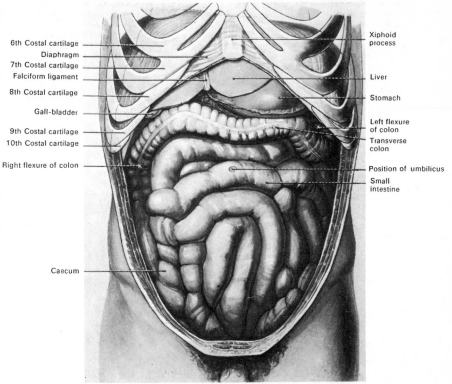

6th Costal cartilage
Diaphragm
7th Costal cartilage
Falciform ligament
8th Costal cartilage
Gall-bladder
9th Costal cartilage
10th Costal cartilage
Right flexure of colon
Caecum

Xiphoid process
Liver
Stomach
Left flexure of colon
Transverse colon
Position of umbilicus
Small intestine

1 – Contents of the abdomen in position, the front wall of the abdomen and the omentum removed. From Cunningham's *Anatomy*. Oxford University Press.

at the sides the protection afforded to the contained organs by the iliac bones and down-sloping ribs is still more effective; but in front the whole extent is protected only by soft tissues. The latter consist of the skin, a varying amount of fat, three layers of broad, flat muscle, another layer of fat, and finally the smooth, thin peritoneum which lines the whole cavity. The absence of rigidity allows of the necessary distension when food is taken into the especially of the pair of muscles running vertically (recti), which are divided into four or five sections by transverse lines; while with advance of age it is quite natural that a certain amount of fat should be deposited on and inside the abdomen.

Contents – The principal contents of the abdominal cavity are the digestive organs, ie. stomach, intestines, and the associated glands the liver and pancreas (plate I and illustration 1). The position of the stomach is above and to the left when the individual is recumbent, but may be much lower in the erect position. The liver lies above and to the right, lying to a large extent under cover of the ribs, and occupying the hollow of the diaphragm, by which alone both it and the stomach are separated from the lungs and heart. Against the back wall on either side lie the kidneys (plate II), protected also to a great extent by the last two ribs; and from the kidneys run the ureters, or urinary ducts, down along the back wall to the bladder in the pelvis. The pancreas lies across the spine between the kidneys, and upon the upper end of each kidney lies a suprarenal gland. High up on the left and partly behind the stomach lies the spleen. The great blood-vessels and nerves, the absorbent vessels and the glands connected with them, lie on the back wall, and the remainder of the space is taken up by the intestines or bowels (see INTESTINE), the large intestine lying in the flanks on either side in front of the kidneys and crossing below the stomach from right to left, while the small intestine hangs from the back wall in coils which fill up the spaces between the other organs. Hanging down from the stomach in front of the bowels is the omentum, or apron, containing a considerable amount of fat, and helping to protect the bowels from cold and injury. In pregnancy the uterus, or womb, as it increases in size, rises up from the pelvis into the abdomen, lifting the coils of the small intestine above it.

The *pelvis* is that portion of the abdomen which lies within the bony pelvis (see BONE), and contains the rectum or end part of the intestine, the bladder, and, in the male the prostate, in the female the uterus, ovaries, and Fallopian tubes.

ABDOMEN, DISEASES OF – (See under STOMACH, DISEASES OF; INTESTINE, DISEASES OF; DIARRHOEA; LIVER, DISEASES OF; PANCREAS, DISEASES OF; KIDNEY, DISEASES OF; BLADDER, DISEASES OF; HERNIA; PERITONITIS; APPENDICITIS; TUMOURS.)

Symptoms – The symptoms of various diseases will be found under the above headings, and only some general symptoms of abdominal disease, or symptoms, the meaning of which is not plain, but which nevertheless point to trouble in definite organs, will be mentioned here.

PAIN – This is a most important symptom, because the internal organs being devoid of ordinary sensation, pain in them generally means a considerable interfer-

ence with structure or function. The *site* of the pain may indicate the organ affected. Thus pain under the ribs on the left, or in the pit of the stomach, generally points to the stomach as being at fault. When it is felt on the right high up, and shoots through to the right shoulder, it indicates trouble connected with the liver or gall-bladder. Pain situated on the right, and low down in the iliac region, may arise from a diseased appendix. On the left, and low down, or at the exit of the bowel, it means some rectal trouble. Finally, pain situated vaguely all over the front of the abdomen, especially round the navel, points to inflammation of the peritoneal lining of the abdomen, or to irregularity in movement of the small intestine.

The *character* of the pain is also important. A dull, aching pain is not generally serious, though, if persistent, it may indicate chronic peritonitis or obstruction. (See PERITONITIS; and INTESTINE, DISEASES OF.) A twisting, griping pain is generally, eg. in babies, due to spasmodic movements of the small intestine, often produced by errors in diet, and called colic. A straining pain with frequent calls to stool indicates irritation low down in the large bowel. The pains of stomach trouble are of varied nature. (See DYSPEPSIA.) Sudden, colicky, agonizing pain is often due to the passage of a gall-stone, if situated high up on the right, shooting through towards the back, or to the passage of a renal calculus, if shooting from the back down into the groin. Pain of a dull character slightly to the right of the pit of the stomach, especially when it is relieved by taking food, suggests some trouble in the duodenum.

TENDERNESS on pressure is generally a sign of inflammation either of an organ situated beneath the tender spot or of the peritoneum. (See APPENDICITIS; PERITONITIS.)

VOMITING is an important symptom. (See VOMITING.) When due to irritation of the stomach, it usually ceases as the contents of this organ are brought up. If it persists, it may be due to some obstruction in the bowels, or may be of nervous origin, eg. in sea-sickness, or brain tumour, and have no direct connection with the abdomen.

DIARRHOEA is another important symptom, and may be of serious import. (See DIARRHOEA.)

SWELLING of the abdomen may be so marked as to call the patient's attention to it. This may be due merely to excessive deposit of fat, especially in elderly people –

for example, in women at the menopause. (See CORPULENCE; DIET.) Enlargement, of course, occurs in pregnancy. The abdomen in habitual constipation may become more distended, partly by accumulation of gas, or the enlargement may be due to chronic obstruction of the bowels. (See CONSTIPATION; and INTESTINE, DISEASES OF.) Finally, a collection of fluid may produce the swelling (see DROPSY; LIVER, DISEASES OF; HEART, DISEASES OF; PERITONITIS), or it may be due to enlargement of a single organ.

INDRAWING of the abdomen occurs in wasting diseases, and also to a marked extent in meningitis. (See MENINGITIS.)

DISTENSION OF THE VEINS on the surface of the abdomen indicates some interference with the circulation in the portal vein or in the inferior vena cava.

VISIBLE MOVEMENTS are sometimes seen, due to the bowels or stomach being distended and contracting forcibly in the attempt to drive their contents onwards. They indicate (unless they are visible merely on account of extreme thinness of the abdominal wall) some obstruction in the bowel or stomach. (See PERISTALSIS.)

The differentiation of abdominal diseases is often one of the most difficult problems with which even an expert has to deal, and frequently it is only after a period of observation, lasting in difficult cases perhaps some weeks, that a diagnosis of approximate accuracy can be arrived at. This is partly due to the difficulty or impossibility of feeling the surface and dimensions of the contained organs, eg. the kidneys, especially in stout persons; partly to the vagueness of symptoms set up in organs which are very little sensitive to even extreme changes in their structure; and partly to the readiness with which the organs change their relative positions, and to the great changes in shape and position often brought about by previous disease.

Treatment – Details of treatment are given under the headings of the various diseases. On the whole, people are rather too much given to regarding abdominal symptoms as trivial and amenable to home treatment. In many a case incurable dyspepsia would have been got rid of in its early stages if its symptoms had not been neglected, and not infrequently patients with acute obstruction of the bowels die because a dose of castor oil was taken when a doctor should have been consulted. In this connection one may say that whenever the three symptoms of (a) abdominal pain, (b) vomiting or retching, and

(c) stoppage of the bowels for a day or two, or stoppage followed by a little diarrhoea, have occurred together, the case demands the attention of a skilled medical adviser. If severe abdominal pain be directly traceable to some dietetic indiscretion, the offending material should be got rid of speedily by an emetic, if it is still in the stomach (see EMETICS); or by a purgative if the symptoms are referable to the bowels (see PURGATIVES). If the pain be griping in character, eg. in babies, relief is often given by pressure; thus nurses often lay their charges stomach downwards across the arm, or adults get some relief by lying face downwards on a pillow. (See COLIC; LEAD-POISONING.) The application of heat, in the form of a hot-water bottle, may also give relief. When the pain is of an agonizing nature, stronger remedies are necessary. (See COLIC.)

ABDOMEN, INJURIES OF – When one considers the exposed nature of the abdomen to the front and the thinness of the wall covering the viscera, it is surprising how seldom blows and crushes damage the contained organs. This is explained by the fact that the firm muscles, which are perhaps half an inch (12 mm) in thickness, offer the same type of protection as would be given by a slab of india-rubber of like thickness tightly stretched, while the fat still further dissipates the effect of violence. When a kick or blow causes rupture of an organ, the violence has generally been unexpected, and the muscles have been surprised in a lax condition. It is true that instantaneous death may follow a comparatively trivial blow on the epigastrium or pit of the stomach, and this is due to shock (see SHOCK) caused by injury to a nerve-plexus situated in the back of the abdomen in that region. Rupture of the liver, kidney, or spleen may occur, with haemorrhage into the surrounding tissues, from severe crushes between railway-carriage buffers, from falls from a height, motor-car accidents, etc.; but these are not necessarily fatal unless some large blood-vessel be torn. Rupture of the bowel occasionally follows a blow or wound and is almost necessarily fatal in a few days, unless the abdomen be opened by a surgeon and the torn bowel stitched within a few hours of the accident.

Persons run over by vehicles are liable to have the bladder ruptured. This occurs especially in the case of children, and it happens only when the bladder is full, or nearly so, of urine. In such a case the inability to pass water soon after the accident, provided that it was not passed for some hours previously, or the passage of blood, indicates the necessity of a speedy operation to stitch the torn bladder.

Straining to lift a weight beyond the strength, or excessive straining at stool, ment, a band which crosses the groin obliquely and divides thigh from abdomen; and two are horizontal: the subcostal plane which passes through the lowest part of the costal margin, and the intertubercular plane which passes through the most outwardly projecting points of the iliac or haunch bones. These

Xiphisternal plane

Tip of 9th costal cartilage

Subcostal plane

Intertubercular plane

Anterior superior iliac spine

2 – Regions of the abdomen. For meanings of letters, see text. From Appleton etc, *Surface and Radiological Anatomy*. W. Heffer and Sons.

may force a loop of the intestine through the muscular part of the abdominal wall, so producing a hernia or rupture. (See HERNIA.)

ABDOMEN, REGIONS OF – For convenience of reference the abdomen is divided into regions by artificial lines (illustration 2). Two are vertical, passing through the middle of the inguinal liga-divide off nine regions named as follows: Epigastrium or pit of the stomach (E), two Hypochondriac regions (H), Umbilical or Navel region (U), two Lumbar or Loin regions (L), Hypogastric region (Hy), and two Iliac regions or Groins (I). The inguinal region on each side is the lower part of the hypogastric region. This contains the inguinal canal which pierces the abdominal wall obliquely.

ABDUCENT NERVE is the sixth nerve rising from the brain and controls the external rectus muscle of the eye, which turns the eye outwards. It is particularly liable to be paralysed in diseases of the nervous system, thus leading to an inward squint.

ABLATION means the removal of any part of the body by a surgical operation.

ABORTIFACIENT is a drug which causes artificial abortion.

ABORTION or MISCARRIAGE, means the separation and expulsion of the contents of the pregnant uterus before the 28th week of pregnancy. The frequency of abortion is not known, but it is estimated that 10 to 15 per cent of pregnancies end in abortion. The common time for abortion to occur is from the 8th to 13th week of pregnancy.

Causes – The cause of the abortion may be found in the mother or in the germ cells, or in some completely extraneous factor.

So far as the mother is concerned, the most common cause is an abnormality of the hormonal balance which controls the course of pregnancy (qv). The main defect is a lack of progesterone (qv). This hormone is secreted by the corpus luteum (qv) in the early weeks of pregnancy and sub-sequently by the placenta (qv). The function of progesterone is to ensure the safe embedding of the fertilized ovum in the mother's uterus (or womb), and then to ensure that the uterus does not start contracting until the time for labour is due. It is thus obvious why a defective supply of progesterone can result in abortion.

Other maternal causes of abortion include disturbances of other endocrine glands, or hormones, such as hypothyroidism, or myxoedema (qv), and diabetes mellitus (qv); high blood pressure; Bright's disease (qv); any acute illness; congenital abnormalities of the uterus, and any severe emotional disturbance.

Two oft-quoted classical causes of abortion are syphilis and drugs. Syphilis is certainly a dangerous disease for a pregnant mother to have, but it is more likely to cause the death of the foetus after the 28th week of pregnancy; and technically this is not an abortion. Several drugs have achieved a popular reputation as abortifacients, or inducers of abortion, but the reputation is usually fallacious. As many a misled woman has found, it is incredibly difficult to induce an abortion by means of drugs in a healthy pregnancy. This even applies to pills containing lead, though there is no doubt that lead can induce an abortion.

Any defect in the germ cells, whether ovum or spermatozoon, may lead to abortion if it is severe enough to cause gross malformation of the embryo.

Finally, reference must be made to criminally induced abortion. This may be attempted in a variety of ways, particularly the introduction of fluids or instruments into the uterus. It is a dangerous practice, as shown by a Ministry of Health investigation into 294 fatal abortions. At least 199 of these were criminal abortions, 105 (53 per cent) of whom died from sepsis. (See also BLIGHTED OVUM.)

Treatment – The treatment depends largely upon whether the abortion is threatened or inevitable. In the case of the former, often a few days' rest in bed is all that is necessary, following which the mother takes particular care at the next two period times. If an abortion is inevitable, the treatment is that of a miniature labour. More complicated, and requiring skilled supervision, is the treatment of what is known as an incomplete abortion (that is, when part of the foetus and/or placenta have been retained in the uterus), and – most dangerous of all – the treatment of a septic abortion.

Therapeutic abortion – Abortion, or termination of pregnancy, is a criminal offence in Britain, but the whole outlook on abortion was changed by the Abortion Act, 1967 which came into force in 1968, and created exceptions to the Offences Against the Persons Act, 1861, which made it an offence 'unlawfully to administer any poison or other noxious thing or to use any instrument or any other means whatsoever with intent to procure a miscarriage', or to supply any such poison or instrument for this purpose. Under the terms of the 1967 Act, a pregnancy can be terminated: in other words, an abortion can be induced by a 'registered medical practitioner if two registered medical practitioners are of the opinion, formed in good faith, (a) that the continuance of the pregnancy would involve risk to the life of the pregnant woman or of injury to the physical or mental health of the pregnant woman or any existing children of her family greater than if the pregnancy were terminated; or (b) that there is a substantial risk that if the child were born it would suffer from such physical or mental abnormalities as to be seriously handicapped'.

In 1977, 132,999 legal abortions were

carried out in England and Wales, compared with 127,904 in 1976 and 169,362 in 1973.

ABRASION means the rubbing off of the surface of the skin or of a mucous membrane due to some mechanical injury. Such injuries, though slight in themselves, are apt to allow entrance of dirt-containing organisms and so to lead to an abscess or some severer form of inflammation.

Treatment – The most effective form of treatment consists in the thorough and immediate cleansing of the wound with soap and water. An antiseptic such as 1 per cent cetrimide can then be applied, and a sterile dry dressing.

ABSCESS is a localized collection of pus. A minute abscess is known as a pustule (see PUSTULE), a diffused production of pus is known as cellulitis or erysipelas (see ERYSIPELAS). An abscess may be acute or chronic.

ABSCESS, ACUTE – An acute abscess is one which develops rapidly within the course of a few days or hours. It is characterized by a definite set of symptoms.

Causes – The direct cause is various bacteria. In a few cases the presence of foreign bodies, such as bullets or splinters, or contact with poisonous plants, such as poison ivy, may produce abscesses, but these foreign bodies, may remain for life buried in the tissues without causing any trouble provided they are not contaminated with bacteria or other micro-organisms.

The micro-organisms most frequently found are *staphylococci*, and next to these *streptococci*, though the latter cause more virulent abscesses, or in general the more serious condition of erysipelas or cellulitis. Other abscess-forming organisms are *Pseudomonas pyocyanea*, which produces blue or greenish pus; and *Escherichia coli*, which lives always in the bowels, probably aiding digestion, and under certain conditions wanders into the surrounding tissues and produces abscesses.

The mere presence of micro-organisms is not sufficient to produce suppuration (see IMMUNITY; and INFECTION); indeed streptococci, which upon occasion produce most disastrous effects, can often be found on the skin and in the skin glands of perfectly healthy individuals. Given the proper micro-organisms in the tissues, whether they will produce abscesses or not depends upon two factors: (1) the virulence of the organism at the time, and (2)

the resisting power of the individual. In the case of bad health, as in diabetes mellitus, fever, Bright's disease, the tissues are less resistant, and cold, injury, or previous disease of a part renders that particular part less able to cope with bacterial invasion. On the other hand, good food, vigorous exercise, and healthy open-air life help to render the individual more or less immune from the ill-effects of these bacteria. They are communicated, principally in a virulent form, from one wound to another; but they live also in the air, in dust, and in water. They enter the body generally by a wound, but may also come through the mucous membrane of the intestine when this is rendered less resistant by conditions such as appendicitis; they may also pass through the mucous membranes of the nose, mouth, respiratory and urinary passages, and cause local abscesses, or even through the skin by way of its minute lubricating glands.

When bacteria have gained access, for example, to a wound, they rapidly multiply, and, by the formation of poisonous substances, irritate the surrounding tissues, and so produce local dilatation of the blood-vessels, slowing of the blood-stream, and exudation of blood corpuscles and fluid. The leucocytes, or white corpuscles of the blood, collect around the invaded area, apparently under some attracting influence of the bacteria (chemotaxis), and destroy the latter either by actually devouring and digesting them (see PHAGOCYTOSIS), or by forming some substances which cause their death. These white corpuscles undergo a granular fatty degeneration, and in turn die, and form the white constituent of the pus (pus corpuscles). Meanwhile, the area where these changes have been taking place has been cut off from communication with the rest of the body by plugging of the blood and lymphatic vessels around it. The tissues of the affected area die and are digested by the action of the white corpuscles, and the cavity so produced is distended by fluid and by the white corpuscles which flock to it in increasing numbers till all bacteria have disappeared. The abscess is shut off from healthy tissue by what is known as the abscess wall. The bacteria may find their way along a vessel to some little distance, where the same process takes place, and these secondary abscess cavities may coalesce with the original one.

Symptoms – The classic symptoms of inflammation are *rubor*, *calor*, *tumor* and *dolor*: ie. redness, warmth, swelling and pain; and, besides these, when the abscess is well developed, a considerable amount of fever, perhaps with delirium, sets in, and the temperature rises to 100° to 104° F (38° to 40° C). When the cavity containing fluid has been formed, a sign, known as fluctuation, can be made out. Later, as the abscess is distended almost to bursting, the skin becomes reddish blue, glazed, and thin; and this is known as 'pointing' of the abscess; or if the abscess is very deep-seated the skin over it becomes swollen, and pits on pressure. The lymphatic glands in the neighbourhood may be swollen and tender in an attempt to stop the bacteria spreading to other parts of the body. Immediately the abscess is opened, or bursts, the pain disappears, the temperature falls rapidly to normal, the elasticity of the tissues around the cavity diminishes its bulk, and the healing of the small space left proceeds rapidly. If, however, the abscess discharge into an internal cavity, such as the bowel or bladder, it may heal very slowly, and the reabsorption of its poisonous products may cause general ill-health for long. When an abscess is deep-seated an important sign for diagnosis is provided by examination of the blood. (See LEUCOCYTOSIS.)

Treatment – As soon as there is evidence that pus has formed, we know that Nature's attempt to destroy the bacteria has been successful, and, as the further formation of pus is designed simply to burst a passage to the exterior, we can relieve pain, stop unnecessary destruction of tissue, and shorten the process by opening the abscess. This is done as soon as there is evidence from fluctuation, redness or pitting of the skin that pus has formed. Previous to this it may be advisable to give a course of injections of penicillin, and these may prevent the formation of an abscess. Nature's efforts may be aided by the application of heat. This has the effect of diminishing the pain; of aiding resolution, if abscess formation is not going to take place; and of hastening the formation of an abscess cavity, and softening the overlying tissues if the latter process has already begun.

When the abscess is opened three things are attended to:

(1) That important structures such as arteries in the neighbourhood are not damaged.

(2) That the opening is as far away as possible from a new source of infection like the mouth or anus.

(3) That the opening is large and so situated that the cavity can drain itself completely; otherwise, if the abscess cavity

be large or irregular, a further collection of pus takes place, and the wound will not heal but forms a sinus (see SINUS); for this reason it may be necessary to make two or more 'counter-openings'.

After the abscess is opened a simple wet dressing, of moist lint covered by gutta-percha tissue, and this again covered by absorbent wool (to absorb the remaining discharge) and a bandage, should be applied and changed daily. If the cavity be large it may be necessary to 'pack' the opening with a strip of gauze or lint, or to insert a drainage tube, so as to ensure healing from the bottom of the cavity. The injection of penicillin into the abscess cavity may be of value in some cases.

Special varieties of acute abscess: ABSCESS IN ABDOMEN – When this occurs in the iliac region it is generally a result of appendicitis (see APPENDICITIS); when in the lumbar region it may be the result of this disease 'pointing' backwards, or may be the result of inflammation in the loose tissue around the kidney (perinephric abscess). In the upper part of the abdomen it is known as a subphrenic abscess, and may be the consequence of ulceration from the stomach or bowels, or of abscess in the liver. All these conditions are very grave.

ABSCESS IN BONE (see BONE, DISEASES OF).

ABSCESS OF BREAST (see BREAST, DISEASES OF).

CEREBRAL AND CEREBELLAR ABSCESS – These are apt to come on suddenly in cases in which the middle ear is diseased, generally after long-standing discharge from the ear. The stoppage of the discharge in such a case is a warning of danger. (See EAR, DISEASES OF.)

ABSCESS IN THE FINGER (see WHITLOW).

ILIAC ABSCESS (see APPENDICITIS).

ABSCESS OF THE JAW (see GUMBOIL).

ABSCESS IN THE KIDNEY (see KIDNEYS, DISEASES OF).

ABSCESS OF THE LUNG may follow pneumonia or the drawing of some foreign body, such as food, down the windpipe. Being deep-seated, its presence may be hard to diagnose. It may burst either into a bronchus, when pus will be spat up, or into the pleural cavity. (See LUNG DISEASES.)

ABSCESS IN THE PLEURAL CAVITY is known as empyema. (See EMPYEMA.)

ABSCESS, CHRONIC – A chronic abscess is one which takes weeks or months for its development. In the majority of cases it is tuberculous.

Causes – Some acute abscesses, instead

7

of bursting, may settle down, become surrounded by dense fibrous tissue, and so form chronic abscesses, but these are rare. Abscesses may form in the liver as a complication of amoebic dysentery. (See DYSENTERY.) The tubercle bacillus, or *Mycobacterium tuberculosis*, as it is now known, however, is generally the cause. How it obtains entrance is still in dispute; in the case of abscesses of the neck it is probably through the throat or tonsil, and in the case of abscesses elsewhere, through the circulation from the lung or intestinal canal, owing to polluted air or food. A common source of infection is milk which has not been boiled or pasteurized. Abscesses arise most commonly from tuberculous deposits in glands or bones, especially in the vertebrae or bones of the spine, the epiphyses or large ends of long bones near a joint, and the ribs. They may start also in the synovial membranes, ie. membranes lining a joint (see JOINT DISEASES), in the loose tissue beneath the skin, quite apart from disease of any other structure, and, not uncommonly, in the testicle.

Symptoms – There is far less in the way of symptoms than in acute abscess. Sometimes the swelling is noticed by accident; it is not hot, red or in general painful, as is an acute abscess. The skin becomes red only a short time before the abscess bursts. If the temperature be taken every four hours it will generally be found that there is a slight rise either in the forenoon or late afternoon. If the abscess be untreated it generally enlarges till it bursts, then a ragged wound is left, infection with other organisms takes place, and the resulting sinus with 'mixed infection' becomes extremely difficult to heal. If such a sinus be large, as in a psoas, or ilio-psoas abscess, it may persist for years, and the patient becomes exhausted by the resulting hectic fever; or waxy disease (see AMYLOIDOSIS) attacks the liver and kidneys, and causes wasting and death.

Character of the pus – The fluid is thin and watery (not thick and white as in an acute abscess) and contains little curdy masses. It is not really 'pus', as pus corpuscles are almost entirely absent, and only fragments of the dead tissues are found under the microscope.

Treatment – For the purpose of discussing treatment it will be assumed that the abscess is tuberculous.

The introduction of the anti-tuberculous drugs, streptomycin (qv), para-aminosalicylic acid (qv), and isoniazid (qv), has revolutionized the outlook in tuberculous abscesses and has removed many of the hazards which attached to them at one time. The general rules for improving the health of the individual and resting the affected part still apply, but the administration of these drugs shortens the period of treatment and convalescence very considerably. Further details will be found under GLANDS; and JOINT DISEASES.

Special varieties of chronic abscess:
ABSCESS OF THE LIVER – This occurs in persons who have been the subject of amoebic dysentery (see DYSENTERY), frequently after returning in apparently fair health to a temperate region where this form of dysentery does not occur. The liver becomes enlarged and tender, and there is a degree of ill-health and slight jaundice. When threatening, it is treated by emetine, rest, and light diet; and when it has formed should be at once operated on, lest it burst into the lung or the peritoneal cavity.

ISCHIO-RECTAL ABSCESS – This forms at the side of the rectum. Whether it bursts or is opened, it is very difficult to keep clean, on account of its position, and so forms a sinus; or, if it opens into the bowel, a fistula. (See FISTULA.) It may occur late in a case of pulmonary tuberculosis, but may also occur as the first manifestation of tuberculosis.

RETROPHARYNGEAL ABSCESS – This is due generally to disease of the spinal column in the neck. It is opened from the side of the neck; otherwise it bursts into the mouth, and the discharges from it lead to rapid falling-off in health, and to death unless efficient treatment is instituted.

ILIO-PSOAS ABSCESS – This arises generally from tuberculous disease of the spinal column in the lumbar region, and, though this may cure itself, the abscess bursts into the sheath of the psoas muscle and passes along the muscle through the iliac region into the thigh, on the inner side of which it generally 'points'. Its early symptoms resemble those of hip-joint disease. (See JOINT DISEASES.) The opening and scraping of such an abscess often require large incisions in the thigh, groin, and lumbar region, and if the wound becomes the seat of mixed infection the resulting sinus may last months or years. Fortunately, the introduction of anti-tuberculous drugs has reduced the risk of this very considerably.

ACTINOMYCOTIC ABSCESS – This is another form of chronic abscess, which occurs about the jaw or mouth. (See ACTINOMYCOSIS.)

ABSINTHISM – Absinthe is a liquor prepared by steeping several herbs, especially anise and wormwood, in alcohol for several days. It is greenish in colour. It was first introduced into France by soldiers stationed in Algiers between 1830 and 1850, for whom it had been prescribed as a febrifuge (qv), and its employment spread thence into other countries. Its use becomes a habit like that of alcohol, but its effects are more demoralizing. Its habitual use brings on tremors and paralysis, in the arms especially, with delusional insanity.

ABSTRACT – This is a dry powder produced by extracting the active principles from a crude drug with strong alcohol, mixing with sugar of milk, and drying. Abstracts are standardized so as to be twice the strength of the crude drug.

ACACIA GUM, or GUM ACACIA, is a gummy exudation from various species of the acacia tree, which, dissolved in water to form mucilage, is used in coughs and sore throat and in states of irritation of the stomach and bowels.

ACANTHOSIS NIGRICANS is a rare disease in which pigmented warty growths appear on the skin in different parts of the body and in the mouth.

ACAPNIA means a condition of diminished carbon dioxide in the blood.

ACARUS – The group of animal parasites which includes *Sarcoptes scabiei*, the cause of the skin disease known as Itch, or Scabies. This parasite used to be known as *Acarus scabiei*. (See ITCH.)

ACCIDENT PREVENTION IN THE HOME – Over 800,000 accidents in the home requiring emergency treatment are estimated to occur each year in England and Wales. In 1974, domestic accidents were responsible for 6,717 deaths in England and Wales. Such accidents in the home are most liable to occur in the young and the old.

In *children* the type of accident varies to a certain extent with age. Choking, and suffocation from food or secretions are the commonest causes of accidents in children under the age of 1 year. This is why there should be no pillow in baby's cot or pram. When learning to walk there is a tendency to fall, and this may result in a serious accident if the fall is into a fire or a full bath. As inquisitiveness develops accidents may occur from pulling a saucepan of hot food off the kitchen stove or from sampling medicines. Prevention of burns is of paramount importance. Under the Heating Appliances (Fireguard) Act 1954 all new gas and electric fires must be guarded, but there are still too many old-fashioned gas and electric fires in use without adequate guards. The fireguard mesh must be small enough to exclude small fingers, and the fireguard must be well away from the heated element. Modern paraffin heaters are self-extinguishing if tilted more than 45 degrees. It is now an offence to sell nightdresses made of readily ignited material. Cotton and rayon and the man-made fibres, Acrilan, Courtelle and Orlon, are easily set on fire. Nylon, Terylene and the heavier woollen fabrics are more resistant. The major fire-risk is the wide-skirted dress, apron and nightdress. Girls as well as boys should wear pyjamas. To prevent children poisoning themselves, all medicines, whether tablets or liquid, must be kept in locked medicine cupboards. A point to be remembered here is that the common practice of parents 'bribing' their children to take their medicine as a sweet may have unfortunate, if not fatal, consequences if the child finds the bottle and demolishes the contents on the ground that they are sweets – as mummy said. All paints, polishes, pesticides, petroleum products, turpentine, garden fertilizers, disinfectants and the like must be kept well out of the reach of prying hands. To avoid burning accidents in the kitchen crawling and toddling children should be firmly banned from the kitchen during cooking operations. Falls on stairs are the most dangerous. These should be avoided by having a gate at the top and bottom of the stairs.

In *old age* falls are the major cause of accidents, and they are particularly dangerous at this age because of the ease with which the limbs are broken. Old bones tend to be fragile (see OSTEOPOROSIS), and a fall in old age that would cause no more than bruising in younger life may well result in a broken arm or leg. Prevention consists predominantly of a well-designed home. Stairs should be shallow, carpeted and have a handrail, or preferably two. There should be no polished floors or worn-out mats. To prevent slipping, mats should have a rubber-backed underlay. There should be no steps leading down into a room. Lighting must be adequate with easily accessible switches. Central heating is essential for winter warmth. The bath should be shallow with a slip mat inside and outside, and there should be handles on each side for ease of getting in and out. To prevent burns, fireguards and fire-resistant clothes are just as essential as in childhood, and smoking in bed should be discouraged. The risk of poisoning can be reduced by ensuring that all medicines are clearly labelled with instructions as to when and in what dosage they are to be taken. In those with failing memory self-administration should be discouraged as the elderly individual may forget that he has already taken his prescribed dose.

At all ages accidents may occur from electric shock due to faulty switches and wiring. Tinkering with electric installations is dangerous – if not fatal, and many fires are due to faulty wiring which has been allowed to age with the house – and the owner. In England in 1976, 59 people died by electric shock in home accidents. In addition, 45 people died in fires involving electrical equipment. Wounds, too, are common, whether caused by knives, tin-openers or razors. These are seldom serious, but severe injuries may be caused by mechanical or powered equipment such as washing machines and mixers in the kitchen or rotary lawnmowers and hedge-cutters in the garden.

All accidents are preventable, it has been said. This may be true in theory, but not in practice. In practice, however, their number could be radically reduced if first aid was a compulsory item in the routine school curriculum. Pending such a move, every parent should look upon an approved course of first aid as an essential preliminary to marriage. Full details of such courses can be obtained from the British Red Cross Society, the St. John Ambulance Association, or the St. Andrew's Ambulance Association. (See FIRST AID.)

ACCOMMODATION is the faculty possessed by the eye of altering its refractive power so that rays of light, whether from a near or distant point, are brought accurately to a focus on the retina. (See EYE.) It is effected by means of the elasticity of the crystalline lens. If the eye be directed towards a distant object the rays of light entering it should be focused exactly on the retina; if now the eye be turned towards an object a few inches off, the elastic, circular ligament, in the centre of which the lens is suspended, is drawn together by the circular ciliary muscle, allowing the lens to become more globular (illustration 3), as it constantly tends to do. The lens becomes therefore of higher power, and the diverging rays from the near object are still brought to a focus on the retina. The amount of power possessed by the eye of thus suiting itself for objects far off and near at hand is known as range of accommodation. At the age of forty-five the lens has lost much of its elasticity, though this change has been gradually proceeding throughout life; and by the age of sixty, even though it be quite clear, it is incapable of this accommodative change in shape; consequently a natural change with advancing years is that persons become unable to read, sew, or do other fine work near at hand without glasses, though for distant vision no such assistance is necessary. This natural change is known as presbyopia (qv).

In addition to this, there are three errors in the refractive power of the eye which may be either present at birth or come on early in life and persist through life, and in which these movements of the lens are not always sufficient to focus the rays of light accurately on the retina. These are astigmatism (see ASTIGMATISM), hypermetropia (see HYPERMETROPIA) or long sight, in which the eyeball is too short, and myopia

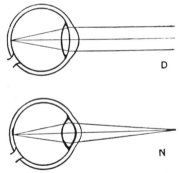

3 – Diagram illustrating resting position of eye for distant vision (D), and increased convexity of lens for vision of a near object (N).

(see MYOPIA) or short sight, in which the eyeball is too long. (See also SPECTACLES.)

ACCOUCHEUR is a physician who specializes in the practice of midwifery.

ACEDAPSONE is a sulphone (qv) which is being used in the treatment of leprosy.

ACETABULUM is the cup-shaped socket on the pelvis in which rests the head of the femur or thigh-bone, the two forming the hip joint. (See HIP JOINT.)

ACETAZOLAMIDE is a drug which acts by inhibiting the enzyme carbonic anhydrase. This enzyme is of great importance in the production of acid and alkaline secretions in the body. Acetazolamide has proved of value as a diuretic and in the treatment of glaucoma.

ACETIC ACID, also called pyroligneous acid, is prepared by the distillation of wood and subsequent separation from tar. It is also synthesized from acetylene. In the pure form it is solid, being then known as glacial acetic acid. It is the active principle of vinegar, which is prepared from wine by the action of a particular ferment discovered by Pasteur. This grows on the surface of the vine, taking from the air oxygen which it gives up to the alcohol of the wine, so producing acetic acid. Weak acetic acid has all the actions of vinegar, and is less expensive. Strong acetic acid is a caustic and irritant poison.
Uses In strong solution acetic acid is used to destroy warts or raise blisters. In cases of excessive sweating the weak acid is of value, because, sponged over the skin, it checks perspiration and produces a sense of grateful coolness; for this purpose a few tablespoonfuls of vinegar may be added to a quart of water. Used similarly it is good for headache.

ACETOHEXAMIDE is one of the oral hypoglycaemic drugs being used in the treatment of diabetes mellitus. It is thought to act by increasing the output of insulin.

ACETONE is a chemical substance found in the urine in wasting conditions like cancer, in diabetes mellitus, in prolonged vomiting, and in acute fevers – especially in children. With it occur in the urine β-hydroxybutyric and acetoacetic acids, particularly in severe cases of diabetes. A large quantity of these acids and of acetone in the urine in diabetes indicates approaching coma. (See also ACIDOSIS.)

ACETYLCHOLINE is one of the substances which mediates the transmission of nerve impulses from one nerve to another, or from a nerve to the organ it acts on such as muscles. Its predominant role is in the parasympathetic nervous system (qv), but it also plays an important part in the transmission of nerve impulses in the brain. Acetylcholine is rapidly destroyed by cholinesterase, an enzyme present in the blood.

ACETYLCYSTEINE is a drug that is used in the treatment of fibrocystic disease of the pancreas (qv) and paracetamol poisoning (qv).

ACETYLSALICYLIC ACID (see ASPIRIN).

ACHALASIA is another term for spasm, but indicates not so much an active spasm of muscle as a failure to relax.

ACHALASIA OF THE CARDIA is a condition in which there is a failure to relax of the muscle fibres round the opening of the gullet, or oesophagus, into the stomach. (See OESOPHAGUS, DISEASES OF.)

ACHLORHYDRIA means an absence of hydrochloric acid from the stomach juice; it occurs in about 4 per cent of healthy people and in several conditions, including pernicious anaemia, carcinoma of the stomach and gastritis.

ACHONDROPLASIA is the name of a form of dwarfing in which the arms and legs are abnormally short and the head large. It is a hereditary condition, and the commonest form of dwarfism. It affects both sexes and, whilst many are stillborn or die soon after birth, those who survive have a normal expectation of life and good health.

ACHORION is the name of the fungus causing favus or honeycomb ringworm. (See RINGWORM.)

ACHYLIA GASTRICA means the complete absence of ferments and of hydrochloric acid from the gastric juice, so that in this condition the food is passed from the stomach in a state of incomplete digestion.

ACIDITY is a vague term, more used in popular language than in scientific medicine, and meaning that the reaction of the blood, or of one or more of the secretions, is less alkaline or more strongly acid than normal, while a considerable number of symptoms is rightly or wrongly attributed to the condition.
The blood in health is alkaline, and an elaborate chemical mechanism keeps the degree of alkalinity remarkably constant. This mechanism hinges largely round the relative amounts in the blood of carbonic acid (H_2CO_3) and sodium bicarbonate $(NaHCO_3)$: $H_2CO_3/NaHCO_3$. By this

and other mechanisms the acids formed in metabolism are neutralized and got rid of through the lungs. These acids are the fixed acids, such as lactic, sulphuric, phosphoric, and carbonic acid which are produced in large amounts daily as a result of tissue activity. The blood in disease never becomes actually acid. except in the terminal stages of life. But the blood may become *less alkaline*, the patient in this state is said to have acidaemia – although the blood is not acid.

ACIDOSIS is a condition in which there is either (i) a production in the body of two abnormal acids – β-hydroxybutyric and acetoacetic acids, or (ii) a diminution in the alkali reserve of the blood.

Causes – The condition is usually due to faulty metabolism of fat which results in the production of β-hydroxybutyric and acetoacetic acids. It occurs in diabetes mellitus when this is either untreated or inadequately treated, starvation, persistent vomiting, and delayed anaesthetic vomiting. It also occurs in the terminal stages of Bright's disease when it is due to failure of the kidneys. A milder form of it may occur in severe fevers, particularly in children. (See also ACETONE.)

Symptoms – General lassitude, vomiting, thirst, restlessness, and the presence of acetone in the urine form the earliest manifestations of the condition. In diabetes a state of coma may ensue and the disease end fatally.

Treatment – The underlying condition must always be treated: eg. if the acidosis is due to diabetes mellitus insulin must be given. For the acidosis, alkalis should be given; eg. bicarbonate of soda, either by mouth, or by injection if there is persistent vomiting or if the patient is unconscious. Glucose should also be given, and adequate fluids.

ACIDS are substances which combine with alkalis to form salts. Most are oxygen compounds, have a sour taste, and turn blue litmus red. They are divided into (*a*) mineral or inorganic, and (*b*) vegetable or organic. In strong solution the mineral acids act upon stomach and bowels as irritant poisons, but small quantities in weak solution aid digestion, diminish the alkalinity of the blood, are excreted in the urine, the acidity of which they increase, act as mild astringents and refrigerants, and check excessive sweating. The action of the organic acids varies, but the best known, ie. acetic, citric, lactic, tartaric, while in strong solution acting like mineral acids, in weaker solution after absorption into the blood become decomposed into carbonates, and have precisely the opposite actions: ie. those of alkalis.

Varieties commonly used – (*a*) *Inorganic*: boracic, or boric, chromic, hydrochloric, hydrobromic, nitric, nitro-hydrochloric, phosphoric, sulphuric, sulphurous.

(*b*) *Organic*: acetic, carbolic, carbonic, citric, gallic, hydrocyanic or prussic, lactic, salicylic, tanic or tannin, tartaric.

Uses – The strong mineral acids, especially chromic and nitric, with pure acetic and carbolic from among the organic acids, are used as caustics to remove outgrowths such as corns, warts, piles, and also to destroy diseased tissue in poisoned wounds and spreading sores. In using them, care must be taken not to let the action extend too far and destroy healthy tissue; they are usually applied on a glass rod, and an alkali, oil, or glycerin should be at hand to apply in case a drop falls on the healthy surface.

Weak acids are given in dyspepsia (see DYSPEPSIA), usually after meals, to stimulate digestion in the stomach. For this action hydrochloric acid (the acid naturally present in the gastric juice), or nitro-hydrochloric acid, is chiefly used.

The astringent action is utilized in excessive sweating. (See also ACETIC ACID.) When the urine is very alkaline there is a tendency to the formation of phosphatic calculi, and catarrh of the bladder is often present; these are relieved by acids among various other substances.

In fevers and in cases in which an increase in the output of urine is desirable, the vegetable acids or their acid salts are given, eg. citrate, tartrate or acetate of potash, because they lessen dryness of the mouth and thirst, cause a feeling of refreshment, stimulate the kidneys and sweat glands, and lower the temperature. In general acidity (see ACIDITY) the vegetable acids are used as indirect alkalis.

For the use of special acids see under ACETIC ACID; CARBOLIC ACID; SALICYLIC ACID, etc.

ACIDS, POISONING BY – Although most acids have an extremely sour and burning taste, which warns a person drinking one of his error before very much is swallowed, several are so much used in commercial processes, and so easily obtained, that accidental and intentional poisoning by acids is not uncommon.

Symptoms – The symptoms produced

are destruction of the skin and mucous membrane about the mouth, great pain in the mouth, throat, and stomach, and sometimes fainting or collapse. There is also later a risk of scarring and contraction of the throat. These are especially the symptoms of poisoning by strong mineral acids, or by citric, or tartaric in large quantities, while several, such as prussic and carbolic, have symptoms peculiar to themselves and not due to irritation. For the treatment of poisoning by these last two see PRUSSIC ACID POISONING and CARBOLIC ACID POISONING.

Treatment – Give large quantities of water by mouth, and if possible add alkalis to it – such as cream of magnesia, bicarbonate of soda, or baking soda. If none of these is immediately available, plaster from the ceiling, whitewash from the walls, or soapy water may be used. These neutralize the acid taken and form harmless salts, and also soothe the irritated mucous membrane. On no account must emetics be given. The patient must be treated for shock. Soothing or demulcent substances, such as milk in oil, or barley water, must also be given.

ACINUS is the name applied to each of the minute sacs of which secreting glands are composed, and which usually cluster round the branches of the gland-duct like grapes on their stem.

ACNE, or ACNE VULGARIS, is a chronic skin disease which affects practically all adolescents. Fortunately, in the vast majority of these it is relatively insignificant and only in about 15 per cent of youngsters is it severe enough to require treatment. It usually begins around puberty, achieves its peak in the late teens, and disappears in the early twenties. By the age of 23, some 5 per cent of people have acne severe enough to need treatment, whilst by the age of 40 this figure is down to 1 per cent. There is a rare form of acne which occurs in baby boys, usually in a family with a strong history of acne. This usually disappears around the age of 5 years. Acne may be induced by certain drugs, including the corticosteroids, lithium, phenytoin, rifampicin, and the iodides and bromides. *Industrial acne* occurs in those exposed to vapours of chlorinated naphthalenes used in insulating cable and in those coming in contact with soluble cutting oils of high boiling points.

Causes – Three main factors are necessary for the development of acne: an in-creased production of sebum (qv); obstruction of the pilosebaceous, or sebaceous, ducts (see SKIN; and SEBACEOUS GLANDS); and the presence of micro-organisms. The activity of the sebaceous glands is controlled by testerone, the male sex hormone, or androgen as it is known. This explains the onset of acne at puberty. In boys the androgen is produced predominantly in the testes as they develop to normal adult activity. In girls it comes predominantly from the adrenal glands. This increased production of sebum, the secretion of the sebaceous glands, is accompanied by blockage of the ducts through which it normally reaches the surface of the skin. It is this accumulation of sebum, which gradually becomes infected with skin micro-organisms, that leads to the formation of the small lumps, or comedones, the characteristic feature of acne. In girls acne tends to flare up in the week preceding menstruation. Sunlight, especially natural sunlight, has a favourable influence on the condition. In some, particularly males who participate in active sports, it tends to be worse on the back after sweating. The influence of diet is non-proven, though fats and sweets, especially chocolate, have been traditionally associated with it. Stress plays a part, and this has been attributed to acne subjects, especially girls, tending to pick their spots during times of strain and thereby exacerbate the condition.

Symptoms — The eruption occurs predominantly on the face, back and chest, the face usually being the most affected. These are the sites of the eruption because they are the areas most richly supplied with sebaceous glands. The eruption consists of little black spots (blackheads or comedones) which indicate the mouths of blocked sebaceous (or pilosebaceous) ducts, hard pimples generally showing one of these blackheads on the top, and little pustules surrounded by a red area of inflammation which gradually grow, burst and then heal. In more severe cases there may be hard lumps, half an inch (12 mm) across, which last for weeks or longer, suppurate, and leave a permanent hardness or scar. The amount of scarring of the skin left after the condition has cleared up depends upon the severity of the eruption, but in the majority of cases it clears completely.

Treatment – In milder cases all that is needed is daily washing of the affected parts. Some recommend detergents instead of soap and water, to degrease the skin. Sulphurated potash lotion applied twice daily by dabbing on with cotton-wool or the finger tips may be helpful. Some recommend the application of an ointment containing retinoic acid (a vitamin A derivative). In more severe cases a course of either tetracycline or erythromycin is given. The usual dose is 250 mg twice daily, but this may be increased, under medical supervision, for resistant cases and maintained for several months. A course of sunlight therapy is often helpful. Natural sunlight is more efficacious than artificial sunlight, but a three-month course of the latter in hospital during the winter often helps. In resistant cases a course of X-rays or grenz rays may be tried. Those with acne should be discouraged from squeezing out comedones with their fingers or so-called comedone expressors. In those who are left with severe scarring a course of dermabrasion (qv) may remove these blemishes.

ACONITE (also known as Wolfsbane, or Blue rocket or Monkshood) is an extremely poisonous plant found in different species all over the world, and largely grown for its appearance in gardens. All parts of the plant are poisonous. The root has been mistaken for horse-radish, although the resemblance, to those who know horse-radish by sight, is not very great. The root of the horse-radish is long, whitish outside, when scraped remains white, and has the well-known pungent odour. Aconite root is short and stumpy, brown, and when scraped the white cut surface speedily turns pinkish; if it be chewed, the tongue in a few minutes tingles, then becomes numb and swollen, and a burning sensation is felt in the mouth. The action of aconitine, its active principle, is produced by smaller doses than in the case of any other drug; accordingly aconite is a favourite homoeopathic remedy.

Uses – Aconite is seldom used at the present day, although in the form of a liniment it is sometimes used externally to relieve pain, sprains and rheumatism. Tincture of aconite, which is still kept in some households, should never be used without the sanction of a doctor.

ACONITE POISONING – This may occur, as stated above, by mistaking the root for horse-radish, by children eating parts of the plant, or by the administration of too large a dose.

Symptoms – There are characteristic symptoms in the mouth (see ACONITE) after chewing parts of the plant. If a large amount of the poison has been taken into

the stomach, vomiting and purging follow after some time. Numbness is felt all over the body. The pulse becomes weak, the breathing laboured, and the face livid. Convulsions may come on, but consciousness is retained.

Treatment – Give plenty of warm water to drink. The poison must be got rid of at once, preferably by washing out the stomach with a solution of tannic acid (6 grams in 4·5 litres [1 gallon]). Alternatively, an emetic may be given, one of the handiest being a tablespoonful of mustard in a cupful of cold water; or, best of all, one or two tablespoonfuls of sal volatile in water, this being also a stimulant. Emetics, however, should not be given if the victim is in a state of collapse. Stimulants, such as leptazol or atropine, may be given by injection. Artificial respiration may be necessary.

ACRIDINE is a colourless crystalline compound occurring in coal-tar. Its formula is $C_{13}H_9N$. From this are derived the valuable acridine dyes or flavines, used as antiseptics.

ACRIFLAVINE is an aniline derivative. It is an orange-red crystalline powder, readily soluble in water, which gives a rich yellow colour to substances brought into contact with it, and in a solution of 1 in 1000 of water, possesses strong antiseptic powers.

ACROCYANOSIS is a condition, occurring especially in young women, in which there is persistent blueness of hands, feet, nose and ears.

ACRODYNIA (see ERYTHROEDEMA).

ACROMEGALY is a chronic disease characterized by increased massiveness of the bones, most noticeable in the jaws, hands and feet. The bones of the chest and elsewhere are also lengthened and thickened so that the whole person becomes more massive. There is also enlargement of the tongue, lips and ears, as well as many of the organs of the body such as the heart and liver, and the skin becomes thick and coarse. It is not uncommon, it having been estimated that in the United Kingdom 100 to 500 new cases occur every year. It is associated with tumours or other disorders causing increase in size of the front part of the pituitary gland (qv) which lies inside the skull on the base of the brain. The condition is due to an excessive secretion by this gland of a substance, known as the growth hormone, which has the effect of stimulating the growth of bones, so that if it begins in early life great stature results – the condition known as gigantism; if later, a thickening of the bones, most noticeable in the hands and feet. The disease advances slowly, and sometimes it stops its progress after the bones are slightly enlarged. High blood pressure is a common complication, as is diabetes mellitus (qv), and many victims of the disease complain of severe, persistent headache. A disorder of vision, involving limitation of the field of vision at its outer sides, is apt to be caused by interference with the optic tracts through the increase in size of the gland in advanced stages of the disease.

Treatment – Surgical removal of the front portion of the pituitary gland is sometimes practised. In other cases treatment consists of irradiation of the gland with X-rays or with radioactive isotopes. Promising results are also being obtained from the use of an ergot alkaloid known as bromocriptine.

ACROMION is the part of the scapula or shoulder blade forming the tip of the shoulder and giving its squareness to the latter. It projects forward from the scapula, and, with the clavicle or collar-bone in front, forms a protecting arch of bone over the shoulder joint.

ACROPARAESTHESIA is a disorder occurring predominantly in middle-aged women in which there are numbness and tingling of the fingers.

ACTH is the commonly used abbreviation for corticotrophin (qv).

ACTINOMYCIN D is an antibiotic isolated from *Streptomyces antibioticus* and *Streptomyces chrysomallus* which has an inhibitory action on neoplastic cells.

ACTINOMYCOSIS is an acute or chronic suppurative disease affecting cattle in which it is known as Woody Tongue, and sometimes found in man.

Causes – The direct cause is the ray-fungus or actinomyces known as *Actinomyces israeli*, which occurs as a commensal (qv) in the mouth. In certain circumstances still rather obscure, but one of which is undoubtedly trauma, such as a fractured jaw or extraction of a tooth, the *A. israeli* becomes active. It then causes hard swellings, abscesses and ulcers, in the pus of which the fungus is found in little yellow balls of a size which can just be made out by the naked eye. These little balls are found to consist of masses of thread-like material matted together, and of club-shaped bodies radiating from a common centre, hence the name of ray-fungus. It used to be thought that the human infection arose from the chewing of straw or grain, or was caught from cattle, but this is now known not to be the case. In over 50 per cent of cases the disease occurs in or about the mouth; in 20 per cent it occurs in the abdomen, and in 15 per cent in the thorax.

Symptoms – These are general bad health, the presence of hard fibrous masses about the mouth or tongue, or in other organs, and the development sooner or later in these masses of abscesses which after bursting form sinuses or ulcers that will not heal.

Treatment – The outlook has been changed completely since the introduction of the antibiotics. The best results are usually obtained with large doses of penicillin, but in some cases chlortetracycline is more effective. Surgical treatment may be required, as in the draining of abscesses.

ACTIVE PRINCIPLES are the portions of a drug which produce its effect, being administered for convenience, or of necessity, with the water, oils, vegetable fibre, etc., which make the bulk of the drug. They are of various chemical nature, but, in general, alkaloids. (See ALKALOIDS.)

ACUPUNCTURE is a traditional Chinese method of treatment by puncture of a part with needles. Its rationale is that disease is a manifestation of a disturbance of Yin and Yang energy in the body, and that acupuncture brings this energy back into balance by what is described as 'the judicious stimulation or depression of the flow of energy in the various meridians'. What is still not clear to the western mind is why needling, which is the essence of acupuncture, should have the effect it is claimed to have. Of its efficacy in skilled Chinese hands, however, there can be no question.

ACUTE DISEASE – A disease is said to be acute in contradistinction to chronic when it comes on rapidly and produces death rapidly, or goes on to speedy recovery, eg. acute bronchitis; or the word is used, though less often, in the sense of severe or sharply painful, eg. acute sciatica, acute neuralgia.

ADDER-BITE (see BITES).

ADDISONIAN ANAEMIA is another term for pernicious anaemia. (See ANAEMIA.)

ADDISON'S DISEASE – This disease, described by Thomas Addison of Guy's Hospital, London, in 1855, consists of a state of anaemia, extreme weakness, low blood pressure, dyspepsia, wasting, pigmentation of the skin and mucous membranes, and subnormal temperature. It is due to disease of the suprarenal glands (qv), resulting in destruction of the cortical section of the gland.

Causes – The condition found after death is generally tuberculosis or atrophy of the suprarenal glands, causing their destruction to a greater or less extent. More rarely it is caused by other diseases, such as cancer of, or haemorrhage into, the glands. The disease destroys the secreting tissue of the glands, especially the cortex, and so checks the formation of the powerful secretion which these glands produce in health, and which is necessary for the proper functions of the body, as for example for the maintenance of the blood pressure and the contractile power of the muscles.

Symptoms – In the words of Addison, the main symptoms are: 'Anaemia, general languor or debility, remarkable feebleness of the heart's action, irritability of the stomach, and a peculiar change of the colour in the skin'. The colour ranges from yellow to dark brown, or even black, and though at first marked on the exposed surface (ie. face and hands), and on regions where pigment occurs naturally (groins, armpits, etc.), it gradually increases in area and in depth of tint. The next most prominent symptom is weakness on the least exertion, with giddiness, noises in the ears, or even fainting when efforts are made. Nausea, vomiting, occasional diarrhoea are also symptoms, and there are palpitation of the heart and feebleness of the pulse. The sufferer in general gets gradually worse, though there may be periods of betterment lasting some months. Untreated the disease rarely lasts longer than three or four years, and it may prove fatal within some months. Sometimes recovery may occur.

Several other diseases cause a limited pigmentation, especially of the face, so that this symptom must not always be taken as a sign of Addison's disease. Such conditions are cirrhosis of the liver, abdominal cancer, menstrual irregularity, exophthalmic goitre; while pregnancy brings on the so-called 'masques des femmes enceintes', which fades after delivery.

Treatment – The outlook in this disease has improved so considerably as a result of substitution therapy that it is now possible for many patients with this disease to lead more or less normal lives. Treatment consists of the regular administration of cortisone (qv). In all cases the administration of common salt is essential, as there is a depletion of this salt in the disease.

ADENINE ARABINOSIDE is an antiviral agent that is proving of value in the treatment of certain forms of herpes. (See HERPES SIMPLEX; and EYE, DISEASES OF.)

ADENITIS means inflammation of a gland. (See LYMPHATICS.)

ADENO- is a prefix denoting relation to a gland or glands.

ADENOIDS (see NOSE, DISEASES OF).

ADENOMA means a benign tumour composed of glandular tissue. It may arise in any part of the body in which glandular tissue occurs: eg. the thyroid gland. It must be differentiated from an adenocarcinoma, which is a malignant tumour composed of glandular tissue. (See TUMOURS.)

ADENOVIRUSES are a group of viruses which cause infections of the upper respiratory tract resembling the common cold, and often referred to as febrile catarrh.

ADHESION – This means the uniting together of structures which should normally be separate and freely movable. It is the result of acute or chronic inflammation. The medium by which the attachment takes place may at first be fibrin (as a result of acute inflammation), but later is, in every case, fibrous tissue either in masses or in bands.

Causes – The most important adhesions are those taking place in serous and joint cavities. When one of these structures becomes inflamed there is a great exudation of fluid into the cavity. From this fluid a solid material separates and becomes deposited upon the smooth surface of the cavity. This solid 'fibrin' should, in the course of recovery, be reabsorbed; but, if the inflammation be very severe, or if there be repeated attacks of it, this absorption does not completely take place, the two layers of fibrin on the opposing surfaces of the cavity stick together, and the united mass is 'organized' into the less absorbable fibrous tissue (see FIBROUS TISSUE). As a result there is restricted movement in the parts concerned; thus in the case of a joint there is ankylosis (see JOINT DISEASES); if the inflammation has been pleurisy the lung becomes adherent to the chest wall; if peritonitis, bands are formed between stomach, bowels, and other abdominal organs.

Symptoms – It is generally difficult to tell, except from the history of an inflammatory attack and from the presence of disordered function of internal organs, that adhesions are present (see PLEURISY; PERITONITIS). Sometimes adhesions between loops of bowels may be very serious and cause obstruction, if an old-standing and rigid fibrous band becomes twisted round a loop of bowel (see INTESTINE, DISEASES OF).

Treatment – While the adhesions are still *fibrinous* one expects complete absorption if the inflammation be speedily subdued. If the adhesions are *fibrous*, and show their presence by interference with the function of the organs concerned, one can seldom expect their complete absorption.

Sometimes, eg. when obstruction of the bowels is due to an adhesion, an immediate operation is necessary, and the adhesion is then divided. Adhesions causing limitation of movement in joints can often be broken down by means of manipulation.

ADHESIVE PLASTERS – These are made by spreading upon some supporting material, such as plain or elastic cloth or plastic film, some sticky substance containing drugs of various sorts. The sticky material consists of a mixture of cohesive and adhesive agents, plasticisers and fillers. The cohesive agents include Para rubber, pale crêpe rubber and smoked sheet rubber, polyisobutylene or other synthetic higher polymers with similar properties. The adhesive agents include various resins such as colophony and its derivatives.

Uses – Plasters are generally useful on account of their power of gripping a part and exerting steady pressure on it. They are sometimes used to obtain the absorbent effect of steady pressure combined with warmth and moisture in the treatment of chronic callous ulcers (see

ULCERS). In this case the plaster is put on in strips, each of which overlaps the last, and has no holes; it must be changed every few days if it. covers an unclean ulcer. Belladonna plaster is used for soothing pain. To support a sprained joint, eg. the ankle, a plaster is often applied in overlapping strips passing round the leg and instep. Plasters of felt are employed to protect corns, bunions, and small sores from abrasion; and 'corn plasters', containing salicylic acid in various strengths, are used to soften and remove corns. (See BLISTERS.)

Mode of application – Most plasters with a rubber basis stick by simply laying the plaster with the adhesive side next to the skin, but some must be warmed. If the plaster be wide, or the surface to be covered be rounded, it is necessary to cut deep notches into the plaster before heating (see illustration 4), and the edges so formed are allowed to overlap or separate.

4 – Diagram showing the method of slitting an adhesive plaster: *a*, to support the breast; *b*, for the back.

Plaster strips used to support the ankle or leg should be applied like a bandage (qv).

ADIPOCERE (see PUTREFACTION).

ADIPOSE TISSUE or FAT is a loose variety of fibrous tissue, in the meshes of which lie cells, each of which is distended by several small drops, or one large drop, of fat. This tissue replaces fibrous tissue when the amount of food taken is in excess of the bodily requirements. (See DIET; CORPULENCE.)

ADIPOSIS DOLOROSA, also known as Dercum's disease, is a condition in which painful masses of fat develop under the skin. It is commoner in women than in men and is thought to be caused by some disturbance of the pituitary gland (qv).

ADOPTION (see CHILD ADOPTION).

ADRENAL GLANDS (see SUPRA-RENAL GLANDS).

ADRENALINE is an extract derived from the suprarenal glands of animals.

17

ADRENERGIC RECEPTORS

(See SUPRARENAL GLANDS.) In the United States Pharmacopoeia it is known as epinephrine. It is also prepared synthetically. When injected it produces the same effect as stimulation of the sympathetic nervous system (qv). Among its important effects are raising of the blood pressure, increasing the amount of glucose in the blood, and constricting the smaller blood-vessels. It is applied directly to wounds on gauze or lint to check haemorrhage. Injected along with some local anaesthetic it permits of painless, bloodless operations being performed on the eye, nose, etc. It is injected hypodermically to relieve asthma, and to stimulate the heart in collapsed conditions. It is also injected as an antidote in the condition of hypoglycaemia, when too large a dose of insulin has been given.

ADRENERGIC RECEPTORS are the sites in the body on which adrenaline (qv) and comparable stimulants of the sympathetic system (qv) act. Drugs which have an adrenaline-like action are described as being adrenergic. It is now known that there are three different types of adrenergic receptors, known as alpha, beta$_1$, and beta$_2$, respectively. Stimulation of alpha receptors leads to constriction of the bronchi, constriction of the blood vessels with consequent rise in blood pressure, and dilatation of the pupils of the eyes. Stimulation of beta$_1$ receptors leads to a rise in heart rate and output of the heart, whilst stimulation of beta$_2$ receptors leads to dilatation of the bronchi. The practical implications of this complicated set-up were soon seized upon, particularly from the point of view of discovering useful new drugs.

For long it had been realized that in certain cases of asthma adrenaline had not the usual beneficial effect of dilating the bronchi during an attack; rather did it make the asthma worse. This, it was found, was due to its acting on both the alpha and beta adrenergic receptors. A derivative, isoprenaline, was therefore produced which acted only on the beta receptors. This had an excellent effect in dilating the bronchi, but unfortunately also affected the heart, speeding it up and increasing its output – an undesirable effect which meant that isoprenaline, still a valuable drug in the treatment of asthma, has to be used with great care. In due course drugs were produced, such as salbutamol, which act predominantly on the beta$_2$ adrenergic receptors in the bronchi and have relatively little effect on the heart.

The converse of this side of the story was the search for what became known as beta adrenoceptor-blocking drugs, or beta-adrenergic blocking drugs. The theoretical argument was that if such drugs could be synthesized, they could be of value in taking the strain off the heart – for example: stress→stimulation of the output of adrenaline→stimulation of the heart→increased work for the heart. A drug that could prevent this train of events would obviously be of value, for example, in the treatment of angina pectoris (qv). And so it proved, and today there is a series of beta adrenergic-blocking drugs which are subserving a most useful purpose, not only in angina pectoris, but also in various other heart conditions such as disorders of rhythm, as well as high blood pressure. They are also proving of value in the treatment of anxiety states by preventing disturbing features such as palpitations. An unexpected dividend is that some of them at least appear to be of help in the treatment of migraine. One of the best known of the group is propranolol (qv). Whilst their full scope is yet to be investigated, they have justifiably been described as 'perhaps the most interesting and useful new group of drugs introduced in the last decade'.

ADULTERATION OF FOOD – The incidence of adulteration of food has decreased considerably during the last century. The procedure for the inspection of food is laid down in the Food and Drugs Act, 1955, which empowers local authorities to appoint public analysts. A 'sampling officer' is an authorized officer of the local authority, and he may purchase any sample of food (or drug) and submit it for analysis to the local public analyst. In making such a purchase the following procedure must be followed, otherwise it will not be possible to obtain a conviction of the seller. After the purchase has been completed the purchaser must immediately inform the vendor that he proposes to have the sample analysed. The article must then be divided into three portions and each portion must be separately packed and sealed. One portion is then handed to the vendor, one is sent to the public analyst, and the third is retained by the purchaser.

Examples of adulteration – MILK – Milk which contains less than 3 per cent of fat or 8·5 per cent of milk solids other than fat is presumed to be adulterated. The addition of the following to milk is prohibited by law: colouring matter, water, dried or condensed milk or any fluid constituted therefrom, skimmed or separated milk, preservatives of any kind, any thickening substance (except cane or beet sugar to cream). The most common forms of adulteration of milk are the addition of water or the removal of fat. The most satisfactory method of deciding whether or not adulteration with water has taken place is the freezing point method. Milk which freezes above $-0.53°$ C can be considered to be adulterated. Even more important is the problem of milk-borne disease. (See MILK.)

BUTTER – No preservative may be added to butter and not more than 16 per cent of moisture is permitted by the legal standard. The two most common forms of adulteration of butter are the addition of other fats, eg. cotton-seed oil, and excessive amounts of water.

MARGARINE must not contain more than 16 per cent of moisture or 10 per cent of butter fat. It must be reinforced with 760 to 940 international units of vitamin A and 80 to 100 international units of vitamin D per ounce.

BREAD is usually fairly pure. (See BREAD.)

FLOUR – All flour intended for human consumption must contain not less than 1·6 mg of iron, 0·24 mg of vitamin B_1, and 1·60 mg of nicotinic acid or nicotinamide per 100 grams, and, except in the case of flour containing the whole of the products derived from the milling of wheat, 235 to 390 mg of powdered chalk per 100 grams. If wheat flour should be adulterated with flour of other grains, eg. barley, maize, rye, these can be easily recognized under the microscope.

BAKING POWDERS consist of an acid salt, such as cream of tartar in acid calcium phosphate, and bicarbonate of soda and starch. They act by virtue of the carbon dioxide they evolve in the presence of moisture. They must yield at least 8 per cent of available carbon dioxide and not more than 1·5 per cent of residual carbon dioxide. Neither must they contain more than 15 parts per million of fluorine. If carelessly prepared, the acid salt may contain an excess of arsenic. They may also contain alum.

EGG SUBSTITUTE POWDERS, to give them their correct designation, are virtually baking powders coloured yellow with turmeric or a coal-tar dye. Lead chromate has occasionally been found in them.

CUSTARD POWDERS usually consist of coloured and flavoured maize starch, but they have been known to contain sago, rice, or potato.

COCOA – There is no standard for cocoa in Great Britain. As sold it usually contains cornflour (or some similar material) and sugar. This is done because pure cocoa is rather indigestible on account of its high fat content. (See COCOA.)

COFFEE, unless bought as beans, is liable to contain chicory. Chicory can be recognized by the fact that in water it sinks and colours the water brown, whereas coffee floats in the water and scarcely stains it. They can also be differentiated under the microscope. (See COFFEE AND TEA.)

TEA – Because of the careful examination to which it is submitted by Customs officers, tea is seldom adulterated now as it used to be in the old days with exhausted leaves, leaves from other sources or from green tea 'faced' with indigo or Prussian blue. Cheap tea may still contain a high proportion of tea dust. Unadulterated tea should contain 1·5 to 5 per cent of theine, the alkaloid to which it owes its stimulating action. (See COFFEE and TEA.)

SUGAR is usually pure. Sometimes flour may be mixed with it, but this can easily be detected by the presence of a sediment when the sugar dissolves. *Brown sugar* is less highly refined cane sugar containing traces of colouring matter. *Demerara sugar*, strictly speaking, is a type of cane sugar originally obtained from the region of Guyana known as Demerara, which is yellowish-brown in colour. Ordinary cane sugar may be adulterated with a synthetic brown dye to simulate brown or demerara sugar.

CHOCOLATES AND SWEETS – Chocolate should contain not less than 10 per cent of ground cocoa nib or 5 per cent of essence of cocoa, to which are added cocoa fat, starch, sugar and milk. Inferior chocolate (usually imported) contains only 2 to 3 per cent of ground cocoa nib; when exposed to a strong light it appears to have a greyish or bluish-grey bloom. Ultra-violet light and X-rays can be used to reveal chemical impurities. Inferior boiled sweets may be contaminated with minute traces of arsenic due to the use of impure glucose instead of sugar. (See CHOCOLATE.)

HONEY may be adulterated with cane sugar or glucose.

JAMS AND MARMALADE are seldom adulterated at the present day. The unofficial standards for jams adopted by the manufacturers are that 'full fruit standard' contains 30 to 45 per cent of fruit, whilst 'lower fruit standard' contains 20 per cent of fruit.

MEAT cannot readily be adulterated except by the sale of unsound or diseased meat. Horseflesh can be distinguished by the fact that it is dark and coarse, has a sickly odour and a soapy feel, and the fat is yellow. As horseflesh contains more glycogen (qv) than oxflesh, the addition of a few drops of a solution of iodine or potassium iodide to a decoction of the flesh will produce a violet coloration.

ARROWROOT may be adulterated with potato starch, rice or wheat flour.

CINNAMON and other similar spices are adulterated with flour and may contain sand.

GROUND GINGER may contain pepper.

PEPPER often contains 1·5 to 3 per cent of sand and grit. This is an example of unavoidable adulteration.

PICKLES, SAUCES AND CHUTNEY often consist principally of vinegar thickened with curry powder, pea-flour and caramel.

MUSTARD is sold mixed with cornflour to keep the mustard grains separate; otherwise it would go solid.

VINEGAR should contain no other acid except acetic acid, no lead or copper and no colouring matter. It has been decided in the courts that non-brewed vinegar containing less than 4 per cent acetic acid is 'not of the nature, substance or quality demanded'. Artificial vinegar is made by diluting acetic acid and it may be coloured with caramel. Sulphuric acid has been used as an adulterant. No preservative may be added to vinegar. It is illegal to describe 'synthetic' or 'artificial' vinegar as 'vinegar'. (See ACETIC ACID.)

ALCOHOLIC BEVERAGES – Whisky may be diluted with water legally; it must not be more than 35 degrees under proof. Some low-grade whiskies may contain potato spirit. Brandy is made from fermented grape juice but inferior brands are made from potato spirit, coloured with burnt sugar and flavoured with various agents, or a little real brandy. Beer may contain arsenic if chemically prepared glucose is used in its manufacture. It may also contain an excessive amount of common salt or excessive preservative: the amount of preservative is limited by Regulations to 70 parts of sulphur dioxide per million. Wines should be made from the fermented juice of the grape. Calcium sulphate is sometimes added to wine to increase its dryness and improve its keeping properties; this is known as 'plastering'. If excess is added, this may lead to the formation of sufficient potassium sulphate to produce a purgative effect. To avoid this, not more than 2 grams of calcium sulphate is permitted per litre in France. Artificial colouring matter, especially logwood, may be added to wine. The only preservative allowed in wine is sulphur dioxide, not exceeding 450 parts per million. There is relatively little tampering with foreign wines in Britain, but fraudulent imitations are sometimes sold under the title of 'British wines': eg. water coloured with cochineal, flavoured with essences and thickened with sugar. Cider, because of its acidity, may become contaminated with lead. (See ALCOHOL.)

Preservatives in food – Preservatives, such as boric acid, borax, formaldehyde, benzoic acid and sulphur dioxide, used to be added often to foodstuffs. Their indiscriminate use led to much trouble and their use is now forbidden by Regulations, with the exception of sulphur dioxide and benzoic acid in specified amounts in specified foods, and sodium or potassium nitrite in ham, bacon, and cooked pickled meat. In the case of cooked pickled meat not more than 200 parts per million may be added. Under these Regulations the term 'preservative' does not include salt, saltpetre, sugar, glycerin, alcohol, vinegar, acetic acid and spices. Up to 70 parts of sulphur dioxide or 120 parts of benzoic acid may be added to sweetened mineral waters, but cordials and fruit juices can contain only up to 350 parts of sulphur dioxide or 800 parts of benzoic acid per million parts. Alcoholic wines are not allowed to contain more than 450 parts of sulphur dioxide per million; for beer the upper limit is 70 parts per million, whilst for cider it is 200 parts per million. Sulphur dioxide is also used in jams and marmalade, the limit being 100 parts per million. Pickles, sauces, and chutney may not contain more than 250 parts of benzoic acid per million. Sausages may have sulphur dioxide added as a preservative (450 parts per million).

AEDES AEGYPTI is the scientific name of the mosquito (illustration 5) which conveys to man (by biting) the viruses of yellow fever and of dengue or 'breakbone fever'. (See DENGUE; and YELLOW FEVER.)

AEGOPHONY is the bleating or punchinello tone given to the voice as heard by auscultation, when there is a small amount of fluid in the pleural cavity.

AERODONTALGIA is the relatively rare form of dental pain occasionally felt

5 – *Aedes aegypti* (female). The transmitter of yellow fever and dengue. From Manson: *Tropical Diseases*. Bailliere Tindall.

in restored or non-vital teeth by those who fly. It is thought that it is caused by expansion of gas entrapped in the pulp canal of the tooth, resulting from the change in altitude.

AEROPHAGY means air-swallowing, and is the name applied to a habit which some persons, especially when suffering from dyspepsia, contract of swallowing mouthfuls of air. This at first gives relief to the discomfort and pain of indigestion, but later prolongs and aggravates it. The resulting breathlessness can be relieved to some extent by taking peppermint water or chloroform water in doses of a tablespoonful, but the chief necessity is to overcome the habit of swallowing air.

AEROSOL is a suspension of very fine liquid (or rarely solid) particles in a gas such as air or oxygen. The size of aerosol particles ranges from 30 micrometres (a micrometre $= \frac{1}{1000}$ millimetre) down to a fraction of a micrometre. The fine mist of an aerosol can be produced by either a hand spray or by a special machine known as a nebulizer. There are three main uses for aerosols in medicine. (i) To destroy pests such as malaria- or yellow-fever-carrying mosquitoes, and lice which transmit typhus. DDT is a usual constituent of such aerosols. (ii) To sterilize premises such as hospital wards, schoolrooms and cinemas, to prevent the spread of airborne droplet infections. The usual constituents of such aerosols are sodium hypochlorite, hexylresorcinol, or propylene glycol. (iii)

To combat diseases of the lungs such as asthma and chronic bronchitis, by producing an aerosol which is inhaled by the patient. Such aerosols may contain one of the drugs used for the relief of an asthmatic attack such as adrenaline or isoprenaline. They should only be used under medical supervision.

AESTHESIOMETER is an instrument for measuring the sensation of touch in a person

AETIOLOGY is the part of medical science dealing with the causes of disease.

AFFUSION is a method of treatment by pouring water upon the body. (See BATHS; COLD, EFFECTS OF; DOUCHES.)

AFIBRINOGENAEMIA is a condition in which the blood is incoagulable as a result of absence of fibrin (qv). It is characterized by haemorrhage. There are two forms: (*a*) a congenital form, and (*b*) an acquired form. The latter may be associated with advanced liver disease, or may occur as a complication of labour. Treatment consists of the intravenous injection of fibrinogen and blood transfusion.

AFTERBIRTH, or PLACENTA, is the name given to the thick, spongy disc-like cake of tissue which connects the embryo with the inner surface of the womb, the embryo otherwise lying free in the amniotic fluid. (See AMNION.) The placenta is mainly a new structure growing with the embryo, but, when it separates, a portion of the inner surface of the womb, called the maternal placenta, comes away with it. It is mainly composed of loops of veins belonging to the embryo, lying in blood-sinuses, in which circulates maternal blood. Thus, though no mixing of the blood of embryo and mother takes place, there is ample opportunity for the exchange of fluids, gases, and the nutriment brought by the mother's blood. The width of the full-sized placenta is about eight inches (20 cm), its thickness one inch (2·5 cm). One surface is rough and studded with villi, which consist of the loops of foetal veins; the other is smooth, and has implanted in its centre the umbilical cord, or navel string, which is about as thick as a finger and 20 inches (50 cm) long, contains two arteries and a vein, enters the foetus at the navel, and forms the sole connection between the bodies of mother and foetus. The name 'afterbirth' is given to the structure because it is expelled from the

21

womb in the third stage of labour (see LABOUR).

AFTERPAINS are pains similar to but feebler than those of labour, occurring in the two or three days following childbirth. **Causes** are generally the presence of a blood-clot or retained piece of placenta which the womb is attempting to expel.

AGAMMAGLOBULINAEMIA is a condition found in children, in which there is no gamma-globulin (qv) in the blood. These children are particularly susceptible to infections as they are unable to form antibodies to the infecting micro-organism.

AGAR, or AGAR-AGAR, is a gelatinous substance prepared from seaweed. It is used in preparing culture-media for use in bacteriological laboratories. It is sometimes given for relieving constipation.

AGE, NATURAL CHANGES IN – The length of life is a characteristic of each species. Thus, senile changes are found in a mouse at 2 years, in a rat at 3 years, in a dog at 12 to 14, in a horse at 30, whilst the allotted years of man are three score years and ten. As age advances, the tissues become more rigid and less elastic. The bones become more brittle. The ligaments are stiffer, so that contortions of the body and limbs, as in gymnastic feats, become impossible. Fat is deposited beneath the skin in middle life with accompanying increase in weight. It may be absorbed again in old age, leaving the skin wrinkled. Deposition of fat also occurs in internal organs, eg. the heart, weakening their activity. The skin becomes thin, is less well lubricated, and its vessels do not react properly to heat and cold, so that cold is more acutely felt. The chief change is in the blood-vessels, the walls of which become first thicker, then more brittle. This means that obstruction (eg. in the coronary arteries that supply the heart muscle with blood) or haemorrhage (eg. into the brain, with apoplexy) more readily occurs. This change is hastened by alcoholic excesses and some diseases, and the extent to which it has occurred is the measure of the interference with the employments of active life, so that it has been said, 'A man is as old as his arteries'. This thickening of the arteries in the brain and consequent narrowing of their calibre, causing a poorer blood-supply to the brain, is one of the chief reasons of mental feebleness in old age. The menopause occurs in women between forty-five and fifty (see MENSTRUATION), and men sometimes about the age of sixty have some months' illness and feebleness, after which strength again returns. Sexual activity tends to diminish but seldom becomes dormant. Loss of elasticity in the lens of the eye brings about the need of spectacles for reading from forty upwards. Another eye change occurs after fifty in the appearance of a whitish ring (arcus senilis) round the cornea, near its edge; this is of no significance. Of more importance is the thickening of the lens known as cataract (qv) which tends to occur after the age of fifty and may so interfere with sight that the lens has to be removed. After sixty the teeth, if still good, may begin to fall out, and the hair whitens. (See also CLIMACTERIC; and EXPECTATION OF LIFE.)

AGENE is nitrogen trichloride and was used for many years as a flour improver and bleacher. As a result of experiments that showed that agene produced hysteria in dogs and some other animals, the British and US governments prohibited the use of agene as a flour improver, substituting chlorine dioxide as an alternative improver.

AGENESIA, or AGENESIS, means incomplete development or the failure of any part or organ of the body to develop normally.

AGGLUTINATION is the adherence together of small bodies in a fluid. Thus, blood corpuscles agglutinate into heaps (rouleaux) when added to the serum of a person belonging to an incompatible blood-group. Bacteria agglutinate into clumps and die when exposed to the presence of antibodies in the blood. This is important in regard to diagnosis of certain diseases due to bacteria. In typhoid fever, for example, the blood of an animal is immunized against typhoid bacilli by repeated injections of these. The blood-serum of the animal, known now as antityphoid serum, is issued to laboratories for use when bacilli are found in the excretions of a patient who is possibly suffering from typhoid fever. The bacilli are exposed to the action of a drop of the serum; if the serum shows the power of agglutinating these bacteria, this forms evidence that the bacteria in question are typhoid bacilli. The reaction may also be carried out in the contrary manner: that is to say, the serum from the blood of a patient, who may be suffering from typhoid fever, but in regard to whom the diagnosis is still a matter of doubt, is added to a drop of fluid containing bacteria known to be typhoid bacilli; if these are agglutinated into clumps by the patient's serum, the patient is then known to be suffering from typhoid fever; if they do not agglutinate, his symptoms are due to some other condition. This reaction for typhoid fever is known as the Widal reaction. Comparable agglutination reactions, using an appropriate serum, are used in the diagnosis of a number of diseases, including glandular fever (when it is known as the Paul-Bunnell reaction), typhus fever (when it is known as the Weil-Felix reaction), undulant fever, and Weil's disease.

AGNOSIA is the term given to the condition in which, in certain diseases of the brain, the patient loses the ability to recognize the character of objects through the senses – touch, taste, sight, hearing.

AGONY is excessive pain associated with struggling.

AGORAPHOBIA means a sense of fear experienced in large open spaces and public places, and is a symptom of psychological disorder. There are said to be 300,000 victims of it in the United Kingdom. Those who suffer from what can be a most distressing condition can obtain help and advice from the Phobic Society, 4 Cheltenham Road, Chorlton cum Hardy, Manchester M21 1QN. (*Tel*: 061–881 1937.)

AGRANULOCYTOSIS is a condition in which the white corpuscles in the blood of the polynuclear or granular variety become greatly lessened in numbers or disappear altogether. This change is found accompanying long-standing suppurative conditions, especially about the throat and mouth, and is a very serious one. It is also caused in some cases by taking such drugs as amidopyrine, thiourea, sulphonamides and chloramphenicol.

AGRAPHIA is the loss of power to express ideas by writing. (See APHASIA.)

AGUE (see MALARIA). The term is also sometimes applied to neuralgia (brow ague) and to a state of tremor of the muscles found in various diseases (such as brass founders' ague).

AGUE CAKE is the old term applied to the enlarged spleen found in malaria.

AIR is of very uniform composition both in towns and country as regards its general constituents. These are:

	per cent
Oxygen	20·94
Nitrogen	78·09
Argon	0·94
Carbonic Acid	0·03

Besides these there are always ozone, minerals and organic matters in small and variable amounts, and more or less water vapour according to the weather. In the air of towns, sulphurous acid and sulphuretted hydrogen are important impurities derived from combustion. After air has been respired once, the oxygen falls by about 4 per cent and the carbonic acid rises to about 4 per cent, while organic matter and water vapour are greatly increased and the air rises in temperature. The cause of the discomfort felt in badly ventilated rooms and crowded halls is associated with the increase in the temperature and moisture of the air, but a high percentage of carbonic acid may be present without causing any noticeable discomfort or appreciable quickening of the respiration. Microbes are found especially in dusty air, and during coughing, sneezing and loud talking they are expelled from the air passages on droplets of moisture. When epidemic diseases such as influenza are rife, infection is apt to be conveyed through the air by these means, especially in badly ventilated and overwarmed rooms. When the amount of carbonic acid present in the air exceeds 0·1 per cent there is usually a distinct sense of 'stuffiness', which forms the best guide as to the necessity for increased ventilation. The continued breathing day after day of a 'stuffy' atmosphere is apt to produce headache, drowsiness, depression, inability to concentrate on work, dryness of the throat and a tendency to 'catch cold' easily, thus resulting in a gradual deterioration of health. Inadequate ventilation has much to do with the onset of pulmonary tuberculosis as well as with infection by other diseases such as influenza and the common cold. (See VENTILATION.)

Uses (see CLIMATE; INHALATIONS; RESPIRATION; VENTILATION).

AIR-BEDS consist of stout rubber perforated in numerous places by rubber tubes which open on the upper and lower surfaces and add strength to the bed. The bed is blown up from one end by means of an automobile or bicycle pump to the desired hardness. Such a bed is both easier for the nurse to manage and more comfortable to the patient than a water-bed.

Uses – In general an air-bed is placed under a bedridden person or one suffering from devitalizing disease of the nervous system, in order to prevent the formation of bed sores, by distributing pressure all over the patient's back. Apart from the tendency to bed sores, a patient who is long confined to bed, who is fevered, or who is much emaciated, derives a sense of great coolness and comfort from an air-bed.

AIR PASSAGES – These are the nose, pharynx or throat (the large cavity behind the nose and mouth), larynx, trachea or windpipe, and bronchi or bronchial tubes. The air, on entering the nose (illustration 6), passes through a high narrow passage on each side, the outer wall of which has three projections (the nasal conchae) which almost touch the dividing septum between the nostrils, thus making on each side three passages or meatuses (illustration 330), in which the air is warmed, moistened, and relieved of particles of dust. (See NOSE.) Mouth-breathing is, accordingly, a bad habit because the air is not prepared for entrance to the lungs. In the pharynx the food and air passages meet and cross.

6 Vertical section through the middle of the head and neck, showing the upper air passages. The passages for air, *a*, are indicated by a pecked line, those for the food, *f*, by a dotted line; *et*, Eustachian tube; *l*, larynx; *w*, windpipe; *t*, tonsil; *to*, tongue; *g*, gullet. For other letters, see illustration 89.

24

The larynx lies in front of the lower part of the pharynx and is the organ where the voice is produced (see VOICE) by aid of the vocal cords. The opening between the cords is called the glottis, and shortly after passing this the air reaches the trachea or wind-pipe, a tube 4 to 5 inches long (10 to 12·5 cm), and ¾ inch (2 cm) wide (illustration 7).

This leads into the chest and divides above the heart into two bronchi, one of which goes to each lung, in which it splits into finer and finer tubes (see LUNGS). The larynx is enclosed in two strong cartilages, the thyroid (of which the most projecting part, the Adam's apple, is a prominent point on the front of the neck) and the cricoid (which can be felt as a hard ring about an inch below). Beneath this, the trachea, which is stiffened by rings of cartilage, so that it is never closed in any position of the body, can be traced down till it disappears behind the breast-bone.

AIR-SICKNESS – The manifestations of this condition are very similar to those of SEA-SICKNESS (qv). The most satisfactory remedy is hyoscine hydrobromide, 1/60 to 1/120 grain (1 to 0·5 mg).

AKINESIA means loss, or impairment, of voluntary movement, or immobility. It is characteristically seen in Parkinsonism (qv).

ALASTRIM, or VARIOLA MINOR, is a form of smallpox which differs from ordinary smallpox in being milder and having a low mortality.

ALBINISM is a state of poverty (or absence) of pigment in the superficial tissues of the body, producing a pale pink colour of the skin, whiteness of the hair, and pinkness of the eye. A person showing these peculiarities is called an albino. It may also occur only in patches.

Causes – It is congenital, existing from birth, though the parents of an albino are not necessarily subjects of albinism. It occurs with a frequency of about 1 in 10,000.

Symptoms – An albino may show nothing remarkable beyond white hair, white delicate skin and pink eyes, but many are physically and mentally feeble. Usually the absence of pigment to screen the eye from bright light gives rise to trouble, and the person has a tendency to inflammation of the eyes. (See EYE, DISEASES OF.)

Treatment – There is no remedy. The eyes should be protected in bright light by wearing dark glasses.

Thyroid cartilage

Cricothyroid ligament

Cricoid cartilage

Trachea

Left bronchus

Right bronchus

Apical bronchus

Apical bronchus

Subapical bronchus

Subapical bronchus

parterial bronchus

Pectoral bronchus

Pectoral bronchus

Lingular bronchus

Hyparterial bronchus

Middle lobe bronchus

Anterior basal
bronchus

Anterior basal
bronchus

Axillary basal
bronchus

Axillary basal
bronchus

Dorsal bronchus

Cardiac bronchus

Posterior basal bronchus

M.C.

7 – The lower air passages. From *Gray's Anatomy*. Longmans.

ALBUMINS are proteins. They enter into the composition of all the tissues of the body. Their characters are that they are soluble in pure water; can be dried into a light, flaky, non-crystalline powder; are coagulated by heat, and precipitated by various agents like nitric acid, tannin, alcohol, or perchloride of mercury.

Varieties – Albumins are generally divided according to their source of origin, as muscle-albumin, milk-albumin, blood- or serum-albumin, egg-albumin, vegetable-albumin, etc. These differ both in chemical reactions and also physiologically, for though serum-albumin occurs in the blood, some albumins, eg. egg-albumin, injected direct into the blood are highly poisonous.

Uses – When taken into the stomach they are all converted into a soluble form by the process of digestion, and are then absorbed into the blood, whence they go to build up the tissues gradually worn out in the activity of the body. (See ALBUMINURIA; BRIGHT'S DISEASE.)

ALBUMINURIA means a condition in which albumin is present in the urine. It is more correctly described as proteinuria, because the other blood proteins are present in the urine as well as albumin, though albumin is far in excess of the others. It is of immense importance because it is often a symptom of serious heart or kidney disease.

Causes – (1) *Kidney disease* is the most important cause of albuminuria, and in some cases the discovery of albuminuria may be the first evidence of such disease. This is why an examination of the urine for the presence of albumin constitutes an essential part of every medical examination. Almost any form of kidney disease will cause albuminuria, but the most frequent form to do this is Bright's disease. In the subacute (or nephrotic) stage of Bright's disease the most marked albuminuria of all may be found. Albuminuria is also found in infections of the kidney (pyelitis) as well as in infections of the bladder (cystitis) and of the urethra (urethritis). The development of albuminuria in pregnancy is always an indication for the individual receiving careful medical treatment, as it may be the first sign of one of the most dangerous complications of pregnancy: toxaemia of pregnancy, Bright's disease, or eclampsia (qv).

(2) *Heart failure* is always accompanied by albuminuria, particularly when the right side of the heart is failing. In severe cases of failure, accompanied by dropsy, the albuminuria may be marked. It is due to congestion of the kidneys.

(3) *Fever* is practically always accompanied by albuminuria, even though there is not actual kidney disease. The albuminuria disappears soon after the temperature becomes normal.

(4) *Drugs and poisons* – These include arsenic, lead, mercury, gold, copaiba, salicylic acid and quinine.

(5) *Anaemia* – A trace of albumin may be found in the urine in severe cases of anaemia.

(6) *Functional or orthostatic albuminuria* – Almost any normal person may have a transitory albuminuria after severe muscular exertion or after a cold bath, and it may occasionally appear after eating a large amount of protein: eg. raw eggs. The form commonly known as *orthostatic* or postural albuminuria is much more common and is of importance because, if the true cause is not recognized, it may be taken as a sign of kidney disease. In the 1914–18 War it was found in 4 per cent of healthy British soldiers, and in an American investigation it was found in 5 per cent of healthy university freshmen. The cause is still doubtful, but it is probably due to temporary congestion of the kidneys caused by adoption of the upright position in individuals with some slight disturbance of the circulation of the blood in the kidneys. At one time it was thought that individuals with this type of albuminuria were more prone to develop Bright's disease later in life than individuals in whom it was not present, but this has now been definitely disproved. The features of this type of albuminuria are that it usually occurs in young people, usually between the ages of 8 and 18 years, and that it is not present while the patient is at rest. Thus, the specimen of urine obtained the first thing in the morning, before the individual gets up, contains no albumin, whilst a specimen obtained later in the day, after the individual has been up and about, will contain albumin.

Albuminuria and Life Assurance – Most companies will not issue a life policy to anyone with permanent albuminuria lest this be due to Bright's disease. Even cases in which no serious disease manifests itself have, if the albuminuria persists, a shorter expectation of life than other people, and so require a higher premium. In cases of doubt, tests to measure the function of the kidney may be carried out. If the tests show normal function, then the albuminuria takes on a much less serious aspect.

Treatment – The treatment is that of the

underlying disease. (See BRIGHT'S DISEASE, etc.) In the case of functional albuminuria due to excessive exercise, cold baths, or excessive ingestion of protein, treatment consists of removal of the cause. Individuals who have orthostatic or postural albuminuria are usually adolescents or young adults who are not in good training, and the treatment consists of getting them into good condition. Unless bathing is found to produce albuminuria, they should be encouraged to have a cold plunge every morning, followed by rapid friction with a towel. 'Early to bed, early to rise' is sound advice for these individuals, in addition to regular exercise in the open air.

ALBUMIN WATER is used for administration as a light form of nourishment to patients with weak digestion or suffering from diarrhoea or some condition in which only very small amounts of food can be borne. To prepare albumin water a raw egg is broken in two on the edge of a cup. The white is allowed to escape by passing the yolk from one half of the shell to the other. The white is then whisked for 10 minutes to a stiff froth, $\frac{1}{2}$ pint (250 ml) of cold water is added, and it is allowed to stand for an hour to dissolve. Lemon juice may be added to flavour, and a cupful may be given at one time.

ALBUMOSE is the term applied to the products of digestion of protein foods, differing from albumin in not being coagulable by heat. Albumose is further converted by digestion into peptone.

ALCOHOL, more correctly ETHYL ALCOHOL, or ETHANOL, is a liquid obtained by the action of yeast on solutions of sugar, especially of grape sugar or glucose. Carbonic acid gas is also formed in the process and escapes. After fermentation of the sugary fluid has taken place, the alcohol is separated from the water by distillation and from the last traces of water by the action of lime, which absorbs the latter. Absolute alcohol contains 99·4 to 100 per cent (by volume) of alcohol. It is a powerful irritant, and even in moderate quantities a poison. Rectified spirit, or spirit of wine, contains 90 per cent of alcohol by volume, and is used to make essences, tinctures and weaker spirits of 80, 70, 60, 50, 45, 25 and 20 per cent strength. Proof spirit contains 57 per cent (by volume) of alcohol. It is called 'proof' spirit, because an old test of its strength was to drench gunpowder with it, set fire

to it, and if the gunpowder was ignited the alcohol stood the proof. The legal definition of proof spirit is 'that which at the temperature of 51° by Fahrenheit's thermometer weighs exactly twelve-thirteenth parts of an equal measure of distilled water'. Spirits are described in terms of so many degrees over or under proof (O.P. or U.P.), depending upon the quantity of distilled water which must be added to, or deducted from, 100 volumes of the sample in order to produce spirit of proof strength. Another method of indicating spirit strength, commonly used on the labels of alcoholic drinks is to give it as a number of degrees, proof spirit being taken as 100 per cent. Thus a spirit said to be 70° would contain 70 per cent of proof spirit: ie. it would be 30° under proof.

Alcohol freezes at a very low temperature, and so is used for thermometers for the Arctic regions. It dissolves many things which water does not dissolve, such as fats, oils and resins. Mixed with wood-spirit, it forms methylated spirit, on which no duty is payable but which is, of course, unfit for drinking. It coagulates the tissues, and so has a hardening effect upon skin, wounds, etc.

Varieties of alcoholic liquors – Spirits and wines sold under various names differ very much in the amount of alcohol contained in different samples under the same name, but table 1 gives a general idea of the percentages of alcohol by volume present in the various forms of beverage. Many of the stronger forms are sold commonly in a more diluted state than that indicated in the table. Some of the weaker wines, on the other hand, are 'fortified' by the addition of spirit to confer on them more stimulating properties.

	per cent
Rum, Whisky	30
Brandy, Gin	30
Liqueurs	15 to 55
Port, Sherry	15 to 16
Madeira	15 to 16
Champagne	10
Burgundy	about 10
Claret	about 9
Moselle, Hock	about 9
Strong ale	about 8
Cider	2 to 3
Beer	2 to 3

Table 1 – Alcoholic content of alcoholic liquors

Various wines, manufactured or home-made, are produced by fermenting mixtures of fruit and sugar: eg. cowslip wine, ginger wine, orange bitters, raisin wine,

27

raspberry wine, red currant wine. The percentage of alcohol in these British wines is usually about 10 or 12, rising in some of the stronger forms to over 20 per cent.

SPIRITS, including *rum* from molasses, *brandy* from wine, *whisky* from malted grain, and *gin* from grain and juniper berries, are prepared by fermentation followed by distillation. They contain in their raw state more or less fusel oil, an oily substance consisting of amyl and butyl alcohols which have a more harmful effect upon the nervous system than ethyl alcohol. These, however, are slowly converted to ethers, which give to long-kept spirit its prized flavour and aroma, and are harmless. Spirits are by law prohibited from being delivered for consumption in Britain until they have been warehoused for at least three years. *Vodka* is just water added to neutral spirits and has practically no odour as it contains none of the ethers or congeners that give the prized flavour and aroma to brandy, whisky and gin.

LIQUEURS are spirits in which have been steeped various spices, leaves and fruits, and which have, in addition to the properties of alcohol, those of the various ingredients.

PORT, SHERRY, MADEIRA, and other Portuguese and Hungarian wines, are known as *fortified wines*, because spirit is added to them for preservation. They are therefore stronger, and containing much unchanged grape-juice have more body and bouquet than those in which the alcohol is simply derived from the grape-juice, which is completely used up in fermentation. They improve by keeping, as the tannin and other harsh-tasting substances separate out gradually as a crust.

CHAMPAGNE and other effervescent wines are white wines to which much sugar has been added after bottling, so that fermentation goes on and carbonic acid gas is produced, which becomes, on long keeping, intimately blended with the wine, and adds greatly to its effect. Hence champagne is more stimulating and its effects more rapid than in the case of other wines much stronger in alcohol.

CLARET, BURGUNDY, MOSELLE, HOCK, and other wines from the northern vineyards, are thin and acidulous from cream of tartar, and so form refreshing drinks with no special virtue beyond the stimulating effect of the alcohol they contain. They are, however, less harmful in gout than the wines with much body, and there is not the same necessity for keeping them many years before using.

BEER, in addition to being weakly alcoholic, contains an infusion of hops which gives it bitterness.

Effects of alcohol – Alcohol, when drunk, is quickly and completely absorbed. About one-fifth of any dose taken is absorbed from the stomach, and almost the whole of the remainder is absorbed in the upper part of the small intestine within two or three hours of having been taken. Very little is excreted by the breath, urine and other channels. This seldom amounts to more than one-twentieth of the quantity swallowed. The remainder is completely used up within twenty-four hours, being oxidized mainly to produce heat. The body can derive one-fifth of the total energy it requires from alcohol, and in this way alcohol spares carbohydrates and fats taken in the food. There is a tendency therefore for both of these to be deposited in the tissues as superfluous fat when alcohol is habitually added to the diet without a decrease of the other food.

With regard to the mental effect of alcohol, this is dependent partly upon its effect on the circulation and partly on its anaesthetic action on the nervous system, dulling small pains and the sense of worry and anxiety. Owing to a similar dulling action upon the higher intellectual faculties, self-criticism and self-control are also to a considerable extent lessened, and this creates the false impression that alcohol is having a stimulating action. Alcohol is not a stimulant, it is a depressant. If a larger dose be taken, the functions of sense perception and skilled movement are to a certain extent dulled and deteriorate, with the result that there is a certain clumsiness of behaviour. The person now begins to make ill-adjusted movements, shows some slurring of speech, and becomes less quick and less capable in performing acts which require decision and promptitude: eg. avoiding a collision when driving a motorcar. In a further stage the intellectual processes of judgment, self-criticism, and self-control are largely suspended and the functions of sense perception and skilled movement become very greatly impaired, until ultimately a heavy sleep or stupor supervenes which lasts until the alcohol absorbed by the nervous system has been oxidized and consumed. There is no proof that alcohol in any dose improves the efficiency with which either skilled or unskilled work can be carried out during the few hours while the alcohol acts.

With regard to the action on digestion, moderate doses of alcohol increase the secretions of the stomach and thus may aid digestion in persons in whom these secretions are defective. Different wines have very varying effect on different persons in this respect, probably on account of the substances other than alcohol which they contain. When alcoholic beverages are taken habitually over long periods, and especially in the more concentrated form of spirits, they exert a pronounced effect of irritation upon the mucous membrane of the stomach and thus lead to chronic indigestion.

With regard to the action of alcohol on respiration and circulation of the blood, moderate doses have practically no effect upon the breathing, although very large doses have a paralysing effect, and when death occurs from alcohol it is brought about by stoppage of the respiration. As to its 'stimulating' action on the circulation, this is in part brought about by the lessening of mental strain induced by its narcotic and sedative action. It is also due in part to its action in dilating the small blood-vessels, and thus reducing the blood-pressure and possibly relieving strain on the heart.

The popular reputation of alcohol as a means of 'warding off cold' is due largely to its power of dilating the superficial blood-vessels and of dulling the sensory nerves of the skin, so that the skin actually becomes warm, while external impressions are not felt. If at the same time as the alcohol is administered, warmth is applied to the surface of the body by hot blankets, hot bottles, etc., the skin becomes more capable of absorbing the external heat and thus the alcohol acts as a restorative.

The official statistics issued by the Registrar General indicate a heavy mortality among persons occupied in the liquor trade, who are known to consume more than the average amount of alcohol. The experience of insurance companies has made them adverse to admitting on ordinary terms persons who are habitual users of alcoholic beverages in large amount.

Alcohol and Driving – During recent years increasing attention has been devoted to the effect of alcohol upon the ability to drive a motor-car. It is now recognized that even quite small amounts of alcohol may be sufficient to impair those standards of watchfulness and efficiency which are vitally important if accidents are to be reduced to a minimum in these days of ever-increasing congestion on the roads and ever-increasing speed of cars. In the seven years, 1970–76, convictions for driving under the influence of drink or drugs doubled – from 25,000 to

50,000, whilst in 1974 and 1975 two in every five motor vehicle drivers and riders aged 16–24 who died in traffic accidents had a blood alcohol concentration above the legal limit.

Careful attention is therefore being given to means of detecting whether or not a car-driver has had sufficient alcohol to interfere with his capacity as a driver. Particular attention has been devoted to means of estimating the amount of alcohol that has been consumed and correlating this with the ability to drive. It is now generally accepted that the amount of alcohol in the blood is a reliable guide, and that this can be estimated directly, or indirectly by estimating the amount of alcohol in the urine or in the expired breath of the individual. The last of these is the most unreliable.

In October 1967, the Road Safety Act came into force, making it an offence for a motorist to drive, attempt to drive, or be in charge of a vehicle if his (or her) blood alcohol level is over 80 mg per 100 millilitres or his (or her) urine alcohol is over 107 mg per 100 millilitres.

These figures must not be taken to mean that it is safe to drive a car if one's blood or urine alcohol is below these levels. Equally dangerous is it to attempt to correlate one's consumption of alcohol with one's blood or urine alcohol levels. The only safe rule is not to drive after drinking.

Uses of Alcohol – *Externally* it is used in the cheap form of methylated spirit to cleanse the skin of oily, fatty, or resinous substances, which water will not remove. Also to harden the skin of the feet before a long walk, or that of the back in persons confined to bed for long periods, and so prevent bed sores (qv).

A whisky pack or brandy pack is an old-fashioned remedy to stimulate infants reduced to a state of collapse by diarrhoea or bronchitis.

Internally there are few, if any, absolute indications for the use of alcohol, and during the last fifty years the use of alcohol as a medicine has declined rapidly.

Alcohol may be of value in stimulating the appetite during convalescence. It is also a useful sedative sometimes in old people, particularly in an individual who is used to taking alcohol regularly in moderation. Its value as a stimulant of the heart is doubtful. There is a certain amount of justification for the use of undiluted whisky or brandy in the treatment of fainting, provided this is not due to some serious condition such as haemorrhage. It should never be given to a patient who is suffering from shock. Champagne and brandy-and-soda have a traditional reputation for the relief of vomiting, including sea-sickness.

The popular habit of taking spirits 'to keep the cold out' is a delusion. Alcohol gives a sense of warmth to the skin by bringing the blood there; but, as the blood is rapidly cooled in cold air, the risk of frostbite and even death by freezing is increased, so that experienced hunters and mountaineers will on no account touch spirits on biting cold days or at high altitudes.

In health, there is no necessity for alcohol, and, as so many persons contract the alcohol habit, it would be well for every one to consider the question carefully before embarking on its habitual use. Even far short of drunkenness its constant use in large quantities certainly shortens life. (See ALCOHOLISM, CHRONIC.)

ALCOHOLISM, ACUTE – This is the condition produced by taking excessive quantities of alcohol over a short period. The effects vary greatly according to the hereditary and nervous constitution of the person concerned, his or her age and social surroundings, and to a great extent with the kind of liquor taken, whether it is taken with food, and whether it has been taken for a long time previously.

Varieties – There are many curious effects produced and phases of character brought to light by the disturbance of mental balance, but the three important forms are ordinary drunkenness, alcoholic mania, and delirium tremens.

Symptoms – ORDINARY DRUNKENNESS is too common to need much description. First the person is brightened, his spirits rise, his conversation is witty, the skin becomes flushed, and there is a general sense of well-being. As he becomes really drunk a phase of depression-excitement comes on: one person becomes angry, resents fancied affronts, and tries to pick quarrels, another becomes melancholy and lugubrious, a third grows maudlin, and weepingly recounts the secrets of his family to perfect strangers, while a fourth type assumes a regal manner and gives away his money and valuables or makes promises which he cannot possibly fulfil: and all lose the controlling power of reason. A third stage is that in which all feeling of shame is lost, and there is dullness of sense and loss of power, the drunk man or woman reeling or falling and rising with difficulty. The fourth stage

is popularly known as 'dead drunk'; the person lies in a state of insensibility, with stertorous breathing and dilated pupils.

ALCOHOLIC MANIA is the form which often affects neurotic young men or women with a family taint of insanity. A state of excitement and fury, leading sometimes to attempts at murder or suicide, comes on after, it may be, only a few glasses of spirits or wine, and lasts some hours or days, without any tendency to dullness or sleep. Some persons who are liable to epileptic attacks have a fit when alcohol is taken even in moderate amount.

DELIRIUM TREMENS is the most serious form, and is popularly known as 'bluedevils', because of the hallucinations accompanying the state. It follows on a long course of drinking which has ended in a bout, or may be brought on by an injury or business worries in a heavy drinker; but it does not follow a single 'spree'. Tremors all over the body, but especially in the hands and tongue, are the first sign of its onset, then complete loss of appetite, sickness, rise of temperature, weak pulse and constant purposeless movements. Finally hallucinations come on; spiders, flies, mice, rats are described on the clothes or floor, or disgusting objects like snakes, toads, and demons; or the bystanders are taken for policemen, hangmen, etc., and the furniture distorts itself into weird shapes. Lastly, delirium of a terrified or raging type comes on, in which there is more or less danger of suicide or homicide. Pneumonia of a serious type is apt to ensue, and if these two be combined the case is usually fatal. When a case of delirium tremens follows upon a very prolonged course of chronic alcoholism the mental state sometimes passes into one of permanent mental feebleness, due to organic changes in the brain. (See also KORSAKOW'S SYNDROME.)

Treatment – Ordinary drunkenness is best treated by letting the person sleep it off, or, if great quantities of alcohol have been rapidly taken, the stomach should be washed out with the stomach-tube. In the second or excited stage, and in alcoholic mania, if the person be uncontrollable, he is to be treated as in *delirium tremens*. In the latter, admission to hospital is necessary, with careful nursing and constant supervision. Paraldehyde is the best sedative in the acute phase, and promising results are being reported from the use of tranquillizers. If any infection, such as pneumonia is present, full doses of antibiotics are given. A high-calorie, highvitamin diet should be given, with particular emphasis on a high intake of vitamin B₁ (thiamine).

ALCOHOLISM, CHRONIC – This is the condition of mind and body produced by taking too much alcohol over long periods. The consumption of alcoholic drink in the United Kingdom over the last decade is shown in table 2. In the last twenty years the average consumption of beer has gone up by 50 per cent, that of spirits has increased threefold, and that of wine fourfold. It is estimated that 33,000,000 of the population of Britain drink alcoholic beverages and that over 300,000 of them are alcoholics. In Scotland it is estimated that around 1 per cent of persons over 15 years of age are the subjects of alcoholism. The annual cost to industry in Britain of absenteeism, accident proneness and inefficiency due to excessive drinking is estimated to be over £35,000,000, and over a third of our prison population is in prison for crimes connected with alcohol. Convictions for drunkenness have nearly doubled in the last twenty years.

Chronic alcoholism is a disease, but it is

	1960	1965	1969
BEER			
Total consumption (million litres)	4526	5026	5512
Consumption per head of population (litres)	85·5	91	98·7
Consumption per head of population aged 15 and over (litres)	111·6	118·3	130
SPIRITS			
Total consumption (million litres)	98	112	112
Consumption per head of population (litres)	1·8	2·1	2
Consumption per head of population aged 15 and over	2·4	2·7	2·6
WINE			
Total consumption (million litres)	122	162	204
Consumption per head of population (litres)	2·3	3	3·7
Consumption per head of population aged 15 and over (litres)	3	3·9	4·8

Table 2 – Consumption of alcoholic drink in the United Kingdom, 1960–1969.

necessary to differentiate between the chronic alcoholic and the excessive drinker. The latter is able to stop drinking if he is given sufficient good reason for doing so, whereas the victim of chronic alcoholism cannot voluntarily abstain for more than a short while. As one expert has put it: 'The regular heavy drinker lives to drink, but the alcoholic *must* drink to live'. According to the World Health Organization, 'alcoholics are those excessive drinkers whose dependence on alcohol has attained such a degree that they show a noticeable mental disturbance or an interference with their bodily and mental health, their interpersonal relations and their smooth economic and social functioning; or who show the prodromal signs of such development. They therefore need treatment'.

Whatever the reason for drinking, the long-continued consumption of alcohol can result in many medical disorders. The most frequent of these is *gastritis* (qv). Indeed, the most common cause of acute and chronic gastritis is over-indulgence in alcohol. Cirrhosis of the liver (see LIVER, DISEASES) is a frequent complication. Injurious effects on the heart from habitual spirit drinking are not uncommon, and there is an increased tendency for alcoholics to suffer from diseases of the arteries (qv). Peripheral neuritis (qv) is also common. In the early stages this manifests itself by pains in the feet and hands, and tenderness in the calves of the legs, followed later by wrist-drop and foot-drop. In severe cases the cranial nerves may be involved and this may be accompanied by blindness. The fiery visage (see ROSACEA) is a well-known sign of the chronic alcoholic. Finally, there may be severe mental disturbance, such as Korsakow's syndrome (qv) and delirium tremens (see ALCOHOLISM, ACUTE).

There are four types of chronic alcoholics: (i) The alcoholic with a good previous personality; about 80 per cent of these make a successful recovery: ie. remain totally abstinent. (ii) The alcoholic whose basic personality is neurotic. About 30 per cent recover, but they are prone to relapse before they finally become abstinent. (iii) The alcoholic whose basic personality is psychotic. The outlook in this group depends entirely upon the psychosis. In a sense they are not true alcoholics, and treatment is aimed primarily at the psychosis. (iv) The alcoholic whose basic personality is psychopathic. The outlook for this group is extremely bad. The woman psychopath is particularly addicted to alcohol, and she often attempts suicide – and often succeeds.

The prognosis is good if the patient has a happy home and a good job to return to. Those who are separated or divorced, or the bachelor living on his own, find it more difficult to maintain sobriety. The patient who seeks help has the best chance to recover. Undergoing treatment simply to pacify or please the marital partner, or to avoid being cut out of a will, is a poor prognostic sign. Patients of poor, or limited, intelligence, are unlikely to respond to treatment. Excessive drinking in early adult life is usually found in the neurotic. Violent abnormal behaviour of young people under the influence of alcohol suggests an underlying psychosis, such as schizophrenia, or epilepsy. Alcoholism developing at the menopause suggests a depressive state; if it develops in later life it suggests a senile depressive state and has a poor prognosis. A feature of the chronic alcoholic is that he has few hobbies, few outside interests, and little interest in other people. His entire life is centred round drinking.

Treatment – To be successful this must practically always be carried out in the first instance in hospital or special clinic. Very few, if any, can be treated at home, and even outpatient treatment is seldom successful without a preliminary period of inpatient treatment.

The essential feature of treatment is the immediate withdrawal of all alcohol over a period not exceeding forty-eight hours. To overcome, or prevent, the inevitable disturbances this causes, the patient is given tranquillizers and intensive vitamin therapy. The disruption of the drinking pattern is then completed either by the so-called vomiting technique, using apomorphine, or by the use of disulfiram. This is a drug which so upsets the patient when he takes alcohol in addition that he develops an aversion to alcohol. An alternative drug, calcium carbimide, is now available which has a similar action.

Once the drinking pattern has been disrupted, the patient then undergoes a course of psychotherapy. Hypnosis is proving particularly useful in this respect. In addition, group therapy is valuable, especially once the patient has recovered and has returned to his normal surroundings. This is the basis of Alcoholics Anonymous, an informal organization of men and women 'for whom alcohol has become a major problem, and who, admitting it, have decided to do something about it'. The address is PO Box 514, 11 Redcliffe Gardens, London, SW10 (Tel: 01–352 9779). Help and advice for the relatives of problem drinkers and alcoholics are available from AL-Anon Family Groups, of which there are now 350 in Britain. Details are available from AL-Anon Family Groups, 61 Great Dover Street, London S.E.1 4YF (Tel: 01–403 0888).

Finally, it must be stressed that there can be no compromise with the alcoholic if he is to be considered cured. Total abstinence is essential for life in every case. There are no exceptions to this rule.

ALCURONIUM is a relaxant drug which is being used by anaesthetists in relatively short operations of around twenty minutes' duration.

ALDOSTERONE is a hormone secreted by the adrenal cortex. It plays an important part in maintaining the electrolyte balance of the body by promoting the reabsorption of sodium and the secretion of potassium by the renal tubules. It is thus of primary importance in controlling the volume of the body fluids.

ALEXIA is another name for word-blindness. (See APHASIA.)

ALGESIMETER is the name of an instrument used in measuring the sensitiveness of areas of the skin.

ALGID is that stage of cholera and malaria in which extreme coldness of the body occurs. (See CHOLERA; MALARIA.)

ALIENIST means an expert in the treatment of insanity.

ALIMENTARY CANAL is the passage along which the food passes, in which it is digested (see DIGESTION), and from which it is absorbed by lymphatics and blood-vessels into the circulation. The canal consists of the mouth, pharynx or throat, oesophagus or gullet, stomach, small intestine, and large intestine, in this order (illustration 8). For details see articles under these heads. The total length of the alimentary canal is about 30 feet (9 metres) in man.

8 – Alimentary canal, *M*, mouth; *Ph*, pharynx; *L*, larynx; *OE*, oesophagus; *S*, stomach; *D*, duodenum, *J*, jejunum, and *I*, ileum, together forming the small intestine; *AV*, appendix, *C*, caecum, *AC*, ascending colon, *HF*, hepatic flexure, *TC*, transverse colon, *SF*, splenic flexure, *DC*, descending colon, *Sg*, sigmoid flexure, *R*, rectum, together forming the large intestine; *G*, gall-bladder; *H*, hepatic ducts; *DC*, common bile-duct; *P*, pancreatic duct.

ALKALI is a substance which neutralizes an acid to form a salt, and turns litmus and other vegetable dyes blue. Alkalis are generally oxides or carbonates of metals.

Varieties – Ammonia, lithia (lithium oxide). potash (potassium hydroxide) and soda (sodium carbonate) are the principal ones; the carbonates of these act as weaker alkalis, and their bicarbonates still weaker. Lime (calcium oxide), magnesia (magnesium oxide), baryta (barium oxide) and strontium are called alkaline earths, and act as alkalis. Substances which in the body are converted into alkalis, such as acetates, citrates and tartrates, are called 'indirect' alkalis. In the body protein substances also act as alkalis, absorbing acids and thus preventing the development of general acidosis.

Uses – In poisoning by acids, one at once administers dilute alkaline solutions (see ACIDS, POISONING BY). Caustic, ie. undiluted, alkalis are used to destroy warts. Bee-stings and insect-bites cause irritation because of an acid injected by the insect, and consequently are relieved by weak alkaline applications. Very weak solutions of sodium or potassium bicarbonate are given internally for bronchitis, when the phlegm is thick. In heartburn, bicarbonate of soda (20 grains [1·2 G.]), or as much as can be comfortably held on a fivepence piece is taken after a meal, to soothe irritation and spasm of the stomach. The largest use of alkalis is in the treatment of duodenal ulcer and other forms of dyspepsia associated with hyperchlorhydria (qv). The most commonly used alkalis for this purpose are magnesium trisilicate, magnesium carbonate and aluminium hydroxide.

ALKALIS, POISONING BY – Persons may drink soap-lye, ammonia, caustic soda, caustic potash, washing soda, pearl ash, spirit of hartshorn, by mistake, and, when this has been done, plenty of water should be given to drink, to which should be added, if available, weak acids such as vinegar, orange juice or lemon juice. Oily substances, such as olive oil, or white of egg, or milk may thereafter be administered. On no account must any attempt be made to make the patient vomit.

ALKALOIDS are substances found commonly in various plants. They are natural nitrogenous organic bases and combine with acids to form crystalline salts. Among alkaloids, morphine was discovered in 1805, strychnine in 1818, quinine and caffeine in 1820, nicotine in 1829, atropine in 1833. Only a few alkaloids occur in the animal kingdom, the outstanding example being adrenaline, which is formed in the medulla of the suprarenal, or adrenal, gland. Alkaloids are often used

33

for medicinal purposes. The name of an alkaloid ends in 'ine' (in Latin ina).

NEUTRAL PRINCIPLES are crystalline substances with actions similar to those of alkaloids but having a neutral reaction. The name of a neutral principle ends in 'in', eg. digitalin, aloin.

The following are the more important alkaloids, with their source plants:

Aconite, from Monkshood.
Atropine, from Belladonna (juice of Deadly Nightshade).
Cocaine, from Coca leaves.
Hyoscine, from Henbane.
Morphine ⎫
Codeine ⎬ from Opium (juice of Poppy).
Thebaine ⎭
Nicotine, from Tobacco.
Physostigmine, from Calabar bean.
Pilocarpine, from Jaborandi leaves.
Quinine ⎫ from Cinchona or Peruvian bark.
Quinidine ⎭
Strychnine, from Nux Vomica seeds.

ALKALOSIS means an increase in the alkalinity of the blood, or, more accurately, a decrease in the concentration of hydrogen ions in the blood. It occurs, for example, in patients who have had large doses of alkalis for the treatment of gastric ulcer.

ALKAPTONURIA (see OCHRONOSIS).

ALKYLATING AGENTS are so named because they alkylate or react with certain biochemical entities, particularly those concerned with the synthesis of nucleic acid. Alkylation is the substitution of an organic grouping in place of another grouping in a molecule.

The importance of the alkylating agents in medicine is that by interfering with the growth of cells they have proved of value in the treatment of various forms of malignant disease. Unfortunately they interfere with the growth of normal cells as well as malignant cells, and this restricts their use to a considerable extent.

Nevertheless several of them, including mustine (qv) and thiotepa (qv) have proved of considerable value in the chemotherapy of malignant disease.

ALLANTIASIS is a name for sausage-poisoning. (See FOOD POISONING.)

ALLANTOIN is a crystallizable substance obtained from allantoic fluid, foetal urine, etc., and also prepared by the oxidation of uric acid. It is used in the treatment of ulcers to stimulate the formation of the surface epithelial layer of the skin.

ALLANTOIS is a vascular structure which, very early in the life of the embryo, grows out from its hind-gut. The end becomes attached to the wall of the womb. It spreads out at the end, becomes stalked, and develops later into the placenta and umbilical cord (see AFTERBIRTH), which forms the only connection between the mother and embryo.

ALLERGEN is the term applied to any substance, usually a protein, which, taken into the body, makes the body hypersensitive or 'allergic' to it. Thus in hay fever the allergen is pollen.

ALLERGY means special sensitiveness of an individual to certain foods, pollens or other products of plants, animal emanations, insect bites, etc., so that in such an individual conditions like asthma, dyspepsia, nettle-rash, hay fever, eczema and headache are produced. The term anaphylaxis is given to a similar serious reaction following the injection of serum. (See ANAPHYLAXIS.) The substances that produce allergy, known as allergens, are generally of protein nature and include such ordinary foods as eggs, milk, flour and potatoes; also strawberries, tomatoes, cauliflower, walnuts, pork, shell-fish, salmon, coffee, etc., as well as colouring agents and preservatives in food; it may also be caused by inhalation of dust from feathers (in pillows), of the hair of horses, dogs or cats, of face powder containing orris root, and of pollen, especially from grasses and certain flowers What happens in allergic individuals is that allergens induce the formation of antibodies. When an allergen comes in contact with its antibody this leads to the release of those substances, such as bradykinin (qv) and histamine (qv), which are responsible for the actual allergic reaction, whether this be asthma, hay fever, eczema or the like.

Symptoms – The reaction in sensitive persons usually appears within a few minutes, but may be delayed for hours. One of the most common effects is nettle-rash or dropsical swellings in various parts; hay fever is another common result; sometimes there is swelling in a joint. Another type of reaction consists in spasmodic contractions of unstriped muscle so that the person affected may become urgently ill with asthma, or may develop spasms in the stomach with painful dyspepsia and vomiting, or in the intestine with symptoms resembling obstruction or severe diarrhoea, or may be troubled by irritability of the bladder. In other cases, neuralgia, headache or attacks of giddiness may come on.

Treatment – It is important to find out the food or other substance to which the individual is sensitive. Sometimes this has been discovered by long personal experience. Skin testing may also be carried out by inoculating into a series of scratches extracts of various foods, etc., likely to cause allergy, and the substance responsible produces a weal (qv) surrounded by redness within a few minutes. When the substance is discovered, it should in future be carefully avoided, or, if it is an ordinary food, the sensitiveness can sometimes be abolished by taking this food constantly in small quantities, very gradually increased. In other cases, particularly of hay fever, it may be possible to desensitize the affected individual by a series of injections of a vaccine made from the substance (eg. pollen) to which he or she is sensitive. Severe symptoms, as in asthma, may be relieved by an injection of adrenaline, 5 to 10 minims (0·3 to 0·6 ml). There is now available a range of antihistamine drugs (qv) which are of value in treating cases in which the cause of the condition cannot be avoided or is not known.

ALLOCHEIRIA is the name for a disorder of sensation in which sensations are referred to the wrong part of the body.

ALLOGRAFT is a piece of tissue or an organ, such as the kidney, transplanted from one to another of the same species: eg, from man to man. It is also known as a homograft.

ALLOPATHY is a term applied sometimes by homoeopathists to the methods used by regular practitioners of medicine and surgery. The term literally means curing by inducing a different kind of action in the body, and is an erroneous designation.

ALLOPURINOL is a drug of value in the treatment of gout. It acts by suppressing the formation of uric acid. It is also being used in treatment of stone in the kidney.

ALOES is the dried juice of a plant which grows in South Africa (*Aloë ferox*) and the West Indies (*A. barbadensis*). It acts as a purgative, and, taken in the evening, it acts next morning. Since it tends to cause griping, it is usually combined with other drugs. (See CONSTIPATION.)

ALOIN is an extract from aloes used in pills; the dose is from $\frac{1}{4}$ to 1 grain (15 to 60 mg).

ALOPECIA is another name for baldness. (See BALDNESS.)

ALOPECIA AREATA is the term given to the disorder in which the hair comes out in patches, resulting in shiny, smooth, bald areas. (See BALDNESS.)

ALPENSTICH is a term applied to pneumonia which is apt to affect persons exposed to the cold of high regions.

ALUM is either potash alum, potassium aluminium sulphate, or ammonia alum (ammonium aluminium sulphate). It is an astringent, and may be used as a powder to rub into abrasions when bleeding will not stop of itself. As an emetic, a teaspoonful of powdered alum may be given in water. A 1 to 4 per cent solution is used as a mouth-wash in stomatitis and pharyngitis, and a 2 per cent solution is useful when applied to the skin in cases of excessive perspiration.

ALUMINIUM is a light whitish metal which is very malleable and ductile and is much used for the manufacture of surgical instruments and as a base for artificial dentures. Aluminium hydroxide is used internally as an antacid and absorbent in dyspepsia. Aluminium powder is used for dusting on the skin around colostomy openings (see COLOSTOMY) to protect the skin.

ALVEOLAR ABSCESS (see GUMBOIL).

ALVEOLITIS means inflammation of the alveoli (see ALVEOLUS) of the lungs.
EXTRINSIC ALLERGIC ALVEOLITIS is the condition induced by the lungs becoming allergic (see ALLERGY) to various factors or substances. It includes bagassosis (qv), farmers' lung (qv), mushroom-workers' lung (qv), budgerigar-fancier's lung and pigeon-breeders' lung (qv). It is characterized by the onset of shortness of breath, tightness of the chest, cough and fever. The onset may be sudden or gradual. Treatment consists of removal of the affected individual from the offending material to which he has become allergic. Corticosteroids (qv) give temporary relief. Desensitization is not a practical proposition.

ALVEOLUS is a term applied to the

sockets of the teeth in the jaw-bone. The term is also applied to the minute divisions of glands and the the air sacs of the lungs.

AMANTADINE is a drug which is being used in the treatment of certain virus infections, and is proving of value in the prevention of certain forms of influenza. It is also used in the treatment of Parkinsonism (qv).

AMAUROSIS is the term applied to blindness in which there is no obvious lesion of the eye, the blindness being caused by disease of the optic nerve, retina or brain, or being due to hysteria.

AMBIVALENCE is the term applied to the psychological state in which a person concurrently hates and loves the same object or person.

AMBLYOPIA means defective vision for which no recognizable cause exists in any part of the eye. It may be due to such causes as defective development, hysteria, excessive use of tobacco or alcohol. The most important form is that associated with squinting (or strabismus), or gross difference in refraction (qv) between the two eyes. It has been estimated that in Britain 5·7 per cent of young adults have amblyopia due to this cause.

AMBULANCE is a vehicle for conveying sick or injured individuals. Under the National Health Service a comprehensive ambulance service is available for the whole country. There is no charge for this except in the case of patients who are being taken to a nursing home or the pay wards of a hospital. The responsibility for arranging for the ambulance rests with the doctor in charge of the patient. In the case of an emergency, eg. an accident or sudden illness in the street, an emergency ambulance service is available and the quickest way of obtaining an ambulance is through the police. The ambulance service is provided by local health authorities, which not only provide their own ambulances but are allowed to provide them through the agency of other bodies, such as the British Red Cross Society.

There is also a Hospital Car Service run by persons who use their own cars to take patients to and from hospital. They are paid an approved mileage allowance by the appropriate local health authority.

AMBULATORY FEVER is one in which the attack is at first so mild that the person keeps on going about as usual. It occurs especially in typhoid fever, and then the sick person forms a source of infection.

AMENORRHOEA is the absence of the menstrual flow during the time of life at which it should occur. (See MENSTRUATION.)

AMENT is an idiot or mentally deficient person – one having no mind.

AMENTIA is the state of being an ament; mental deficiency from failure of the mind to develop normally.

AMETHOCAINE is a powerful local anaesthetic which is used when a prolonged effect is required. It is also used as a spinal anaesthetic.

AMETROPIA means an error in the refractive power of the eye so that images are not properly focused on the retina. It may occur as long-sightedness (hypermetropia), short-sightedness (myopia), or astigmatism, or as a combination of either of the first two with astigmatism. It is corrected by appropriate lenses.

AMIDOPYRINE, or PYRAMIDON, is an analgesic and antipyretic remedy, which is seldom used now because of the risk of its causing agranulocytosis (qv).

AMIKACIN is a semi-synthetic derivative of kanamycin (qv) which is proving of value in the treatment of infections caused by micro-organisms resistant to gentamicin (qv) and tobramycin (qv).

AMILORIDE is a diuretic that acts without causing excessive loss of potassium.

AMINACRINE HYDROCHLORIDE is a derivative of acridine and is used as a local antiseptic.

AMINES are substances derived from ammonia or amino-acids (qv) which play an important part in the working of the body, including the brain and the circulatory system. They include adrenaline (qv), noradrenaline (qv) and histamine (qv). (See also MONOAMINE OXIDASE INHIBITORS.)

AMINO-ACID is the name given to the ultimate products of digestion of protein foods and from which the protein materials of the body are again built up. They are organic acids in which one or more hydrogen atoms have been replaced by the chemical group NH$_2$. (See PROTEIN.)

AMINOCAPROIC ACID is one of a group of drugs introduced for the control of bleeding. These drugs act by inhibiting what is known as the fibrinolytic system. This is a complex system which helps to maintain the coagulation mechanism of the blood in such a state that clotting of the blood only occurs when it is necessary. Thus, if fibrinolysis is prevented then the blood will clot more easily and bleeding will stop.

AMINOMETRADINE is a synthetic, non-mercurial diuretic which is effective when taken by mouth.

AMINOPHYLLINE is the name given to a combination of theophylline and ethylenediamine. It has a fourfold use: (*a*) as a diuretic; (*b*) in the treatment of angina pectoris by virtue of its action in improving the blood supply to the heart muscle; (*c*) in the treatment of bronchial asthma; (*d*) in the treatment of Cheyne-Stokes respiration.

AMINOPTERIN is an antimetabolite (qv) which is proving of value in the treatment of acute leukaemia (qv).

AMITRIPTYLINE is one of the antidepressant drugs. It has also been used in the treatment of severe hiccup.

AMMONIA is a pungent gas formed by heating a mixture of sal-ammoniac and quicklime. Dissolved in water it forms the well-known spirits of hartshorn, or liquor ammoniae. It is given off slowly from carbonate of ammonia, which is used as smelling salts. Carbonate of ammonia is the chief ingredient in aromatic spirits of ammonia or sal volatile. In chloride of ammonia or sal-ammoniac it is fixed. (For ammonia poisoning, see ALKALIS, POISONING BY.)

Uses – Externally, strong ammonia produces blistering. For bee-stings, weak ammonia is applied locally to relieve the pain. (See ALKALI.) Internally it is a powerful stimulant, and, therefore, a teaspoonful of sal volatile in water is given, or smelling salts are applied to the nose, when fainting threatens. The chloride and the carbonate of ammonia are used as expectorants (qv), whilst the former is also a diuretic (qv).

AMNESIA means loss of memory.

AMNIOCENTESIS is the process whereby a sample of amniotic fluid is obtained in order to carry out the process of examination known as amnioscopy (qv). It involves inserting a needle through the abdominal wall into the uterus usually between the 12th and 16th week of pregnancy, and withdrawing a sample of the amniotic fluid (see AMNION).

AMNION is the tough fibrous membrane which lines the cavity of the womb during pregnancy, and contains from one to two pints (0·5 to 1 litre) of fluid in which the embryo floats. It is formed from the ovum along with the embryo, and in labour the part of it at the mouth of the womb forms the 'bag of waters'. (See LABOUR.) When a child is 'born with a caul', the caul is a piece of amnion.

AMNIOSCOPY is the method whereby the fluid in the amniotic sac (see AMNION) can be assessed without interfering with the course of pregnancy. It is of value in determining whether the foetus is distressed and therefore whether or not labour should be induced, and also in finding out whether the foetus, or unborn child, is suffering from certain congenital diseases, such as mongolism. It is also possible to say what is the sex of the child.

AMNIOPLASTIN is the name given to the membrane prepared from the AMNION (qv) and used in surgery to prevent, for example, the brain adhering to the skull after operations on it. The amnioplastin is placed between the skull and the brain. It is also wrapped round nerves which have been operated on, to prevent their being bound down by scar tissue.

AMODIAQUINE is a member of the 4-aminoquinoline series of substances, and is used in the prevention, and treatment, of malaria.

AMOEBA is the name applied to a minute protozoan organism consisting of a single cell, in which is a nucleus surrounded by protoplasm that changes its shape as the protozoon progresses or absorbs nourishment. Several varieties are found under different conditions within the human body, these forms being known as entamoebae. One variety, *Entamoeba coli* (illustration 9), is found in the large intestine of man without any associated disease: another, *Entamoeba gingivalis*, is found in

37

AMOEBIASIS

9 – *Entamoeba coli*, unencysted. 1, ectoplasm; 2, endoplasm; 3, nucleus; 4, karyosome; 5, vacuoles; 6, ingested bacteria. From Blacklock and Southwell, *A Guide to Human Parasitology*. H. K. Lewis & Co. Ltd.

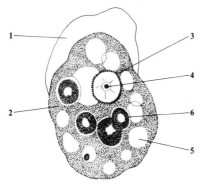

10 – *Entamoeba histolytica*, unencysted. 1, ectoplasm; 2, endoplasm; 3, nucleus; 4, karyosome; 5, vacuoles; 6, ingested red blood cells. From Blacklock and Southwell, *A Guide to Human Parasitology*. H. K. Lewis & Co. Ltd.

the sockets of the teeth associated with pyorrhoea; another, *Entamoeba histolytica* (illustration 10), is the causative organism of amoebic dysentery (see DYSENTERY). Other forms are found in the genital organs.

AMOEBIASIS (see DYSENTERY).

AMOXYCILLIN (see PENICILLIN).

AMPHETAMINES are a group of drugs closely related to adrenaline and act by stimulating the sympathetic nervous system. There are now more than fifty preparations of amphetamine substances.

On being inhaled, they constrict the blood-vessels in the nose and so ease the congestion or 'stuffiness' of nasal catarrh. Their indiscriminate use for this purpose is harmful and they should only be used under medical supervision. When taken by mouth they have a profound stimulating effect on the brain, producing a sense of well-being and confidence and increasing the capacity for mental work. This effect, however, is temporary, and its use for this purpose, except under medical supervision, is fraught with danger.

By virtue of the fact that they inhibit appetite, they rapidly achieved a widespread reputation for slimming purposes. In view of the risks attached to their continued use, they are now seldom used for this purpose. Indeed there is growing evidence that the dangers of the amphetamines including the risk of becoming addicted to them, far outweigh their advantages.

AMPHORIC is an adjective denoting the kind of breathing heard over a cavity in the lung. The sound is like that made by blowing over the mouth of a narrow-necked vase.

AMPHOTERICIN is a mixture of antifungal substances derived from *Streptomyces nodosus*, which is proving of value in the treatment of certain of the diseases classified under the heading of mycosis (qv). It is, however, a very toxic substance and is therefore only used in those infections in which the outlook is otherwise hopeless.

AMPICILLIN (see PENICILLIN).

AMPOULE is a small glass container having one end drawn out into a point capable of being sealed so as to preserve its contents sterile. It is used for containing solutions for hypodermic injection.

AMPUTATION means the severing of any limb or part completely from the body. In the case of organs other than limbs the word excision is generally used. An amputation through a joint without sawing of bone is called a disarticulation.

Objects of amputation – In the great majority of cases a limb is amputated because it has been damaged beyond the hope of recovery. It is not always easy to say at once that a limb should, or should not, be removed after an injury, but the three chief points are, as to whether (1) extensive portions of muscle, skin, and bone are so crushed and torn as to make their death and separation inevitable; (2) the great nerves and blood-vessels are divided so as to destroy the vitality of the limb; and (3) the laceration is so extensive,

38

or involves joint cavities so as to render cleansing of the wound impossible and endanger the patient from blood-poisoning (qv) due to septic absorption. Often after gunshot wounds, crushes in machinery, or railway accidents, where a decision cannot be made at once, the injured limb is cleaned (blood-vessels tied, sinews stitched, etc.), and a careful watch maintained for some days to see if healing will take place. This is done especially in the case of the hand, where every fragment of tissue is valuable because of the delicate movements the upper limb executes, and where, fortunately, circulation by anastomosis is good. (See ANASTOMOSIS.) But in the lower limbs, the chief point is to have a small scar and a sound stump, so that the weight of the body can be borne, and therefore a few inches of length are, if necessary, sacrificed and amputation oftener performed. The more common sites of amputation in the lower limbs are shown in illustration 11. Site 4 is used for injuries in which the whole forefoot is mangled and for severe deformities of the foot. Site 3, or midleg amputation, is the site of selection for injuries around the ankle, while sites 2 and 1 are reserved for more extensive injuries.

Not infrequently, when bones or joints are diseased, especially with persistent discharges, or when gangrene has taken place, amputation of part of a limb is necessary. Another object of amputation is to remove malignant tumours entirely, such as those in the foot. Still another case for amputation is where a limb is paralysed completely, and a more useful artificial substitute can be fashioned. Owing to improvements in surgery which have taken place in recent years, many injured limbs can now be saved which previously would have required to be amputated.

Methods of amputation – When a limb is to be amputated, it is elevated to empty it of blood as far as possible, then a tight or elastic band called a tourniquet is applied, to prevent bleeding; and, the limb being cut off by one of the following methods, the cut ends of the blood-vessels are ligatured, the tourniquet removed, the muscles and sinews stitched over the bone, and finally the edges of the skin stitched together. Thus there may be almost no blood lost. The *circular method* is one in which skin, muscles or flesh, and bone are cut or sawn at successively higher levels, so that the skin meets afterwards over the other tissues. It is an old method, and, being rapid, was used before the days of anaesthesia. In the *elliptical method* the

11 Sites for amputation: (1) supracondylar, (2) at knee joint, (3) midleg, (4) Syme's. From Illingworth, *A Short Textbook of Surgery*, 9th edition. Churchill Livingstone.

tissues are divided in the form of an oblique circle, so that one side of the cut is much lower down the limb than the other. This has the advantage of bringing the resulting scar over to one side of the limb, and thus providing a better covering for the end of the sawn bone.

The *flap method* is one in which a large flap of skin and fibrous tissue is carefully dissected up from the underlying muscles, and, after the limb is removed, laid across the cut surface and stitched at its sides and end. Only one flap may be made, or more often two, which meet end to end and side to side. Sometimes the flap consists of muscle as well as of skin, and occasionally a slice of bone with its covering membrane is included in the flap so as to produce a broad surface of bone when the flap is turned into its final position, and thus to form a better support in the case of lower-limb amputations. The flap method is that most frequently used, partly because with it the scar does not fall opposite the end of the bone, and also because a limb seldom being injured at the same level all round, the formation of a flap enables a larger part to be saved.

Shrinkage of the stump continues for two to six months after amputation and obviously a permanent artificial limb (qv), or prosthesis as it is now known, cannot be fitted until such shrinkage is complete. This delay has many practical disadvantages, and it is now the general practice to start physiotherapy immediately after the operation and to start the patient walking with a temporary prosthesis within a week.

AMYLASE is an enzyme (qv) in pancreatic juice which facilitates the conversion of starch to maltose. (See PANCREAS.)

AMYL NITRITE is a volatile, oily liquid prepared by the action of nitric and nitrous acids upon amyl alcohol. It resembles other nitrites in its power of relieving spasms and dilating blood-vessels, and it acts with great rapidity when inhaled, producing its effects in a few seconds. (See NITROGLYCERIN.)

AMYLOBARBITONE, or AMYTAL, is one of the barbiturate group of drugs. Its approximate duration of action is 6 to 8 hours. The dose is 100 to 200 mg.

AMYLOIDOSIS, or WAXY DISEASE, is the condition in which deposits of complex protein, known as amyloid, are found in various parts of the body. It is a degenerative condition resulting from various causes such as chronic infection, including tuberculosis and rheumatoid arthritis.

AMYLOSE is the name applied to any carbohydrate of the starch group.

AMYLUM is another name for starch.

AMYOTROPHIC LATERAL SCLEROSIS is a disease of the nervous system in which, as a result of degeneration of nerve cells in the spine and brain, there is progressive wasting of the muscles of the body, with spastic paralysis. It is a form of Motor Neutrone Disease. (See PARALYSIS.)

AMYOTROPHY means atrophy or loss of substance of a muscle.

ANAEMIA is the condition characterized by inadequate red blood cells and/or haemoglobin in the blood. It is considered to exist if haemoglobin levels are below 13 grams per 100 ml in males and below 12 grams per 100 ml in adult non-pregnant women. No simple classification of anaemia can be wholly accurate, but the most useful method is to divide anaemias into: (*a*) microcytic hypochromic anaemia, (*b*) megaloblastic hyperchromic anaemia, (*c*) aplastic anaemia, (*d*)

haemolytic anaemia. In Britain, anaemia is much more common among women than in men. Thus, around 10 per cent of girls have anaemia at the age of 15, whilst in adult life the incidence is over 30 per cent between the ages of 30 and 40, around 20 per cent at 50, and around 30 per cent at 70. Among men the incidence is under 5 per cent until the age of 50, and it then rises to 20 per cent at the age of 70. Ninety per cent of all cases of anaemia in Britain are microcytic, 7 per cent are macrocytic, and 3 per cent are haemolytic or aplastic. (See also SICKLE-CELL ANAEMIA; and THALASSAEMIA.)

MICROCYTIC HYPOCHROMIC ANAEMIA – This corresponds to a large extent with what used to be known as 'secondary anaemia'. It takes its name from the characteristic changes in the blood.

Causes – (1) *Loss of blood.* (*a*) As a result of trauma. This is perhaps the simplest example of all, when, as a result of an accident involving a large artery, there is severe haemorrhage.

(*b*) Menstruation. The regular monthly loss of blood which women sustain as a result of menstruation always puts a strain on the blood-forming organs. If this loss is excessive, then over a period of time it may lead to quite severe anaemia.

(*c*) Child-birth. A considerable amount of blood is always lost at child-birth, and if this is severe, or if the woman was anaemic during pregnancy, a severe degree of anaemia may develop.

(*d*) Bleeding from the gastro-intestinal tract. The best example here is anaemia due to 'bleeding piles' (see PILES). Such bleeding, even though slight, if maintained over a long period of time, is a common cause of anaemia in both men and women. The haemorrhage may be more acute and occur from a duodenal or gastric ulcer, when it is known as haematemesis (qv).

(*e*) Certain blood diseases, such as purpura (qv) and haemophilia (qv), which are characterized by bleeding.

(2) *Defective blood formation* – (*a*) This is the main cause of anaemia in infections. The organism responsible for the infection has a deleterious effect upon the blood-forming organs, just as it does upon other parts of the body.

(*b*) Toxins. In conditions such as chronic Bright's disease and uraemia there is a severe anaemia due to the effect of the disease upon blood formation.

(*c*) Drugs. Certain drugs, such as lead, depress blood formation.

(3) *Inadequate intake of iron* – The daily requirement of iron for an adult is 12 mg,

and 15 to 20 mg during pregnancy. This is well covered by an ordinary diet, so that by itself it is not a common cause. But if there is a steady loss of blood, as a result of heavy menstrual loss or 'bleeding piles', the intake of iron in the diet may not be sufficient to maintain adequate formation of haemoglobin.

(4) *Inadequate absorption of iron* – This may occur in diseases of the stomach or bowels: eg. ulcerative colitis.

In many cases the anaemia is found to be due to a combination of two or more of these causes. A severe form of this anaemia in women, known as CHLOROSIS, used to be common, but it is seldom seen nowadays.

Symptoms – These depend upon whether the anaemia is sudden in onset, as in severe haemorrhage, or gradual. In all cases, however, the striking sign is pallor, the depth of which depends upon the severity of the anaemia. The colour of the skin may be misleading, except in cases due to severe haemorrhage, as the skin of many people is normally pale. The best guide is the colour of the internal lining of the eyelid. When the onset of the anaemia is sudden the patient complains of weakness and giddiness, and he loses consciousness if he tries to stand or sit up. The breathing is rapid and distressed, the pulse is rapid, and the blood-pressure is low. The tongue is often sore (glossitis), and the nails of the fingers may be brittle and concave instead of convex (koilonychia). In some cases, particularly in women, the Plummer-Vinson syndrome is present. This consists of difficulty in swallowing and may be accompanied by huskiness; in these cases glossitis is also present. There may be slight enlargement of the spleen, and there is usually some diminution in gastric acidity.

Changes in the blood – The characteristic change is a diminution in both the haemoglobin and the red cell content of the blood. There is a relatively greater fall in the haemoglobin than in the red cell count, so that the colour index is less than unity. The colour index is the percentage of haemoglobin stated in terms of the amount contained in each red cell. In health it is 1·0 (or unity). If the blood is examined under a microscope the red cells are seen to be paler and smaller than normal. These small red cells are known as microcytes.

Treatment consists primarily of giving sufficient iron by mouth to restore, and then maintain, a normal blood picture. The main iron preparation now used is

Ferrous Sulphate, 3 grains (200 mg), thrice daily after meals. When the blood picture has become normal, the dosage is gradually reduced. A preparation of iron is now available which can be given intravenously, but this is only used in cases which do not respond to iron given by mouth, or in cases in which it is essential to obtain a quick response.

If, of course, there is haemorrhage, this must be arrested, and if the loss of blood has been severe it may be necessary to give a blood transfusion. Care must be taken to ensure that the patient is having an adequate diet and a period of rest in hospital, followed by a holiday, is often beneficial. If there is any underlying toxic or infective condition, this, of course, must be adequately treated.

MEGALOBLASTIC HYPERCHROMIC ANAEMIA – There are various forms of anaemia of this type, such as those due to nutritional defects and those associated with excessive destruction of red cells in the body, but the most important is that known as PERNICIOUS ANAEMIA.

PERNICIOUS ANAEMIA, or ADDISONIAN ANAEMIA, is found in all civilized countries. Up until about fifty years ago its cause was unknown and it was an invariably fatal disease. In 1926, two Americans, G. R. Minot and W. P. Murphy, reported that pernicious anaemia responded to treatment with liver. This discovery ranks in importance with that of insulin in the treatment of diabetes mellitus. This form of treatment is based upon the now well-proved fact that pernicious anaemia is due to lack of what is known as the *intrinsic factor*. For the formation of normal red blood corpuscles a substance known as the extrinsic factor is necessary. The efficient absorption of this factor into the body is dependent on the presence of intrinsic factor which is produced normally by the mucosa lining the distal part of the stomach. It is the inability of the patient to produce the intrinsic factor that leads to the onset of pernicious anaemia. In a normal person with adequate amounts of intrinsic factor, approximately 70 per cent of the extrinsic factor (which is vitamin B_{12} and is present in meat and other foods) in the daily diet is absorbed into the body. In patients with pernicious anaemia, however, less than 2 per cent is absorbed.

Symptoms – Pernicious anaemia is a disease of middle age, being rare under the age of 40 years. It affects both men and women. The onset is usually insidious, so that the anaemia is usually well developed before medical advice is sought. In addition to the general symptoms and signs already described in the section on microcytic anaemia, the important features of pernicious anaemia are as follows. The patient, who is often prematurely grey-haired, has a characteristic lemon-yellow complexion. The tongue is often sore and appears thinner, smoother, and redder than usual – a condition which makes it very like that of a dog. There is often soreness and excoriation of the corners of the mouth – a condition known as cheilosis. There may be slight enlargement of the spleen. There is a complete absence of free hydrochloric acid in the stomach, even after the injection of histamine; this is one of the most important points in the diagnosis of pernicious anaemia.

One of the most serious complications of pernicious anaemia is a disease with the cumbersome title of SUBACUTE COMBINED DEGENERATION OF THE CORD. This, as the name indicates, is a degenerative condition of the spinal cord, and the importance of recognizing its onset is that it can be cured by adequate treatment of the anaemia. Its early manifestations are a sensation of tingling or 'pins and needles' in the legs, accompanied by stiffness. Later, if untreated, the stiffness becomes progressively worse, finally leading to paralysis.

Changes in the blood – The important finding in the blood is an anaemia in which there is a relatively greater diminution in the number of red cells than in the haemoglobin content of each cell, so that the colour index is 1·0 or more. The red cells are larger than normal, ie. megalocytes, and they appear to be redder than normal. They also vary in shape (*poikilocytosis*) and in size (*anisocytosis*). Occasionally a few primitive red cells (normoblasts) may be found. The total white cell count is diminished: ie. there is leucopenia. The final diagnosis depends upon an examination of the bone marrow, which is found to contain many very primitive red cells: ie. megaloblasts.

Treatment consists of the administration of vitamin B_{12} in the form of hydroxocobalamin. It is given by injection. Preparations are available which can be given by mouth, but the general consensus of expert opinion is that these are not satisfactory for efficient control of the disease. The dosage usually depends mainly upon the severity of the anaemia, but there is also considerable personal variation in different patients, so that treatment must be supervised by a physician and checked by repeated examinations of the

blood. It must always be remembered that a patient with pernicious anaemia requires to take vitamin B_{12} for the rest of his life.

APLASTIC ANAEMIA is a disease in which the red blood corpuscles are very greatly reduced and in which no attempt appears to be made in the bone marrow towards their regeneration. The cause in many cases is not known, but in rather less than half the cases the condition is due to some toxic substance, such as benzol or certain drugs, or ionizing radiations. The patient becomes very pale, with a tendency to haemorrhages under the skin and mucous membranes, and the temperature may at times be raised. The red blood corpuscles diminish steadily in numbers. Treatment consists primarily of regular blood transfusions. Although the disease is often fatal, the outlook has improved in recent years. About 25 per cent of patients recover when adequately treated, and others survive for several years. In severe cases promising results are being reported from the use of bone marrow transplantation.

HAEMOLYTIC ANAEMIA results from the excessive destruction or haemolysis (qv) of the red blood cells. This haemolysis may be due to undue fragility of the red blood cells, when the condition is known as congenital haemolytic anaemia, or acholuric jaundice. Another important form is haemolytic disease of the newborn (qv). In other cases it is due to transfusion with incompatible blood. (See TRANSFUSION OF BLOOD.)

ANAEROBE is the term applied to bacteria having the power to live without air. Such organisms are found growing freely, deep in the soil, as, for example, the tetanus bacillus.

ANAESTHESIA means loss of the power of feeling. The word is applied either to loss over a limited area of skin produced by certain nervous diseases, by freezing, or by local anaesthetic drugs such as procaine, or to a total loss of feeling and consciousness, in the state produced by chloroform, ether and similar drugs. When only loss of the sense of pain is meant, without loss of the sense of touch, the correct term is analgesia.

ANAESTHETICS are drugs and other measures which produce insensibility to external impressions.

Historical – Although it is mainly owing to the researches of distinguished chemists and physicians in the last century that anaesthesia has come to occupy the foremost place it now does in medicine, there is abundant evidence to show that it is a practice of great antiquity. Besides the mention by Homer of the anaesthetic effects of nepenthe, and the reference by Herodotus to the practice of the Scythians of inhaling the vapours of a certain kind of hemp to produce intoxication, the employment of anaesthetics in surgery by the use of mandrake is particularly noted by Dioscorides and Pliny. It also appears, from an old Chinese manuscript, that a physician named Hoa-tho, who lived in the third century, gave his patients a preparation of hemp, whereby they were rendered insensible during the performance of surgical operations. Mandrake was extensively used as an anaesthetic by Hugo de Lucca, who practised in the thirteenth century. The soporific effects of mandrake are remarked by Shakespeare, who also makes frequent mention of anaesthetizing draughts, the composition of which is not specified.

In 1800, Sir Humphry Davy, experimenting on nitrous oxide gas, discovered its anaesthetic properties, and described the effects it had on himself when inhaled with the view of relieving local pain. He suggested its employment in surgery, but his suggestion remained unheeded for nearly half a century.

The inhalation of sulphuric ether for the relief of asthma and other lung affections had been employed by Dr Pearson, of Birmingham, as early as 1785; in 1818, Faraday showed that the inhalation of the vapour of sulphuric ether produced anaesthetic effects similar to those of nitrous oxide gas; and this property of ether was confirmed by the American physicians, Godman (1822), Jackson (1833), Wood and Bache (1834).

These observations, however, appear to have been regarded as mere scientific curiosities till December 1844, when Dr Horace Wells, a dentist of Hartford, Connecticut, underwent in his own person the operation of tooth extraction while rendered insensible by nitrous oxide gas. On September 30, 1846, Dr Morton, a dentist of Boston, employed the vapour of sulphuric ether to procure general anaesthesia in a case of tooth extraction, and thereafter administered it with complete success in cases requiring surgical operation. This great achievement marked a new era in surgery. Operations were performed in America in numerous instances under ether inhalation, the result being to establish more firmly its value as a

successful anaesthetic. The news of the discovery reached England on December 17, 1846. On December 19, Mr Robinson, a dentist in London, and on the 21st, Mr Liston, the eminent surgeon, operated on patients anaesthetized by ether; and the practice soon became general both in Great Britain and on the Continent.

Sir James Y. Simpson, of Edinburgh, was the first to apply anaesthesia by ether in midwifery practice. This he did on January 19, 1847, and he subsequently employed ether inhalation in numerous cases of both easy and difficult parturition, an account of which he published, containing much important information.

These observations excited great interest in the medical world, and led to the extensive employment of ether inhalation till November 15, 1847, when Simpson announced his discovery of the anaesthetic properties of chloroform (the trial of which had been suggested to him by Mr Waldie, a chemist of Liverpool). He proposed it as a substitute for sulphuric ether, which for a time it almost completely displaced for anaesthetic purposes in Britain. In America, however, ether remained the favourite drug for this object. In 1858, Dr Snow, of London, published a work, *On Chloroform and other Anaesthetics*, which was the first attempt to place the whole subject on a scientific basis. The number of fatalities which took place during the administration of various anaesthetics had by this time begun to attract attention, and mechanical inhalers designed to prevent the administration of too concentrated a vapour were invented by Clover in 1862 and Junker in 1867.

Experiments with various other drugs were made by other men, and during the period 1860–70 a movement, starting in the United States, took place in favour of nitrous oxide, or 'laughing-gas', for dental work, and this anaesthetic, firmly installed towards the end of the decade for tooth extractions and other short operations, has never gone out of use, being reckoned one of the safest anaesthetics we possess. In 1876, Clover introduced an apparatus whereby nitrous oxide and ether could be inhaled in succession, and as the initial stages of ether administration are difficult and unpleasant, and are obviated by beginning with the gas, this instrument and method proved of great usefulness.

Choice of anaesthetic – At the present day there is a large range of anaesthetics to choose from. Many of these require complicated apparatus for their administration (illustration 12), whilst others are potentially dangerous unless used by an experienced anaesthetist. The choice of anaesthetic in any one particular case often requires considerable judgment, and, except with a highly skilled anaesthetist, the sound working rule is that the doctor should use the anaesthetic of which he has had most experience. In the case of the general practitioner called upon in an emergency to administer an anaesthetic for a surgical operation, this usually means ether or chloroform.

The following is a useful classification of the present range of anaesthetics.

VOLATILE ANAESTHETICS – These include ether, chloroform, nitrous oxide, ethyl chloride, vinyl ether,

anaesthesia: ie. when the anaesthetic is introduced directly into the lungs by means of a tube passed into the trachea. Endotracheal anaesthesia is employed in operations in the head or neck where a mask or any other anaesthetic apparatus would get in the way of the surgeon. Ethyl chloride is seldom used to maintain anaesthesia; it is more commonly used to induce anaesthesia, especially in children.

BASAL NARCOTICS – These are used to induce anaesthesia, without any distress to the patient, preliminary to the use of some other anaesthetic, under the influence of which the operation in question is to be carried out. In practice they have removed many of the terrors of anaes-

12 – A modern machine for administering anaesthetic. British Oxygen Co. Ltd.

trichloroethylene, cyclopropane and halothane. The last four should only be used by anaesthetists experienced in their use. Mixtures of chloroform and ether are sometimes used. Nitrous oxide has two great advantages: the patient recovers quickly from the anaesthetic, and there is relatively little nausea and vomiting. Its use for major surgical operations, however, requires considerable skill and special apparatus, and for this purpose therefore it can only be used by an experienced anaesthetist. It is now tending to be replaced by cyclopropane. Nitrous oxide is an excellent anaesthetic for minor surgical operations, for dentistry, and in midwifery, but in the first of these it is tending to be replaced by the basal narcotics. It is often used in endotracheal

thesia, so far as the patient is concerned, as they induce loss of consciousness so quickly and painlessly. It is seldom safe to use these basal narcotics to produce a degree of anaesthesia which is sufficient to permit of operations being performed without the addition of some other anaesthetic. They are given either per rectum or intravenously. Thiopentone sodium is the one most commonly used at the present day.

STEROID ANAESTHETICS – Some years ago it was discovered that a state of anaesthesia could be induced by large doses of steroid hormones. A derivative of one of these hormones has now been prepared in which the anaesthetic action can be obtained without the hormone action. This preparation, known as hydroxydione, is given intravenously and appears to have certain advantages over other anaesthetics.

LOCAL ANAESTHETICS are given by injection to induce loss of sensation in the area to be operated upon, without any general loss of consciousness. For major operations they are more commonly used on the Continent than in this country. Cocaine was the first local anaesthetic to be used, but on account of its toxic properties it has been almost entirely replaced by synthetic preparations. These include procaine hydrochloride, lignocaine and cinchocaine hydrochloride.

SPINAL ANAESTHETICS are used when it is considered inadvisable to induce general anaesthesia and local anaesthesia is contraindicated. Their two main advantages are that they can be used in patients with diseases of the lung in whom a general anaesthetic may lead to complications, and that they produce excellent relaxation of the muscles. The same anaesthetics are used for inducing local anaesthesia, with the exception of cocaine, which is never used as a spinal anaesthetic. The solution is injected into the spinal canal by the same technique as in use for lumbar puncture (qv).

EPIDURAL ANAESTHESIA is a form of anaesthesia predominantly used to relieve the severity of labour pains. It is induced by the injection of a local anaesthetic such as lignocaine into the extradural space (see SPINAL CORD).

Stages of anaesthesia – Whatever be the anaesthetic employed, the effects are much the same, though some symptoms are more prominent with one anaesthetic, others with another, and in the case of basal narcotics the initial stages are hurried over and the patient plunged almost at once into deep unconsciousness.

STAGE I – There is great rapidity of thought, but disturbance of judgment and power of control. Giddiness, tingling, and other peculiar or pleasant sensations are felt. The patient may be emotional, or may sing, shout or struggle, and then passes off into a dreamy state, with partial loss of sensation. The heart's action becomes stronger and the pupils dilate.

STAGE II – There is complete loss of consciousness. The speech becomes unintelligible, changing to a mere muttering. There may be muscular spasms of various sorts, also coughing, retching and possibly vomiting. The pupils become small.

STAGE III – There is absolute unconsciousness and complete muscular relaxation, and in this stage surgical operations

are performed. The heart's action is weakened, most reflex movements abolished, and the pupil dilates again but is still capable of contracting when the eyelid is raised so that light enters the eye.

STAGE IV – This is the stage of danger, the breathing becomes shallow, the face pallid or livid, the heart weak and irregular, and the pupils widely dilated. If the anaesthetic be not at once removed, breathing and pulse then stop and the person dies.

Uses of anaesthetics – The most evident use of anaesthetics is to relieve the pain of surgical operations and of convulsive diseases. Their use has made possible much more prolonged and delicate operations than could be performed upon the conscious and suffering body. An anaesthetic is also an aid in diagnosis, particularly of abdominal conditions, producing muscular relaxation and allowing the free handling of painful regions. Anaesthetics are also used in medical practice to quiet violent spasmodic states, as in the uraemia of Bright's disease, in a succession of epileptic fits, in lock-jaw, and in strychnine poisoning. (For the use of local anaesthetics, see ANALGESICS.) (See also CURARE.)

ANALEPTIC means a restorative medicine, or one which acts as a stimulant of the central nervous system: for example caffeine.

ANALGESIA means loss of the power to feel pain without loss of consciousness: eg. in some nervous diseases or due to some drugs. (See also AUDIOANALGESIA.)

ANALGESICS are drugs or other measures which cause temporary loss of the sense of pain without unconsciousness and without necessarily loss of the sense of touch. Some act generally on the brain or the nerves to dull pain which is already present (see ANODYNES); others act locally, such as cocaine, benzocaine, procaine and the process of freezing, which are used to prevent pain which would otherwise necessarily be caused by operations. In a position between that of a general anaesthetic and a local analgesic stand drugs such as morphine and scopolamine which are used for the production of a torpid, semi-insensible state like that sometimes used in child-birth (see TWILIGHT SLEEP).

Uses – Local insensibility to pain may be produced in a considerable variety of ways, but most of these fall into one of four classes: (1) infiltration of the region to be operated upon by a solution of the analgesic drug; (2) injection of the solution into or near the nerve trunks which convey the sensations of the part; (3) painting, spraying, or rubbing the surface, especially of mucous membrane, with the drug; and (4) the application of intense cold.

The first drug to be used for local anaesthesia or analgesia in operations was cocaine, which has certain disadvantages in that it is destroyed by boiling and that it readily causes symptoms of poisoning, so that it cannot be safely used in doses over $\frac{1}{2}$ grain (30 mg). Procaine, which is an artificially prepared substance, has largely displaced cocaine because it is many times less poisonous and so can be used in larger doses. Amethocaine is largely used for spinal analgesia. One of the most widely used local anaesthetics at the present moment is lignocaine. Quinine and urea hydrochloride has been employed as an analgesic in cases in which a prolonged effect is desired, as its results last for several days.

When *infiltration analgesia* is employed, a weak solution of procaine is generally used to which a small amount of adrenaline is added. A long hypodermic needle is used to inject this solution in large quantity (several ounces) into and especially around the part upon which the operation is to be performed. By this means tumours can be removed, the abdomen opened, and similar serious operations, which do not involve great shock to the patient and in which general unconsciousness is not desirable, can be performed.

When general loss of sensation in a region is to be brought about by injecting a nerve trunk or its neighbourhood, stronger solutions (eg. procaine 2 per cent) are used in similar quantities. The large nerves of a limb are sometimes treated in this way for the prevention of the shock caused by a severe operation, even when a general anaesthetic is also employed. This method is much used for painless tooth extraction. The two methods of infiltration and regional analgesia are often combined: for example, to perform amputations below the knee or elbow or in removal of a goitre.

Another way of applying the injection method is by *spinal analgesia*, in which sensation is abolished temporarily in the lower limbs by injection of the drug into the spinal canal.

The *surface application* of analgesics is in general only useful in cases in which operations are to be performed upon mucous membranes, such as those of the nose or throat, where cocaine and benzamine can readily be applied by painting or spraying.

A transitory analgesia is produced by *freezing* the skin. This is usually effected by spraying a small area with ethyl chloride, which very quickly evaporates, with the production of intense cold.

ANALYSIS means a separation into component parts by determination of the chemical constituents of a substance. The process of analysis is carried out by various means: eg. chromatographic analysis by means of the adsorption column; colorimetric analysis by means of various colour tests; densimetric analysis by estimation of the specific gravity; gasometric analysis by estimating the different gases given off in some process; polariscope analysis by means of the polariscope; volumetric analysis by measuring volumes of liquids. Analysis is also sometimes used as an abbreviation for psycho-analysis (qv).

ANAMNESIS is the term applied to the statement of the past history of some particular case of disease.

ANAPHYLAXIS is a condition of excessive sensitiveness exhibited by certain persons or animals to the injection of foreign material into their tissues. A common example is the pain, swelling, eruption, feverishness and general prostration which occasionally follow the injection of serum containing diphtheria or tetanus antitoxin. An example of a slighter form of anaphylaxis is afforded by persons who suffer from nettle-rash, asthma, and similar symptoms when they take some food of which their system is intolerant, or by other persons who present similar symptoms when exposed to the emanations of certain animals, eg. horses, cats or fowls. There is an acute form, fortunately rare, known as anaphylactic shock which may occur within minutes of the injection of certain drugs or vaccines to which the injected individual is hypersensitive. It is characterized by severe shortness of breath, marked fall in blood pressure and acute urticaria (qv). Treatment consists of the immediate intramuscular injection of adrenaline (qv). (See ALLERGY.)

ANAPLASIA means the state in which a body cell loses its distinctive characters and takes on a more primitive form; it occurs, for example, in cancer, when cells proliferate rapidly.

ANASARCA is a condition of general dropsy.

ANASTOMOSIS is a term describing the means by which circulation is carried on when large vessels are narrowed or closed, as by pressure. In the limbs, especially around joints, and in internal organs, small arteries open freely into their neighbours to form a network from which the smallest vessels carry off the blood. By this means pressure from one side, or even the ligature of the main artery to a limb, is prevented from stopping the flow of blood to any part, because so soon as one artery is closed, the other arteries of the limb dilate, through relaxation of their muscle fibres, and the supply of blood passes on as before, but by new channels. Anastomosis is also a term describing the joining together (by operation) of any two parts of the alimentary tract or of blood-vessels such as the arteries and veins.

ANATOMY is the science which deals with the structure of the bodies of men and animals. Brief descriptions of the anatomy of each important organ are given under the headings of the various organs. It is studied by dissection of bodies specially bequeathed for the purpose or of the bodies of those who die in hospitals and similar institutions, unclaimed by relatives.

ANATOXIN is another name for toxoid (qv).

ANCROD is an enzyme (qv) present in the venom of the Malayan pit viper which destroys the fibrinogen in blood and thereby prevents the blood clotting. In other words it is an anticoagulant (qv).

ANCYLOSTOMIASIS is the parasitic infestation caused by two nematodes, *Ancylostoma duodenale* and *Necator americanus*, perhaps better known as the hookworm. The former is also known as the tunnel-worm on account of the ravages it caused among the men at work on the St Gotthard tunnel. They produce great anaemia, debility, and cardiac weakness, sometimes leading to death. The disease is widespread in the tropics and subtropics, as well as certain mines in Europe. *Ancylostoma duodenale* occurs in the Far East, the Mediterranean littoral and the Middle East, whilst *Necator americanus* is found in East, West and Central Africa, Central and South America and the Far East. In recent years these geographical demarcations have been largely broken down. The worms are about $\frac{1}{2}$ inch (12 mm) in length and inhabit the upper part of the small intestine, often in great numbers; here they embed themselves in the mucous membrane lining the bowel. In certain parts of India it is so common that about 75 per cent of the population are said to be affected; it is also very common in Egypt. The worms embedded in the small intestine produce an enormous number of eggs which pass from the body in the stools; the embryos, finding their way into water, mud, or damp earth, develop rapidly and can maintain their vitality for weeks or months, if moisture be present. In the insanitary conditions so widespread in the areas where the disease occurs, the embryos gain access to the human host through the skin – usually the feet. They may also gain access through the drinking of polluted water. Ultimately, through the blood-stream and the lungs, they gain access to the intestine, where they develop. The disease is a very serious one, partly in consequence of the numbers of persons prevented from working by the debility it causes, and partly because death in such debilitated persons is not uncommon.

Treatment — The most effective remedies are tetrachloroethylene, bephenium hydroxynaphthoate, pyrantel embonate, and mebendazole. The anaemia which always accompanies chronic infestation with ancylostoma also requires intensive treatment. This consists of one or more of the following: iron, liver extract, the vitamin B complex, and a high protein diet.

ANDROGEN is the general term for any one of a group of hormones which govern the development of the sexual organs and the secondary sexual characteristics of the male.

ANENCEPHALY is the term given to the condition in which a child is born with a defect of the skull and absence of the brain. (See SPINA BIFIDA.)

ANEURINE is an alternative name for vitamin B_1. (See THIAMINE.)

ANEURYSM means a dilatation upon an artery, due to yielding of the vessel-wall and gradual stretching by the pressure of the blood.

Varieties – There are several ways of classifying aneurysms. With reference to structure, they have been separated into *true aneurysms*, in which the vessel-wall is merely thinned and stretched but still intact, and *false aneurysms*, in which the wall has been thinned away till all the coats of the artery (see ARTERIES) have given way, and the blood is enclosed only by the greatly thickened fibrous tissues surrounding the artery. With reference to shape, they are called *fusiform* when the artery is dilated all round for some distance, this form being common on the thoracic aorta; *sacculated* when a spot on one side has been pushed out gradually to form a sort of pouch, which is the usual form when medium-sized arteries are affected; *dissecting* when the inner coat has given way somewhat suddenly and blood has passed between the coats and torn its way some distance along the vessel wall; *miliary* when the aneurysm is very small and looks like a millet seed on the side of the vessel, which is a form often found on the vessels in the brain. An *arteriovenous aneurysm* is one where there is a communication between an artery and a vein.

Causes – The two main factors responsible for the formation of an aneurysm are (1) strain; (2) weakening of the wall of the artery. The latter is the more important. No amount of strain, whether due to a raised blood-pressure or to muscular effort, will lead to aneurysm formation unless there is some local weakening of the wall of the artery. The two most important causes of weakening of the arterial wall are syphilis and atheroma (qv). Practically all aneurysms of the thoracic aorta are due to syphilis. Atheroma is the more common cause of aneurysms in the abdominal aorta. Aneurysms may also be due to loss of the support provided by the surrounding tissues, eg. in the lungs, where an aneurysm may form in one of the branches of the pulmonary artery as a result of destruction of the surrounding tissue by tuberculosis. Occasionally they may be due to congenital defects in the arterial wall: the most common site for such aneurysms is the circle of Willis (qv) at the base of the brain. More rarely they may arise as a result of repeated small trauma and strain in exposed arteries, such as the popliteal artery, which have not much support from the surrounding tissues; popliteal aneurysms were more common in the old coaching days among those who spent most of their working lives on horseback. Small aneurysms, known as *mycotic* aneurysms, may also arise in cases of severe sepsis, as a result of infection of the arterial wall. Aneurysms are more common in men than in women, and particularly among those who indulge in hard physical labour, such as labourers and stevedores.

Symptoms – These vary greatly with the size and position of the aneurysm, but there are some which are characteristic of all forms. The *type of person* who suffers is usually a man in his forties or fifties, who has had an arduous or irregular life and has often indulged in high living. There may be other signs of arterial disease, such as cirrhotic Bright's disease (see BRIGHT'S DISEASE), or a previous apoplexy. If the aneurysm be in a limb, a round *swelling* is noticed, perhaps as large as a walnut or Mandarin orange, which expands and diminishes with each heart-beat. The swelling is generally painless, and the skin over it is unchanged (unlike an abscess). Aneurysms rarely occur farther from the trunk than the elbow or knee. If the aneurysm be internal it is situated upon a great vessel, and is often very large in size before it causes any definite symptoms, which are mainly due to interference with surrounding organs. *Pain* is felt only when the swelling presses upon nerves, upon the air passages, causing great breathlessness, or upon bone, wearing it gradually away. In the latter case pain may be agonizing, although in early cases it is not infrequently taken for mere rheumatic pain. *Breathlessness* or *difficulty in swallowing* may occur where there is a large thoracic aneurysm, from pressure on the windpipe or gullet, also *cough* of a barking, irritating nature, and changes in the voice, from irritation or paralysis of the left recurrent laryngeal nerve. In thoracic and abdominal aneurysm there may be a *bulging* in the upper part of chest or abdomen, as the case may be, which can be felt to throb when one hand is placed on it in front and the other on the back; in a later stage pulsation can also be seen. The *aneurysmal tippet* is the name given to a network of dilated veins which appears upon the chest and shoulders, owing to obstruction of the circulation through the great veins, by a thoracic aneurysm. *Swelling of the skin* or oedema is found with all aneurysms sooner or later from the same cause. Many other signs, such as inequality of the pupils, difference in the pulse on the two sides of the body, and murmurs heard over the swelling, are present in different aneurysms, but can be appreciated only by the trained observer.

Aneurysm is a serious disease: it is apt to cause great interference with other organs; it may at any time burst and cause sudden death from bleeding into the loose tissues or cavities of the body; it is a sign that the arteries are extensively diseased, and the person unfit for active work. The duration of life is generally only a few years, although it may be prolonged for twenty if the aneurysm fills up with clot, which forms a natural method of cure.

Treatment – (*a*) – MEDICAL – Although the aneurysm tends constantly to increase in size, another tendency is for the blood in contact with the unhealthy wall to clot. If this be encouraged, the aneurysm may become a solid mass, which practically may be looked on as a cure, because there is no more tendency to grow or to burst. To this end the circulation must be quieted by rest in bed, freedom from worry, and a bland diet. Potassium iodide is often of value, particularly if the aneurysm is syphilitic in origin, and in cases due to this cause penicillin is given.

(*b*) SURGICAL – Tremendous advances have been achieved in recent years in the surgical treatment of aneurysms. In many cases, as in aneurysms of arteries in the limbs, all that is required is to ligature the artery above and below the aneurysm, the circulation to the limb being maintained by anastomosis (qv) of the other arteries in the limb. In the case of other major arteries, such as the aorta, the aneurysm is replaced by a graft so that the circulation through the artery can be maintained. This graft may consist of a piece of an artery removed from a cadaver, or of synthetic material such as orlon.

ANGINA means literally choking, and is a term applied to swellings of the throat or other cause of difficulty in breathing, as *tonsillar angina* or quinsy, *laryngeal angina* or laryngitis, *membranous angina* or croup, *anginal scarlatina* or scarlet fever with abscesses round the throat.

ANGINA PECTORIS is a term applied to a violent paroxysm of painful sensations in the chest, arising for the most part in connection with disease of the coronary arteries.

Causes – Angina pectoris is generally held to be due to an inadequate blood-supply to the myocardium: ie. the heart muscle. The myocardium receives its blood-supply through the coronary arteries. Thus angina pectoris may be due to spasm of the coronary arteries or to narrowing of the lumen of these arteries as a result of arteriosclerosis (qv) or atheroma (qv). It is probably seldom due to spasm alone. In the majority of cases it is due either to spasm plus arteriosclerosis (or atheroma) or to arteriosclerosis (or atheroma). Occasionally the defective blood-supply may be the result of disease of the first part of the aorta or of the aortic valve. Because of its association with coronary artery disease, angina pectoris is predominantly a disease of middle age and is more common in men than in women.

Symptoms – The characteristic feature of angina pectoris is the occurrence of pain behind the chest-bone, arising as a result of exertion and relieved by rest. This pain often spreads into the left arm. The amount of exertion necessary to induce the pain varies considerably, and to a certain extent gives some idea of the severity of the condition. Thus, it may only occur on hurrying, whilst in other cases the blood-supply to the myocardium may be so defective that the least exertion, eg. turning over in bed, may be sufficient to induce a severe paroxysm of pain. Aggravating factors are exposure to cold, or exertion immediately following a meal. The paroxysm of pain seldom lasts for more than a few minutes, provided the affected individual remains at complete rest. In most instances the pain is so severe that the affected individual is unable to continue any exertion. Occasionally it is accompanied by a feeling of impending dissolution, often referred to as *angor animi*: this is more prevalent in the Latin races than in the more phlegmatic Anglo-Saxon.

Treatment – The aim of treatment is to prevent the occurrence of pain by persuading the patient to restrict his activities. Thus, he should always rest for at least half an hour after a meal. He should always be warmly clad when he goes out of doors in cold weather. In more severe cases his bedroom should be on the ground floor and should be warmed in the winter. He should always allow himself plenty of time so that he never needs to hurry. If he is overweight he should restrict his diet so as to bring his weight down. Even with all these precautions, attacks of pain may still occur, and for the relief of these glyceryl trinitrate tablets B.P., or trinitrin tablets as they are also known, each containing 500 micrograms, are the most satisfactory. A tablet should be placed in the mouth, as soon as pain is felt, and allowed to melt in the mouth. It should not be swallowed intact, as this delays the onset of relief. Most patients with angina pectoris carry a small supply of these tablets about with them wherever they go, so that they are always available for immediate use. An alternative form of treatment is amyl nitrite, which is supplied in the form of small glass 'perles'. One of these, held in a handkerchief, is broken between the fingers and the contents then inhaled. Whilst usually as effective as trinitrin tablets, amyl nitrite is more liable to produce unpleasant side-effects such as headache and giddiness. Both these preparations bring relief in angina pectoris by virtue of the fact that they cause vasodilatation of the coronary arteries and thereby improve the blood-supply to the myocardium.

Many surgical operations have been recommended for the relief of angina pectoris but few, if any, of them have lived up to the original claims made for them. Recently, however, promising results have been reported with severe cases which were resistant to all forms of medicinal relief, by a grafting operation bypassing the blockage in the coronary arteries. Time will tell whether it is any more effective than its predecessors.

ANGIOCARDIOGRAPHY means X-raying of the heart after injection of a radio-opaque substance.

ANGIOGRAPHY means rendering the blood-vessels visible on an X-ray film by injecting into them a radio-opaque substance. In the case of arteries this is known as *arteriography*; the corresponding term for veins being *venography* or *phlebography*. This procedure demonstrates whether there is any narrowing of the lumen of the vessel.

ANGIOMA is a tumour composed of blood-vessels. (See TUMOUR and NAEVUS.)

ANGIONEUROTIC OEDEMA is a condition of localized dropsy, similar in many ways to nettle-rash. The precise cause is not known. (See NETTLE-RASH.)

ANGITIS, or ANGIITIS, means inflammation of a vessel such as a blood-vessel, lymph-vessel, or bile-duct.

ÅNGSTRÖM UNIT (called after Swedish physicist) is a measurement of length and equals $\frac{1}{10000}$ micrometre, or one-hundred-millionth of a centimetre. It is represented by the symbol Å and is used to give the length of electro-magnetic waves.

ANHYDRAEMIA is the term used to describe an abnormal loss of water from the blood.

ANIDROSIS is the condition in which there is an abnormal diminution in the secretion of sweat.

ANISE, or ANISEED, is the dried fruit of *Pimpinella anisum*, from which is obtained a volatile oil used as a flavouring agent in some mixtures, as a mild expectorant, and as a remedy for colic in children. (See OILS.)

ANISINDIONE is one of the newer anticoagulants which is active when taken by mouth. Its maximum effect occurs in about 36 hours, and its action passes off within 48 hours of cessation of treatment. (See also ANTICOAGULANTS.)

ANKLE is the joint between the leg bones (tibia and fibula) above, and the talus (the Roman dice-bone) below. It is a very strong joint with powerful ligaments binding the bones together at either side, many sinews running over it, and bony projections from the leg bones, which form large bosses on either side, called the outer and inner malleoli, extending about half an inch (12 mm) below the actual joint. Two common injuries near the ankle are a sprain, on the inner side, consisting of tearing of the internal ligament; and fracture of the fibula (Pott's fracture) on the outer side. (See also JOINT DISEASES.)

ANKYLOSING SPONDYLITIS (see SPINE, DISEASES AND INJURIES OF).

ANKYLOSIS is a term meaning the condition of a joint in which the movements are restricted by fibrous bands, or by malformation, or by actual union of the bones. (See JOINT DISEASES.)

ANKYLOSTOMA (see ANCYLOSTOMA).

ANODYNES are curative measures which soothe pain. They act by removing the cause of pain, by soothing the irritated nerves of the painful part, or by paralysing the part of the brain by which the painful impression is received. Substances which destroy the power of feeling altogether are called anaesthetics (qv), those which destroy only the power of feeling pain are analgesics (qv).

Varieties – Alkaline applications are anodynes to bee-stings. Prolonged application of either cold or heat is an anodyne in inflammation. Chloroform, camphor and menthol are local anodynes, while internally various synthetic products like aspirin soothe pain in distant parts.

Uses – Opium is the oldest and most

powerful anodyne, but can only be used in cases of excessive pain, because of its tendency to habit-formation. Barbiturates dull pain, but with it the mental faculties, so that they also interfere with the performance of everyday duties. Aspirin and paracetamol seem to have the power of dulling only that part of the brain which perceives the pain, and so are most suitable in slighter pains which do not incapacitate though they interfere with ordinary duties. (For further details, see NEURALGIA; HEADACHE; INFLAMMATION; and the various drugs named.)

13 – *Anopheles gambiae*. The most dangerous malaria-carrier in Africa. From Manson's *Tropical Diseases*. Baillière Tindall.

ANOPHELES is the generic name of a widely distributed group of mosquitoes, certain species of which transmit to man the infecting agent of malaria (illustration 13). *Anopheles maculipennis* and *A. bifurcatus* are both found in England and can both transmit the malaria parasite.

ANOREXIA means loss of appetite. (See APPETITE.)

ANOREXIA NERVOSA (see APPETITE).

ANOREXIANT DRUGS are drugs which reduce appetite. Many of them are synthetic sympathomimetic amines – ie. produce effects simulating those produced by stimulation of the sympathetic nerves. Typical examples are amphetamine (qv), chlorphentermine (qv) and phenmetrazine (qv). In no circumstances should they ever be used except under strict medical supervision.

ANOSMIA means loss of sense of smell. (See NOSE, DISEASES OF.)

ANOXAEMIA means reduction of the oxygen content of the blood below normal limits.

ANOXIA is the term applied to that state in which the body tissues have an inadequate supply of oxygen. This may be because the blood in the lungs does not receive enough oxygen, or because there is not enough blood to receive the oxygen, or because the blood stagnates in the body.

ANTABUSE (see DISULFIRAM).

ANTACIDS are medicines which correct acidity, either general or stomachic. (See ACIDITY; ALKALI; DYSPEPSIA.)

ANTE- is a prefix meaning before or forwards.

ANTEFLEXION means the abnormal forward curvature of an organ in which the upper part is sharply bent forward. The term is especially applied to forward displacement of the uterus.

ANTENATAL is a term applied to conditions occurring before birth. It is used with reference both to mother and child. (For Antenatal Clinics, see MATERNITY AND CHILD WELFARE.)

ANTEVERSION is the term applied to the forward tilting of an organ, especially of the uterus.

ANTHELMINTICS are substances which cause the death or expulsion of parasitic worms. (See PARASITES.)

ANTHRACOSIS is the change which takes place in the lungs and bronchial glands of coal miners, and others, who inhale coal dust constantly. The lungs are amazingly efficient in coping with this problem. During a working lifetime a coal-miner may inhale around 5000 grams of dust, but at post-mortem examination it is rare to find more than about 40 grams in his lungs. The affected tissues change in colour from greyish pink to jet black, owing to loading with minute carbon particles. This fine form of dust appears to be almost devoid of any harmful effect.

ANTHRAX is a very serious disease occurring in sheep and cattle, and in those who tend them or handle the skins and fleeces, even long after removal of the latter from the animals. It has also broken out occasionally in epidemics among wool-sorters or cattle-tenders. In 1973, three cases were notified in England, one of which proved fatal. It is sometimes referred to as malignant pustule, wool-sorters' disease, splenic fever of animals or murrain.

Causes – The cause is a bacillus (*B. anthracis*) which grows in long chains and produces spores of great vitality. These spores retain their life for years, in dried skins and fleeces; they are not destroyed by boiling, freezing, 5 per cent carbolic lotion, or, like many bacilli, by the gastric juice. The disease is communicated from a diseased animal to a crack in the skin, eg. of a shepherd or butcher, or from contact with contaminated skins or fleeces. Nowadays skins are handled wet, but if they are allowed to dry so that dust laden with spores is inhaled by the workers an internal form of the disease results. Instances have occurred of the disease being conveyed on shaving brushes made from bristles of diseased animals.

Symptoms – (*a*) EXTERNAL FORM. – This is the 'malignant pustule'. After inoculation of some small wound, a few hours or days elapse, and then a red, inflamed swelling appears, which grows larger till it covers half the face or the breadth of the arm, as the case may be. Upon its summit appears a bleb of pus, which bursts and leaves a black scab, perhaps half an inch (12 mm) wide. At the same time there is great prostration and fever. The inflammation may last ten days or so, when it slowly subsides and the patient recovers, if surviving the fever and prostration.

(*b*) INTERNAL FORM – This takes the form of pneumonia with haemorrhages, when the spores have been drawn into the lungs, or of ulcers of the stomach and intestines, with gangrene of the spleen, when they have been swallowed. It is usually fatal in two or three days.

Treatment – Prevention is most important by disinfecting all hides, wool and hair coming from areas of the world, such as the Middle and Far East, where the disease is commonly found. All hides should be handled wet, so that spores cannot be present in dust; for the internal form is four times as fatal as the external. The hands of workmen must be carefully washed before eating, and working clothes changed. By these means the number of deaths from anthrax, in the English woollen manufacturing districts has been reduced to a tenth of the number that occurred fifty years ago, before the disease was understood. An efficient vaccine is now available. Treatment consists of the administration of large doses of penicillin or of one of the tetracyclines. There is also an antiserum which can be given in addition to penicillin. If there is a pustule, this is kept clean, but must not be cauterized or incised.

ANTI- is a prefix meaning against.

ANTIBIOTIC is the term used to describe any antibacterial agent derived from micro-organisms, such as penicillin, streptomycin, chloramphenicol and chlortetracycline.

ANTIBODIES are substances in the blood which destroy or neutralize various toxins or 'bodies' (eg. bacteria), known generally as antigens. The antibodies are formed, usually, as a result of the introduction into the body of the antigens to which they are antagonistic, as in all infectious diseases.

ANTICOAGULANTS are drugs which prevent coagulation of the blood. The main ones now in use are heparin (qv), anisindione (qv), cyclocoumarol (qv), dicoumarol (qv), ethyl biscoumacetate (qv), phenindione (qv) and warfarin (qv). Patients who are on anticoagulants require to be under medical supervision, and it is now usual for them to receive from their doctors an Anticoagulant Card with instructions about the use of whatever anticoagulant drug they may be taking.

ANTIDEPRESSANTS are drugs which relieve depression by a direct antagonizing action on the depression. They include drugs such as imipramine and phenelzine.

ANTIDOTES are remedies which neutralize the effects of poisons. Thus acids have alkalis as antidote and vice versa.

ANTIGEN is the term applied to a substance which causes the formation of antibodies: that is bodies which act in opposition to poisons formed in the body or introduced from outside.

ANTIHISTAMINE DRUGS are drugs which antagonize the action of histamine (qv) and are therefore of value in the treatment of certain allergic conditions such as hay fever, nettlerash, and certain forms of eczema.

APPROVED NAME	PROPRIETARY NAME
Group I. *Least Sedative*	
Antazoline	Anstitin
Chlorcyclizine	Di-Paralene
	Histantin
Chlorpheniramine	Piriton
Phenindamine	Theophorin
Triprolidine	Actidil
Group II. *Moderate Sedative*	
Dimenhydrinate	Dramamine
Mepyramine	Anthisan
Promethazine	Avomine
theoclate	
Tripelennamine	Pyribenzamine
Group III. *Highly Sedative*	
Diphenhydramine	Benadryl
Promethazine	Phenergan

Table 3 – Classification of
antihistamine drugs

A selection of those available in Great Britain is given in table 3, where they are classified according to their sedative effect. This classification has been used because the degree of sedation produced by the drug, through its action on the central nervous system, is often the deciding factor in selecting the preparation to be used in a given case. It should be noted that those in Group III are also liable to cause a dry mouth and blurring of the vision, just as hyoscine does.

ANTIKETOGENIC is the term applied to foods and remedies which prevent or decrease the formation of ketones: ie. bodies related to acetone.

ANTIMETABOLITES are a group of drugs which have been introduced for the treatment of certain forms of malignant disease. Chemically, they closely resemble substances (or metabolites) which are essential for the life and growth of cells. When introduced into the body they are 'mistaken', so to speak, by the cell for the corresponding metabolite, thereby preventing the cell from making use of the metabolite, or substance, which is essential for its growth. By this means the life of the cell is affected and it ultimately dies.

ANTIMONY is the name applied to a metal and also to its sulphide, a black powder found in nature. The tartrate of potassium and antimony is commonly known as tartar emetic in reference to its chief property. The preparations of antimony are all irritants; hence in large doses they are poisons, producing vomiting,

purging, and also paralysis of the heart and nervous system. In moderate amounts they stimulate secretions from the bronchial tubes, intestine and skin, and thus ease cough, move the bowels, and cause free perspiration.

Antidote – Dimercaprol (qv) is the antidote to antimony. Should a poisonous amount be taken by mouth the stomach should be washed out with strong tea. Failing this, calcium hydroxide or magnesium oxide should be used for this purpose.

Uses – Once a popular constituent, in the form of antimonial wine and James's powder (antimonial powder), of preparations for the treatment of fever and bronchitis, antimony is only used now in the treatment of certain tropical diseases such as kala-azar and schistosomiasis. For this purpose either the trivalent or pentavalent salts are used. These include antimony lithium thiomalate, antimony sodium tartrate, antimony potassium tartrate, sodium antimonylgluconate, stibocaptate and stibophen.

ANTIPERISTALSIS is a term meaning a movement in the bowels and stomach by which the food and other contents are passed upwards, instead of in the proper direction. (See PERISTALSIS.)

ANTIPHLOGISTICS is an old term meaning remedies used against inflammation, fever, and similar conditions.

ANTIPYRETICS are measures used to reduce temperature in fever.

Varieties – Cold-sponging, wet-pack, baths and diaphoretic drugs such as quinine, salicylate of soda, and aspirin.

Uses (*see under above headings*).

ANTISEPTICS are substances which have the property of preventing or arresting putrefaction in dead animal or vegetable matter. The access of air, together with a moderate amount of warmth and of moisture, is necessary for the occurrence of the putrefactive changes, which consist essentially in the breaking up of the complex organic material, and the formation of new and simpler combinations among its constituent elements. During the process, various gases and vapours are evolved, and the lower forms of animal and vegetable life are observed to grow and multiply in the putrefying substance. The exciting causes of putrefaction depend upon the growth and activity of micro-organisms (see BACTERIOLOGY). The changes which take place in a wound when organisms gain entrance to it and

53

flourish upon its discharges are collectively known as sepsis or septic processes (see ABSCESS).

Varieties – By exclusion of the air, or even by covering from germ-laden dust, dead matter that does not already contain bacteria may be kept intact for an indefinite time, as shown in the method of preserving meat by hermetically sealing the jars, after destruction of all germs by heat. Again, the preservative influence of a low temperature is well known; extreme cold is a powerful antiseptic, as proved in the case of the frozen mammoths of northern Asia. Furthermore, the abstraction of moisture will prevent corruption in dead material. In warm and dry climates, animal food may be preserved by exposure to the sun. In the ancient practice of embalming the dead, which is the earliest illustration of the systematic use of antiseptics, the moister portions of the body were removed before the preservative agents were added. The action of direct sunlight is highly destructive to bacteria, having more effect upon some kinds than others.

For practical purposes reliance is chiefly placed on heat and chemical substances which destroy bacteria. Many substances which are strong antiseptics are of little practical use, either because they produce changes in the fluids with which they come in contact of such a nature as to hinder their further action, or because they are too irritating or too destructive when they come in contact with the tissues of the body. Further, some antiseptics act strongly upon certain organisms and less effectively upon others, so that the value of an antiseptic varies in different circumstances.

HEAT is one of the most effective antiseptics and may be applied at a temperature of 100° to 150°C. Dry articles to be disinfected may be brought into contact with steam under pressure, or more simple articles to be preserved from decomposition or sterilized may be boiled for a short period. This method is, however, obviously inapplicable to the living body and to many fragile articles.

BORIC ACID is a weak antiseptic which is used because of its unirritating qualities. It may be used up to the full strength at which it dissolves in cold water: ie. 1 part in 20 of water.

CARBOLIC ACID, originally introduced by Lord Lister, is a powerful antiseptic: 1 part in 100 of water will in the course of some hours kill most bacteria. Up to a strength of 1 part in 20 of water it may be brought in contact with tissues for a short time, but even this strength is dangerous for prolonged application.

MERCURIC SALTS are among the most powerful antiseptics. Perchloride of mercury (mercuric chloride) may be used for washing the hands in a strength of 1 in 1000 of water. For vaginal douching, it may be used in a strength of 1 in 100,000. Even in the strength of 1 part in 100,000 of water it kills almost all bacteria in a few minutes. The cyanide of mercury is also used, either in lotions of similar strength, or by saturating lint, gauze, or wool for application to wounds. The disadvantage of mercuric salts is that though very powerful they are highly irritating, and secondly, that they are precipitated and rendered useless by the proteins of discharges with which they come in contact.

CRESOL, TRICRESOL, or CRESYLIC ACID, is a mixture of substances obtained from coal-tar, which is less poisonous than carbolic acid. Various preparations sold under propretary names, such as CREOLIN, CYLLIN, JEYES' FLUID, ACROSYL, and IZAL, are of similar nature and widely used. They are all dark oily liquids which form a white milky emulsion in water. LYSOL and some others contain fluid soap which aids their cleansing and penetrating action. They are all useful general disinfectants for hospital and domestic use. TAR WATER is a popular antiseptic often used because of the cresols and similar substances that it contains.

HYDROGEN PEROXIDE has the double merit of being a strong antiseptic and at the same time non-irritating. It may be freely applied to mucous membranes in the full pharmacopoeial strength, although, even when considerably diluted with water, it is still a powerful germicide. It is essential that it should be fresh, as it rapidly deteriorates by losing oxygen.

IODINE is a strong antiseptic and is specially used in the form of weak solution of iodine (2·5 per cent strength).

IODOFORM has the power of checking septic changes when discharges come in contact with it, probably by its power of giving off iodine. It is sometimes used to impregnate gauze for filling abscesses and other cavities.

CHLORINE GAS is a powerful antiseptic. It is used for the sterilization of water supplies, either as the gas or in the form of chlorinated lime (bleaching powder). CHLORINATED LIME, which gives off chlorine gas, is much used to disinfect drains. Chlorine has the disadvantage of being very irritating and of bleaching and destroying many substances, eg. cloth, leather, with which it comes in contact.

HYPOCHLOROUS ACID, under such names as EUSOL, DAKIN'S SOLUTION, is effective for septic wounds.

SULPHUR DIOXIDE is highly antiseptic. It is used as a food preservative, and also for the disinfection of rooms by fumigation.

FORMALDEHYDE is one of the more powerful antiseptics, and dissolved in water is used as a spray for disinfection of walls and furniture. It is also used in throat lozenges. It is excessively irritating, and therefore cannot be used as an antiseptic for application to the tissues.

POTASSIUM PERMANGANATE is an antiseptic on account of its oxidizing properties. It is used in strengths of 1 part in 4000 of water or weaker as a gargle, douche and as a wash for the hands.

ACRIFLAVINE, PROFLAVINE, and other aniline dyes as well as BRILLIANT GREEN, have a powerful action as antiseptics, and have also a gentle stimulating action on the tissues. They can be used in a strength of 1 part in 1000 of normal saline, and they can be mixed with various other antiseptics without detriment.

ALCOHOL is a powerful antiseptic, and, like ETHER, is used for removing septic matter and grease from the skin.

NITRATE OF SILVER is a powerful antiseptic used for lotions, eye drops, etc., in the strength of 1 part in 500 or 1000 of water. Other silver salts which are less irritating to the tissues are used in a similar way.

SALTS OF COPPER, SALTS OF IRON, SALTS OF LEAD, CHLORIDE OF ZINC, and compounds of most of the heavy metals act as strong antiseptics, but most of them, on account of their irritating or poisonous action, are not readily applicable for this purpose.

BALSAM OF TOLU, BALSAM OF PERU, and other aromatic substances are mild antiseptics.

CETRIMIDE, a mixture of alkyl ammonium bromides, is most effective for cleaning and disinfecting wounds and as a first-aid dressing in burns. It is also suitable for disinfecting utensils.

CHLORHEXIDINE has proved particularly valuable in obstetric practice, as a skin disinfectant, and in the treatment of burns.

CHLOROXYLENOL is non-irritating and is widely used in obstetric practice.

HEXACHLOROPHANE is a widely used antiseptic, one of the advantages of which is that it retains its activity in the presence of soap. It is therefore often used in soaps and creams in a concentration of 1 to 2 per cent.

CLIOQUINOL is an iodine-containing preparation used in the form of a cream, lotion or ointment – the treatment of skin infections. The usual strength is 3 per cent. It stains clothing and linen yellow.

POLYNOXYLIN is a condensation product of formaldehyde and urea used as a cream (10 per cent) in the treatment of infections of the skin.

POVIDONE-IODINE slowly liberates iodine on contact with the skin. As an ointment it is used in the treatment of infections of the skin.

Uses – Antiseptics act in various ways. Some of them kill bacteria by drying them: eg. common salt and syrup used as preservatives extract water from bacteria and thus kill them; other antiseptics kill bacteria by oxidation: eg. hydrogen peroxide, potassium permanganate; others coagulate the fluids in and around bacteria: eg. perchloride of mercury; and still others act as bacterial poisons: eg. cresol. The practice of using antiseptics has been in vogue for thousands of years. Thus cedar oil, tar and resins were in use among the Egyptians. Pitch, copper salts, vinegar, etc., were used for wounds by the Romans, while the fumes of sulphur for purification and salt as a preservative of food have been employed from the earliest times. Many of the stronger and more irritating antiseptics are now used as disinfectants (see DISINFECTION).

The methods of applying antisepsis or, as it should more correctly be described, asepsis (qv) in surgery are as follows. The sterilization of the hands of all those participating in an operation varies with the instructions of individual surgeons, but in essence is based upon washing the hands and arms up to the elbows under hot running water, using a sterile nail-brush and some antiseptic such as hexachlorophane soap, for at least five minutes. The hands are then immersed in an alcoholic solution, such as 75 per cent isopropyl alcohol. The skin of the patient is prepared by shaving, followed by a bath using some antiseptic soap. This is often done the day before the operation, and the area to be operated on is then covered by a dressing. On the operating table, and immediately before the operation, a wide stretch of skin in the operation area is cleaned by the antiseptic of the surgeon's choice, usually iodine but always coloured so that the cleansed area is clearly defined. Instruments and dressings are sterilized in autoclaves (qv).

By these means it is ensured that no germs can come in contact with the operation wound. To make doubly sure that such infection should not occur, all modern hospitals are equipped with a Central Sterile Supply Department (CSSD) which supplies all the sterilized material, such as dressings and instruments, required throughout the hospital, whether in operating theatres, wards or casualty departments.

ANTISPASMODICS (see SPASMO-LYTICS).

ANTITOXINS, ANTITOXIC SERUM (see SERUM THERAPY).

ANTIVENINE, or ANTIVENOM, is the name given to SNAKE VENOM ANTISERUM, which is produced by the injection of snake venom into animals in small but increasing doses. In course of time the animal becomes immune to the particular venom injected, and the antiserum prepared from its serum is effective in neutralizing venom injected by the bite of a snake of the same species. No antiserum effective against all venoms is available. The custom is for each country to prepare antisera able to neutralize the venoms of indigenous snakes. The antivenom active against the venom of the adder is known as Zagreb antivenom. To be of any use, it must be administered as soon as possible after the snake bite. (See BITES, STINGS AND POISONED WOUNDS.)

ANTROSTOMY is the term applied to the operation in which an opening is made through the nose into the maxillary antrum. (See ANTRUM.)

ANTRUM means a natural hollow or cavity.

The *maxillary antrum* is now known as the maxillary sinus (see SINUS).

The *mastoid antrum* is situated in the mastoid process, the mass of bone felt behind the ear. It may become the seat of an abscess in cases of suppuration of the middle ear (see EAR, DISEASES OF).

The *pyloric antrum* is the part of the stomach immediately preceding the pylorus (qv).

ANURIA is a condition in which no urine is voided. (See BRIGHT'S DISEASE; URINE.)

ANUS is the opening at the lower end of the bowel. It is kept closed by two muscles, the external and internal sphincters. The latter is a muscular ring which extends about an inch (25 mm) up the bowel, is nearly $\frac{1}{4}$ inch (6 mm) thick, and is kept constantly contracted by the action of a nerve centre in the spinal cord. Constipation is sometimes due to its failure to relax. In disease of the spinal cord the muscle may be paralysed, and inability to retain the motions results.

ANUS, DISEASES OF (see RECTUM, DISEASES OF).

AORTA is the large vessel which opens out of the left ventricle of the heart and carries blood to all the body (illustration 14). It is about $1\frac{1}{2}$ feet (45 cm) long and 1 inch (2.5 cm) wide. Like other arteries it possesses three coats, of which the middle one is much the thickest. This consists partly of muscle fibre, but is mainly composed of an elastic substance, called elastin. The aorta passes first to the right, and lies nearest the surface behind the end of the second right rib-cartilage; then it curves backwards and to the left, passes down behind the left lung close to the backbone, and through an opening in the diaphragm into the abdomen, where it divides, at the level of the navel, into the two common iliac arteries, which carry blood to the lower limbs. Its branches, in order, are: two coronary arteries to the heart wall; the brachiocephalic, left

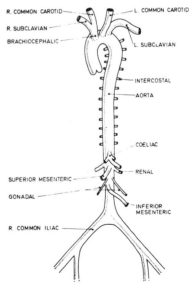

14 – Main branches of the aorta. From Passmore and Robson, *A Companion to Medical Studies.* Blackwell Scientific Publications.

common carotid, and left subclavian arteries to the head, neck and upper limbs; several small branches to the oesophagus, bronchi, and other organs of the chest; nine pairs of intercostal arteries which run round the body between the ribs; one pair of subcostal arteries which is in series with the intercostal arteries; four (or five) lumbar arteries to the muscles of the loins; coeliac trunk to the stomach, liver and pancreas; two mesenteric arteries to the bowels; and suprarenal, renal and testicular arteries to the suprarenal body, kidney, and testicle on each side. From the termination of the aorta rises a small branch, the median sacral artery, which runs down into the pelvis, and may, in a sense, be regarded as the continuation of the aorta. In the female the ovarian arteries replace the testicular.

The chief diseases of the aorta are atheroma and aneurysm. (See ARTERIES, DISEASES OF; ANEURYSM; and COARCTATION OF THE AORTA.)

AORTITIS means a degenerative condition of the lining of the aorta. It is usually produced by syphilis.

AORTOGRAPHY is the technique of rendering the aorta visible in an X-ray film by injecting a radio-opaque substance into it. (See also ANGIOGRAPHY.)

APERIENTS are medicines which produce a natural movement of the bowels. (See CONSTIPATION; and PURGATIVES.)

APEX is the pointed portion of any organ which has a conical shape. The apex of each lung reaches about one and a half or two inches (3·5 to 5·0 cm) above the collar-bone into the neck. In health the apex of the heart can be felt below the fifth rib immediately inside the nipple.

APGAR SCORE is a method of assessing a baby's condition at birth, in which a value of 0, 1 or 2 is given to each of five signs: colour, heart-rate, muscle tone, respiratory (or breathing) effort, and the response to stimulation. A total score of 10 is satisfactory.

APHAKIA is a term which means absence of the lens of the eye.

APHASIA means a loss of the power of speech, due to injury to the centres which govern this act in the brain. The higher of these centres, which have to do with forming the ideas of speech, putting words together in sentences, and governing the movements of mouth, tongue and larynx, lie on the surface of the cerebral hemispheres, especially of the left; while the lower centres, which directly bring the muscles of the voice organs into action, under superintendence of the higher ones, are in the medulla or hind brain.

Causes – The cause is destruction of a portion of the brain, including one of these higher centres, owing to rupture of a blood-vessel, and haemorrhage into the brain tissue; or owing to blocking of a blood-vessel by an embolus (see EMBOLISM), or by clotting of the blood on the diseased wall of a vessel (see THROMBOSIS), any one of which cuts off the supply of blood to the part concerned. The causes are thus the same as in apoplexy (ie a stroke), and aphasia may be one of the symptoms of an apoplectic seizure, especially when the right side of the body is paralysed, or may occur by itself, according to the extent of brain involved. Other diseases, such as tumours, may also be the cause, the important factor being interference with the functions of certain definite areas of the brain.

Varieties – It was first pointed out by Broca that the inferior frontal gyrus (illustration 15) on the left side of the brain in right-handed persons, and vice versa in left-handed persons, is, after death, found to be diseased in those who have, in life,

15 – Diagram showing areas upon the left surface of the cerebrum associated with definite functions. CS, central sulcus; LS, lateral sulcus.

suffered from inability to speak, although the intelligence and powers of silent reading and of writing may have remained. Such a condition is known as *motor aphasia*. But the state is generally more complicated. In addition to Broca's speech area, which governs the movements of the tongue, mouth and larynx that frame words to express ideas, there is a centre in the middle frontal gyrus of the left side, which regulates the power of writing intelligibly, and disease of this region produces loss of power to write rationally, even though the hand remains quite able to hold a pen, this condition being known as *agraphia*. These two forms involve loss of power of *production* of speech and writing, but there are corresponding losses of power of *perception* known as *word blindness* and *word deafness*, the two conditions being grouped together as *sensory aphasia*. In the former of these the afflicted person is unable to read correctly, though his vision is perfect, and he may be able to spell and even to write, though not to read what he writes. This condition is due to disease in the angular gyrus. In word deafness the disability consists in failure to understand what is said, and, though the sufferer hears perfectly, the sounds are to him like those of a foreign tongue which he does not understand; in this case the disease lies in the superior temporal gyrus. There are still more complicated forms in which the disease affects, not the surface of the brain, but the strands of nerve fibres, which run from one centre to another and reduce the working of the whole arrangement to a system.

Symptoms – The disorder generally follows an attack of apoplexy and exists along with some paralysis on the right side of the body. *Aphasia* may come on suddenly and last only a few hours or days, being due then to a passing congestion of the brain, or to a block in the circulation, which is later swept away. Generally it is permanent, and, naturally, a person with aphasia has always some mental impairment. Sometimes he is absolutely without the power of speech, though often a few interjections, like 'Oh dear', 'Yes', or 'No', or meaningless sounds, or even oaths, can be pronounced. When the condition is one of *sensory aphasia*, names of persons, of places, even of the commonest household articles, are forgotten, a cat is called 'a brush', a bell 'a pen', and so forth, or the person gives meaningless answers to questions, so that conversation becomes very slow or quite impossible.

Treatment – This is as in apoplexy, of which the condition often forms a part (see APOPLEXY). The condition is seldom much improved if it has lasted more than a week without betterment. But in some cases, after the haemorrhage or other cause is long past, brilliant results are achieved by teaching the afflicted person to read and speak just as one would teach a child, a new part of the brain apparently being educated.

APHONIA means loss of voice. It is caused by some disorder in the throat or in the nerves proceeding to the throat muscles, or by hysteria. (See VOICE.)

APHTHAE (see THRUSH).

APNOEA means stoppage of breathing, such as occurs when the blood is artificially supplied with too much oxygen; for example, by taking several deep breaths in quick succession. (See ASPHYXIA.)

APO- is a prefix implying separation or derivation from.

APOMORPHINE is a crystalline alkaloid closely related to morphine and having a powerful emetic action. Apomorphine hydrochloride is given hypodermically in doses of 2 to 8 mg in cases of poisoning in which the patient is unable to swallow or a very rapid emetic action is desired. It is also used in the treatment of alcoholism.

APONEUROSIS is the term applied to the white fibrous membrane which serves as an investment for the muscles and which covers the skull beneath the scalp.

APOPLEXY is a term introduced by Hippocrates, meaning a stroke of sudden insensibility or of bodily disablement connected with some diseased condition of the brain.

Causes – In persons who are the subject of heart disease, a clot may form in the cavities or on a valve of the heart, and being carried away by the blood-stream may lodge in a vessel of the brain so as to form a plug which prevents blood from reaching the part supplied by the vessel in question. The occurrence of this *embolism* is absolutely sudden and produces all the symptoms of apoplexy. When it occurs, the prospect of improvement is better than when the apoplectic symptoms are due to haemorrhage. In elderly people whose blood-vessels are extensively diseased and whose circulation is feeble, a type of apoplexy, of more gradual onset, may appear in consequence of the blood clotting in the interior of the vessels, this process being known as *thrombosis*.

The most important occasion of apoplexy is *haemorrhage* into the brain by the rupture of blood-vessels. The blood-vessels of the brain, like those in other parts of the body, are liable to undergo degenerative changes after middle life. These changes affect the minute arteries as well as the larger vessels, rendering their texture fragile, and at the same time impairing their function in maintaining the healthy nutrition of the brain. Hence, in the immediate vicinity of the diseased blood-vessels the substance of the brain itself undergoes degeneration and becomes softened. The small vessels having thus lost the natural support of the surrounding tissues, and being here and there distended into aneurysms by disease, are liable to give way, and blood escapes into the brain. The haemorrhage may be slight in amount and in parts of the brain where its presence gives rise to little disturbance; but where a large blood-vessel has ruptured, and more especially where the blood has been extravasated in or around the important structures at the base of the brain, the result is a stroke or apoplexy, as described below, and death not infrequently follows within a short period. In favourable cases, in which a certain measure of recovery takes place, the effused blood undergoes gradual absorption, or becomes enveloped in a sort of capsule formed by the surrounding brain substance, and ceases to cause further disturbance. But even in such cases some degree of paralysis remains. Moreover, the nutrition of the brain is so impaired as to render probable a recurrence of the haemorrhage, and thus the danger to life, as is well known, increases with each successive attack.

From what has been stated, it will be observed that apoplexy is usually a disease of advanced life. Nevertheless it may occur at any period of life, and cases of true apoplexy in very young children have, for example, sometimes followed whooping-cough. It is more common in men than in women. What has from early times been described as the apoplectic habit of body, consisting of a stout build, a short neck, and florid complexion, is now generally discredited, it being admitted that apoplexy occurs about as often in thin and spare persons who present no such peculiarity of conformation. A hereditary tendency is acknowledged as one of the predisposing causes of apoplexy. Important contributory factors are progressive disease of the kidneys, degenerative changes in the heart and blood-vessels and raised blood-pressure. With respect to the exciting causes of a stroke of apoplexy, it may be stated generally that whatever tends directly or indirectly to increase the tension within the cerebral blood-vessels may bring on an attack. Hence, such causes as immoderate eating or drinking, severe exertion of body or mind, violent emotions, much stooping, overheated rooms, over-exposure to the sun, and sudden shocks to the body, may precipitate the attack in a susceptible individual. Many cases in elderly people occur while some violent exertion is being made, such as hurrying to catch a train or during straining at stool.

Symptoms – Apoplectic attacks vary both as regards their intensity, the particular symptoms shown, and the after-effects, but well-marked cases present the following symptoms. The person attacked becomes, more or less suddenly, deprived of consciousness and all power of voluntary motion. He lies as if in a deep sleep, with a flushed face, a slow pulse, stertorous breathing, accompanied with puffing of the cheeks during expiration, and with the pupils of the eyes insensible to light and contracted or unequal. This state in many respects resembles the coma of narcotic poisoning, and is unfortunately too often mistaken by unskilled persons for alcoholic intoxication. The symptoms and history of the case, however, are usually sufficient to enable a medical man to form a correct diagnosis.

The presence of complete paralysis down one or other side is a point which in general differentiates apoplexy from narcotic poisoning and alcoholic intoxication, the paralysis being demonstrable even during unconsciousness by lifting the limbs and noting the characteristic suddenness and helplessness with which those on the affected side fall when not supported. The fact that in either of the last-named conditions the person can generally be partially roused, while in apoplexy unconsciousness is complete, is also valuable. Assistance is also gained by observing the state of the pupils, which are usually unequal, whereas in narcotic poisoning they are usually much contracted, while in alcoholic intoxication they are widely dilated.

In this condition of insensibility death may occur within a few hours, or there may be a gradual return to consciousness, in which case it is usually found that the result of the attack remains in the form of paralysis of one side of the body (hemiplegia), while occasionally there may also be noticed some impairment of the mental powers, pointing to damage done to the brain. (See PARALYSIS; and APHASIA.)

An attack of apoplexy may occur without unconsciousness, a sudden paralysis of one side of the body being the only manifestation. Occasionally, when the haemorrhage takes place gently, the symptoms are gradually developed over a period of several hours (*ingravescent apoplexy*). Sometimes premonitory symptoms occur. Persistent headache of a dull throbbing character, a sense of fullness in the head, vomiting, giddiness, noises in the ears, slight confusion of mind, and numbness of a limb or of one side of the body are among the more important premonitory symptoms; and these may exist for a variable length of time before the attack comes on. Such symptoms, especially in a person known to be gouty or the subject of high blood-pressure with or without kidney disease, at or beyond middle life, indicate danger of an apoplectic seizure.

The effects of a stroke or apoplexy, as regards the paralysis which remains after the immediate attack is over, are described under *Hemiplegia* in the article on PARALYSIS. The dangerous period of an apoplectic attack is during the first two or three days and especially during the first twenty-four hours, when the haemorrhage in the brain may be increased or even started again, after it has ceased, by injudicious disturbance of the patient, such as may be caused by his removal to a distance. A certain amount of danger remains for a period of three weeks or thereabout while the process of absorption and organization of the blood clot is taking place. During this period also such improvement in the patient's condition of paralysis as will take place reaches almost its full extent.

Treatment – A knowledge of these facts is of the utmost importance in the treatment of apoplexy, as obviously much can be done in the way of warding off a stroke when it appears to threaten, and of preventing a recurrence in cases where there have been previous attacks. With respect to the treatment of apoplexy, it must be admitted that little can be done during the state of unconsciousness, apart from skilled nursing. The great importance of absolute quiet, with the body in the recumbent position and the head supported on a low pillow, cannot be too strongly emphasized. Care must be taken that the patient receive nothing of a stimulant nature, which would tend to raise the general blood-pressure and increase the haemorrhage in the brain. If the blood-pressure is very high, the administration of hypotensive drugs may be of value. (See ESSENTIAL HYPERTENSION.)

The patient must be carefully watched, and symptoms treated as they arise. When consciousness returns care and quietness are necessary to prevent recurrence of the haemorrhage. The diet must be light for some time after the attack, and the period of convalescence should be prolonged. In the after-treatment of the resulting paralysis much may be done to prevent stiffness and to preserve the power of the muscles in the weakened limbs by physiotherapy, including exercises, massage and electrical treatment, and continuing reassurance.

APOSTEMA is an old term for abscess.

APOTHECARIES' WEIGHT (see WEIGHTS AND MEASURES).

APPENDICECTOMY, or appendectomy, is the operation for the removal of the appendix vermiformis.

APPENDICITIS is the name of an inflammatory disease starting in the vermiform appendix. (See APPENDIX.)

Varieties – The disease is classified in many ways with regard to its treatment and its anatomical characters. First of all, one must separate the *acute* from the *chronic* or *relapsing form*. In the latter the person affected is troubled by repeated slight attacks of pain in the right iliac region, perhaps never bad enough to keep him from moderate work, but sufficient to be a burden; or there is a sense of constant indefinable weakness and discomfort in this situation. In some cases the slightly inflamed appendix undergoes at times spasmodic, painful contractions: the so-called *appendicular colic*. This may be associated with the presence of concretions in the interior of the appendix or with adhesions between it and neighbouring parts. In other cases the inflammatory process is so mild that no symptoms directly referable to the appendix ever occur, but the patient suffers from constipation, indigestion, or general abdominal discomfort produced in a reflex manner by the disturbance of the appendix. The *acute form* is that which is usually known as an 'attack of appendicitis'. Unless adequately and properly treated, this form may proceed to two very serious forms. *Gangrenous appendicitis* is one in which the inflammation is so intense that the appendix sloughs away, and the bowels communicate, through the opening, with the peritoneal cavity. The other form is *suppurative appendicitis*, in which the inflammation is not quite so severe but the appendix becomes the centre of an abscess. Both of these latter forms are extremely dangerous to life and are often very sudden in their development. It is for this reason that the vast majority of cases of acute appendicitis are operated upon as soon as possible.

Causes – Acute appendicitis is the most common abdominal surgical emergency – certainly in western civilization. It occurs at all ages, but is most common in the first twenty years of life. It tends to be more common in males than in females. The precise cause is not known, but the condition is usually due to a combination of infection and obstruction. What probably happens in most cases is that the appendix becomes obstructed. This may be due to a small mass of faeces accumulating in the appendix or to kinking of the appendix. The contents of the obstructed appendix being infective, the whole appendix rapidly becomes infected, with the dire consequences already described, unless immediate skilled surgical treatment is available.

The widespread popular idea that grape-seeds, apple-pips, and similar small objects have a special faculty for finding out the appendix, lodging there, and setting up appendicitis, is fallacious. Though such objects are found there occasionally, these cases are exceptional, and the small masses of hardened faeces or minute concretions of lime, which are common, are a result of, rather than the cause of, the appendicitis.

Symptoms – An attack of appendicitis comes on as a rule suddenly, without the early feelings of languor and malaise common to most acute diseases. The principal symptoms are four in number: (*a*) sudden pain in the abdomen, often vague in situation at first, but usually settling in the right iliac region. It is generally very severe, and the patient has to lie constantly on his back with the right leg drawn up. (*b*) Disturbance of the digestive functions, consisting in loss of appetite, nausea, often vomiting, and constipation, which has usually been present for a day or two. (*c*) Tenderness to touch in the right iliac region, which in very many cases has its point of greatest intensity defined with curious exactitude at a point called Munro's or M'Burney's point, situated about halfway between the spine of the iliac bone and the navel. (*d*) Fever of a moderate amount, generally about 102° F (39° C). The first three of these occur with varying intensity in other diseases of the abdomen, in which, however, fever is uncommon. Distinct resistance and hardness of the muscles in the right lower quarter of the abdomen can be made out on pressure, and swelling is usually visible in the right iliac region after two or three days. In *gangrenous appendicitis* the symptoms are extreme, the fever high, and death may come on with startling rapidity, if an operation be not performed. In *suppurative appendicitis* an abscess forms with marked swelling, though rarely before the end of the first week, and this also calls for operation.

In some cases an attack is very slight, the bowels around become matted together, an abscess collects in the cavity so formed, and only when it comes near the surface is the condition diagnosed.

Treatment – In no circumstances should a purgative be given. A patient with acute appendicitis seen within thirty-six hours of the onset should be operated on forthwith, the mortality in the hands of good surgeons being very low: around 0·25 per cent. If the case is seen after forty-eight hours of the onset and improvement has set in, some surgeons recommend postponement of the operation until the inflammation has completely subsided; others hold that operation should be done at once. If operation is refused or impossible, the patient should be kept quiet in bed, be given only water by mouth, and perhaps have an injection of morphine. If the case is one of gangrenous appendicitis immediate operation is the only possible course; for the great danger of the disease consists in the production of a general peritonitis through the escape of bacteria and putrescent material in large amount from the interior of the appendix. (See PERITONITIS.)

APPENDICOSTOMY is the term describing the operation whereby an artificial opening is made into the appendix vermiformis, through which the bowel may be irrigated in certain diseases of the colon.

APPENDIX is a term applied to appendages of several hollow organs. The epiploic appendices are a number of tags of fat hanging from the outer surface of the large intestine. The appendices of the larynx are two pouches, one on either side between the false and true vocal cords. The term appendix is most commonly applied to the vermiform appendix of the large intestine (illustration 16). It is a tubular prolongation of the large intes-

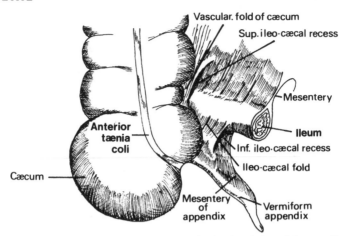

16 – Part of the bowel situated in the right iliac region showing the relations of the appendix to the ileum (the last part of the small intestine) and the caecum (the first part of the large intestine). The anterior taenia is one of the three bands of longitudinal muscle fibres which run along the entire length of the large intestine. From Cunningham. *Textbook of Anatomy*. Oxford University Press.

tine with an average length of 9 or 10 cm and a width of 6 mm. It lies in the right lower corner of the abdomen and has peritoneal, muscular and mucous coats similar to those of the rest of the intestine.

APPETITE is the craving for the food necessary to maintain the body and to supply it with sufficient energy to carry on its functions. The ultimate cause of appetite is a question of supply and demand in the muscles and various organs, but the proximate cause is doubtful. Unlike hunger, it is probably an acquired, rather than an inborn, sensation. Thus, a new-born infant experiences hunger, but probably not appetite. Whatever other factors may be concerned, the tone of the stomach is of importance. This is supported by the fact that in conditions associated with poor appetite the tone of the stomach is poor, whilst in conditions such as duodenal ulcer which are characterized by a good, or even excessive appetite, the stomach is often hypertonic. Important factors in stimulating appetite are anticipation and the sight and smell of well-cooked food. Just as, conversely, the sight or smell of badly cooked food may remove all desire for food. Undoubtedly a good appetite is necessary to good digestion, and a perfectly healthy taste and appetite ought to be both a guide to the suitability of foods and a gauge of the amount required. Like every other bodily function, appetite may be out of order. It

may be depraved, and may indicate quite unsuitable articles of diet, from toasted cheese in dyspeptics, who know by experience that such an article upsets their digestion, to cinders, hair, pebbles, etc., in the condition known as *pica*, which occurs sometimes during pregnancy, in children, in hysteria, and often in mental disorders. The two chief disorders, however, are excessive increase of appetite and diminution or loss of appetite.

Excessive appetite may be simply a bad habit, due to habitual over-indulgence in good food, and resulting in gout, obesity, etc., according to the other habits and constitution of the person. It may also be a sign of diabetes mellitus or thyrotoxicosis.

Diminished appetite is a sign common to almost all diseases causing general weakness, because the activity of the stomach and the secretion of gastric juice fail early when vital power is low. It is the most common sign of dyspepsia due to gastritis (see DYSPEPSIA) and of cancer of the stomach. In some cases it is a manifestation of stress or strain such as domestic worry or difficulties at work. Indeed, appetite seems to be particularly susceptible to emotional disturbances.

There is one condition known as *anorexia nervosa*, in which the sufferer, usually a young woman, sleeps little, eats almost nothing, but is constantly exerting energy upon some favourite pursuit; this condition is liable to end in a total nervous breakdown. Many of these young women have developed a phobia about putting on weight, and a severe psychological disorder underlies the physical condition. Treatment is difficult and usually consists of psychotherapy combined with a tranquillizer such as chlorpromazine.

Diminished appetite in feverish states is a salutary thing, as the digestive functions are reduced in power, and people in these circumstances should restrict themselves to a light diet, consisting mainly of milk and fruit juices, and should rest quietly at the same time.

APPROVED NAMES is the term used for names devised or selected by the *British Pharmacopoeia* Commission for new drugs. The intention is that if any of the drugs to which these Approved Names are applied should eventually be included in the *British Pharmacopoeia* the Approved Name should be its official title. The issue of an Approved Name, however, does not imply that the substance will necessarily be included in the *British Pharmacopoeia* or that the Commission is prepared to recommend the use of the substance.

APRAXIA means loss of power to carry out regulated movements.

APYREXIA means absence of fever.

ARACHIS OIL, also known as peanut oil, is the oil expressed from the seeds of *Arachis hypogoea.* It is sometimes used to replace olive oil when the latter is in short supply. It is commonly used as the vehicle for the intramuscular injection of drugs: eg. penicillin.

ARACHNOID MEMBRANE is one of the membranes covering the brain and spinal cord (see BRAIN). Arachnoiditis is the name applied to inflammation of this membrane.

ARBOVIRUSES are a group of viruses, of which there are around 200, which are transmitted to man by arthropods. They include the viruses of dengue (qv) and yellow fever (qv) which are transmitted by mosquitoes.

ARC EYE, or SNOW BLINDNESS, is the excruciatingly painful condition caused by excessive exposure to ultra-violet radiation. Treatment consists of the application of a local anaesthetic and of homatropine, and then bandaging the eyes for twenty-four hours.

ARCUS SENILIS is the white line which appears round the cornea of the eye with advancing years. (See AGE, NATURAL CHANGES IN.)

ARENAVIRUSES are a group of viruses, so called because under the electron microscope they have a sand-sprinkled (Latin, *arenosus*) appearance. Among the diseases in man for which they are responsible are lassa fever (qv) in West Africa, Argentinian haemorrhagic fever (mortality rate 3 to 15 per cent), a similar disease in Bolivia (mortality rate 18 per cent), and lymphocytic choriomeningitis, in which deaths are uncommon.

AREOLA literally means a small space, and is the term applied to the red or dusky ring round the nipple, or round an inflamed part. Increase in the duskiness of the areola on the breast is an important early sign of pregnancy.

ARGENTUM is the Latin word for silver.

ARGYLL ROBERTSON PUPIL is a condition (described originally by Dr Argyll Robertson) in which the pupils contract when the eyes converge on a near object, but fail to contract when a bright light falls on the eye. It is found in several diseases, especially in locomotor ataxia and general paralysis of the insane.

ARGYRIA means the effect produced by taking silver salts over a long period, and consists of a deep duskiness of the skin, especially of the exposed parts.

ARGYROL (see SILVER)

ARM is the part of the upper limb between the shoulder and elbow, but is generally taken to include also the forearm and shoulder regions. The upper limb is attached to the body by the strong pectoral muscles in front and by several powerful muscles springing from the spine and ribs behind. The great mobility of the shoulder is largely due to the fact that the only contact with the bones of the trunk takes place between the collar-bone and the upper end of the sternum or breast-bone, the shoulder-blade sliding freely between the muscles of the back as the arm is raised and lowered. The bones of the arm (see illustration 83 on page 127) are the clavicle or collar-bone and the scapula or shoulder-blade lying at the upper part of the chest, the humerus, a single bone in the upper arm, and the radius and ulna lying side by side in the forearm. Eight small bones compose the wrist (or carpus) and connect the hand with the lower end of the radius.

The shoulder-joint is of the ball-and-socket variety, the head of the humerus resting against the glenoid cavity of the shoulder-blade. The elbow is a hinged joint formed at the lower end of the humerus above, while the ulna forms the chief part of the joint below, the radius resting lightly against the humerus. When the hand is rotated so as to lie palm up or back up, the radius in the first case lies alongside the ulna and in the latter crosses over it. The chief muscle which bends the elbow is the biceps in front of the upper arm, while the triceps lying behind straightens the limb (see illustrations 315, 316 on pages 604–605). A group of muscles attached at the inner side of the elbow act to bend the wrist and fingers; another group of muscles attached to the outer side of the elbow have the general action of straightening and bending backwards the wrist and fingers.

One large artery (brachial artery) runs down the inner side of the upper arm, corresponding to the seam of the coat sleeve in position (illustration 17). At the elbow this divides into two branches, the radial and ulnar arteries. The radial artery can be felt pulsating near the wrist and is generally known as the pulse. The ulnar artery lies to the inner side of the forearm, deeply imbedded in muscles. A large group of nerves lies at the inner side of the armpit, and these nerves run downwards to supply the muscles and skin of the arm. The ulnar nerve can readily be felt behind the inner side of the elbow, where it is exposed to bruising and is popularly known as the 'funny bone'. The large radial nerve runs down the back of the upper arm and the outer side of the forearm. At the back of the upper arm it is often damaged, leading then to the condition known as drop-wrist (qv), in which the hand hangs helpless and cannot be raised.

The collar-bone, by reason of its exposed position, is liable to fracture from falls on the shoulder, and the radius is often broken by falls on the palm of the hand. The shoulder-joint, on account of its great mobility, is prone to be dislocated in twists of the upper arm, but the elbow-joint is seldom injured. A small bursa or cavity lies between the skin and the end of the ulna at the point of the elbow, and this is often inflamed as the result of injury, and in the same way as the bursa in front of the knee is affected in the condition known as housemaid's knee. (See BURSITIS.)

ARMENIAN BOLE is a pale reddish earth used in tooth powders and sometimes administered internally for irritable conditions of the stomach.

ARMPIT, or AXILLA, is the pyramidal hollow between the upper arm and chest, bounded in front by the pectoral or breast muscles, behind by the shoulder-blade and its muscles, and running up to a point beneath the collar-bone. It contains the axillary vessels and nerves which run to the arm, also much fatty tissue, many sweat glands and lymphatic glands. The latter are important, because in poisoned wounds of the arm they may become inflamed, resulting in abscess; and still more, because in cancer of the breast they become infected with cancer, and have to be removed with the breast. Wounds in the armpit are dangerous on the outer, front, and back walls, because large blood vessels run there.

ARNICA is a medicine derived from *Arnica montana*, a plant of the Western United States and Europe. The tincture of arnica is used as a domestic remedy. Externally the tincture is used as a lotion for application to sprains and bruises, which it relieves by virtue of its weakly irritant action. It is seldom used internally, though sometimes it is given to stimulate digestion.

ARRHYTHMIA means any variation from the normal regular rhythm of the heart-beat. The condition is produced by some affection interfering with the mechanism which controls the beating of the heart, and includes the following disorders: sinus arrhythmia, atrial (or auricular) fibrillation, atrial flutter, heart block, extrasystole, pulsus alternans, and paroxysmal tachycardia. (See HEART DISEASES.)

ARROW POISON (see BITES, etc.).

ARROWROOT is a West Indian plant (*Maranta arundinacea*). As sold, it is a white powder, consisting of almost pure starch, derived from the root of the plant. It is much used as an invalid food, because the particular form of the starch renders it easy of digestion, but it must, of course, be combined with other forms of nourishment. (See FARINACEOUS FOODS.)

ARSENIC is a metal, but is better known by its oxide, white arsenic, by two arsenites of copper, Scheele's green and emerald green, and by two sulphides of arsenic, orpiment or king's yellow, and realgar. It is extensively used in dyeworks, in the manufacture of chemicals, in making enamel, in hardening shot and type, in fly-papers, sheep-dips, yellow and green paints, and is further given to horses to improve their coat. Applied pure, it is a strong germicide and caustic, and in large doses is a powerful irritant to stomach and intestines. When taken over long periods, larger and larger doses can be tolerated, till at last a quantity many times the poisonous dose has no apparent ill-effect. In some parts of the world, as among the mountaineers of Styria, its use has become a habit, and in these people it produces a sense of well-being and greater capacity for sustaining fatigue.

ARSENIC POISONING may be acute or chronic.

Acute – The symptoms are violent purging, vomiting, and great prostration. The treatment is to give an emetic, followed by soothing drinks like milk, gruel, and the like.

Chronic poisoning occurs among dyers and paperhangers, or from contamination of food by, or other contact with, green or yellow paint, or wall-paper containing arsenic. It may also occur in those taking so-called tonics containing arsenic. The symptoms are irritability of the eyes and throat, with cough, tendency to sickness, diarrhoea, prostration, and skin eruptions, and often headache, tremors, paralyses, and other nervous signs (see NEURITIS). The treatment is first of all discovery and removal of the source of poisoning, after which one must wait till the arsenic has been gradually expelled from the system by help of fresh air, good food, and tonics. Persons who have been subjects of arsenic poisoning may be left in a debilitated condition with weak digestion and symptoms of neuritis lasting several years.

In both acute and chronic arsenical poisoning, in addition to the measures outlined, a course of dimercaprol (qv) is now given. This is the most efficient known antidote to arsenic.

ARTERIES are vessels which convey blood away from the heart to the tissues of the body, limbs, and internal organs. In the case of most arteries, the blood has been purified by passing through the lungs, and is consequently bright red in colour, but in the pulmonary arteries which convey it to the lungs it is impure, dark, and like the blood in veins.

The arterial system begins at the left ventricle of the heart with the aorta (see AORTA), which gives off branches that subdivide into smaller and smaller vessels, the final divisions, called arterioles, being microscopic, and ending in a network of capillaries, which perforate the tissues like the pores of a sponge, and bathe them in blood that is collected and brought back to the heart by veins. (See CIRCULATION.)

The chief arteries after the *aorta* and its branches (see AORTA) are: (1) the *common carotid* (illustration 17), running up each side of the neck and dividing into *internal carotid* to the brain, and *external carotid* to the neck and face; (2) the *subclavian* to each arm, continued (illustration 18) by the *axillary* in the armpit, and the *brachial* along the inner side of the arm, dividing at the elbow into the *radial* and the *ulnar*, which unite across the palm of the hand in arches that give branches to the fingers; (3) the two *common iliacs* (illustration 17), in which the aorta ends, each of which divides into the *internal iliac* (illustration 18) to the organs in the pelvis, and the *external iliac* to the lower limb, continued by the *femoral* in the thigh, and the *popliteal* behind the knee, dividing into the *anterior* and *posterior tibial* arteries to the front and back of the leg. The latter passes behind the inner ankle to the sole of the foot, where it forms arches similar to those in the hand, and supplies the foot and toes by *plantar branches*.

Structure – The arteries are highly elastic, dilating at each heart-beat as blood is driven into them, and forcing it on by their resiliency (see PULSE). Every artery has *three coats* (illustration 20): (*a*) the outer or adventitia, consisting of ordinary strong fibrous tissue; (*b*) the middle or media, consisting of muscular fibres supported by elastic fibres, which in some of the larger arteries form distinct membranes; and (*c*) the inner or intima, consisting of a layer of yellow elastic tissue on whose inner surface rests a layer of smooth plate-like endothelial cells, over which flows the blood. In the larger arteries the muscle of the middle coat is largely replaced by elastic fibres, which render the artery still more expansile and elastic. When an artery is cut across, the muscular coat instantly shrinks, drawing the cut end within the fibrous sheath that surrounds the artery, and bunching it up, so that a very small hole is left to be closed by blood-clot. (See HAEMORRHAGE.)

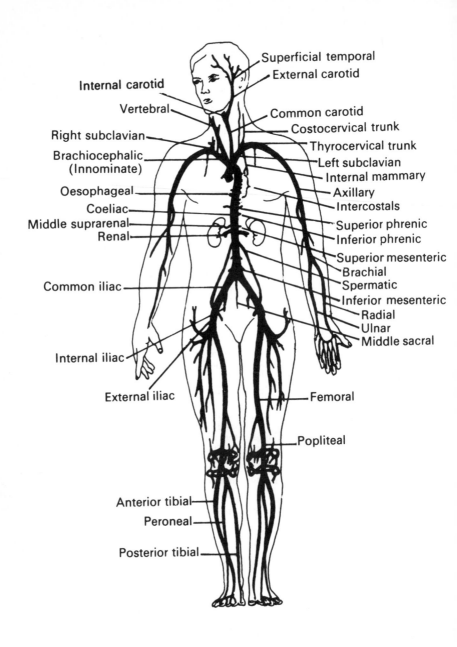

Internal carotid

Superficial temporal
External carotid

Vertebral

Common carotid
Costocervical trunk

Right subclavian

Thyrocervical trunk

Brachiocephalic
(Innominate)

Left subclavian
Internal mammary

Oesophageal

Axillary

Coeliac

Intercostals

Middle suprarenal

Superior phrenic

Renal

Inferior phrenic

Superior mesenteric
Brachial
Spermatic

Common iliac

Inferior mesenteric
Radial
Ulnar
Middle sacral

Internal iliac

External iliac

Femoral

Popliteal

Anterior tibial
Peroneal

Posterior tibial

17 – The chief arteries of the body.

18 — The arteries of the upper limb, anterior view (left) and posterior view (right).

19 – The arteries of the lower limb, anterior view (left) and posterior view (right).

ARTERIES, DISEASES OF – *Arterio-sclerosis*, which is a condition of thickening and rigidity involving predominantly the middle coat of medium-sized arteries, occurs as a natural change in old age. In some individuals, however, the change occurs earlier. Hence the old adage that a man is as old as his arteries. The cause is still obscure, but certain facts are well established, even though they may only be predisposing factors. There is a hereditary tendency, and this is most marked in cases in which it develops at a relatively early age. There is a definite association with high blood-pressure in many cases, but arteriosclerosis can occur without a high whilst if the arteries to the legs and feet are involved, gangrene may occur.

Atherosclerosis is a condition characterized by the presence in the inner coat, or intima, of arteries of the degenerative condition known as atheroma. This manifests itself by nodes, or plaques, of yellowish material containing a high proportion of cholesterol (qv) and other lipids (qv). As these plaques enlarge, and the intima increases in thickness, the lumen of the artery becomes smaller and smaller. In due course the lumen of the artery may be so narrowed that it becomes blocked. If this occurs in the coronary arteries, which supply the heart muscle, the result is the

20 – Diagram to show the structure of an artery. *A*, lumen of artery lined with endothelial cells; *B*, elastic membrane; *C*, muscular coat, or media; *D*, adventitia; *E*, capillary supplying adventitia with blood. From Hill, *Manual of Human Physiology*. Edward Arnold & Co.

blood-pressure. It is much more common in patients with diabetes mellitus than in individuals without this disease. It is also a common finding in gout. The traditional association with alcoholism and lead poisoning is not so certain. The distribution of arteriosclerosis throughout the arterial tree varies considerably. It may give rise to no symptoms, and only does so if it involves certain arteries. Thus, if it involves the arteries to the brain, the individual is liable to have a stroke; if it involves the coronary arteries which nourish the muscle of the heart, it may result in angina pectoris or a coronary thrombosis; if the arteries of the kidney are involved, a form of Bright's disease may develop;

all too common coronary thrombosis. If it occurs in the arteries in the brain it causes a stroke. The cause of atherosclerosis is not known, but one factor is the consumption of excessive saturated fats.

Following on atheroma, plates of lime may form in the arteries, or these vessels may, in extreme states, be changed into brittle calcareous tubes, very liable to tearing from slight injuries. When this condition occurs in older people, it is confined to the middle coat and is accompanied by marked calcification; it is known as *Mönckeberg's sclerosis*.

Syphilis and other inflammatory diseases may bring about an *obliterative inflammation*, in which the internal coat becomes greatly thickened (*endarteritis*) and in which the artery is more or less completely blocked. This leads to very serious effects, particularly in the case of arteries supplying the heart and brain. (See also THROMBOANGIITIS OBLITERANS; ANEURYSM.)

ARTERIOGRAPHY (see ANGIO-GRAPHY).

ARTERIOLE is a small artery.

ARTERIO-VENOUS ANEURYSM is an abnormal communication between an artery and a vein. It is usually the result of an injury, such as a stab or a gunshot wound, which involves both a neighbouring artery and vein.

ARTERITIS means inflammation of an artery.

ARTHRITIS means inflammation of a joint or joints. The chief forms are osteoarthritis (or osteoarthrosis, as it is now known), rheumatoid, gouty, gonorrhoeal, tuberculous, and traumatic. (See JOINTS, DISEASES OF; GONORRHOEA; GOUT; and RHEUMATISM.)

ARTHROPATHY is a term applied to any form of joint disease.

ARTHROPLASTY is the term applied to the operation for the making of a new joint, or the loosening of a fixed or stiff joint.

ARTHROPODS are segmented invertebrates with jointed legs. They include a wide range of organisms, such as scorpions, mites, ticks, spiders and centipedes.

ARTICULAR means anything connected with a joint: eg. articular rheumatism.

ARTICULATION is a term employed in two senses in medicine, either meaning the enunciation of words and sentences or meaning a joint.

ARTIFICIAL INSEMINATION is the introduction of semen into the vagina by artificial means. It has long been used in animal breeding, and of recent years has been used to an increasing extent in human beings in an attempt to allow a married woman to become pregnant who cannot do so by the normal method.

There are two forms of artificial insemination: AIH and AID. In AIH (artificial insemination by the husband) the semen is obtained from the husband. In AID (artificial insemination by a donor) the semen is obtained from a man other than the woman's husband. The former is used when the husband can produce healthy semen but is unable to impregnate his wife; the latter (AID) when the husband is sterile. (See INFERTILITY.)

ARTIFICIAL KIDNEY (see KIDNEY, ARTIFICIAL).

ARTIFICIAL LIMBS AND OTHER PARTS – It is often necessary, for aesthetic or practical reasons, to replace part of the body, lost by injury or disease, with more or less efficient copies of the original, or prostheses as they are now known. From ancient times this has been the case: Herodotus speaks of a man with a wooden foot; the Romans carried the manufacture of limbs to a high degree of efficiency, as witnessed by a leg, the oldest known artificial limb in existence, neatly formed of thin bronze plates, leather and iron, found in a tomb at Capua and dating from around 300 BC; the Etruscans fashioned gold teeth five centuries before the Christian era; Goetz von Berlichingen (1480–1562), to supply his lost right hand, had one made of iron and thus became known as Goetz of the Iron Hand; and Ambroise Paré, who wrote on surgery in the sixteenth century, has a chapter upon artificial limbs. From then there was little advance until 1800 when James Potts, of London, patented an artificial leg made of two hollow wooden cones with a steel knee joint and a wooden ankle joint. It became known as the Anglesey leg after its owner, the Marquis of Anglesey and, with few modifications, remained the basis of British designs until the 1914–1918 War. Since the 1939–45 War there have been striking advances, particularly in artificial hands, as the result of the introduction of electronics and myoelectric means of control.

Arms – Owing to the very delicate movements which the upper limb has to carry out, it is never amputated if there is any possibility of its being of any use. When amputation is decided upon, as little as possible of the arm is removed. Great strides have been made in the provision of artificial arms and hands (illustration 21), and it is now found that 50 per cent efficiency can be obtained when the amputation has been above the elbow, and 75 per cent efficiency when it is below the elbow.

69

ARTIFICIAL RESPIRATION

Appliances are now available which allow an individual who has lost an arm to engage in carpentry, many branches of engineering, and the electrical trades. Such an individual can also write, shoot, play golf and cricket, and even fly-fish.

Legs – An artificial substitute can come much nearer to the usefulness of the original in the lower than in the upper limb. As a result of experience gained in the two World Wars artificial lower limbs are now so efficient that the individual often suffers little disability. This applies particularly to amputations below the knee, but even in the case of amputations high in the thigh many individuals can often resume their old occupations. In addition, they can often ride a bicycle or a horse, or drive a motor car, whilst in the field of recreation,

Teeth – Where a single tooth is false it is often fitted by a gold peg to the fang of the lost natural one. Where a number are fitted, a plate, either adhering accurately to the gum by suction, or attached to neighbouring teeth by 'crown and bridge work', is employed to carry them. It has been found that in the case of elaborate artificial attachments to roots of teeth suppurative processes of a harmful nature are apt to take place. Less dental work is therefore done at the present day in the form of 'crowning' teeth and attaching artificial teeth by pegs than was formerly carried out.

Nose – The making of a new nose is the oldest known operation in plastic surgery, Hindu records of such operations dating back to 1000 BC. Loss of a nose may be

21 – A typical modern artificial hand (*left*), and a myoelectric hand (*above*) fitted to a below-elbow socket, with electrodes fitted.

tennis and golf are quite normal pastimes. One of the great secrets of success in the fitting of artificial limbs is to restore the patient's morale and to stimulate his sense of independence.

Eyes – Artificial eyes are worn both for appearance and to protect the socket from dust, though, of course, vision is impossible. They are made of glass or plastic, and are thin shells of a boat-shape, representing the front half of the eye which has been removed. The stump which is left has still the eye-muscles in it, and so the artificial eye still has the power of moving with the other, though to a less extent, and it is often difficult for this reason to tell at a short distance that a person has a false eye. A glass eye has to be replaced by a new one every year. Plastic eyes have the advantage of being more comfortable to wear, and more durable and of being unbreakable.

due to eroding disease, war wounds, gunshot wounds or dog bites, whilst in Asia additional causes are dacoity or, in women, punishment for marital infidelity. In essence the operation is the same as that practised a thousand years before Christ: namely the use of a skin graft, brought down from the forehead. Alternative sources of the skin graft today are skin from the arm, chest or abdomen. As a means of support the new nose is built round a graft of bone or of cartilage from the ear.

ARTIFICIAL RESPIRATION (see DROWNING, RECOVERY FROM).

ARYTENOID is the name applied to two cartilages in the larynx.

ASAFETIDA is a gum resin of unpleasant odour, obtained from the root of

70

Ferula foetida, and popularly known as Devil's Dung. It used to be given as an expectorant to increase the secretion of mucus in the air-passages or as an antispasmodic in colic with flatulence.

ASBESTOSIS is a form of pneumoconiosis (qv), but its main hazard is the risk of cancer of the lung or pleura, or sometimes of the ovary. It is caused by the inhalation of asbestos dust, either in the mining or quarrying of it, or in one of the many industries in which it is used: eg. as an insulating material, in the making of paper, cardboard and brake linings.

ASCARIASIS is the disease produced by infestation with the roundworm, *Ascaris lumbricoides* (illustration 22), also known as the maw-worm. Superficially it resembles a large earthworm. The male measures about 7 inches (17 cm) and the female 9 inches (23 cm) in length. It is a dirt disease, most prevalent where sanitation and cleanliness are lacking, particularly in

22 – *Ascaris lumbricoides*. Worms from patient after treatment. (*Clinical Tropical Diseases*, A. R. D. Adams and B. G. Maegraith, Blackwell Scientific Publications. Photo: J. Brady)

the tropics and subtropics. Consumption of food contaminated by the ova (eggs), especially salad vegetables, is the commonest cause of infection. In children, infection is commonly acquired by crawling or playing on contaminated earth, and then sucking their fingers. After a complicated life-cycle in the body the adult worms end up in the intestines, whence they may be passed in the stools. A light infection may cause no symptoms. A heavy infection may lead to colic, or even obstruction of the gut.

Occasionally a worm may wander into the stomach and be vomited up.

Treatment consists of the administration of levamisole, a piperazine derivative, pyrantel embonate, or mebendazole.

ASCITES means dropsical swelling of the abdomen. (See DROPSY.)

ASCORBIC ACID is a substance present in various natural sources such as fruits and vegetables, or synthetically prepared. (See VITAMIN.)

ASEPSIS is a term, used in distinction from 'antisepsis', to mean that principle in surgery by which, instead of strong germicides like corrosive sublimate or carbolic acid being applied to wounds, all the dressings, sponges, and instruments used are sterilized by steaming, boiling, or dry heat. Thin, sterilized, india-rubber gloves are worn by surgeons and prevent risk of infection from the hands. Aseptic surgery has the advantage that the germ-destroying activity of the tissues and their healing power after wounds are not lessened by antiseptics which decrease the vitality of the tissues. Healing is therefore surer and more rapid after an aseptic operation. (See also ANTISEPTICS.)

ASPARAGINASE is an enzyme that breaks down the amino-acid, asparagine. This is of no significance to most cells in the body as they can make asparagine from simpler constituents. Certain tumours, however, are unable to do this and therefore, if they cannot receive ready-made supplies of the amino-acid, they die. It is on this basis that asparaginase is proving of promise in the treatment of tumours which, by the administration of asparaginase, are deprived of an essential metabolite – and perish.

ASPERGILLOSIS is a disease caused by invasion of the lung by the fungus, *Aspergillus fumigatus*. The infection is acquired by inhalation of air-borne spores of the fungus which settle and grow in damaged parts of the lung such as healed tuberculous cavities, abscesses, or the dilated bronchi or bronchiectasis (qv).

ASPERGILLUS is the name applied to a group of fungi including the common moulds. Several of these are capable of infecting the lungs and producing a disease resembling pulmonary tuberculosis.

ASPHYXIA means literally absence of pulse, but is the name given to the whole series of symptoms which follow stoppage of breathing and of the heart's action.

Causes – For practical consideration, by far the most important cause is *drowning*. Human beings are not adapted to extract the oxygen dissolved in water – first, because the amount is only one-third of that required to supply the needs of the processes of diffusion which take place in the lungs; and, secondly, because the air or fluid taken in through the mouth must return the same way, there being no second opening and rapid constant stream like that by which in fishes a great quantity of water passes over the gills in a short time. *Blockage of the air passages* occurs in some diseases, such as croup, diphtheria, swelling of the throat due to wounds or inflammation, asthma (to a partial extent), tumours in the chest (causing slow asphyxia), and the external conditions of suffocation and strangling. *Poisonous gases* also cause asphyxia. Carbonic acid gas in excessive amount in the air, due to the breathing of a number of individuals in a small space, as in the Black Hole of Calcutta, or to the fumes given off in fermentation vats, has often caused death. Carbon monoxide gas is still more deadly, and in the form of 'water gas', or when it is given off, for example, by a stove or charcoal brazier in a badly ventilated room, has killed many persons during sleep. (See CARBON MONOXIDE.) Several gases, such as sulphurous acid (from burning sulphur), ammonia, and chlorine (from bleaching-powder), cause involuntary closure of the entrance to the larynx, and thus prevent breathing. Other gases, such as nitrous oxide (or laughing-gas), chloroform, and ether, in poisonous quantity, cause stoppage of breathing by paralysing the respiration centre in the brain.

Symptoms – In the vast majority of cases death from asphyxia is due to insufficiency of oxygen supplied to the blood. The first signs – apart from instinctive efforts to escape from the cause, such as the struggles of a drowning man – are rapid pulse and gasping for breath. Next comes great increase in the pressure of the blood, causing throbbing in the head, with lividity or blueness of the skin, due to failure of aeration of the blood, followed by still greater struggles for breath and by general convulsions. In this stage, the veins and right side of the heart become overfilled with blood, owing to stoppage of the circulation, which follows contraction of the minute arteries all over the body

from the irritation of the impure blood in them. Accordingly, the heart becomes over-distended and gradually weaker, a paralytic stage sets in, and all struggling and breathing slowly cease. When, on the other hand, asphyxia is due to charcoal fumes, coal-gas, and other narcotic influences, there is no convulsive stage, and death ensues gently and may occur in the course of sleep. After death, the right side of the heart, the large veins, and the pulmonary artery are found distended by blood, and this blood is fluid instead of in clots, as it is after a gradual death. These are the chief signs of death by asphyxia, but each cause produces distinguishing signs of its own.

Treatment – So long as the heart continues to beat, recovery may be looked for under prompt treatment. The one essential of treatment is to get the impure blood aerated by artificial respiration. Besides this, the feeble circulation can be helped by various methods. (See under DROWNING, RECOVERY FROM.) When the heart is very feeble or even stopped, the face extremely blue, and the veins of the neck and arms swollen, the person's life may possibly be saved by opening a vein in the arm or neck, and so allowing some blood to escape and the heart to contract again.

ASPHYXIA NEONATORUM is imperfect breathing in the new-born infant. It has been estimated that it plays a part in about half the deaths which occur during the first month of life. The main causes are serious illness of the mother during the latter months of pregnancy, anaesthetics or analgesics given to the mother during labour, prolonged labour, obstruction to the circulation in the umbilical cord, obstruction of the infant's air passages, intracranial haemorrhage, and congenital heart disease.

ASPIRATION means the withdrawal of fluid or gases from the natural cavities of the body or from cavities produced by disease. It may be performed either for curative purposes, or, very often, a small amount is drawn off for diagnosis of the nature or origin of the fluid.

Uses – *Dropsy* used to be one of the most common conditions requiring its application, but since the introduction of efficient diuretics (qv) it is much less frequently required. When in the abdomen, dropsy which persists in spite of the administration of diuretics can be relieved by means of a metal tube or cannula about the size of a small quill, which is provided with a sharp point or trocar capable of being drawn out. After careful cleansing of the skin, and having ensured that the bladder is empty, the trocar and cannula are plunged boldly into the lower part of the abdomen. There is practically no pain, and only a local anaesthetic is necessary. After the cannula, with the trocar inserted in it, has been pushed through the skin the trocar is withdrawn, leaving the tube in place. To this tube is attached an india-rubber tube leading to a bottle, which is air-tight, and in which a vacuum can be produced by a hand air-pump. The fluid is drawn out into the bottle, and 1, 2 or more litres may be withdrawn at one time. When the dropsy is in the legs, Southey's tubes are still occasionally used. Here the cannula is very fine, and has about a yard of fine india-rubber tubing attached, which draws the water slowly off (in the course of several hours) by siphon action. *Pleurisy with effusion* is another condition requiring aspiration, and a litre or more of fluid may be drawn off by an aspirator or a large syringe and needle. *Chronic abscesses* and *tuberculous joints* may call for its use, the operation being done with a small syringe and hollow needle. *Pericarditis* with effusion is another condition in which aspiration is sometimes performed. The spinal canal is aspirated by the operation of lumbar puncture. (See LUMBAR PUNCTURE.) In children the ventricles of the brain are sometimes similarly relieved from excess of fluid by piercing the fontanelle (soft spot) on the infant's head. (See HYDROCEPHALUS.)

ASPIRIN, or ACETYLSALICYLIC ACID, is a white crystalline powder which is used like sodium salicylate as a remedy for rheumatism, chorea, neuralgia, etc., also to reduce fever in infectious diseases. It has some action in relieving pain and producing sleep and is therefore often used for headache and slighter degrees of insomnia. The dose is 5 to 15 grains (300 mg to 1 G).

ASPIRIN POISONING may not be common in relation to the vast amounts that are consumed every year, but nevertheless it is a worrying problem.

In ordinary doses it may induce bleeding from the stomach. This is usually quite mild, but it can be severe. In small doses it can produce a severe allergic reaction in individuals who are sensitive to it. This takes the form of asthma and angioneurotic oedema.

When an overdose is taken there is marked over-breathing, sweating and vomiting. Later the individual becomes restless and irritable, and there may be convulsions before consciousness is finally lost.

Treatment – The stomach should be washed out, preferably with an alkaline solution, and a litre of 5 per cent sodium bicarbonate should be left in the stomach. If there has been much loss of fluid by sweating and vomiting, fluids may need to be given intravenously. In severe cases oxygen may need to be administered.

ASTASIA-ABASIA is the term applied to the condition in which a person is unable, because of defective will-power, to stand or to walk.

ASTEREOGNOSIS means the loss of the capacity to recognize the nature of an object by feeling it, and indicates a lesion (eg. tumour) of the brain.

ASTHENIA means want of strength. (See DEBILITY.)

ASTHENOPIA means a sense of weakness in the eyes, coming on when they are used. As a rule it is due to long-sightedness, slight inflammation, or weakness of the muscles that move the eyes. (See VISION.)

ASTHMA is a disorder of respiration characterized by severe paroxysms of difficult breathing, usually followed by a period of complete relief, with recurrence of the attacks at more or less frequent intervals. The term is often incorrectly employed in reference to states of embarrassed respiration, which are plainly due to permanent organic disease within the chest, and which have none of the distinctive characters of true asthma.

Cause – Asthma is an allergic reaction which manifests itself by spasmodic contraction of the smaller bronchial tubes (see ALLERGY). It is this narrowing of the bronchial tubes, often accentuated by swelling of the lining epithelium, that is responsible for the great difficulty in breathing which is the characteristic feature of the condition. There is a large number of substances to which the asthmatic subject may be hypersensitive, contact with which is responsible for an attack. These include pollens; the emanations of certain animals such as cats, dogs, horses; house dust; certain articles of diet; bacteria. In recent years increasing attention has been drawn to the importance of the house-dust mite, *Dermatophagoides*, as a cause. Fifty per cent of asthmatics in Japan are said to be allergic to butterflies. The discovery of the substance to which the individual is susceptible may sometimes be difficult. Thus, it may be noted that attacks of asthma occur when the patient goes to bed, and it may be found that these occur because he is susceptible to horse hair, with which the pillow is filled. In other instances the difficulty may be due to the fact that the individual is hypersensitive to more than one substance. In many cases the specific susceptibility of the individual may be enhanced by some non-specific conditions, such as emotional disturbance, worry, indigestion or an infection such as a sore throat or a 'cold in the head'. There is another group of asthmatic subjects in whom the asthma is due to sensitization to bacteria responsible for some chronic or repeated infection. For instance, an individual who is subject to repeated attacks of tonsillitis, sinusitis, or nasal catarrh may become sensitized to the causative organism, so that whenever he becomes infected with this organism he is liable to develop attacks of asthma. The reason why asthma does not develop in all such individuals subject to repeated infections, is that such attacks only occur in the individual who has the tendency to develop hypersensitivity. This tendency is usually hereditary, and it will often be found that the asthmatic subject suffers from other allergic conditions such as hay fever and urticaria (or nettle-rash). Asthma is more common in males than in females, and the first attack usually occurs in childhood. It is estimated that around 1 in 20 schoolchildren suffer from the disease. In England, in the year June 30, 1974, to May 31, 1975, the number of days of certified incapacity for sickness and invalidity benefits due to asthma was 1,689,000 for men and 556,000 for women.

There is a form of asthma which may not develop until later in life. This occurs in individuals who suffer from chronic bronchitis. A certain proportion of these people ultimately become sensitized to the organisms responsible for their chronic bronchitis, and this sensitization may not develop until middle age.

Two other conditions to which the term asthma is applied must be carefully differentiated from the condition that has just been described. These are *cardiac asthma* and *renal asthma*. The former consists of sudden attacks of shortness of breath while the patient is resting; it is a grave sign, as it is due to severe heart failure. Renal asthma, which is probably similar in causation to cardiac asthma, occurs in the terminal stages of chronic Bright's disease, and, again, is a sign of extremely grave significance.

Symptoms – The onset of an attack of asthma is usually sudden, although there may exist certain premonitory symptoms which warn the sufferer of its approach, such as a feeling of discomfort, drowsiness, irritability, and depression of spirits. The period when the asthmatic paroxysm comes on is generally during the night, or rather in the early hours of morning. The patient then awakes in a state of great anxiety and alarm, with a sense of weight and tightness across the chest, which he feels himself unable to expand with freedom. Respiration is performed with great difficulty, and is accompanied by wheezing noises. His distress rapidly increases, and he can no longer retain the recumbent position, but gets up, and sits or stands with his shoulders raised, his head thrown back, and his whole body heaving with his desperate efforts to breathe. His countenance is pale or livid, and wet with perspiration, while his extremities are cold; his pulse is rapid, and may be irregular or intermitting. All his clothing must be loose about him; he cannot bear to be touched, and the very presence of others around him seems to aggravate his distress. His one desire is to breathe fresh air; and he will place himself by an open window and sit for hours in the middle of the night, unmindful of the exposure. The paroxysm, after continuing for a variable length of time, often extending over many hours, begins to abate, the breathing becomes easier, and the subsidence of the attack is often marked by the occurrence of coughing with expectoration.

After the cessation of the attack the patient appears to be, and feels, comparatively well. In cases of long standing, however, the subject of asthma comes to bear permanent evidence of its effects. He is easily put out of breath on exertion and he requires to lie with his head elevated, circumstances to be ascribed to organic changes in the chest, which oft-recurring attacks of asthma are liable to induce (see EMPHYSEMA). The asthmatic paroxysms, although occasionally periodic, do not generally observe any regularity in their return. They may recur each successive night for several days, or there may be no return for many weeks or months, this being to a large extent dependent on a renewal of the exciting cause.

Treatment – The treatment of asthma consists in the employment of remedies to allay the paroxysms, and in the adoption of measures likely to prevent their recurrence. During the attack the patient should be placed in as favourable circumstances for breathing as practicable. He usually selects the position easiest for himself. Abundance of air should be admitted to the apartment, and he should be interfered with as little as possible. The household remedial agents employed with the view of relieving the paroxysms are numerous, and only a few of the more important of them can be mentioned. Much value is attached by some to the smoking of stramonium and even tobacco smoking appears in some instances to give relief. The fumes of nitre-paper (blotting-paper prepared by being dipped in a saturated solution of nitre and dried) burnt in the apartment may succeed in mitigating the paroxysm. (See NITRE.) Glass capsules containing amyl nitrite, which are crushed and held beneath the nostrils, sometimes give relief in bad cases; so too does the tincture of lobelia. Coffee is a popular and useful remedy, but, to do good, the infusion must be very strong, and taken on an empty stomach. Dry cupping of the back, and placing of the hands in very hot water contained in basins placed at the side of the bed, are other household remedies.

In the majority of cases, however, certain drugs are required which should only be taken under medical supervision. These include adrenaline (by injection), ephedrine, aminophylline, isoprenaline, salbutamol, terburaline, and sodium cromoglycate. The latter two are often taken by means of inhalation. In severe cases, corticotrophin, or one of the cortisone group of drugs, is often of value.

To prevent the recurrence of the paroxysms special care must be taken by the sufferer to avoid those influences, whether connected with locality or mode of life, which his experience may have proved to have been the occasion of former attacks. Particularly must care be taken to avoid exposure to those influences apt to bring on bronchitis. Breathing exercises are often of value in reducing the frequency of attacks. In the group of cases found to be due to a particular animal emanation or article of diet, care should be taken to avoid this cause. Thus in those cases due to the house-dust mite preventive measures include daily vacuum-cleaning of the bedroom, the use of synthetic bedding material which should be washed frequently and the enclosure of the mattress in an impervious cover. The sensitiveness of the individual can sometimes be diminished by a course of treatment by vaccine prepared from the bacteria present in his expectoration.

The possibility that psychological factors may be responsible, in part at least, should always be borne in mind, and, if present, they should be dealt with if possible. Hypnosis is of value in some cases.

ASTIGMATISM is an error of refraction in the eye due to the cornea (the clear membrane in front of the eye) being unequally curved in different directions, so that rays of light in different meridians cannot be brought to a focus together on the retina. The curvature, instead of being globular, is egg-shaped, longer in one axis than the other. The condition causes objects to seem distorted and out of place, a ball for instance looking like an egg, a circle like an ellipse. The condition is remedied by suitable spectacles of which one surface forms part of a cylinder. (See SPECTACLES.)

ASYNERGIA means the absence of harmonious and co-ordinated movements between muscles having opposite actions – eg. the flexors and extensors of a joint – and is a sign of disease of the nervous system.

ASYSTOLE means arrest of the action of the heart.

ATARACTIC is the term used to describe drugs which induce peace of mind. For all practical purposes it is synonymous with tranquillizer (qv). It has never been widely adopted in Britain.

ATAVISM means the principle of inheritance of disease or bodily characters from grandparents or remoter ancestors, the parents not having been affected by these.

ATAXIA means loss of power of governing movements, though the power necessary to make the movements is still present. Thus an ataxic person may have a good grip in each hand but be unable to do any fine movements with the fingers, or, if the ataxia be in the legs, he throws these about a great deal in walking, though he can lift the legs and take steps quite well. This is due to a sensory defect. (See FRIEDRICH'S ATAXIA and LOCOMOTOR ATAXIA.)

ATELECTASIS means collapse of a part of the lung, or failure of the lung to expand at birth.

ATENOTOL is a drug that is proving of value in the treatment of high blood pressure. One of its practical advantages is that only one dose a day need be taken.

ATHEROMA is a degenerative change in the inner and middle coats of arteries. (See ARTERIES, DISEASES OF.)

ATHEROSCLEROSIS is a form of arteriosclerosis (qv), in which there is fatty degeneration of the middle coat of the arterial wall.

ATHETOSIS is the name for slow, involuntary, writhing, and repeated movements of the hands and feet, caused by disease of the brain.

ATHLETE'S FOOT is a somewhat loose term applied to a skin eruption on the foot, usually between the toes. It is commonly due to ringworm (qv), but may be due to other infections, or merely excessive sweating of the feet.

ATLAS is the name applied to the first cervical vertebra. (See SPINAL COLUMN.)

ATONY means want of tone or vigour in muscles and other organs.

ATOPY is a form of hypersensitivity characterized, amongst other features, by a familial tendency.

ATRESIA means the absence of a natural opening, or closure of it by a membrane. Thus atresia may be found in new-born infants preventing the bowels from moving, and, in young girls after puberty, absence of the menstrual flow may be due to such a malformation.

ATRIUM is the name now given to the two upper cavities of the heart. These used to be known as the auricles of the heart. The term is also applied to the part of the ear immediately internal to the drum of the ear. (Plural: ATRIA.)

ATROPHY is a term in medicine used to describe a state of wasting due to some interference with the function of healthy nutrition. It is essential for the maintenance of health that a due relation exist between the processes of waste and repair, so that the one may not be in excess of the other. When the appropriation of nutriment exceeds the waste, hypertrophy or increase in bulk of the tissues takes place. (See HYPERTROPHY.) When, on the other hand, the supply of nutritive matter is suspended or diminished, or when the power of assimilation is impaired, atrophy or wasting is the result. Thus the whole body becomes atrophied in many diseases; and in old age every part of the frame, with the exception of the heart, undergoes atrophic change. Atrophy may, however, affect single organs or parts of the body, irrespective of the general state of nutrition, and this may be brought about in a variety of ways. One of the most frequently observed of such instances is atrophy from disuse, or cessation of function.

Thus, when a limb is deprived of the natural power of motion, either by paralysis or by painful joint disease, atrophy of all its tissues sooner or later takes place. This form of atrophy is likewise well exemplified in the case of those organs and structures of the body which subserve important ends during foetal life, but which, ceasing to be necessary after birth, undergo a sort of natural atrophy, such as the thymus gland, and certain vessels specially concerned in the foetal circulation. The ovaries, after the child-bearing period, become shrunken.

Atrophy of a part may also be caused by interruption to its normal blood supply, as in the case of the ligature or obstruction of an artery. Again, long-standing disease, by affecting the nutrition of an organ and by inducing the deposit of morbid products, may result in atrophy, as frequently happens in affections of the liver and kidneys. Parts that are subjected to continuous pressure are liable to become atrophied, as is sometimes seen in internal organs which have been compressed by tumours or other morbid growths, and as was well illustrated in the case of the feet of Chinese ladies, which were prevented from growing by persistent compression exercised from birth.

Atrophy may manifest itself simply by loss of substance; on the other hand, it is often found to co-exist with degenerative changes and the formation of fibrous or fatty growth, so that the part may not be reduced in bulk, although atrophied as regards its proper structure. Thus, in the case of the heart, when affected with fatty degeneration, there is atrophy of the proper muscular texture, but this, being largely replaced by fatty material, the organ may undergo no diminution in volume, but may, on the contrary, be increased in size. Atrophy is usually a gradual and slow process, but sometimes it proceeds rapidly. In the disease known by the name of *acute yellow atrophy of the liver*, that organ undergoes such rapidly destructive change as results in its shrinking to half, or one-third, of its normal size in the course of a few days.

The term *progressive muscular atrophy* (*wasting* or *creeping palsy*) is applied to an affection of the muscular system, which is characterized by the atrophy and subsequent paralysis of certain muscles, or groups of muscles, and is associated with morbid changes in the anterior part of the grey matter in the spinal cord. This disease begins insidiously, and is often first observed to affect the muscles of one hand, generally the right. Gradually other muscles in the arms and legs become affected in a similar manner, their atrophy being attended with a corresponding diminution in power. (See PROGRESSIVE MUSCULAR ATROPHY *under* PARALYSIS.)

The term *idiopathic muscular atrophy* (also known as *muscular dystrophy*) is applied to a somewhat similar condition affecting young people in whom a progressive degeneration of the muscles occurs. In this condition no change is found in the nervous system after death, the cause apparently acting directly upon the muscles. (See MUSCLES, DISEASES OF.)

ATROPINE is the active principle of belladonna, the juice of the deadly nightshade. Because of its action in dilating the pupils it was at one time used as a cosmetic to give the eyes a full, lustrous appearance. In addition to this effect, it temporarily impairs vision by paralysing accommodative power. (See ACCOMMODATION.) It has the effect of checking the activity of almost all the glands of the body, including the sweat glands of the skin and the salivary glands in the mouth. It relieves spasm by paralysing nerves in the muscle of the intestine, bile-ducts, bladder, stomach, etc. It has the power, in moderate doses, of markedly increasing the rate of the heart-beats, though by very large doses the heart, along with all other muscles, is paralysed and stopped.

Uses – Externally, liniment of belladonna is used in neuralgia, and other painful conditions. Plaster of belladonna is used in muscular rheumatism. To the breasts, a plaster of belladonna is applied to stop the milk formation in threatened abscess. It is doubtful, however, whether the belladonna in either the liniment or the plaster is of any real value. In eye troubles, atropine drops are used to dilate the pupil for more thorough examination of the interior of the eye, or to draw the iris away from wounds and ulcers on the centre of the eye; they also soothe the pain due to light falling on an inflamed eye, and are further used to paralyse the ciliary muscle and so prevent accommodative changes in the eye while the eye is being examined with the ophthalmoscope (qv). Belladonna is employed in coughmixtures for bronchitis and whoopingcough to dry up the mucus and check spasmodic coughing. In renal colic, gallstone colic, and other agonizing spasmodic conditions, atropine is given along with morphine by hypodermic injection. It is also used to decrease the amount of gastric secretion in peptic ulcer. It has been used as an antidote in opium poisoning and to muscarine, the poisonous principle of some toadstools.

ATROPINE METHONITRATE is a derivative of atropine, which is particularly used in the treatment of congenital pyloric stenosis (see STOMACH, DISEASES OF), and which quite often overcomes the stenosis so effectively that operation is not necessary.

ATROPINE or BELLADONNA POISONING – This may occur from children eating the berries or leaves of the deadly nightshade (see BERRIES, POISONOUS). The warning symptoms are: (1) great dryness of the mouth and throat, (2) wide dilatation of the pupils, (3) increased rate of the heart's action. There is sickness later, and the poisoned person has an excited delirium with, at the same time, bodily languor and weakness. If the dose has been very large, paralysis, unconsciousness, and gradual stoppage of heart and breathing ensue.

Treatment – The swallowed material should be got rid of by washing out the stomach or by giving an emetic. If breathing becomes feeble, artificial respiration must be performed. The patient should be given plenty to drink and be made to pass water frequently, as the poison is excreted by the kidneys, and may otherwise be reabsorbed.

AUDIOANALGESIA is a method of relieving the pains of childbirth. It is produced by the patient listening through headphones to a combination of white sound and high-fidelity music. The intensity of the sound is controlled by the woman herself according to the intensity of her pain. Experience suggests that the method is successful in women who are well adapted, like music and have some understanding of labour and delivery.

AUDIOMETRY is the testing of hearing.

AUDITORY NERVE (see VESTIBULO-COCHLEAR NERVE).

AURA is a peculiar feeling which persons, subject to epileptic seizures, have just before the onset of an attack. It may be a sensation of a cold breeze, a peculiar smell, a vision of some animal or person, an undefinable sense of disgust, or the like, but it is very important for persons who experience it, because it gives warning that a fit is coming and may enable a place of safety or seclusion to be reached.

AURAL DISEASES (see EAR, DISEASES OF).

AUREOMYCIN (see CHLORTETRA-CYCLINE).

AURICLE is a term applied both to the pinna or flap of the ear and also to the ear-shaped tip of the atrium of the heart.

23 – Electric auriscope. The battery is situated in the handle.

AURISCOPE is an instrument for examining the ear. The source of illumination may be incorporated in the instrument, as in the electric auriscope (illustration 23), or it may be an independent light which is reflected into the ear by means of a forehead mirror.

AURISTILLAE are ear-drops.

AURUM is the Latin name for gold.

AUSCULTATION is a term in medicine applied to the method employed by physicians for determining, by the sense of hearing, the condition of certain internal organs. The ancient physicians appear to have practised a kind of auscultation, by which they were able to detect the presence of air or fluids in the cavities of the chest and abdomen.

In 1819, the distinguished French physician, Laennec, introduced the method of auscultation by means of the stethoscope with which his name stands permanently associated. For some time previously, physicians, more especially in the hospitals of Paris, had been in the habit of applying the ear over the region of the heart for the purpose of listening to the sounds of that organ, and it was in the employment of this method that Laennec conceived the idea that these sounds might be better conveyed through the medium of some solid body interposed between his ear and the patient's chest. He accordingly, by way of experiment, rolled up a quire of paper into the form of a cylinder and applied it in the manner just mentioned, when he found that he was able to perceive the action of the heart more distinctly than he had ever been able to do by the immediate application of his ear. He thence inferred that not merely the heart's sounds, but also those of other organs of the chest might be brought within reach of the ear by some such instrument. He therefore had constructed the wooden cylinder, or stethoscope, which bears his name. This instrument was subsequently modified by Piorry to the form of a thin narrow cylinder, about 7 inches (18 cm) long, with an expansion at one end for applying to the chest, and a more or less flattened surface at the other for the ear of the listener.

The binaural stethoscope (illustration 24), consisting of a small expanded chest-piece and two flexible tubes with ivory or vulcanite ends that fit tightly into the ears of the observer, is the type now generally used. This form is in some ways more convenient to use, though the sounds are no more clearly heard than with Piorry's instrument, and, in some cases, are less distinct, as the conduction of sound by the flexible tubes is entirely aerial. Various modifications of the binaural stethoscope have been introduced, such as the phonendoscope, in which the place of the chestpiece is taken by a small drum. An electrical stethoscope has been devised, through which, by the help of a microphone, telephone, and electric valves, the beating of the heart, murmurs, etc., may be heard at a distance from the patient with any desired intensity.

The numerous conditions affecting the lungs can be recognized and discriminated

24 – Binaural stethoscope.

from each other by means of auscultation and the stethoscope. The same holds good in the case of the heart, whose varied and often complex forms of disease can, by auscultation, be identified with striking accuracy. But in addition to these, its main uses, auscultation is found to render assistance in the investigation of many obscure internal affections, such as aneurysms and certain diseases of the oesophagus and stomach. To the accoucheur the stethoscope yields valuable aid in the detection of some forms of uterine tumours, and especially in the diagnosis of pregnancy – the auscultatory evidence afforded by the sounds of the foetal heart being one of the most reliable of the many signs of pregnancy and giving valuable information concerning the viability of the foetus.

AUTO- is a prefix meaning self.

AUTISM, or INFANTILE AUTISM, is an abnormality of early childhood development characterized by inability to develop relationships with people and by poverty of language. There is a failure to develop social relationships, with a tendency to self-isolation. In the vast majority of cases the cause is unknown, but in some instances it may be associated with brain damage. It occurs in around 4 per 10,000 school children. The onset is usually insidious from birth, or may follow a period of one year's or two years' normal development.

The most characteristic feature of the condition is the child's impaired emotional contact with people, strikingly demonstrated by gaze-avoidance, the child refusing to look people straight in the face. The child is aloof, and there is little communication with other people. The second characteristic feature is the lack of language development. The child either never develops language at all, or loses what speech he had developed. There is impaired understanding of what other people say, repetition of what is said to him, and reversal of pronouns, the child, for example, referring to himself as 'you' and not 'I'. In addition, there are repetitive movements, such as jumping, flicking of the fingers and grimacing, as well as obsessional habits such as insisting on his food being always served in a certain manner, or insisting on wearing certain clothes. If these obsessions are not respected, there may be screaming attacks. Yet another feature is that these children tend to pay no attention to what is said to them. Intellectual ability ranges from severely subnormal to normal.

The outlook for these children is not very promising. The best results are obtained in those with a relatively high intelligence quotient. Another good sign is the presence of useful language at the age of 5 years. The earlier treatment is begun, therefore, the better. There is nothing specific about this. It is all aimed at trying to gain, and maintain, emotional contact with the child, a process which depends as much as anything on the patience, understanding and sincerity of the parents. Parents of autistic children can obtain help and guidance from the National Society for Autistic Children, 1a Golders Green Road, London NW11 8EA.

AUTOCLAVE – This is one of the most effective ways of ensuring that material, eg. surgical dressings, is completely sterilized and that even the most resistant bacteria with which it may be contaminated, are destroyed. Its use is based upon the fact that water boils when its vapour pressure is equal to the pressure of the surrounding atmosphere. This means that if the pressure inside a closed vessel be increased, the temperature at which water inside the vessel boils, will rise above 100 C. By adjusting the pressure, almost any temperature for the boiling of the water will be obtained. This is now one of the most widely used methods of sterilization in hospitals and laboratories.

AUTOGENOUS means self-generated and is the term applied to products which arise within the body. It is applied to bacterial vaccines manufactured from the organisms found in discharges from the body and used for the treatment of the person from whom the bacteria were derived.

AUTO-IMMUNITY is the process whereby an individual develops antibodies to his own tissues. Normally an individual does not develop antibodies to his own tissues, but only to invaders of the body such as micro-organisms. The precise reason why some individuals develop this unfortunate propensity is still obscure but it is proving a fruitful line of investigation into the cause of some diseases of hitherto unknown origin.

AUTO-INTOXICATION means literally self-poisoning, and is any condition of poisoning brought about by substances formed in or by the body.

AUTOLYSIS means the disintegration and softening of dead cells brought about by enzymes in the cells themselves.

AUTOMATISM means the performance of acts without conscious will, as, for example, after an attack of epilepsy or concussion of the brain. In such conditions the person may perform acts of which he is neither conscious at the time nor has any memory afterwards. It is especially liable to occur when persons suffering from epilepsy, mental subnormality, or concussion consume alcoholic liquors. It may also occur following the taking of barbiturates or psychedelic drugs (qv). There are, however, other cases in which there are no such precipitating factors. Thus it may occur following hypnosis, mental stress or strain, or conditions such as fugues (qv) or somnabulism (see SLEEP). The condition is of considerable importance from a legal point of view, because acts done in this state, and for which the person committing them is not responsible, may be of a criminal nature.

AUTONOMIC NERVOUS SYSTEM is the term applied to that part of the nervous system which regulates the functions of some of the internal organs independently of the will power. It consists of two main divisions – the SYMPATHETIC and the PARASYMPATHETIC SYSTEMS (qv).

AUTOPSY means a post-mortem examination, or the examination of the internal organs of a dead body. (See NECROPSY.)

AUTO-SUGGESTION is the term applied to a peculiar mental state, which sometimes occurs after accidents, in which the will and judgment are partially perverted, so that slight or temporary injuries are greatly exaggerated in the imagination, and the person believes himself to be affected by some serious disability. Examples of this are found in paralysed and insensitive limbs following some minor bruise, for example in a railway accident, and the blindness, deafness, or inability to speak, which sometimes followed concussion in soldiers, especially when the injury was received in the dark. This state is also called 'traumatic suggestion'. The condition often approaches very near to, or is mingled with, the condition of malingering, in which the person consciously suggests to himself or produces some disability from an ulterior motive, as, for example, in some of the prolonged cases of disability following a trifling injury for which a person is in receipt of compensation. The term is also applied to the reverse process, by which, either as a result of suggestion by another person, or suggestion applied by the will power of the person affected, a cure of such a condition is accomplished.

AVERSION THERAPY is a form of psychological treatment in which such an unpleasant response is induced to his psychological aberration that the patient decides to give it up. Thus the victim of alcoholism is given a drug that makes the subsequent drinking of alcoholic liquors so unpleasant by inducing nausea and vomiting that he decides to give up drinking. (See ALCOHOLISM, CHRONIC; and DISULFIRAM.) Another commonly used method of inducing aversion is an electric shock. Aversion therapy is proving of value in the treatment of alcoholism, drug addiction, sexual deviations, such as transvestism, and compulsive gambling.

AVITAMINOSIS is the term applied to the condition of a human being or an animal deprived of one or more vitamins.

AVOMINE is the trade name for promethazine theoclate, which is widely, and successfully, used as a remedy for travel sickness.

AXILLA is the anatomical name for the armpit. (See ARMPIT.)

AXIS is the name applied to the second cervical vertebra. (See SPINAL COLUMN.)

AZAPROPAZONE is a drug that is proving of value in the relief of pain and stiffness in rheumatoid arthritis and other rheumatic diseases.

AZATHIOPRINE is a cytotoxic and an immunosuppressive drug. In the first of these capacities it is proving of value in the treatment of acute leukaemia. As an immunosuppressive agent, by reducing the antibody response of the body it is proving of value in facilitating the success of transplant operations by reducing the chances of the transplanted organ, eg. the kidney, being rejected by the body. It is also proving of value in the treatment of ulcerative colitis.

AZOOSPERMIA is the condition characterized by lack of spermatozoa in the semen.

AZOTAEMIA means the presence of urea and other nitrogenous bodies in greater concentration than normal in the blood. The condition is generally associated with advanced types of kidney disease.

AZOTE is another name for nitrogen.

B

BABINSKI REFLEX is the name applied to an abnormal response of the plantar reflex. When a sharp body is drawn along the sole of the foot, instead of the toes bending down towards the sole as usual, the great toe is turned upwards and the other toes tend to spread apart. This response may be obtained in normal infants, but after the age of about two years its presence indicates some severe disturbance in the upper part of the central nervous system.

BACILLI are micro-organisms which are rod-like in form. (See under BACTERIOLOGY.)

BACITRACIN is a polypeptide antibiotic derived from *Bacillus licheniformis*. It is active against the same range of bacteria as penicillin.

BACK – The back consists mainly of the spinal column and hinder parts of the ribs, and the wide-spreading iliac or haunch bones with the sacrum below. The bones are covered by thick and powerful muscles, which above support and move the head and which below pass round the flanks and downwards into the lower limbs. The skin covering the back is not very sensitive and is not greatly subject to painful conditions. The powerful muscles, of which the chief is the erector spinae, are much subject to minor injuries, the result of twists and strains, and also to rheumatic affections (see LUMBAGO). Diseases and injuries of the spinal column and spinal cord are of a very serious nature (see SPINAL COLUMN ; and SPINAL CORD).

BACKACHE is a symptom of many diseases. In addition to being the result of local causes, pain referred to the back is often due to disease or disorder in deep-seated organs.

Causes – (*a*) LOCAL – *Lumbago* (qv), or a rheumatic condition in the muscles or nerves of the loins, which may be of a chronic aching nature, or may come on suddenly, feeling like a blow, is the commonest cause. In a certain number of cases the cause is a prolapsed intervertebral disc (qv). A similar condition is often set up by unwonted exercise of these muscles in golfing, gardening, and the like. *Weakness* in growing boys or girls may cause a feeling of extreme weariness every day, and may be associated with lateral curvature

of the spine, if not attended to. *Spinal disease* sometimes causes backache, and is associated with rigidity of the back, and often with great tenderness to the touch, with or without any deformity. Stiffness with pain sometimes follows some long-continued fever which has led to weakness in the back, especially found after typhoid fever. It is also a not uncommon sequel to influenza. A state of permanent stiffness is sometimes found in old people in whom the spine has become the seat of chronic rheumatic changes leading to the formation of bony outgrowths between the different vertebrae. (See OSTEOARTHROSIS.)

(*b*) INDIRECT – *Kidney disease* is sometimes a cause of pain in the loins. All sorts of *pelvic trouble* in women, such as menstrual disorders, prolapse of the womb, and ovarian inflammation and tumours, are accompanied by a dull, dragging-down pain in the back. *Gallstones* sometimes cause an acute pain high up near the right shoulder. *Stomach ulcers* may cause a pain above the level of the last rib and close to the left side of the spine. Backache may also be one of the first symptoms of *smallpox*, and of several other febrile diseases.

Treatment – This is of course the treatment of the disease causing the pain. When the pain is due to a local cause, such as lumbago, the loins must be kept warm by extra clothing or a flannel belt. Heat, most easily applied in the form of a rubber hot water bottle, gives relief as does massage, ironing with a flat-iron through a piece of cloth, and, in acute cases, application of mustard leaf. Weakness in young persons is rectified by gymnastics, callisthenics and other forms of exercise, with regular daily periods of rest, and the careful avoidance of stooping or a twisted position at lessons. Perhaps the best exercise of all for strengthening the muscles of the back is the use of a skipping-rope.

BACLOFEN is a muscle-relaxing drug that is proving of value in relieving the spasm of muscles in some cases of multiple sclerosis (qv).

BACTERAEMIA is the term given to the condition in which bacteria are present in the bloodstream.

BACTERIA is a term which, strictly speaking, means small micro-organisms of a simple primitive form, but the word is now vaguely used to cover a great variety of low microscopic forms of plant life. It is equivalent to terms such as 'germs', 'microbes', 'micro-organisms'.

BACTERICIDE strictly means anything which kills bacteria, but is usually applied to drugs and antiseptics which do this. Hence BACTERICIDAL.

BACTERIOLOGY is the branch of biological science concerned with the study of the lowest forms of plant life, particularly of those which cause disease in men and animals, and putrefaction. It is now tending to be replaced by the more general term, microbiology. (For details on INFECTION; IMMUNITY; ANTISEPTICS; VACCINATION; SERUM THERAPY; and OPSONINS, see these headings.) Although bacteria had been noticed about 1687 by Leeuwenhoek and others after the introduction of the microscope, they were not definitely associated with disease until the nineteenth century. Goodsir, in 1842, described *sarcinae* in the stomach, and Davaine in 1865 noticed the large organisms of anthrax, but Pasteur was the first, about 1865, to make a complete study of the manner in which micro-organisms multiply and produce disease. He was followed by Koch, who in 1876 worked out the complete life-history and spore formation of the bacillus of anthrax. In 1877, Koch published his methods of staining films of bacteria; in 1878 his great memoir on the cause of infectious diseases, describing those kinds of bacteria which produce suppuration in wounds; and in 1881 his method of obtaining pure cultures of different organisms. Koch's methods founded the science of bacteriology, and with little change they are still in use.

Classification of micro-organisms – If we include the viruses the micro-organisms of the vegetable kingdom which cause disease may be grouped as follows: (1) *Moulds*, of which penicillium, the green cheese-mould, and mucor, a white mould, are examples. These grow on leather, bread, and in fact anything of a nutritious nature which happens to be damp, their spores floating everywhere in the air. One mould is sometimes a cause of pneumonia, another causes disease in salmon, and others produce the various forms of ringworm. (2) *Yeasts*, of which one is of great importance as being the producer of alcohol. (3) *Bacteria* proper. These are again divided, mainly owing to their shape, into *cocci*, which are round; *bacilli*, long,

slender rods; *spirilla*, curved or wavy. They have secondary names according to some physical property, such as the power of producing colour, as *Staphylococcus aureus*, which appears under the microscope in grape-like clusters, produces pus in the body, and grows in golden-yellow masses when artificially cultivated. *Streptococci* are cocci arranged in chains; *diplococci* occur in pairs. (4) *Rickettsiae*, named after the bacteriologist Ricketts, are disease-causing micro-organisms, coccal or rod-shaped, and intermediate in size between bacteria and viruses. Rickettsiae are the infecting agents in typhus and typhus-like fevers, and also of trench fever. *Rickettsiae prowazekii*, the infecting agent of typhus, is conveyed to man by infected lice. Other rickettsial infections – such as Rocky Mountain fever – are conveyed by ticks or fleas. (5) *Viruses* are living agents which cause disease and are so minute that they pass through porcelain filters impassable by ordinary bacteria and cannot be seen with ordinary microscopic methods (ultramicroscopic). They appear to be living crystals of protein, and cause such diseases as poliomyelitis, measles, mumps, chickenpox, the common cold, and influenza.

Properties of bacteria – MOTION – It is doubtful if cocci have this power, but most of the bacilli and spirilla move rapidly and freely, either by quick contortions similar to those of a fish-tail, or by beating the fluid in which they lie by flagella, long whip-like lashes, with which many, such as the bacillus of typhoid fever and the spirillum of cholera, are provided. This power of movement is of immense importance in the spread of disease. The movements become more active if the temperature is raised. Bacteria are attracted to certain substances and repelled by others, this property being known as *positive* and *negative chemotaxis*.

SIZE – It is difficult at first to grasp the extreme smallness of these bodies. Many thousands of them may lie upon the smallest visible speck of dust. The round forms or cocci are between 0·5 and 1·5 micrometres in breadth. The bacillus of anthrax, much the largest disease-producing bacillus, is less than 8 micrometres in length, and most of the bacilli are only 0·25 micrometre or a little more, in breadth.

REPRODUCTION – The moulds have special filaments which produce hundreds of spores, and the yeasts give off little buds from their surface which produce new chains of yeast, but most of the simpler bacteria multiply by growing in size and then splitting into two. As a result of this, long chains are formed in which the individuals lie end to end, or masses, in which they lie side by side. A bacterium may grow and split in about half an hour, with the result that, given favourable circumstances of warmth, food, etc., a single bacterium could, in the course of twenty-four hours, produce nearly 300,000,000,000,000,000 individuals. Fortunately such favourable circumstances are seldom completely attained in nature. Another important method of reproduction possessed by some bacilli, such as that of anthrax, is by spores. Each bacillus produces only one spore, which, however, is much more tenacious of life than the bacillus and often capable of surviving after being boiled, or after drying for months or years. Each spore again produces a bacillus when it alights in a suitable germinating ground.

Effects of growth – Bacteria produce disease by means of toxins, which are products injurious to the tissues. They are classified into two main groups. Most of them are *endotoxins*. These are toxins that are retained within the bacterial cells, and the bacteria produce their ill-effects wherever they may be in the body. Thus, in pneumonia, due to the pneumococcus which tends to congregate in the lungs, the brunt of the attack from the toxins falls on the lungs, producing the typical signs of consolidation. (See PNEUMONIA.) The other group of toxins is that known as *exotoxins*. These are toxins that pass out from the bacteria into the surrounding medium and then circulate throughout the body, the bacteria themselves tending to 'stay put'. The best example of this type of toxin is that of the bacillus responsible for diphtheria, in which the bacillus tends to congregate on the tonsils while the exotoxin it produces circulates round the body, damaging particularly the cells of the heart.

Some bacilli produce acids by their growth, such as that which turns milk sour. Alcohol, as is well known, is the product of the activity of yeast. Many bacteria also produce brilliant pigments of red, yellow, blue, green, or purple colour, such as the *Bacillus prodigiosus*, which turns milk red, and the *Pseudomona pyocyanea*, which produces blue pus in abscesses. Many bacteria produce gases from the substances in which they develop such as sulphuretted hydrogen, carbon dioxide, marsh gas. Others in the colon play a useful and necessary part in digestion although from time to time when other factors come into play they can produce untoward results such as appendicitis, peritonitis, and other diseases in the neighbourhood of the bowels. Many of the actions of bacteria depend upon ferments which are produced by them and exercise a complicated action. These ferments are sometimes set free in the fluid surrounding the bacteria, and sometimes retained for a time within the bacteria themselves. Most bacteria produce substances which finally stop their growth and activity, checking the excessive growth of, and finally killing their respective bacteria. Some microorganisms are particularly prone to digest themselves: the process known as autolysis (qv).

Conditions of growth – FOOD – Some bacteria live by taking carbon dioxide and nitrogen from the air and producing complex organic substances in their growth, so that these bacteria are of great importance in some of the operations of farming. Most, however, break down the complex plant and animal bodies into simpler substances. All require some moisture for their growth. Some bacteria are readily killed by drying, thus the vibrio of cholera is killed by two or three hours of drying, but the ordinary bacteria of suppuration may be dried for at least several days, and anthrax spores still survive after drying for several years. A few bacteria live best, or only, in living bodies, being then called parasitic, or, if they produce disease, pathogenic. Others live only in dead matter, and are called saprophytic. The substances on which they grow best are gelatinous or starchy matters containing a little soluble animal substance, like peptone, and a trace of salts, or in fluids like broth, containing much animal or vegetable matter.

WARMTH – The bacteria of putrefaction flourish best at the ordinary temperature found inside a house: ie. about 20° C; the disease-producing bacteria at the temperature of the body: ie. 37° C. Freezing, though it stops growth for the time, does not kill most bacteria, which afterwards take on new activity; but a process of thawing and freezing repeated several times in succession kills all organisms. Boiling, on the other hand, is more deadly to them, and, if continued for a few minutes, kills most bacteria, though not their spores. The latter are killed by superheated steam at 120° C. Dry heat can be survived at much higher temperatures. A satisfactory method of destruction is intermittent exposure of sterilizing dishes, instruments, and the like at 100° C for twenty to forty-five minutes on each of three successive days. These are exposed to steam rising from boiling water, in a Koch or Arnold's sterilizer, or, equally efficiently, in an ordinary pot with a lid. This kills all bacteria. Next day they are similarly treated, when any spores which have been present have developed into bacteria, and these are likewise killed. A third application of steam, on the day again following, renders certain the freedom from spores and bacteria.

LIGHT – Bacteria develop best in the dark, though some produce their special effects only when exposed to light. Direct sunlight stops their growth, and exposure for several hours to the full light of the sun kills most bacteria, notably those of plague and tuberculosis. The effect of sunlight is increased by dryness, and it has been found, for example, that even anthrax spores, which possess greater vitality than almost any other bacteria, are killed when dried and exposed to sunlight for one and a half hours, although, if moisture is present, a much longer exposure to sunlight is necessary. The effect is still further increased by heat, so that bacteria live for a very short time only in hot, dry, and sunshiny localities. Electric light has a similar, although weaker, action, the violet rays being most powerful in killing bacteria, but the X-rays have very little effect in checking bacterial growth.

AIR – Most bacteria grow with or without fresh air. A certain amount of fresh air is necessary to rapid putrefaction, but a very free supply, and certainly the presence of pure oxygen, tends to destroy bacteria. Bacteria, such as those of tetanus (lock-jaw) and of gas gangrene, can develop only deep in the earth or in deep wounds where oxygen is absent, and these are known as anaerobic bacteria.

Relation to disease – The first bacterium stated to be connected with disease was the anthrax bacillus. Since the introduction of modern bacteriological methods, about 1880, a great number of bacteria responsible for disease have been demonstrated. The proof that a bacterium is the direct cause of any disease depends upon the fulfilment of three conditions laid down by Koch: (1) that the bacterium be always found in the body or its discharges when a certain disease is present; (2) that the bacterium can be isolated and cultivated under laboratory conditions and thus freed from other possible causes of the disease; and (3) that on the inoculation of a healthy man or animal with a culture of the bacterium,

which is now free from any possible contamination, symptoms of the original disease appear in the animal inoculated. Thus complete proof has been obtained in the case of a large number of diseases, while in the case of other diseases for some technical reason, such as that the organism cannot be grown in the laboratory or because no animal can be found to suffer typically from the disease, an absolute proof of the connection between the disease and the organism is so far wanting.

Among the diseases which have been definitely shown to be due to particular organisms are the following.

ACUTE INFLAMMATION AND SUPPURATION – Localized inflammation may be due to a great variety of organisms, of which the various *staphylococci* and *streptococci* are the chief. Staphylococci are the most common agents in producing infections of the skin, with pus formation, such as skin pustules, boils, carbuncles, styes and impetigo. They are also liable to infect wounds. Streptococci also cause infections of the skin, including erysipelas. They are also a common cause of cellulitis, tonsillitis, otitis media and puerperal fever, as well as scarlet fever. They are also a causative factor in rheumatic fever and acute glomerulonephritis. One form of streptococcus is the cause of subacute bacterial endocarditis. Streptococci commonly produce more deep-seated, serious, and spreading diseases, such as erysipelas. They also occur in broncho-pneumonia and ulcerative endocarditis. The streptococcus is a common cause of tonsillitis, is responsible for puerperal fever, often starts infection of wounds (especially those sustained in war), and indeed may attack any part of the body, resulting in such conditions as peritonitis, meningitis, empyema. Suppuration may also be produced by several bacteria mentioned below as associated with particular diseases.

PNEUMONIA of the acute lobar type is usually due to the pneumococcus or *Diplococcus pneumoniae*. This organism is of several different types, types I and II being much the most common, while type III is found in about 12 per cent of cases of pneumonia. A few cases of pneumonia are due to the *streptococcus*, *Haemophilus influenzae* and the *pneumobacillus*, or *Klebsiella pneumoniae* as it is now known. There is also a form of pneumonia, known as primary atypical pneumonia, which is due to a virus.

CEREBROSPINAL FEVER – This disease is due to the *Meningococcus*, which occurs in four types. It appears to gain entrance to the body through the nasal passages, where it is frequently found even in people who do not suffer from the disease.

RHEUMATIC FEVER is commonly associated with a haemolytic streptococcus.

SCARLET FEVER and some allied infections are due to a haemolytic streptococcus.

GONORRHOEA is due to a diplococcus – the gonococcus – which is found to a large extent inside the cells of the discharge.

SYPHILIS is caused by a minute spiral-shaped organism, or spirochaete, known as *Treponema pallidum*. Other diseases due to different varieties of spirochaetes are RELAPSING FEVER, YAWS, SPIROCHAETAL JAUNDICE, and RAT-BITE FEVER.

TUBERCULOSIS is due to one or other of two mycobacteria, known as the human and the bovine types. Tuberculosis in the lung is almost always caused by the human type, while abdominal tuberculosis, as well as tuberculosis of bones and joints, found in children, is due in many cases to the bovine type derived from milk, and tuberculosis of the glands in young children is due to the latter type. Other types of *Mycobacteria tuberculosis* cause similar diseases in birds and fish, while closely allied bacilli are found subsisting in grass.

LEPROSY is caused by the *Mycobacterium leprae* which presents certain close resemblances to the mycobacterium of tuberculosis.

GLANDERS, or FARCY, is caused by *Loefflerella mallei*.

ACTINOMYCOSIS, or WOODY TONGUE, is caused by *Actinomyces israeli*, which is one of a genus of micro-organisms known as actinomyces. The MADURA FOOT OF INDIA is caused by an organism belonging to a closely associated genus.

ANTHRAX, or WOOLSORTERS' DISEASE, is due to a relatively large organism, the *Bacillus anthracis*, which produces spores that may retain their vitality when dried for several years.

TYPHOID FEVER and the group of diseases related to it, such as paratyphoid fever A and B, bacillary dysentery, and forms of food poisoning, are due to *Salmonella typhi*, *Salmonella paratyphi*, and *Shigella sonnei*, and a number of other organisms which resemble one another considerably in their mode of growth, cultural characters, and, broadly speaking, in the effects which they produce on the intestine and the body generally.

DIPHTHERIA is due to the *Bacillus diphtheriae* (or *Corynebacterium diphtheriae*,

as it is now known), which is often found in the throat of healthy persons, but which in susceptible persons produces a very severe type of surface inflammation with general toxic effects throughout the body.

TETANUS, or LOCK-JAW, is produced by the *Bacillus tetani* (or *Clostridium tetani*, as it is now known), which is an anaerobic bacillus growing especially deep in the soil or in dung-heaps. It produces spores which, like those of anthrax, are extremely tenacious of life.

GAS GANGRENE is a disease produced by various anaerobic bacilli, especially the *Bacillus welchii* (or *Clostridium welchii*), which grow deep in highly cultivated soil, and, like the tetanus bacillus, cause infection when such soil is disturbed.

CHOLERA is due to the cholera vibrio, an organism of S-shaped appearance which is very readily destroyed by drying or by weak antiseptics.

PLAGUE is caused by a rod-shaped bacillus, *Yersinia pestis*, which is transmitted to man through rodents and fleas.

INFLUENZA is due to a virus. Three specific viruses have, so far, been isolated, and others that may take part in the infection are under investigation. At one time it was thought that influenza was due to the *Haemophilus influenzae* (Pfeiffer's bacillus), but it is now known that this is only one of the secondarily infecting organisms that are often found in influenza.

WHOOPING-COUGH is due to a minute oval bacterium, the *Haemophilus pertussis*, or *Bordetella pertussis* as it is now known.

MALTA FEVER is due to a minute coccus, the *Brucella melitensis*.

MALARIA is due to an organism known as the *Plasmodium*. Three different but closely related types cause the three varieties of malaria. The plasmodia belong to a group of micro-organisms known as protozoa. Other diseases which are due to protozoa are: AMOEBIC DYSENTERY, due to the *Entamoeba histolytica*; SLEEPING SICKNESS, due to the *Trypanosoma gambiense*; KALA-AZAR, due to the *Leishmania donovani*, and other closely allied diseases.

TYPHUS FEVER, and the group of diseases associated with it, are caused by a genus of bacteria known as Rickettsiae. These are transmitted to man by lice, ticks or mites. A closely associated genus of bacteria known as Coxiella is responsible for Q fever.

Study of bacteria – It is impossible to go more than very briefly into the highly technical methods employed in a bacteriological laboratory. The material to be examined must be collected in such a way as to prevent contamination by organisms from outside sources, eg. the skin or the air. For example, in collecting matter from the throat to find if the *Corynebacterium diphtheriae* is present, a glass tube plugged with cotton-wool and containing a cotton-wool swab at the end of a piece of wire is used. The throat is rubbed with the swab, which is then carefully withdrawn, reinserted in the tube, and sent to the laboratory. When the urine is to be examined for the presence of bacteria, it is carefully collected into a sterile bottle closed with a sterilized stopper and similarly sent to the laboratory. Similar precautions are taken in the case of material from other sources. The bacteriological methods used fall into four groups.

(1) EXAMINATION BY THE MICROSCOPE – If bacteria are placed in a little fluid upon a glass slide and examined with the aid of a microscope, they appear when magnified some hundreds of times as clear, transparent, often quickly moving particles or lines. For careful observation they must be killed by heat or by some powerful chemical substance, and thereafter stained with appropriate reagents. These are usually aniline dyes of different colours; and the bacteria of different diseases, apart from their size, shape, and general appearance, can often be recognized from the way in which they become stained or fail to stain with certain dyes. Methylene blue is a simple dye generally used for all bacteria. The *Mycobacterium tuberculosis* is distinguished by the peculiar tenacity with which it retains the red fuchsin stain when treated by sulphuric acid and spirit, while from other bacteria this dye can be readily extracted by these reagents. The majority of bacteria are stained a deep purple colour by Gram's stain (successive application of gentian-violet, iodine, and alcohol), but some are readily recognized by being negative to this stain: eg. the gonococcus, meningococcus, and the *Salmonella typhi*. Neisser's stain is much used for the recognition of *Corynebacterium diphtheriae*; it consists of two stains (methylene blue and Bismarck brown) which stain this bacillus in a characteristic variegated manner. Many other bacteria have similar special staining properties by which they can be recognized without further trouble.

(2) CULTIVATION – In general, however, it is not possible to identify an organism with certainty, simply by its appearance, even if suitably stained, and the changes

which its growth in large masses produces upon various nutrient substances contained in glass culture tubes must also be observed. In doing this the first necessity is to prepare a nutrient medium and place it in flat covered plates or in glass tubes of which the open end is plugged with a piece of cotton-wool so as to exclude organisms that might enter from the air, while freely admitting the air itself. These tubes and their contents must be carefully sterilized in the manner already indicated; they are then inoculated, by means of a previously sterilized platinum needle or a glass rod, with material containing the organism which it is desired to study; and are finally placed inside an incubator maintained day and night at the temperature of the body. After being incubated for several days the bacteria have multiplied so as to form colonies easily visible to the naked eye, and from these, small fragments are removed by the platinum needle, stained, and microscopically examined.

Among the nutrient substances on which bacteria are grown in the laboratory, the chief are broth, gelatin, agar, potato, and milk. The turbidity produced in broth after some days' growth, the power to liquefy gelatin, the colours produced on the surface of agar or of cut potato, and the curdling of milk form distinctive characters of different bacteria. Again, various sugars may be added to these substances and the bacteria are thus divided into classes according to their power of fermenting the sugar as they grow. The formation of acid by other bacteria is tested by adding to the tubes litmus or some other reagent which changes its colour when acidified, and the development of gas-bubbles is also an important distinguishing mark.

Some bacteria (known as anaerobic bacteria) fail to grow unless the oxygen be extracted from the tubes in which they are placed or an atmosphere of hydrogen gas be provided by means of a special apparatus.

Since many different types of bacteria are as a rule mingled together in the discharge from a diseased part of the body, it becomes necessary to separate these and to obtain for study cultures of each, free from contamination by the others. For this separation, the organisms are either grown upon a medium to which have been added substances that destroy some kinds of bacteria while sparing others; or they are diluted by mixture with a large quantity of sterile fluid, and, drops of this being stroked over the surface of some nutrient material lying on a broad covered glass plate (Petri dish), the individual bacteria produce within a few days widely separated colonies that can be seen by the naked eye and removed for further examination.

(3) AGGLUTINATION OR PRECIPITATION is a method much used for the identification of certain bacteria (see AGGLUTINATION). It is usually performed by making a uniform emulsion with water of the bacteria to be identified, and then adding a drop of this emulsion to a drop of immune serum on a microscopic slide. Various stock sera are kept in the laboratory, and one of these is chosen corresponding to the disease to which the bacterium is supposed to belong. If the bacteria on microscopic examination are seen to clump together under the action of the serum, this identifies the bacteria as belonging to the disease from which the serum has been prepared. If the bacteria do not clump, the same process is carried out with another serum until the appropriate serum is found. The same process may be carried out without microscopic examination by placing the bacterial emulsion in small test tubes and adding drops of the sera to these. Precipitation of the bacteria to the bottom of the tube can be seen to take place in a tube containing the corresponding bacteria and serum. This method is much used, for instance, in identifying the meningococcus, and the causative micro-organisms of typhoid and paratyphoid fevers.

(4) INOCULATION OF ANIMALS – For the purpose of making certain which of the many kinds of bacteria derived from a case of disease is its actual cause, or in some instances when the bacteria are so few in number or so difficult to cultivate that they cannot be found, it becomes necessary to inoculate animals like mice, guinea-pigs, or rabbits with material containing the bacteria, in order, if possible, to reproduce the disease. This inoculation is effected through pricking the skin or puncturing the abdomen by means of a needle and syringe charged with the material in question. Subsequently the animal is killed and its organs examined for signs of the disease.

BACTERIOPHAGE is an agent which affects growing bacteria so as to break them up and destroy them. It is now known to be a virus.

BACTERIOSTATIC – Bringing bacteria to a standstill by preventing their nourishment and growth.

BACTERIURIA means the presence of bacteria in the urine, usually a sign of infection in the kidneys, bladder, or urethra.

BAGASSOSIS is an industrial lung disease occurring in those who work with bagasse, which is the name given to the broken sugar cane after sugar has been extracted from it. Bagasse, which contains 6 per cent silica, is used in board-making. The inhalation of dust causes an acute lung affection, and subsequently in some cases a chronic lung disease. (See ALVEOLITIS.)

BAL is the abbreviation for BRITISH ANTI-LEWISITE. (See DIMERCAPROL.)

BALANITIS means inflammation of the parts covered by the prepuce.

BALANTIDIASIS is a form of dysentery caused by a protozoa known as *Balantidium coli*, a common parasite in pigs, which are usually the source of infection. It responds to metronidazole.

BALBUTIES is a medical term for stammering or stuttering.

BALDNESS is generally partial and slowly progressive, and is so universal that it may be looked on as a natural change in age. There is a gradual depletion in hair on the head with age: eg., from an average of 615 per square centimetre at the age of 20 to 30 to 485 at 30 to 50 years of age. It is most common in Caucasoids, less so in Negroes and least common in Mongoloids. It may also occur rapidly in patches, or even every hair on the body may be lost, in the disease called alopecia areata.

Causes – Certain *serious diseases* are associated with partial loss of hair as one of their symptoms; but these diseases are of so much greater importance that the thinness of hair is not taken account of, and as a rule remedies itself as these diseases wear off. Such diseases are acute fevers, myxoedema, syphilis, influenza, anaemia, and great anxiety or nervous shock. Baldness is, to a considerable extent, hereditary, and it is generally preceded for some years by seborrhoeic eczema, a condition of dandruff on the scalp. If it first appears relatively early in life – the twenties or early thirties in men – it is likely to be rapidly progressive and total baldness can be expected within a few years. If it does not set in until later life it tends to progress much less rapidly. In women it seldom tends to be rapidly progressive even though it begins to appear relatively early and actual baldness seldom appears until late middle age, and not always then. Every day, in the healthy scalp, a certain number of hairs reach the end of their existence, and are combed out, being replaced in time by others growing up from below. Each hair-follicle in this way produces many hairs in the course of a person's life, but, if the change is too rapid, the hairs become gradually finer, then downy, until finally the hair-producing power of the follicle wears out. This rapid change is due to the eczematous condition of the scalp. Many skin diseases, like lupus, erysipelas, ringworm, which leave a hardened condition of the scalp behind them, cause baldness, and such cases are made worse by the various stimulating hair washes sold for baldness. Other causes include excessive exposure to ultra-violet light as in prolonged sun-bathing, and certain cosmetic procedures such as bleaching, permanent waving, and hair straightening. It can also result from certain hairstyles which impose a mechanical strain on the hair such as the 'ponytail', and by wearing of hair rollers, particularly in bed at night.

Treatment – There is little that can be done to prevent baldness in those disposed to it, but certain measures may slow up the process. Thus, hard hats should not be worn. Indeed, there is much to be said for not wearing a hat at all. No hard brush or sharp comb should be used, as their irritation induces dandruff. The head should be frequently washed, say once a week, preferably using a superfatted soap. Tincture of quillaia (1 in 20) has an old reputation as an excellent shampoo, as has a whipped-up egg. The latter two are sometimes combined, as in the 'egg shampoo', with the following recipe. Beat up the yolk of two eggs in a glass of warm water or half a litre of tincture of quillaia. Strain through a sieve with a fine mesh and apply with a small sponge. Then rinse and dry the hair. The hair should be always thoroughly dried after washing, and, if it remains hard and brittle, a little hair-oil composed of lanolin (1 part) and sesame oil (16 parts) may be applied. If baldness is definitely appearing, the hair may be cut short and bay rum or spirit used daily to wash the scalp. This treatment makes the hair hard and bristly, and removes all dandruff. In people who prefer to wear the hair longer, the head may be washed daily, till the hair ceases coming out, with either Hebra's soap, consisting of green soap (2 parts), rectified

spirit (1 part), filtered and perfumed, or a tablespoonful of soap spirit (*British Pharmaceutical Codex*) in a pint (0·5 litre) of hot water. After washing, the soap must be thoroughly rinsed out and the hair dried, and oiled as above. A pomade consisting of tannin 60 minims (4 ml), lanolin 360 minims (24 ml), sesame oil 120 minims (8 ml) is also good for checking the loss of hair. Perchloride of mercury is one of the best substances for removing dandruff, either in a wash containing 5 ounces (142 ml) of water, 1 ounce (28·5 ml) of eau-de-Cologne, and 1 grain (60 mg) of perchloride of mercury, or in a pomade like that given above, to which 2 or 3 grains (120 or 180 mg) of the perchloride of mercury may be added. Many vaunted hair restorers contain either a little Goulard's water (qv) or, more generally, tincture of cantharides or Spanish fly, 60 minims (4 ml) of vinegar of cantharides being used in 1 ounce (28·5 ml) of spirit to dab on the scalp, coupled with the washing mentioned above. As in the case of disease or defect in any part of the body, attention must be paid to maintaining as high a standard of general health, and healthy living, as possible. Healthy living will not cure or prevent baldness in those born to develop it, but it may well postpone or slow up the process. It is certainly just as effective and much cheaper, than many of the vaunted 'cures' foisted on the public by enterprising advertisers.

ALOPECIA AREATA, or patchy baldness, is common on the scalp, but may affect the hair all over the body. It occurs principally in adolescents and young adults. The cause is not known. It is doubtful whether treatment makes any difference. The hair regrows spontaneously in the vast majority of cases, though sometimes lighter in colour, or even white. Ultra-violet light is beneficial in some cases. The more extensive the areas of baldness, and the more often it recurs, the worse the outlook for regrowth of the hair.

BALNEOLOGY is the department of medical science which deals with the giving of baths. (See BATHS.)

BALSAMS are substances which contain resins and benzoic acid. Balsam of Peru, balsam of tolu, and Friars' balsam (compound tincture of benzoin) are the chief. They are given internally for colds, and aid expectoration, while locally they are used to cover abrasions and stimulate ulcers. Friars' balsam, one teaspoonful, inhaled from a jug of boiling water, is of value in the alleviation of the common cold. Balsam of Peru is given internally in doses of 5 to 15 drops with beaten-up egg; balsam of tolu is similarly administered in doses of 5 to 15 grains (300 mg to 1 G), or is given as the more familiar syrup of tolu in doses of one teaspoonful.

BANDAGES are pieces of material used to support injured parts or to retain dressings in position. The material they are made of includes cotton, calico, gauze, linen, muslin, net, flannel, flannelette, domette crepe, elastic and rubber.

Types – *Triangular bandages* are made by taking a piece of calico 1 yard (1 metre) square and cutting it across cornerwise to form two triangles (illustration 25). The cut side of each is called the 'base', and the opposite right-hand corner is called the 'point'. *Roller bandages* are usually made of open-wove cotton. They are made up in various lengths, and vary in width from half-an-inch to eight inches (12 mm to 20 cm). *Crepe bandages* are elastic cotton bandages which have a one-way stretch. *Domette bandages* are made of a variety of soft elastic flannel. *Elastic bandages* are now available in various forms, their main purpose being to provide firm support as in the treatment of varicose veins. *Plaster of Paris bandages* are bandages impregnated with calcium sulphate, and used as a form of splint. (See PLASTER OF PARIS.) Two recent forms of bandages are being used to an increasing extent: Netelast and Tubegauz. *Netelast* is an elasticated net of cellular cotton and elastic in a wide-mesh tubular net (illustrations 61, 62). Its great advantage is that it can be applied easily and quickly, can be washed and sterilized, and is available in different sizes. *Tubegauz* consists of seamless, circular cotton tubular material (illustration 63), which can be applied easily and quickly to any part of the body.

Uses – *Triangular bandages* are used in first aid, ambulance work, and whenever an easily applied temporary bandage is wanted, either singly or two together. It can be used for almost any part of the body, but is merely a covering intended to retain a dressing, and does not exert much pressure.

A triangular bandage may be applied in one of three forms (illustration 25): (*a*) *open* as a triangle, sometimes with a hem turned over at the base, according to the size of the part to be covered; (*b*) *folded broad*, with the point turned in twice towards the centre of the base; and (*c*) *folded narrow*, like a cravat, the point being turned in three times. These bandages are of great use for first aid and for military work, as they take up little room, can be readily applied, and can be taken off easily without disturbing the injured part. Their mode of application is readily seen from the accompanying illustrations.

The flat hand may be covered in by a bandage similar to that for the foot (illustration 38), the wrist being placed on the centre of the base and the fingers towards the point, which is turned back over them; the ends are folded in and tied off round the wrist.

Bandages similar to those shown for the arm and elbow (illustrations 28, 30) may be applied to the leg and knee of a person who is not going about; but in walking, triangular bandages applied to these parts are apt to slip down.

The knots of all triangular bandages should be reef-knots, which are much more easily undone than the other form. It is essential that they should always be tied on the outer side of a limb, or in such a position that they can be easily removed without disturbing the injured part.

The uses of the triangular bandage in the treatment of fractures are described under FRACTURES. (See also SLINGS.)

Roller Bandages – The chief methods of applying roller bandages are: *Simple spiral*, in which the bandage circles up the limb, each turn overlapping half of that preceding. This is used for a cylindrical part of the body like the lower limb (illustration 43). *Spiral with reverses*, in which the bandage is turned sharply over on itself at each circle so as to lie smooth when the circles tend to separate widely. It is used for conical parts like the forearm or calf (illustration 42). *Figure of 8*, in which the bandage loops alternately round two parts of the body. It is used to cover a projection or hollow such as the shoulder or armpit, by looping round trunk and arm alternately. *Spica*, which is used for a joint, the turns covering one another completely in the bend of the joint, and separating partly over the prominence like the arrangement in a coat-of-mail (illustrations 47, 55, 56). It is simply a modified figure of 8. *Trefoil* is a bandage applied to the head, and is the same in principle as the figure of 8, though it has three loops instead of two (illustrations 50, 51). *Capeline* is another bandage for the head (illustration 49).

In applying a roller bandage the first circle must be firmly fixed by covering it completely with the next to prevent slip-

(*continued on page 100*)

25 — Triangular bandage unfolded and folded.

28 – Bandage for arm. Triangle folded broad is carried three times round and tied.

26 – Bandage for shoulder. Two triangles: one folded into sling for wrist; the second open with point on neck and ends tied round arm.

27 – Bandage for open hand. Triangle is folded narrow; centre is placed on palm of hand; ends are carried round to back, crossed, carried round wrist twice, and tied.

29 – Bandage for closed fist, in which a roll of cotton-wool, lint, etc., is grasped. Four stages.

91

30 – Bandage for elbow. Triangle folded broad is laid with centre on elbow; ends are crossed in front, carried round forearm, crossed again in front, carried round upper arm, and tied.

32 – Bandage for groin. Two triangles, folded narrow and tied end to end.

31 – Bandage to cover the chest. One triangle: the point is laid over one shoulder, the ends are carried round the sides and tied over the same shoulder-blade; the longer of the two ends is carried up and tied to the point; a, front; b, back. To cover the back the same bandage is used with knots in front.

33 – Bandage for hip. Two triangles: one folded narrow and tied round waist; the other with point on the side and ends tied round thigh; a, first stage; b, finished.

35 – Bandage for eye. Triangle folded narrow; centre is placed over the eye, and carried round head, crossed, carried forwards, and tied.

36 – Bandage for lower jaw. Two triangles folded narrow; place one with centre below, the other with centre in front of the chin. The former is tied above, the latter behind, head. The ends of both are finally tied together.

34 – Bandage for head. (a) Triangle with a hem turned up on base is placed with centre of base on forehead and point on back of neck; (b) ends are carried behind head, crossed on neck, carried forward, and tied on forehead; (c) point is finally pinned up. Three stages.

37 – Bandage for side of head. Triangle folded narrow; centre is placed over one ear, one end carried over top of head, the other beneath chin; the two turn round one another above ear, and are then carried round forehead and back of head and tied over centre of forehead.

93

40 – Bandage to support the breasts. A wide bandage is used. After each pair of turns beneath the breasts a circle to fix is taken round the waist.

38 – Bandage for foot. Foot is placed on triangle with heel near the centre of base; ends are folded over three times to lie along side of heel; point is turned up over front of ankle, ends tied round ankle, and point is finally pinned down over the knot. *a*, First stage; *b*, second stage; *c*, finished.

41 – Bandage for the knee (spica). The dotted outline shows the beginning of bandage.

39 – Bandage to fix a dressing on the chest, and cover in the arm. In actual practice a wider bandage would be used, and the turns would overlap. For clearness they are here shown separated.

42 – Spiral with reverses for leg.

43 – Simple spiral for lower limb.

44 – Bandage coveringe heel. First turn covers heel, second and third bind down its loose edges; fourth and fifth bind down the loose edges of second and third.

45 – Method of 'fixing' bandage firmly for application to foot.

46 – Spiral with reverses for thigh.

47 – Ascending spica for groin.

48 – Commencement of descending spica for groin. In the ascending spica the bandage runs up across the front of the thigh and each turn is higher than the one before. In the descending spica the turns across the thigh run down and each turn is at a lower level than its predecessor. The body turns pass round the pelvis, not round the waist. When both groins are to be bandaged, a turn of ascending spica on one alternates with a turn of descending spica on the other; after each pair of turns a complete circular turn is made round the pelvis.

49 – Capeline bandage for head. Two bandages are stitched end to end. The bandage is rolled off one to the other till one roller is half as large again as the other. The larger part circles round the head close above the eyebrows and ears, and low down on the back of the head, binding down at each turn a strip of the other, which passes alternately backward and forward on either side.

50 – Bandage for head (trefoil). This consists essentially of three turns repeated in order. *a* shows commencement on the nape of the neck and first turn; *b* shows second and third turns, the bandage next passing below chin and round to nape of neck; *c* shows the gradual covering in of head; and *d* a further stage. To fix all, a final turn in the position of the first should be made low down on the nape of the neck behind and close above the eyebrows front.

53 – Bandage for eye; turns pass alternately round forehead and down over eye.

51 – Same bandage (trefoil) from the other side. Shows that the vertical turns pass behind the ear on one side, in front of it on the other. When bandage is used to cover in one ear, the first turn should pass round the other side of the head, as shown. This bandage cannot be used to cover in the part of the head shown bare in illustration 48 *d*, for which the capelline bandage or a four-tailed bandage may be used.

54 – Spiral with reverses for hand and forearm.

52 – Simple spiral for arm.

55 – Spica for elbow.

56 – Spica for shoulder or armpit.

57 – Method of 'fixing' bandage before commencing spiral with reverses for hand.

58 – Bandage for closed fist, in which a pad or wool should be placed. There are alternate loops round wrist and round knuckles. Four stages.

61 – A Netelast tubular net being used to retain a dressing on the head. Roussel Laboratories Ltd.

59 – Bandage for finger. It starts round wrist for the purpose of fixing, passes in an open spiral down to the point of the finger (1), then upwards again as a spiral with reverse at each turn (2), and ends round wrist.

62 – A colostomy night belt with Netelast, holes for the legs having been cut in the net. Roussel Laboratories Ltd.

60 – Two special bandages. *a*, T-bandage; *b*, many-tailed bandage; the central strip is placed behind the part to be bandaged, and the numbers indicate the order in which the 'tails' of the bandage are applied.

63 – Tubegauz applied to thumb and fingers. Seton Products Ltd.

ping; or a still better method of fixing consists in taking a figure of 8 turn round the limb, as shown in illustrations 45 and 57, and covering this with the subsequent turns of the bandage. The bandage must pass upwards or the limb will become blue owing to the blood in the superficial veins being pressed backwards towards the extremity of the limb. It should cross the front of the limb from within outwards in order to give more room for making reverses towards the outer side.

Where skin surfaces come into contact, one should be separated from the other by cotton-wool, as otherwise moisture accumulates and the surfaces readily become abraded. This should be done, for example, between the fingers, behind the ear, in the armpit, and underneath the breasts. In order to make the bandage lie smoothly it is important in applying it that the head of the bandage should always, except in reversing, remain in contact with the part that is being bandaged, round which it is simply rolled.

Bandages of special shape are used for certain parts of the body. The *four-tailed bandage* is made for the jaw or the crown of the head by tearing a 4-foot (1·2-metre) strip of roller bandage up the middle from both ends, leaving 4 inches (10 cm) untorn in the centre; it is applied in the same manner as the two triangular bandages shown in illustration 36. The *T-shaped bandage* (illustration 60) for the fork is made by stitching the middle of a 4-foot (1·2-metre) strip of roller bandage to the end of a similar strip which is torn up the middle for the greater part of its length;

the untorn strip forms a waist belt, the divided part passes down through the fork and its ends are pinned to the part that forms the waist belt. The *many-tailed* bandage (illustration 60) for the abdomen is made by stitching a strip of roller bandage down the middle of several 4-foot (1·2-metre) strips, each of which overlaps one-half of that below; shorter strips are used for fractured or painful limbs.

BANTI'S DISEASE (see SPLENIC ANAEMIA).

BARAGNOSIS means the inability on the part of a patient to recognize that an object placed in the hand has weight, a condition due to disease of the brain.

BARANY'S TEST is a test for gauging the efficiency of the balancing mechanism (the vestibular apparatus) by applying hot or cold air or water to the external ear.

BARBER'S ITCH (see SYCOSIS).

BARBITONE, is one of the barbiturate group of drugs. It has a prolonged action, lasting for 10 to 20 hours. The dose is 300 to 600 milligrams (5 to 10 grains). Caution must be exercised in taking barbitone or any of its derivatives, because of the danger of over-dosage, and of habit-formation.

BARBITURATES – The barbiturate drugs are all derivatives of barbituric acid, so called because it was first prepared on St Barbara's Day (1899). They form one of

	British Pharmacopoeia Name	Proprietary Name	Dose	Approximate Duration of Action in Hours
Long acting	Phenobarbitone	Luminal	30 to 120 mg	12 to 24
	Phenobarbitone sodium		60 to 200 mg by injection	12 to 24
	Barbitone		250 to 500 mg	10 to 20
	Barbitone sodium	Medinal	250 to 500 mg	8 to 16
Intermediate acting	Butobarbitone	Soneryl	100 to 200 mg	8 to 10
	Amylobarbitone	Amytal	100 to 200 mg	6 to 8
	Amylobarbitone sodium	Sodium amytal	100 to 200 mg	6 to 8
	Pentobarbitone sodium	Nembutal	100 to 200 mg	6 to 8
Short acting	Cyclobarbitone	Phanodorm	200 to 400 mg	4 to 6
	Quinalbarbitone sodium	Seconal sodium	100 to 200 mg	4 to 6

Table 4 – Dosage and duration of action of the barbiturates

the most extensive series of sedative, hypnotic, and anaesthetic drugs at present in use. The more important ones, with their duration of action and dosage, are listed in table 4.

BARIUM SULPHATE is a heavy white powder used in X-ray diagnosis. The mass of barium forms an opaque shadow and shows the outline of the cavity in which it lies. Thus the physician can see the size and position of the stomach in an X-ray photograph, or can trace a meal in its passage through the bowels.

BARLEY-WATER is a beverage made by allowing 2 ounces (57 G) of pearly barley to simmer for two hours with a quart (1 litre) of water, then adding sugar and lemon to flavour, and straining.

BARRIER CREAMS are substances applied to the skin before work to prevent damage to the skin by irritants handled at work. They are also used in medicine: eg. for the prevention of bedsores and napkin rashes.

There are three main types of barrier creams: –

A **dust barrier** to protect the skin against sensitizing dusts and against substances which, if absorbed, will produce systemic poisoning.

A **water-repellent barrier** for those whose hands are constantly exposed to water, alkalis, and water-soluble oils.

An **oil-repellent or water-miscible barrier**, which is a protective against oils, greases and solvents, and which facilitates their removal without the use of abrasives or oil solvents.

The following formulae, prepared by the barrier substances subcommittee of the *British Pharmacopoeia Codex* revision committee are now in wide use:

Dust barrier:

Casein (Rennet finely powdered)	3
Sodium alginate	2
Glycerin	6
Stearic acid	10
Triethanolamine	1·55
Chlorocresol	0·2
Phenol	0·5
Distilled water	to 100

Water-repellent barrier:

Hard paraffin	25
Soft paraffin	11·75
Liquid paraffin	3·5
Cetostearyl alcohol	5
Triethanolamine	0·7
Stearic acid	1·8
Chlorocresol	0·2
Distilled water	to 100

Water-repellent barrier:

Kaolin (sterilized)	20
Fuller's earth (200 mesh)	3
Hard soap (powdered)	12
Glycerin	6
Stearic acid	2
Sodium chloride	1
Chlorocresol	0·2
Phenol	0·5
Distilled water	to 100

Skin-conditioning cream:

Monostearin, self-emulsifying	10
Glycerin	6
Triethanolamine ricinoleate	1
Wool alcohols	6
Chlorocresol	0·2
Oleyl alcohol	3
Distilled water	to 100

The skin-conditioning cream is used after work if the hands are dry and degreased.

Silicones (qv), which are water repellent, are being used increasingly as barrier creams.

The hands should be clean and dry before applying a barrier cream. The cream should be applied sparingly to the whole of the hands, and not just rubbed into the palms. It is essential to coat the backs of the hands, paying special attention to the sides of the fingers and the webs between. The cream should be well rubbed into the nail folds and under the free edges of the nails. To get the full value from silicone creams, they should be applied twice daily for ten days before exposing the hands to irritants; after this a once-daily application should be sufficient.

A point which is being increasingly emphasized by the experts is that the use of barrier creams must not be allowed to lead to any slackening in the attention paid to other more important protective measures, such as standards of cleanliness in workshops and the wearing of protective clothing.

BARRIER NURSING is the nursing of a patient suffering from an infectious disease in such a way that the risk of his passing on the disease to others is effectively reduced. Thus, precautions are taken to ensure that all infective matter, such as stools, urine, sputum, discharge from wounds, and anything that may be contaminated by such infective matter, such as nurses' uniforms, bedding and towels are so treated that they will not convey the infection. (See NURSING.)

BASAL METABOLISM (see METABOL-ISM).

BASEDOW'S DISEASE is another name for exophthalmic goitre or Graves' disease. (See GOITRE.)

BASILIC VEIN is the prominent vein which runs from near the bend of the elbow upwards along the inner side of the upper arm. It is generally the vein opened in venesection for blood-letting.

BASILICON OINTMENT is an old name for an ointment of resin, lard, wax, and almond oil.

BASOPHILIA is a term applied to the bluish appearance under the microscope of immature red blood corpuscles when stained by certain dyes. This appearance, with the blue areas collected in points, is seen in lead poisoning and the condition is called punctate basophilia. The term basophilia may also mean an increase in the numbers of basophil cells in the blood.

BAT EARS is the term commonly applied to prominent ears. The condition may be familial, but this is by no means the rule. Strapping the ears firmly back has no effect and is merely a waste of time and an embarrassment to the child. In cases in which the condition is proving a definite embarrassment to the child, it can be rectified by plastic surgery.

BATHER'S ITCH, also called SWIMMER'S ITCH, WATER ITCH, and SCHISTOSOME DERMATITIS, is the term given to a blotchy rash on the skin occurring in those bathing in water which is infested with the larvae of certain trematode worms known as *Schistosomes* (see SCHISTOSOMIASIS). The worm is parasitic in snails. The skin rash is caused by penetration of the skin by the free-swimming larval cercaria. Bather's itch is common in many parts of the world, including USA, Canada, Central and South America, Australasia, Malaysia and Japan. It has also been found in Wales, France, and Germany.

BATHS – The main action of water on the skin is as a vehicle for heat, and baths act largely either by extracting heat from, or adding to, the body. The sweat glands of the skin excrete some 30 ounces (850 ml) of water daily, containing about one-twentieth part of the nitrogenous waste of the body, and their excretory activity may be greatly increased by baths of high temperature. Baths also exert a mechanical effect by virtue of the fact that water is slightly denser than the human body and therefore causes the body to float on its surface. They also exert an important psychological effect, the heat of a warm bath and the buoyancy of the water allowing a paralysed patient to perform movements of which he thought he was no longer capable. (See also SAUNA.)

The elderly, infirm and handicapped often find considerable difficulty getting into or out of a bath. For them the procedure shown in illustration 64 is recommended.

A. WATER BATHS – (1) COLD – This is a bath about 60° F or 16° C (cold tap temperature). It should be taken while the body is warm, and its daily use is a healthy habit. The average person should go straight from bed to a plunge bath of the above temperature; or, if preferred, a warm bath of about 100° F or 38° C may be first taken, and then a cold douche or sponge from the cold-water tap. The cold bath should last from a few seconds to two minutes, and the warm bath preceding it up to ten minutes. The bather should rub himself vigorously in both baths, and must at once rub himself dry with a coarse towel and quickly dress. During drying the skin becomes rosy, and a delightful warm glow comes on and lasts several hours. Persons whose blood-vessels do not react properly to changes of temperature are apt to suffer one or other of two things after a bath. The 'reaction' is due to a quick contraction, followed by a moderate dilatation of the blood-vessels in the skin, and in persons with poor 'tone' of the arteries, either an excessive dilatation follows a hot bath, which the cold bath cannot overcome, and the blood being unduly cooled in the full vessels of the skin, a 'chill' results; or the vessels contract too firmly after the cold bath, so that cold hands and feet result. The latter can be got over by taking the cold bath in two stages, first a tepid bath on getting out of bed, and then a sponge or douche from the cold tap. Even the weakest person may get part of the benefits of a cold bath without any ill effect, by taking a tepid bath at 90° F or 32° C, and cooling it down by running in tap water in the course of five minutes to 75° F or 24° C, rubbing the body and legs vigorously all the while, or having them rubbed, and afterwards drying rapidly. Very cold baths must be avoided by those with a tendency to apoplexy.

(2) TEPID – A tepid bath is one slightly below the body temperature: ie. about

64 – Fill the bath, which should have a slip mat, to the required amount and temperature and then turn off the taps. Step into the bath *facing the end opposite to the taps* (**a**). Go down on hands in the bath water (**b**). Slide around (**c**) – either to the right or left, whichever is found to be easier – into a sitting position. You will now be sitting in the bath in the normal position facing the taps (**d**). It is of help in controlling this turn around if a foot is placed against the vertical end of the bath to act as a pivot. When bathing is over, first let the bath water run away; then reverse the procedure by turning round on to hands and knees (**b**), stand up, and step out onto a non-skid bathmat.

90° F or 32° C. It is the convenient temperature for large baths. Prolonged tepid baths have a soothing effect. The patient is placed in a bath at 95° F or 35° C, and cooled down slowly to about 92° F or 33·3° C.

(3) WARM – A warm bath is one ranging from about the body temperature, 99° F or 37° C, to about 110° F or 43° C. Water at 115° F (46° C) can just be borne by the hand, but not by the whole body. A warm bath quickens the pulse, and lowers the blood-pressure. It also causes free perspiration. A warm bath of about 104° F (40° C) for ten or fifteen minutes, followed by a cold douche, in the robust, is one of the best means of preventing the stiffness which follows prolonged muscular effort. But very warm baths are dangerous to those suffering from disease of the heart.

B. VAPOUR BATHS – (1) AROMATIC – The patient sits in a special box, his head protruding through a hole in the lid, while steam from water containing fir-balsam, lavender, etc., circulates round him. Beyond acting as a hot bath this form is of no therapeutic value.

(2) RUSSIAN BATHS have much the same effect as warm-water baths. The bath is generally taken in a room which is filled with vapour, but as good an effect may be

obtained from a cabinet, or a tent of blankets, in which the patient sits on a chair some inches over boiling water. In a vapour bath 120° F (49° C) can be borne readily, and the person should remain in the vapour until he breaks into a copious perspiration, usually in about fifteen or twenty minutes. Subsequently a cold douche or bath should be taken, according to the state of his 'reaction'. In Russia it is a common practice immediately after the vapour bath to pour a stream of ice-cold water all over the surface of the body.

C. DRY BATHS – (1) HOT-AIR BATHS may be taken as the TURKISH or ROMAN bath, in a specially constructed building heated by pipes in the walls, with tepid room, hot room, washing room, and cooling room, through which the bather goes in succession. A hot bath may also be taken in an electric-light cabinet, where the person sits exposed to brilliant light and heat till he sweats copiously, when he takes a cold-water bath.

Such a bath may also be given in bed, the patient lying under a curved wire shield. In hospitals the under-surface of the shield is provided with numerous electric-light bulbs which speedily raise the temperature of the enclosed air to a high degree (illustration 65).

The duration of a Roman bath is about

two hours, and it leaves a feeling of great freshness. In either of these baths one may lose 6 pounds (2·7 kg) at one time by sweating. They are useful for reducing weight, and for rheumatism.

The electric-light bath can be given in bed, the lights being underneath a curved shield, 5 feet (152 cm) long, which covers the patient, and there are also smaller shields for single limbs. A dry temperature of 200° F (93° C) can be borne without discomfort for a quarter of an hour, and has excellent results in chronic rheumatism, rheumatoid arthritis and sciatica. When a sick person is being treated by

65 – Radiant heat bath with electric-light bulbs under curved asbestos shield to cover patient.

such a high temperature bath, it is necessary that his pulse should be frequently examined, in case the heart's action should become enfeebled.

(2) SAND BATHS are used for rheumatic conditions, the sand being made very hot to purify it, and heaped on the patient when moderately cool.

(3) WAX BATHS are also used for rheumatic aches and pains. Paraffin wax with a melting point of around 115° F (46° C) is placed in a thermostatically controlled tank. The affected hand, or hands, is then dipped in the molten wax about ten times until it is well coated with wax. It is then wrapped in wax-proof paper in a plastic bag and wrapped in a towel for about twenty minutes. The wax is then removed.

With care the method can be used at home, the wax being melted in a double saucepan on an electric stove. Because of its inflammability it must not be heated over a naked flame.

D. MEDICINAL BATHS – (1) ALKALINE BATHS are used to soften the skin in certain skin diseases like general eczema. Six ounces (170 G) of washing soda are added to 30 gallons (135 litres) of tepid water.

(2) BRAN BATHS are used to soothe general irritation of the skin. Four pounds (1·8 kg) of bran are boiled and the liquor added to a tepid bath, in which the patient soaks for half an hour.

(3) PEAT and MUD BATHS are used generally for rheumatism at various spas. The patient is covered with a layer of warmed mud, such as fango, lies in it for perhaps twenty minutes, and is then washed clean by a cold douche. Such baths can be taken at a much higher temperature than water baths (102° to 112° F (39° to 44° C)).

(4) MUSTARD BATHS are used for the feet to check colds, and for the whole body as a good general stimulant. For this, a handful of mustard is made into a paste with cold water and stirred into the warm bath.

(5) PINE-NEEDLE BATHS are pleasant and stimulating. They are prepared by adding to a tepid bath the water in which several pounds of fresh pine needles have been boiled.

(6) SEA-WATER BATHS are best taken in the sea. Brine baths are found at various spas. Failing that, about 9 pounds (4 kg) of common salt are added to 30 gallons (135 litres) of water. The effect is very stimulating. Such baths are used in cases of chronic rheumatism. They are also of value in the treatment of the so-called decubitus ulcers which are liable to occur in patients with spinal cord injuries. The recommended strength for this purpose is 5 per cent crude rock salt and 2·5 per cent magnesium sulphate.

(7) CARBONIC ACID BATHS are used for their stimulating effect upon the skin and upon the body generally. They may be administered by the aid of water which is naturally effervescent, as at Royat, St Moritz, Spa, and Marienbad, where they are specially in vogue for the treatment of heart disorders; or the carbonic acid may be allowed to escape from cylinders in the bath-water; or weak formic acid is mixed with the water in which small cotton bags of washing soda are placed. Such effervescent baths, especially when taken warm, have a marked action in increasing

the circulation in the skin and diminishing general arterial blood-pressure.

(8) FOAM BATHS, contain some soapy substance such as an extract of quillaia bark, or some detergent preparation, which on stirring produces a copious froth. They usually contain also some substance which adds to the frothy effect by development of carbonic acid gas, and they then have the effects mentioned above under carbonic acid baths.

(9) SULPHUR BATHS are used for the presence in the water of sulphuretted hydrogen, which not only stimulates the skin but is to some extent absorbed. The bath may be prepared artificially by adding from $\frac{1}{4}$ to $\frac{1}{2}$ pound (112 to 224 G) of sulphuret of potassium or of yellow sulphur to 30 gallons (135 litres) of hot water. Sulphur baths are specially used in the treatment of skin diseases and in rheumatism.

(10) SITZ BATHS are baths in which only the hips and buttocks are immersed.

(11) SALINE BATHS are baths which are isotonic (qv): ie. contain 9 grams of sodium chloride to 1 litre of water. They are a refreshing, convenient and relatively pain-free way of managing large or awkwardly placed wounds on the limbs or trunk, which are septic and contain purulent material which needs to be removed to speed up the healing process.

E. ELECTRIC BATHS may be given in earthenware, stone or wooden baths. The bath is filled with tepid water, in which the patient lies. An electrode hangs in the water at either end, not touching the patient, and a moderate current is passed through the water. This bath is used in cases of debility and neurasthenia. (See ELECTRICITY IN MEDICINE.)

BCG VACCINE – BCG (*Bacillus Calmette-Guérin*) vaccine, which was introduced in France in 1908, is the only vaccine that has produced significant immunity against the tubercle bacillus and at the same time has proved safe enough for use in human subjects. The original work of Calmette and Guérin has now been amply confirmed by investigators in many parts of the world. There are two main indications for the use of BCG vaccine: (*a*) for the protection of new-born infants or children exposed to special risks of infection; (*b*) for the immunization of adolescents or young adults, such as nurses, who are known to have developed no natural immunity to tuberculosis and who are exposed to particularly heavy infections. (See IMMUNITY.)

BEANS are widely used as a source of food. In the western world they include the kidney bean, or French bean (*Phaseolus vulgaris*) which is the now popular 'baked bean', the scarlet runner bean (*Phaseolus multiflorus*), haricot beans, navy beans and pea beans. In the East, and particularly in China, the most widely eaten bean is the soya bean (*Glycine hispida*) which has twice the protein content of most other pulses. Modern methods have now been evolved whereby it can be converted into an acceptable imitation of meat. It is also a constituent of the vegetable milk substitutes being used in the developing countries of Africa, South America and Asia. (See PULSES; SOYA BEANS.)

BEAT ELBOW, BEAT HAND, and BEAT KNEE are terms applied by miners to an inflamed condition with swelling of the elbow, hand or knee. The condition is particularly common in miners, but occurs in other trades also from constant pressure and the ingraining of particles of dirt, caused by the constant use of a tool or pressure in resting on the joints at work. The condition sometimes proceeds to suppuration, but usually subsides under soothing and antiseptic applications.

BECLOMETHASONE DIPRO-PIONATE is a corticosteroid that is proving of value as a cream or ointment in the treatment of certain skin diseases. It is also of value by inhalation in the treatment of asthma and hay fever, and by insertion into the nose in the treatment of perennial rhinitis. (See NOSE, DISEASES OF.)

BED – The bed used in cases of sickness should consist of an iron *frame* of at least 6 feet (183 cm) in length and 3 feet 3 inches to 3 feet 6 inches (99 to 107 cm) in width, and should be provided with a stiff *wire mattress*. A piece of canvas or felt, fixed to the mattress, should form a *mattress cover* to prevent rusting of the wire. Upon this is a mattress of wool, hair, latex, or rubber or plastic foam, or it may have interior springs. The mattress should have a loose cover of cotton, which can be washed from time to time as required, or a plastic or polythene cover. Over the mattress is placed a sheet which is tucked in firmly beneath the mattress all round to form the *under sheet*. The bed is completed by the *upper sheet* and *blankets*, varying in number according to the season of the year, and by a light *bedcover*. Two thin *pillows*, each covered by a linen or cotton pillow-slip, should be supplied, but it is important both in health and in disease that the support for the head should not be too high, and the pillows should simply be sufficient to fill up the distance between the head and shoulder when the patient lies on the side.

The bed should stand with its head towards the wall and the foot towards the centre of the room or ward, and there should be a free passage up either side for access by the attendants. In some diseases and injuries the bed requires special modification. In all cases confined to bed for longer than a few days a *draw sheet* is required. The draw sheet is formed as follows: An ordinary sheet is folded lengthwise so that the folded sheet is sufficiently wide to extend from the patient's shoulders to behind the knees. Between the folds of this is placed a mackintosh sheet one yard (0·9 metre) square, or it is often more convenient to place the mackintosh sheet beneath the draw sheet, directly upon the under sheet. This folded sheet is pushed at one end under the mattress, carried across the bed, and the superfluous length is folded up and pushed out of the way under the mattress at the other side. From time to time the sheet is pulled through beneath the patient towards the shorter end, thus bringing a fresh piece of sheet beneath the back. In *rheumatic fever* and other conditions in which the patient perspires profusely, the patient lies directly upon and is covered by a blanket, as the woollen material absorbs the perspiration better than sheets. In cases of *fracture* of a lower limb it is necessary to make the bed more rigid, and for this purpose boards are placed across the wire mattress. In cases of *bronchitis* it is frequently necessary to erect a tent over the bed, to cut off draughts or to retain a moist atmosphere produced by a steam kettle. This can be effected by a light screen placed round the bed and covered with a blanket (illustration 92).

In cases of paralysis, prolonged fever, and other *devitalizing conditions*, the patient may require to be placed upon a mattress which supports his body evenly instead of allowing pressure to come upon its most projecting parts. For this purpose a *water-bed* (qv) may be employed, or, better, an *air-bed* (qv). The water-bed is filled with warm water after it is placed upon the mattress, and care is taken to expel all bubbles of air by stroking it with the hand towards the inlet through which the water is poured. The air-bed is much more easily managed, and is pumped up by an ordinary bicycle pump from time to

time without the necessity of removing the patient. The under sheet is laid directly on top of the water-bed, or air-bed.

A *bed rest* must sometimes be provided for patients unable to breathe comfortably in a recumbent position, or in order to change the position from time to time of a patient permanently confined to bed. For this purpose, four or five pillows may be placed behind the patient's back or, preferably, a rest, consisting of a horizontal part hinged to a cane-backed rest resembling the back of a chair and supported on a strut, is used and furnished with a couple of pillows. In order to give a still further change of position, a *bed table* may be used. This is supported on four legs some 3 feet 6 inches (107 cm) high and is of sufficient width (about 4 feet (120 cm)) to enable each pair of legs to stand on either side of the bed. Upon this the patient can lean forward.

BED BUG, or *Cimex lectularius* (illustration 66), is a wingless, blood-sucking insect, parasitic on man. It is a flat, rusty brown insect, 5 mm long and 3 mm wide, with an offensive, never forgotten smell, which cannot fly. The average life is 3 to 6 months, but it can live for a year without food. The bed bug remains hidden during the day in cracks in walls and floors, and

66 – The female bed bug, magnified twice.

in beds. It does not transmit any known disease. Eggs hatch out into larvae in 6 to 10 days, which become adult within about 12 weeks. A temperature of 44°C kills the adult in an hour. Various agents have been used to disinfect premises, such as sulphur dioxide, ethylene oxide mixed with carbon dioxide, hydrogen cyanide and heavy naphtha, but a solution of DDT in kerosene is the most effective disinfecting agent.

BED CHANGING – Two methods are adopted for changing the bed-clothes without removing the sick person from the bed. One of these, called medical changing, is generally applicable when the upper part of the body or head is affected. The other, known as surgical changing, is generally used when the lower part of the body is affected or when the lower limbs are the site of fracture or similar disability.

67 – Sheet changing, first stage.

68 – Patient turned on right side and sheets rolled against his back.

69 – Patient turned on left side, and sheet rolls pulled through beneath him to be spread out.

MEDICAL CHANGING – The bed-clothes are first removed until the patient is covered only by a blanket and the upper sheet (illustration 67). The patient is then turned upon one side (right) near the right edge of the bed (illustration 68). The soiled sheet with the draw sheet is then rolled up lengthwise from the right edge of the bed until the roll lies against the patient's back. The fresh sheet is made into a roll lengthwise; one edge is tucked in under the right edge of the mattress and the sheet is unrolled across the bed towards the left until the roll lies alongside the roll of soiled sheet. The patient is next turned on the back and then on the left side near the left-hand side of the bed (illustration 69).

He now lies upon the unrolled portion of the fresh sheet. The soiled sheet, which now lies behind his back, is pulled off the bed and the roll of fresh sheet is unrolled and its edge tucked beneath the left-hand edge of the mattress. During this procedure the patient remains covered by the upper sheet and a blanket. A fresh draw sheet is introduced by similar procedure. Finally, the pillows are placed in fresh pillow-slips.

SURGICAL CHANGING – In some cases the under sheet is more conveniently changed from the top or bottom of the bed. To do this the edges of the soiled sheet are pulled out all round from under the edges of the mattress. The sheet is then pulled down under the patient's hips, and, finally, from under the legs. The fresh sheet is now rolled up from top and bottom to the middle, and the double roll is pushed through from the side of the bed beneath the patient's hips while an attendant raises these slightly from the bed. By gently easing up the patient's shoulders the upper half of the sheet is unrolled and tucked in at the top of the mattress, and by similarly elevating his legs slightly the lower half is unrolled and tucked in at the foot of the bed.

CHANGING DRAW SHEET – When it is necessary to insert a fresh draw sheet, the draw sheet is folded up as in the method for changing the under sheet and is introduced either by rolling the patient over or slightly elevating his hips. When the draw sheet requires to be replaced frequently, it is more convenient to place the square of mackintosh on the under sheet and to insert the draw sheet above it separately.

CHANGING NIGHTDRESS – When it is necessary to change the nightdress of a person confined to bed, the fresh nightdress should be warmed; one arm is then slipped out of the soiled nightdress and inserted into the corresponding sleeve of the fresh nightdress. The soiled nightdress is then slipped over the patient's head and removed, and the fresh one is slipped on and arranged. This should be carried out without removing the upper sheet and blankets. In the case of patients too ill to be much disturbed, the nightdress may conveniently be slit down the back.

BED SORES or PRESSURE SORES, are areas of inflamed skin, tending to ulcerate, which appear upon the body or limbs of those long confined to bed, and especially of those much weakened by disease.

Causes – Sores seldom occur in vigorous persons confined to bed by a fractured limb or other minor cause. They appear in those who have not much fat between bones and skin, in the aged, in those suffering from prostrating weakness, and especially in those whose nervous system is at fault and the nutrition of whose skin is consequently impaired: for example in a person with a fractured spine, or with degeneration of the spinal cord. The direct cause may be wrinkles left in the bedclothes, discharges allowed to soil the invalid's back, and want of daily observation of the places where sores are likely to form.

Symptoms – Very often the invalid feels no pain; sometimes he complains only of a hard place or wrinkle in the bed-clothes. The sites where sores commonly form are where the bones show plainly through the skin in the lower part of the back, on the heels, on the haunch, on one ankle, on the elbows, or on the shoulder blades. At first, for one or two days, there is redness of the skin over a prominence, which quickly turns blue and dusky. Then a black slough forms, and comes away, leaving a raw surface, which widens if not carefully treated.

Treatment – The best treatment is preventive, by keeping the patient's back scrupulously clean and dry, by washing it daily with soap and water, sponging it with spirit in order to dry and harden the skin, and, finally, dusting it with a powder of zinc oxide or boric acid (or instead of using spirit and dusting powder, the skin may be preserved by rubbing in daily a little zinc oxide ointment); by examining night and morning for any sign of redness; and especially by changing the invalid's position, so as to relieve the various prominences from constant pressure. The twice-daily smearing of the skin with barrier creams (qv) containing silicone, such as dimethicone cream, is proving of value. The regular administration of vitamin C (qv) is also of value.

If redness appear over a prominent part, this must be wrapped in dry cotton-wool and the patient at once put on an air ring or air-bed. Superficial sores are treated with 1 per cent gentian violet, or zinc and castor-oil cream. Deeper sores can be treated with cetrimide. When a black, hard slough is forming, and the surface is breaking, infection is almost invariably present and the type of dressing must be changed. Among those that have been recommended are: cod-liver oil; picric acid solutions; tannic acid solutions; eusol; one of the flavine group of antiseptics, eg. proflavine, flavazole. Irradiation of the affected area with ultra-violet light has also been used, in addition to one of these dressings. Whatever dressing is used, sloughs (qv) are removed as they become loosened. When the area has become clean again, a return is made to dry dressings.

BEEF-TEA forms a valuable stimulant for invalids, but has no food value whatsoever.

To prepare beef-tea take 1 pound (455 G) of lean beef, cut into shreds, and place it in a jar with 1 pint (570 ml) of cold water. Allow to stand for about half an hour, then tightly cover the jar and place it in a saucepan of water. Heat gradually, but for the first hour do not allow the temperature to exceed 167° F (75° C). From time to time stir the mixture and squeeze the lumps of meat against the side of the jar. At the end of an hour bring the mixture to the boil and then remove it at once from the stove. The beef-tea is then poured off, not strained. The residue is then squeezed firmly with a wooden spoon in a coarse strainer and the juice so obtained added to the tea, which is then set aside to cool. The fat which settles on the top is removed with a warm spoon. Beef-tea is usually administered in quantities of one teacupful at a time: ie. 5 or 6 ounces (140 to 170 ml).

BEER (see ALCOHOL).

BEE STINGS (see BITES).

BEETROOT, or GARDEN BEET, is a vegetable mainly eaten cold as a constituent of a salad. It contains 2·8 grams of carbohydrate, 0·5 gram of protein and a trace of fat, in addition to 8·5 mg of calcium and 0·2 mg of iron, per ounce.

BELLADONNA (see ATROPINE).

BELL'S PARALYSIS is paralysis of the muscles of the face on one or both sides, causing inability to close the eye, to smile, to show the teeth, and the like, on the affected side. The paralysis is due to damage of the seventh or facial nerve. When due to inflammation, it is often temporary, and complete recovery may ensue, but when due to a wound in front of the ear, to fracture of the base of the skull, or to a stroke of apoplexy, it is apt to be permanent, although apoplectic paralysis of the face is more favourable for recovery than that due to injury. (See PARALYSIS.)

BELTS AND BINDERS are commonly worn, not only as articles of dress, but as supports and curative agents.

Uses – Flannel binders give great comfort in cases of lumbago when worn next to the skin. Persons of all ages, with weak and easily tired backs, get great support from wearing a broad belt round the waist. When, however, the upper part of the body is subject to great muscular efforts, as in athletes and navvies, it is a great mistake to encircle the waist tightly with a narrow belt, which ought to run round in the hollow on either side between the summit of the haunch-bone and the hip-joint, and so give full play to the abdominal muscles and those of the loins. Elderly persons who have a large, flabby abdomen often suffer from a form of dyspepsia due to want of support of the abdominal organs, which is relieved by wearing a broad, shaped belt round the lower part of the abdomen, or corsets with such a belt attached. This abdominal belt should be tight in its lower part, and loose above the navel, to allow free movement of the stomach in digestion, and not interfere with breathing.

BEMEGRIDE is a drug which antagonizes the hypnotic and respiratory depressant action of the barbiturates, and has proved of value in the treatment of barbiturate poisoning.

BENDS (see CAISSON DISEASE).

BENNETT'S FRACTURE, so-called after an Irish surgeon, Edward Hallaran Bennett (1837–1907), is a longitudinal fracture of the first metacarpal bone, which also involves the carpo-metacarpal joint.

BENZEDRINE is a proprietary name for amphetamine sulphate (see AMPHETAMINE).

BENZENE HEXACHLORIDE is an insecticide which acts more rapidly than DDT but not for such a long time. When first sprayed it is 10 times as toxic to insects as DDT, but its action wears off in 3 to 4 months, whereas that of DDT will persist for up to a year.

BENZHEXOL is a drug that is proving of value in the treatment of Parkinsonism (qv).

BENZOCAINE is a white powder with soothing properties used as a sedative for inflamed and painful surfaces.

BENZODIAZEPINES are a group of minor tranquillizers, or anxiolytic sedatives, as they are sometimes known, which are concerned with the control of emotion, and also have an anticonvulsant action. They include chlordiazepoxide (qv), diazepam (qv) and nitrazepam (qv).

BENZOIC ACID is an antiseptic. It, or benzoate of sodium, is still given internally in cases of infection along the urinary tract, especially in inflammation of the bladder with decomposition of the urine. Other acids are neutralized in the blood, but benzoic acid is excreted as hippuric acid and acidifies the urine. It is also used as a preservative in certain foodstuffs and beverages: eg. fruit cordials, pickles.

BENZOIN is a balsamic resin, which is an ingredient of inhalations used in the treatment of bronchitis and common colds. The most widely used of these is Friars' balsam. (See BALSAMS.)

BENZOTHIADIAZINES, or THIAZIDES, are a group of diuretics which are effective when taken by mouth. They act by virtue of inhibiting the reabsorption of sodium and chloride in the renal tubules. They also have a blood-pressure-lowering effect. Chlorothiazide was the first member of this group to be introduced, but is now being replaced by hydrochlorothiazide. Another widely used member of this important group of drugs is bendrofluazide.

BENZYL BENZOATE is widely used as a lotion in the treatment of scabies (qv)

BENZYLPENICILLIN (see PENICILLIN).

BERGER RHYTHM is the term applied to normal rhythmical changes of electric potential in the brain. The electrical 'waves' can be recorded graphically as in the electro-encephalogram (qv). A person with epilepsy has abnormal waves.

BERIBERI, called by the Japanese KARKÉ, is a disease found in Japan, Malaysia, China, Manila, Fiji Islands, India, West Africa, Western Australia and round the Gulf of Mexico, and consists in inflammation of the nerves all over the body. (See NEURITIS.)

Causes – It is found among those living in certain parts of the tropics, whose diet consists mainly of highly milled rice. It also occurs in Newfoundland and Labrador, where the inhabitants' main item of diet is white wheaten flour. In both groups of population the removal of the husk of rice and of the wheat berry leaves the diet very deficient in vitamin B_1 (thiamine). It is the lack of this vitamin that causes the trouble.

Symptoms – The affected person becomes, first of all, for some days feverish and weak; then, though feeling better in general health, he gradually develops symptoms of paralysis, especially of the hands and feet, dropsy, palpitation of the heart and loss of sensation in large areas of the skin, especially about the legs. These pass off, in general, in the course of some weeks, and the sufferer gradually recovers health, or occasionally he gets worse and dies from heart failure.

Treatment – The treatment required is large doses of vitamin B_1 (thiamine) (qv), plenty of nourishing food, and complete rest.

BERKEFELD FILTER is a candle-shaped filter made of diatomaceous earth. It restrains ordinary bacteria but lets through viruses.

BERRIES, POISONOUS – As most berries in Britain are either red or blackish in colour when ripe, their colour is one of the simplest ways of distinguishing them.

Black poisonous berries – One of the most poisonous of these is the *deadly nightshade* (*Atropa belladonna*) (illustration 70). Three berries are sufficient to kill a child. Ripening from July onwards, they are dull black in colour, often as large as a small marble, and surrounded by a persistent withered calyx. The plant usually grows in semi-shaded sites and is up to three feet (1 metre) in height. Even more poisonous, but fortunately less common, is the *baneberry* (*Actaea spicata*) which grows in woods on limestone in Yorkshire, Lancashire and Westmorland. The berries are nearly a quarter of an inch (6 mm) in diameter and grow on stems one or two feet (30 to 60 cm) long. More common is *Herb Paris* (*Paris quadrifolia*), which grows in semi-shaded sites, and has stems up to two feet (60 cm) high. The berries are up to a quarter of an inch (6 mm) in diameter and contain 16 to 20 dark-coloured seeds. The *buckthorn* (*Rhamnus cathartica*) and the *alder buckthorn* (*Rhamnus frangula*) (illustration 71) are shrubs up to 20 feet (6 metres) in height which grow in woody thickets on peaty soil. The berries grow in clusters and are about the size of blackcurrants. Each berry contains four seeds. Only on unpruned *privets* (*Ligustrum vulgare* (illustration 72) and *Ligustrum ovaliform*) are berries found in quantity. About the size of a pea, the berry has two chambers inside, usually with one or two seeds in each. These berries have caused fatal poisoning in children. The *cherry laurel* (*Prunus laurocerasus*), commonly grown in gardens and parks, produces in late summer small berries very like small black cherries except that the fruit stalk is short and rigid and the berries, up to about twelve in number, are borne along a common stalk 4 inches (10 cm) long. The *spurge laurel*

70 – Atropa belladonna.

71 – Rhamnus frangula.

72 – Ligustrum vulgare.

74 – Solanum dulcamara.

(*Daphne laureola*), which grows sparingly in woodlands in England, produces egg-shaped blue-black berries on stems which grow to about four feet (1·25 metres) in height. The *ivy* (*Hedera helix*) (illustration 73) produces berries about the size of a pea which ripen in early spring.

Red poisonous berries – These are even more dangerous because their colour is so much more attractive to children. The *woody nightshade* or *bittersweet* (*Solanum dulcamara*) (illustration 74), which is common in South and Central England, is a straggling plant which bears clusters of six to eight bright-red translucent berries. These are very like redcurrants except

that there is no tuft of old flower parts at the upper end of the fruit and they contain numerous seeds, compared with the six or eight in the redcurrant. The *white bryony* (*Bryonia dioica*) is another scrambling plant of the wayside and wasteland. It is most commonly found in Southern England and is almost entirely absent in the North. The berry is dull scarlet in colour, about a centimetre in diameter and contains three to six large flat, yellow-and-black mottled berries. The *black bryony* (*Tamus communis*) (illustration 75) is another straggling plant. The berries are bright crimson in colour and grow in small bunches. Superficially they are like

73 – Hedera helix.

75 – Tamus communis.

76 – Arum maculatum.

redcurrants. The *cuckoo-pint* or *lords and ladies* (*Arum maculatum*) (illustration 76), which grows in damp woodlands, sometimes in hedgerows, especially on basic soils, produces bright-red berries which ripen from August onwards. The berries, about the size of a pea, grow in clusters of eight to twenty at the upper end of a sturdy, naked, green stem about six to nine inches (15 to 22 cm) long, and bear three small marks at the apex and usually contain three brownish, rough-coated seeds. The *dwarf baytree* (*Daphne mezereum*) (illustration 77), which is usually cultivated in gardens because of its heavily scented, pink or purplish flowers from

77 – Daphne mezereum.

January onwards, bears small clusters of red berries from August onwards. They may be mistaken for redcurrants but can be distinguished by the lack of a tuft of withered flower parts at the upper end of the fruit. The berry of the *yew* (*Taxus baccata*) (illustration 78), which grows naturally in Southern Britain, and is planted widely elsewhere for ornament, ripens from August onwards. The pale, half-inch-long (12 mm) seed is half submerged in a soft, red, juicy cup. This fleshy cup, which has a sickly sweet taste, is not particularly poisonous, but the seed is highly poisonous.

For fuller details the reader is referred to *Bulletin 161. British Poisonous Plants*, published by the Ministry of Agriculture and Fisheries, and obtainable from Her Majesty's Stationery Office.

[The nine illustrations in this section are reproduced by courtesy of L. Reeve & Co. Ltd., from *Illustrations of the British Flora*, fifth edition, by W. H. Fitch and W. G. Smith.]

78 – Taxus baccata.

BERYLLIOSIS is a disease of the lungs caused by the inhalation of particles of beryllium oxide.

BETAMETHASONE is a corticosteroid (qv) which has an action comparable to that of prednisolone, but in much lower dosage. In the form of BETAMETHASONE VALERATE it is used as an application to the skin as an ointment, cream or lotion.

BETATRON (see RADIOTHERAPY).

BETHANIDINE is a hypotensive drug which acts by blocking the sympathetic nervous system.

BEZOAR is a concretion found in the stomach and intestines of animals, especially goats, which was formerly used as a remedy against poisoning. It is also occasionally found in man.

BICARBONATE OF SODA, or BAKING SODA (see ALKALI).

BIDET is a fixed sitz-bath raised on legs which is used for administering douches and enemas.

BIGUANIDES are a group of chemical substances which act as oral hypoglycaemic agents (that is, reduce the level of the blood sugar when given by mouth), and are proving of value in the treatment of diabetes mellitus. They include metformin (qv) and phenformin (qv). Their precise mode of action is not known, but they appear to increase the using up of glucose either directly or indirectly by facilitating the action of insulin. (See DIABETES MELLITUS.)

BILE is a thick, bitter, golden-brown or greenish-yellow fluid, secreted by the liver, and stored in the gall-bladder. It consists of water, mucus, pigments (bilirubin and biliverdin), salts of three complex acids (cholic, chenodeoxycholic and deoxycholic acids), cholesterol and some mineral salts, and it is discharged through the bile-ducts into the intestine, a few inches below the opening from the stomach. This discharge is constant, but is much increased shortly after food is taken, and again, some hours later, when the food is digested. Bile is partly an excretion of waste material thrown out by the liver, partly a secretion endowed with some functions in digestion, especially that of fats, and it further aids the absorption of nourishment from the food passing down the bowels, and prevents excessive decomposition by destroying various micro-organisms. About a pint to a quart (0·5 to 1 litre) is secreted daily in man, but the greater part of this is reabsorbed with the food, passes into the blood, and ultimately circulates back to the liver, to be again excreted, and so on.

Jaundice is a condition in which the flow of bile becomes obstructed, so that the bile is not poured into the intestine, but circulates in the blood. As a consequence, the bile pigments are deposited in the tissues, and the skin becomes yellow or olive-green, while, at the same time, the stools become grey or white and the urine dark. (See JAUNDICE.)

Bilious headache, or biliousness, is a vague term, applied either to migraine (see HEADACHE) or to the headache and vomiting which occur in acute catarrh of the stomach set up by errors in diet. (See DYSPEPSIA.)

Vomiting of bile occurs in the two last-named conditions, and is also a sign of obstruction of the bowels, but bile may be brought up in any case of persistent vomiting or retching.

BILHARZIASIS is another name for schistosomiasis (qv).

BILIRUBIN is the chief pigment in human bile. It is derived from haemoglobin (qv) which is the red pigment of the red blood corpuscles. The site of manufracture of bilirubin is the reticulo-endothelial system (qv). When bile is passed into the intestine from the gall-bladder, part of the bilirubin is converted into stercobilin and excreted in the faeces. The remainder is reabsorbed into the blood-stream, and of this portion the bulk goes back to the liver to be re-excreted into the bile, whilst a small proportion is excreted in the urine as urobilinogen.

BILIVERDIN is the chief pigment of bile in herbivora and birds. It is a precursor of bilirubin in the production of the latter from haemoglobin, and there is a small amount in human bile.

BINOVULAR TWINS is the term applied to twins who result from the fertilization of two separate ova.

BIOCHEMISTRY means the chemistry of living organisms and of vital processes.

BIOFEEDBACK is a technique whereby an auditory or visual stimulus follows on from a physiological response. Thus, a subject's electrocardiogram (qv) may be monitored, and a signal passed back to the subject indicating his heart rate: eg, a red light if the rate is between fifty and sixty beats a minute; a green light if it is between sixty and seventy a minute. Once the subject has learned to discriminate between these two rates he can then learn to control his heart rate. How this is learned is not clear, but it is claimed that by this biofeedback it is possible to control the heart rate and blood pressure, relax spastic muscles, and even bring migraine under control.

BIOPSY means the removal and examination of tissue from the living body for diagnostic purposes. For example, a piece of a tumour may be cut out and examined to determine whether it is cancerous.

BIOTIN is one of the dozen or so vitamins included in the vitamin B complex. It is found in liver, eggs, and meat, and it is also synthesized by bacteria in the gut. Absorption from the gut is prevented by avidin, a constituent of egg-white. The daily requirement is small: a fraction of a milligram daily. Gross deficiency results in disturbances of the skin, a smooth tongue and lassitude.

BIPP is a colloquial term used to designate an antiseptic and soothing paste applied to wounds and consisting of bismuth subnitrate, iodoform and paraffin. It was much used in the war of 1914–18.

BIRD FANCIER'S LUNG (see PIGEON BREEDER'S LUNG).

BIRTH (see LABOUR) – The average length of a child at birth is about 21 inches (53 cm), and the weight 7 pounds (3·2 kg). A *stillborn* child is 'any child which has issued forth from its mother after the twenty-eighth week of pregnancy and which did not at any time after being completely expelled from its mother breathe or show any other sign of life'. *Premature birth* is one which takes place before the natural time (see PREMATURE BIRTH), but in which the child is capable of surviving. A birth which takes place so prematurely that the child must necessarily die is known as an abortion or *miscarriage* (see MISCARRIAGE).

BIRTH-MARKS are of various kinds. The most common are port-wine marks (see NAEVUS). Pigment spots are found, very often raised above the surface and more or less hairy, being then called moles (see MOLES).

BISACODYL is a laxative which acts by stimulation of the nerve endings in the colon by direct contact with the mucous lining.

BISMUTH is a metal, of which the carbonate, subnitrate, salicylate, subgallate and oxychloride are used in medicine.
Uses – In irritative and painful conditions of the stomach or of the bowels, eg. when diarrhoea or vomiting is present, they have a sedative action. The salicylate of bismuth especially is used to check diarrhoea, the usual medicinal dose of it or of the subnitrate being about 20 grains (1·2 G). Given internally, bismuth salts turn the stools black. The subgallate is used in the form of suppositories in the treatment of haemorrhoids.

Externally, as dusting powder, they are used, both as a cosmetic and in eczema and other moist conditions of the skin, being commonly mixed, in equal proportions, with starch powder or oxide of zinc, or both.

BITES AND STINGS – Bites of animals are in general to be treated as punctured or lacerated wounds (see WOUNDS), but as animals' teeth are, in general, foul, suppuration is very apt to arise if the bite be deep. The bite of some reptiles, scorpions, spiders, etc., causes definite symptoms of poisoning, while, after the bites of several animals, especially the wolf and the dog, there is often a risk of rabies. Wounds which are *septic*, ie. poisoned by bacteria, are dealt with in the section on WOUNDS.

Dog bites in Britain are treated by washing (not scrubbing) the bite with soap and water, and then applying hydrogen peroxide or cetrimide. The bite is then covered with a dressing. Penicillin is also given as a rule, and measures taken to prevent tetanus. More active treatment is required if there is possible risk of rabies (qv).

Snake bites are not necessarily poisonous, for not only are many snakes harmless, but persons can, like the snake-charmers of India, render themselves immune by the injection under the skin of gradually increasing doses of the poison. It is estimated that the annual death rate from snake bites, throughout the world, is 25,000 to 35,000, of which 20,000 to 25,000 occur in India. In Europe there are probably only 2 or 3 fatal cases every year. The last fatal case reported in England and Wales occurred in 1957, and in the previous fifty years only seven deaths due to snake bite had been reported. There was a fatal case in Scotland in 1975. In the five years up to 1974 the Regional Poisons Treatment Centre at Edinburgh Royal Infirmary had inquires about six children and five adults bitten by adders; none died.

The principal poisonous snakes belong to the viper and cobra families, and all inject their poison through a pair of grooved or hollow teeth connected with poison glands. These include in Asia the cobra, the king cobra, the krait, the deboia and the phoorsa; in America the rattlesnake, the copperhead, and the moccasin; in South America the fer-de-lance and the coral snake; in Africa cobras, vipers and the puff-adder; and in Australia the death-adder, tiger snake, copperhead, brown snake and black snake. The sea snakes of the Pacific and Indian Oceans are almost all poisonous. The only poisonous snake in Britain is the adder (*Vipera berus*). It is chiefly found in Scotland, Dartmoor and the New Forest. It is not found in Ireland. In a not inconsiderable number of cases of adder bite the victim is to blame as he has attempted to handle or torment the snake. Adders are not aggressive and usually try to get out of the way of humans. This they should be allowed to do without any let or hindrance.

The symptoms of snake-poisoning are swelling and paralysis of the bitten part, with general depression, palpitation, difficulty of breathing, faintness and later paralysis and convulsions, followed, in severe cases, by death. These symptoms appear within fifteen minutes to an hour after the bite. After the bite of a deboia or of one of the rattlesnakes very severe suppuration may occur in the neighbourhood of the bite in people who recover.

Treatment of an adder bite in Britain consists of immobilizing the limb by splinting, washing the wound with water, and giving an analgesic to relieve the pain. Medical advice should then be sought immediately, no matter how mild may appear to be the immediate effects of the bite. Expert opinion is divided as to whether or not antivenine (qv) should be given. Outside Britain, where the consequences can be much more serious, treatment consists of applying a tourniquet between the bite and the body, to prevent the poison being absorbed into the body. This should be released for a few seconds every fifteen minutes, in order to prevent gangrene. The bite should then be sucked vigorously for five-minute periods at frequent intervals. A serum known as *antivenine* (qv) is available as an antidote against many snake bites, and this should be injected intravenously in liberal amounts as soon as possible. Antivenoms are also becoming available which are active against the venoms of individual snakes, such as the carpet viper (*Echis carinatus*) which is widely distributed in Northern Africa, the Middle East, Pakistan, India and Sri Lanka. The individual should also be treated as for shock, ie. resting quietly, kept warm, and given a blood transfusion and oxygen if necessary. As stimulants, sal volatile, strong tea, or coffee may be given, *not* alcohol.

Poisonous fishes exist in most tropical waters, especially around the islands of the Pacific and Indian Oceans, and their venom may be conveyed to man either by poisonous stings or by their bite. The action of the poison is mostly a depressing one upon the heart, and in the case of some of the tropical fishes convulsions and even death may be produced.

Weever fish (known as bishop fish in Cornwall), which are found on Atlantic coasts, as well as on sandy Mediterranean coasts, have poisonous spines which can cause painful wounds – usually in the feet. As the poison is destroyed by heat, the affected foot should be repeatedly bathed in water as hot as the victim can tolerate. A wise precaution is to wear suitable footwear when paddling or bathing.

Jelly-fish around British shores are fairly harmless, with the exception of the so-called Portuguese Man-of-War which occasionally invades our coasts. It has been described as looking 'rather like a pale blue Cornish pastie with a dark line down its back', and has tentacles up to 40 feet (13 metres) in length. The first thing to do in treatment is to withdraw the tentacle if it is still in the skin but this must not be done with the naked hand without the risk of being stung. A glove of wet sand, however, will usually give sufficient protection. The affected part should then be sprayed or gently washed with methylated spirit. Antihistamine preparations may also be helpful, either applied locally as a cream or, in more serious cases, given by mouth or by injection.

The stings of the much more dangerous jelly-fish found in North Australian and Pacific and Indian waters may prove fatal unless immediate medical attention is available.

Sea-urchins are a hazard, particularly to skin divers, because of their spines. The main culprit is *Paracentrobus lividus*, a sea urchin found on rocks in the Mediterranean, the Atlantic coasts of France and Spain, and the south coast of England. It has a black body, 1 to 2 inches (2·5 to 5 cm) in diameter, covered with sharp, purple articulated spines an inch (2·5 cm) long. The most severe injuries occur from treading on, or diving on to, collections of them on rocks. This produces a severe burning pain. Prevention consists of avoiding rocky shores when swimming or diving. First-aid treatment consists of removal of the spines as soon as possible. This may require the use of a local anaesthetic or anaesthetizing the skin with ethyl chloride (qv). Once removed, an antiseptic dressing

BITOSCANATE

should be applied to the affected area until the wound heals. If not removed, the spine may result in a small tender cyst and, if this is burst as a result of pressure on it, there may be a recurrence of severe burning pain.

Toads and salamanders secrete a milky fluid from the skin of the back which is irritating locally, and which, in small animals and weakly children, is said to kill if introduced by a wound.

Centipedes, scorpions and tarantulas (large tropical spiders) kill their prey by poison, and can inflict a very painful, though probably seldom fatal, bite on human beings. The treatment is to apply a ligature as for snake bite at once, and to suck the wound or wash it well with a strong solution of permanganate of potassium. Some other substances have also a reputation as antidotes, such as ammonia, spirit of camphor, tobacco juice, turpentine, and camphor and chloral rubbed up together. An antitoxic serum has been prepared for use against scorpion bite in Egypt. If an abscess forms it is treated like an abscess from any other cause.

Harvest-bugs, fleas, ticks, lice and mosquitoes often cause great irritation of the skin by their bite. Harvest-bugs may bury themselves in the skin and have to be picked out with a needle. Dimethyl phthallate applied to the skin or clothing is an effective repellent. Human beings vary much in their susceptibility to flea bites. The best preventive is dimethyl phthalate. Failing this, smearing the skin with oil of pennyroyal or oil of lavender is helpful, or dusting the underwear and socks with pyrethrum powder, menthol or camphor. Ticks are common parasites of household pets in Britain but seldom attack human beings. In Scotland, however, bites by sheep ticks are accepted as a natural minor hazard of life. The best preventive is dimethyl phthalate or diethyltoluamide. It may be dislodged from the skin by applying the lighted end of a cigarette or the hot end of a match that has just been lit and blown out, or covering it with alcohol, petrol or petroleum jelly. Once bitten, calamine lotion relieves the itching. Lice may be got rid of, if in the hair, by the application of a 2 per cent emulsion of DDT. They may be got rid of from the clothes by baking these in an oven or fumigating with burning sulphur for several hours, or by the use of DDT. (See also under INSECTS IN RELATION TO DISEASE.) Bites by mosquitoes or bugs are soothed by bathing with salt water, by painting with sal volatile or calamine lotion, or by applying an antihistamine cream or ointment. They may be prevented by smearing the skin with dimethyl phthalate (qv), or, if this is not available, camphor water, lime juice or one of the oils of pennyroyal, lavender, cloves or cinnamon.

Trombicula autumnalis is the harvest mite. It is also known as red bug and chigger. It is found in the fields in the autumn and attacks man by crawling up the legs. Measuring 1 × 1·5 mm, it can pass through ordinary clothing. It produces local redness and itching. Relief from the itching is obtained by bathing the affected part with weak ammonia or baking soda, or calamine lotion with or without the addition of 0·5 to 1 per cent phenol. Bites may be prevented by the use of an insect-repellent cream containing dimethyl phthalate and diethyltoluamide which is obtainable from most chemists without a prescription.

Ants, bees, wasps and hornets cause great irritation by the stings with which they are provided. Those of ants are allayed by eau-de-Cologne, vinegar or lemon juice. Bees sometimes leave a part of their sting as well as poison in the skin, and this should be looked for first of all and carefully wiped out. The sting of a wasp in the throat, the insect having been taken into the mouth in biting a fruit, has caused death owing to rapid swelling, which blocks the air passage. In England and Wales, in the ten-year period, 1962–71, there were 47 deaths due to insect stings: wasps were responsible for 33, and bees for 11; in three the insect was not identified. Most of these deaths were due to stings in the throat. For bee stings the treatment is the dabbing on of ammonia, bicarbonate of soda or washing blue. For wasp and hornet stings a weak acid, such as vinegar or lemon juice, is said to be better.

Hairy-caterpillars, by brittle, poisoned hairs, cause an itchy red rash after contact. It is relieved by vinegar or olive oil.

Nettle stings are relieved by bruised dock leaves or raw onion juice.

BITOSCANATE is a drug that is proving of value in the treatment of hookworm infestations. (See FILARIASIS.)

BITTERS are among the oldest of drugs still prescribed. Wormwood, probably the oldest of them all, though never prescribed as such today, being one of the main constituents of absinthe (qv), is mentioned in the Papyrus Ebers from a tomb in Thebes (1500 BC), and bitters are referred to in the Hippocratic writings (*circa* 400 BC). They are alcoholic extracts of herbs used to stimulate the appetite and to a lesser extent as flavours for tonics and other remedies. There are three main groups of bitters:

(*1*) *SIMPLE BITTERS* – These are used to stimulate appetite and the action of the stomach, and they include calumba, gentian (qv) and quassia (qv).

(*2*) *AROMATIC BITTERS* – These combine the property of bitterness with that of aromatic volatile oils, and are commonly used as flavours and carminatives (qv). They include cardamom (qv) and orange.

(*3*) *INCIDENTAL BITTERS* – These are drugs which act as bitters, but this action is incidental to more important therapeutic effects. These include aloes (qv), quinine (qv) and strychnine (nux vomica). (See STRYCHNINE.)

The precise action of bitters is not known, and the modern tendency in medicine is to look upon them as a remnant of the days when medicine was more of an art than a science. Granted that the wise thing is to try and find out the cause of any loss of appetite, but often this is not possible. It is in these circumstances that bitters, which are definitely known to increase gastric secretion, often have a beneficial effect in improving the individual's interest in food. Whether or not this is psychological may be open to question but, whatever the reason, if it results in an individual's appetite improving, then something has been achieved.

BLACK DEATH is an old name for plague. (See PLAGUE.)

BLACKFAT TOBACCO DISEASE is a form of pneumonia caused by the smoking of blackfat tobacco, a tobacco flavoured with a mineral oil known as canopus oil. It is a popular tobacco in the West Indies and West Africa, but to date cases of blackfat tobacco disease have only been reported in Guyana.

BLACK DRAUGHT is a powerful purgative preparation, known also as compound senna mixture, and containing Epsom salts, senna and liquorice. The dose is two to three tablespoonfuls.

BLACK DROP is another name for laudanum or tincture of opium. (See OPIUM.)

BLACKHEADS (see ACNE).

BLACK MOTIONS are passed when there is great constipation, and when bismuth or iron is being taken; but the most important cause is blood changed by the digestive processes, and proceeding from ulceration somewhere in the stomach or bowels.

BLACK VOMIT is due to the presence of blood in the stomach. There may be dark masses, as in yellow fever, or a small amount of black sediment like coffee-grounds, as in ulcer of the stomach.

BLACKWATER FEVER is an acute illness characterized by haemoglobinuria ('black water'), jaundice, fever, vomiting, anaemia, and severe haemolysis. It is associated with malignant tertian malaria, and occurs in Central Africa, India and the Far East.

Although the precise cause is still obscure, it is known that the disease may be precipitated in malarial subjects by the taking of quinine or by exposure to cold, by fatigue, and by trauma. Predisposing factors include exposure by non-immune individuals to virulent strains of the malarial parasite and irregular and inadequate treatment of such infections. The mortality rate usually varies between 10 and 20 per cent, but may be as high as 40 per cent.

Symptoms – These are fever, rigor, nausea, bilious vomiting, epigastric discomfort, jaundice and the passage of pinkish, red or port-wine coloured urine – haemoglobinuria. The spleen and liver are enlarged and tender. After a few hours the temperature falls, there is profuse sweating, and the skin becomes jaundiced. Mild cases may recover in a day or two. Severe cases have a succession of attacks.

Treatment – This consists in (1) absolute rest in bed; (2) administration of plenty of alkaline fluids; (3) glucose given intravenously (and sodium bicarbonate if necessary); (4) blood transfusion, and subsequent remedies for anaemia. Recent evidence suggests that corticosteroids are of value. Careful nursing is most important.

BLADDERS are sacs formed of muscular and fibrous tissue and lined by a mucous membrane, which is united loosely to the muscular coat, so as to allow freely of increase and decrease in the contained cavity. Bladders are designed to contain some secretion or excretion, and communicate with the exterior by a narrow opening through which their contents can be discharged. In man there are two, the *gall-bladder* and the *urinary bladder*.

GALL-BLADDER – This is situated under the liver in the upper part of the abdomen, and its function is to store the bile, which it discharges into the intestine by the bile duct. For further details, see LIVER.

URINARY BLADDER – This is situated in the pelvis, in front of the last part of the bowel. The bladder, in the full state, rises up into the abdomen and holds about a pint (570 ml) of urine. Two fine tubes, called the ureters, lead into the bladder, one from each kidney; and the urethra, a tube as wide as a lead pencil when distended. leads from it to the exterior, a distance of $1\frac{1}{2}$ inches (4 cm) in the female and 8 inches (20 cm) in the male.

Structure – The wall of the bladder is similar in structure to that of the bowels, and consists of four coats. The inner surface is lined by a soft mucous membrane covered by epithelial cells of irregular shape. This is attached to the muscular coat by a loose, fibrous, sub-mucous coat, in which run numerous blood-vessels. In the muscular coat the muscle fibres are arranged in several layers, and run in various directions, thereby adding greatly to the strength of the wall. On its upper and back part, the bladder possesses a covering of serous membrane, formed by part of the general peritoneal lining of the abdominal cavity, but this outermost coat does not extend down to the base of the bladder, where the latter lies in close contact with the other pelvic organs. The bladder is suspended in position by numerous ligaments, four of which are fibrous bands, while the remaining five are formed by thickened portions of the peritoneum. The base of the bladder is directed downwards and backwards, and in this part are the three openings of the ureters and urethra. The exit from the bladder is kept closed by a muscular ring, which is relaxed every time water is passed.

BLADDER, DISEASES OF – For diseases of the gall-bladder see GALL-BLADDER. (See also URINE.)

The urinary bladder is subject to several diseases, but, partly owing to its inaccessibility, as it lies deep in the pelvis behind the pubic bones, partly owing to general ignorance as to its site and functions, symptoms set up in it are often attributed to the bowels and other organs. Diseased conditions in it are diagnosed in part by the symptoms they set up, in part by chemical and microscopical examination of the urine, and in the more obscure conditions by means of the cystoscope. The *cystoscope* consists of a narrow metal tube fitted up as a telescope, and bearing at its end a small electric lamp by which the cavity is lighted up. The instrument is introduced through the urethra, and shows any tumour or ulcer which may exist, and also whether blood in the urine comes from the bladder wall or runs out of the ureters from the kidneys. (See CYSTOSCOPE.) *Sounding* is another process, consisting in the introduction of a curved solid metal rod, when the presence of a stone is suspected, against which the sound can be felt or heard to strike. *Catheters* are tubes about the thickness of quills, which are made of metal, vulcanite, india-rubber, etc., and are used to draw off the water when it is not possible to expel this voluntarily, or, when the bladder is to be washed out for some diseased condition. (See CATHETERS.) The following are some of the chief diseased conditions:

CYSTITIS, or INFLAMMATION OF THE BLADDER – **Causes** – Bacteria live readily in the urine but they do not multiply in the healthy bladder. When some cause is present to weaken the bladder wall, or, when bacteria are introduced in large numbers, for example on a dirty catheter, they multiply inside this organ and set up inflammation.

There may be direct infection from neighbouring organs, as the urethra in gonorrhoea. Any cause that prevents the free voiding of the urine, such as stricture or narrowing of the urethra, or enlargement of the prostate gland at the outlet of the bladder, which is a common occurrence in elderly men, may produce a chronic form of cystitis. In women it is commonly associated with prolapse of the womb. A stone, if present, is apt by its irritation to do the same. One of the most frequent organisms found in the urine in cases of cystitis is the common colon bacillus (or *Escherichia coli*, as it is now known). Tuberculous cystitis may be found, due to the *Mycobacterium tuberculosis* which produces a chronic ulcer on the bladder wall. Another very chronic form is caused by the schistosome, a small parasitic worm which may settle in the minute blood-vessels of the bladder wall. This form is very common in Egypt and South Africa. (See SCHISTOSOMIASIS.)

Symptoms – Pain in the region of the bladder or in the small of the back, frequency of making water, and a condition of bad smell, turbidity and whitish sediment in the urine, are the chief facts noticed by the sufferer. In acute cases there may be high temperature and shivering fits. In the chronic form the very frequent desire to pass small quantities of urine is the most marked symptom.

Treatment – Rest in bed and hot applications, like rubber hot water bottles to the lower part of the abdomen, along with simple diet and large quantities of bland fluid, such as barley water, to drink, may be all that is necessary. Large doses of potassium citrate are also helpful, usually combined in a mixture with tincture of hyoscyamus. In the majority of cases, however, it is necessary to give drugs that will destroy the causative organism. In practice this means one of the sulphonamides or antibiotics. The choice is dependent upon which organism is responsible for the infection, and this is determined by submitting a specimen of urine to bacteriological investigation.

STONE, or CALCULUS, in the bladder may be of any size up to that of a hen's or goose's egg, or even larger. The largest one ever seen in England, in 1809, is said to have weighed 2¾ pounds (1·36 kg). An almost equally large one, weighing 2½ pounds (1·13 kg) was removed in a London hospital in 1975. There are three varieties of stone: (*a*) URATIC, associated with acidity (see ACIDITY) or with the gouty constitution; (*b*) OXALIC, composed of oxalate of lime, and often associated with a nervous dyspeptic type of temperament; (*c*) PHOSPHATIC, which occur in long-standing cases of inflammation of the bladder, accompanied by constant demomposition of the urine. This is the most common type of stone found in the bladder.

Symptoms – The symptoms of inflammation of the bladder, together with discomfort on movement, and sudden pain immediately after the passing of water, are those generally found.

Treatment – Although control of the diet may reduce the tendency to the formation of stones in the bladder, the only method of treatment once they have formed is surgical removal. In spite of many vaunted claims, there is no drug known which can remove, or dissolve, stones in the bladder. In 1739 a secret remedy sold by Mrs Joanna Stephens was considered so effectual in stones that the secret was bought by the British Government for £5000. It was found to consist of calcined egg shells, soap and aromatic bitters – that is, its essentials were lime, phosphates and alkalies. Surgical removal

of the stone (or stones) is carried out by either *litholapaxy* or *lithotomy*. Litholapaxy consists of passing into the bladder through the urethra an instrument known as a lithotrite which crushes the stone, after which the small pieces are removed through the urethra. The advantage of this method is that no incision is required and the patient is only laid up for one or two days. If the stone is larger than 2 inches (5 cm) in diameter, however, or if there are too many stones present, lithotomy has to be performed: ie. the bladder is opened through an incision in the lower abdominal wall and the stone (or stones) are removed in this way.

TUMOURS in the bladder are often the cause of large quantities of bright blood being passed with the urine. For their removal the bladder is opened through the lower part of the abdomen. Some respond well to radio-active isotopes. (See ISOTOPE.)

RUPTURE of the bladder may occur in old men who have long suffered from difficulty in passing water and cystitis, or in healthy persons owing to a blow or crush. (See ABDOMEN, INJURIES OF.)

BLAUD'S PILL is a pill containing carbonate of iron, used in the treatment of anaemia.

BLEEDER is a term applied to persons in whom it is difficult to stop bleeding when some small wound has been sustained. (See HAEMOPHILIA.)

BLEEDING (see HAEMORRHAGE; and BLOOD-LETTING).

BLENORRHOEA means an excessive discharge of mucus or slimy material from a surface, such as that of the eye, nose, bowel, etc. The word catarrh is used with the same meaning, but also includes the idea of inflammation as the cause of such discharge.

BLEOMYCIN is an antibiotic, obtained from *Streptomyces verticillus*, that is being used with a certain amount of success in the treatment of cancer of the upper part of the gut, the genital tract and lymphomas.

BLEPHARITIS means inflammation of the eyelids. (See EYE DISEASES AND INJURIES.)

BLEPHAROSPASM means spasm of the eyelids.

BLIGHTED OVUM, or BLIGHTED FOETUS, is the term used to describe a condition in which apparently normal development of the embryo and its surrounding membranes continues for a short time and then the embryo dies, leaving the membranes alive for a little longer. The causes are not clear but are assumed to be either defects (possibly hereditary) in the ovum or fertilizing sperm, or some fault in the mother's womb. (See ABORTION; and FOETUS.)

BLINDNESS – In the National Assistance Act, 1948, a 'blind person' is defined as one 'so blind as to be unable to perform any work for which eyesight is essential'. In the case of children, the term 'blind' includes not only the totally blind, but also those who cannot be taught by visual methods which make use of large print, blackboard writing, or lenses for magnifying ordinary print. At December 31, 1967, the number of registered blind, according to these definitions, in England and Wales was 102,597. These included 12 infants aged under one year, 381 children aged one to four years, 1778 aged five to fifteen, and 71,807 adults aged 65 and over. Among the 2210 blind persons under the age of 65, registered in 1967, the commonest cause was diabetes mellitus, which was responsible for 14·7 per cent of cases. Next in order of frequency came myopia (13·8 per cent), optic atrophy (10·8 per cent), glaucoma (7·8 per cent), cataract (6 per cent). Congenital syphilis was responsible for 1·4 per cent. The latest available figures show that at March 31, 1977, 112,935 people were registered as blind in England, Wales and Northern Ireland, while at March 31, 1974, there were 10,063 in Scotland. (See also VISION.)

Any blind person, or his or her relatives, can obtain help and advice from the Royal National Institute for the Blind, 224–228 Great Portland Street, London, WIN 6AA.

BLIND SPOT (see EYE).

BLISTERS AND COUNTER-IRRITANTS – These are employed in cases of both acute and chronic inflammation, on the principle that irritation of the skin causes congestion of the parts immediately below the skin, while it relieves congestion of deep-seated organs through an action upon the nerves that regulate the size of the minute blood-vessels.

Varieties – Substances so employed are spoken of generally as counter-irritants, and divided into *rubefacients*, or substances which merely redden the skin and cause it to peel off; and *vesicants*, or blistering applications, when, in addition, they produce a collection of fluid under the horny layer of the skin; but there is no sharp division between them, most rubefacients producing blisters if left on long enough. The chief *rubefacients* are: mustard, turpentine, cajuput oil, capsicum, tincture of iodine and liniments of ammonia, chloroform, etc., and of *vesicants* we have cantharides or Spanish fly, pure acetic acid, ammonia and chloroform.

The CAUTERY is also used for this purpose. (See CAUTERY.)

Uses – MILDER COUNTER-IRRITANTS are used in cases of bronchitis, congestion of the stomach with vomiting, vague rheumatic pain, sprains and when a prolonged application is desired, so that some swelling or thickening due to chronic inflammation may be absorbed, or some continued pain lessened.

BLISTERS are used (1) to subdue severer forms of pain and inflammation, for example, in pleurisy, pericarditis and sciatica, in which case they are applied a little distance away from the seat of pain; and (2) to promote absorption of thickenings and effusions in joints, etc., in which case the blister is applied to the skin immediately over the affected part.

How to apply a blister or counter-irritant – *Mustard* is made into a paste and spread on muslin or brown paper, and so applied directly to the skin for twenty to thirty minutes, until a warm glow is felt. Mustard leaves can also be purchased and similarly used after moistening. If a more powerful action be desired, mustard may be dusted thickly over the surface of a linseed-meal poultice, and this applied for a similar length of time. After-redness is less if muslin has been placed between the mustard and the skin.

One must be careful not to apply mustard too long in weak persons and children, or a slough may result. For a milder effect the paste may be made with equal quantities of mustard and flour. The skin should be sponged with warm water, dried, and anointed with a little Simple Ointment BP after the mustard is removed.

Turpentine and *cajuput oil* are generally sprinkled, about a teaspoonful at a time, upon flannel cloths, which are then wrung out of hot water, and used for pain in the abdomen or back. (See POULTICES and FOMENTATIONS.)

Tincture of iodine is usually painted on the skin once or twice a day till the cuticle comes off in flakes, but just short of blistering. It is used over joints.

Cantharides blisters are produced by painting on Liquor Epispasticus (blistering fluid), or by applying cantharides plaster, but are never used today in Britain because of their dangers, though they are still in use in some European countries.

Acetic acid, ammonia, and *chloroform* are used by soaking a piece of lint of the required size in one of these fluids, applying it, and covering with a watch-glass till the blister rises.

BLOOD is the fluid which circulates through the arteries, capillaries, and veins, exchanging fluid and gases with the bodily tissues. The latter receive the products absorbed from the food and the oxygen taken up by the blood in its passage through the lungs, while the blood removes from the tissues carbon dioxide to discharge it in the lungs, and various waste products, of which it rids itself in its passage through the kidneys.

millimetre of blood, the blood of women containing slightly fewer than that of men. The *white corpuscles* are of several different kinds, and wander through the walls of the small blood-vessels, upon occasion, into the tissues; here they have many functions to perform, of which the chief are the repair of wounds, the absorption of foreign bodies, and the destruction of bacteria; their dead bodies form, when in large numbers, the matter or pus of abscesses. Their number is less than 1 to 500 of the red corpuscles. They are bigger than the red blood cells, ranging in diameter from around 10 to 15 micrometres. The chief varieties of white corpuscles are those with a single large nucleus (monocytes), those with a nucleus consisting of several variously shaped parts (polymorphonuclear), and small corpuscles resembling those formed in the lymphatic glands (lymphocytes). They are also classed according to whether the granules they contain stain with a blue alkaline dye (basophil) or with a red acid dye (eosinophil). The *blood platelets* are extremely minute, and play some important part in clotting. The range of the normal blood count is shown in table 5.

Red corpuscles: Men	4·5 to 6·5 million per c.mm
Red corpuscles: Women	4·0 to 5·5 million per c.mm
Haemoglobin: Men	13·5 to 18 G. per 100 ml
Haemoglobin: Women	12·0 to 16 G. per 100 ml
White corpuscles	4000 to 10,000 per c.mm
Neutrophils	2500 to 7000 per c.mm
Eosinophils	50 to 400 per c.mm
Basophils	20 to 200 per c.mm
Lymphocytes	1500 to 3000 per c.mm
Monocytes	200 to 800 per c.mm
Platelets	150,000 to 500,000 per c.mm

Table 5 – Range of normal blood count.

Composition – The blood consists, in addition to the fluid, of minute bodies, or corpuscles. These are of three kinds: red corpuscles, white corpuscles and blood platelets. In the *fluid* are dissolved the various salts and proteins which nourish the tissues (see also LYMPH), and also the waste products, such as uric acid, destined for removal from the body. The *red corpuscles* act as the carriers of oxygen; each is a disc, with an average diameter of 7·2 micrometres (about $\frac{1}{3000}$ inch), hollowed out on either surface, and contains a substance called haemoglobin, which acts as a medium of interchange between the oxygen of the air in the lungs, and the tissues requiring it. Each red blood corpuscle, or erythrocyte as it is technically known, contains about 600 million haemoglobin molecules. There are about 5,000,000 red corpuscles in every cubic

Examination of blood – The corpuscles of the blood may be counted. For this purpose a minute drop is drawn up into a special graduated tube provided with a bulb in which the blood is mixed with a suitable diluting fluid. A drop of this diluted blood is blown out upon a special glass slide on which have been ruled with a diamond a number of lines that divide the surface into areas of a 400th square millimetre in size. A cover glass is then lowered upon the drop and so supported on a raised glass rim that a definite distance (0·1 millimetre) separates it from the ruled surface. The slide is then placed under a microscope, the average number of corpuscles that have settled on each square is counted, and thus the number in one four-thousandth of a cubic millimetre is ascertained.

The haemoglobin is estimated by taking

a drop in a fine measured tube, diluting it with distilled water in a graduated tube till it assumes the same tint as a known standard, and then, by reading off the amount of water added, the percentage of haemoglobin is obtained.

Dried films are also prepared by smearing the blood on slides and staining these, usually with aniline dyes, methylene blue, and eosin dissolved in methyl alcohol; in these dried films the corpuscles can be examined by a high magnifying power and a differential count can be made of the various forms.

Formation of blood – The average life of a red blood corpuscle is about 120 days. To renew the wear and tear, as well as to make good losses by wounds, constant manufacture is going on in the marrow of butes foodstuffs, such as sugar and proteins absorbed from the intestine and elaborated by various glands; and it forms a general medium of communication between organs that are chemically interdependent; for example, carrying to the stomach the materials for the gastric juice, to the muscles ferments formed in the pancreas, etc., and absorbing secretions needed for the general purposes of the body, like those of the thyroid gland and suprarenal glands.

BLOOD, DISEASES OF (see ANAEMIA; and LEUKAEMIA).

BLOOD GROUPS – People are divided into four main groups in respect of a certain reaction of the blood. This

79 – Section of blood clot, showing network of strings of fibrin. Magnified 400 times. From Schafer's *Histology*. Longman.

the bones, in some glands, and also probably in the spleen, the daily turnover of haemoglobin being about 6·5 grams.

Amount of blood – In health this is around 85 millilitres per kilogram (2·2 pounds) of body weight, or 9 per cent ($\frac{1}{11}$th) of the weight of the body.

Clotting of blood occurs when blood is shed, and is due to the formation of threads of fibrin (illustration 79), which, as it shrinks, squeezes out from its interstices a clear, faintly straw-coloured fluid – serum. (For details of clotting, see COAGULATION.)

Functions of blood – The red corpuscles act as oxygen carriers; the white corpuscles have mainly a defensive action against the onset of infection. The fluid of the blood carries in solution various waste-products such as carbon dioxide to be exhaled by the lungs, urea and salts to be removed by the kidneys; also it distri-

depends upon the capacity of the serum of one person's blood to agglutinate the red blood corpuscles of another's in certain circumstances. The reaction depends on antigens, known as agglutinogens, in the red corpuscles and antibodies, known as agglutinins, in the serum. There are two of each, the agglutinogens being known as A and B. Anyone's blood corpuscles may have (1) no agglutinogens, (2) agglutinogen A, (3) agglutinogen B, (4) agglutinogens A and B: these are the four groups (table 6).

Group	Agglutinogens in the corpuscles	Agglutinins in the plasma	Frequency in Great Britain
AB	A and B	None	2 per cent
A	A	Anti-B	46 per cent
B	B	Anti-A	8 per cent
O	Neither A nor B	Anti-A and Anti B	44 per cent

Table 6 – The four main blood groups.

The practical importance is that, in blood transfusion, the person giving and the person receiving the blood must belong to the same blood group, or a dangerous reaction will take place from the agglutination that occurs when blood of a different group is present.

Rhesus factor – In addition to these A and B agglutinogens (or antigens) there is another one known as the Rhesus (or Rh) factor, so named because there is a similar antigen in the red blood corpuscles of the Rhesus monkey. About 84 per cent of the population have this Rh factor in their blood and are therefore known as 'Rh-positive'. The remaining 16 per cent who do not possess the factor are known as 'Rh-negative'.

The practical importance of the Rh factor is that, unlike the A and B agglutinogens, there are no naturally occurring Rh antibodies, but such antibodies may develop in an Rh-negative person if the Rh antigen is introduced into his or her circulation. This can occur (*a*) if an Rh-negative person is given a transfusion of Rh-positive blood, (*b*) if an Rh-negative mother married to an Rh-positive husband becomes pregnant and the foetus is Rh-positive. If this happens, the mother develops Rh antibodies which can pass into the foetal circulation, where they react with the baby's Rh antigen and cause haemolytic disease of the foetus and newborn. This means that the child may be stillborn or become jaundiced shortly after birth (see HAEMOLYTIC DISEASE OF THE NEWBORN).

As about one in six expectant mothers is Rh-negative, this explains why a blood-group examination is now considered an essential part of the antenatal examination of a pregnant woman. It also explains why Rh-positive blood should never be transfused to an Rh-negative girl or woman.

BLOODLESSNESS (see ANAEMIA).

BLOOD-LETTING

was a practice much in vogue for various ailments a century ago. Indeed, many people had themselves bled regularly for the purpose of avoiding the bad health consequent on over-eating and over-drinking. It came, in time, to be so much abused – many sick people undoubtedly having died, not of the original disease, but of the excessive bleeding practised for its cure – that it fell into almost complete disuse. Certain conditions are, however, benefited by withdrawing blood either from the affected part or from the general circulation. The chief methods of blood-letting are three in number.

Vein puncture is employed when it is desired to obtain a small quantity of blood for analysis or the performance of various tests. For this purpose a hollow hypodermic needle is pushed into a vein, one of those at the bend of the elbow usually being chosen, while pressure by a band or by the fingers is exerted on the veins in the upper arm. If it is desired to obtain the serum of the blood, the blood is run off into a test tube and allowed to clot. If the blood is required for analysis, clotting may be prevented by adding to the tube, before the blood is drawn off, a few crystals of potassium oxalate or potassium citrate.

Venesection consists in the opening of a vein, usually, owing to its superficial position, one of the veins just above the bend of the elbow. After the desired amount has flowed out, a pad and tight bandage are used to stop the bleeding. This method is of use in certain cases of acute heart failure, when life may depend upon quickly and temporarily relieving the strain on the heart. It is also used in the treatment of polycythaemia (qv).

Cupping was at one time used either as dry-cupping to draw blood to the surface, or as wet-cupping to withdraw blood from a congested area. (See CUPPING.)

Leeches were formerly used to draw blood. After they are removed, bleeding is generally free, and may be encouraged, if desired, by warm poultices. They are seldom used at the present day.

BLOOD-POISONING

is a serious condition, and is known as septicaemia or pyaemia, according as the sufferer is simply poisoned by micro-organisms circulating in the blood, or as he develops, in addition, abscesses at different points over his body, owing to bacteria deposited from the blood. There is a milder form called sapraemia, in which the person becomes fevered and ill owing to the absorption of foul or putrid substances from the bowels or from wounds, but is not dangerously affected, and there is a chronic form called 'hectic fever', in which constant absorption of poisonous material takes place from cavities in the lungs, from diseased bones, etc. (see TUBERCULOSIS).

Causes – Wounds or inflamed areas, especially in bones, joints and veins, may be invaded by specially virulent bacteria, or, owing to great constitutional weakness of the person, for example, in alcoholics or diabetics, the bacteria may find a specially congenial soil for their growth. Women after delivery are specially liable to infection – the condition known as puerperal fever – but this is much less common nowadays as a result of more efficient methods of prevention.

Symptoms – In septicaemia very high temperature, followed speedily by death, may be the only sign. In pyaemia there are, in addition, shivering (rigor), profuse sweating, pains in the joints and muscles and the signs of abscesses at different points, which may last over days or weeks.

Treatment – The introduction of antiseptic surgery by Lord Lister immensely reduced the frequency of blood-poisoning, but the position has been improved out of all recognition by the introduction of the sulphonamides and antibiotics. Which of these should be used in a given case depends upon the causative organism, but in the majority of cases penicillin given intramuscularly is the treatment of choice. Active surgical treatment by amputation, opening of abscesses, antiseptic douches, etc., according to circumstances, may also be necessary.

BLOOD-PRESSURE is the name given to the pressure that must be applied to an artery, say in the arm, in order to stop the pulse in the vessel beyond the point of pressure. It is generally assumed to be equivalent to the pressure to which the blood is subjected by the force of the heart and the elasticity of the vessels, but it is also dependent on the thickness and hardness of the vessel wall, and on the volume of blood thrown out of the heart at each beat.

The blood-pressure is greatest at each heart-beat (systolic pressure) and falls somewhat between the beats (diastolic pressure). The systolic pressure in children is equal to that of a mercury column about 100 mm high, in young adults about 120, and it tends to increase with advancing age as the arteries get thicker and harder, but this is by no means always the case.

The blood-pressure is raised temporarily by exposure to cold, and permanently by kidney disease, by some disorders of the ductless glands, and in the condition known as essential hypertension (qv). A blood-pressure of 180 is not uncommon in cases of chronic kidney disease, and it may, in advanced cases, be as high as 250 or occasionally even 300 mm. Mental worry combined with lack of sufficient exercise has also an important effect in producing raised blood-pressure.

The pressure is below the normal as the result of warmth, eg. after a hot bath, as well as in exhaustion, weakening diseases, fevers and generally in heart failure.

The blood-pressure may be estimated roughly by the pressure with which it is necessary to apply the finger at the wrist in order to obliterate the pulse. It is more exactly measured by means of an instrument known as the *sphygmomanometer*. This consists of a flat rubber bag which is strapped round the arm, and the interior of which communicates by two tubes with either a pressure gauge or a mercury manometer, and with a hand pump. The bag is pumped up so as to constrict the arm, and the systolic pressure is taken as that at which the pulse disappears as felt at the wrist or as heard in the artery at the bend of the elbow.

An abnormally high blood-pressure is often accompanied by disease of the arteries, so that persons with greatly raised pressure are specially liable to apoplexy. In cases associated with advanced disease of the kidneys, the heightened blood-pressure is to some extent a salutary matter, because the circulation of the blood through the diminished vessels of the kidneys is thereby increased. In such a case the general health of the patient is better while the pressure remains moderately high, and if it be reduced too much by drugs and other means the general health deteriorates.

BLOOD-SPITTING (see EXPECTORATION; and HAEMOPTYSIS).

BLOOD TRANSFUSION (see TRANSFUSION OF BLOOD).

'BLOWING' OF CANS means the presence of gas in cans of food, the gas resulting from putrefaction or fermentation of the food, or from the action of fruit on the metal of the container, producing hydrogen. The ends of the can or tin bulge and give a tympanitic note on percussion. The food in such cans should not be eaten.

BLUE DISEASE is a popular term for cyanosis. (See CYANOSIS.)

BLUE PILL, or MERCURY PILL, is a purgative. It contains mercury and liquorice. It is also said to stimulate the activity of the liver. The dose is from 4 to 8 grains (250 to 500 mg).

BLUE STONE is copper sulphate.

BOILS, or FURUNCLES, are small areas of inflammation starting in the roots of hairs, and due to the growth of a micro-organism (generally that known as a staphylococcus). When a large number of boils form close together at one time the mass is called a carbuncle.

Causes – The essential cause is bacterial. Diabetics and the subjects of Bright's disease are specially troubled with boils, so that anyone liable to recurrence of boils should submit himself to medical examination in case he may be suffering from one of these diseases. Persons who eat too much food, or who are recovering from an exhausting illness, are also liable to them. Friction, which irritates the hair roots, is an important cause, and therefore boils are commonest on the back of the neck, on the forearm, and on the leg, while those who row or ride have them about the buttocks.

Symptoms – A red swelling forms round a hair, and causes a good deal of irritation and scratching. It gets larger for some days, being, as a rule, not very painful, unless subject to chafing. When, however, the boil begins on the head, in the ear, or in the nose, where the tissues will not stretch readily, the pain may be very great. Even after two or three days the swelling may slowly subside, and the inflammation gradually pass off, the boil being said to 'abort'. In most cases, about the sixth or seventh day the top of the boil breaks, and some thin fluid, and perhaps matter, oozes out. The yellowish core, consisting of a small mass of dead tissue, is now seen occupying the interior of the boil, and this comes away about a couple of days later, after which the boil speedily heals. If the boil be not treated, however, the first is apt to be followed by a crop of others in the neighbourhood, owing to the discharge from the first boil infecting other hairs. There is a special danger in boils of the upper lip and nose; for these may lead to inflammation within the head. Generally a boil, though its presence causes great annoyance, does not lead to fever or other general symptoms. But in boils of the ear, or about the face, there may be high temperature and great prostration, which are serious signs. Carbuncles are exhausting, and, in old people, very dangerous.

Treatment – At first the boil should be kept as still as possible, and to this end a piece of antiseptic sticking-plaster with a small hole cut in the centre, through which any discharge can pass, may be applied over the boil and kept in position for several days, when the boil very often aborts. Another method to prevent boils coming to a head is to paint the boil and a small area of skin round it night and morning for several days with strong tincture of iodine (10 per cent). If, however, the boil is painful, or if it is proceeding to suppuration, hot fomentations should be applied, or magnesium sulphate paste. Magnesium sulphate paste is very effective, but must be freshly made. Carbuncles, painful boils and boils about the lip and nose may become very dangerous and should on no account be squeezed or fingered. As penicillin is so effective against staphylococcal infection, it has proved of value in the treatment of severe boils and carbuncles. General treatment in the form of good food, and avoidance of alcohol is also necessary. The taking of yeast is said to be of value. New boils are more effectively prevented from forming by rubbing powdered boric acid gently into the skin around the old boil twice a day after washing and drying. In recurrent cases a course of injections of a specially made vaccine or of toxoid may be of value.

BONE forms the framework upon which the rest of the body is built up. The bones are generally called the skeleton, though this term also includes the cartilages which join the ribs to the breast-bone, protect the larynx, etc.

Structure of bone – Bone is composed partly of fibrous tissue, partly of bone earth (phosphate and carbonate of lime), intimately mixed together. As the bones of a child are composed to the extent of about two-thirds of fibrous tissue, whilst those of the aged contain two-thirds of bone earth, one readily understands the toughness of the former and the brittleness of the latter. One speaks of *dense bone*, of which the shafts of the limb bones are composed, the bone being a hard tube surrounded by a membrane, the periosteum, and enclosing a fatty substance, the marrow; and of *cancellous bone*, which forms the short bones and the ends of long bones, in which a fine lace-work of bone fills up the whole interior, enclosing marrow in its meshes. The marrow (qv) of the smaller bones is of great importance. It is red in colour, and in it red blood corpuscles are formed. Even the densest bone is tunnelled by fine canals (Haversian canals) in which run small blood-vessels, nerves and lymphatics, for the maintenance and repair of the bone (illustration 80). Round these Haversian canals the bone is arranged in circular plates called lamellae, the lamellae being separated

80 – Transverse section of dried bone. The open spaces are Haversian canals surrounded by lamellae. Magnified by about 200.

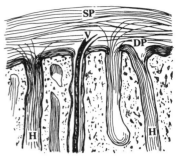

82 – Surface of a growing bone. *SP*, Superficial fibrous layer of periosteum; *DP*, deep cellular layer forming bone; *V*, blood-vessel entering the bone; *HH*, Haversian canals. Magnified by about 200.

from one another by clefts, known as lacunae, in which single bone-cells are contained. Even the lamellae are pierced by fine tubes known as canaliculi lodging processes of these cells. Each lamella is composed of very fine interlacing fibres.

Growth of bones – Bones grow in thickness from the fibrous tissue and lime salts laid down by cells in their substance (illustrations 81, 82); while the long bones grow in length from a plate of cartilage (epiphyseal cartilage) which runs across the bone about half an inch or more from its ends, and which on one surface is also constantly forming bone till the bone ceases to lengthen about the age of sixteen or eighteen. The existence of this cartilage is important to bear in mind, because in children an injury to it may lead to diminished growth of the limb.

Repair of bone is effected by cells of microscopic size: some called osteoblasts, elaborating the materials brought by the blood, and laying down strands of fibrous tissue, between which bone earth is later deposited; while other cells, known as osteoclasts, dissolve and break up dead or damaged bone. When a fracture has occurred, and the broken ends have been brought into contact, these are surrounded by a mass of blood at first; this is partly absorbed and partly organized by these cells, first into fibrous tissue and later into bone. The mass surrounding the fractured ends is called the callus, and for some months it forms a distinct thickening, which is gradually smoothed away, leaving the bone as before the fracture. If the ends have not been brought accurately in contact a permanent thickening results.

Varieties of bones – Apart from the structural varieties, bones fall into four classes: (*a*) long bones like those of the limbs; (*b*) short bones composed of cancel-

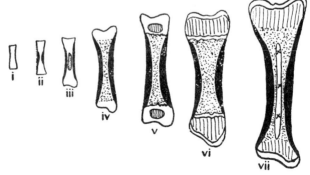

81 – Diagram to show growth of a long bone. Cartilage, white. Subperiosteal bone, black. Other sites of bone formation, dotted and vertical lines. (i) Shows the original cartilage model and successive drawings show the development of the bone until in (vi) the only cartilage left is that at the ends of the bone. In (vii) X indicates the bone marrow cavity. From Schafer, *Essentials of Histology* (after Mathias Duval). Longmans, Green & Co., Ltd.

Skull

Cervical vertebrae

First and second
thoracic vertebrae

Clavicle

Scapula

Sternum

Humerus

Eleventh and twelfth
thoracic vertebrae

Lumbar vertebrae

Hip bone

Radius

Sacrum

Coccyx

Ulna

Carpus

Metacarpals

Phalanges

Femur

Patella

Tibia

Fibula

Tarsus

Metatarsals

Phalanges

s.w.w

Sesamoid
83 – Human skeleton. From *Gray's Anatomy*. Longman.

BONE

lous tissue like those of the wrist and the ankle; (c) flat bones like those of the skull; (d) irregular bones like those of the face or the vertebrae of the spinal column (or backbone).

The skeleton consists of over 200 bones (illustration 83). It is divided into an AXIAL part, consisting of the skull, the vertebral column, the ribs with their cartilages, and the breast-bone; and an APPENDICULAR portion consisting of the four limbs. The hyoid bone in the neck, together with the cartilages protecting the larynx and windpipe, may be described as the VISCERAL skeleton.

AXIAL SKELETON – The *skull* (illustration 81) consists of the cranium, which has eight bones, viz. occipital, two parietal, two temporal, one frontal, ethmoid, and sphenoid; and of the face, which has fourteen bones, viz. two maxillae or upper jaw-bones and one lower jaw-bone, two malar or cheek bones, two nasal, two lacrimal, two turbinal, two palate bones, and one vomer bone. (For further details, see SKULL.) The *vertebral column* (illustration 86) consists of seven vertebrae in the cervical or neck region, twelve dorsal vertebrae, five vertebrae in the lumbar or loin region, the sacrum or sacral bone (a mass formed of five vertebrae fused together and forming the back part of the *pelvis*, which is closed at the sides by the haunch-bones), and finally the coccyx (four small vertebrae representing the tail of lower animals). The vertebral column has four curves: the first forwards in the neck, the second backwards in the dorsal region, the third forward in the loins, and the lowest, involving the sacrum and coccyx, backwards. These are associated with the erect attitude, develop after a child learns to walk, and have the effect of diminishing jars and shocks before these reach internal organs, much as carriage springs protect the contents of a vehicle from injury. This is still further aided by discs of cartilage placed between each pair of vertebrae. Each vertebra (illustration 86) has a solid part, the body in front, and behind this a ring of bone, the series of rings one above another forming a bony canal, up which runs the spinal cord to pass through an opening in the skull at the upper end of the canal and there join the brain. (For further details, see SPINAL COLUMN.) The *ribs*, twelve in number, on each side, are attached behind to the twelve dorsal vertebrae, while in front they end a few inches away from the breast-bone, but are con-

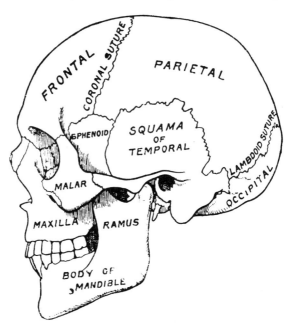

84 – Side view of skull. From Hill, *Manual of Human Physiology.* Edward Arnold & Co.

85 (*above*) – Human dorsal vertebra seen from above. K, body of vertebra; R, neural ring enclosing the spinal cord; B.B, notches by which the nerves emerge; D, spinous process; Qu,Qu, transverse processes; G,G, articular processes for the vertebra above; Rg,Rg, those for the head of the corresponding ribs.

86 (*left*) – The spinal column. C7, cervical; D12 dorsal; L5, lumbar vertebrae; S5, sacrum; Coc4, coccyx; C,C, the twelve ribs of the left side; Ps,Ms,Xs, three parts of the sternum; V,V, vertical axis of the spine showing its four curves.

tinued forwards by cartilages. Of these the upper seven reach the breast-bone, these ribs being called true ribs, the next three are joined each to the cartilage above it, while the last two have their ends free and are called floating ribs. The *breast-bone*, or sternum, is shaped something like a short sword, about 6 inches (15 cm) long, and rather over an inch (2·5 cm) wide.

APPENDICULAR SKELETON – The *upper limb* consists of the shoulder region and three segments – the upper arm, the forearm, and the wrist with the hand, separated from each other by joints. In the shoulder lie the clavicle or collar-bone (which is immediately beneath the skin, and forms a prominent object on the front of the neck), and the scapula or shoulder-blade behind the chest. In the upper arm is a single bone, the humerus. In the forearm are two bones, the radius and ulna; the radius, in the movements of alternately turning the hand palm up and back up (called, respectively, supination and pronation), rotating round the ulna, which re-

mains fixed. In the carpus or wrist are eight small bones – the scaphoid, lunate, triquetral, pisiform, trapezium, trapezoid, capitate, and hamate. In the hand proper are five bones called metacarpals, upon which are set the four fingers, each containing the three bones known as phalanges, and the thumb with two phalanges.

The *lower limb* consists similarly of the region of the haunch and three segments – the thigh, the leg, and the foot. The haunch-bone is a large flat bone made up of three – the ilium, the ischium, and the pubis, fused together, and forms the side of the pelvis or basin which encloses some of the abdominal organs. The thigh contains the femur, and the leg contains two bones – the tibia and fibula. In the tarsus are seven bones: the talus (which forms part of the ankle joint), the calcaneus or heel-bone, the navicular, the lateral, intermediate, and medial cuneiforms, and the cuboid. These bones are so shaped as to form a distinct arch in the foot both from before back and from side to side. Finally, as in the hand, there are five metatarsals and fourteen phalanges, of which the great toe has two, the other toes three each.

Besides these named bones there are others sometimes found in sinews called sesamoid bones, while the numbers of the regular bones may be increased by extra ribs or diminished by the fusion together of two or more bones.

BONE, DISEASES OF – Owing to the fact that most bones are deeply buried in the muscles, and that they contain in their earthy matter so much indifferent material, diseases in the bones are both apt to escape notice for a long time, and are actually much slower in their progress than similar diseases in other organs.

ACUTE INFLAMMATION is the disease which produces the most rapid effects. It is divided into acute *periostitis*, or inflammation of the surface of the bone and its enveloping membrane; acute *osteitis*, or inflammation of the bony substance itself; and acute *osteomyelitis*, or inflammation in the bone and its central cavity. Of these three conditions, osteomyelitis is by far the most important.

Causes – Osteomyelitis is usually due to infection with the *Staphylococcus aureus*. There is usually a history of a fall or a knock involving the affected limb. The disease is predominantly one of childhood.

Symptoms – In the slighter forms there is pain with tenderness to touch over a bone, which on examination is found swollen, but there are no general symptoms. In more serious cases severe pain comes on suddenly in a limb, one day perhaps after a slight accident. There is much fever, the temperature rising to 104° or 105° F (40° or 40·5° C), and often shivering, and at night delirium. After two or three days the limb becomes swollen, hot, and tender to touch, and still later the skin becomes inflamed and red. If the condition be not treated, general blood poisoning may result, or abscesses may form in other parts, and death may follow.

Treatment – As the *Staphylococcus aureus* is one of the organisms most sensitive to penicillin, the introduction of penicillin has revolutionized the treatment. Instead of being a condition practically always demanding operation and often causing prolonged invalidism, it can now be controlled by penicillin within a short space of time. The earlier treatment with penicillin is instituted, the better the results. Unless penicillin is given at an early stage, it may still be necessary to operate to remove any part of the bone that has been completely destroyed as a result of the infection. Such a dead portion of bone is known as a sequestrum (qv).

CHRONIC INFLAMMATION includes several quite distinct conditions, viz. abscess, necrosis, and exostosis, these conditions usually being due to injury, syphilis, or tuberculosis.

ABSCESS occurs generally in boys about the age of fourteen or fifteen, and the bone usually affected is one of those in the lower limb. The cause is either some local injury or local tuberculous disease.

Symptoms – There is a painful swelling on the bone usually at the outer or inner side of the knee, and the temperature of the limb may be raised. The pain is generally worse at night and may prevent sleep. This may persist for months or years unless efficiently treated.

Treatment – The treatment is surgical, by having the abscess opened, and the administration of the appropriate antibiotic.

NECROSIS means death of a bone. As already stated, it generally follows acute bone inflammation. It also follows severe fractures, occurs from contact with phosphorus (see OCCUPATIONAL DISEASES), in syphilis, and occasionally at the end of some severe infectious disease like typhoid fever.

Symptoms – Usually in the course of suppuration a passage is burst to the exterior, and remains as a constantly discharging sinus. At the bottom of this lies the dead bone or sequestrum, and an operation must be performed for its removal. Usually about three to six months elapse after the original injury before it is loose and ready for removal. If it be not removed the sinus continues to discharge and amyloidosis (qv) of various internal organs may develop.

EXOSTOSIS is an outgrowth upon a bone, which may be produced by long-continued irritation: eg. the bony growths on the inner side of the knee of those who ride much; or may be a symptom of syphilis; or may be of the nature of a tumour. (See below.)

SYPHILITIC DISEASE of bone in the secondary stage of this disease takes the form of nodes or swellings due to localized inflammation of the periosteal membrane, and in the tertiary stage there are often areas of great hardening with necrosis of pieces of bone.

TUBERCULOUS DISEASE in bone as a rule occurs in young people, but it is also found now and then in a person well up in years (senile tuberculosis). It may occur (a) in the bones of the hand or foot, in which case several may be affected; (b) in the ends of the long bones, when it is very apt to lead to disease of the neighbouring joint; (c) in the vertebrae, where it often results in curvature of the spine, or produces a chronic abscess. (See ABSCESS, CHRONIC.) Caries is the name given to a crumbling condition of the bone produced by this or any other disease.

Symptoms – Generally the health is not first-rate and there may be a history of tuberculosis in other organs. There is generally pain, tenderness, and swelling of the affected part. The whole limb, when a toe or finger is affected, may feel hot. Later the skin may get red and thin and a chronic abscess form and burst, leaving a sinus. Or the condition may heal, leaving the bone only a little thickened. The progress is in any case slow, lasting many weeks or months.

Treatment – The administration of anti-tuberculous drugs is all-important. Rest to the part affected, general exercise of the body in the fresh air, and good food are necessary. When the skin threatens to break, this should be anticipated by an operation, in which the diseased bone, etc., is all scraped away, or even amputation may be advisable in very bad cases. (See further under JOINTS, DISEASES OF.)

TUMOURS – CHONDROMA, a small tumour of cartilage and bone, grows sometimes under the nail of a finger or toe, and causes a good deal of pain and annoyance. It is easily removed, generally by splitting the nail, and does not return. CANCER rarely if ever begins in a bone, though secondary cancers commonly develop inside bones; for example cancer of the breast may be followed by secondary cancer in the bone of the arm or elsewhere. SARCOMA is a tumour sometimes found, especially in the larger bones, causing the bone to break readily, or dilating it to a great size; amputation is necessary for its removal.

RICKETS is a disease of childhood in which the bones do not harden as they ought to do. (See RICKETS.)

ACROMEGALY is a disease in which the bones enlarge in size. (See ACROMEGALY.)

OSTEITIS is a general term applied to inflammatory conditions of bone. It includes *osteitis deformans* (qv), in which the long bones become curved and the skull thickened; also *osteitis fibrosa cystica generalisata* (qv), in which bones become

weakened as a result of the presence of cysts.

OSTEOMALACIA is a disease characterized by a gradual loss of lime salts in the bones, so that these become soft and lose their proper form. It is due to lack of vitamin D and of calcium in the diet. (See OSTEOMALACIA.)

OSTEOPOROSIS is a condition characterized by rarefaction and brittleness of bone due to lack of calcium. (See OSTEOPOROSIS.)

OSTEOGENESIS IMPERFECTA is a hereditary disease of bone, characterized by extreme fragility of the skeleton (See OSTEOGENESIS IMPERFECTA.)

FIBROUS DYSPLASIA is a rare disease in which areas of bone are replaced by fibrous tissue. (See FIBROUS DYSPLASIA; and FIBROUS TISSUE.)

BORAX, or BIBORATE OF SODA, acts in much the same ways as boric acid, but has not its acid reaction.

Uses – Its chief use is in the form of a lotion (about 1 part to 30 of water) in all forms of itching and chapping of the skin. In thrush (qv) and other forms of irritation about the mouth in children the honey of borax, smeared on several times a day, is very soothing. To clean the mouth as well as soothe it, borax in honey wiped over the gums and tongue is very efficient. As in the case of boric acid, it should not be used in infants and young children.

BORBORYGMUS means flatulence in the bowels.

BORIC ACID, or BORACIC ACID, is found in volcanic districts, or is prepared from borax. It is a mild antiseptic.

Uses – It is used for dressing wounds, either dusted on as powder or in a lotion (1 part in 30). This lotion, mixed with an equal quantity of warm water, makes an extremely good eyewash for painful and inflamed eyes. Lint is sold ready soaked in boric lotion, dried, and generally dyed pink; it requires only to be dipped in water and applied. Offensive perspiration of the feet is checked by dipping the stockings in boric lotion and drying them before wearing. Because of the risk of toxic effects it should not be used in infants and young children.

BORNHOLM DISEASE, also known as devil's grip, and epidemic myalgia, is an acute infective disease due to Coxsackie viruses (qv), and characterized by the abrupt onset of pain around the lower margin of the ribs, headache, and fever. It occurs in epidemics, usually during warm weather, and it is more common in young people than the old. The illness usually lasts seven to ten days. It is practically never fatal. The disease is named after the island of Bornholm in the Baltic, where several epidemics have been described.

BOROGLYCERIN is a clear unctuous antiseptic, made by dissolving boric acid crystals in glycerin while hot.

BOTULISM is a term applied to a rare type of food-poisoning caused by the toxin arising from the presence in improperly preserved foods of the *Clostridium botulinum*. The first symptoms come on a few hours after the food has been taken and consist of vomiting, abdominal pain, and difficulty of vision. Later, nervous symptoms consisting of double vision, drooping of the eyelids, weakness of the facial muscles, dilatation of the pupils, and difficulty in swallowing and breathing appear. The prognosis is extremely grave, the mortality rate being higher than 50 per cent. Fortunately, the condition is rare in Britain. There have only been 21 cases this century in seven different incidents, with 12 deaths. Since the outbreak at Loch Maree in 1922, when eight fishermen died of the disease after eating sandwiches containing duck paste, sixteen cases have occurred in the United Kingdom (table 7), with two deaths: one from the 1949 incident, and one from the 1978 incident.

Year	No. of cases	Causes
1922	8	Duck paste (Loch Maree)
1932	2	Rabbit and pigeon broth
1934	1	Jugged hare
1935	2	Vegetarian nut brawn
	1	Home-made pie
1949	5	Macaroni cheese
1955	1	Pickled fish from Mauritius
1978	4	Tinned salmon

Table 7 – Recorded incidents of botulism in the United Kingdom since 1922.

During this period several outbreaks of botulism have been reported in Britain, especially in water fowl, broiler chickens, ferrets and mink. Very occasionally it may occur as a result of contamination of a wound by *Clostridium botulinum*. Recently cases have been reported in USA, and one in Britain, of botulism in infants due to the spontaneous formation of botulinum toxin in the infant's gut.

Treatment – An antitoxic serum is available, and this should be given, along with full doses of antibiotics. Because of the nervous signs, such as difficulty in swallowing, skilled nursing is essential.

BOUGIES are solid instruments for introduction into natural passages in the body either in order to apply medicaments which they contain or with which they are coated, or, more usually, in order to dilate a narrow part or stricture of the passage. Thus we have, for example, urethral bougies, oesophageal bougies, rectal bougies, made usually of flexible rubber or, in the case of the urethra, of steel.

BOUILLON is a broth or soup prepared from meat. It is much used in various food preparations and also as a medium for cultivating organisms in bacteriological laboratories.

BOULIMIA, or BULIMIA, means exaggerated appetite. (See APPETITE.)

BOWELS (see INTESTINE).

BOW LEGS, or GENU VARUM, may be due to an abnormal posture of the limbs in the womb before birth. It often corrects itself, but in more severe or persistent cases, correction may be necessary by means of manipulation, the wearing of a plaster cast, or operation. In the first few years of life, however, a certain amount of bowing of the legs, associated with a tendency to pigeon-toe, may be quite normal and corrects itself as the child grows older. In older children it may be due to bone diseases, such as rickets (*qv*). Correction of the deformity may be assisted by the wearing of strong shoes with arch support and an outer sole wedge.

BOXING INJURIES rank eighth in frequency among sports injuries. During the 1973–74 season there were 2963 contests under the auspices of the London Amateur Boxing Association. The injuries recorded in these contests were as follows:

Cuts round the eye	36
Fractured thumbs	3
Sprained thumbs	4
Strained groin muscle	1
Concussion	12
Cut lips	2
Fractured metacarpal bone	2
Cut ear	1
Haematomas	3
Fractured jaw	2
Dislocated shoulder	1
Cut forehead	2
Retrograde amnesia	1
Epistaxis	1

According to the 'Report on the Medical Aspects of Boxing' issued by the Committee on Boxing of the Royal College of Physicians of London in October 1969, of 224 ex-professional boxers examined, 37 showed evidence of brain damage which was disabling in thirteen. Commenting on this, the report says: 'This prevalence rate of 17 per cent indicates that one in six of the boxers studied showed evidence of some damage to their nervous systems attributable to boxing but probably only a third of these were affected severely enough to be recognized as "punch drunk"'. The report also notes that 'the Committee has had discussions with members, including medical officers of the British Boxing Board of Control and appreciate that professional boxing under their auspices is, today, closely and carefully controlled. It is therefore not possible to draw conclusions about the risk of brain damage in professional boxing today'. Apart from the death of a young Romanian boxer in 1975, there has been no death in amateur boxing in Great Britain during the last three years, but a British amateur boxer died in The Netherlands in 1972, following a cerebral haemorrhage. In the United States of America, in 1962, two boxers died after professional fights and two after amateur bouts, compared with 32 killed in football and six in baseball. In 1978, an Italian professional boxer died of a cerebral haemorrhage. It has been estimated that there have been 500 boxing fatalities this century.

The commonest boxing injury is simple nose-bleeding. This can easily be stopped by sitting the boxer upright, pinching the nose, and applying a cold sponge. If it persists after the bout, the nose is plugged with adrenaline gauze or adrenaline-soaked cotton-wool. In the case of abrasions on the face and head, bleeding is stopped by firm pressure. The wound is then bathed with warm saline, and this is followed by application of 1 per cent cetrimide, and then a light dusting with sulphathiazole powder.

Many boxing injuries can be prevented by the wearing of bandages over the metacarpals, the use of gum shields and laceless gloves weighing 8 ounces (225 grams), and by having a 'Sorbo' rubber covering under the canvas of the ring.

BRACHIAL means 'belonging to the upper arm'. There are, for example, a brachial artery, and a brachial plexus of nerves through which run all the nerves to the arm. The brachial plexus lies along the outer side of the armpit, and is liable to be damaged in dislocation at the shoulder.

BRACHYCEPHALIC means short-headed and is a term applied to skulls the breadth of which is at least four-fifths of the length. BRACHYCEPHALY is a characteristic of the Alpine race.

BRACHYDACTYLY is a term applied to the conditions in which the fingers or toes are abnormally short.

BRADYCARDIA means slowness of the beating of the heart with corresponding slowness of the pulse (below 60 per minute). (See HEART DISEASES.)

BRADYKINESIA is a term used to describe the condition in which the movements of the body and limbs are abnormally slow.

BRADYKININ is a substance derived from plasma proteins, which plays an important role in many of the reactions of the body, including inflammation (qv). Its prime action is in producing dilatation of arteries and veins. It has also been described as 'the most powerful pain-producing agent known'.

BRAIDISM, after James Braid, who introduced it into medicine, is another name for hypnotism. (See HYPNOTISM.)

BRAIN – The brain and spinal cord together form the central nervous system, the twelve nerves passing on each side from the brain, and the thirty-one from the cord being called the peripheral nervous system, while the complex chains of nerves and ganglia lying within the chest and abdomen, and acting to a large extent independently of the other two systems, though closely connected with them, make up the autonomic system, and govern the activity of the viscera.

Divisions – The brain in its simplest form in lowly vertebrate animals is a thickened part at the front end of the spinal cord, developed in order to govern the organs of special sense, viz. smell, sight, hearing, and taste, lodged near at hand. Higher in the scale, in fishes for example, there are marked bulgings of nervous matter forming the fore-brain, the mid-brain, and the hind-brain, and that part connected with the nerves of the eyes appears to be the highest governing part. In man, however, the part in front of this is specially developed, and not only forms

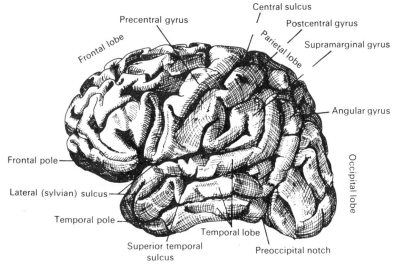

Central sulcus
Precentral gyrus
Postcentral gyrus
Supramarginal gyrus
Frontal lobe
Parietal lobe
Angular gyrus
Frontal pole
Occipital lobe
Lateral (sylvian) sulcus
Temporal pole
Temporal lobe
Superior temporal sulcus
Preoccipital notch

87 – Side view of the brain.

the great bulk of the entire brain, but governs the activities of the rest. This part is called the cerebrum (illustrations 87, 88, 89).

THE CEREBRUM forms the great bulk of the brain in amount and consists of two cerebral hemispheres which occupy the entire vault of the cranium and are incompletely separated from one another by a deep median cleft, the longitudinal cerebral fissure. At the bottom of this cleft the two hemispheres are united by a thick band of some 200 million transverse nerve fibres: the corpus callosum. Other clefts or fissures, or sulci as they are now known, make deep impressions, dividing the cerebrum into lobes. Of these the chief are the lateral sulcus and the central sulcus. The lobes of the cerebrum are the frontal lobe in the forehead region, the parietal lobe on the side and upper part of the brain, the occipital lobe to the back, and the temporal lobe lying just above the region of the ear.

Numbers of shallower infoldings of the surface called furrows or sulci separate raised areas called convolutions or gyri. The outer $\frac{1}{8}$ inch (3 mm) or thereabouts of the cerebral hemispheres consists of grey matter largely made up of ganglion cells, while in the deeper part the white matter consists of medullated nerve fibres connecting different parts of the surface and passing down to the lower parts of the brain. Among the white matter lie several

rounded masses of grey matter, the lentiform and caudate nuclei. In the centre of each cerebral hemisphere is an irregular cavity, the lateral ventricle, each of which communicates with that on the other side and behind with the 3rd ventricle through a small opening, the interventricular foramen, or foramen of Monro.

THE BASAL NUCLEI consist of two large masses of grey matter imbedded in the base of the cerebral hemispheres in man, but forming the chief part of the brain in many of the animals. Between these masses lies the 3rd ventricle, from which the infundibulum, a funnel-shaped process, projects downwards into the pituitary body, and above lies the pineal gland. This region includes the important hypothalamus.

THE MID-BRAIN, or mesencephalon, is a stalk about $\frac{3}{4}$ inch (20 mm) long connecting the cerebrum with the hind-brain. Down its centre lies a tube, the cerebral aqueduct, or aqueduct of Sylvius, connecting the 3rd and 4th ventricles. Above this aqueduct lie the corpora quadrigemina, and beneath it are the crura cerebri, strong bands of white matter in which important nerve fibres pass downwards from the cerebrum.

THE PONS is a mass of nerve fibres, some of which run crosswise and others are the continuation of the crura cerebri downwards.

THE CEREBELLUM lies towards the back,

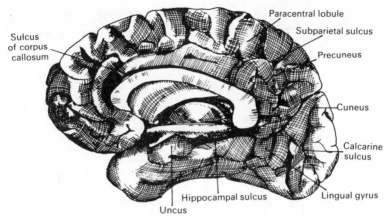

Paracentral lobule
Subparietal sulcus
Precuneus
Sulcus of corpus callosum
Cuneus
Calcarine sulcus
Lingual gyrus
Hippocampal sulcus
Uncus

88 – Vertical section through the middle of the brain.

underneath the occipital lobes of the cerebrum.

THE MEDULLA OBLONGATA, is the lowest part of the brain, in structure resembling the spinal cord, with white matter on the surface and grey matter in its interior. This is continuous through the large opening in the skull, foramen magnum, with the spinal cord. Between the medulla, pons, and cerebellum lies the 4th ventricle of the brain.

Structure – The brain is made up of grey and white matter. In the cerebrum and cerebellum the grey matter is arranged mainly in a layer on the surface, though both have certain grey masses imbedded in the white matter. In the other parts the grey matter is found in definite masses called nuclei, from which the nerves spring. The grey matter consists mainly of cells in which all the activities of the brain begin. These cells vary considerably in size and shape in different parts of the brain, though all give off a number of processes, some of which form nerve fibres. The cells on the surface of the cerebral hemispheres, for example, are very numerous, being set in layers five or six deep (illustration 90). In shape these cells are pyramidal, giving off processes from the apex, from the centre of the base, and from various projections elsewhere on the cell. The grey matter is everywhere penetrated by a rich supply of blood-vessels, and the nerve cells and blood-vessels are supported in a fine network of fibres, known as neuroglia. The white matter consists of nerve fibres, each of which is attached, at one end, to a cell in the grey matter, while, at the other end, it splits up into a tree-like structure round another cell in another part of the grey matter in the brain or spinal cord. The fibres have insulating sheaths of a fatty material, which, in the mass, gives the white matter its colour, and they convey messages from one part of the brain to the other (association fibres), or, grouped into bundles, leave the brain as nerves, or pass

89 – Vertical section through the middle of the head and neck. *Ch*, Cerebellum; *CC*, corpus callosum; *FC*, falx cerebri, the process of dura mater lying between the two cerebral hemispheres; *H*, pituitary body; *M*, medulla oblongata; *P*, pons; *Sp.c*, spinal cord; *v*, vertebral column. For other letters, see illustration 6.

135

90 – Vertical section through the cerebral cortex of the frontal region, showing the pyramidal cells and their processes.

down into the spinal cord, where they end near, and exert a control upon, cells from which in turn spring the nerves to the body. Both grey and white matter are bound together by a felt-work called neuroglia. The general arrangement of fibres can be best understood by describing the course of a motor nerve fibre. Arising in a cell on the surface in front of the central sulcus, such a fibre passes inwards towards the centre of the cerebral hemisphere, the collected mass of fibres as they lie between the lentiform nucleus and optic thalamus being known as the internal capsule. Hence the fibre passes down through the crus cerebri, giving off various small connecting fibres as it passes downwards. After passing through the pons it reaches the medulla, and at this point crosses to the opposite side (decussation of the pyramids). Entering the spinal cord, it passes downwards to end finally in a series of branches (arborization) which meet and touch (synapse) similar branches from one or more of the cells in the grey matter of the cord (see SPINAL CORD).

Size – The weight of the average male brain is 49 ounces (1·4 kg), ranging from 1·24 to 1·68 kg, of the female brain 44 ounces (1·25 kg), ranging from 1·13 to 1·51

kg, but brains have been found as heavy as 65 ounces (1·8 kg). The maximum mass of brain tissue is reached at the age of 20, and then decreases steadily.

Functions – The cerebrum is associated with the intellectual faculties in man, and also exerts a guiding influence over the rest of the nervous system. It is not, however, necessary to actual life. If the cerebrum of a frog be destroyed it still breathes and its heart beats, it can hop if pinched, and swim if put in water, but when left alone it sits still till it perishes. If the same happens to a pigeon it can fly when thrown in the air, and can alight, but it does not fly away when threatened, nor will it take food, having lost even the instinct to preserve life. If, on the other hand, the cerebellum of a pigeon be destroyed, the bird cannot maintain its balance, the cerebellum being concerned in the regulation of muscular movements and in preserving the equilibrium of the body.

Plato recognized three mental faculties, which he placed, respectively, in the liver, heart, and brain, these organs being supposed to secrete the 'animal spirits' appropriate to each faculty; and this view was accepted by the medical writers of antiquity. In the Middle Ages the Arabian physicians, however, following Galen's opinion, placed the different mental faculties in the several ventricles of the brain, this theory being adopted by Duns Scotus, Thomas of Aquino, and referred to by Burton in his *Anatomy of Melancholy*.

Descartes (1596–1650) had the fanciful idea that the pineal body was the seat of the mind, though this structure is now supposed to be the vestige of a third eye. After his time it was fancied that the whole brain must act together in every process, from the fact that, in cases of severe injury to the head, much substance can be lost from some parts of the brain without impairment of any one definite function or memory.

But it is now known that definite areas of the surface are associated with definite functions. The earliest systematic attempt to localize the functions of the brain to certain areas was made by Gall and Spurzheim, who founded the system of phrenology in the first quarter of the nineteenth century. Although this system was proved to be wrong both as regards the functions of the brain and the philosophic analysis of mental processes, the criticism it called forth gave a great impetus to the attempt to localize the functions of the brain in definite spots. Between 1820 and 1840 it became established that, in persons who have lost the power of speech during life, the brain shows some disease in the left frontal lobe after death, and in 1861 Broca made the first definite discovery in cerebral localization, by proving that the faculty of speech is governed by a centre in the region of the inferior frontal gyrus, named (after him) Broca's convolution. His discovery was followed later by the important observation of Hughlings Jackson that certain forms of epilepsy, associated with movements beginning in a definite limb, are caused by disease affecting the part of the brain that borders on the central sulcus, and this discovery was confirmed and extended by many experimenters and physicians. Fritsch, Hitzig, Ferrier, Sherrington, Grünbaum and others have shown that definite areas near the central sulcus are associated with the movement of definite parts (illustration 91). Further, the occipital lobes are

91 – Diagram showing areas upon the left surface of the cerebrum associated with definite functions. cs, central sulcus; ls, lateral sulcus.

associated with the sense of sight, the temporal lobe with hearing, and the inner surface of the same lobe with taste and smell. The purely intellectual faculties are probably associated with the frontal lobes, which seem to govern nothing else. The cerebellum has to do with the powers of balancing and of regulating movements. The medulla and pons have important functions, governing many of the processes most essential to life, eg. those of respiration, rate of the heart, swallowing, vomiting, and giving off all the nerves which arise from the brain, except the first four.

Membranes – The brain is separated from the skull by three membranes: the dura mater, a thick fibrous membrane; the arachnoid mater, a more delicate structure; and the pia mater, adhering to the surface of the brain, and containing the blood-vessels which nourish it. Between each pair is a space containing

fluid on which the brain floats as on a water-bed. The fluid beneath the arachnoid membrane mixes with that inside the ventricles through a small opening in the 4th ventricle, called the median aperture, or foramen of Magendie.

These fluid arrangements have a great influence in preserving the brain from injury.

Nerves – The nerves which come off the brain are twelve in number:

I.	Olfactory, to the nose (smell).
II.	Optic, to the eye (sight).
III.	Oculomotor ⎫
IV.	Trochlear ⎬ to eye-muscles.
VI.	Abducent ⎭
V.	Trigeminal, to skin of face.
VII.	Facial, to muscles of face.
VIII.	Vestibulocochlear, to ear (hearing and balancing).
IX.	Glossopharyngeal, to tongue (taste).
X.	Vagus, to heart, larynx, lungs, and stomach.
XI.	Spinal accessory, to muscles in neck.
XII.	Hypoglossal, to muscles of tongue.

Blood-vessels – Four vessels carry blood to the brain: two internal carotid arteries in front, and two vertebral arteries behind. These communicate to form a circle (circle of Willis) inside the skull, so that if one be blocked the others, by dilating, supply its place. The chief branch of the internal carotid artery on each side is the middle cerebral, and this gives off a small but very important branch which pierces the base of the brain and supplies the region of the internal capsule with blood. The chief importance of this vessel lies in the fact that the blood in it is under specially high pressure, owing to its close connection with the carotid artery, so that haemorrhage from it is liable to occur and thus give rise to apoplexy. Two veins, the internal cerebral veins, bring the blood away from the interior of the brain, but most of the small veins come to the surface and open into large venous sinuses, which run in grooves in the skull, and finally pour their blood into the internal jugular vein that accompanies the carotid artery on each side of the neck.

BRAIN, DISEASES AND INJURIES OF – The signs of brain disease are in general indirect, being manifested by some defect in sensation or in the power of action, or by some peculiarity of conduct. The symptoms are more fully discussed under NERVOUS DISEASES. (See also APHASIA; APOPLEXY; ENCEPHALITIS; EPILEPSY; HEADACHE; HYDROCEPHALUS; MENINGITIS; MENTAL ILLNESS; PARALYSIS.) The following are some of the conditions more exclusively connected with the brain.

ABSCESS is a very serious condition. It results from wounds of the scalp which suppurate and in which the inflammatory matter does not get free exit, or from suppurating ear disease, in which the discharge from the ear has been stopped. The symptoms are rather vague, but sooner or later there are severe headache and vomiting, with rise of temperature, and often some interference with vision. When the abscess lies in the temporal lobe the temperature is often below normal. The treatment should be prevention, by keeping every scalp wound clean, and by having every case of discharging ear disease under medical supervision (see EAR, DISEASES OF). When it is recognized that an abscess has occurred in the brain, it is customary to trephine the skull and evacuate the abscess, after which recovery often takes place.

ANAEMIA OF THE BRAIN is the cause of fainting when suddenly brought on by weakness of the heart's action. Anaemia of a more chronic type is a cause of sleeplessness in elderly persons, accompanied by weakness of mental power and drowsiness during working hours. It also causes headache, giddiness, and ringing in the ears.

COMPRESSION OF THE BRAIN may be caused by the growth of a tumour in the brain, a collection of blood between the brain and skull from injury of the membranes, or suppuration in the same locality from a neglected scalp wound or fracture of the skull. Unconsciousness coming on some hours after a blow on the side of the head is generally due to a fracture tearing one of the arteries in the membranes and producing a large clot between the skull and brain. The symptoms are vague, but, in addition to unconsciousness, there are generally difficulty of breathing, feeble pulse, and paralysis down one side of the body. The treatment is trephining of the skull (see TREPHINING).

CONCUSSION is a bruising of part of the brain as the result of a blow on the head (generally at the back) or a severe shake of the body. Cases vary in severity from mere giddiness and headache for an hour or two, to complete loss of consciousness lasting for weeks, and include those curious instances of lost memory for facts or even for personal identity which have been much used by novelists. The person lies unconscious and can be roused with difficulty. If he answers questions at all he does so irrelevantly, and shows great

irritability of temper, going off to sleep again at once. He lies turned away from the light, with his knees drawn up on the body. Consciousness and convalescence come on very gradually, and for months there may be loss of memory, bad temper, and great susceptibility to the effects of alcohol. Recovery is generally good, but a tendency to epilepsy may remain. The treatment is complete rest in a darkened room, with careful nursing to ensure that no complications develop in the lungs and to prevent the development of bed sores. The urine may need to be drawn off. Once consciousness is regained, there should be a prolonged period of rest in order to prevent persisting or recurring headaches.

BRAIN FEVER is a popular name for several conditions. One is a state of prostration following some severe mental strain, which is not very serious and passes off in the course of a few weeks of rest. Another condition known under this name is encephalitis lethargica, also known popularly as 'sleepy sickness', in which inflammatory changes accompanied by oedema and haemorrhages take place in parts of the brain, causing a serious and often fatal disorder. (See ENCEPHALITIS LETHARGICA.) Another condition often called by this name is inflammation of the membranes of the brain, or meningitis, which occurs most commonly in children and which may be a very dangerous disease (see MENINGITIS).

HAEMORRHAGE into the brain causes apoplexy. (See APOPLEXY.)

LACERATION of the brain may occur in fracture of the skull. When the injury affects the upper part of the cerebrum, it is not of so great importance as the fact of whether the wound is kept clean and free from suppuration, although near the central sulcus damage to the brain may result in paralysis of a limb. When it occurs at the base of the skull serious injury of the brain is apt to result, often ending in death (see FRACTURES).

SOFTENING of the brain is a term used in a strictly scientific sense and in a popular sense. In the former case an actual area of brain tissue softens owing to its blood supply being cut off by plugging of its blood-vessels, or in consequence of some long-standing inflammatory process. The symptoms are then those of apoplexy, though not so sudden as if the cause were haemorrhage. In the popular sense, when persons, who have been the subjects of gout, alcoholism, or syphilis, especially elderly persons, become gradually dull in intellect, drowsy, absent-minded, emotional, and finally demented, because of their diseased blood-vessels diminishing the blood supply to, and causing deterioration of, the brain, these symptoms are also attributed to 'softening of the brain'.

TUMOURS of the brain produce very insidious and very complex symptoms, depending on the region they affect. Among the general symptoms are headache, giddiness, vomiting independent of food, and tenderness of the head on pressure. Blindness and mental symptoms come on later, owing to rise of pressure inside the skull. Sometimes these tumours are tuberculous or syphilitic in origin, when the general treatment for these diseases may be of some help. In other cases, little good can be done, except palliation of the pain and other symptoms – sometimes by trephining to relieve the pressure. Occasionally a tumour produces definite 'localizing' symptoms indicating its position in the brain. In such cases an operation may be performed for the complete and successful removal of the tumour, or it may be treated with radio-isotopes (see ISOTOPES). As a result of advances in neurosurgery and in nuclear medicine, it is becoming possible to deal successfully with an increasing number of tumours of the brain.

BRAN is the meal derived from the outer covering of a cereal grain. It contains little or no carbohydrate, and is mainly used to provide roughage (qv) in certain cases of constipation.

BRANDY (see ALCOHOL).

BREAD is one of the cheapest of foods: hence its popularity throughout the ages as the 'staff of life'. It is also highly digestible and absorbable, and contains a reasonable amount of protein. In Britain it is made almost exclusively from wheat flour. The wheat germ is made up of bran (13 per cent), inner endosperm (83 per

cent), outer endosperm (2 per cent), germ (1 per cent), and scutellum (1 per cent), and each 100 grams contains 9 grams of protein, 2·5 grams of fat, 70 grams of carbohydrate, 36 mg of calcium, 3 mg of iron, and 295 micrograms of thiamine (vitamin B_1). These are approximate figures as the precise amounts vary depending upon the type of wheat used. Unfortunately, the flour made from the wheat grain is too indigestible for most human beings. This 100 per cent wholemeal flour is therefore refined by modern milling processes, in the course of which much of the roughage is removed. In low-extraction flour the bran, germ, scutellum and outer layer of endosperm are all removed. The disadvantage of this from the nutritional point of view is that it involves the loss of much of the iron, calcium and vitamin content of the flour (table 8). This loss is relatively slight with 85 per cent extraction, as at this level the germ and scutellum are still retained, and therefore most of the thiamine and iron.

The controversy still rages between the protagonists of high-extraction and those of low-extraction flour. Nutritionally there is no doubt as to the superiority of the former, particularly so far as the vitamin B content is concerned. Some of the other apparent nutritional advantages are counterbalanced by the fact that high-extraction flour is less digestible than 70 per cent extraction flour – which is the normal level of commercial milling. Much of the edge has been taken out of the controversy by the Government regulation, whereby all flour intended for human consumption must be so reinforced that it shall contain not less than 1·65 mg of iron, 0·24 mg of thiamine, and 1·6 mg of nicotinic acid or nicotinamade (one of the vitamin B constituents) per 100 grams, and, except in the case of flour containing the whole of the products derived from the milling of bread, 235 to 390 mg of powdered chalk per 100 grams.

The making of bread, with its spongy

	Thiamine	Nicotinic acid	Pantothenic acid	Riboflavin	Pyridoxine
	mg	mg	mg	mg	mg
Whole wheat flour	0·40	5·0	1·5	0·16	0·40

Percentage of vitamin remaining

Extraction rate per cent					
85	89	39	76	52	44
80	63	32	58	47	27
70	20	23	49	33	16

Table 8 – The vitamin content per 100 grams of whole wheat flour and the percentage retained in flour of different extraction rates texture, from flour is due to the latter containing gluten, the mixture of proteins that constitutes the nitrogenous content of flour. Gluten produces the dough which when blown up by the carbon dioxide released as a result of the fermentation of yeast, remains in the form of a sponge. It is because of this high content of gluten that wheat makes much better bread than other cereals. Rye comes next to wheat as a bread-making grain, but its low content of gluten makes the bread moist and dense, and those not used to it find it rather sour. A typical example of rye bread is the black bread so popular in parts of Europe. Maize contains no gluten and therefore maize meal cannot be used alone to make bread. It can, however, be baked into cakes, and outside Britain is often mixed with wheat flour to make bread. Barley, too, contains little gluten and therefore produces a heavy dough. Mixed with wheat flour, however, it produces a quite acceptable bread. The same applies to oatmeal.

The average nutritional value of the bread made from the current reinforced 70 per cent wheat flour per 100 grams is 8 grams per cent protein, 1·5 grams per cent fat, 53 grams per cent available carbohydrate. 90 mg per cent calcium, 1·8 mg per cent iron, giving a calorie value of 240. When bread is toasted, water is driven off and the calorie value therefore rises – to around 300 Calories per 100 grams. The increased digestibility of toast is due to the fact that it is chewed more effectively than bread. Conversely the traditional indigestibility of new bread is due to its moisture making it difficult to chew, and it is therefore swallowed before it has soaked up much saliva.

BREAK-BONE FEVER is another name for dengue (qv).

BREASTS, or MAMMARY GLANDS, are found in the most highly developed class of animals, called the Mammalia, for the purpose of suckling the young. As a rule they are confined to the female sex, though the male has rudimentary nipples, and, even in man, individuals occur in the male sex who have well-developed glands and have been known to produce milk. These glands are developed in the front of the chest, and, in the full-grown female, extend from the second to the sixth or seventh rib, being at the centre about 2 inches (5 cm) thick. There is usually one on each side, but small supplementary breasts are occasionally found in the armpit or low down

on the abdomen. In the centre is a dark patch, called the areola, which surrounds the nipple. This areola darkens during pregnancy. This, together with enlargement of the whole breast and dilatation of its veins, forms an important and early sign of this condition. In structure each breast consists of from twelve to twenty compartments, each of which contains a system of branching tubes lined by cells that form the fatty and fluid materials composing the milk. In each section the tubes open on the surface of the nipple by a single small tube, or duct, of which therefore there are twelve to twenty in all. Between these gland tubes lie muscle fibres (which give the breasts their firmness), fibrous tissue, and fat (which is specially plentiful in elderly women).

BREASTS, DISEASES OF – These glands go through great changes during the course of life, becoming considerably enlarged about the age of puberty, afterwards congested at each monthly period, then undergoing great development during pregnancy, so as to be double the usual size during the time of suckling, and finally, with advancing years, undergoing gradual absorption, though, in stout persons, their actual size increases from deposit of fat.

ACUTE INFLAMMATION, or MASTITIS, *AND ABSCESS* – **Causes** – This is most common during the period of suckling a child, and particularly during the first two months. The infection usually reaches the breast from the nipple, as a result of cracks of the nipple and lack of cleanliness. Another common cause is an indrawn nipple. Passing congestion, producing swelling and tenderness, sometimes appears in boys or girls at the time of puberty, but rarely goes on to abscess formation.

Symptoms – Discomfort in some part of the breast, with increased hardness and fullness, usually towards the lower edge, is first noticed, and, if treatment be then begun, the majority of cases do not go on to an abscess. If the condition remains untreated, definite pain next comes on, especially when the infant sucks, along with redness, swelling, and heat, the general signs of abscess. Finally, the skin over one spot, usually about a couple of inches from the nipple, turns purple, and here the abscess bursts.

Treatment – It is essential that every care should be taken to prevent infection of the breast, by scrupulous attention to cleansing of the breast during the later stages of pregnancy and during suckling. This is best done by careful washing with soap and water; scrubbing with a brush is usually unnecessary. If the nipples are retracted during pregnancy, they should be drawn out every day. During suckling, the nipples should be carefully cleaned with sterile (ie. boiled) water each time the baby is put to the breast.

If, in spite of these precautions, the breast becomes hard, tender, or congested, suckling should be suspended on the affected side, and the breast firmly bandaged over by a large pad of cotton-wool. The affected breast should be emptied by gentle expression, or this may be done by a breast pump. The common practice today is to start using an antibiotic, usually penicillin, at a very early stage as this reduces the risk of abscess formation. If an abscess forms, it is opened and drained. In severe cases in which it is necessary to wean the baby, the secretion of milk is stopped by taking one of the oestrogenic hormones: eg. stilboestrol (qv).

CHRONIC INFLAMMATION, or MASTITIS, may take the form of a chronic abscess, but, more commonly, it consists of simple swelling and pain in one part of the breast, often erroneously believed by the affected person to be cancer.

Symptoms – This condition is not due to infection, but to some disturbance of the normal control of the breast exerted by the ovaries and the pituitary gland. It occurs with increasing frequency after the age of 30 years, and is more liable to occur in women who have borne children. Pain is the principal symptom. This is worse just before the monthly period or during the early days of the period. It may be confined to one part of the breast or may involve the whole breast. Both breasts may be involved. One or more swellings may be seen or felt in the breast.

Treatment – The condition is made much worse by the patient allowing her mind to dwell on it and by constant handling of the swelling, so that when the breast is completely covered up and supported by a well-fitting brassière, complete recovery may speedily take place. The first essential, however, is that medical advice is sought, to decide whether or not the pain and swelling are due to cancer of the breast.

NEURALGIA may be very painful during pregnancy, in pelvic disorders, or in general troubles like anaemia and rheumatism. It is treated like neuralgia elsewhere.

CRACKED NIPPLES are sometimes very troublesome. For their treatment see under Acute Inflammation. When there is a chronic eczematous condition, a nipple-shield should be applied and fixed with plaster or tapes.

TUMOURS – In consequence of the fact that the breast is one of the organs most frequently attacked by cancer, many women render themselves unnecessarily unhappy over some swelling in the breast, taking for cancer what is often simply chronic inflammation, or a cyst or adenoma, the two latter being common non-malignant growths. In every case, immediately a woman discovers a small nodule in her breast she should consult a doctor. If the swelling is not cancer – and usually it is not – her mind will be relieved, and the treatment, whether by operation or not, will not in general necessitate the removal of the breast. If cancer be present, then the earlier an operation be done the more chance there is of a complete cure. (See MASTECTOMY.)

BREATH, DISORDERS OF – The composition of the breath and the changes that air undergoes when it is breathed are described under AIR; the manner in which breathing is affected is described under RESPIRATION. (See also BREATHLESSNESS; CHEST DISEASES; LUNG DISEASES.)

BAD BREATH, or HALITOSIS, is sometimes extremely unpleasant to those around the subject of the trouble, although the smell may be extremely foul without the person himself being conscious of it.

Causes – Frequent causes are bad teeth, infections of the gums (eg. Vincent's angina), chronic tonsillitis, and indigestion. Besides these, an excessively foetid condition is caused by bronchiectasis (qv), by ulceration about the bones of the nose, and by a disease of the nose, known as ozoena, in which crusts constantly form there (see NOSE, DISEASES OF).

Treatment – Careful attention to the hygiene of the mouth is the first essential (see TEETH), or the dental treatment of any defective teeth or infection of the gums. Tonsillectomy may be required if the tonsils are chronically inflamed. In one form of tonsillitis, small cheesy pellets of secretion collect in the hollows of the tonsils and putrefy; the tendency to this is lessened by gargling daily (see GARGLES). Indigestion with furred tongue is also credited with being a frequent cause of bad breath (see DYSPEPSIA). The smell may be temporarily relieved by placing a small drop of some essential oil, such as cloves, occasionally on the tongue, or by various scented sweets, or by means of a mouth wash containing one teaspoonful of concentrated peppermint water B P, and one teaspoonful of salt in 8 ounces (200 millilitres) of water.

BREATH-HOLDING – Breath-holding attacks are not uncommon in infants and toddlers. They are characterized by the child suddenly stopping breathing in the midst of a bout of crying evoked by pain, some emotional upset, or loss of temper. The breath may be held so long that the child goes blue in the face. The attack is never fatal and the condition disappears spontaneously after the age of 3 to 5 years, but once a child has acquired the habit it may recur quite often.

The attacks require no treatment as recovery is spontaneous and rapid. In no circumstances should the parents dramatize the situation by slapping, pinching, or drenching the child with water.

BREATHING (see RESPIRATION).

BREATHLESSNESS may be due to any condition which renders the blood impure or deficient in oxygen, and which therefore produces excessive involuntary efforts to gain more air.

Causes – Many diseased *conditions of the lungs* diminish the area available for breathing: eg. pneumonia, tuberculosis, emphysema, bronchitis, collections of fluid in the pleural cavities, and pressure by a tumour or aneurysm.

Pleurisy causes short, rapid breathing to avoid the pain of deep inspiration.

Narrowing of the air passages may produce sudden and alarming attacks of difficult breathing, especially among children: eg. in laryngismus, croup, asthma, and diphtheria (see these headings).

Almost all *affections of the heart* cause breathlessness when the person undergoes any special exertion.

Anaemia is a frequent cause.

Obesity is often associated with shortness of breath.

Among the *general diseases* which may interfere with breathing, the uraemia of Bright's disease and the coma which may occur in diabetes mellitus must be noted.

Treatment – In young girls who become breathless on very slight exertion the treatment is generally that for bloodlessness. (See ANAEMIA.) For the treatment of breathlessness in stout people, see CORPULENCE. In all conditions of breath-

lessness due to disease of a lung, the patient finds most ease in breathing when he lies upon the affected side. In most inflammatory conditions of the air passages much relief is gained from steam inhalations. The subjects of heart disease, if able to go about, should not unduly exert themselves, and are benefited by one of the forms of treatment mentioned under HEART DISEASES. Persons confined to bed by a heart affection are often unable to lie down, and must be provided with a comfortable bed-rest. Their difficulty of breathing is often due to bronchitis (see BRONCHITIS), or to collection of fluid in the chest (see DROPSY), which requires special and energetic treatment. For breathlessness with lividity, oxygen inhalation is often usefully employed.

BRETYLIUM TOSYLATE is one of the drugs introduced for the treatment for hypertension. It acts by inhibiting sympathetic nerve action.

BRIGHT'S DISEASE is a term applied to a class of diseases of the kidneys which have as their most common symptom the presence of albumin in the urine, and often also the presence of dropsy. These associated symptoms, in connection with kidney disease, were first described in 1827 by Dr Richard Bright. Since that time the subject has been investigated by many able physicians, and it is now well established that the above-named symptoms may be dependent on various causes. (See ALBUMINURIA.) Further, one or both of these symptoms may be absent in cases of Bright's disease which are readily recognizable as such from other symptoms.

There is still considerable confusion in the classification of this group of diseases but, speaking generally, it may be said that the terms nephritis or glomerulonephritis are synonymous with Bright's disease, and that these are subdivided into:

Acute Bright's Disease or Acute Glomerulonephritis.

Subacute Bright's Disease or Subacute Glomerulonephritis.

Chronic Bright's Disease or Chronic Glomerulonephritis.

ACUTE BRIGHT'S DISEASE (ACUTE GLOMERULONEPHRITIS).

Cause – This is a disease predominantly of childhood. It is practically always associated with an infection of the throat, tonsils, sinuses, or some other part of the upper respiratory tract by the haemolytic streptococcus. As this is the causative organism of scarlet fever and of erysipelas, acute glomerulonephritis may also occur in association with these two diseases. The first signs of kidney involvement usually occur 7–21 days after the original infection with the haemolytic streptococcus. In view of this fact, taken in conjunction with the fact that no infecting organism is ever found in the urine or in the kidneys, it is now assumed that glomerulonephritis is an allergic reaction on the part of the kidneys to the haemolytic streptococcus. Predisposing factors are exposure to cold or general poor health, but it will often be found that the condition occurs in a previously healthy child without any warning apart from the fact that he has had a 'sore throat' for some days. In this form of the disease the kidneys are red, swollen, and congested. There is a diffuse congestion of the blood-vessels throughout the kidneys, and this results in degeneration and swelling of the lining cells of the glomeruli. Later the renal tubules are involved. These damaged lining cells of the glomeruli and the tubules are passed in the urine, and, glued together in the inflammatory process with red blood corpuscles, they unite to form casts of the renal tubules through which they have passed.

There is another form of acute glomerulonephritis in which there is a less diffuse involvement of the kidneys – what is sometimes termed acute focal glomerulonephritis. This occurs in conditions such as subacute bacterial endocarditis (qv), in which small clots (or emboli) are discharged from the damaged heart valve, and some of these emboli lodge in the kidneys.

Symptoms – The symptoms to which the condition gives rise are usually of a severe character, although frequently cases of acute Bright's disease, occurring, for example, in the course of scarlet fever, are so mild as to escape notice at the time, and only cause trouble when the condition becomes chronic in later life. Vomiting often ushers in the attack; pain in the back of a moderate degree is also a common symptom, and there is often for the first day or two a slight febrile disturbance. Dropsy, varying in degree from slight puffiness under the eyes to an accumulation of fluid distending the body cavities and causing serious embarrassment to respiration, is a common accompaniment. The digestion is almost invariably disordered, the appetite is poor, and the patient is troubled with headache. There is

also a rise in the blood-pressure. The urine is reduced in quantity, is of dark, smoky, or blood-stained colour, and, when it is tested, is found to contain a large amount of albumin, while under the microscope blood corpuscles with hyaline and epithelial casts, as already mentioned, are found in abundance.

This state of acute inflammation, if very severe, may lead to stoppage of the excretion of the urine to such an extent that waste products accumulate in the blood and paralyse vital activity. Death is then generally preceded by severe headache followed by unconsciousness and often by convulsions, a condition known as acute uraemia. Even in extreme cases, however, energetic treatment may save the patient's life. Death may also result from heart failure. More frequently the acute disease partially subsides and gradually results in the establishment of subacute or chronic Bright's disease. In other cases an arrest of the inflammatory action occurs, the urine increases in amount, the blood and later the albumin and other abnormal constituents disappear from the urine, the dropsy subsides, the strength returns, and the disease entirely disappears.

Treatment – The greatest care must be taken of a person showing for the first time the symptoms of acute Bright's disease, because, although the condition is seldom fatal in a first attack, if it be allowed to pass on to the chronic form the person must in future live the life of a semi-invalid, or, at all events, is greatly limited in the extent of his activities. The patient must remain in the equable temperature of bed, carefully protected from all chance of chill. During the acute phase of the disease the diet should be light and there should be some restriction of the fluid intake. Unless the daily output of urine is very low, however, it is seldom advisable to restrict the fluid intake to much less than two pints (1 litre) daily. At first the diet should consist principally of milk and glucose drinks flavoured with fruit juices. As the condition improves, the diet should be gradually supplemented by the addition of milk puddings, jelly, bread and butter, and steamed fish. Although restriction of protein is not now considered as essential as it used to be, meat should not be given during the first few weeks.

If kidney function ceases, as judged by the inability of the patient to pass any urine, then the time has come for the use of haemodialysis, or the artificial kidney (qv) as it is known.

When dropsy is a troublesome feature, the abolition of salt from the diet and the substitution of salt-free bread and of potatoes, fresh butter, fruit, and green vegetables for the milk is recommended by some authorities. During the period of convalescence care must be exercised in the avoidance of animal food in large quantity, of alcoholic stimulants, and of chills to the surface of the body. Ideally, the patient should be kept in bed until the urine has become normal again but in those cases which do not clear completely this is obviously impracticable. The general rule in these circumstances is that the patient is allowed up and about under careful control once the function of the kidneys, as judged by standard tests, ceases to improve. A change for a time to a dry, warm climate is often beneficial.

SUBACUTE BRIGHT'S DISEASE (SUBACUTE GLOMERULONEPHRITIS) may occur as a direct sequel of the acute stage of the disease, the patient passing direct from the acute to the subacute phase. In other cases the transition is more gradual: the patient never recovers completely from the acute phase, and over a period of months, or even years, gradually passes into the subacute stage. In yet another small group of cases subacute glomerulonephritis appears to develop without any preceding acute glomerulonephritis. The probable explanation of these cases is that the acute stage has been so mild as to be overlooked, but the pathological process has been present all the time, gradually producing extensive enough changes in the kidney to result in all the typical signs and symptoms of subacute glomerulonephritis. The brunt of the process in this stage falls on the renal tubules, which are the site of marked degenerative changes, resulting in swelling and desquamation of the lining cells. The kidneys are large and white. The urine contains large amounts of albumin, many fatty and hyaline casts, but practically no blood.

This stage of Bright's disease is sometimes referred to as the nephrotic stage, nephrosis being a term introduced by Muller in 1905 to designate a degenerative lesion confined to the kidney tubules.

Symptoms – The characteristic features are dropsy, which may be generalized and include ascites (fluid in the abdomen) and effusions in the pleural cavity; pallor, which is partly due to anaemia and partly due to the subcutaneous oedema; normal or low blood-pressure; diminution in the daily output of urine, and marked albuminuria. Indeed, there are few other conditions in which such gross albuminuria is found. Unlike the acute stage, there is little or no blood in the urine, and the nitrogenous contents of the blood are only slightly raised in amount, if at all. The protein content of the blood is much decreased owing to the steady loss of protein in the urine, and this hypoproteinaemia, as it is called, is one of the principal causes of the dropsy. Patients in this stage of Bright's disease are very susceptible to infections, especially of the lungs and the intestines, and such an infection may be responsible for a fatal termination.

Treatment – The essentials of treatment are rest in bed, relief of the oedema (or dropsy) and alleviation of the anaemia. As the oedema is primarily due to a deficient concentration of protein in the blood. treatment should consist of a high protein diet: ie. one containing 100–120 grams of protein daily. The less salt the diet contains the better, but a 'salt-free' diet is most unpalatable. If the dropsy does not respond to such a diet, then diuretics should be administered: urea, mersalyl, chlorothiazide, or theophylline ethylenediamine (aminophylline). Full doses of iron are given to relieve the anaemia. In certain cases the administration of cortisone, or one of its analogues, is of value.

CHRONIC BRIGHT'S DISEASE (CHRONIC GLOMERULONEPHRITIS) is the final stage of the disease. It may follow directly upon the subacute stage, or may arise as a result of repeated recurrence of the acute stage. In other cases there may be a long period intervening between the subacute and the chronic stage, whilst in others again there may be no history of previous kidney disease. Here the probable explanation is that the original stages of the disease have been so slight as to be overlooked. The kidneys in this stage are small, contracted, and usually white in appearance because of the diminution in the number of active blood-vessels. This characteristic appearance is due to gradual replacement of the active kidney tissue by fibrous, or scar, tissue. It should be pointed out that a similar condition, both pathologically and clinically, may arise as a result of long-continued degenerative changes in the kidneys produced by arterial disease. This is the condition now commonly referred to as *nephrosclerosis*.

Symptoms – These vary considerably, depending upon the stage the changes in the kidney have reached. In the early stages they may be similar to those of the subacute stage, but gradually the blood-pressure tends to rise, the albuminuria decreases in amount, the dropsy diminishes (until heart failure sets in), and the nitrogenous contents of the blood (eg. urea) increase. Because of the inability of the kidneys to concentrate the urine, the specific gravity of the urine falls to 1005 (or less) and there is not the normal variation between the concentration of the urine voided during the night and that voided during the day. Very often in the later stages the patient complains of symptoms not apparently directly connected with the kidney: eg. headache, shortness of breath, failing vision, loss of appetite, indigestion, or even apoplexy. Many of these symptoms are due to the associated arteriosclerosis or high blood-pressure. The dimness of vision is due to retinitis, which arises as a result of arteriosclerosis of the retinal artery. The apoplexy is a result of arteriosclerosis of the arteries supplying the brain. This may lead to blockage of the arteries (cerebral thrombosis) or rupture of the arteries (cerebral haemorrhage). If the patient does not die of some intercurrent infection, heart failure, or a stroke, the final stage is uraemia (qv).

Treatment – As the condition is incurable, the treatment is palliative: ie. it is directed to relieving as much as possible the strain on the kidneys and the heart. Thus the patient should lead as quiet and as sheltered a life as possible, preferably in a warm, dry climate. He should avoid exposure to cold and damp, and in the winter should always be warmly clad. A certain amount of quiet exercise should be encouraged, except when there are exacerbations of the condition; these are indications for a period of rest in bed. The diet should not contain too much protein, but it is a mistake to impose too rigid restrictions. The appetite is often poor and requires stimulating rather than the reverse. Condiments, spices, strong tea and coffee should be avoided. Alcohol in moderation, especially in the form of spirits and light wines, does no harm. If signs of heart failure develop, then digitalis should be given. Dropsy may be so marked as to require treatment, and here theophylline ethylenediamine (aminophylline) is the safest diuretic. If this fails, then a diuretic such as chlorothiazide or frusemide may be given, but its use must be carefully controlled. Sedatives are often required, and of these the barbiturates are usually the most effective: eg. phenobarbitone. In some cases chloralamide or chloral hydrate may be more effective. Iron

should be given if there is any anaemia, but the anaemia in chronic glomerulonephritis is very resistant to treatment. If constipation is troublesome, some mild laxative should be given, such as liquid paraffin, bisacodyl or a senna preparation.

BROMHEXINE is an expectorant (qv) which is proving of value in the treatment of asthma and chronic bronchitis.

BROMIDES are salts of bromine. The bromides of potassium, sodium, strontium, and ammonium are used in medicine. They act chiefly by depressing activity, and dull sensibility of the brain.

Uses – Introduced to clinical medicine just over a hundred years ago, the bromides were for long the standard treatment of epilepsy. For this purpose they have now been largely replaced by the barbiturates, or more recent anticonvulsant drugs, but they are still of value in occasional cases of epilepsy which do not respond satisfactorily to the newer drugs. Their other use is as an occasional sedative in mild cases of insomnia: either alone in a dosage of 10 to 20 grains (0·6 to 1·2 G), or in combination with chloral hydrate. They have the disadvantage of tending to produce an eruption, especially about the face. (See BROMISM.) As a result of taking bromides for a long time some people may show symptoms of a disturbed balance of mind, which pass off when the drug is omitted.

BROMIDROSIS means the excretion of evil-smelling perspiration. (See PERSPIRATION, DISORDERS OF.)

BROMISM is the name given to a group of symptoms consisting of acne on the face, mental dullness, sleepiness, weakness, unsteady gait, and bad breath, which shows that too much bromide is being taken.

BROMPHENIRAMINE MALEATE is an antihistamine preparation.

BROMOCRIPTINE is an ergot (qv) alkaloid which is being successfully used in the treatment of acromegaly (qv). It is also proving of value in the treatment of Parkinsonism (qv), the suppression of lactation (qv), and the pain in the breast that sometimes precedes menstruation.

BROMPTON MIXTURE is a prescription of somewhat variable constituents, but consisting basically of morphine, cocaine and whisky (or rum) which for long has had a high reputation as a most effective pain-reliever, particularly in the terminal stages of painful diseases such as cancer.

BRONCHIAL TUBES (see AIR PASSAGES; BRONCHUS; LUNGS).

BRONCHIECTASIS is a condition characterized by dilatation of the bronchi. This is the result as a rule of infection of the bronchial tree leading to obstruction of the bronchi. As a result of the obstruction the affected individual cannot get rid of the secretions in the bronchi beyond the obstruction. This accumulates and becomes infected and gradually weakens the wall of the bronchi which dilate and become an increasingly large deposit of infected material. The initial infection may be due to bacterial or viral pneumonia or the infection of the lungs complicating measles or whooping-cough. Other causes are obstruction of the bronchi by tuberculosis, cancer of the lung or the inhalation into the lungs of a foreign body, such as a tooth during dental extraction. It usually starts in childhood but may not manifest itself until adult life. It manifests itself by the coughing up of large amounts of putrid, foul-tasting, foul-smelling expectoration, which may contain blood. The condition is not immediately dangerous to life, but as a rule it results in a gradual deterioration of health, with night sweats, clubbing of the fingers and toes (see CLUBBING), and an aggravated form of chronic bronchitis.

Treatment consists of getting rid of the accumulated secretion in the dilated bronchi by means of what is known as postural drainage. This consists of the patient lying on the affected side over the edge of the bed with a pillow under him, and the head well down, so as to drain the affected area. This allows the infected secretion to drain to the trachea (or windpipe) whence it is coughed up. This should be carried out for a quarter of an hour night and morning. It helps to increase the amount of secretion got rid of if a relative or friend percusses, or firmly taps, on the chest over the affected area. At the same time the patient should take deep breaths and cough firmly to dislodge the secretion and get rid of it. Should there be a flare-up of the condition, as there often is, this postural drainage should be done four times a day. If the odour is particularly unpleasant, this may be kept in check by inhalations of creosote, or by vaporizing creosote and other aromatic substances in steam near the bed. If there should be a flare-up of the condition due to infection, this is controlled by antibiotics. If the condition is localized to one lobe of the lung, then an operation (lobectomy) may be performed to remove the affected lung. Patients with bronchiectasis should be immunized against influenza every autumn, should not smoke, and should ensure that they have a well-balanced diet and as much fresh air as possible.

BRONCHIOLECTASIS is the term applied to the morbid dilatation of the bronchioles as a result of disease of their walls.

BRONCHIOLES is the term applied to the finest divisions of the bronchial tubes.

BRONCHIOLITIS is a name sometimes applied to bronchitis affecting the finest bronchial tubes, also known as capillary bronchitis.

BRONCHITIS means inflammation of the mucous membrane of the bronchial tubes. Well known as one of the most common hazards of the climate of Great Britain, bronchitis exists in either an *acute* or a *chronic* form.

(*a*) *ACUTE BRONCHITIS*, like other inflammatory affections of the chest, often develops following exposure to cold, particularly if accompanied with damp, or sudden change from a heated to a cool atmosphere. It may also arise as the result of inhaling irritating dust or vapours. The exciting cause is infection of the bronchial tree with one or more of the catarrh-producing organisms, and great numbers of these bacteria are commonly found in the expectoration.

Symptoms – The symptoms vary according to the severity of the attack, and more especially according to the extent to which the inflammatory action spreads in the bronchial tubes. The disease usually manifests itself at first in the form of catarrh, or the common cold; but the accompanying feverishness and general constitutional disturbance proclaim the attack to be something more severe, and symptoms denoting the onset of bronchitis soon present themselves. A short, painful, dry cough, accompanied with rapid and wheezing respiration, a feeling of rawness and pain in the throat and behind the breast-bone, and of oppression or tightness throughout the chest, mark the early stages of the disease.

After a few days, expectoration begins

to come with the cough, at first scanty and viscid or frothy, but soon becoming copious and of purulent character. In general, after free expectoration has been established the more urgent and distressing symptoms abate; and, while the cough may persist for a length of time, often extending to three or four weeks, in the majority of instances convalescence advances, and the patient is ultimately restored to health, although not infrequently a tendency is left to a recurrence of the disease on exposure to its exciting causes.

When the ear or the stethoscope is applied to the chest of a person suffering from such an attack as that just described, there are heard in the earlier stages snoring or cooing sounds, mixed up with others of wheezing or fine whistling quality, accompanying respiration. These are named dry sounds or rhonchi, and they are occasionally so abundant and distinct as to convey their vibrations to the hand applied to the chest, as well as to be audible to a bystander at some distance. As the disease progresses these sounds become to a large extent replaced by others of crackling or bubbling character, which are termed moist sounds or crepitations. Both these kinds of abnormal sounds are readily explained by a reference to the pathological condition of the parts. One of the first effects of inflammation upon the bronchial mucous membrane is to cause some degree of swelling, which, together with the presence of a tough secretion closely adhering to it, tends to narrow the tubes. The respired air as it passes through the narrowed tubes gives rise to the dry or sonorous breath sounds, the coarser being generated in the large, and the finer or wheezing sounds in the small divisions of the bronchi. Before long, however, the discharge from the bronchial mucous membrane becomes more abundant and less glutinous, and accumulates in the tubes till dislodged by coughing. The respired air, as it passes through this fluid, causes the moist *râles*, or crepitations, above described. In most instances both moist and dry sounds are heard abundantly in the same case, since different portions of the bronchial tubes are affected at different times in the course of the disease.

Such are briefly the main characteristics presented by an ordinary attack of acute bronchitis running a favourable course.

The case, however, is very different when the inflammation spreads into, or when it primarily affects, the minute ram-

ifications of the bronchial tubes which are in immediate relation to the air-cells of the lungs, giving rise to that form of the disease known as *capillary bronchitis*. When this takes place all the symptoms already detailed become greatly intensified, and the outlook becomes much more serious in consequence of the interruption to the entrance of air into the lungs, and thus to the due aeration of the blood. Indeed the condition may become indistinguishable from bronchopneumonia. The feverishness and restlessness increase, the cough becomes incessant, the breathing extremely rapid and laboured, the nostrils dilating with each effort, and evidence of impending suffocation appears. The surface of the body is pale or dusky, the lips are livid, while breathing becomes increasingly difficult and is attended with suffocative paroxysms which render the recumbent posture impossible. Unless speedy relief is obtained by coughing and expectoration, the patient's strength gives way, somnolence and delirium set in, and death ensues. All this may be brought about in a few days, and such cases, particularly among the very young or the aged, sometimes prove fatal within forty-eight hours.

In addition to the auscultatory signs present in ordinary bronchitis, there generally exist in this form of the disease abundant fine crepitations at the bases of both lungs; and the appearance of these organs after death shows the minute bronchi and many of the air-cells to be filled with matter similar to that which had been expectorated, and which has thus acted as a mechanical hindrance to the entrance of the air and caused death by asphyxia.

Acute bronchitis is pre-eminently dangerous at the extremes of life, and mortality statistics show it to be one of the most fatal of the diseases of those periods. This is to be explained not only by the well-recognized fact that all acute diseases tell with great severity on the feeble frames alike of infants and aged people, but more particularly by the tendency which bronchitis undoubtedly has, in them, to assume the capillary form, and, when it does so, to prove quickly fatal. The importance therefore of early attention to the slightest evidence of bronchitis among the very young or the aged can scarcely be overrated.

Bronchitis is also apt to be very severe when it occurs in persons who are addicted to intemperance. Again, in those who suffer from any disease affecting directly or indirectly the respiratory functions, such as tuberculosis or heart disease, the supervention of an attack of acute bronchitis is an alarming complication, increasing, as it necessarily does, the embarrassment of breathing. The same remark is applicable to those numerous instances of its occurrence in children who are, or have been, suffering from such diseases as have always associated with them a certain degree of bronchial irritation, such as measles and whooping-cough.

One other source of danger of a special character in bronchitis remains to be mentioned: collapse of the lung. Occasionally a branch of a bronchial tube becomes plugged up with secretion, so that the area of the lung to which this branch brings air ceases to be inflated on inspiration. The small quantity of air imprisoned in the portion of lung gradually escapes, but no fresh air enters, and the part collapses and becomes of solid consistence. Increased difficulty of breathing is the result, and when a large portion of lung is affected by the plugging up of a large bronchus, a fatal result may rapidly follow, the danger being specially great in the case of children. Fortunately, the obstruction may sometimes be removed by vigorous coughing, and relief is then obtained.

Treatment – In those mild cases which are more of the nature of a simple catarrh little else will be found necessary than confinement in a warm room, or in bed, for a few days, and the use of light diet, together with warm diluent drinks, warm milk being specially beneficial. Additional measures are called for when the disease is more markedly developed. Either penicillin or one of the sulphonamides should be given. In the early stages of the disease, when the cough is harsh and unproductive, linctuses give considerable relief. Sedatives are also usually required at night: eg. chloralamide or phenobarbitone. Opium or morphine must never be given to a patient with bronchitis, because of its depressant effect upon the respiratory centre. In the later stages of the disease, as the cough becomes looser, expectorants (qv) are of value. From the outset of the attack the employment of warm applications to the chest, in the form of an electric pad, medicated wool, or a rubber hot-water bottle, affords great relief. In children, rubbing the chest with some stimulating liniment such as camphorated oil has a similar effect.

In the earlier stages few remedial measures are of greater value than the frequent inhalation of steam. This is accomplished readily enough in the case of adults by the use of an inhaler or simply by breathing over an open-mouthed vessel containing boiling water. In children, in whom this plan cannot be carried out in the same manner, there is in general no difficulty in surrounding them with an atmosphere of steam by erecting over the bed or cot a tent, formed by a screen and blanket,

92 – Bronchitis tent and steam kettle.

under which can be led the orifice of a tin kettle heated by a spirit lamp or electric heater, and provided with a spout 2 or 3 feet (60 or 90 cm) long (illustration 92). Various drugs of soothing or expectorant qualities, such as tincture of benzoin and menthol, can also be added to the water in the kettle, or poured upon a sponge which is placed in the end of the spout, and so inhaled in the steam (See INHALATION.)

When the bronchitis is of the capillary form, the great object is to overcome the infection as quickly as possible by means of full doses of the sulphonamides, penicillin, or one of the other antibiotics, to maintain the patient's strength, and to endeavour to secure the expulsion of the morbid secretion from the fine bronchi (see POSTURAL DRAINAGE). In addition to the remedies already mentioned, oxygen may be called for.

(*b*) *CHRONIC BRONCHITIS* –
Causes – This form of the disease may arise as the result of repeated attacks of the acute form, or it may exist altogether independently. It occurs more often among persons advanced in life than among the young, although no age is exempt from it.

It is one of the most common causes of death in this country and is much more common than in any other country (table 9). Hence its international reputation as

Country	Number of deaths	Death rate per 100,000 population
England and Wales	31,862	66·2
West Germany	10,465	17·5
France	2,251	4·6
Hungary	654	6·4
USA	6,151	3·1
Japan	5,288	5·4
Australia	2,586	22·4

Table 9 – A comparison of the death rate from bronchitis in seven different countries in 1966

the 'English disease'. Whilst there is probably a constitutional predisposition to the disease, there are in addition six important contributory factors:

(1) Exposure to irritant dust, smoke or fumes either as an occupational hazard or as part of the atmospheric pollution prevalent in industrial areas.

(2) Excessive cigarette smoking.

(3) Bad housing.

(4) A cold, damp, foggy climate.

(5) Obesity.

(6) Recurring respiratory infections.

The usual history of this form of bronchitis is that of a cough recurring during the colder seasons of the year, and in its earlier stages, departing entirely in summer, so that it is often called 'winter cough'. In many persons subject to it, however, attacks are apt to be excited at any time by very slight causes, such as changes in the weather; and in advanced cases of the disease the cough is seldom altogether absent.

Chronic bronchitis may arise secondarily to some other ailment. This is especially the case in heart disease, in which it often proves a serious complication.

Symptoms – The symptoms and auscultatory signs of chronic bronchitis are on the whole similar to those pertaining to the acute form, except that the febrile disturbance and pain are much less marked. The cough is usually more troublesome in the morning than during the day. There is usually free and copious expectoration of a thin frothy fluid, and occasionally this is so abundant as to constitute what is termed bronchorrhoea.

Chronic bronchitis leads to alterations of structure in the affected bronchial tubes, their mucous membrane becoming thickened or even ulcerated, while occasionally permanent dilatation of the bronchi takes place, often accompanied with profuse foetid expectoration. In long-standing cases of chronic bronchitis, the nutrition of the lungs becomes impaired, and dilatation of the air-sacs (emphysema) and other complications result, giving rise to more or less constant breathlessness and leading to deformity of the chest (barrel-shaped chest). Chronic bronchitis is liable, in some instances, particularly when accompanied with loss of flesh and strength, to be mistaken for tuberculosis; but, whilst this is a possibility which must always be borne in mind, particularly in the elderly, the physician who carefully regards the history of the case and observes the physical signs and symptoms, will in general be able to distinguish the one disease from the other. In this, too, the examination of the sputum for the presence of the tubercle bacillus is of great importance, the discovery of this organism at once indicating the tuberculous nature of the malady.

Chronic bronchitis does not often prove directly fatal, nor is it necessarily inconsistent with long life. Its chief danger lies in the tendency to intercurrent acute attacks, particularly in the aged; and in this manner it is a disturbingly common cause of death.

Treatment – The treatment to be adopted in chronic bronchitis depends upon the severity of the case, the age of the patient, and the presence or absence of complications. Attention to the general health is a matter of prime importance in all cases, more particularly among persons whose work entails exposure. As severe bronchitis is seldom found in one who has never smoked, smoking – certainly of cigarettes – should be given up. If the victim is overweight, he should take steps to get his weight down. In those aggravated forms of chronic bronchitis in which the slightest exposure to cold air brings on fresh attacks, it may become necessary, where circumstances permit, to enjoin confinement to a warm room, or removal to a more genial climate during the winter months.

When expectoration is difficult, such remedies as squill combined with carbonate of ammonia may prove useful. Alternatively, particularly for the troublesome cough with which the individual with chronic bronchitis tends to awaken in the morning, a hot drink, or an alkaline mixture such as the Compound Sodium Chloride Mixture of the British Pharmaceutical Codex 1973, may be effective. The inhalation of vapour containing Friars' balsam or menthol is often followed by marked benefit in this way.

The value of antibiotics in chronic bronchitis is still undecided. Some recommend their routine use every winter, whilst others contend that this is unnecessary and not without its drawbacks. In many cases infection plays a relatively unimportant part, and for such patients antibiotics are obviously of little value, and treatment must consist of the general measures outlined above. In the presence of infection, as exemplified by a purulent sputum and/or the finding of antibiotic-sensitive organisms in the sputum, antibiotics may be of great value.

Acute attacks of the disease, which are so apt to arise in the chronic form, must be dealt with on the principles already indicated in treating of acute bronchitis.

BRONCHOGRAPHY means rendering the outline of the bronchial tree visible on an X-ray film by means of the injection of a radio-opaque substance through the larynx. This is a simple procedure carried out under general anaesthesia and allows the accurate location of, for example, a lung abscess, bronchiectasis (qv), or a tumour in the lung.

BRONCHOPHONY means the resonance of the voice as heard by auscultation over the site of the large bronchial tubes, and, in diseased conditions, conveyed beyond these by cavities or solidification of parts of the lung.

BRONCHO-PNEUMONIA (see PNEUMONIA).

BRONCHOSCOPE is an instrument constructed on the principle of the telescope, which on introduction into the mouth is passed down through the larynx and windpipe and enables the observer to see the interior of the larger bronchial tubes.

BRONCHUS, or bronchial tube, is the name applied to tubes into which the windpipe divides, one going to either lung. The name is also applied to the divisions of these tubes distributed throughout the lungs, the smallest being called bronchioles (illustration 93).

BRONZED SKIN is one of the symptoms of Addison's disease. (See ADDISON'S DISEASE.)

BROW AGUE is a term used to denote both frontal neuralgia or tic douloureux (see NEURALGIA) and migraine or megrim (see MIGRAINE).

93 – The larynx, windpipe, bronchial tubes, and lungs: L, larynx; T, thyroid cartilage; C, cricoid cartilage; Tr, trachea splitting at B into the two bronchi; a, apex of each lung; b, base of each lung.

BRUCELLA ABORTUS is a bacterium closely related to *Brucella melitensis*, the causative organism of Malta or undulant fever. *Br. abortus* causes infectious abortion in cattle, and is excreted in cow's milk, whence it finds its way into the human intestinal tract, giving rise to the most troublesome disease, undulant fever.

BRUCELLA MELITENSIS is the name of a bacterium present in the milk of the goats of Malta and causing Malta or undulant fever among those drinking the milk. Undulant fever is common along the shores of the Mediterranean.

BRUCELLOSIS, also known as UNDULANT FEVER, MALTA FEVER, MEDITERRANEAN FEVER, ROCK FEVER, NEAPOLITAN FEVER, and LEVANT FEVER, is a long-continued fever which occurs principally on the shores and islands of the Mediterranean, but is found also in many other countries.

Causes – In Malta and the Mediterranean littoral the causative organism is the *Brucella melitensis* which is conveyed in goat's milk. In Great Britain, the USA, and South Africa, the causative organism is the *Brucella abortus*, which is conveyed in cow's milk. This is the organism which is responsible for contagious abortion in cattle. In Great Britain it is largely an occupational disease. Thus, in 1974, 70 per cent of the cases occurred in farm workers, 10 per cent in veterinary surgeons, and 6 per cent in abattoir workers. Ten per cent probably acquired it from drinking un-pasteurized milk. It is now prescribed as an industrial disease (see OCCUPATIONAL DISEASES), and insured persons who contract the disease at work can claim industrial injuries benefit.

The number of recorded cases in England, Wales and Scotland in recent years is shown in the accompanying table, which demonstrates the relatively high incidence in Scotland.

Year	England	Scotland
1967	221	188
1968	203	305
1969	198	292
1970	324	325
1971	221	392
1973	217	
1974	162	
1975		113

Table 10 – No. of cases of brucellosis in England and Scotland, 1967–75.

Symptoms – The characteristic features of the disease are fever, drenching sweats necessitating a change of night attire and bed linen, pains in the joints and back, and headache. The temperature is usually undulating. There are, however, many atypical cases, and the diagnosis may be difficult. The liver and spleen may be enlarged. The diagnosis is confirmed by the finding of *Br. abortus*, or antibodies to it, in the blood. Recovery and convalescence tend to be slow.

Treatment – Treatment is directed towards relieving the sleeplessness, the pain in the joints, and other symptoms. The condition responds well to one of the tetracycline antibiotics, and also to gentamicin, and co-trimoxazole, but relapse is all too common. In chronic cases a combination of streptomycin and one of the tetracyclines is often more effective.

Prevention – It can be prevented by boiling or pasteurizing all milk used for human consumption. A compulsory eradication programme is now in force, with a view to ensuring that in due course it may be possible to bring the disease under control, as in Scandinavia, the Netherlands, Switzerland and Canada where the disease has disappeared following the eradication of the disease in animals. In Malta it has practically been abolished by ceasing to use goats' milk.

BRUISES, or CONTUSIONS, are more or less extensive injuries of the deeper parts of the skin and underlying tissues, accompanied generally by outpouring of blood from damaged vessels, but unattended by corresponding open wounds.

Varieties – An extensive bruise may be accompanied by a wound, in which case the injury is known as a contused wound. (See WOUNDS.)

The simplest type of bruise is one in which only the deeper layers of the skin are damaged, causing a slight bluish discoloration due to the tearing of minute vessels and the escape of blood into the cellular spaces of the skin. As the result of a severe blow, the muscles may be bruised and torn without any wound in the skin, and the resulting effusion of blood may cause a large swelling which sometimes, though not usually, results in the formation of an abscess. When a bone is bruised, as by a kick on the shin or by a fall upon the knee or elbow, changes similar to those which follow an actual fracture are produced and a permanent thickening of the bone may result. Bruises of this type are of great importance, because an effusion of blood into the cavity of a joint leads to stiffness lasting some weeks, which, if absorption of the blood be not complete, may remain in some degree permanent owing to the formation of adhesions (see ADHESIONS; and JOINTS, DISEASES OF). Further, it is held by many authorities that some slight injury of this nature is sometimes the starting-point of the tuberculous disease which attacks the bones of children. Severe bruises of internal organs, as from a crush or run-over accident, sometimes occur even when the skin has escaped injury and shows no mark (see ABDOMEN, INJURIES OF). Bruising of the brain or spinal cord occasionally occurs in consequence of a severe shaking, as in a railway accident, and is known as concussion (see BRAIN, DISEASES OF).

Appearance of a bruise – The extent of a bruise and the depth of its tint depend upon the amount of blood which has escaped from the vessels, and this again varies according to the violence of the blow and peculiarities of the person injured. In some diseases, like haemophilia and scurvy, extensive bruises are produced by little or no violence. Sometimes a bruise is so sharply limited that it gives a distinct impression of the instrument with which it has been inflicted, whilst in other cases the blood runs downwards and produces a black mark at some distance from the injured part, as seen, for example, in the blackness beneath the eye which may follow an injury of the forehead or temple.

The colour of a bruise is at first black or

bluish, later becoming brown, and finally changing to yellow, which fades away as alterations take place in, and absorption occurs of, the blood pigment. (See HAEMATOIDIN AND HAEMIN.) The time occupied in disappearance of a bruise depends largely upon the amount of blood effused, but in moderate bruises ten days or a fortnight must elapse before the injury ceases to be noticeable.

Treatment of slight bruises consists chiefly in preventing the effusion of blood after an injury. This is done by firm pressure over the site for three to five minutes. This may be followed by cold compresses firmly fixed in position by suitable bandages. Ice may also be applied with good results. If it be not convenient to apply cold, various astringent substances may be used in the form of evaporating lotions kept in contact with the part for eight or ten hours; thus a cloth may be wrung out in Goulard's water and applied to the bruise, or the skin may be painted with hazeline or tincture of arnica. In painful bruises one of the best applications is lead and opium lotion. (See GOULARD'S WATER.) The injured part, if a limb, should be elevated in a sling or on a couch.

Mere surface bruises and abrasions are benefited by application of hazeline. If the skin be much ruffled or ingrained with dirt the affected area should be well washed with hot water and soap, and then with some antiseptic such as cetrimide. It may then be advisable to cover the area with an adhesive plastic dressing for a day or so.

BRUIT and MURMUR are words used to describe abnormal sounds heard in connection with the heart, arteries, and veins on auscultation.

BRUXISM is the term applied to teeth grinding (qv).

BUBO means a swelling of a lymphatic gland in the groin in venereal disease or in plague. (See PLAGUE.)

BUCHU is a remedy derived from the leaves of *Agathosma betulina* and similar plants. It contains volatile oil and mucilage and is administered in inflammatory conditions of the bladder.

BUDGERIGAR – FANCIER'S LUNG is a form of extrinsic allergic alveolitis, resulting from sensitization to budgerigars, or parakeets as they are known in North America. Skin tests have revealed sensitization to the birds' droppings and/or serum. As it is estimated that budgerigars are kept in 5–6 million homes in Britain, current figures suggest that anything up to 900 per 100,000 of the population are exposed to the risk of developing this condition. (See ALVEOLITIS.)

BUERGER'S DISEASE (see THROMBOANGIITIS OBLITERANS).

BULIMIA means insatiable appetite.

BULLA is another word for blister.

BUMETANIDE is a diuretic (qv) which is active when taken by mouth. It acts quickly – within half-an-hour – and its action is over in a few hours.

BUNDLE OF HIS, or atrioventricular bundle, is a bundle of special muscle fibres which pass from the atria to the ventricles of the heart and which form the pathway for the impulse which makes the ventricles contract, the impulse originating in the part of the atria known as the sinuatrial node.

BUNIONS (see CORNS AND BUNIONS).

BUNIONETTES (see CORNS AND BUNIONS).

BUPIVACAINE is a local anaesthetic.

BURKITT'S LYMPHOMA (see LYMPHOMA).

BURNING FEET is a syndrome (qv) characterized by a burning sensation in the soles of the feet. It is rare in temperate climes but widespread in India and the Far East. The precise cause is not known, but it is undoubtedly associated with malnutrition, and lack of one or more components of the vitamin B complex is the likeliest cause.

BURNING MOUTH is a common complaint. It is most commonly associated with faulty dentures. (See TEETH, DISEASES OF.) Other causes include infections of the mouth. (See MOUTH, DISEASES OF.) It is a not uncommon complaint at the time of the menopause and diabetic subjects are liable to complain of it, especially if their diabetes is not under control. Vitamin deficiency, particularly of certain members of the vitamin B complex, may be responsible. It may be due to a fungal infection following the administration of antibiotics.

BURNS and SCALDS – Burns are injuries caused by dry heat, scalds by moist heat, but the two are similar in symptoms and treatment. Severe burns are also caused by contact with electric wires, and by the action of acids and other chemicals. The burn caused by chemicals differs from a burn by fire only in the fact that the outcome is more favourable, because the chemical destroys the bacteria on the part, so that less suppuration follows.

Severe and extensive burns are most frequently produced by the clothes, for example, of a child, catching fire. This applies especially to cotton garments, which blaze up quickly. It should be remembered that such a flame can immediately be extinguished by making the individual lie on the floor so that the

is much pain, but healing occurs without a scar.

3RD DEGREE – The scarf-skin or epidermis is all peeled off, and the true skin below is in part destroyed, so as to expose the endings of the sensory nerves. This is a very painful form of burn, and a scar follows on healing.

4TH DEGREE – The entire skin of an area is destroyed, with its nerves, so that there is much less pain than in the last form. A scar forms, later contracts, and may produce great deformity.

5TH DEGREE – The muscles also are burned, and still greater deformity follows.

6TH DEGREE – A whole limb is charred. It separates as in gangrene.

In practice, however, today burns are referred to as either *superficial* (or partial

94 – The structure of the skin in relation to the depth of a burn. A-A: Partial-thickness burn. This will heal in 7 to 10 days. B-B: Partial-thickness burn. This will usually heal within 3 weeks. C-C and D-D: Full-thickness burn which will require grafting.

flames are uppermost, and wrapping him in a rug, mat, or blanket. As prevention is always better than cure, particular care should always be exercised with fires and kettles or pots of boiling water in houses where there are young children or old people. Equally important is it that children's night-clothes and frocks be made of non-inflammable material. Pyjamas are also much safer than nightdresses. Severe scalds are usually produced by escape of steam in boiler explosions.

Degrees of burns – The French surgeon Dupuytren divided burns into six degrees, according to their depth.

1ST DEGREE – There is simply redness. Such burns may be painful for a day or two. Similar effects are produced by prolonged exposure to sunlight and to X-rays.

2ND DEGREE – There is great redness, and the surface is raised up in blebs. There

thickness) burns when there is sufficient skin tissue left to ensure regrowth of skin over the burned site; and *deep* (or full thickness) when the skin is totally destroyed and grafting will be necessary (illustration 94).

Symptoms – Whilst many domestic burns are minor and insignificant, more severe burns and scalds can prove to be very dangerous to life. The main danger is due to shock (qv). This arises as a result of loss of fluid from the circulating blood at the site of the burn. This loss of fluid leads to a fall in the volume of the circulating blood. As the maintenance of an adequate blood volume is essential to life, the body attempts to compensate for this loss by withdrawing fluid from the uninjured areas of the body into the circulation. This, however, in turn, if carried too far begins to affect the viability of the body cells, and, as a sequel, essential body cells, such as those of the liver and kidneys, begin to suffer, and the liver and kidneys cease to function properly. This will show itself by the development of jaundice (qv) and the appearance of albumin in the urine. (See ALBUMINURIA.) In addition, the circulation begins to fail with a resultant lack of oxygen (see ANOXIA) in the tissues, and the victim becomes cyanosed (see CYANOSIS), restless and collapsed and, in some cases, death ensues. In addition, there is a strong risk of infection occurring. Particularly is this the case with

95 – The 'rule of nine' for assessing the extent of a burn or scald in relation to the surface area of the body.

severe burns which leave a large raw surface exposed and very vulnerable to any micro-organisms. The combination of shock and infection can all too often be life-threatening unless expert treatment is immediately available.

The immediate outcome of a burn is largely determined by its extent. This is of more significance than the depth of the burn. To assess the extent of a burn in relation to the surface of the body, what is known as the Rule of Nine (illustration 95) has been evolved. From the figure it will be seen that the head and each arm cover 9 per cent of the body surface, whilst the front of the body, the back of the body,

154

and each leg each cover 18 per cent, with the perineum accounting for the remaining 1 per cent. The greater the extent of the burn, the more seriously ill will the victim become from loss of fluid from his circulation, and therefore the more prompt should be his removal to hospital for expert treatment. The depth of the burn, unless this is very great and reaches the 5th or 6th degree, is mainly of import when the question arises as to how much surgical treatment, including skin grafting, will be required.

Treatment – This depends upon the severity of the burn. In the case of quite minor burns or scalds, all that may be necessary if they are seen immediately is to hold the part under cold running water until the pain is relieved. Cooling is one of the most effective ways of relieving the pain of a burn. If the burn involves the distal part of a limb, eg. the hand and forearm, one of the most effective ways of relieving pain is to immerse the burned part in lukewarm water and add cold water until the pain disappears. As the water warms and pain returns more cold water is added. After some three to four hours, pain will not reappear on warming, and the burn may be dressed in the usual way. Thereafter a simple dressing – eg. a piece of sterile gauze covered by cotton-wool, and on top of this a bandage or a piece of Elastoplast – should be applied. The part should be kept at rest and the dressing kept quite dry until healing takes place. Blisters should be pierced with a sterile needle, but the skin should not be cut away. No ointment or oil should be applied, and an antiseptic is not usually necessary.

In slightly more severe burns or scalds, it is probably advisable to use some antiseptic dressing. These are the cases which should be taken to a doctor – whether a general practitioner, a factory doctor, or a casualty officer in hospital. There is still no general consensus of expert opinion as to the best 'antiseptic' to use. Among those recommended are chlorhexidine, and antibiotics such as bacitracin, neomycin and polymixin. An alternative is to use a Tulle Gras dressing which has been impregnated with a suitable antibiotic. One of the many methods recommended is to apply a cream containing chlorhexidine and ligno-caine (which has the double advantage of being both antiseptic and pain-relieving), covering this with a Tulle Gras dressing, covered in turn by cotton-wool and a crêpe bandage. To ensure that the burn is completely sealed off the ends of the dressing are completely sealed with zinc oxide plaster. The dressing is left on for four or five days before being changed unless the burn becomes painful or there is any evidence of infection (such as redness, swelling and pain), when it is changed immediately.

In the case of severe burns and scalds, the only sound rule is immediate removal to hospital. Unless there is any need for immediate resuscitation, such as artificial respiration, or attention to other injuries there may be, such as fractures or haemorrhage, nothing should be done on the spot to the patient except to make sure that he is as comfortable as possible and to keep him warm, and to cover the burn with a sterile (or clean) cloth such as a sheet, pillow-cases, or towels wrung out in cold water. If pain is severe, morphine should be given – usually intravenously. Once the victim is in hospital, the primary decision is as to the extent of the burn, and whether or not a transfusion is necessary. If the burn is more than 9 per cent of the body surface in extent, a transfusion is called for. The precise treatment of the burn varies from hospital to hospital, but the essential is to prevent infection if this has not already occurred, or, if it has, to bring it under control as quickly as possible. A high-protein diet, with ample fluids, is also necessary to compensate for all the protein that has been lost along with the fluid from the circulation. The process of healing is slow and tedious in the case of extensive burns, and involves careful nursing, the maintenance of morale, physiotherapy and occupational therapy. A vital decision is as to whether skin grafting is required, and when this should be initiated.

So far as the ultimate outcome is concerned, the main factor, as has already been noted, is the extent of the burn. The greater this is, the worse the outlook. The outlook is also poor in infants and old people.

Chemical Burns – Phenol or lysol can be washed off promptly before they do much damage. Acid or alkali burns should be neutralized by washing them repeatedly with sodium bicarbonate or 1 per cent acetic acid, respectively. Alternatively, the following buffer solution may be used for either acid or alkali burns: monobasic potassium phosphate (70 grams), dibasic sodium phosphate (70 grams) in 850 millilitres of water.

BURSAE are natural hollows in the fibrous tissues, lined by smooth cells and containing a little fluid. They are situated at points where there is much pressure or friction, and their purpose is to allow free movement without stretching or straining the tissues: for example, on the knee-cap or the point of the elbow, and, generally speaking, where one muscle rubs against another or against a bone. They develop also beneath corns and bunions, or where a bone comes to press in an unwonted manner on the skin.

BURSITIS means inflammation within a bursa. Acute bursitis is of the nature of an abscess, being produced by injury of a bursa, especially on the knee or elbow, when the prominent part of the joint becomes swollen, hot, painful, and red. It is treated as an abscess. (See ABSCESS.)

Chronic bursitis is due to too much movement of, or pressure on, a bursa. For example, the condition of housemaid's knee is a chronic inflammation of the patellar bursa in front of the knee, due to too much kneeling. This condition may consist of either a collection of fluid in the bursa, or, less frequently, in thickening of its walls, producing in either case an elastic swelling over the joint, with pain. In the former case, resting the limb, with counter-irritation (see BLISTERS) over the swelling, or injection of some irritant substance into its interior, forms the treatment; in the latter case, removal by operation.

Chronic bursitis about the sinews round the wrist and ankle is generally called a ganglion. (See GANGLION.)

BUSULPHAN is a preparation allied to the nitrogen mustard group of compounds (qv), with an action on dividing cells similar to that of irradiation. It is proving of value in the treatment of chronic myeloid leukaemia.

BUTTER (see DIET).

BUTYROPHENONES are a group of drugs, including haloperidol, which are proving to be effective in the treatment of psychotic illness.

BYSSINOSIS is a pneumoconiosis (qv), or chronic inflammatory thickening of the lung tissue, due to the inhalation of dust in textile factories. It is found chiefly among cotton and flax workers and, to a lesser extent, among workers in soft hemp. It is rare or absent in workers in jute and the hard fibres of hemp and sisal. In 1976, in England, 102 new cases were diagnosed in the cotton and flax industries.

C

CABBAGE is a vegetable much used in Great Britain. It contains about 5 per cent of carbohydrates, the remainder being largely indigestible vegetable fibre and water. It is a good source of vitamin C (see DIET).

CACAO is the name given to the seeds of *Theobroma cacao*, which yield cocoa, chocolate, and cocoa butter.

CACHET means an oval capsule, generally made of rice paper, for enclosing a dose of unpleasant medicine. Cachets are softened by moistening with water prior to swallowing.

CACHEXIA is the feeble state produced by serious disease, such as cancer.

CACOLET is the name given to a chair suspended from a pack-saddle for transporting wounded.

CADAVERIC RIGIDITY is the stiffness which comes on after death. (See DEATH, SIGNS OF.)

CAECUM is the dilated commencement of the large intestine lying in the right lower corner of the abdomen. Into it the small intestine and the appendix vermiformis open, and it is continued upwards through the right flank as the ascending colon.

CAESAREAN SECTION means the delivery of a child by opening the abdomen and womb from in front. It is supposed to get its name from the traditional, but unproven, story that Julius Caesar was so delivered. It is performed when delivery by the natural passage is undesirable because of the risk to mother and child: for example, because of bony deformity of the pelvis; also when the mother has died just before labour, so as to save the child.

CAFFEINE is a white crystalline substance obtained from coffee, of which it is the active principle. Its main actions are as a cerebral stimulant, a cardiac stimulant, and as a diuretic. It is also of value in some cases of asthma. It is a constituent of many tablets for the relief of headache, usually combined with aspirin and paracetamol. Granular effervescent citrate of caffeine forms a useful, non-intoxicating stimulant in headache due to tiredness.

CAISSON DISEASE, or COMPRESSED AIR ILLNESS, affects workers in compressed air, such as underwater divers and workers in caissons. Its chief symptoms are pains in the joints and limbs (bends), pain in the stomach, headache and dizziness, and paralysis. Sudden death may occur. The condition is caused by the accumulation of bubbles of nitrogen in different parts of the body.

CAJUPUT OIL is a green oil with a camphor-like smell, used for rubbing over painful joints. Spirit of cajuput in teaspoonful doses is useful for severe colic.

CALABAR BEAN is another name for physostigmine (qv).

CALAMINE, or CARBONATE OF ZINC, is a mild astringent used, as calamine lotion, to soothe and protect the skin in many conditions such as eczema and urticaria.

CALCANEUS is the name of the heel-bone or os calcis.

CALCICOSIS is the term applied to disease of the lung caused by the inhalation of marble dust by marble-cutters.

CALCIFEROL, or VITAMIN D_2, is a crystalline substance extracted from irradiated ergosterol, and has the same action as vitamin D. (See VITAMIN.)

CALCIFICATION is the process of deposit of lime salts. This occurs in old scars, as, for example, in the scars left by healed tuberculosis.

CALCITONIN is a hormone produced by the thyroid gland (qv) which lowers the concentration of calcium in the blood.

CALCIUM is the metallic element present in chalk and other forms of lime. The chief preparations used in medicine are calcium carbonate (chalk), calcium chloride, calcium gluconate, calcium hydroxide (slaked lime), liquor of calcium hydroxide (lime-water), calcium lactate, and calcium phosphate (see LIME). Although still commonly used in the treatment of chilblains, there is little evidence that calcium is of any real value in this condition. Calcium gluconate is freely soluble in water and is used in conditions in which calcium should be given by injection.

Calcium is a most important element in diet, and the chief sources of it are milk and cheese. Calcium is especially needed by the growing child and the pregnant and nursing mother.

The recommended daily intakes of calcium are: 500 mg for children, 700 mg for adolescents, 500–900 mg for adults and 1200 mg for pregnant or nursing mothers.

CALCIUM CARBIMIDE is a drug used in the treatment of alcoholism that has the same action as disulfiram (qv) but produces a milder reaction.

CALCULI is the general name given to concretions in, for example, the bladder, kidneys, gall-bladder.

CALIBRE is a talking book service which is available to all blind and handicapped people who can supply a doctor's certificate certifying that they are unable to read printed books in the normal way. Its catalogue contains over 370 books for adults and over 250 for children, and additions are being made at the rate of around three a week. Full details can be obtained from Calibre, Wendover, Aylesbury, Bucks HP22 6PQ.

CALLIPER SPLINT is one that is applied to the broken leg in such a way that in walking the weight of the body is taken by the hip bone and not by the foot.

CALLOSITIES are thickenings of the outer skin or cuticle. (See CORNS.)

CALLOUS ULCER (see ULCER).

CALLUS is the new tissue formed round the ends of a broken bone. (See FRACTURES.)

CALOMEL, or SUBCHLORIDE OF MERCURY, is not to be confounded with corrosive sublimate or perchloride of mercury, a far more active drug and deadly poison. It is a powerful purgative. (See MERCURY.)

CALORIE is the name applied to a unit of energy. Two units are called by this name. The small calorie, or gram calorie, is the amount of heat required to raise one gram of water one degree cen-

tigrade in temperature. The large Calorie or kilocalorie, which is used in the study of dietetics and physiological processes, is the amount of heat required to raise one kilogram of water one degree centigrade in temperature. The number of Calories required to carry on the processes necessary for life and body warmth, such as the beating of the heart, the movements of the chest in breathing, and the chemical activities of the secreting glands, is, for an adult person of ordinary weight, somewhere in the neighbourhood of 1600 Calories. For ordinary sedentary occupations an individual requires about 2500 Calories, for light muscular work slightly over 3000 Calories, and for hard continuous labour about 4000 Calories daily.

Under the International System of Units (SI) (see WEIGHTS AND MEASURES) the kilocalorie has been replaced by the joule, the abbreviation for which is J.1 kilocalorie = 4186·8 J. As the term calorie, however, is so well established in medical writing, it is proposed to retain it in this edition. Conversion from Calories (or kilocalories) is made by multiplying by 4·186, but a factor of 4·2 is simpler and accurate enough for all practical purposes.

CALUMBA is a bitter. (See BITTERS.)

CALVARIA, is another name for the skull cap or vault of the head.

CALX is another name for lime or chalk. It is an old term for the heel.

CALYX means a cup-shaped cavity, the term being especially applied to the recesses of the pelvis of the kidney.

CAMPHINE is another name for oil of turpentine.

CAMPHOR is a solid, crystalline, oily substance distilled from the wood of a species of laurel grown in Japan and Formosa, or made synthetically. It is sold in the form of cubes, or in powder known as flowers of camphor.

Uses – Externally, it is often placed among bed-clothes to keep off fleas, lice, and other insect pests, but for this purpose it has now been largely replaced by the much more efficient DDT (qv). In gout, and various painful skin conditions, it is rubbed up with menthol, thymol or salol to form an oily liquid which can be smeared over the surface with great relief. Liniment of camphor and camphorated oil (1 ounce [28·5 G] of camphor in 8 ounces [228 ml] of olive oil) is likewise useful in painful conditions or as a mild counter-irritant to produce a warm glow when rubbed into the chest in bronchitis and similar conditions.

Internally, spirit of camphor in 5 to 30 drop doses and camphor water in table-spoonful doses are used to relieve spasms like hiccup and colic, and to ward off colds in the head.

Dissolved in oil camphor is sometimes used by hypodermic injection in the treatment of serious heart failure, but this practice has died out in Britain.

CANALICULUS means a small channel, and is applied to (*a*) the minute passage leading from the lacrimal pore on each eyelid to the lacrimal sac on the side of the nose; (*b*) any one of the minute canals in bone.

CANCELLOUS is a term applied to loose bony tissues as found in the ends of the long bones.

CANCER, CARCINOMA and SARCOMA are general names for forms of tumour to which the term 'malignant' is applied. They are differentiated from benign tumours by four principal criteria: (1) They are not encapsulated, or surrounded by a capsule, and they invade and destroy the tissues in which they arise. (2) They have an unlimited power of disorderly reproduction, quite unlike the orderly way in which the healthy cells of an organ are reproduced. (3) Their cells usually show some loss of differentiation of structure and tend to become more like primitive cells. (4) They are capable of producing metastases, or secondary growths, at a distance from the parent, or primary, tumour. Cancer or carcinoma is composed mainly of epithelial cells, or cells similar to those of skin or of the mucous membrane lining the stomach and bowels, or of secreting glands; but these cells are imperfect in form and arrangement (illustration 96), although they generally retain their characters sufficiently to allow of the organ from which they have come being recognized when a section of the cancer is examined under the microscope (illustration 97). A sarcoma is a tumour developing in the connective tissue of bones, muscles, sinews, etc., and in structure resembling imperfect connective tissue (illustration 98). Sarcoma is less common than cancer in the proportion of

158

about one case of the former to twenty of the latter.

Cancers are classified mainly according to the structure they present on microscopic examination. A cancer growing on skin surface is generally known as an EPITHELIOMA. A cancer arising in the stomach or intestine and presenting an appearance resembling imperfectly formed gland tubules is known as ADENOCARCINOMA. A cancer composed almost entirely of cells without supporting tissue is known as a SOFT CANCER. One in which the cells are much compressed and obliterated by development of fibrous tissue is known as a HARD or SCIRRHUS CANCER; these occur particularly in the breast. Various degenerations also occur in cancers, such as

96 – Scanning electron micrograph of human cancer cells, magnified 1500 times. (Photo: Imperial Cancer Research Fund, reproduced on cover of *Nature*, 25.5.78)

glue-like degeneration (COLLOID CANCER), cystic degeneration, calcareous degeneration. Sarcoma is classified into ROUND-CELLED SARCOMA, SPINDLE-CELLED SARCOMA, etc., according to the microscopic appearances.

Causes – The cause of malignant growths is still undiscovered. Many theories have been advanced, and, considering the fact that cancer is gradually becoming more frequent, it has become of great importance to establish the nature of the cause as a first step towards prevention and treatment. Much has been done in the last few years by various cancer research laboratories to increase our knowledge as to the distribution of cancer in the animal kingdom and among different races, and also to study the mode of spread and conditions of growth in this

97 – Microscopic section of cancer of the breast, showing columns of cancer cells (1) surrounded by fibrous tissue (2).

98 – Small round-celled sarcoma of muscle. (1) sarcoma cells, (2) muscle fibres. Both from Kettle's *Pathology of Tumours.* H. K. Lewis & Co. Ltd.

disease. It has been found that cancers occur in animals as well as among human beings, and that no race is exempt from the disease.

It has been found by experiments on animals that cancer can be transferred directly from one animal to another by inoculating a healthy animal with a small piece of cancerous tissue, and it has further been found that, when transferred in this way through a long succession of animals, the type of cancer produced remains always the same. An important step was taken by the Japanese workers who found that cancer could be produced in experimental animals by painting the skin with

tar. British workers then isolated the actual chemical substance in tar which produces the cancer, and it was found that this substance is chemically similar to substances present in the healthy body. Does some chemical twist take place and make these normal substances carcinogenic or cancer-producing? Another important factor to be investigated is infection. Many micro-organisms have been incriminated, but the only one that has stood the test of serious investigation is the virus. For example, there is a type of cancer in fowls which is caused by a virus. There is, however, no present evidence that any human cancer is caused by a virus, though viruses are associated with lymphoma (qv). It is also possible that viruses may play a part in the development of some forms of acute leukaemia (qv), of cancer of the breast and of cancer of the cervix uteri, as well as some sarcomas. Another factor in the causation of cancer is the influence of the hormones of the ductless glands. It appears, for example, that the female sex hormone has an effect on the development of breast cancer. Still another factor is heredity. All this, and other work, suggest that cancer is not one disease with one cause, but an abnormal reaction of the tissues to a variety of exciting agents. Some scientists have supposed that no external cause is necessary, but that in early or embryonic life parts of the developing body come to rest, only to start sudden and irregular growth at a later period of life. The structure of some cancers, in which a cancerous growth develops in one part of the body resembling an embryonic structure or some other organ at a distance, lends support to this view.

Several factors are important considerations in the origin of the disease.

OCCUPATION – With the increasing complexity of many industrial processes, evidence is accumulating as to the risk of some of these processes inducing cancer. Thus it is now known that workers with asbestos, vinyl chloride and certain rubber-manufacturing processes, as well as some wool workers, run a higher risk of developing cancer than other members of the community. (See OCCUPATIONAL DISEASES.)

INJURY – Smoking a clay pipe has been observed to bring on cancer of the lip, constant alcoholic indulgence to favour cancer of the throat and stomach, while a scar, eg. of an old ulcer, may be the starting-point. Chimney-sweeps, paraffin workers, and workers in some other special employments have a great liability to cancer of the skin, apparently from long-continued irritation. It has also been found by experiments on animals that the prolonged application of tar to an area of skin may result ultimately in development of cancer. There does not seem any reason to suppose that cancer follows mechanical damage caused by a blow or wound, although there is ground for the belief that sarcoma occasionally follows some severe injury, such as fracture of a bone.

LOCALITY – There are undoubtedly wide variations in the incidence of cancer in different parts of the country, apart from the fact that death rates for a given age are higher in urban than in rural areas.

The explanation of these geographical differences is still not known.

HEREDITY – Although, strictly speaking, there is no evidence that, in man, cancer is inherited, there is a growing volume of evidence that there may be a familial tendency to develop cancer. Thus, it has been shown that women with carcinoma of the breast or of the uterus have a larger proportion of female relatives with such cancers than would be expected in women in general.

AGE – Cancer is rare before adolescence, the commonest age being between fifty and sixty years. Although cancer is tending to increase in prevalence, there appears from the returns of the Registrar General for England to be no tendency for the number of persons affected below the age of forty-five years to rise, and cancer is now more a disease of old age than formerly. Sarcoma is commoner in younger persons.

SEX – In 1977, in England, the deaths from malignant disease in men were 63,234, compared with 54,531 in women. These figures correspond to a crude death-rate per million living of 2800 males and 2294 females. There is a marked difference in the site of cancer in the two sexes. Thus, in males the most commonly involved site is the lungs, followed by the gastro-intestinal tract and the prostate. In women, on the other hand, the breasts and uterus account for one-third of all cancers. The lungs and the larynx are much less commonly involved among women than among men.

INCIDENCE – In Great Britain in 1970, 171,595 cases of cancer were registered: an incidence rate of approximately 32 for every 10,000 persons of the population. What this means is that around three out of every ten persons will have contracted cancer at some time in their lives and that two of these three people will die from cancer while the third will die from some other cause.

Symptoms – These vary according to the organs with which the growth interferes. Thus cancer of the stomach tends to cause dyspepsia and, it may be, severe pain; cancer in the bowels is apt to lead to gradually increasing obstruction, which may produce either diarrhoea or constipation; cancer affecting the jaw is apt to set up neuralgia; when the growth originates in the womb, flooding is one of the principal early symptoms; when pressure is exercised upon a vein, dropsy results, and so forth. When the growth takes place on the surface there is a hard swelling, which in time is liable to break down and ulcerate. In all cases, the growth tends to spread by the lymphatic vessels, and the glands in the neighbourhood soon become affected by secondary growths if the original one be not speedily removed. This applies especially to cancer, and is one reason why cancer is so liable to return after apparently complete removal. Sarcoma tends less to spread along the lymphatic vessels, but occasionally minute fragments are carried away to distant organs in the circulating blood. When a cancer begins to ulcerate by invading the skin or an internal mucous membrane, a state of poor health and weakness, called cachexia, results. The duration of symptoms of cancer is extremely variable. When the stomach is affected, these seldom last much longer than six months. When the breast is affected, the duration may be very much longer, especially if the main part of the growth has been removed, and life is then often prolonged for many years. The same applies to cancer of the rectum, when an artificial opening is made so that the growth is not irritated by the passage over it of intestinal contents.

Mortality – Cancer now stands second in importance as a cause of death, having in England, in 1977 caused 117,765 deaths as compared with 145,089 due to ischaemic heart disease, while tuberculosis accounted for 898, bronchitis and pneumonia, for 70,543 and vascular lesions of the nervous system, including cerebral haemorrhage, for 68,291.

About 140,000 new cases of cancer are reported in England and Wales each year, which is equivalent to 29 per 10,000 population. Deaths from cancer accounted for 22 per cent of all deaths in England in 1977. In the same year out of every 100 cancer deaths in men the site of the cancer was the lung in 40, the stomach in 10 and the intestine in 11. In women the most common site was the breast (20), followed by the lung (12), the stomach (8), and the uterus and the cervix of the uterus (6).

The increase in cancer is partly explained by the fact that diagnosis is now more precise and many deaths are registered as due to cancer which formerly would have been attributed to 'old age', 'obstruction of the bowels', etc.; and partly by the fact that more people now reach the ages at which cancer prevails.

Treatment – It should be strongly urged that any person finding a hard swelling under the skin should consult a surgeon. In the event of the swelling not being

cancer, mental relief will be gained; and if it be cancer, there is at an early stage the chance of the only completely successful remedy at present known: that is thorough removal. The improvement of modern surgical technique and early diagnosis lead now to the possibility of operations which greatly prolong the life of persons affected by cancer, and in some cases permit of permanent recovery. This is admirably demonstrated in Table 11, which shows the percentage of patients surviving five years after operation for cancer. Thus it will be seen, for example, that in the case of cancer of the breast, 78 per cent of those diagnosed and treated at an early stage of the disease were alive and well without any signs of cancer five years later, compared with only 6 per cent not diagnosed and treated until a later stage.

	Diagnosed and treated early	Diagnosed and treated late
Breast	78	6
Larynx	88	20
Mouth	69	11
Skin	90	14
Cervix uteri	82	3

Table 11 – Percentage of patients with cancer of different parts of the body alive and well with no signs of cancer five years after treatment.

In the case of certain internal cancers, e.g. of the stomach, attempts at complete removal have not, taking all cases together, attained a great measure of success, but much can be done in the way of operations designed for relief of symptoms, which thus prolong life. Much greater success has attended modern operations for complete removal of cancer of the breast and the womb.

Many 'cures' have from time to time been vaunted, such as arsenic paste, turpentine, injections of trypsin, adrenaline and lead salts, but these have all proved useless on trial. In many cases much benefit accrues from combined treatment by surgery, X-rays, and radium. (See RADIUM, also RADIOTHERAPY under X-RAYS.) Radioactive isotopes are also proving of value in many cases. (See ISOTOPES.)

The most recent development in the treatment of cancer, is chemotherapy. Several chemical substances have been discovered to have an effect on malignant tumours. The major problem here is that, though there are now over thirty anticancer drugs, most of them not only damage or kill cancer cells, but also have a harmful effect on the normal cells of the body. They are therefore potentially dangerous and must be used with the greatest of care. Even so there are now at least ten types of cancer which can be cured by chemotherapy in a proportion of patients. These include some of the leukaemias (qv), Hodgkin's disease (qv), choriocarcinoma (qv), and some forms of cancer in childhood.

In the terminal care of patients with inoperable cancer the three essentials are loving care, good nursing and the administration of adequate doses of pain-relieving drugs. This is a regime that can put considerable strain on the relatives should the patient be nursed at home. Such relatives who are finding the strain too great will obtain valuable help and advice from either The Marie Curie Memorial Foundation, 124 Sloane Street, London SW1X 9BP; or The National Society for Cancer Relief, Michael Sobell House, 30 Dorset Square, London NW1.

CANCRUM ORIS, also called WATER CANKER or NOMA, is a gangrenous ulcer about the mouth which affects weakly children, especially after some severe disease, such as measles. It is due to the growth of bacteria in the tissues.

CANDIDIASIS, or CANDIDOSES, is the infection caused by *Candida albicans*. The infection may occur in the mouth, where it is known as thrush (qv), lungs, intestine, vagina, skin or nails.

CANDIDICIN is an antibiotic produced by a strain of *Streptomyces griseus*, which is proving of value in the treatment of certain fungal infections such as moniliasis (qv).

CANINE TEETH, or EYE-TEETH, (see TEETH).

CANITIES is the term applies to whitening or greying of the hair.

CANKER is a name applied to small ulcers which form about the mouth and lips as the result of some local irritation, eg. a jagged tooth, or in a condition of dyspepsia and deteriorated general health. (See MOUTH, DISEASES OF.)

CANNABIS INDICA, consists of the flowering tops of *Cannabis sativa*. (See DRUG ADDICTION.)

CANNED FOOD – The canning of food has increased tremendously of recent years, and indeed it is difficult to imagine the modern civilized world without canned food. Originally popularized in the United States of America, it had to overcome considerable prejudice in Great Britain. Such prejudice still persists to a certain extent, but, irrespective of the merits of the controversy of fresh versus preserved food, it must be recognized that the advantages of canned food far outweigh the disadvantages. Modern methods of canning are so efficient that not only is the purity of the food preserved but its nutritional value is retained. There is, of course, some loss of vitamin content but this has been much reduced of recent years. Indeed there is probably less loss of vitamins in canning than in the average domestic cooking. The further great advantage of canning is that it makes available to many people foodstuffs which otherwise they would either never be able to obtain or could only obtain at certain seasons of the year.

Methods of canning vary according to the foodstuff, but the two essentials of all canning processes are (1) heat treatment of the food and (2) expulsion of all air, after which the can is hermetically sealed. One of the major problems in canning is achieving the optimum temperature that will kill all bacteria but will not affect the nutritive value of the food or spoil its taste. A step to cope with this problem is the introduction of aseptic canning, in which the food is sterilized before it is sealed in sterilized cans. Many canned foods will keep for long periods: eg. canned fish, meat preparations and soups will keep for five years, whilst canned vegetables will keep for two years. These, however, are safe figures. Cans of up to 20 years of age have been found to be in good condition, and the contents quite edible.

Dangers of canned food – Outbreaks of food poisoning due to canned food are rare unless the food is contaminated after the container is opened, though, as Aberdeen learned to its cost, outbreaks of typhoid fever can occur as a result of the contamination of the contents of cans cooled in contaminated water. In 1960–63 (inclusive), in England and Wales, 63 of the 749 outbreaks of food poisoning, for which information was available, were due to canned food: canned meat on 44 occasions, canned fish on 13 occasions, and canned vegetables on six occasions. The organism most commonly responsible was the staphylococcus. In other cases decomposition of canned fish or meat may occur due to faulty cans, whilst the acid in fruits or vegetables may lead to erosion of faulty tinplate or soldering, with contamination of the foodstuff with tin or lead.

Examination of canned food – Most cases of poisoning with canned food could be avoided if cans were examined before use. Canned food is carefully inspected either in the canning factory if made in this country or at the port of entry if imported. About 1·5 per cent of canned meat is rejected in this country. It is a sound rule never to buy a canned food which does not bear a manufacturer's name. Another sound rule is that good cans usually contain good food. Any can which is leaking should be immediately discarded, and much rusting should be regarded with suspicion. 'Blowing', or bulging of the ends of the can, is the most important sign of a faulty can, but this must be differentiated from the bulging of one side of a can due to an indentation in

Uses – Its only use is for blistering (see BLISTERS), and it may be applied as a plaster, in a paste, or painted on in ethereal solution called liquor epispasticus but it is seldom used now.

CANTHUS is the name applied to the angle at either end of the aperture between the eyelids.

CAPILLARIES are the minute vessels which join the ends of the arteries to the commencement of the veins. Their walls consist of a single layer of fine, flat transparent cells, bound together at the edges (illustration 99), and the vessels form a mesh-work all through the tissues of the body, bathing the latter in blood with only the thin capillary wall interposed, through which gases and fluids readily pass. These vessels are less than $\frac{1}{1000}$ inch (0·025 mm) in width. (See CIRCULATION OF THE BLOOD.)

99 – A diagram to show the arrangement of the endothelial cells fitting together to form the wall of a capillary. From *Hewer's Textbook of Histology*. William Heinemann, Ltd.

the opposite side. Tapping of a sound can should produce a dull note; if the note is drum-like, this suggests gas-formation in the can due to decomposition. Shaking should produce no sound in a can of meat, but this test, of course, is of no value in the case of canned fruit, which contains syrup. If on opening the can an unpleasant or a stale odour is noted, or if, in the case of meat, there is a loss of firmness of the contents or a fading of the colour, the contents should be discarded.

CANNULA, or CANULA, is a tube for insertion into the body, designed to fit tightly round a trocar, a sharp pointed instrument which is withdrawn from the cannula after insertion, so that fluid may run out through the latter.

CANTHARIDES, or SPANISH FLY, is a powder made of the body and wings of a dried beetle, *Cantharis vesicatoria*, which inhabits Spain, Italy, Sicily and Southern Russia.

Action – It is an irritant, first, to the part with which it is brought in contact, and, secondly, to the genital and urinary organs by which it is discharged from the body.

CAPREOMYCIN is an antibiotic derived from *Streptomyces capreolus*, which is proving of value in the treatment of tuberculosis.

CAPSICUM, or CAYENNE PEPPER, consists of small orange-coloured pods containing whitish seeds. It is irritating when applied either internally or to the skin.

Uses – Externally the powdered pepper is used in an ointment, or in the form of 'Chillie paste', to rub over sprains and bruises, the discoloration of which it helps to remove. Internally, tincture of capsicum is given for some forms of dyspepsia, and is said to be useful (in 15-drop doses before meals) to allay the craving for alcohol.

CAPSULE is a term used in several senses in medicine. The term is applied to a soluble case, usually of gelatine, for enclosing small doses of unpleasant medicine. *Enteric-coated capsules,* which have been largely superseded by enteric-coated tablets, are capsules treated in such a manner that the ingredients do not come in contact with the acid stomach contents but are only released when the capsule disintegrates in the alkaline contents of the intestine.

163

The term is also applied to the fibrous or membranous envelope of various organs, as of the spleen, liver or kidney. It is also applied to the ligamentous bag surrounding various joints and attached by its edge to the bones on either side.

CAPUT MEDUSAE is the term describing the abnormally dilated veins that form round the umbilicus in cirrhosis of the liver.

CAPUT SUCCEDANEUM is the temporary swelling which is sometimes found on the head of the new-born infant. It is due to oedema in and around the scalp, caused by pressure on the head as the child is born. It is of no significance and quickly disappears spontaneously.

CARAWAY FRUIT, generally called caraway seed, is used to prepare caraway water and caraway oil. A tablespoonful of the former or 2 drops of the latter on sugar is useful for checking colic, griping pains in children, and flatulence.

CARBACHOL is a drug which stimulates the parasympathetic nervous system. It is given, for example, for paralysis of the gut and for retention of urine due to atony.

CARBAMAZEPINE is a drug which is proving of value in the treatment of trigeminal neuralgia (see TRIGEMINAL NEURALGIA). It is also of value in the treatment of certain cases of epilepsy. Because of its occasional action in causing aplastic anaemia and jaundice it must only be used under careful medical supervision.

CARBENICILLIN (see PENICILLIN).

CARBENOXOLONE is a derivative of glycyrrhetinic acid, the active principle of liquorice, which is proving of value in the treatment of gastric ulcer.

CARBIMAZOLE is at present one of the most widely used drugs in the treatment of hyperthyroidism. It acts by interfering with the synthesis of thyroid hormone in the thyroid gland.

CARBOHYDRATE is the term applied to an organic substance in which the hydrogen and oxygen are usually in the proportion to form water. Carbohydrates are all, chemically considered, derivatives of simple forms of sugar and are classified as monosaccharides (eg. glucose), disaccharides (eg. cane sugar), polysaccharides

(eg. starch). Many of the cheaper and most important foods are included in this group, which comprises sugars, starches, celluloses and gums. When one of these foods is digested, it is converted into a simple kind of sugar and absorbed in this form. In the disease known as diabetes mellitus (qv), the most marked feature consists of an inability on the part of the tissues to assimilate and utilize the carbohydrate material. Each gram of carbohydrate is capable of furnishing slightly over 4 Calories of energy. (See DIET.)

CARBOLIC ACID, or PHENOL, is a coal-tar preparation, first introduced into medicine by Lord Lister.

Action – Carbolic acid first paralyses and then destroys all forms of life, having a specially destructive action upon lowly organisms like bacteria. It has a softening action upon tissues, pus, etc., and it also vaporizes readily, so that it has much greater penetrating power than alcohol, perchloride of mercury, and other powerful antiseptics, which have a hardening action that retards their germicidal power. It dulls pain when applied to an inflamed part, by benumbing the nerves around.

It must never be forgotten that pure carbolic acid, or even a weak lotion too long applied, may painlessly kill the skin and cause it to slough. This effect is lessened by smearing the damaged part with glycerin or with oil.

Internally it has similar actions, and even in moderate doses it is a poison, being first of all an irritant and on absorption a narcotic.

Carbolic acid is used as a standard antiseptic for comparison of the power of other substances to kill germs.

Uses – Because of the risk of producing gangrene or ulceration, carbolic acid must never be used in a compress or dressing on the skin. In the pure form it is sometimes used as a cauterizing agent to sterilize septic areas. In the pure form it is also used in minute amounts in the treatment of ulcers of the cornea. In very weak solution it is used as a throat gargle. As a $2\frac{1}{2}$ per cent solution in glycerin it is useful in treatment of infections of the ear. A further use is in the treatment of haemorrhoids and varicose veins. As a 1 per cent lotion it is of value in the treatment of itching conditions of the skin.

As a disinfectant 1 in 20 of water (or 5 per cent) is the convenient strength, and is used to put in the bottom of the sputum-dish of consumptives, to steep the sheets soiled by typhoid-fever cases, to swab the floors and walls of sickrooms. Lysol is now more commonly used for this purpose.

CARBOLIC ACID POISONING may be due to accident or suicide. No bottle containing carbolic lotion should ever be kept near other medicine bottles, as a few teaspoonfuls may cause death.

Carbolic acid poisoning may also come on slowly through gradual absorption from dressings by a wound. The urine generally is black for a day or two before the case gets serious.

Symptoms – If the acid has been swallowed there is a sense of burning about the mouth and throat, followed by numbness, and the skin and mucous membrane of the mouth show white where the acid has touched them. Unconsciousness and stupor soon come on, and death follows usually in a few hours.

Treatment – Olive oil, or any fatty substance like milk or cream, should be administered at once, and the stomach washed out or emptied by an emetic in several tumblerfuls of tepid water. Large doses are also given internally of Epsom salts or sulphate of magnesium, which combines with the carbolic acid and renders it harmless.

CARBON (see CHARCOAL).

CARBON DIOXIDE SNOW is formed when carbon dioxide (CO_2), stored under pressure in a cylinder, is allowed to escape through a small nozzle. This sudden expansion lowers its temperature to about -70 C and the CO_2 is obtained as a white powder or 'snow', which is then compressed into a cake or tube for application to the skin. It is a most effective method of freezing a localized area, and is commonly used in the treatment of warts (qv).

CARBONIC ACID, or CARBON DIOXIDE, is the gas formed by the tissues and exhaled by the lungs (see AIR and VENTILATION). It effervesces from aerated waters and sparkling wines, and is used in baths for stimulation to the skin (see BATHS). Carbon dioxide in cylinders, combined with oxygen, is used to control breathing in anaesthesia and in cases of carbon monoxide poisoning.

CARBON MONOXIDE is a colourless and odourless gas, the presence of which in a room is undetectable by the occupants. Hence its danger because it has 300 times the affinity for oxygen that haemoglobin (qv) has. It converts haemoglobin into carboxyhaemoglobin, and thereby deprives the tissues of the body of oxygen, as there is no haemoglobin left to pick up oxygen in the lungs and carry it throughout the body. Being odourless the unfortunate occupants of the room – or garage – have no idea that they are breathing it, and therefore they cannot take avoiding action by turning off the source of the carbon monoxide or getting out into fresh air. The result is that they become unconscious in the contaminated atmosphere and, all too often, by the time they are found, they are dead. Carbon monoxide has a special action on the ganglia at the base of the brain, and, if sufficient amounts are inhaled, permanent destructive changes occur in this vital part of the nervous system. What makes carbon monoxide poisoning all the more dangerous is its insidious onset, which so impairs the mental faculties at an early stage that, in the words of one expert, 'the person affected may be brought to the very verge of unconsciousness without appreciating in the least degree that anything is wrong'. Hitherto one of the commonest causes of carbon monoxide has been coal gas, particularly if inadequately combusted in a badly ventilated room, as in a water heater in a bathroom, but this risk is being brought under control in Britain as a result of the introduction of so-called natural gas, which contains no carbon monoxide. This, however, does not mean that natural gas is absolutely safe in this respect. It still suffers from the defect of all carbon-containing fuel, whether coal, oil, coke, wood, or manufactured (or town) gas or natural gas. This is that when burned in the absence of sufficient oxygen, or, whenever, for any reason, combustion is incomplete, carbon monoxide is formed. In the case of gas the risk is particularly high with water heaters in inadequately ventilated bathrooms, and with portable gas fires. The gas industry no longer permits the use or sale of the latter, but unfortunately there are still an unknown number in use. Anyone who owns such a portable gas fire should get rid of it at once. So far as gas water heaters in bathrooms are concerned, it is essential to ensure that it has a flue and that this is adequate and is neither blocked nor faulty. Three golden rules recommended by one of the British Gas Boards for the use of gas water heaters are:

1. Do not block any permanent means of ventilation, eg. an air-vent.

CARBON TETRACHLORIDE

Degree of saturation of haemoglobin with carbon monoxide

Per cent	*Signs and symptoms*
0 to 10	No symptoms
10 to 20	Tightness across the forehead Possibly headache Flushed skin Yawning
20 to 30	Headache Dizziness Palpitations on exercise
30 to 40	Severe headache Weakness Dizziness Nausea Collapse (possibly)
40 to 50	As above, with increased respiratory rate and pulse rate, and more possibility of collapse
50 to 60	Syncope Coma Cheyne-Stokes' respiration
60 to 70	Coma Weakened action of the heart and breathing Death imminent or actually takes place
70 to 80	Respiratory failure Death
90	Immediate arrest of the heart

Table 12 – The manifestations of carbon monoxide poisoning, according to the amount of carbon monoxide in the blood. The limit of safety is 18 to 20 per cent.

2. Leave the window or door open while the water heater is in use.

3. Turn off the gas before entering the bath.

The same care about maintaining adequate ventilation must be observed with all forms of heating derived from carbon-containing fuel, as listed above. Perhaps the greatest risk in this respect today is from the use of oil heaters in rooms in which all sources of ventilation, such as windows and ventilators, have, for all practical purposes, been hermetically sealed. This is one of the major reasons why deaths in the home from carbon monoxide poisoning, other than piped gas, have increased fivefold in the last two decades. Coke braziers are yet another recurring cause of carbon monoxide poisoning. Not the least important, however, in this automobile-ridden age is the exhaust gas of petrol vehicles. This is why the engine of a car must *never* be switched on in a garage unless the garage doors are open, and the car must be run out into the open air the moment the engine has been started. A further useful precaution is always to run the car into a garage nose first, so that the exhaust pipe is jutting out towards the open air. The main manifesta-

tions of carbon monoxide poisoning are shown in table 12. One of the most striking signs of carbon monoxide poisoning is the cherry-red appearance of the victim's face. This is due to the large amount of carboxy-haemoglobin in the blood.

Treatment of carbon monoxide poisoning consists of the immediate removal of the victim into the open air, followed by artificial respiration (qv) and, if available, the inhalation of oxygen and carbon dioxide. In this context 'immediate' means 'instant'. Speed is the essence of success, and may literally make all the difference between life and death. Artificial respiration should be given by the Schafer method, and the mixture of oxygen and carbon dioxide should contain 5 per cent of carbon dioxide. If the victim has been unconscious, he must rest in bed for the next twenty-four hours; otherwise there is a liability for him to collapse. Such collapse is particularly likely to occur on exertion.

CARBON TETRACHLORIDE is a colourless liquid with a strong odour, used against hookworms and other parasites in doses of 30 to 60 minims (2 to 4 ml),

166

though to a decreasing extent as it is replaced by more effective remedies.

CARBOXYHAEMOGLOBINAEMIA is the term applied to the state of the blood in carbon monoxide poisoning, in which this gas combines with the haemoglobin, displacing oxygen from it. (See CARBON MONOXIDE.)

CARBROMAL is a white powder with soporific action, given in doses of 5 to 15 grains (300 mg to 1 G).

CARBUNCLE like a boil, is an infection of a hair follicle and sebaceous gland or of a sweat gland, but unlike a boil it does not remain localized but spreads more deeply. The infecting organism is usually a staphylococcus. (See BOILS; and KIDNEYS, DISEASES OF.)

CARCINOGENESIS is the means or method whereby the changes responsible for the induction of cancer are brought about.

CARCINOMA is another name for cancer (qv).

CARDAMOM, AROMATIC TINCTURE OF, is a bright red fluid, prepared from the seeds of *Elettaria cardamomum*, useful to relieve spasm and flatulence, and much used to colour medicines. (see CARMINATIVES.)

CARDIA is a term applied to the upper opening of the stomach which lies immediately behind the heart.

CARDIAC DISEASE (see HEART DISEASES).

CARDIAC MASSAGE is the procedure used to restart the action of the heart if it is suddenly arrested. For long the only recognized method of doing this was by opening the chest wall and massaging the heart directly by hand. This is perfectly feasible if the heart stops beating during an operation. Elsewhere, however, it is seldom a practicable proposition.

Recently it has been shown that in many cases the arrested heart can be made to start beating again by rhythmic compression of the chest wall.

This is done by placing the patient on a hard surface – a table or the floor – and then placing the heel of the hand over the lower part of the sternum and compressing the chest wall firmly, but not too

forcibly, at the rate of 60 to 80 times a minute. At the same time artificial respiration must be started by the mouth-to-mouth method. (See DROWNING, RECOVERY FROM.)

CARDIAC PACEMAKER – The rate and rhythm of the heart are controlled by a small collection of specialized nervous tissue known as the sinuatrial node, situated at the base of the heart (see HEART). This is the natural pacemaker of the heart – or cardiac pacemaker. When the impulse sent out by this pacemaker cannot reach all parts of the heart (a condition known as heart-block), the heart either stops or contracts in an irregular manner. (See HEART DISEASES.)

In these cases the natural pacemaker can be replaced by an artificial pacemaker which, for all practical purposes, is a battery which stimulates the heart and allows it to beat at normal speeds. Most pacemakers are powered by mercury cells. Batteries powered by lithium-iodide batteries are also available, as well as an isotope-powered one, the potential longevity of which is 20 to 30 years, compared with two years for mercury batteries and 10 years for lithium batteries. The majority of cardiac pacemaker units are normally adjusted to deliver 65 to 75 impulses a minute. The pacemaker is either fixed to the outside of the chest or implanted in the armpit, and connected to an electrode catheter which is passed through the main vein in the neck. into the heart.

Under the Motor Vehicles (Driving Licences) Amendment Regulations 1973. which came into force on January 1, 1974. patients with heart disease whose condition has been brought under control by the fitting of a pacemaker can be given a licence to drive provided they satisfy the following conditions: (a) that their driving vehicle is not likely to be a source of danger to the public: (b) that the applicant has made adequate arrangements to receive regular medical supervision by a cardiologist throughout the currency of the licence and is complying with these arrangements.

CARDIOANGIOGRAPHY means rendering the outline of the heart visible on an X-ray film by injecting a radio-opaque substance into it.

CARDIOLOGY is the term applied to that branch of medical science devoted to the study of the diseases of the heart.

CARDIOMYOPATHY is a form of heart disease of unknown origin. It may occur at any age and is an affection of the heart muscle. It presents in a variety of forms. One may be the cause of sudden death in young people. In another there are signs of heart failure including dropsy (qv).

CARDIOSPASM means the spasmodic contraction of the muscle surrounding the opening of the oesophagus into the stomach: also termed ACHALASIA OF THE CARDIA. (See OESOPHAGUS, DISEASES OF.)

CARFECILLIN (see PENICILLIN).

CARIES is a process of gradual decay in bones, analogous to ulceration in the soft tissues. (See BONE, DISEASES OF; and TEETH, DISEASES OF.)

CARLSBAD SALT is the salt derived from Carlsbad water, with aperient properties. An artificial Carlsbad salt can be prepared by taking sodium sulphate 55 parts, potassium sulphate 1 part, sodium chloride 10 parts, sodium bicarbonate 35 parts, and mixing. If 90 grains (6 G) be added to 1 pint (500 ml) of water, a fluid closely resembling the natural Carlsbad water is obtained.

CARMINATIVES are preparations to relieve flatulence, and any resulting griping, by the bringing up of wind, or eructation (qv). Their essential constituent is an aromatic volatile oil, usually of vegetable extraction. As in the case of bitters, their precise mode of action is not known, but in practice, when swallowed, they induce a pleasant taste which may be accompanied by an increased flow of saliva. This is followed by a sensation of warmth as they are swallowed, and sooner or later there ensues the bringing up of wind. There is a large variety of carminatives, many of which are referred to elsewhere, such as caraway, cardamon, chamomile, cinnamon, cloves, dill, ginger, nutmeg and peppermint. Most of them are now used more for their flavouring effects either in medicine or in the kitchen, but, again as in the case of bitters, if used in moderation in correct dosage, they can undoubtedly help the individual to renew his or her interest in food, and thereby increase, or at least restore, his interest in life. Whether this is accompanied by the bringing up of wind is incidental.

CARNEOUS MOLE is an ovum which has died in the early months of pregnancy.

It usually requires no treatment and evacuates itself.

CAROTENE is a colouring matter of carrots, other plants, butter and yolk of egg, and is the precursor of vitamin A, which is formed from carotene in the liver. (See VITAMIN.)

CAROTID BODY is a small reddish-brown structure measuring 5 to 7 × 2·5 to 4 millimetres, situated one on each side of the neck, where the carotid artery divides into the internal and external carotid arteries (illustration 17). Its main function is in controlling breathing so that an adequate supply of oxygen is maintained to the tissues of the body.

CARPAL TUNNEL SYNDROME is a condition characterized by attacks of pain and tingling in the first three or four fingers of one or both hands, which usually occur at night. It is caused by pressure on the median nerve as it passes under the strong ligament that lies across the front of the wrist. It often responds to rest induced by fixing the wrist in a plaster splint. If it does not respond to this treatment, the pressure is relieved by surgical division of the compressing ligament.

CARPUS is the Latin term for the wrist, composed of eight small bones firmly joined together with ligaments, but capable of a certain amount of sliding movement over one another. (See WRIST.)

CARRAGEEN, or IRISH MOSS, is derived from the sea-weed, *Chondrus crispus*. It is pleasantly soothing and in the form of a jelly is sometimes added to an invalid diet. Half an ounce (14 G) of the moss is added to $1\frac{1}{2}$ pints (850 ml) of water and boiled down to 1 pint (500 ml). Its main dietetic value is on account of the iron, calcium, and iodine which it contains.

CARRIERS OF DISEASE (see INFECTION).

CARTILAGE is a hard but pliant substance forming parts of the skeleton, eg. the cartilages of the ribs, of the larynx and of the ears. Microscopically, cartilage is found to consist of cells arranged in twos or in rows, and embedded in a ground-glass-like material devoid of blood-vessels and nerves (illustrations 100, 101). The end of every long bone has a smooth layer of cartilage on it where it forms a joint with

100 – Diagram to show division of cartilage cells. From *Hewer's Textbook of Histology*. William Heinemann, Ltd.

101 – Vertical section of articular cartilage covering end of tibia. Magnified 30 times, *a*, *b*, *c*, groups of cartilage cells embedded in matrix; *d*, layer of calcified cartilage; *e*, bone. From Schafer, *Essentials of Histology*. Longmans.

other bones (articular cartilage), and in young persons up to about the age of sixteen there is a plate of cartilage (epiphyseal cartilage) running right across the bone about half an inch (12 mm) from each end. The latter, by constantly thickening and changing into bone, causes the increase in length of the bone. (See BONE.) In some situations there is found a combination of cartilage and fibrous tissue, as in the discs between the vertebrae of the spine. This fibro-cartilage, as it is known, combines the pliability of fibrous tissue with the elasticity of cartilage. The bones of fishes are mostly formed of cartilage. Cartilage when boiled for a long time yields a substance like gelatine. (For cartilages of the knee, see KNEE.)

CARUNCLE is the name applied to any small fleshy eminence, whether normal or abnormal.

CASCARA SAGRADA is the bark derived from *Rhamnus purshiana*, or *Rhamnus frangula*, from which a liquid and a solid extract of powerful purgative action are prepared. The full dose for one administration is $\frac{1}{2}$ to 1 teaspoonful of the liquid extract or $1\frac{1}{2}$ to 4 grains (100 to 250 mg) of the solid. But it is best taken in small doses of 5 or 10 drops of

169

the fluid extract after each meal, or night and morning; gradually this may be decreased and finally left off, the bowels continuing regular in action. The elixir of cascara is a pleasanter preparation, of which the dose is ½ to 1 teaspoonful.

CASCARILLA is an aromatic bitter tonic derived from the bark of *Croton eluteria* (see BITTERS). The dry bark has been used as a substitute for tobacco during attempts to break off the habit of smoking.

CASEATION is a process which takes place in the tissues in tuberculosis and some other chronic diseases. The central part of a diseased area, instead of changing into pus and so forming an abscess, changes to a firm cheese-like mass which may next be absorbed or may be converted into calcareous deposit and fibrous tissue, and so healing results with the formation of a scar.

CASEIN is that part of milk which forms cheese or curds. It is produced by the union of a substance, caseinogen, dissolved in the milk, with lime salts also dissolved in the milk, the union being produced by the action of rennin, a ferment from the stomach of the calf. The same change occurs in the human stomach as the first step in the digestion of milk, and therefore when milk is vomited curdled it merely shows that digestion has begun.

CASTOR OIL is a thick colourless oil pressed from the seeds of *Ricinis communis*, the castor-oil plant. Owing to its general action over the whole intestine it is perhaps the best purgative for a single administration, though, in consequence of the fact that its action is often followed by slight constipation, it is unsuitable for frequently repeated use.

The dose for an adult is from one teaspoonful to two tablespoonfuls. To a child one year old a teaspoonful may be given. To help to disguise its nauseous flavour, the cup in which it is given should be scalded out with hot water, of which a little remains in the bottom; the oil is next poured in, and upon it a little brandy or whisky in the case of an adult. The oil may be then swallowed without leaving too much taste behind. In the case of a child, lemon juice may be substituted for the brandy or whisky.

CASTRATION is the term applied to an operation for removal of the testicles or ovaries.

CASTS of hollow organs are found in various diseases. Membranous casts of the air passages are found in diphtheria and in one form of bronchitis, and are sometimes coughed up entire. Casts of the interior of the bowels are passed in cases of mucous colitis associated with constipation, and casts of the microscopic tubules in the kidneys passed in the urine form one of the surest signs of Bright's disease.

CATALEPSY is a term applied to a nervous affection characterized by the sudden suspension of sensation and volition, accompanied by a peculiar rigidity of the whole, or of certain muscles, of the body. The subjects of catalepsy are in most instances females of highly nervous or hysterical temperament. The exciting cause of an attack is usually mental emotion operating either suddenly, as in the case of a fright, or more gradually in the way of prolonged depression. Sometimes the typical features of the disease are exhibited in a state of complete insensibility, together with a statue-like appearance of the body, which will retain any attitude it may be made to assume during the continuance of the attack. In this condition the whole organic and vital functions appear to be reduced to the lowest possible limit consistent with life, and to such a degree as to simulate actual death. The attack may be of short duration, passing off within a few minutes. It may, however, last for many hours, and in rare instances persist for several days; and it is conceivable that in such cases the appearances presented might be mistaken for real death, as is alleged to have happened occasionally. Catalepsy is sometimes associated with epilepsy and with grave forms of mental disease. From what has been stated it follows that the successful treatment of such a disease as catalepsy must depend upon the due recognition of both its corporeal and mental relations. (See ECSTASY; HYSTERIA; SLEEP.)

CATAMENIA is another term for menstruation.

CATAPHORESIS is the term applied to a method of treatment by introduction of medicine through the unbroken skin by means of an electric current. (See IONIZATION.)

CATAPLASM is another name for poultice.

CATAPLEXY is the term applied to a condition in which the patient has a sudden attack of muscular weakness affecting the whole body. (See also NARCO-LEPSY.)

CATARACT is an opacity of the crystalline lens of the eye, more or less completely obscuring vision.

Causes and varieties – The most common form is *senile cataract*, which begins about the age of fifty in eyes which may have been perfectly healthy. In every eye, the lens from childhood onward slowly hardens and loses its power of focusing for near objects. In the cataractous eye there is a special hardening and rapid shrinking at the centre of the lens, which leads to splitting up and gradual disintegration of the lens, with consequent loss of transparency. Senile cataract, then, has nothing to do with loss of general health, or with disease of the rest of the eye. *Cataract in children* may be found at birth, and there may or may not be other disease of the eye, so that the result of operation is not so promising. *Diabetic cataract* appears sometimes in persons suffering from diabetes mellitus. *Black cataract* is one in which the lens is black in colour, due to deposition of pigment. *Partial cataracts* of various forms occur, obscuring vision in one direction but not requiring operation. *Posterior cortical cataract* is one at the back of the lens, and is a rare form which is important because it follows disease in the back of the eye, and, though there is impairment of vision, this is not due to the cataract or cured by its removal. It comes on in fairly young persons.

Cataract from injury (*traumatic cataract*) is caused by almost any wound of the lens, and sometimes by severe blows on the eye. *Heat* (*infra-red*) *cataract* occurs in glass-workers who have long been engaged in glass manufacture, and in certain iron-workers. *Irradiation cataract* is caused by X-rays, radium, or nuclear energy. *Electric cataract* may develop rapidly after the passage through the body of a powerful electric current.

Symptoms – The first thing noticed is the appearance of motes in the vision, not floating, like those seen by almost every healthy eye against a white background, but stationary.

Bright objects are seen multiplied, especially bright lights at a distance in the dark. A moderate degree of shortsight-edness may come on, which is relieved for a time by spectacles. Gradually increasing blindness is the most apparent symptom, and in the early stages the person may be less blind in the dusk than in bright light, because, the centre only of the lens being affected, a clear part round the edge admits the rays of light when the pupil, ie. the opening in the iris, dilates, as it does in dull light.

Finally, when the cataract is well advanced, it becomes visible to by-standers as a ground-glass-like mass filling up the pupil.

Treatment – No medicines or eye-washes or ointments are of any use against cataract. Atropine drops, which dilate the pupil, are much resorted to by quacks, because their use is followed for a time by better vision, for the reason just given. The cataract is unaffected by such applications, and can be removed only by operation. This is performed when the cataract reaches the stage of interfering with vision to an extent that prevents the reading of newsprint. There is a great variety of operations, but the chief are *extracapsular extraction* of the lens by opening the anterior capsule and expressing the lens through the pupil and hooking it out; *intracapsular extraction* by grasping the anterior capsule with toothless forceps and gently tearing away the capsule so that the entire cataract enclosed in its intact membranes comes away. The operation is usually done under a local anaesthetic and is safe and successful even in very old persons, though demanding great skill. Patients are usually allowed out of bed on the second or third postoperative day, and the stay in hospital is usually less than a fortnight.

The latest advance in the treatment of cataract is the insertion of acrylic lenses within the eye after extraction of the cataract. This gives the patient much better sight than did the old operation.

Sometimes after an operation for cataract disappointment is experienced because the sight is not restored. In such cases the retina also is diseased, and though the removal of the cataract admits light to the eye, the defective retina is unable to perceive objects clearly. To avoid this disappointment the eyes should be carefully examined by an expert before the cataract becomes sufficiently dense to obscure the back of the eye.

CATARRH is a term employed to describe a state of irritation of the mucous membranes, particularly those of the air passages, associated with a copious secretion of mucus. This complaint, so prevalent in damp and cold weather, usually begins as a nasal catarrh or coryza, with a feeling of weight about the forehead and some difficulty in breathing through the nose, increased on lying down. Fits of sneezing, accompanied with a profuse watery discharge from the nostrils and eyes, soon follow, while the sense of smell and to some extent that of taste become considerably impaired. There is usually present some amount of sore throat and of bronchial irritation, causing hoarseness and cough. Sometimes the vocal apparatus becomes so much inflamed (laryngeal catarrh) that temporary loss of voice results. There is always more or less feverishness and discomfort, and often an extreme sensitiveness to cold. After two or three days the symptoms begin to abate, the discharge from the nostrils and chest becoming thicker and of purulent character, and producing when dislodged considerable relief to the breathing. On the other hand, the catarrh may assume a more severe aspect and pass into some form of pulmonary inflammation. (See BRONCHITIS; and CHILLS AND COLDS.)

The term catarrh is also applied to describe a state of irritation, accompanied by abnormal secretion of mucus, in the stomach (see DYSPEPSIA), in the bowels (see DIARRHOEA; and INTESTINE, DISEASES OF), in the bladder (see Cystitis under BLADDER DISEASES), and in other mucous surfaces.

CATATONIA is a term applied to a symptom of mental disease in which the patient remains rigidly in the same position, behaving very much like a statue. Catatonia minor is a term applied to the group of symptoms occurring in the mental disease, schizophrenia, in which the patient shows peculiar mannerisms, continuing to repeat the same words or actions. (See MENTAL ILLNESS.)

CATECHOLAMINES are substances produced in the body from the dietary amino-acids (qv), phenylalanine and tyrosine. They include adrenaline (qv) and noradrenaline (qv).

CATECHU is a reddish extract from the leaves of the *Uncaria gambier*, containing much tannin and acting as an astringent. Compound catechu powder, containing catechu, kino, rhatany, cinnamon and nutmeg, and tincture of catechu is given in diarrhoea, and catechu lozenges are useful in relaxed sore throat.

CATGUT is used in surgery for tying cut arteries and stitching wounds. It is made from the fibrous coat of the intestines of animals, especially of the sheep, requires very careful purification, and in the tissues is gradually absorbed – in about five to ten days – as it is itself an animal substance. Hardened catgut is catgut which has been treated with a suitable hardening agent to prolong the time taken for it to be absorbed; catgut hardened by treatment with chromium compounds is known as chromicized catgut.

CATHARTICS are substances which produce an evacuation of the bowels. (See PURGATIVES.)

CATHETERS are hollow tubes used for passing into various organs of the body, either for investigational purposes or to give some form of treatment.

Varieties – *Cardiac catheters* are introduced through a vein in the arm and passed into the heart in order to diagnose some of the more obscure forms of congenital heart disease, and often as a preliminary to operating on the heart. *Endotracheal catheters* are used to pass down the trachea into the lungs, usually in the course of administering anaesthetics (qv). *Eustachian catheters* are small catheters that are passed along the floor of the nose into the Eustachian tube (qv) in order to inflate the ear. *Nasal catheters* are tubes passed through the nose into the stomach to feed a patient who cannot swallow: so-called nasal feeding. *Rectal catheters* are catheters passed into the rectum in order to give injections. *Suprapubic catheters* are catheters passed into the bladder through an incision in the lower abdominal wall just above the pubis, either to allow urine to drain away from the bladder, or to wash out an infected bladder. *Ureteric catheters* are small catheters that are passed up the ureter into the pelvis of the kidney, usually to determine the state of the kidney, either by obtaining a sample of urine direct from the kidney or to inject a radio-opaque substance preliminary to X-raying the kidney. (See PYELOGRAPHY.) *Urethral catheters* are catheters that are passed along the urethra into the bladder, either to draw off urine or to wash out the bladder (illustration 102). It is these last three types of catheters that are most extensively used, and will now be described in detail.

Urethral catheters may be made of plastic, rubber, gum elastic (or silkweb),

102 – Apparatus for washing out the bladder.

silver or glass. Plastic and rubber catheters are now those most widely used. They may be straight or bent. The straight catheters have the eye near the tip, which is solid in order to make introduction of the catheter easier. The bent catheters have one or two bends, which makes it easier to pass them in a patient with an enlarged prostate. There is also an olive-headed catheter, which has a moulded tip to make it easier to pass the catheter through a urethra which has a stricture. A whistle-tipped catheter has an open tip, and is used when there is a risk of the catheter becoming obstructed as may happen, for instance, if there is much bleeding with large clots of blood. Indwelling, self-retaining catheters are used when a catheter needs to be left in for some time. They have a small balloon at the tip which, when inflated, keeps the catheter in position and prevents its coming out. *Suprapubic catheters*, which are not now used as much as at one time, are larger than urethral catheters and are usually made of rubber. *Ureteric catheters* are long, thin and graduated. They are made of terylene base, nylon web, gum elastic, or plastic on nylon web.

Sterilization – The cleaning and sterilization of catheters is of paramount importance. After use, catheters must be carefully cleaned at once. This is done by rinsing them through with running water, and then syringing through with cetrimide. The outside is then well washed with soap and water. Rubber, silver and glass catheters are sterilized by being placed in boiling water. Once the water has again come to the boil, the catheter is boiled for ten minutes. Plastic (vinyl) catheters can be sterilized by boiling, or by autoclaving at 250° F (120° C) at 15 pounds pressure for fifteen minutes, after which they must be removed at once from the autoclave. Gum elastic catheters are difficult to sterilize, which is one reason why they are being given up. The introduction of disposable catheters, which are only used once and then discarded, has led to their being used to an increasing extent. They are sterilized by gamma radiation.

Uses – The use of any form of catheterization of the bladder, whether urethral, ureteric or suprapubic, must be made under the strictest possible sterile conditions. Not only must the catheter be sterilized, but the hands of those passing the

173

catheter must be prepared with the same care as for a surgical operation, and the opening of the urethra must be sterilized with the utmost care so as to avoid passing any infection into the bladder. The greatest gentleness must be exercised in introducing the catheter. This applies particularly in passing a urethral catheter in men, in whom the urethra is so much longer than in women.

CAT-SCRATCH FEVER is a disease, probably due to a virus, which is characterized by enlargement of the glands. In spite of the name, there is a history of a cat scratch in only about half the cases; in others the infection is acquired through a puncture of the skin by a splinter or thorn. The glandular swelling is usually slight and of short duration, but in some cases may go on to abscess formation which requires aspiration. The infection is not controlled by penicillin.

CAUL (see AMNION).

CAUSTICS and CAUTERIES are used to burn diseased tissues, the former by chemical action, the latter by their high temperature.
Varieties – The chief chemical caustics in use are acetic, lactic, chromic, carbolic and nitric acids, caustic soda and caustic potash, arsenic in paste, and nitrate of

rheumatic pains, etc. (see BLISTERS). The galvanocautery is used to reduce inflamed tissues about the nose and throat. The Paquelin's cautery was at one time much in vogue for removal of small growths, conversion of foul ulcers and poisoned wounds into healthy burns, and operations upon very vascular organs like haemorrhoids.

CAVERNOUS BREATHING indicates a peculiar quality of the respiratory sounds heard on auscultation over a cavity in the lung.

CEFOXITIN is a semi-synthetic antibiotic, given by injection, which is proving of value in the treatment of infections due to Gram-negative micro-organisms such as *Proteus* which are resistant to many other antibiotics.

CELLS are the microscopic particles which build up the tissues, of which they are the smallest structural divisions.
Every cell (illustration 103) consists essentially of a cell-body of soft albuminous material called protoplasm, in which lies a kernel or nucleus which seems to direct all the activities of the cell. Within the nucleus may be seen a minute body, the nucleolus; and there may or may not be a cell-envelope around all. (See also MITOCHONDRIA.)

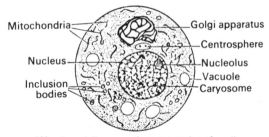

Mitochondria — Golgi apparatus
Centrosphere
Nucleus — Nucleolus
Vacuole
Inclusion bodies — Caryosome

103 – A semi-diagrammatic representation of a cell.

silver or lunar caustic. Of cauteries there are Corrigan's button cautery, the electro-cautery, consisting of a platinum point heated by an electric current, the galvano-cautery, in which a wire is heated with a galvanic current, and Paquelin's cautery, which has a hollow metal point kept hot by benzine constantly blown into it, and diathermy (see DIATHERMY).
Uses – Caustics are used to destroy warts, small tumours, etc. The cautery is used, mildly heated, as a counter-irritant instead of a blister in sciatica, neuralgia,

Cells vary much in size, ranging in the human body from $\frac{1}{10000}$ inch (0·0025 mm) to about $\frac{1}{1000}$ inch (0·025 mm). But the egg of a hen is still a simple cell, though enormously distended by food material.
All animals and plants consist at first of a single cell (the egg-cell, or *ovum*), which begins to develop when fertilized by the sperm-cell derived from the opposite sex. Development begins by a division into two new cells, then into four, and so on till a large mass is formed. These cells then arrange themselves into layers, and form

various tubes, rods, and masses which represent in the embryo the organs of the fully developed animal. (See FOETUS.)

When the individual organs have been laid down on a scaffolding of cells, these gradually change in shape and in chemical composition. The cells in the nervous system send out long processes to form the nerves, those in the muscles become long and striped in appearance, and those which form fat become filled with fat droplets which distend the cells. Further, they begin to produce, between one another, the substances which give the various tissues their special character. Thus, in the future bones, some cells deposit lime salts, and others form cartilage; while, in tendons, they produce long white fibres of a gelatinous substance. In some organs the cells change little: thus the liver consists of columns of large cells packed together, while many cells, like the white blood corpuscles, retain their primitive characters almost entire.

Thus cells are the active agents in forming the body, and they have a similar function in repairing its wear and tear. Tumours (qv), and especially malignant tumours, have a highly cellular structure, the cells being of an embryonic type, or, at best, forming poor imitations of the tissues in which they grow.

CELLULAR TISSUE is an old name for the loose fibrous tissue which forms, so to speak, packing between the skin and muscles and round the different organs.

CELLULITIS means an inflammation taking place in cellular tissue. (See ABSCESS; and ERYSIPELAS.)

CELLULOSE is a carbohydrate substance forming the skeleton of most plant structures. It is colourless, transparent, insoluble in water and is practically unaffected by digestion. In vegetable foods it therefore adds to the bulk, but it is of no value as a food-stuff. It is found in practically a pure state in cotton-wool.

CELLULOSE PHOSPHATE is a drug which prevents the absorption of calcium from the gut. For this reason it is used in patients with a high level of calcium in the urine (hypercalciuria) to prevent the formation of stones in the kidneys, and also for the treatment of stones in the kidneys in such patients.

CEMENT BURNS arise as a result of prolonged contact of the skin with builders' cement. They are due to quicklime which constitutes 65 per cent of cement. As they are chemical, and not thermal, burns, the victim feels no immediate pain and therefore allows the contact to persist. The precautions that should be taken include adequate protection of the hands and feet, and avoidance of prolonged contact of the skin with cement.

CENSOR is a term applied to the mental influence which prevents certain subconscious thoughts and wishes from coming into consciousness unless they are disguised so as to be unrecognizable.

CENTENARIANS (see EXPECTATION OF LIFE).

CENTRE is a term applied to a collection of nerve cells which give off nerve fibres and control some particular function: eg. the speech centre and the vision centre in the brain.

CEPHALOSPORINS have been described as 'a valuable and versatile group of broad-spectrum, non-toxic antibiotics'. Most of them available at the moment are semi-synthetic derivatives of cephalosporin C, an antibiotic originally derived from a sewage out-fall in Sardinia. They include cephaloridine, cephalothin, cephalexin, cephradine, and cephalozin. The term is sometimes used to include a group of semi-synthetic antibiotics with a comparable range of antibacterial action, but derived from a species of streptomyces. Strictly speaking this group, which includes cefoxitin, should be described as cephamycins. The indications for the use of individual members of the group vary. Some are active when given by mouth. Some have to be given by injection. One of their valuable features is that they are sometimes active against micro-organisms that have become resistant to penicillin, such as the gonococcus.

CERATE is a medicinal preparation, intended for external application, made with a basis consisting of wax in whole or in part which can be spread on the skin without melting: eg. camphor cerate, compound menthol cerate.

CERCOMONAS is the term applied to a genus of minute protozoan animals found in the intestine and other cavities of man and animals. One form is said to be responsible for occasional cases of diarrhoea.

CEREAL is the term applied to any plant of the nature of grass bearing an edible seed. The important cereals are wheat, oats, barley, maize, rice and millet. Along with these are usually included tapioca (derived from the cassava plant), sago (derived from the pith of the sago palm) and arrowroot (derived from the root of a West Indian plant), all of which consist almost entirely of starch. Semolina, farola and macaroni are preparations of wheat.

Cereals consist predominantly of carbohydrate, their general composition being:

	per cent
Water	10 to 12
Protein	10 to 12
Carbohydrate	65 to 75
Fat	0·5 to 8
Mineral matter	2

Table 13 – Composition of cereals.

They are therefore an excellent source of energy, and indeed can be regarded as the mainstay of civilization. On the other hand, their deficiency in protein and fat means that to provide a balanced diet, they must be supplemented by other foods rich in protein and fat, such as meat, milk and eggs. The percentage composition of the more important cereals is as follows:

	Water	Protein	Fat	Carbohydrate	Cellulose	Ash
Wheat	12·0	11·0	1·7	71·2	2·2	1·9
Oatmeal	7·2	14·2	7·3	65·9	3·5	1·9
Barley	12·3	10·1	1·9	69·5	3·8	2·4
Rye	11·0	10·2	2·3	72·3	2·1	2·1
Maize	12·5	9·7	5·4	68·9	2·0	1·5
Rice (polished)	12·4	6·9	0·4	79·4	0·4	0·5
Millet	12·3	10·4	3·9	68·3	2·9	2·2
Buckwheat	13·0	10·2	2·2	61·3	11·1	2·2

Table 14 – Composition of certain cereals.

Wheat is mainly used in the form of bread (qv). The reason why other cereals, with the exception of rye, are not used for bread-making is that they do not contain gluten, a protein which becomes viscid and adhesive when mixed with water. In the process of producing white flour much of the vitamin B complex, the iron and the calcium is lost, so that, from the nutritional point of view, wholemeal bread should be eaten. *Rye* is the other great bread-making cereal of the world. Compared with wheat-flour, rye-flour is deficient in protein. Preparations such as Ryvita are made from crushed whole rye. *Oats* are used in the form of oatmeal for human consumption. Although oats and oatmeal are among the richest of cereals from the point of view of analysis, in practice when taken as porridge they are not particularly nutritious. This is because of the large amount of water in porridge: eg. a 7-oz helping of porridge will contain only 3–4 oz of oatmeal (ie. 90 Calories). It is the milk (and sugar) taken as a rule with porridge which enhances its food value. *Maize*, a staple article of diet in America, compares favourably with other cereals as a source of energy. In Great Britain it is used mainly in the form of *cornflour* and custard powder, in the preparation of which practically all the protein and the fat in the maize is removed. *Barley* is now used more for malting and for fodder than for human consumption. The barley water (qv) so popular in the sick-room is merely a pleasant drink and is of practically no value as a food; it contains over 99 per cent of water. *Rice*, the staple article of diet in the East, is the poorest of all cereals in fat and protein. On the other hand, because of the small amount of cellulose it contains, it is almost completely absorbed during the course of digestion. This renders it a useful food in certain diseases of the alimentary tract.

CEREBELLUM AND CEREBRUM (see BRAIN).

CEREBRAL PALSY is the term used to describe a group of conditions characterized by varying degrees of paralysis and occurring in infancy or early childhood. In some 80 per cent of cases this takes the form of spastic paralysis: hence the lay description of them as 'spastics'. The incidence is believed to be around 2 or 2·5 per 1000 of the childhood community. In the majority of cases the abnormality dates from before birth or occurs during birth. Among the pre-natal factors are some genetic malformation of the brain, a congenital defect of the brain, or some adverse effect on the foetal brain as by infection during pregnancy. Among the factors during birth that may be responsible are trauma to the child or prolonged lack of oxygen such as can occur during a difficult labour. This last factor is considered by some to be the most important single factor. In some 10 to 15 per cent of cases the condition is acquired after birth, when it may be due to kernicterus (qv), infection of the brain, cerebral thrombosis or embolism, or trauma. The congenital form is commoner in boys than girls, and a high proportion of the cases are first-born children.

The disease manifests itself in many

ways. The victim may be spastic or flaccid, or the slow, writhing involuntary movements, known as athetosis, may be the predominant feature. These involuntary movements often disappear during sleep and may be controlled, or even abolished, in some cases by training the child to relax. The paralysis varies tremendously. It may involve the limbs on one side of the body (hemiplegia), both lower limbs (paraplegia), or all four limbs (tetraplegia). Mental subnormality is not uncommon.

The outlook for life is good, only the more severely affected cases dying in infancy. Although there is no cure, much can be done to help these unfortunate children, particularly if the condition is detected at an early stage. Little can be done to help those who have severe mental subnormality, but much can be done for those with normal intelligence by team work, giving attention to education, physiotherapy, occupational therapy and speech training. In this way many of these handicapped children are now reaching adult life as useful members of the community. Much help in dealing with these children can be obtained from the Spastics Society, 12 Park Crescent, London W1N 4EQ.

CEREBROSPINAL FEVER is another name for cerebrospinal meningitis. (See under MENINGITIS.)

CEREBROSPINAL FLUID is the fluid within the ventricles of the brain and bathing its surface and that of the spinal cord. It is normally under a pressure of 60 to 150 mm of water and contains 0 to 5 lymphocytes per c.mm. In each 100 millilitres of cerebrospinal fluid there are normally between 10 to 20 mg of protein (mostly albumin), 50 to 80 mg of glucose, and 725 to 750 mg of chlorides.

CERECLOTH means linen or cotton cloth impregnated with wax and made antiseptic for use in dressing wounds.

CEREVISIA is the Latin name for yeast.

CERUMEN is the name for the wax-like secretion found in the external ear.

CERVICAL means anything pertaining to the neck, or to the neck of the womb.

CERVICITIS means inflammation of the cervix uteri or neck of the womb.

CERVIX UTERI is the neck of the womb or uterus and is placed partly above and partly within the vagina. (See UTERUS.)

CETRARIA, or ICELAND MOSS, is a substance used in the form of decoctions, jellies or lozenges in irritable states of the mouth and throat.

CETRIMIDE (also known as CETAVLON) is the official name for a mixture of alkyl ammonium bromides. It is a potent antiseptic, and as a 1 per cent solution is used for cleaning and disinfecting wounds, and in the first-aid treatment of burns. As it is also a detergent, it is particularly useful for cleaning the skin, and also for cleansing and disinfecting greasy and infected bowls and baths.

CHAFING OF THE SKIN occurs in infants at the natural folds, eg. groins, armpits, elbows, where two moist surfaces constantly rub one another; in stout elderly people at similar positions; and generally where the clothes cause friction or pressure, as in the armpits or on the feet of those who walk great distances.

To prevent chafing the folds of the skin should be kept specially clean by washing with warm water and super-fatted soap, carefully dried, and then dusted with fuller's earth or any dusting-powder, such as a mixture of starch, zinc oxide and subnitrate of bismuth in equal parts.

CHAGAS' DISEASE, or American trypanosomiasis, is a disease widespread in Central and South America, and caused by the *Trypanosoma cruzi*. The disease is transmitted by the biting bugs, *Panstrongylus megistus* and *Triatoma infestans*. It occurs in an acute and a chronic form. The former, which is most common in children, practically always affects the heart, and the prognosis is poor. The chronic form is commonest in adolescents and young adults and the outcome depends upon the extent to which the heart is involved. There is no effective drug treatment. (See also SLEEPING SICKNESS.)

CHALAZION is a small swelling of the eyelid, formed by the distension of a gland with secretion.

CHALICOSIS is a term applied to a disorder of the lungs found among stonecutters, and due to the inhalation of fine particles of stone.

CHALK is calcium carbonate.

CHALK-STONES (see GOUT).

CHALYBEATE tonics or waters are those containing salts of iron. (See IRON.)

CHAMOMILE TEA is a bitter made by infusing half an ounce (14 G) of dried chamomile flowers in half a pint (280 ml) of boiling water for fifteen minutes and then straining. It is used cold in wineglassful doses.

CHANCRE means the primary lesion of syphilis.

CHANCROID means a soft or non-syphilitic venereal sore. It is caused by a micro-organism known as *Haemophilus ducreyi*. It is usually acquired by sexual contact, and responds well to treatment with sulphadimidine (qv).

CHANGE OF LIFE (see CLIMACTERIC; and MENSTRUATION).

CHAPPED HANDS occur in cold weather, when the activity of the sweat and sebaceous glands is reduced and there is therefore less natural protection of the skin. If the hands are then degreased by prolonged immersion in soapy water, and afterwards exposed to cold air, the skin becomes inelastic and cracks.
Prevention – A mop should be used for washing up, and household rubber gloves worn when using strong bleaching solutions, ammonia or degreasing compounds for cleaning ovens. A barrier cream (qv), such as petroleum jelly or lanolin, may be used, but most housewives find these too greasy. A more effective, and less greasy barrier cream is the *British Pharmacopoeia* Oily Cream. Adequate drying of the hands is essential, and the hands should be protected from cold weather so far as possible.
Treatment – Once chapping has occurred, a cream, such as the Oily Cream just mentioned or another *British Pharmacopoeia* preparation, Aqueous Cream, should be applied every night at bedtime. After it has been applied, the hands should be covered with thin cotton gloves. The painful cracks which are so liable to form at the fingertips are best treated with a paint consisting of equal parts of tincture of benzoin and collodion.

CHAPPED LIPS (see LIPS).

CHAPPED NIPPLES (see BREASTS).

CHARCOAL as used in medicine is a black powder prepared from vegetable matter such as sawdust, peat, cellulose residues and coconut shells by carbonization and activation. Its medicinal value is a result of its ability to absorb both gases and chemicals. It is available in the form of a powder, granules, tablets or biscuits.
Uses – Its traditional use is in the treatment of flatulence in a dose of 4 grams, on the principle that it absorbs the intestinal gases, but its value in this role is doubtful. It is also used in the treatment of poisoning with many drugs such as aspirin, paracetamol, barbiturates and morphine, all of which it absorbs. Here the dosage is much higher – up to 50 grams in water. A strawberry-flavoured preparation is now available which makes it more palatable and easier to administer to children. This is supplied as a powder containing 20 grams in a 200-millilitre bottle. The powder is stable for several years. When needed, the bottle is filled with water and the suspension swallowed. Another traditional use is as a deodorizing application to foul ulcers.

CHARCOT-LEYDEN CRYSTALS are sharp crystals found in the sputum of those suffering from asthma, and of those affected by some blood diseases.

CHARCOT'S DISEASE is the name applied to a swelling and disorganization of the joints which comes on late in locomotor ataxia (qv).

CHARPIE is linen waste, formerly used to absorb discharges, but now replaced by absorbent cotton-wool.

CHAULMOOGRA OIL, or HYDNO-CARPUS OIL, is a volatile oil obtained from the seeds of an Asiatic shrub, *Hydnocarpus wightiana*, which was at one time widely used in the treatment of leprosy. It has now been largely replaced by sulphones and other drugs.

CHEILOSIS is the term applied to an eczematous condition of the lips, especially at the angles of the mouth, and believed to be due to deficiency in the diet of one of the vitamins in the vitamin B complex – riboflavin. ANGULAR STOMA-TITIS and PERLÈCHE are other terms used to describe the condition, which may be associated with a red, sore tongue; fine desquamation at the junction of nose and lip, just inside the nose, and in the ears; eczema of the scrotum and perineum.

CHEIROPOMPHOLYX is the term applied to a disease of the skin in which little blisters filled with clear fluid suddenly appear on the hands and fingers. (See also POMPHOLYX.)

CHEMOSIS means swelling of the conjunctival membrane that covers the white of the eye.

CHEMOTAXIS means the property possessed by certain cells of attracting or repelling other cells.

CHEMOTHERAPY means the treatment of disease by chemical substances. In the modern sense it dates from the discovery by Paul Ehrlich, in 1910, of the action of Salvarsan ('606') in destroying the spirochaete of syphilis. This organic arsenical preparation revolutionized the treatment of syphilis. The next great advance in chemotherapy was the introduction of the sulphonamides in 1935. Just as Salvarsan had revolutionized the treatment of syphilis so did the sulphonamides revolutionize the treatment of infections with the streptococcus, pneumococcus, gonococcus and similar organisms. They remained supreme in the treatment of such infections as septicaemia, pneumonia, and certain forms of meningitis, until the introduction of penicillin during the 1939–45 War. Subsequently a series of new antibiotics (qv) have been discovered, including streptomycin, chloramphenicol and the tetracyclines.

Chemotherapy has also played an important rôle in tropical medicine: eg. mepacrine and proguanil for the treatment of malaria; the amidines in the treatment of sleeping sickness in man, and the sulphones in the treatment of leprosy.

CHENODEOXYCHOLIC ACID is one of the bile acids (see BILE), which is used in the treatment of cholesterol gallstones (see GALL-BLADDER, DISEASES OF).

CHENOPODIUM OIL, distilled from American wormseed, is used in the treatment of roundworms and hookworms in doses of 3 to 15 minims (0·2 to 1 ml).

CHEST, or THORAX, is the upper part of the trunk. It is enclosed by the breast-bone and rib-cartilages in front, by the twelve ribs at each side, and by the hinder parts of these along with the spinal column behind. Above, it is continued by an opening a few inches wide, through which pass the windpipe, gullet and large blood-

104 – Chest with the skin and muscles removed from the front, showing the position of heart and lungs. *H*, Heart; *LL*, left lung; *RL*, right lung; *W*, windpipe; *L*, liver; *S*, stomach.

vessels, into the root of the neck; while, below, its cavity is separated from that of the abdomen by a thin dome-shaped plate of muscle, the diaphragm or midriff. Between each pair of ribs lie two thin muscular layers, the intercostal muscles, which fill up the spaces between the ribs, and move the chest wall in respiration. Its outlines are further covered and moulded behind by four layers of muscles, sometimes several inches thick, and by the shoulder-blade with its muscles, and in front by the two pectoral muscles which pass from the ribs to the upper arm. Further, there is a more or less plentiful layer of fat beneath the skin, and in this fat lie the breasts, extending in the female from the second rib down to the seventh.

Contents – The chest contains the lungs illustration 104), one on each side, with the end of the windpipe, which divides into right and left bronchial tubes, to the two lungs; the heart in the middle and projecting on the left almost to the nipple, with the great vessels which carry blood from and to it; the gullet, which passes down on the left side of the spinal column to enter the abdomen through an opening in the diaphragm; the thoracic duct of the absorbent system, which runs up to enter a vein in the neck; and various important nerves which control the contained organs. Each lung is enclosed in a smooth, double membrane, the pleura (see LUNGS), and the heart in a similar membrane, the pericardium.

CHEST, DEFORMITIES OF – The healthy chest is gently rounded all over, its contour being still more rounded in women by the breasts, and in transverse outline it should present an oval shape slightly flattened behind and having a proportion of about 10 to 7·5 between its side-to-side and front-to-back measurements. The angle at the lower end of the breast-bone formed between the edges of the rib cartilages of the two sides should be about four-fifths of a right angle. An interval of about two inches should exist between the twelfth rib and the haunch-bone. The circumference varies from 33 inches (84 cm) for a man of 5 feet (152 cm) in height to about 40 inches (102 cm) for a man of 6 feet (183 cm).

Long chest is one in which the shoulders slope downwards, the ribs incline downwards as they come forwards more than they should do, the lower ribs touch or almost touch the haunch-bones, and the circumference is small. Further, the neck is long, the throat prominent, and the shoulder-blades stand out behind, the chest for this reason being also called the winged or alar chest. Traditionally, this form is said to predispose to tuberculosis and other lung diseases, probably because the lungs are never properly expanded, but this long chest can be much improved and the circumference rapidly increased by proper exercises.

Flat chest is often a consequence of lung diseases, and flatness is sometimes found along with too great length. In this form, the ribs and their cartilages grow too straight in front, so that the chest loses in fullness. This form is partly curable in youth by exercises.

Barrel chest is one in which the ribs are too horizontal, the shoulders raised, and the chest short. It is the opposite in every respect of the long chest. The curves of the chest resemble those of a barrel and the ribs the hoops. This form is due to too great expansion of the lungs, especially in the disease called emphysema. The chest being blown out almost to its full capacity at expiration, inspiration is made very laborious.

Rickety chest is due to rickets in early life, and usually the head and other bones

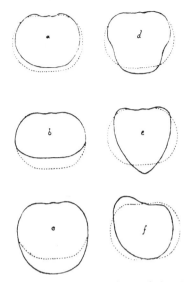

105 – Outline of various forms of chest in transverse section, the dotted line in each case showing the normal shape. *a*, long chest; *b*, flat chest; *c*, barrel-shaped; *d*, rickety chest; *e*, pigeon breast; *f*, bulged chest in curvature of the spine.

are also affected. (See RICKETS.) There is a hollow down each side owing to the yielding of the soft growing ribs in early life under the pressure of the atmosphere. There is, however, a protrusion of the front of the chest, so that the lungs are not pressed on, or specially liable to disease. Frequently the chest shows, down each side, a row of nodules placed at the junction of the ribs with their cartilages, and known as the 'rickety rosary'. Sometimes the lower part of the chest is much bulged out from moulding over the liver and other abdominal organs.

Pigeon breast is one in which the cross-section of the chest becomes triangular, the breast-bone forming a sort of keel in front, like that in the pigeon's breast. It is due to the ribs becoming straightened so as to push the breast-bone straight forwards, and is caused by some obstacle to the entrance of air in early life.

Bulging of the chest may be due to curvature of the spine, which makes a projection behind, and consequently, the chest being shortened, causes the breast-bone to bend on itself and project in front. When the spine twists to one side, that side becomes flattened, the other side bulging and the contained organs being pushed into it.

Hollowing of the chest is found in many conditions. In tuberculosis, when the lung becomes chronically solidified in its upper part, and later probably develops a cavity, it shrinks, and the chest wall to some extent falls in beneath the collar-bone. In pleurisy of long standing the lung is apt to collapse, ie. undergo a shrinking process and lose its air spaces, so that the whole chest wall of that side sinks inwards under atmospheric pressure.

CHEST DEVELOPMENT is of great practical importance in view of the fact that persons with long and flat chests suffer more often from serious lung disease than those who have good chest capacity. The art of full breathing also confers a feeling of exhilaration upon those who practise it, and adds ease to the carriage of the body. Many persons, debarred from entering one of the public services through having too small a chest circumference, owe this largely to a faulty manner of carrying the chest, the ribs being allowed to droop and the shoulders to slope downwards and forwards, although one or two inches might be added to the girth in a few days or weeks by proper exercises. The muscles which come into action in taking a breath fall into two classes: (1) the muscles of ordinary inspiration, including the diaphragm, and the intercostal muscles, which suspend one rib from that next above it; and (2) the muscles of forced inspiration, including most of the muscles of the neck, the shoulder and the abdomen, which come into play in taking an extra deep breath.

The lungs rise a distance of half an inch to one and a half inches (12 to 36 mm) above the collar-bone into the root of the neck, and this portion is little expanded except in forced breathing. It is here that tuberculosis is liable to make its first appearance, and, though cause and effect are not quite clear, there can be little doubt that the deficient expansion, and consequently sluggish circulation, play an important part in this location of the disease.

Although violent exercise like football has an indirect influence in expanding the chest by necessitating deep breathing, other forms of athletics add mainly to the size and strength of the muscles on the chest without increasing its capacity. Probably the only exercise which attains the latter thoroughly is forced breathing.

Every one, whether of athletic build or not, may practise this by the following three movements (illustration 106). These should be carried out night and morning, with the upper part of the body bare, or covered only by a loose or elastic undervest:

(*a*) The person standing erect holds the hands in front of him, backs upwards, on a level with his hips. As he begins to breathe

106 – Movements for expansion of the chest.

he raises them till, at the end of an inspiration, they are straight above his head. As he breathes out he lets them slowly fall to their former position. This he repeats with each breath, making the breaths as deep as possible.

(*b*) Standing with the hands by the sides, palms forwards, he raises them away from the sides as he breathes in, to the same position as in the first movement, and lets them descend slowly outwards as he breathes out.

(*c*) Standing with elbows bent, the thumbs pressed against the upper part of the chest, and the finger-tips of opposite hands touching, he carries the arms outwards and as far backwards as possible, keeping them always on a level with the shoulders, as he draws a deep breath, and brings them forwards again as he breathes out.

In performing these movements a light pair of dumb-bells (not exceeding 2 pounds (900 grams) each) may, if desired, be used, and the movements will then be a better exercise for the arm muscles.

It is of the utmost importance that the movements should be slow: not quicker than six to the minute, and preferably about three per minute, and each movement should be a conscious effort, not made automatically. If each movement be performed twenty times, a fair amount of exercise will be obtained in about a quarter of an hour.

Further, the person should cultivate the habit of breathing deeply at all times, and of standing, sitting or walking with the shoulders well braced back, so as to take the weight of the shoulder blade and upper limb off the expansile part of the chest.

CHEST DISEASES (see LUNGS, DISEASES OF; HEART DISEASE; ANEURYSM; ANGINA PECTORIS; PLEURISY; PNEUMONIA; BRONCHITIS; TUBERCULOSIS) – Chest diseases are of special importance, because the lungs and heart are perhaps the most important organs in the body, and are especially difficult to treat, as these are the only organs which cannot rest for a few minutes without death becoming imminent. Further, they are so closely placed and so intimately associated by the circulation of the blood, that when one suffers from disease, either acute or chronic, the other is rarely unaffected.

Symptoms – Owing to the rigid nature of the chest wall, changes in the enclosed organs rarely become visible to the eye. *Pain* is a very important symptom. Very

severe pain may, it is true, be caused by muscular rheumatism in the chest wall (the condition called pleurodynia) or by neuralgia, but when of a stabbing character and felt at the end of every breath it suggests pleurisy as a cause. Pain about the heart may be caused by indigestion, but if severe, and especially if brought on by exertion, seldom is found without some slight or serious heart disease. An agonizing spasm of the heart, often coupled with a feeling of impending death, is known as angina pectoris (see ANGINA PECTORIS). Severe persistent pain of a boring character is suggestive of an aneurysm (see ANEURYSM). *Expectoration* of blood may occur both in heart and in lung disease, and various other characters are noteworthy in the sputum (see EXPECTORATION). *Breathlessness* is an important sign of lung and heart diseases (see BREATHLESSNESS). *Other organs* are prone to be affected by disease of either heart or lungs; thus in tuberculosis the digestive system sometimes gives the first sign of ill-health, and in heart disease congestion of the liver, or swelling of the feet, may be for long the main trouble. *Cough* is one of the best-known symptoms of lung mischief, either of tuberculosis or of bronchitis, but it may be due to irritation of other parts of the respiratory system, or even of the stomach.

Treatment – Rest is the most important factor in the treatment of all chest conditions, because, when the body is quiet, the circulation of the blood becomes slower, the rate of pulse and respiration slackens, and so the heart and lungs have a partial rest. Pain is soothed by the application of hot-water bottles, or counter-irritants to the chest. Fresh air is specially necessary in lung disease (see TUBERCULOSIS). Infections are controlled by the sulphonamides or antibiotics. Various drugs called expectorants are given to act upon the lungs, or similar drugs are inhaled (see EXPECTORANTS; and INHALATIONS). Oxygen is much used both in affections of the heart and of the lungs. In the case of the heart, there are several drugs by which the action of this organ can be slowed, or quickened, or made more regular: for example, digitalis.

CHEST INJURIES – Injuries due to moderate violence are not usually serious, resulting generally in muscular bruises or in fractured rib (see FRACTURES). If the ribs do not penetrate the lung, union and recovery are rapid, but, if the lung be injured, various complications, such as emphysema, effusion of blood and entrance of air into the pleural cavity, abscess in the lung, traumatic pneumonia, may ensue. Penetrating wounds of the lungs, as by a bullet or stab, are apt to lead to similar complications, but do not necessarily produce serious effects unless a large vessel be severed. Simple fractures of ribs may be serious in old people, and bronchitis often follows their occurrence. Wounds of the heart are generally at once fatal from haemorrhage, but this organ has been so seriously injured as to require stitching, and yet recovery has ensued.

CHEYNE-STOKES' BREATHING is a type of breathing seen in some serious nervous affections, such as brain tumours and apoplexy, and also in the case of persons with advanced disease of the heart or kidneys. When well marked it is a sign that death is impending, though milder degrees of it do not carry such a serious implication in elderly patients. The breathing gets very faint for a short time, then gradually deepens till full expirations are taken for a few seconds, and then gradually dies away to another quiet period, again increasing in depth after a few seconds and so on in cycles (illustration 107).

feverish or has a slight shivering, or may feel more severely ill with vomiting and pains in the back and legs. Almost at the same time, and at all events within twenty-four hours, an eruption consisting of red pimples which quickly change into vesicles filled with clear fluid appears on the back and chest, sometimes about the forehead, and less frequently on the limbs. These vesicles during the second day may show a change of their contents to turbid, purulent fluid and within a day or two they burst, or, at all events, shrivel up and become covered with brownish crusts. An important point of difference between this eruption and that of smallpox is that these vesicles keep on appearing for several days, so that vesicles are seen at all stages of development, whilst in those of smallpox all parts of the rash are at the same stage at one time. In a slight case there may be only eight or ten of these vesicles, or there may be several hundreds. The small crusts have all dried up and fallen off in little more than a week and recovery is almost always complete.

Treatment – The child must be isolated from susceptible children for a week from the appearance of the rash or until all the

107 – Tracing of Cheyne-Stokes' breathing. The upper curve shows the oxygen saturation of the blood. When this falls to a certain level (↑) breathing is stimulated and the oxygen saturation rises again. When it reaches a certain level breathing diminishes or ceases (↓). From Bell, Davidson and Elmslie-Smith, *Textbook of Physiology and Biochemistry*, 8th edition, 1972. Churchill Livingstone.

CHICKENPOX, or VARICELLA, is an acute contagious disease predominantly of children, though it may occur at any age, characterized by feverishness and an eruption on the skin.

Causes – The disease occurs in epidemics affecting especially children under the age of ten years. It has no connection with smallpox, to which it bears a superficial resemblance. It is due to a virus, and the condition is an extremely infectious one from child to child.

Symptoms – There is an incubation period of fourteen to twenty-one days after infection, and then the child becomes

vesicles are dry, but there is no need to wait until the scabs have separated. A patient need not be confined to bed unless the temperature is raised, but he should be kept in one room. If the rash appear on the face, care must be taken to prevent scratching or pock marks may remain. Calamine lotion or a simple dusting powder relieves the itchiness. No other treatment beyond isolation is required.

CHICORY (see ADULTERATION OF FOOD).

CHIGGER is another name for the harvest mite (see PARASITES).

CHILBLAIN, or ERYTHEMA PERNIO, is an inflamed condition of the skin of the hands or feet, or even of the ears, occurring in persons of defective circulation and in those of poor health.

Causes – Chilblains are found especially in childhood and adolescence. Underfeeding, poor clothing and a defective circulation favour their appearance. Persons who suffer from them have habitually cold and numb hands and feet, and are subject to chills and colds in the head. In these persons, tight boots often are sufficient to bring on chilblains of the feet, and warming the hands at the fire when they are cold produces chilblains on the fingers, the skin becoming engorged with blood in consequence of the irritation or warmth, and later losing its vitality.

Symptoms – There are three stages in the development of a chilblain:

(1) The skin, usually of the little toe, the outer side of the foot, or the inner side of the hand, becomes purple and very itchy.

(2) Blebs, containing a thin yellow fluid, form on this discoloured area, which becomes very painful.

(3) These blebs break and leave behind an ulcerated surface very difficult to heal.

True chilblains should not be confounded with a cracked or chapped condition of the hands, feet, lips, or ears brought on by cold wind, or washing with hot water during cold weather in persons of robust constitution but delicate skin.

Treatment – Preventive treatment is the best. Good food and warm clothing improve the general condition upon which chilblains depend. Regular exercise, and a cold or modified cold bath every day (see BATHS) improve the circulation. The person liable to chilblains should wear wide boots and thick woollen socks in winter, and, before going into the open air, should always pull on a pair of woollen gloves. Garters and constrictions round the wrist or ankle, which interfere with the circulation, should be abolished, and india-rubber shoes should not be worn. If the hands and feet are cold they should be rubbed for warmth, not held before the fire. In the first stage the chilblain may be rubbed with hazeline snow or cream, or painted with tincture of iodine. Carefully controlled irradiation with ultra-violet light from a carbon-arc lamp is often beneficial. Voyagers to the Arctic regions rub the part with a mixture of whisky and soap. In the second and third stages some simple ointment, like boracic, and a dressing of wool are best, or the part may be painted with compound tincture of benzoin.

CHILD ADOPTION – In Great Britain around 2·5 per cent of all liveborn infants, or 25,000 per annum, are legally adopted. Adoption and illegitimacy are closely inter-related. In England and Wales 80 per cent, and in Scotland 90 per cent, of adopted children are illegitimate. Conversely, in England and Wales 30 per cent, and in Scotland nearly 40 per cent, of illegitimate children are adopted. The majority of parents who adopt children are between 25 and 35 years of age, and only some 10 per cent are 40 or over. A mother cannot give formal consent to the placement of her infant until the baby is 6 weeks old, although informal placement may take place earlier. Thereafter there must be a probation period of three months before court proceedings can take place. Thus, few adoptions can be formally legalized before the age of 6 months. Sixty per cent of all adoptions are completed by the end of the first year, and nearly three-quarters by the end of the second year.

Adoption can be carried out in three ways. (i) Through an adoption agency; this accounts for approximately 70 per cent of adoptions. (ii) By the mother directly placing the infant with adoptive parents; this accounts for nearly 30 per cent of adoptions. A high proportion of such adoptions are adoptions by the mother (now married) of her own baby or adoption by her relatives. (iii) Through a third party acting as an intermediary between mother and adoptive parents; this accounts for only 1 to 3 per cent of all adoptions. Of infants who are legally adopted, some 72 per cent are adopted by non-relatives, and 28 per cent by relatives.

There are two types of registered adoption agency: the voluntary adoption society, and the local authority acting as an adoption agency. In England and Wales approximately two-thirds of agency placements are carried out by voluntary societies and one-third by local authorities. In Scotland the proportions are approximately equal. For many years voluntary societies have had a national organization: the Standing Conference of Societies Registered for Adoption. This has now been replaced by a national organization: the Association of British Adoption Agencies, which includes both voluntary adoption societies and local authorities acting as adoption agencies. Its address is: 4 Southampton Row, London WC1B 4AA (tel. no: 01-242 8951).

CHILD-CROWING is another name for laryngismus. (See LARYNGISMUS.)

CHILDREN, FEEDING OF (see INFANT FEEDING).

CHILDREN, PECULIARITIES OF – The fact that children cannot put into words, or cannot correctly estimate, the nature of troubles and pains from which they suffer, coupled with the great importance of remedying as early in life as possible any physical or mental defect, or any bad habit, makes the observation of their peculiarities of great importance.

Activity – For some weeks after an infant is born the only signs of intelligence, apart from the performance of the merely animal functions, consist in *constant movements* of the lips, head, and limbs. The fingers are constantly opened and shut, the legs drawn up and down, and the lips pouted, while the child is awake; and the vigour of these movements gives a good idea of the vitality of the child. At about the third or fourth month the child should begin to develop the power of attention, as shown by his staring fixedly at any bright or moving object presented to him and ceasing other movements while his attention is so engaged. During the sixth month teething begins. A delay in teething is one of the signs of rickets (see TEETH). About the end of the first year of life the child should be gaining the power to stand and walk (see GAIT).

Crying in early childhood is a manifestation of either pain, or hunger, or discomfort. The most common pain is that known as 'gripes' and associated with indigestion, in which the cry is of a wailing character, with a note of ill-temper (see COLIC). In head pain the cry is of a sharp, piercing nature. In older children frowning is a common symptom of headache, especially when it is due to eye-strain (see VISION, DISORDERS OF).

Temperature is not much of a guide to disease in children, because the temperature-regulating mechanism is easily thrown out of gear.

Fullness under the eyes may be a symptom of Bright's disease.

An open mouth in breathing, especially when deafness and shortness of breath accompany it, is usually due to enlargement of the tonsils and adenoids in the throat. A child so affected is generally found to snore when asleep. (See NOSE, DISEASES OF.) Accompanying these symptoms in older children we find broadening of the bridge of the nose, narrow nostrils, and often narrowing of the roof of the mouth with projecting front teeth.

The expression of the face is often of great importance. Brain disease causes contractions of the facial muscles producing the appearance of emotions quite foreign to childhood, and causing the deep lines which, in middle-aged persons, are supposed to denote character. The head, too, is often drawn back in such a case, and the back arched. Deep hollowing of the eyes during an attack of gastroenteritis (qv) and vomiting is a grave sign, indicating great exhaustion. The size of the cranium is large in children compared with that of the face. At birth the proportion is about eight to one, though the face rapidly grows in size. On the top of the head is the fontanelle or soft spot, which at birth is about a square inch in size, and gradually closes as the bones grow till, at the end of the second year, it should have disappeared. Premature closure, with narrowing of the forehead, is often, though not necessarily, associated with mental deficiency. Late closure, with the development of a lofty, 'intellectual'-looking forehead, is one of the signs of rickets.

Bad postures in children, such as standing on one leg, stooping at the shoulders, and leaning the left elbow on the table at lessons, should be discouraged as tending to produce deformities. The latter habit may produce considerable curvature of the spine and defective development of one side of the chest.

Nervousness may show itself by twitching movements of hands and feet, and a shy, nervous child is apt to be unintentionally clumsy. Twitchings and grimaces may show the beginning of St. Vitus's dance, and children are apt to be punished for these quite involuntary peculiarities, such punishment only aggravating the condition. Grinning on every occasion, however, shows a want of control over the muscles of expression, and indicates a low-class brain and necessity for careful upbringing. Convulsions in young children are due to many causes (see CONVULSIONS), and when some nervous disease is the cause they form a serious symptom. Although much more common in children, they are not by any means as grave as fits of similar severity in adults. The involuntary or unconscious passing of urine, or enuresis (see NOCTURNAL ENURESIS), showing itself generally by wetting of the bed, is usually a bad habit in a nervous child and capable of correction by careful psychological treatment, but is occasionally due to physical conditions needing correction.

Bad habits in children include such actions as persistent sucking of the thumb or tongue, biting the nails, rolling or nodding the head in a rhythmic manner, knocking the head violently on the pillow, rhythmic swaying of the body, eating of dirt. These habits all consist in a morbid exaggeration of some normal action which has an extraordinary fascination for the children who practise it. They should be corrected at an early stage, firmly yet tactfully and without any fuss, by checking the child and making him carry out some other activity on each occasion when the habit is noticed. Advice should be sought at a child-guidance clinic or from the family doctor if the habit persists.

Left-handedness is often taken for a sign of stupidity, and children are punished when they do not use the right. This is a great mistake, because the condition is due to the fact that the side of the brain governing the left hand has developed in advance of the other. The child may, however, be taught to do certain things with the right hand, and so attain a condition of ambidexterity.

The teaching of children should not be forced before the age of seven, and up to this age should be directed rather to teaching habits of study, orderliness, and regularity. The teaching of good habits should begin at birth. This may be done, for example, in the matter of feeding. The periods at which the child is to be fed having been determined upon, these should be adhered to, despite the child's crying. It is astonishing how soon the child accepts this discipline and ceases to cry for food at irregular times. Present-day teaching in the kindergarten and primary schools is directed towards instructing children how to observe and study rather than towards cramming them with facts. After the age of seven is reached, the child's brain is quite capable of enduring some fatigue, and regular lessons should be begun, or the child will learn idle, loafing habits. It has been calculated that an intelligent 6-year-old child knows the meaning of around 13,000 words. Two years later this figure has more than doubled.

Sleep should be longer the younger the child, and nervous children should have a specially good allowance. Table 15 (see second column), gives approximately the minimum periods of sleep at different ages.

These, however, it must be stressed, are merely approximations. Some children can do with relatively little sleep and will lie quite happily in bed for an hour or more before falling asleep, whilst they may waken relatively early in the morning. Rigid rules therefore cannot be laid down. The important thing is that the child is put

	Hours a Day
During first year	20
During second year	14–16
From second to fourth year	12–14
From fourth to sixth year	10–12
From sixth to twelfth year	10
From twelfth to sixteenth year	9

Table 15 – Minimum requirements of sleep at different ages.

to bed at a reasonable hour and learns to amuse himself there, without attention, until he falls asleep.

CHILLS and COLDS form a subject of some importance because, although in general trivial ailments, on occasion they are the prelude to serious diseases.

Causes – The so-called 'common cold' may follow some chill to the surface, such as exposure to a draught of cold air, breathing in a foggy atmosphere, wetting of the feet on a cold day, sudden immersion in water, some persons being specially liable after one of these to develop a catarrh of the respiratory passages and feverish state. These, however, are only predisposing factors, and the primary cause is a virus. Often a 'cold in the head' runs through all the members of a family or school or a group of persons employed together, and such an 'infectious cold' is due to the causative virus passed from one person to another by sneezing or coughing.

Varieties and symptoms – A cold in the head with catarrh of the nose is known to every one; the catarrh sometimes extending up into the frontal sinuses and causing a severe browache, or involving the maxillary sinuses (see SINUS) and causing face-ache, or even spreading up the Eustachian tubes and causing inflammation of the middle ear with painful earache. Generally, these secondary affections disappear as the cold gets well, but suppuration may result in these various cavities, most commonly in the middle ear, though seldom in the frontal sinus. When the throat is the part affected, inflammation of the tonsils may result. (See TONSILLITIS.) In persons who use the voice much, or in those who indulge overmuch in alcohol, the larynx is a weak point, and laryngitis, with huskiness or even temporary loss of voice, is the common result of a chill. The cold may affect the respiratory passages farther down and bronchitis then results, or if the surfaces of the air spaces in the lungs be inflamed, pneumonia is the condition produced. When the air passages from the larynx downwards contain mucus, coughing results, this being a series of involuntary explosive expirations designed to force the irritating substance up into the mouth, from which it is spat out. Some persons have a liability, as the result of a chill, to catarrh not of the respiratory, but of the alimentary system, as shown by ensuing dyspepsia or diarrhoea. It should be remembered that a so-called 'cold' is the commencement of several infectious and serious diseases, such as measles, whooping-cough, influenza, and tuberculosis. Medical advice should therefore be sought whenever this apparently trivial malady lasts more than a few weeks. Finally a chilly sensation is a frequent accompaniment of some nervous shock either of a severe nature or even of some minor type.

Treatment – There is very little one can do in the treatment of a cold. Most people have their pet remedies, and most of these are harmless. On 'catching a cold', with a temperature above normal, the best thing to do is to go to bed and stay there at least 24 hours, if not two days. In this way the course of the cold will be cut short, and at the same time the sufferer will not be exposing other people to his infection. The best way to prevent colds is to isolate the infected by keeping them in bed. Vaccines seem to be ineffectual in the prevention of colds.

CHIMERA is an organism, whether plant, animal or human being, in which there are at least two kinds of tissue differing in their genetic constitution. In recent years it has become possible to combine together two embryos (qv) at a very early stage of development so that they develop as a single individual. Such an animal, which thus can have four parents, instead of two, is an example of a chimera.

CHINCOUGH is another name for whooping-cough. (See WHOOPING-COUGH.)

CHIRAGRA is an ancient term applied to gout affecting the hand.

CHIRETTA, or CHIRATA, is a favourite bitter, resembling gentian. (See BITTERS.)

CHIROPODIST is the name applied to one who treats corns, bunions, and other minor affections of the hands and feet.

CHIROPRACTOR is a term applied to a person who practises chiropractic, which is a system of adjustment by hand of supposed minor displacements of the spinal column in order to relieve pressure upon the nerves issuing at the intervertebral foramina. The essential fallacy of this system lies in the fact that the foramina for the exit of the spinal nerves are so large that pressure upon these nerves is only possible in gross displacements caused by very severe injury or disease.

CHIRURGEON is an obsolete method of spelling surgeon.

CHLAMYDIA is a genus of microorganisms which include those responsible for non-specific urethritis (qv), ornithosis (qv), psittacosis (qv), and trachoma (qv). They are also widespread in birds and animals.

CHLOASMA is a condition in which brown blotches appear, especially on the face. It occurs chiefly in pregnant women, in whom the spots fade after delivery. It also tends to occur in the menopause.

CHLORALAMIDE is a crystalline powder with faintly bitter taste which is generally regarded as a safe hypnotic. It is given in doses of 15 to 45 grains (1 to 3 G).

CHLORAL HYDRATE is a substance which when taken internally in moderate doses, produces sound, dreamless, refreshing sleep, like natural sleep. It acts rapidly, within about half-an-hour, and its effect lasts for about eight hours. It is, however, dangerous in large doses, and persons taking it frequently may contract a habit for it. It should not be taken in conjunction with alcohol. In safe doses it does not lessen pain appreciably, as opium does, and so will not cure sleeplessness due to this cause. In dangerous doses it paralyses and slows the heart, slows respiration, and reduces body temperature.

Uses – It is given in doses of 5 to 20 grains (300 mg to 1·2 G), or in the form of syrup of chloral, a teaspoonful, but should only be taken under medical observation. It is particularly useful in children (as the syrup) and in old people. *Externally* chloral is an antiseptic, and a lotion of strength 8 grains (500 mg) of chloral to each ounce (28·5 ml) of water is used for cleansing unhealthy ulcers, and some forms of eczema. Chloral and camphor, rubbed together in equal parts, form a clear fluid, as do chloral and menthol, and either of these is useful for painting on to the skin in cases of neuralgia or of gouty pain.

187

CHLORAL POISONING is by no means infrequent, because, the sleep-producing effect of the drug passing off after repeated administrations, the sleepless person is apt to increase the dose too far.

Symptoms – Occasionally, though seldom, there is gastric pain and sickness after a large dose. Usually the result is a speedy and deep sleep, passing gradually into coma, the pulse growing feebler, and the respirations embarrassed till death peacefully ensues.

Treatment – The patient must be persistently irritated and roused as in opium poisoning. The stomach should be at once emptied by stomach tube or emetic. The extremities of the body must be kept warm, and stimulants given. Leptazol and ephedrine are said to be useful. Artificial respiration may be needed.

CHLORAMBUCIL is a derivative of nitrogen mustard (qv), which is proving of value in the treatment of chronic lymphatic leukaemia (qv) and Hodgkin's disease (qv). It is given by mouth.

CHLORAMINE is a white powder with powerful antiseptic action, which is non-irritant and non-poisonous.

CHLORAMPHENICOL is an antibiotic derived from a soil organism, *Streptomyces venezuelae*. It is also prepared synthetically. It is active against a wide range of organisms, but its most striking feature is its activity against certain rickettsiae (qv). It has proved effective in the treatment of typhus, scrub typhus, Rocky Mountain spotted fever, typhoid and paratyphoid fevers. Its activity against certain organisms not susceptible to the sulphonamides and penicillin is proving of value. Particularly is this true of its use in the treatment of meningitis due to *H. influenzae*. It is given by mouth.

It is an antibiotic, however, that must be administered with discrimination because in certain individuals it may cause aplastic anaemia (qv), particularly if given for too long a period or in repeated courses.

CHLORDANE is an insecticide which has been used successfully against flies and mosquitoes resistant to DDT, and for the control of ticks and mites. It requires special handling as it is toxic to man when applied to the skin.

CHLORDIAZEPOXIDE, the proprietary name of which is LIBRIUM, is a widely used anti-anxiety drug.

CHLORETONE, or CHLORBUTOL, is a white powder with an odour like camphor. Applied to the surface of the skin or mucous membrane it has a soothing and antiseptic effect, and internally it acts as a hypnotic.

CHLORHEXIDINE, also known as HIBITANE, is an antiseptic which has a bacteriostatic action against many bacteria.

CHLORINATED LIME, also known as CHLORIDE OF LIME, is a white powder made by passing chlorine gas over slaked lime. Chlorine is a greenish gas, heavier than air, with a pungent, choking smell, and highly poisonous to all forms of bacterial life. By virtue of its power to give off chlorine, chlorinated lime is a powerful bleaching agent and disinfectant, especially when mixed with an acid. To disinfect rooms, chlorinated lime may be mixed with an equal bulk of water acidulated with sulphuric acid, and exposed on flat dishes for some hours. To disinfect water-closets and drains, 1 pound (450 G) of the chlorinated lime may be mixed with a gallon (4·5 litres) of water and poured down the drain.

To disinfect swimming baths it should be added in such an amount that the free chlorine, after combining with any organic matter in the water, is left in a concentration of 0·25 to 1 part per million parts of water. It is an efficient disinfectant for drinking water when added in the proportion of 1 ounce to 2000 gallons (28·3 grammes to 9000 litres). The residual taste of chlorine can be removed by adding a small crystal of sodium thiosulphate, about the size of a grain of rice, to a quart jug of water.

CHLORINE (see CHLORINATED LIME, and SODIUM HYPOCHLORITE).

CHLORMERODRIN is a mercurial diuretic which is active when given by mouth. (See DIURETICS.)

CHLORMETHIAZOLE is a tranquillizer that is proving of value in switching barbiturate-addicted individuals on to a safer hypnotic such as nitrazepam.

CHLORODYNE is another name for the *British Pharmaceutical Codex* preparation known as Chloroform and Morphine Tincture, which contains morphine hydrochloride. The dose is 0·3 to 0·6 millilitre. It is a useful soothing remedy in diarrhoea.

CHLOROFORM is a colourless, volatile liquid, half as heavy again as water, and, unlike ether, non-inflammable. It was discovered by Liebig in 1831, and is a compound of carbon, hydrogen, and chlorine. It does not dissolve to a large amount in water, but mixes readily with alcohol or ether. It dissolves sulphur, phosphorus, fats, resins, and most substances which contain a large proportion of carbon; it is therefore very useful as a cleansing agent. It was introduced into medicine in 1847 by Sir J. Y. Simpson, who was then in search of a substance which could produce unconsciousness for operative purposes more conveniently than ether, introduced a short time previously by Morton in America. (See ANAESTHETICS.)

Uses – Chloroform is used as a solvent of fats, resins, etc., in many chemical processes.

Externally as the liniment of chloroform it is a useful application for rheumatic and similar pains, having both a soothing and a mildly counter-irritant action.

Internally its chief use is by inhalation to produce insensibility to pain during surgical operations, in painful and convulsive diseases such as gall-stone colic, and during child-birth. By mouth, small doses have also the effect of relieving vomiting, especially in seasickness. For this purpose 1 to 5 drops may be taken on a lump of sugar. Spirit of chloroform is a frequent component of cough and digestive mixtures, for its stimulating and soothing effects upon the interior of the stomach and bronchial tubes.

CHLOROMA, or GREEN CANCER, is the name of a disease in which greenish growths appear under the skin, and in which a change takes place in the blood resembling that in leukaemia.

CHLOROMYCETIN is another name for CHLORAMPHENICOL (qv).

CHLOROPHYLL is the name of the green colouring matter of plants. Its main use is as a colouring agent, principally for soaps, oils and fats. It is also being found of value as a deodorant dressing to remove, or diminish, the unpleasant odour of heavily infected sores and wounds.

CHLOROQUINE, which is a 4-aminoquinoline, was introduced during the 1939–45 War for the treatment of malaria. It has also been found of value in the treatment of amoebic abscess in the liver, of the skin condition known as chronic discoid lupus erythematosus, and of rheumatoid arthritis.

CHLOROSIS is a form of anaemia which receives its name from the yellow or faintly greenish-grey complexion of those suffering from it. Very common before the 1914–18 War, it is scarcely ever seen now. (See ANAEMIA.)

CHLOROTHIAZIDE is a potent benzothiadiazine (qv) diuretic which is active when taken by mouth. It has also a blood-pressure-lowering effect when used in conjunction with other hypotensive drugs.

CHLOROTRIANISENE is a synthetic oestrogen (qv) which is active when taken by mouth.

CHLOROXYLENOL, or DETTOL, is an antiseptic which is used for treating cuts, abrasions, and wounds. It is also widely used in obstetric practice. It is only slightly soluble in water (1 in 3000).

CHLORPHENTERMINE is a synthetic amphetamine derivative which is proving of value in the management of obesity.

CHLORPROMAZINE is chemically related to the antihistamine drug, promethazine. It is one of the so-called 'tranquillizers' (qv), and is being used extensively in psychiatry on account of its action in calming psychotic activity without producing undue general depression or clouding of consciousness.

CHLORPROPAMIDE is one of the new oral hypoglycaemic agents. It is a sulphonamide derivative. As it has a prolonged action, it need only be given once a day. It is said to be more effective than tolbutamide (qv). Those taking chlorpropamide should bear in mind that in around 10 per cent of people it causes undue sensitivity to alcohol, resulting in severe flushing of the face, headache and a feeling of intoxication. (See also DIABETES MELLITUS.)

CHLORTETRACYCLINE, also known as aureomycin, is an antibiotic derived from a soil organism, *Streptomyces aureofaciens*. (See TETRACYCLINES.)

CHOCOLATE is a solid substance made by grinding cocoa nibs to powder and mixing with a large amount of sugar and some flavouring substance, such as vanilla. It consists, roughly, half of sugar, starch, and protein, and half of a fat known as cocoa-butter, with small quantities of water and salts, and about 1 per cent of theobromine, an alkaloid of stimulating properties similar to those of tea and coffee.

Chocolate has been used in England since the time of Charles II, when it was very popular. It forms a compact and easily carried food, suitable for sustaining hard labour and for protecting against cold. The energy value of chocolate is about 600 Calories per 100 grams.

CHOKE-DAMP (see DAMP).

CHOKING is the process which results from an obstruction to breathing situated in the larynx (see AIR PASSAGES). It may occur as the result of disease causing swelling round the glottis (the entrance to the larynx), or of some nervous disorders that interfere with the regulation of the muscles which open and shut the larynx, but generally it is due to the irritation of a piece of food or other substance introduced by the mouth, which provokes coughing but only partly interferes with breathing. In the act of swallowing, all food passes over the top of the larynx, and, as a preliminary to swallowing, the glottis is automatically closed by approximation of the sides of the larynx at their upper edge, over which the bolus of food is shot into the gullet (illustration 108). When, as the result of some nervous disease, such as a form of paralysis of the mouth and throat muscles, or simply of an attempt to speak or laugh during eating, this preliminary closure is not complete, a piece of food is apt to lodge in, or some fluid to trickle down into, the larynx. The mucous membrane lining the upper part of the latter being specially sensitive, coughing results in order to expel the cause of irritation. At the same time, if the foreign body be of any size, lividity of the face appears, due to partial suffocation (see ASPHYXIA).

Treatment – If coughing be vigorous the choking person should be let alone, a glass of water being put within his reach, because a gulp of cold water often dislodges the particle, and, at all events, stimulates more vigorous coughing. The choking person should take slow, deep inspirations, which do not force the particle farther in (as sudden catchings of the breath between the coughs do), and which produce more powerful coughs. If

108 – Vertical section through the middle of the head and neck, showing the upper air passages. The passages for air *a*, are indicated by a heavy dotted line, those for the food *f*, by a fainter line; *et*, Eustachian tube; *l*, larynx; *w*, windpipe; *t*, tonsil; *to*, tongue; *g*, gullet. (For other letters, see illustration 89.)

the coughing be weak, one or two strong blows with the palm of the hand over either shoulder blade, timed to coincide with coughs aid the effect of the coughing. In the case of a child the patient may be held up by the legs, when the substance causing the obstruction is more readily dislodged.

If this fails to dislodge the foreign body, what is known as the Heimlich manœuvre should be tried. If the victim is standing or sitting, stand behind him and wrap your arms round his waist. Grasp the closed fist of the bottom hand with the other hand, and place the thumb side of the first against the abdomen slightly above the navel and below the ribs. Then press your fist against the abdomen with a quick upward thrust. Repeat several times if necessary. If the victim is lying down, whether semi-conscious or unconscious, kneel astride his hips facing him. With one hand on top of the other, place the heel of the bottom hand on the abdomen slightly above the navel and below the ribs. Press into the abdomen with a quick upward thrust. Repeat several times if necessary. Should the victim vomit, turn him quickly on his side and wipe out his mouth to prevent him inhaling the vomited material The essence of the manœuvre is the quick upward thrust, which quite often causes the foreign body to shoot out of the mouth.

If this fails, an attempt should be made to remove the foreign body as follows. The bystander should pass his right forefinger along the side of the patient's tongue, forcing the teeth apart first, if necessary, with a knife handle, and keeping them apart by the fingers of the other hand with a napkin rolled round them. The forefinger should be passed as far down the throat as possible, its point then turned towards the middle line and hooked forwards towards the root of the tongue. After a few attempts the foreign body will very likely be dislodged and pulled up into the mouth.

Sometimes, however, the foreign body may be too small to catch; for example, death has been recorded in consequence of a fragment of cabbage leaf which lay over the opening of the larynx like a valve, completely preventing the entrance of air. As the opening is only a slit about a quarter of an inch (6 mm) from side to side and less than an inch (25 mm) from before backwards, such an accident may readily happen. In this case, if the sufferer be livid and unconscious, and if no medical man be obtained within five minutes, someone at hand may undertake to open the larynx below the obstruction, and admit air to the lungs, but, on account of its dangers, this is suitable only in extremest cases. For this purpose a sharp-pointed knife, such as a penknife, should be taken, the prominent Adam's apple in front of the neck felt for, and the knife pushed boldly into the throat at a point half an inch (12 mm) below the prominence (in a full-grown person). The knife must be pushed in exactly in the middle line, straight backwards to the depth of half an inch (12 mm), and the cut extended half an inch (12 mm) downwards. After this, artificial respiration (see DROWNING) may be necessary, and, if there be any bleeding from the wound in the neck, a bystander should press gently with his finger on the edge from which it comes, at the same time pressing the edges of the wound apart so as to allow the air to enter. By this procedure, lives have been saved when the obstruction could not be dislodged through the mouth.

CHOLAEMIA is a vague term applied to conditions in which the bile is not excreted from the body to its usual extent, but circulates in the blood. (See JAUNDICE.)

CHOLAGOGUES are substances which increase the flow of bile by stimulating evacuation of the gall-bladder. The great majority of these act only by increasing the activity of the digestive organs, and so producing a flow of bile already stored up in the gall-bladder. Substances which stimulate the liver to secrete more bile are known as CHOLERETICS.

Varieties and uses – Among the cholagogues are blue pill, calomel, aloes, ipecacuanha, rhubarb, and Epsom salts. The only choleretics are bile and bile salts.

CHOLANGIOGRAPHY is the term applied to the process whereby the bile ducts and the gall-bladder are rendered radio-opaque and therefore visible on an X-ray film. (See IOPANOIC ACID; SODIUM DIATRIZOATE.)

CHOLANGITIS is the term applied to inflammation of the bile ducts.

CHOLECYSTECTOMY means the removal of the gall-bladder by operation.

CHOLECYSTITIS means inflammation of the gall-bladder (qv).

CHOLECYSTOGRAPHY is the term applied to the process whereby the gall-bladder is rendered radio-opaque and therefore visible on an X-ray film. (See IOPANOIC ACID; SODIUM DIATRIZOATE.)

CHOLELITHIASIS means the presence of gall-stones in the bile-ducts and/or in the gall-bladder. (See GALL-STONES.)

CHOLERA belongs originally to Asia, more particularly to India and Bangladesh, where epidemics are known to have occurred at various times for several centuries. It was not, however, till 1817 that the attention of European physicians was specially directed to the disease by the outbreak of a violent epidemic of cholera at Jessore in Bengal. This was followed by its rapid spread over a large portion of British India, where it caused immense destruction of life among both natives and Europeans. By 1823 it had extended into Asia Minor and Russia in Asia, and it continued to advance steadily though slowly westwards, and spread onwards to England, appearing in Sunderland in October 1831, and in London in January 1832. The disease subsequently spread through North and Central America, reaching even to the military posts on the upper Mississippi. In 1835 it was general throughout North Africa, after which this epidemic disappeared.

CHOLERA

About the year 1841 another great epidemic of cholera appeared in India and China, and soon began to extend in the direction traversed by the former, but involving a still wider area. This epidemic appears to have been even more deadly than the former, especially as regards Great Britain and France.

A third great outbreak of cholera took place in the East in 1850, entering Europe in 1853. It was specially severe throughout both North and South America.

A fourth epidemic visited Europe again in 1865 66, but was on the whole less extensive and destructive than its predecessors. In 1884, and again in 1892 and 1893, there were outbreaks in the middle of Europe, the last one being specially severe in Hamburg and some other cities, but, apart from occasional cases brought by ship, there has been no epidemic in Britain or in the United States for many years.

In 1977, a world total of 60,000 cases of cholera was notified, affecting thirty-four countries, including several around the Eastern Mediterranean, and two imported cases were notified in England.

Causes – The cause of the disease is the *Vibrio cholerae*, or comma-bacillus, discovered by Koch. This organism is constantly found in the discharges from the bowels of those suffering from the disease. The most important mode of transmission is by means of contaminated water, but the infection is also conveyed by flies, which contaminate food with infected faeces. The crowding which occurs under conditions of war and famine also favours epidemics.

Symptoms – The incubation period is a few hours to five days. The disease varies in severity from mild cases which do not feel ill enough to take to bed, to cases which are fatal within twenty-four hours. Over 90 per cent of cases, however, are of the so-called *Cholera gravis* type, in which three stages are recognized.

The *first stage*, which lasts for three to twelve hours, is of sudden onset with painless diarrhoea and vomiting. The stools rapidly become frequent and copious, resembling rice-water and containing flakes of fibrin. This is soon followed by agonizing cramps, first in the limbs and then in the abdomen. The patient complains bitterly of thirst and becomes restless and exhausted, with cold bluish skin, sunken eyeballs, and husky voice. The pulse is weak and the temperature taken in the rectum is 101° to 104° F (38.3° to 40° C).

The *second stage* is termed the stage of collapse or algid stage. The symptoms now advance with rapidity. The signs of collapse increase. The surface of the body becomes colder and assumes a dusky blue or purple hue, the skin is dry and wrinkled, indicating the intense draining away, in the evacuations, of the fluids of the body. The features are pinched and the eyes more deeply sunken, the pulse at the wrist is imperceptible, and the voice is reduced to a hoarse whisper (the 'vox cholerica'). There may be complete suppression of the urine.

In this condition, death often takes place in less than one day, but, in epidemics, cases are sometimes observed in which the collapse is so sudden and complete as to prove fatal in one or two hours without any great amount of previous purging or vomiting. In most instances the mental faculties are comparatively unaffected, although in the later stages there is generally more or less apathy.

Reaction may, however, take place, and this constitutes the *third stage*. It consists in the arrest of the alarming symptoms of the second stage, and the gradual but evident improvement in the patient's condition. The pulse returns, the surface assumes a natural hue, and the bodily heat is restored. Before long, the vomiting ceases, and, though diarrhoea may continue for a time, it is not of a severe character and soon subsides, as do also the cramps. The urine may remain suppressed for some time, and on returning is often found to be albuminous.

Even in this stage, however, the danger is not past, for relapses sometimes occur which speedily prove fatal; while, again, the reaction may be of imperfect character, and there may succeed an exhausting fever (the so-called *typhoid stage* of cholera), which may greatly retard recovery, and under which the patient may sink at a period even as late as two or three weeks from the start of the illness.

The death-rate varies tremendously: from over 50 per cent in epidemics to around 5 per cent among patients who have received adequate treatment. The outcome is worst in children and old people. Many mild cases are probably never detected in countries where the disease is epidemic.

The bodies of persons dying of cholera are found to remain long warm, and the temperature may even rise after death. Muscular contractions have been observed to take place after death, so that the position of the limbs may become altered.

Treatment – PREVENTIVE TREATMENT –

When cholera threatens to invade any place, however favourably circumstanced as to its hygienic condition, increased vigilance will be requisite on the part of those entrusted with the care of the public health. Cholera may be introduced into a community by one or more individuals who have themselves only suffered from the first or milder stage of the disease (cholera diarrhoea), since the discharges from the bowels abound in the infective organisms, and, where sanitary arrangements are deficient, may readily contaminate the water of a locality.

Where suspicion attaches to the water, it should be boiled or chlorinated before being used; milk should also be boiled. Water and food should be protected against pollution with flies, and houses should be fly-proofed. Instructions should be issued by the authorities warning all persons against the use of unwholesome food, unripe fruit, and excesses of every kind, and recommending early application for medical advice where there is any tendency to diarrhoea. The discharges from cholera patients should be treated, as soon as passed, with strong disinfectants (see DISINFECTION), and special care should be taken that they are not disposed of in places where they can contaminate drinking-water. In 1893 Haffkine introduced a vaccine for preventive inoculation against cholera, and this seems to afford a certain amount of protection over a period of some months.

CURATIVE TREATMENT – Strict rest in bed is essential. All but a small percentage of cases can now be treated successfully by the administration by mouth of electrolyte solutions. This can be accomplished effectively and economically by the distribution of packets containing pre-weighed amounts of glucose, sodium chloride, potassium chloride and sodium bicarbonate to be added to measured volumes of boiled water in hospital, local treatment centres and, most importantly, in the home, even in the most rural and underdeveloped areas. In severe cases an intravenous infusion is necessary. The infusion fluid consists of two volumes of isotonic sodium chloride (0.9 per cent) plus one volume of sodium lactate (1·75 per cent) or sodium bicarbonate (1·4 per cent). An alternative is the so-called Dacca solution:

Sodium chloride	5 grams	
Sodium bicarbonate	4 grams	
Potassium chloride	1 gram	
Water	to 1 litre	

A blood-pressure below 70 mm of mercury, especially if there is associated cyanosis, restlessness, cramps, and cold extremities, is an indication for immediate transfusion with isotonic saline solution.

Chemotherapy is useful only in reducing the period during which the vibrio remains in the stool. For this purpose, chloramphenicol, chlortetracycline, or one of the insoluble sulphonamides (eg. sulphaguanidine) should be used.

CHOLESTEROL is a sterol, which is one of a class of solid alcohols; these are waxy materials derived from animal and vegetable tissues. It is widely distributed throughout the body, being especially abundant in the brain, nervous tissue, adrenal glands and skin. It is also found in egg yolk and gall-stones. It plays an important role in the body, being essential for the production of the sex hormones, as well as the repair of membranes. It is also the source from which bile acids are manufactured. The total amount in the body of a man weighing 70 kilograms (10 stones) is around 140 grams, and the amount present in the blood is 150 to 250 milligrams per 100 millilitres.

A high blood-cholesterol level – that is, one over 300 mg per 100 ml – is undesirable as there appears to be a correlation between a high blood cholesterol and atheroma (qv), the form of arterial degenerative disease associated with coronary thrombosis and high blood-pressure. This is well exemplified in diabetes mellitus (qv) and myxoedema (qv), two diseases in which there is a high blood cholesterol, sometimes going as high as 700 mg per 100 ml; patients with these diseases are known to be particularly prone to arterial disease. There is also a familial disease known as hypercholesterolaemia, in which members of affected families have a blood cholesterol of around 600 mg per 100 ml, or more, and are particularly liable to premature degenerative disease of the arteries.

The rising incidence of arterial disease in western countries in recent years has drawn attention to this relationship between high levels of cholesterol in the blood and arterial disease. The available evidence indicates that there is a relationship between blood-cholesterol levels and the amount of fat consumed. Thus, in Cape Town it has been shown that in men aged 45 the mean blood-cholesterol level was 234 mg per 100 ml in the European community and 166 mg per 100 ml in the

Bantu community, and this was correlated with the basic difference between the diets of the two communities: 40 per cent of the calories in the European's diet was fat, compared with 20 per cent or less in the Bantu's diet. The suggestion was therefore made that the rising incidence of coronary heart disease, and other manifestations of arterial disease, such as high blood-pressure and strokes, might be arrested by persuading those living in western communities, such as Western Europe and USA, to eat less fat. One of the troubles is that the blood-cholesterol level bears little relationship with the amount of cholesterol consumed, most of the cholesterol in the body being produced by the body itself. Thus, it has been reported that even eating ten eggs, and eggs are the only rich source of cholesterol in the diet, does not usually raise the level of cholesterol in the blood.

On the other hand, it has been shown that diets containing fats with a high proportion of what are known as saturated fatty acids raise the blood-cholesterol level, whereas those with fats containing a high proportion of unsaturated fatty acids lower it. Fats with a high proportion of fatty acids include animal fats such as butter, dripping and the like, whereas the fatty acids with a high proportion of unsaturated fatty acids are predominantly vegetable oils such as olive oil, corn oil, and sunflower oil. The recommendation therefore is that people should reduce their consumption of 'saturated' fats and concentrate on 'unsaturated' fats. Unfortunately, what should have been kept as a straight scientific investigation has become bedevilled with emotional overtones, and it is difficult to give an objective scientific opinion on the present status of the controversy. There is little doubt that there is a tendency to eat too much animal fat today. Here, as elsewhere, the golden rule is moderation in all things. It is also generally admitted that, if an individual's blood cholesterol is on the high side, even if he is not suffering from diseases such as diabetes mellitus, then it is wise for him to curtail his intake of saturated fats, just as he should aim at avoiding obesity. The same probably applies to a man who has had a coronary thrombosis. Whether there is any need to go further than this is problematical, and much more scientific investigation will be necessary before the medical profession is justified in recommending any striking alteration in our eating habits – except, as already noted, to advise moderation in all things.

CHOLESTYRAMINE is a drug that is proving of value in the treatment of the pruritus, or itching (qv), which occurs in association with jaundice. This it does by 'binding' the bile salts in the gut and so preventing their being reabsorbed into the bloodstream, where their excess in jaundice is responsible for the itching. It is also proving useful in reducing the level of cholesterol and triglycerides in the blood and thereby, like clofibrate (qv), helping to reduce the incidence of coronary artery heart disease. (See CORONARY THROMBOSIS.)

CHOLINE, is one of the many constituents of the vitamin B complex. Lack of it in the experimental animal produces a fatty liver. It is found in egg-yolk, liver, and meat. The probable daily human requirement is 500 mg, an amount amply covered by the ordinary diet.

CHONDROMA is a tumour composed in part of cartilage. (See TUMOURS.)

CHORDOTOMY is the term applied to the operation of cutting the nerves in the spinal cord which convey the sensation of pain to the brain. This operation is done for the relief of severe and intractable pain.

CHOREA, or ST VITUS'S DANCE, is the name applied to a disorder of the nervous system occurring for the most part in children, and characterized mainly by involuntary jerking movements of the muscles. The name, St Vitus's dance, was originally applied to those remarkable epidemic outbursts of combined mental and physical excitement which for a time prevailed among the inhabitants of some parts of Germany in the Middle Ages. It is stated that sufferers from this dancing mania were wont to resort to the chapels of St Vitus, the saint believed to possess the power of curing them. The name was transferred to the disease at present under consideration, with which it has evidently nothing to do, and the original application has been to a great extent lost sight of. The term, SYDENHAM'S CHOREA, is also applied to this disorder to distinguish it from Huntington's chorea, a disease of hereditary nature which appears late in life and is accompanied by mental defects.

Causes – Chorea is a condition resulting from involvement of the central nervous system by the same factor (or factors) as are responsible for acute rheumatism (qv). It is more common in girls than in boys, in the proportion of 3 : 1. Like acute rheumatism it is rare under the age of 3 years and uncommon under the age of 5 years. There is no definite evidence that it is hereditary, but it is more likely to occur in excitable, intelligent, ambitious children than in the phlegmatic child. There may be a history of some precipitating factor such as a fright or worry over an impending examination. It forms an occasional but rare complication of pregnancy.

Although chorea is the manifestation of acute rheumatism which is most likely to occur without manifestations of rheumatism elsewhere, the main importance of chorea is that about one-third of children who develop it show evidence of rheumatism elsewhere in the body, and usually in the heart. Recurrences occur in about one-third of the cases, usually within a year of the first attack. Such recurrences are more common in girls than in boys. If the heart is not involved in the first attack, it is unlikely to be affected in recurrent attacks.

Symptoms – The characteristic features are: (1) involuntary, purposeless, incoordinated movements; (2) weakness of voluntary movements; (3) loss of precision of movement; (4) psychological disturbances. The symptoms are usually preceded by changes in the temper and disposition, the child becoming sad, irritable and emotional, while at the same time the general health is impaired. The first thing indicative of the disease is a certain awkwardness or fidgetiness of manner, together with restlessness, the child being evidently unable to continue quiet, but frequently moving the limbs into different positions. In walking, too, slight dragging of one limb may be noticed. The convulsive muscular movements usually show themselves first in one part, such as an arm or a leg, and in most instances they may remain localized to that limited extent, whilst in all cases there is a tendency for the disorderly symptoms to be more marked on one side than on the other. The child when standing or sitting is never still, but is constantly changing the position of the body or limbs in consequence of the sudden and incoordinate action of muscles or groups of them. These symptoms are aggravated when purposive movements are attempted, or when the child is watched. Sometimes the disorder is first noticed owing to the frequency with which the child drops cups, plates and similar articles. Speech is affected, and the taking of food becomes a matter of difficulty. When the tongue is protruded, it comes out in a jerky manner, and is im-

mediately withdrawn, the jaws at the same time closing suddenly and sometimes with considerable force. The heart may be affected as in acute rheumatism, and this may lay the foundation of permanent heart disease (see HEART DISEASES). Usually, there is a remission of the symptoms during sleep.

This disease occasionally assumes a very acute and aggravated form, in which the disorderly movements are so violent as to render the patient liable to be injured and to necessitate forcible control of the limbs or the employment of anaesthetics to produce unconsciousness. Such cases are rare but of very grave character, if, as is common, they are accompanied with sleeplessness, and they may prove fatal by exhaustion. In the great majority of cases, however, complete recovery is to be anticipated sooner or later, the symptoms usually continuing for from one to two months, or even sometimes longer.

Treatment – The first step in treatment is to provide the patient with complete physical and mental rest. Under suitable conditions the disease tends to recover of itself. These conditions, however, are all-important, and embrace the proper feeding of the child with a full nutritious diet, the absence of all sources of excitement and annoyance, such as being laughed at or mocked by other children, and the removal of any causes of irritation and of irregularities in the general health. Confinement to bed is necessary – usually for four to six weeks. Of medicinal remedies the most serviceable are sodium salicylate and aspirin, especially the latter. After recovery the general health of the child should for a long time receive attention, and care should be taken to guard against excitement, excessive study or any exhausting condition, physical or mental.

In the rare instances of the acute form of this malady, where the convulsive movements are unceasing and violent, the only measures available are the use of full doses of chloral, or injections of hyoscine or morphine. It is these cases which tend to end fatally. (See also HUNTINGTON'S CHOREA.)

CHORIOCARCINOMA is a form of cancer affecting the chorion (qv), in which particularly impressive results are being obtained from the use of methotrexate.

CHORION is the name applied to the more external of the two foetal membranes. (See AFTERBIRTH.)

195

CHOROID, or CHORIOID, is the middle of the three coats of the eye, and consists chiefly of blood-vessels, which effect the nourishment of this organ. (See EYE.)

CHOROIDITIS means inflammation of the choroid coat of the eye, and is sometimes associated with inflammation of the iris. (See EYE, DISEASES OF; IRITIS; and VISION.) It may be syphilitic or tuberculous in origin, or it may be due to infection with some other micro-organism. It may also be allergic in origin. In its early stages it may produce no symptoms. When well advanced, it produces inflammation in the retina, when the condition is known as chorioretinitis, and then causes interference with sight in various ways, such as dark spots in the field of vision, loss of vision for particular colours. Its effects vary greatly, according to the position of the inflamed patches, for wide stretches of inflammation may occur situated towards the front of the eye without causing much interference with vision, whilst a very small patch, occurring on or near the macula, or spot of clearest vision in the centre of the back of the eye (see EYE), may cause great visual defect. The condition is easily detected by examination with the ophthalmoscope, even in the early stages; but, though treatment retards, or completely stops, the progress of the disease, little improvement in vision is to be expected.

CHRISTMAS DISEASE is a hereditary disorder of blood coagulation which can only be distinguished from haemophilia (qv) by laboratory tests. It is so called after the surname of the first case reported in this country. About one out of every ten patients clinically diagnosed as haemophilia has in fact Christmas disease. It is due to lack in the blood of what is known as Factor IX.

CHROMAFFIN is a term applied to certain cells and organs in the body, such as part of the adrenal glands, which have a peculiar affinity for chrome salts. These cells and tissues generally are supposed to secrete substances which have an important action in maintaining the tone and elasticity of the blood-vessels and muscles.

CHROMIC ACID is used in several industries, particularly in chromium plating. Unless precautions are taken it may lead to dermatitis of the hands, arms, chest and face. It may also cause deep ulcers, especially of the nasal septum and knuckles.

Uses – The chief medicinal use of chromic acid is as a caustic for the treatment of warts and indolent ulcers. It is also sometimes used in a 2 or 3 per cent solution for the treatment of sweating feet.

CHROMOSOMES are the rod-shaped bodies to be found in the nucleus of every cell in the body. They contain the genes, or hereditary elements, which establish the characteristics of an individual. They occur in pairs, and human beings possess forty-six, made up of twenty-three pairs (illustration 109). The number of chromosomes is specific for each species of animal. (See HEREDITY; and SEX CHROMOSOMES.)

CHRYSAROBIN, or GOA POWDER, is a substance got from Brazil, being a concretion which forms on the stems of the *Araroba* plant, powdered and purified. It is used in various skin diseases, especially psoriasis, either in the form of an ointment or plaster, or made into a paste with vinegar. Whilst efficacious, it has the drawback that it stains the clothes a deep violet colour. These stains, however, may be removed with benzol or weak chlorinated lime in water.

CHYLE is the name given to the milky fluid which is absorbed by the lymphatic vessels of the intestine. The absorbed portion consists of fats in very fine emulsion, like milk, so that these vessels receive the name of lacteals (L. *lac*, milk). This absorbed chyle mixes with the lymph and is discharged into the thoracic duct, a vessel as large as a quill, which passes up through the chest to open into the jugular vein on the left side of the neck, where the chyle mixes with the blood.

CHYLURIA means the passage of chyme (qv) in the urine. This results in the passing of a milky-looking urine. It is one of the manifestations of filariasis (qv), where it is due to obstruction of the lymphatics (qv) by the causative parasite.

CHYME is the name given to the partly digested food as it issues from the stomach into the intestine. It is very acid and grey in colour, containing salts and sugars in solution, and the animal food softened into a semi-liquid mass. It is next converted into chyle.

CHYMOPAPAIN is an enzyme (qv) obtained from the paw-paw, which is being used in the treatment of prolapsed intervertebral discs (qv). When injected into the disc it dissolves it.

109 – Chromosomes of a healthy male. *The Practitioner.*

CICATRIX is another word for scar.

CIDER is an alcoholic beverage made from apples. (See ALCOHOL.)

CILIA is a term applied to minute, lash-like processes which are seen with the aid of the microscope upon the cells covering certain mucous membranes: eg. the trachea (or windpipe) and nose and which maintain movement in the fluid passing over these membranes. They are also found on certain bacteria which have the power of rapid movement.

CIMETIDINE is a drug that is proving of value in the treatment of duodenal ulcer. It acts by reducing the hyperacidity of the gastric juice.

CIMEX LECTULARIUS (see BED BUG; and PARASITES).

CINCHONA is the general name for several trees in the bark of which quinine is found. This bark is also known as Jesuit's bark, having been brought first to notice by Spanish priests in South America and brought to Europe first by the Countess of Cinchon, wife of the Viceroy of Peru, in 1640. The red cinchona bark is that which contains most quinine, and from which it is usually prepared. (See QUININE.) Various extracts and tinctures are made direct from cinchona bark, and used in place of quinine.

CINNAMON is the bark of *Cinnamomum zeylanicum,* a species of laurel grown in Sri Lanka (Ceylon). It has a stimulating action upon the stomach, and assists digestion; hence its use as a condiment. It is also an antispasmodic.

Uses – In flatulent dyspepsia and in sea-sickness, cinnamon powder (10 grains (600 mg)) is very useful. For the same purposes, or for relieving griping, four drops of oil of cinnamon may be taken on sugar, or one tablespoonful of cinnamon water (distilled) may be similarly used.

CIRCLE OF WILLIS, or CIRCULUS ARTERIOSUS, is a circle of arteries at the base of the brain, which is formed by the

CIRCULATION OF THE BLOOD

junction of the basilar, posterior cerebral, internal carotid and anterior cerebral arteries. Congenital defects may occur in these arteries and lead to the formation of aneurysms (qv).

CIRCULATION OF THE BLOOD – This principle was demonstrated for the first time by William Harvey in 1628. The proof of the facts of circulation was one of the most important discoveries in medical science. Before Harvey's discovery the generally accepted view was that the arteries contained a mixture of air and 'vital spirits', with only an accidental admixture of blood, and that the heart by its motions alternately sucked in more air through the pores of the skin and those of the lungs, and through the same channels expelled 'fuliginous vapours'. The 'vital spirits' were assumed to be manufactured by the heart and to be the origin of all activity, whilst the 'fuliginous vapours' were a form of smoke resulting from the bodily motions. The blood in the veins was supposed to be derived from the liver, which absorbed the 'juices of the food', and to ebb and flow in and out of the various organs for their nourishment. Harvey proved, first of all, mainly by the examination of living animals, that the arteries contain only blood. Secondly, he showed by three main propositions that this blood must go round from arteries to veins in a continuous circuit. (1) The quantity of blood passing from the veins into the heart in the course of a whole day is so great that it is quite impossible it could all be manufactured from the food. (2) The blood in the arteries passes in a constant stream to all the members of the body, and does not return by the same route. (3) The blood in the veins flows incessantly to the heart, and does not ebb and flow, as is shown by the valves in veins and in the heart, and by the fact that veins when pressed on do not fill from above. Having proved these points, he assumed there must be 'pores in the flesh' through which the blood 'percolated' from the ends of the arteries to the commencements of the veins. The last link in the evidence was supplied some thirty years later by Malpighi, an Italian scientist, who with the help of the microscope showed these 'pores' to be the minute vessels now called capillaries.

The course of the circulation is as follows (illustration 110): The veins pour their blood, coming from the head, trunk, limbs and abdominal organs, into the right atrium of the heart. This contracts and

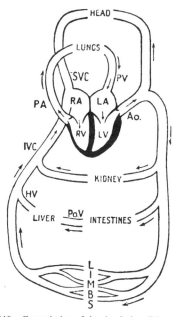

110 – General plan of the circulation. PA, pulmonary artery. PV, pulmonary vein. LA, left atrium. LV, left ventricle. Ao, aorta. PoV, portal vein. HV, hepatic vein. IVC, inferior vena cava. SVC, superior vena cava. RA, right atrium. RV, right ventricle. From Bell, Davidson and Scarborough, *Textbook of Physiology and Biochemistry*. E. & S. Livingstone Ltd.

drives the blood into the right ventricle, which then forces the blood into the lungs by way of the pulmonary artery. Here it is contained in thin-walled capillaries, over which the air plays freely, and through which gases pass readily out and in. The blood gives off carbon dioxide (CO_2) and takes up oxygen (see RESPIRATION), and passes on by the pulmonary veins to the left atrium of the heart. The left atrium expels it into the left ventricle, which forces it on into the aorta, by which it is distributed all over the body. Passing through capillaries in the various tissues (illustration 111) it enters the veins, which ultimately unite into two great veins, the superior and the inferior vena cava, these emptying into the right atrium. This complete circle is accomplished by any particular drop of blood in about half a minute.

In one part of the body there is a further complication. The veins coming from the bowels, charged with food material and other products, split up, and their blood undergoes a second capillary circulation

198

Arteriole

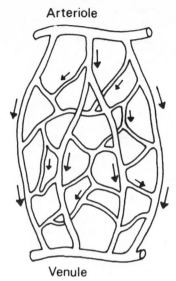

Venule

111 – Diagram of the capillary bed. The direction of the blood flow is shown by the arrows.

aorta. The latter is known as the ductus arteriosus. At birth all these extra vessels and connections close and rapidly shrivel up.

112 – Diagram of the heart opened from in front to show the action of the valves. *RA*, right atrium; *RV*, right ventricle; *P*, pulmonary artery; *LA*, left atrium; *LV*, left ventricle; *A*, aorta.

through the liver. Here it is relieved of some food material and purified, and then passes into the inferior vena cava, and so to the right atrium. This is known as the portal circulation.

The circle is maintained always in one direction by four valves, situated one at the outlet from each cavity of the heart (illustration 112). (See HEART.)

The blood in the arteries going to the body generally is bright red, that in the veins dull red in colour, owing to the former being charged with oxygen, the latter with carbon dioxide (see RESPIRATION). For the same reason the blood in the pulmonary artery is dark, that in the pulmonary veins bright. There is no direct communication between the right and left sides of the heart, the blood passing from the right ventricle to the left atrium through the lungs.

In the embryo, before birth, the course of circulation is somewhat different, owing to the fact that no nourishment comes from the bowels nor air into the lungs. Accordingly, two large arteries pass out of the navel, and convey blood to be changed by contact with maternal blood (see AFTER-BIRTH), while a large vein brings this blood back again. There are also communications between the right and left atria, and between pulmonary artery and

CIRCULATION, DISORDERS OF – The steady maintenance of the circulation depends upon two factors: (1) the power and regularity of the heart; and (2) the condition of the walls of the vessels, especially of the small arteries. The arteries are not rigid tubes, nor are they merely elastic tubes of a definite size, for each vessel has the power of dilating and contracting within wide limits, so as to let a larger or smaller stream of blood pass through. These motions are controlled by constricting and dilating nerves governed by the nervous system, and upon the action of these, more than upon the heart, depends the state of circulation in various parts. For example, when cold strikes the skin the constrictor nerves are stimulated, the vessels contract, and the blood is driven from the skin, which becomes pallid. On the other hand, blushing is due to loss of control by these nerves over the vessels, or, when the redness is extreme, to stimulation of the dilating nerves by some emotion powerfully affecting the nervous system. Similar changes occur, under other conditions, in all the organs.

Causes and symptoms – *Inflammation* in its early stages is associated with great redness and swelling, due to excessive inflow of blood to the inflamed part through widely dilated arteries. *Con-*

199

gestion is a condition sometimes due to inflammation, sometimes to an obstruction to the veins which should carry off the blood, or very often to the feebleness of the heart, which cannot drive the blood upwards from dependent parts like the feet, or like the back portions of the lungs in bed-ridden persons. In old persons with diseased vessels, in which blood-clots are liable to form, congestion of the brain readily takes place from such obstructions. In weak persons, or those exhausted by illness, lying constantly on the back, congestion of the lungs is very apt to come on. Congestion of the lungs with bronchitis, and congestion of the liver and stomach with various disorders of digestion, are common results of valvular disease of the heart (see HEART DISEASES). *Dropsy* and *varicose veins* are similar disorders often due to obstruction to veins. Dropsy is also a usual result of heart disease and of kidney disease (see DROPSY; and VEINS, DISEASES OF). *Bloodlessness* of parts is a disorder in the opposite direction, due to spasm and extreme narrowing of arteries (see RAYNAUD'S DISEASE). A local blanching often precedes *chilblains*, which occur in persons of sluggish circulation. *Cold feet and hands*, especially at night, form a milder variety of the same condition. *Insomnia* in elderly persons is sometimes due to disordered circulation in the brain, because the vessels are extremely narrowed by disease.

Treatment – Where any failure of the heart is present, the case is treated by various cardiac drugs, by rest, and by graduated exercises. Some cases of disordered circulation depending on the vessels are benefited by cold baths (see BATHS) and daily vigorous exercises, while good diet, warm clothing and tonics are of importance for their cure. (See also CHILBLAIN.)

CIRCUMCISION means the cutting round and removal of the foreskin. It is performed as a religious rite among many tribes, notably by the Jews. It is seldom required on medical grounds, but has acquired a cultural reputation among the mothers of the United States of America.

CIRRHOSIS, or FIBROSIS, is a diseased condition, in which the proper tissue is replaced by fibrous tissue similar to scar tissue. The name cirrhosis was originally given by Laennec to the disease as occurring in the liver, because of its yellow colour. (See LIVER DISEASES.)

CIRSOID ANEURYSM is the term applied to the condition in which a group of arteries become abnormally dilated and tortuous.

CITRIC ACID is the acid which gives their sharp taste to lemons, limes, unripe oranges, currants and raspberries. It is practically identical in action and appearance with tartaric acid, which is obtained from grapes and other fruits, although the two differ in chemical composition. It is similar also to malic acid, found in apples, pears and the berries of the mountain ash.

Uses – These vegetable acids and their salts (citrates and tartrates) are changed, on absorption into the blood, into alkaline substances, and act therefore to correct acidity (see ACIDITY). The acids themselves have the power of allaying thirst by stimulating the flow of saliva, and also of creating a feeling of coolness. For both these reasons they are much used for cooling drinks in fever. When, in addition, the stomach is irritable, they are best taken in the form of effervescing drinks, which soothe this organ.

For feverish conditions a few slices of lemon may be put in a tumbler of drinking water, or 'Imperial Drink' made as follows: To one pint (500 ml) of cold water add a teaspoonful of cream of tartar, a squeeze of lemon and two lumps of sugar.

For an effervescing draught, 20 grains (1·2 G) of citric acid or the juice of one fresh lemon may be mixed with a large wineglassful of water; 30 grains (2 G) of bicarbonate of potash or 24 grains (1·6 G) of bicarbonate of soda (ie. about as much baking soda as will lie heaped up on a 5-pence-piece) are dissolved in another wineglassful of water; a third wineglassful of water is sweetened with sugar; the contents of the three wine glasses are mixed just before drinking.

CITRINE OINTMENT, or NITRATE OF MERCURY OINTMENT, is used for stimulating sluggish ulcers, and also, diluted with olive oil, in cases of eczema.

CLAUSTROPHOBIA means the fear of being in a confined space, or the fear experienced while in it.

CLAVICLE is another name for the collar-bone (qv).

CLAVUS is a form of neuralgia about the head, often found in hysterical persons and others, compared by them to the pain of driving in a nail (see NEURALGIA). The term is also applied to a corn, or thickening of the horny epithelium upon the foot (see CORNS).

CLAW-FOOT, or PES CAVUS, is a familial deformity of the foot characterized by an abnormally high arch of the foot accompanied by shortening of the foot, clawing of the toes and inversion, or turning inwards of the foot and heel. Its main effect is to impair the resilience of the foot resulting in a stiff gait and aching pain. Milder cases are treated with special shoes fitted with a sponge rubber insole. More severe cases may require surgical treatment.

CLAW-HAND is a condition of bending and wasting of the hand and fingers, especially of the ring and little fingers. The condition is generally due to paralysis of the ulnar nerve. A somewhat similar condition is produced by contraction of the fibrous tissues in the palm of the hand, partly due to rheumatic changes and partly to injury caused by the constant pressure of a tool against the palm of the hand. (See DUPUYTREN'S CONTRACTURE.)

CLAW-TOES (see CLAW-FOOT).

CLEANLINESS (see ASEPSIS; ANTISEPTICS; BATHS; DISINFECTION).

CLEFT FOOT is a rare congenital abnormality characterized by the absence of one or more toes and a deep central cleft that divides the foot into two. It is sometimes known as lobster foot or lobster claw. It may be accompanied by other congenital defects, such as cleft hand, absent permanent teeth, cleft lip and palate, absence of the nails, and defects of the eye.

CLEFT HAND is a rare congenital abnormality characterized by the absence of one or more fingers and a deep central cleft that divides the hand into two. It is sometimes known as lobster hand. It may be accompanied by other congenital defects, such as cleft foot, absent permanent teeth, cleft lip and palate, absence of the nails and defects of the eye.

CLEFT PALATE is the term applied to a fissure of the roof of the mouth sometimes present at birth and very often combined with hare-lip. (See PALATE, MALFORMATIONS OF.)

CLERGYMAN'S SORE THROAT is the name given to a complication of throat ailments, which gradually comes on in those who do much public speaking, and who possess weak vocal organs. Persons who suffer from it, as a rule, produce the voice badly, using the throat as a resonating chamber instead of gaining the full volume of the voice by keeping the lungs expanded. Speaking, accordingly, is performed with great effort, the more so as the muscles of the larynx and throat soon become tired. The mucous membrane of the throat and even of the nose becomes congested, and catarrh follows on very slight provocation, chronic laryngitis, and pharyngitis being set up. Still greater vocal efforts of an incorrect kind being made to overcome the consequent huskiness and feebleness, the condition gets inevitably worse and worse, till public speaking may become an utter impossibility.

Treatment – The first essential is to obtain correct voice-production, by expansion of the chest (see CHEST, DEVELOPMENT OF), and by a course of lessons on elocution from a good teacher (see VOICE AND SPEECH). The affected person must also get out of the bad habit of straining the throat in speaking. Secondly, the mucous membrane of the throat must be got back to its original state by such measures as gargles of potassium chlorate, or of common salt and baking soda (one teaspoonful of each in a tumblerful of cold water), or of aromatic substances, painting the throat with tincture of iodine or glycerin of tannin, and similar procedures. When the chronic inflammatory condition has proceeded further, and has set up considerable laryngitis and pharyngitis, the case should be under the care of a throat specialist, for local astringent applications to the larynx, throat and nose are necessary, or even the reduction of swollen mucous membrane by the cautery. In advanced stages, complete rest of the voice may be essential, and a change to some climate where the air is warm, moderately moist, and free from dust, may be advisable. Such a climate is found along the south coast of England, on the Mediterranean shores, or in Florida.

CLICKING FINGER is a condition in middle-aged people in which the victim finds on wakening in the morning that he or she cannot straighten the ring or middle finger spontaneously, but only by a special effort, when it suddenly straightens with a painful click. Hence the name. In due course the finger remains bent at all times unless a special effort is made to straighten it with the other hand. The condition is due to a swelling developing in one of the tendons of the affected finger and, if the tendon sheath is slit open surgically, the condition is relieved. Many cases recover spontaneously if the patient is prepared to wait.

CLICKING THUMB is a comparable condition sometimes found in the new-born baby, and occasionally in adults. In the baby, surgery should not be resorted to, as the condition practically always clears up spontaneously. In the adult it can be such a nuisance that it should probably be operated on at a fairly early stage.

CLIMACTERIC was a word originally applied to the end of certain epochs or stages in the life of an individual, at which some great change was supposed to take place. Thus the Greeks supposed the whole body was renewed every seven years, and looked upon certain of these periods as of special importance. There is some justification for such a view, since fourteen is the age about which puberty, ie. the commencement of sexual activity, appears; about twenty-one full sexual maturity is usually attained, which renders this the most approved age for marriage, and the age at which legal majority was once fixed in most countries; at or after forty-two there takes place in women the 'grand climacteric', when menstruation and the power of bearing children ceases; whilst about sixty-three there sometimes appears in men a transitory enfeeblement to which the name of 'climacteric' has also been given, and a Hebrew writer has fixed the utmost span of robust life at 'threescore years and ten'. (See also MENOPAUSE.)

CLIMATE IN RELATION TO DISEASE – Climate is of great medical importance, both because various diseases are found in one part of the world and not in others, so that it becomes necessary to know the reasons for this difference, and because removal of a diseased person to new conditions of air, warmth, moisture and the like, is often a valuable means of cure.

The broad division of climates is into hot, temperate and cold climates, but before considering these it is of interest to note some of the extremes of climate to which man is exposed. The highest temperature ever recorded was 58°C (136°F) at Azizia in Libya in September 1922, while the lowest ever recorded was −88°C at Vostok in Antarctica in August 1920, which holds the record for the lowest average of the warmest month in the year (−33°C). The record for the highest average of the coldest month is held by

Dallol in Ethiopia (31°C). The highest annual total rainfall was recorded in Cherrapunji in India in 1860–61 (26,467 mm [1053 inches]). The lowest annual mean is 0·5 mm (0·02 inch) at Wadi Halfa which has the record for the highest mean annual sunshine (4300 hours), compared with the lowest (500 hours) on Laurie Island.

(*a*) **Hot climates** are generally considered as extending to about 35° from the equator, and possessing an average temperature throughout the year of about 84° F (29° C). In the Southern Hemisphere, Monte Video, Cape Town and Sydney lie just at the edge of this band, while north of the equator the limit divides the northern from the southern states of North America, skirts the south of Algeria, the north of India, and excludes Japan from the hot region. Generally speaking, there are, in this region, a wet and a dry season, but near the equator, two wet and two dry seasons.

(*b*) **Temperate climates** are those from about 35° to 55° of latitude, and have a mean temperature of about 38° F (3·3° C) in winter and 68° F (31° C) in summer. These regions include the northern states of USA, the south of Canada, Central and Southern Europe, and, in the East, Japan.

(*c*) **Cold climates** are those from 55° latitude to the poles. The cold is much modified, however, in some localities by ocean currents, so that Scotland, at the same latitude as Labrador, enjoys a temperate though moist climate, the surrounding seas and air being warmed by the Gulf Stream.

But, in estimating the effect of climate, far more than mere distance from the equator has to be considered. The degree of moisture in the air and presence of the sea near at hand, the rarefaction of the air in consequence of altitude, the difference between night and day temperatures, and the presence or absence of dust and bacteria are all of vital importance. For these reasons climates are classed into four subvarieties: (1) seaboard and ocean climates; (2) inland low climates; (3) mountain climates; (4) dry climates.

(1) *SEABOARD AND OCEAN CLIMATES* – The important features of these climates are the large amount of moisture in the air, the relatively high content of oxygen compared with mountain air, and the presence of salt and iodine. The air of the high seas is also free from dust and bacteria, a point of great importance in lung diseases. Further, large expanses of water warm and cool more slowly than the earth, so that a seaboard climate tends

to be more uniform than inland climates. The cases for which seaside air is most suitable are those convalescent from acute diseases, and those worn out by business or social worries. Holidays at the seaside, especially if the holidays be perforce short, as a rule benefit the jaded dweller in towns more than any other form of 'change of air', although, for the youthful and vigorous, mountain air is often better.

Perhaps the mildest climate in existence is that of the Mediterranean shores from Spain to Greece on the north, and in Algeria, Morocco and Tunisia on the south. The proper time to seek this part is from October to May, so as to avoid the colder northern winter.

Ocean voyages are specially valuable for patients who are convalescent from pulmonary tuberculosis. Various other chronic lung diseases benefit from a long voyage, and so do those persons broken down by over-work. One of the best voyages for English people is that to Australia or New Zealand, which takes over one month, and on which the patient experiences a variety of climates with corresponding stimulation to the system. By leaving England in the late autumn and returning in the late spring, the patient escapes the winter altogether, and has two or three months at the Antipodes, which should be spent in the mountains of Australia or New Zealand. In going to Australia, one should choose a cabin on the port side, and, in returning, one to starboard, for, by this means, the cool breeze is secured both ways. From the United States of America the usual voyage is to the West Indies and thence across to Europe, and back. Another good variety of climate is got by the voyage in which call is made at Lisbon, Teneriffe, Rio de Janeiro, Montevideo, and often a North American port.

(2) *INLAND LOW CLIMATES* include most of the health resorts to which people go in order to drink mineral waters. The general character of inland climates is the great variation between the summer and winter temperature, but, as most of these places are resorted to only in the open part of the year, the climate goes often by the vague name of 'relaxing', in contradistinction to the 'bracing' climate of mountains. In such a climate, the moistness and density of the air, the warmth, and the absence of stimulating sea breezes combine to reduce the pressure at which life is carried on, to diminish the appetite, and to give the organs which discharge waste products from the body a

better chance to carry out their functions. This is aided by the various waters peculiar to these spas. The diseases for which this type of climate is most suitable are rheumatism, gout, skin diseases and other chronic constitutional troubles. Examples of this climate are given by Harrogate, Bath and the watering-places of the Rhine basin. Diseases of the heart and other parts of the circulatory system are treated at some of the less relaxing of these resorts, such as Nauheim, where graduated exercises aid the restful action of the climate.

113 – Bracing and relaxing climates in England and Wales. From Melvyn Howe, *Man, Environment and Disease in Britain.* David and Charles.

(3) *MOUNTAIN CLIMATES* have, as their chief character, the rarity of the air, by reason of which the breathing and heart-beats are increased in rate, and a feeling of buoyancy and increased strength given to the whole system. Further, the air is drier and less laden with dust and bacteria, and there is greater difference between the day and night and between the sun and shade temperatures than at lower levels. Accordingly the mountains are suitable for persons who, though overworked and broken-down, are young and of good physique; for those who are young but delicate, disposed to lung disease, and who have outgrown their strength; for those also who suffer from chronic lung diseases with a certain

203

amount of fever, and for whom sea-voyages are unsuitable. But for the weak and aged, for those with heart diseases, and for those with kidney diseases, mountain climates are unsuitable.

(4) *DRY CLIMATES OR DESERT CLIMATES* combine warmth and dryness. In addition, the air is relatively clear of bacteria, though apt to be dusty, and the nights are cold. Such climates are found in Egypt, Australia, some of the Western States of the USA, and, in a milder degree, on the Pampas of South America and the tablelands of Cape Province in South Africa. These are suited especially for chronic rheumatism and chest diseases.

CLINICAL means literally 'belonging to a bed', but the word is used to denote anything associated with the practical study or observation of sick persons, as clinical medicine, clinical thermometers.

CLINICS (see MATERNITY AND CHILD WELFARE).

CLOFAZIMINE is a drug used in the treatment of certain cases of leprosy.

CLOFIBRATE is the *British Pharmacopoeia* name for a drug which reduces the level of cholesterol (qv) and triglycerides in the blood. It is being used in the treatment of coronary artery heart disease on the principle that, if it reduces the level of cholesterol and triglycerides in the blood, it should reduce the incidence of coronary artery heart disease. (See CORONARY THROMBOSIS.)

CLOMIPHENE is a drug that stimulates ovulation, or the production of ova, through the medium of the pituitary gland. It is thus being used in the treatment of female infertility. One of its hazards is that, if given in too big doses, it may produce multiple births.

CLOMIPRAMINE is an antidepressant drug.

CLOMOCYCLINE is one of the tetracyclines (qv).

CLONAZEPAM is a drug that is proving of value in some cases of epilepsy, and in the restless legs syndrome (qv).

CLONIC is a word applied to short spasmodic movements.

CLONIDINE is a drug originally introduced for the treatment of high blood-pressure. It is also proving of value in the prevention of attacks of migraine. If it is used in the treatment of high blood-pressure, its use must not be stopped abruptly as this may result in a sudden rise of blood pressure within a matter of hours to a dangerously high level. This is not likely to arise with the smaller doses used in the treatment of migraine.

CLONING, from the Greek *klon* meaning a cutting such as is used to propagate plants, is essentially a form of asexual reproduction. It has been successfully achieved in rabbits in which the eggs are tively big, and the initial stages have been achieved – rabbits in which the eggs are only one-thousandth of the size of those of the frog. In essence the technique consists of destroying the nucleus of the egg and replacing it with the nucleus from a body cell of the same species – either a male or a female. This provides the egg with a full complement of chromosomes (qv) and it starts to divide and grow just as it would if it had retained its nucleus and been fertilized with a spermatozoon. The vital difference is that the embryo resulting from this cloning process owes nothing genetically to the female egg. It is identical in every respect with the animal from which the introduced nucleus was obtained – or, as it has been said, a carbon copy of it.

CLOPAMIDE is a diuretic which is proving of value in the treatment of oedema due to heart disease, cirrhosis of the liver and nephrosis.

CLOT is the term applied to any semi-solid mass of blood, lymph or other body fluid. Clotting in the blood is due to the formation of strings of fibrin produced by the action of a ferment (illustration 115). Milk clots in a similar manner in the stomach when exposed to the action of the ferment rennin. Clotting occurs naturally when blood is shed and comes in contact with tissues outside the blood-vessels. It occurs also at times in diseased vessels (*thrombosis*), producing serious effects upon the organs supplied by these vessels. Clots also form sometimes in the heart when the circulation is feeble and irregular. (See COAGULATION; EMBOLISM; THROMBOSIS.)

CLOTHING – The textile fibres from which clothing material is made can be divided into two main types: natural fibres and man-made fibres.

Natural fibres, in turn, can be classified into three main categories according to their origin: vegetable origin, animal origin and mineral origin. Fibres of vegetable origin include flax and cotton. Those of animal origin include wool and hair, silk, fur and leather. Those of mineral origin include asbestos. *Linen*, one of the oldest of textile fabrics, having been used for making fabrics in the times of the Pharoahs, is derived from flax. It has good moisture-absorbing properties, stands up well to washing, and has a cool sensation because of its smooth surface. It is highly combustible. Its cool feel disappears soon after a linen garment is put on, and this sensation is not felt under warm conditions. A further practical disadvantage is that its attractive appearance soon vanishes under the stress and strain of wear and sweating. The most widely used of all textile fibres, is derived from the cotton plant. There are various varieties, *sea island cotton* being one of the top grades. *Mercerized cotton* is cotton which has been treated with a strong solution of caustic soda to increase its capacity to absorb moisture, its lustre and its dyeing qualities. In addition to absorbing moisture, cotton is strong, stands up to vigorous washing, but is highly inflammable. Its ability to absorb and transmit moisture, combined with the fact that it can be made into a lightweight smooth fabric, makes it suitable for hot-weather clothes. Flannelette and Winceyette are cotton material which has been raised or 'fluffed' on one or both sides. They are warm but highly inflammable. *Wool*, derived from sheep, provides 90 per cent of the world's production of animal fibres. It absorbs moisture better than any other textile fibre, is easily affected by alkalis and must therefore be washed with care, but it is not very inflammable. Because of its crimp, or wavy structure, wool provides a fabric which is ideal for warm clothing. *Hair* fibres used in clothing material, apart from wool, include: *Mohair*, the hair of the angora goat. *Cashmere*, the hair of the cashmere goat, which is particularly fine and soft. *Camel*, the coarse outer hair being made into blankets, and the soft undercoat into fibres for coats and the like. *Silk*, the filament produced by the larvae of the silkworm, absorbs moisture, and is more inflammable than wool, but less so than cotton. It is expensive but, as one writer has expressed it, 'having a luxurious handle and appearance, it has for cen-

turies been in much demand combining warmth, softness, suppleness and glamour in one clothing material'. *Asbestos*, a mineral rock, has been the source of textile fibres for centuries. The lamps of the vestal virgins are said to have had an asbestos wick. As it is incombustible, and fibres dervied from it have a high resistance to transfer of heat, it is used to make fire-protective clothing and curtains.

Man-made fibres, like natural fibres, are built up of long chain molecules. There are two groups of such fibres, depending upon their origin: *regenerated fibres*, in which the material already exists in nature; *synthetic fibres*, in which the material is manufactured from chemical elements. *Rayon*, or what used, erroneously, to be known as artificial silk, is basically cellulose. The most widely used form is viscose rayon, which is made from wood pulp and cotton linters. It absorbs moisture well, but is highly combustible. *Cellulose esters* consist of chemically modified cellulose. The fabrics produced from them are less moisture-absorbing than viscose rayon, but more flame-resistant; in this latter respect being comparable to silk. One form has drip-drying properties. *Synthetic fibres* are produced from the group of plastics resistant to heat (thermoplastics). They differ from natural fibres and materials in being moth-resistant, lightweight, not taking up much moisture and not shrinking or deforming, and therefore having drip-drying properties. They melt on exposure to sufficient heat, but do not burn easily. They include an ever-enlarging group of fibres, with a multiplicity of trade names. Only a few can be mentioned here. *Nylon*, the first synthetic fibre to be produced, is derived from coal and petroleum. Although its moisture-absorbing properties are not high, they are greater than most of the other synthetic fibres. Like synthetic fibres in general, it is prone to accumulate electrostatic charges. Its high strength and elasticity, combined with its plasticity, allow it to be heat-set to a permanent shape, making it a high favourite for women's stockings. *Terylene* is a polyester made from polyethylene terephthalate. It has a poor ability to absorb moisture and therefore dries quickly after washing. As it has what is technically known as 'good abrasion resistance', it is widely used to make shirts, trousers and, blended with other fibres, suits. *Orlon*, which is made from polymers or copolymers of acrylonitrile, is as inflammable as cotton or viscose rayon. It is now used particularly in the fashion knitwear field, often blended with other fibres.

General considerations – Material, or fabric, however, is not the only factor to be taken into consideration in deciding on the right clothing. Colour, for example, has an important influence on the coolness of clothing, quite apart from the material. If the body be exposed to the sun's rays clad in black or dark blue, more than twice the amount of heat is absorbed than would be absorbed if the clothing were of the same material but white in colour. Thus, white clothes are twice as cool as black or blue material in the heat of summer. Red stands about half-way between, whilst yellow is almost as cool as white. The texture of the material has also much to do with the warmth it maintains. So-called cellular underclothing is much warmer than the same weight of closely woven material. This is because the intervening air in the interstices of the material is a worse conductor of heat than the material. For the same reason, a single garment is not as warm as two single garments, each of half its thickness, which have a layer of air between them. Another factor to be borne in mind is that loose-fitting underwear is both more comfortable and warmer than tight-fitting underwear.

Corsets are of doubtful value. For young and healthy women they are quite unnecessary. The feeling of limpness felt when they are discarded is simply begotten of their constant use. There are few more certain ways of engendering flabbiness of the abdominal muscles than by wearing corsets. On the other hand, for middle-aged and elderly women, with flabby abdominal walls, partly the result of putting on weight, a well-fitting corset can be one of the most comforting pieces of wearing apparel.

Boots and shoes are often the most ill-fitting item of clothing, using the term in the widest sense, worn by any section of the community, especially women and children. Boots have largely gone out of fashion – and rightly so, except for certain games and mountaineering. There is also much to be said for a well-fitting pair of boots for the 'hiker' who indulges in long walks day after day and over rough country.

Non-inflammability is one of the most important factors, if not the most important, to be borne in mind in buying clothes for children and old people. This applies particularly to night clothes. Thus, children should wear pyjamas, whether girls or boys. Nightgowns are much more likely to come in contact with an open flame. Progress in fire-proofing of material is making slow progress, but, on the other hand, the synthetic, man-made materials now on the market are largely fire-proof, or at least flame-proof, which is the main thing. Any responsible shops selling clothes today will be able to give full and accurate information concerning the non-inflammability of the material they are selling. If not, the purchaser should go elsewhere.

CLOTRIMAZOLE is a drug that is proving of value in the treatment of certain fungal or yeast infections, such as aspergillosis (qv) and cryptococcosis (qv).

CLOVES are the unexpanded flower-buds of a species of myrtle, *Eugenia caryophyllus*, from the Indian Archipelago. Oil of cloves is an antiseptic, checks griping, and masks bad breath. It may be taken in doses of 2 or 3 drops on a lump of sugar, or one tablespoonful of infusion of cloves may be similarly used. Cotton-wool dipped in clove oil and put in a hollow tooth relieves toothache temporarily.

CLOXACILLIN (See PENICILLIN.)

CLUBBING is the term applied to the thickening and broadening of the finger tips and, less commonly, the tips of the toes, that occurs in certain chronic diseases of the lungs and heart. The cause is not known.

CLUB-FOOT, or TALIPES, is a deformity in which the foot is permanently twisted at the ankle-joint, so that the sole no longer rests on the ground in standing.
Varieties – The foot can be twisted in

114 – Bilateral congenital *talipes equinovarus*. Left foot is more severely affected and head of *talus* meets floor on lateral side of foot, where a callosity will form if disorder remains uncorrected. (Photo by courtesy of Mrs. N. E. Shaw, reproduced in *British Medical Journal*, 22,1,77)

four directions. The heel may be pulled up so that the person walks on his toes (*talipes equinus*), or the toes may be bent up so that he walks on his heel only (*talipes calcaneus*), or the sole may look inwards so that he walks on the outer edge of the foot (*talipes varus*), or outwards so that he walks on the inside of the foot (*talipes valgus*). These are usually combined, the heel being drawn up and the sole turned inwards (*equino-varus*) or the heel resting on the ground and the sole looking outwards (*talipes calcaneo-valgus*). A more important division is into those cases in which the deformity exists at birth, which are generally at first fairly easily rectified; and 'into those cases which are acquired later in life as the result of some disease, which do not yield to such simple treatment.

Causes – The cases found at birth are due to some arrest of development resulting in a congenital deformity (talipes equino-varus), or some faulty position of the foetus in the womb (talipes calcaneo-valgus). *Talipes equino-varus* occurs in about 1 per 1000 live births, is twice as common in boys as in girls, and in half the cases involves both feet. Children of affected parents are more likely to have club-foot than those of non-affected parents. Those which are acquired later may be caused by some spasm in the muscles of the one side of the leg (cerebral palsy), or by paralysis of the muscles on the side of the leg away from the deformity (poliomyelitis), or by rigidity due to the scar following a burn or inflammation.

Treatment – *Talipes calcaneo-valgus*, which is almost always due to a faulty position of the foot in the womb, and often involves both feet, responds well as a rule

to manipulation. All that is required in most cases is that the affected part should be moulded into the *equino-varus* position each time mother attends to the babe. It is only in the more severe cases that the foot may need to be strapped into the correct position, or fixed in this position in plaster of Paris for a few weeks. The ultimate result is excellent, but there may be a tendency for the condition to relapse when the child starts walking. This is controlled by a wedge on the heel of the shoe. *Talipes equino-varus* is the most important of all forms of club-foot, and treatment depends upon the cause. If it is due to a congenital deformity, the baby must be referred to a specialist as soon as possible. The sooner treatment is begun the better. This consists of stretching and strapping under medical supervision, the baby being seen regularly by the doctor who does the re-strapping as the foot comes into the normal situation, and the mother being taught to stretch the foot regularly between visits to the clinic. In the more severe cases an operation may be needed if the condition has not responded to non-surgical treatment by the age of 2 or 3 months. In the cases which develop as a result of disease or injury after birth, treatment consists of splinting, strengthening the weakened muscles by massage and electrical stimulation. In the more severe cases operation for transplanting tendons may be necessary.

CLYSTER is another name for enema.

COAGULATION of the blood is the process whereby bleeding (or haemorrhage) is normally arrested in the body.

115 – Section of blood clot, showing network of strings of fibrin. Magnified 400 times. From Schafer, *Histology*. Longmans.

207

The process is summarized in the following diagram:

PROTHROMBIN + CALCIUM + THROMBOPLASTIN
|
THROMBIN + FIBRINOGEN
|
FIBRIN

Prothrombin and calcium are normally present in the blood. Thromboplastin is an enzyme which is normally found in the blood platelets and in tissue cells. When bleeding occurs from a blood-vessel there is always some damage to tissue cells and to the blood platelets. As a result of this damage, thromboplastin is released and comes in contact with the prothrombin and calcium in the blood. In the presence of thromboplastin and calcium prothrombin is converted into thrombin, which in turn interacts with fibrinogen, a protein always present in the blood, to form fibrin. Fibrin consists of needle-shaped crystals, which, with the assistance of the blood platelets, form a fine network (illustration 115) in which the blood corpuscles become enmeshed. This meshwork, or clot as it is known, gradually retracts until it forms a tight mass which prevents any further bleeding. It will thus be seen that clotting, or coagulation, does not occur in the healthy blood-vessel because there is no thromboplastin present. There is now evidence suggesting that there is an antithrombin substance present in the blood in small amounts, and that this substance antagonizes any small amounts of thrombin that may be formed as a result of small amounts of thromboplastin being released.

COAGULUM is the Latin term for a clot.

COAL-MINER'S LUNG (see ANTHRACOSIS).

COARCTATION OF THE AORTA is a narrowing of the aorta in the vicinity of the insertion of the ductus arteriosus. It is a congenital abnormality. Satisfactory results are now obtained from surgical treatment.

COBALAMINS – The cobalamins are a group of substances which have an enzyme action (see ENZYME) and are essential for normal growth and nutrition. (See also CYANOCOBALAMIN; and HYDROXOCOBALAMIN.)

COBALT–60 is a radioactive isotope which is being used as a substitute for radium and high-voltage X-rays in the treatment of malignant disease (illustration 350). (See RADIOTHERAPY.)

COBALT EDETATE is an antidote for prussic acid poisoning (qv).

COCAINE–Coca leaves are obtained from two South American plants, *Erythroxylum coca* and *Erythroxylum truxillense*, and contain an alkaloid, Cocaine, which has marked effects as a stimulant, and, locally applied, as an anaesthetic by paralysing nerves of sensation. The dried leaves have been used from time immemorial by the South American Indians, who chew them mixed with a little lime. Their effect is to dull the mucous surfaces of mouth and stomach, with which the saliva, produced by chewing them, comes into contact, thus blunting, for long periods, all feeling of hunger. The cocaine, being absorbed, produces on the central nervous system a stimulating effect, so that all sense of fatigue and breathlessness vanishes for the time. It was by the use of coca that the Indian post-runners of South America were able to achieve their extraordinary feats of endurance, using half an ounce or thereabout of the leaves daily. The continued use of the drug, however, results in emaciation, loss of memory, sleeplessness and general breakdown. (See DRUG ADDICTION.)

Uses – Before the serious effects that result from its habitual use were realized the drug was sometimes used by hunters, travellers and others to relieve exhaustion and breathlessness in climbing mountains, to steady the nerves, and to dull hunger. The chief use in medicine is by local application to dull pain. Internally it is prescribed along with morphine or heroin for the relief of pain in advanced cancer. (See BROMPTON MIXTURE.) Here the risk of addiction is a secondary consideration. Otherwise it is practically only used in the treatment of diseases of the eye, and diseases of the ear, nose and throat. In the eye it is used as an anaesthetic in the form of eye-drops containing 2 per cent of cocaine hydrochloride. It is also used in the form of lamellae, each of which contains 0·65 mg of cocaine hydrochloride, to induce anaesthesia of the eye. A 5 per cent spray solution is used to anaesthetize the throat and nose, whilst pastilles and lozenges containing 1·5 to 10 mg are used to reduce irritation of the throat and hoarseness. Artificial chemical compounds closely allied to cocaine are injected hypodermically in order to render painless small operations, such as amputation of the fingers, and by injection into the spinal canal to enable major operations to be done on the lower limbs without pain. (See PROCAINE HYDROCHLORIDE.)

COCCUS is the name applied to a rounded form of bacterium. (See BACTERIOLOGY.)

COCCYDYNIA, or COCCYGODYNIA, means the sensation of severe pain in the coccyx.

COCCYX is the lower end of the spinal column, resembling a bird's beak and consisting of four nodules of bone, which represent vertebrae, and correspond to the tail in lower animals. They are deeply buried in the muscles in man, but in occasional cases they project backwards, and are surrounded by a fold of skin, so as to form an actual tail.

COCHLEA is the part of the inner ear concerned with hearing. (See EAR.)

COCILLANA is the bark of *Guarea rusbyi*, a South American plant with properties similar to those of ipecacuanha. It is used as a remedy in coughs.

COCOA, or CACAO, is a powder derived from a tropical plant, *Theobroma cacao*, first brought to Europe by Columbus. It bears a fruit containing pulp in which are embedded seeds, each as large as a bean. The seeds are fermented for some days, then roasted to loosen their husk, after which the two halves of each are pressed out as cocoa-nibs. The nibs consist, half of a fat called cocoa-butter, and half of albuminous material, starch, tannin, gum and water in varying proportions. There is an alkaloid named theobromine, very similar to the caffeine of tea and coffee, present to the amount of 1 per cent, which gives to cocoa and chocolate their stimulating properties. Of tannin, there is about half the amount that is present in tea leaves. The 'soluble-cocoa', sold for domestic use, has much of the fat removed, and consists about one-half of sugar and starchy material, one-quarter of fat, one-fifth of albuminous material, and of moisture, salts, etc., in small amounts. The cocoas of different makers are all very similar. When made with milk and sugar, cocoa forms a valuable food. As it contains little tannin, it is sometimes tolerated by a weak stomach better than tea. (For uses, see CHOCOLATE.)

CODEINE is one of the active principles of opium (qv). In the form of codeine phosphate it is widely prescribed for the relief of a useless, irritative cough, and also along with aspirin for the relief of headaches and rheumatic pains. It tends to be somewhat constipating.

COD-LIVER OIL is made by purification of the oil pressed from the fresh liver of the cod (*Gadus callarius*). Its principal value in medicine arises out of its high content of vitamin D, the vitamin used in the prevention and treatment of rickets. The official cod-liver oil of the *British Pharmacopoeia* contains not less than 85 international units of vitamin D per gram. Cod-liver oil is also a rich source of vitamin A, the official cod-liver oil of the *British Pharmacopoeia* containing not less than 600 units of vitamin-A activity per gram. The protective dose of vitamin D for infants and children is around 400 international units daily. This is best given in the form of cod-liver oil itself. It is sometimes objected that the taste is so unpleasant that an infant or child will not take it. Experience has shown, however, that if the oil is given from the second week of life there is seldom any real difficulty in persuading the infant to take it. The only practical objection to its use is the aesthetic one should any be spilt on baby's clothes – and healthy babies do tend to dribble and splutter. Should it be preferred to give it in a more palatable form, it may be given as cod-liver oil emulsion or cod-liver oil and malt. The amount of cod-liver oil in some of these preparations, however, varies considerably, and if they are used, care must be taken to ensure that the child is receiving sufficient of the oil.

There are some who contend that cod-liver oil and malt is a useful remedy in the treatment of chronic bronchitis.

COELIAC DISEASE is a wasting disease of childhood in which there is inability to absorb fat from the intestines; there is therefore an excess of fat in the stools. It is the result of a constitutional intolerance of gluten (a constituent of wheat flour) which damages the lining membrane of the small intestine. This in turn interferes with the absorption of fat. Treatment is by means of a gluten-free diet. People with coeliac disease, or parents or guardians of coeliac children can obtain help and guidance from the Coeliac Society, P.O. Box 181, London, NW2 2QY. (See also GLUTEN; and MALABSORPTION SYNDROME.)

COELIOSCOPY is the term applied to a method of viewing the interior of the abdomen in patients in whom a tumour or some other condition requiring operation may be present but cannot with certainty be diagnosed. The examination is carried out by making a minute opening under local anaesthesia, and inserting an instrument bearing an electric lamp and telescopic lenses like that for examining the bladder (cystoscope) into the abdominal cavity. Certain of the abdominal organs can then be directly inspected in turn.

COFFEE and TEA – Tea was introduced into Europe in 1610, but for long was so expensive that its use did not become general till during the course of the last century. Coffee, introduced rather later, has become the general beverage among the Latin and Teuton races, while tea has become the favourite with the whole British stock.

Coffee is a bean, obtained from the seed of a plant, *Coffea arabica*, originally hailing from Arabia, and now cultivated in tropical climes all round the world. Tea is the leaf of a plant, *Camellia thea*, brought first from China and now cultivated in Japan, India, Ceylon and Uganda. It contains caffeine (qv) or theine, and tannic acid (or tannin), in addition to vegetable fibre, albuminous matters and volatile oils. It is these volatile oils which give 'China' and 'Indian' tea their characteristic aroma and flavour. Caffeine also gives their stimulating properties to *maté*, or Paraguay tea, derived from the leaves of *Ilex paraguariensis*, and to kola, derived from the seeds of *Cola acuminata*, a West African plant. Tea-leaves contain from 2 to 4 per cent caffeine while coffee-berries have about half that amount. As to tannic acid, tea-leaves have about 10 per cent, and coffee-berries half this amount. But as regards the liquids, since coffee is made about twice as strong as tea in general, a strong teacupful of either will contain nearly two grains (120 mg) of caffeine and over three grains (180 mg) of tannic acid. Coffee is sometimes adulterated with chicory (see ADULTERATION OF FOOD), which has no virtue beyond imparting a dark colour to the mixture and changing its flavour somewhat.

COITUS is sexual intercourse. *Coitus interruptus* (see CONTRACEPTION).

COLCHICUM, the bulb of *Colchicum autumnale*, or meadow-saffron, has long been used as a remedy for gout. How it acts is not quite certain.

Uses – Its main use is in gout, for which colchicine, the active principle of colchicum, in doses of 0·5 mg every one or two hours until the pain is relieved, followed by 0·5 mg thrice daily for about a week, is the form generally employed. Demecolcine, a derivative of colchicine, is sometimes of value in the treatment of chronic myelogenous leukaemia.

COLD, INJURIES FROM (see CHILBLAIN; FROST-BITE; HYPOTHERMIA; also CHILLS AND COLDS).

COLD, USES OF – The application of cold to the surface of the body is capable of influencing the progress of disease in deep-seated parts to a considerable extent by acting on the blood at the surface, or through the nerves which end in the skin. Cold is applied for five chief purposes:

(*a*) **To subdue pain** – In headache, a wet cloth to the forehead, or sponging with an evaporating mixture of vinegar and water, or eau-de-Cologne and water, is a well-known remedy. Sprains, if treated by holding the injured joint at once under running water, are much relieved. Later on, however, cold applications do harm, rather than good, by preventing the absorption of the effused blood. The pain of pleurisy may also be relieved by the application of an ice-bag to the side. Small operations may be done painlessly after freezing the skin of the part by spraying ethyl chloride over it.

(*b*) **To lessen inflammation** – Ice-bags are used in inflammatory conditions to prevent the formation of an abscess. In meningitis, or inflammation of the membranes of the brain, they often give some relief when applied to the head.

(*c*) **To reduce high temperature** – In any fever, sponging the arms and legs, one by one, with tepid water, is harmless and often very soothing. When the temperature runs very high, eg. to 105° or 107° F (40·5 to 41·8° C), wrapping the patient in a wet sheet and rubbing it with ice, or by putting him in a cold bath may be lifesaving. (See also under TYPHOID FEVER; and WET PACK.)

(*d*) **To stop haemorrhage** – In cases of increasing haemorrhage under the skin, for example, a bruised and blackening eye or a sprain, the amount of bleeding, and consequent discoloration, are lessened by applying compresses containing ice or some cooling lotion.

(*e*) **As a general stimulant** – Some

diseases are systematically treated in certain countries by cold bathing: for example, typhoid fever. Others are benefited by an alternation of hot and cold bathing: for example, chronic rheumatism. In general debility, one of the best curative agents is the daily cold bath. (See BATHS.)

(See also HYPOTHERMIA; and CRYOSURGERY.)

COLDS (see CHILLS AND COLDS).

COLECTOMY is the operation for removing the colon.

COLIC – By this term is generally understood an attack of spasmodic pain in the abdomen.

SIMPLE COLIC commonly arises from the presence in the alimentary canal of some indigestible matter, which excites spasmodic contraction of the muscular coats of the intestines. The pain of colic is relieved by pressure over the abdomen, and there is no attendant fever – points which are of importance in distinguishing it from inflammation.

Attacks of this form of colic may occur in connection with a variety of causes other than that above mentioned: eg. from accumulations of faeculent matter in the intestines in the case of those who suffer from habitual constipation; as an accompaniment of nervous ailments and not infrequently as the result of exposure to cold and damp, particularly where the feet become chilled, as in walking through snow. Similar attacks of colic are apt to occur in infants, especially those who are fed artificially; and in such cases it will generally be found that a temporary change of diet will be necessary. The duration of an attack of simple colic is seldom long, and in general no ill consequences follow from it. It is, however, not free from risk, especially that of sudden obstruction of the bowel from twisting, or invagination of one part within another (intussusception) during the spasmodic seizure, giving rise to a very grave condition. Colic is also a serious symptom when due to obstruction of the bowel by a tumour or similar condition. (See INTESTINE, DISEASES OF; INTUSSUSCEPTION.)

LEAD COLIC (*Syn,* painters' colic, *colica Pictonum,* Devonshire colic, dry belly-ache) is due to the absorption of lead into the system. This disease had been observed and described long before its cause was discovered. Its occurrence in an epidemic form among the inhabitants of Poitou was recorded by Francis Citois, in 1617, and the disease was thereafter termed *colica Pictonum.* It was supposed to be due to the acidity of the native wines, but it was afterwards found to depend on lead contained in them. About the middle of the eighteenth century this disease, which had long been known to prevail in Devonshire, was carefully investigated by Sir George Baker, who traced it to the contamination of the native beverage, cider, with lead, either accidentally from the lead-work of the vats and other apparatus for preparing the liquor, or from its being sweetened with litharge. (See LEAD-POISONING.)

BILIARY COLIC and *RENAL COLIC* are the terms applied to that violent pain which is produced, in the one case where a biliary calculus or gall-stone passes down from the gall-bladder into the intestine, and in the other where a renal calculus descends from the kidney along the ureter into the bladder. (See GALL-STONES; and KIDNEY, DISEASES OF.)

Treatment – The treatment of colic consists in means to relieve the spasmodic pain, and in the removal, where possible, of the cause upon which it depends. When the attack appears to depend on accumulations of irritating matter in the alimentary canal, a brisk purgative, such as castor oil, will, in addition, be called for. It must be borne in mind that abdominal pain may indicate the onset of acute appendicitis or be a sign of, say, perforation of a peptic ulcer: in such cases purgatives must on no account be given.

Pressure upon the abdomen may relieve the pain partially if not completely. This may be effected, in the case of a baby, by laying him face downwards across the nurse's arm, and in the case of older people by laying a hot-water bottle upon the abdomen, or by lying face downward upon a folded-up pillow. The various substances known as carminatives or antispasmodics (see ANTISPASMODICS) also aid in giving relief.

COLISTIN is an antibiotic isolated from the soil organism, *Bacillus polymyxa* var. *colistinus.* It is active against many Gram-negative organisms, and is proving of value in the treatment of gastrointestinal and genito-urinary infections.

COLITIS means inflammation of the colon, the first part of the large intestine. *Mucous colitis,* once a fashionable disease, is now recognized not to be a form of colitis and has been named *mucomembranous colic,* or *spastic* or *irritable colon.* It is caused by painful spasms of the colon and occurs in nervous types of individuals. Treatment consists of dealing with the underlying nervous condition, the avoidance of all aperients, and a full diet without an excess of roughage. *Acute catarrhal colitis* occurs as part of an acute gastroenteritis, usually due to food poisoning. The treatment is as for acute diarrhoea (qv). *Chronic catarrhal colitis* is usually due to the abuse of aperients and purgatives.

ULCERATIVE COLITIS is the most important form of colitis. It is an acute condition, the cause of which is not known. Although apparently precipitated at times by exposure to cold or damp or by dietetic indiscretions, these are not the primary cause. It is predominantly a disease of young adults. Once an individual has had the disease, he is very liable to relapses.

Symptoms – The onset may be sudden or insidious. In the acute form there is severe diarrhoea and the patient may pass up to twenty stools a day. The stools, which may be small in quantity, are fluid and contain blood, pus and mucus. There is always fever, which runs an irregular course. In other cases the patient first notices some irregularity of the movement of the bowels, with the passage of blood. This becomes gradually more marked. There is seldom actual pain except immediately prior to the passage of a stool, but there is always a varying amount of abdominal discomfort. The constant diarrhoea leads to emaciation and weakness, and there is always a well-marked anaemia. The acute form may be rapidly fatal, but as a rule the acute phase passes into a chronic stage. The chronic form is liable to run a prolonged course, and the majority of cases are subject to relapses for many years.

Treatment – Rest in bed is essential during the acute stage and as long as there is fever. The diarrhoea is controlled by mixtures containing bismuth salts and opium, and by starch and opium enemas. The diet should be bland and nourishing and should contain a minimum of roughage: ie. a low-residue diet (see DIETS). The anaemia which is always present is treated by means of iron preparations. In some cases it may be necessary to use surgical measures to control the condition; by removing more or less of the affected colon. In many cases excellent results are obtained from the use of cortisone or its analogues; indeed, this, along with sulphasalazine (qv), has become the basic treatment. Another drug proving useful in this condition is

azathioprine (qv). Once a patient has recovered and is back to work again, it is essential for him to remain on a low-residue diet, and to be particularly careful in avoiding unnecessary exposure to cold and damp; otherwise the condition is liable to recur. In the prevention of recurrences, sulphasalazine is proving most effective.

COLLAGEN is the most abundant protein in the body. It is the major structural component of many parts of the body and occurs in many different forms. Thus it exists as thick fibres in skin and tendons. It is also an important constituent of the heart and blood vessels. With calcium salts it provides the rigid structure of bone. It also occurs as a delicate structure in the cornea of the eye, and in what is known as the basement membrane of many tissues including the glomeruli of the kidneys and the capsule of the lens of the eye. Long regarded as an inert substance with a purely mechanical function, it is now realized that it is an active living material which plays a part in many diseases, hereditary and otherwise. On boiling it is converted into gelatin.

COLLAGEN DISEASES is a term used to describe a group of diseases, including acute rheumatism and rheumatoid arthritis, which are characterized by changes in the collagen of the tissues. The precise cause of these changes is not known, but they are probably a sensitization reaction to an unknown toxin, and they respond to cortisone and corticotrophin.

COLLAPSE is a condition of extreme weakness of all the bodily powers, and especially of the nervous system. It forms the termination of many severe diseases, such as cholera, typhoid fever, irritant poisoning. It is closely allied to the condition of surgical shock, but, whilst in collapse from the conditions mentioned the chief feature is feebleness of the heart's action, in shock there are numerous other prominent symptoms. (See SHOCK.)

Symptoms – The face is pale and drawn, the forehead sometimes covered with cold sweat, the eyes sunken and glassy. The voice is weak, the breathing shallow, and the pulse rapid and feeble or imperceptible. The temperature is usually reduced to 96 or 97 F (35·6 or 36·1 C). Generally the patient lies on his back, paying no attention to what is proceeding around him.

Treatment – The patient should be allowed to lie quietly on his back in a darkened room, well covered, and surrounded by hot bottles to maintain the body heat. Stimulants are also necessary.

COLLAPSE THERAPY is the term applied to the method of treating diseases of the lung by bringing about collapse of the diseased part through removing the supporting ribs (thoracoplasty), or introducing air into the pleural cavity (artificial pneumothorax).

COLLAR-BONE, or CLAVICLE (illustration 116), is the bone which runs from the upper end of the breast-bone towards the tip of the shoulder across the root of the neck. It serves to support the upper limb, to keep it out from the side, and to give breadth to the shoulders. The bone is shaped like an 'ƒ' with two curves, which give it increased strength. It is, however, very liable to be broken by falls on the hand or on the shoulder, and is the most frequently fractured bone in the body. (See FRACTURES.)

pyroxylin, with colophony, castor oil and alcohol (90 per cent) in solvent ether. It should be kept in a well-sealed container. Being relatively elastic, it does not crack through the movements of the skin. *Salicylic acid collodion* contains 12 per cent of salicylic acid.

Uses – Collodion is mainly used as a covering for wounds, after these have been cleaned. The objection to its use is that, if a wound, or the surface round it, be not absolutely clean, the discharges from the wound are retained by the collodion, and may carry infection deeply into the tissues. *Salicylic acid collodion* is sometimes used in the treatment of corns and warts.

Mode of application – The wound having been cleaned thoroughly, dried, and all bleeding stopped, collodion is painted over it with a camel-hair brush. Before this has time to dry, a very thin film of cotton-wool is laid on it and painted down with more collodion. Then another film of cotton-wool, followed by collodion, and so on till five or six layers

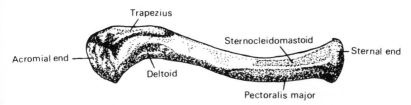

116 – The right clavicle: superior aspect. *Gray's Anatomy*, 35th edition, 1973. Longman.

COLLARGOL is a form of colloidal silver which mixes readily with water and any albuminous fluids, and has an antiseptic action. It is used especially for application to the eyes in inflammatory conditions.

COLLATERAL CIRCULATION (see ANASTOMOSIS).

COLLES'S FRACTURE is a fracture of the lower end of the radius close to the wrist, caused usually by a fall forwards on the palm of the hand, in which the lower fragment is displaced backwards.

COLLODIONS consist basically of a thick, colourless, syrupy liquid, made by dissolving gun-cotton (pyroxylin) in a mixture of ether and alcohol or with acetone. When painted on the skin the solvent evaporates, leaving a tough film behind. *Flexible collodion,* or collodion as it is often referred to, contains 1·6 per cent of

of each have been applied, successful application depending on the films of wool being as thin as possible, and upon each layer being applied before that beneath it has had time to dry completely.

COLLOID is the name given to a type of cancer of internal organs, in which a glue-like substance collects in the interior of the tumour. The term is also applied to substances existing in a colloidal solution, and to the viscid iodine-containing material in the spaces of the thyroid gland.

COLLOIDAL SOLUTIONS are solutions in which a substance very finely divided into particles is suspended in another substance, as, for example, metals like silver and iron suspended in the form of minute particles in water or glycerin. The two constituents of the colloidal solution are called phases – the particles known as the internal phase, and the medium in which they are suspended, the

213

continuous or external phase. The term, suspensoid, is applied to colloids in which the particles consist of pure solid, and the term, emulsoid, is applied to those in which the particles absorb some of the liquid in which they are suspended.

COLLYRIUM means an eye-lotion.

COLOBOMA simply means a defect, but its use is usually restricted to congenital defects of the eye. These may involve, the lens, the iris, the retina or the eyelid.

COLOCYNTH, or BITTER APPLE, is the fruit of a species of cucumber, *Citrullus colocynthis*, growing on the Mediterranean shores. The dried white pulp is a powerful purgative. It is administered usually as colocynth and hyoscyamus pill.

COLON is the first part of the large intestine. (See INTESTINE.)

COLONOSCOPE is an instrument for viewing the interior of the colon. It is made of fibre glass which ensures flexibility, and incorporates a system of lenses for magnification and a lighting system.

COLOPHONY is another name for rosin (qv).

COLOSTOMY is the operation for the establishment of an artificial opening into the colon. This acts as an artificial anus. The operation is carried out when there is an obstruction in the colon or rectum that cannot be overcome, or in cases, such as cancer of the rectum in which the rectum and part of the colon have to be removed. Such a colostomy opening can be trained to function in such a way that the patient can carry on a normal life, eating a more or less normal diet. Anyone wishing help or advice in the practical management of a colostomy should get in touch with the Colostomy Welfare Group, 38–39 Eccleston Square, London, SW1V 1PB. (Tel.: 01-828 5175.)

COLOSTRUM is the first fluid secreted by the mammary glands for two or three days after childbirth. It contains less casein and more albumin than ordinary milk.

COLOUR BLINDNESS (see VISION, DISORDERS OF).

COLOUR INDEX is one of the criteria used in assessing the degree and type of anaemia. It signifies the percentage of haemoglobin in terms of the amount contained in each red blood corpuscle. (See ANAEMIA.)

COLPITIS is a term applied to inflammation of the vagina. (See WHITES.)

COLPOMICROSCOPY is a refinement of colposcopy (qv), whereby it is possible to examine the cervix uteri under a magnification of 270 by the insertion of a microscope tube into the vagina.

COLPORRHAPHY is a term applied to an operation designed to strengthen the pelvic floor in cases of prolapse of the uterus.

COLPOSCOPY is the method of examining the vagina and cervix by means of the binocular instrument known as the colposcope. It is proving of particular value in the early detection of cancer of the cervix.

COLTSFOOT is the name given to the leaves of *Tussilago farfara* or *Tussilago petasites*, the butter burr, used in the form of a decoction for the treatment of coughs.

COMA is a state of profound unconsciousness, in which not only can the sufferer not be roused, but there are not even reflex movements when the skin is pinched, the eyeball touched, etc. The breathing is generally stertorous, but deep, and the heart's action is strong. The cause of coma is usually apoplexy, but it may also be due to high fever, diabetes mellitus, Bright's disease, alcohol, epilepsy, cerebral tumour, meningitis, injury to the head, overdose of insulin, carbon monoxide poisoning, poisoning from opium and other narcotic drugs. If the condition does not begin to pass off in twenty-four hours, death is generally near at hand. (See UNCONSCIOUSNESS.)

COMEDONES (see ACNE).

COMMENSAL is the term applied to micro-organisms which live in or on the body (eg. in the gut or respiratory tract, or on the skin) without doing any harm to the individual.

COMMISSURE means a joining, and is a term applied to strands of nerve fibres which join one side of the brain to the other, to the band joining one optic nerve to the other, to the junctions of the lips at the corners of the mouth, etc.

COMMOTIO CEREBRI is another term for concussion of the brain.

COMPENSATION is a term applied to the counterbalancing of some defect of structure or function by some other special bodily development. The body possesses a remarkable power of adapting itself to even serious defects, so that disability due to these passes off after a time. The term is most often applied to the ability possessed by the heart to increase in size, and therefore in power, when the need for greater pumping action arises in consequence of a defective valve or some other abnormality in the circulation. A heart in this condition is, however, more liable to be prejudicially affected by strains and diseased processes, and the term 'failure of compensation' is applied to the symptoms that result when this power becomes temporarily insufficient.

COMPLEMENT is a normal constituent of blood serum which plays an important part in the antibody-antigen reaction which is the basis of many immunity processes. (See IMMUNITY.)

COMPLEX is the term applied to a combination of various actions or symptoms. The term is particularly applied to a set of symptoms occurring together in mental disease with such regularity as to receive a special name.

COMPLEXION (see ACNE; SKIN DISEASES; SUNBURN).

COMPOSITOR'S DISEASE is a form of lead poisoning which occasionally attacks those who handle type. (See LEAD POISONING.)

COMPRESS is the name given to a pad of linen or flannel wrung out of water and bound to the body. It is generally wrung out of cold water, and may be covered with a piece of waterproof. It is used to subdue pain or inflammation. (See COLD.) A hot compress is generally called a fomentation. (See FOMENTATIONS.)

COMPRESSED AIR ILLNESS (see CAISSON DISEASE).

CONCEPTION signifies the complex set of changes which occur in the ovum and in the body of the mother at the beginning of pregnancy. The precise moment of conception is that at which the male element, or spermatozoon, and the female element, or ovum, fuse together. (See FOETUS.)

CONCRETIONS are masses of various sizes and substances which form in many of the tissues and smaller cavities of the body, in certain circumstances.

Varieties and causes – There is a special liability to the deposit of lime salts in damaged or degenerating tissues. The reason for this is probably much the same as that for the similar deposit from hard water inside kettles and boilers. The tissues in question being inactive do not produce sufficient carbon dioxide to keep dissolved the lime salts in the fluids circulating past and through them. Accordingly, healed-up areas in the lungs, which have been the seat of tuberculosis, the remains of dead parasites and other foreign bodies, degenerated blood-vessels, tumours and scars generally, are apt to have lime deposited in and around them till masses of considerable size are formed. The tartar on the teeth, some stones in the bladder, and the calculi sometimes found in the ducts of salivary glands in the cheek or beneath the tongue, are examples of a similar deposit of lime and phosphates, due to the action of bacteria.

Hair-balls, which are common in the stomachs of lower animals that lick themselves, occur sometimes in mentally deranged patients who have a habit of chewing their hair, and may reach the size of walnuts or larger. (See also BEZOAR.)

Various glands produce secretions, which, by a gradual process of sedimentation build up solid masses in the ducts of these glands. Examples of this are found in the gall-stones, formed of cholesterin separated from the bile, in the uratic stones found in the kidney or bladder of persons suffering from acidity, in the plugs of hardened wax which often give trouble in the ear, and in the cheese-like masses which accumulate in the tonsils and give rise to foetor of the breath.

Gout is a disease in which the pain is due to sharp uratic crystals which are deposited on the surfaces of joints, the same crystals being deposited in other tissues also, at a later stage of the disease, so that large solid masses called 'chalk-stones' are ultimately formed. (See GOUT.)

CONCUSSION OF THE BRAIN (see BRAIN).

CONDIMENTS (see DIET).

CONDURANGO is the dried stem

215

bark of *Marsdenia condurango*, a South American plant which is used as a bitter tonic.

CONDYLE is the name given to a rounded prominence at the end of a bone: for example, the prominences at the outer and inner sides of the knee on the thighbone (or femur). The projecting part of a condyle is sometimes known as an *epicondyle*, as in the case of the condyle at the lower end of the humerus (qv) where the epicondyles form the prominences on the outer and inner side of the elbow.

CONDYLOMA means a localized, rounded swelling of mucous membrane about the opening of the bowel, and the genital organs, sometimes known as 'genital warts' or 'ano-genital warts'. There are two main forms of them: *Condyloma latum*, which is syphilitic in origin, and *Condyloma acuminatum*, which often occurs in association with venereal disease, but is only indirectly due to it, being primarily a virus infection.

CONDY'S FLUID is a powerful disinfectant containing permanganates. (For its action and uses, see PERMANGANATE OF POTASSIUM.)

CONFECTIONS, also known as conserves and electuaries, form a method of prescribing certain bulky drugs mixed into a paste with sugar or honey. The best-known confections are those of senna and sulphur, both of which are aperient in action. Compound confection of guaiacum, better known as 'Chelsea Pensioner', is an old remedy for constipation and rheumatic pains in elderly people, having received its name from the success of its use among the men of that hospital. It contains guaiacum resin, rhubarb, potassium acid tartrate, nutmeg, sublimed sulphur and honey. The dose of all these confections is about a teaspoonful or more.

CONGENITAL deformities, diseases, etc., are those which are either present at birth, or which, being transmitted direct from the parents, show themselves some time after birth.

CONGESTION means the accumulation of blood in a part due to over-filling of its blood-vessels. The condition may be due to some weakness of the circulation (see CIRCULATION, DISORDERS OF), but as a rule is one of the early signs of inflammation (see ABSCESS; INFLAMMATION).

CONGESTION TREATMENT is a method sometimes used to stimulate the process of repair in both acute and chronic states of inflammation. It depends upon the principle that when the blood-vessels of an inflamed part are artificially dilated the number, and consequently the activity, of phagocytes (see PHAGOCYTOSIS) are increased. The congestion is brought about either by obstructing the return of blood (eg. in a limb) by means of an elastic bandage, or by diminishing the atmospheric pressure in the case of flat or outlying parts (eg. the back or the finger) by means of a suction cup or cylinder from which a rubber tube leads to a suction pump.

CONIUM (see HEMLOCK).

CONJUGATE DEVIATION is the term for describing the persistent and involuntary turning of both eyes in any one direction, and is a sign of a lesion in the brain.

CONJUNCTIVA is the membrane which covers the front of the eye. Beginning at the edge of the lower lid, it clothes the inner surface of that lid, and, at the line where the latter joins the cheek, forms a shallow pocket and passes on to the eyeball. Covering the front of the ball it then passes forward to the upper lid, forming a much deeper pocket between this lid and the ball, and so down to the margin of the upper lid, where it meets the skin. The membrane is transparent, especially over the centre of the eye, where a specialized portion, the cornea, admits light to the interior. The 'white' of the eye is formed by the sclerotic or outer coat of the eyeball shining through the conjunctiva. The membrane is richly supplied with nerves of sensation, and is extremely sensitive, so that the slightest touch produces a reflex closure of the lids. (See EYE.)

CONJUNCTIVITIS means inflammation of the conjunctiva. (See EYE DISEASES.)

CONOVID (see NORETHYNODREL).

CONSOLIDATION is a term applied to solidification of an organ, especially of a lung. The consolidation may be of a permanent nature due to formation of fibrous tissue, or may be temporary, as in acute pneumonia.

CONSTIPATION, or COSTIVENESS, means a condition in which the bowels are opened too seldom or incompletely, the motions as a consequence being dry and hard. It should, however, be borne in mind that, though most persons have in health one daily movement of the bowels, some perform this act twice, while in others a motion once in two or more days is perfectly natural. Constipation is a chronic condition, and must be carefully distinguished from acute obstruction of the bowels, a much more serious condition. (See INTESTINE, DISEASES OF.) Great variations, however, take place in colour (see STOOLS), in amount, and in consistence, according to the nature and quantity of the food and drink taken.

Causes – The uncommon causes of constipation are mechanical – that is, obstruction by stricture of the bowel, by tumour, by adhesive bands. The common causes are (1) habit, (2) 'a greedy colon', which absorbs water too quickly, (3) a spastic colon, the muscle of which remains in a state of spasm, (4) lack of tone of the colon muscle, sometimes because of too little vitamin B_1 in the diet, (5) a diet which has not enough 'roughage' in it to stimulate the intestine to activity. Of these, habit is probably most important. Constant neglect to respond to the sensation in the rectum which indicates that it is full and needs emptying leads to retention of faeces, which become dry and hard. The condition is aggravated by the use of purgatives.

Symptoms and effects – The stools are, as is well known, dark, hard, and passed with difficulty, and in small amount. In severe, persistent cases there may be swelling of the abdomen, from the retention of large masses of the remnants from digestion. Colic may occur in long-standing cases, in which the accumulation in the lower part of the bowel is beginning to affect the rest of the gut. Piles, which are a cause of increasing constipation, are often brought on by inattention to the bowels to begin with. Headache and lassitude may be present, but this is largely due to the pressure of the accumulated faeces in the rectum, not to any so-called toxic effect.

Treatment – Assuming that there is no organic cause, such as tumour or other source of mechanical obstruction, the most important matter is the regulation of the daily habits. The person concerned should take a certain amount of exercise daily. Above all things, a habit of opening the bowels, at the same time every day, should be cultivated; a definite hour should be fixed, preferably after a meal,

and best after breakfast, and, no matter whether there be a sensation that the bowels will move or not, the attempt should unfailingly be made. The diet is of importance. On the whole, in cases of constipation this errs in being too concentrated and too unirritating. As a rule, the diet should be changed to include oatmeal porridge, brown bread, green vegetables, and fruit, especially fruit like prunes or brambles, which have a large indigestible residue, while a considerable amount of fluid should be taken. The juice of an orange or grapefruit, or a glass of water, first thing in the morning may help.

The use of aperients and purgatives has usually exaggerated the condition, and as a general rule should be given up.

CONSTITUTION, or DIATHESIS, means the general condition of the body, especially with reference to its liability to certain diseases. A sound constitution is one in which the structure and functions of the various parts and organs are so evenly maintained that there is no apparent liability to any disease. The term 'constitutional' is sometimes vaguely applied to diseases which present knowledge does not permit of our attributing to any definite organ or system. A constitution such as the gouty constitution may be inherited, or it may develop as the result of improper food, habits and environment. On the other hand, a hereditary tendency towards some disease may be gradually eliminated by a careful and regular life.

CONSUMPTION (see TUBERCULOSIS).

CONTACT LENSES are lenses shaped to fit the eyeball. They fit in direct contact with the eye, behind the eyelids, and move with the eye. Their advantages, compared with spectacles, are twofold: optical and cosmetic. In certain disturbances of vision they provide better results than do ordinary spectacles. They are invisible, except on close examination, and are therefore preferred by some people: eg. actors and actresses. Other advantages they possess are that they cannot be knocked off, and can therefore be worn for even strenuous sports, such as football, and that they do not steam in a warm, moist atmosphere. On the other hand, some people find them troublesome to wear for more than a few hours at a time. They require careful fitting, and should therefore only be worn on the recommendation of an experienced ophthalmologist.

217

CONTAGION means the principle of spread of disease by direct contact with the body of an affected person, while by infection is meant the spread through the air or by other distant means.

CONTINUED FEVERS are typhus, typhoid and relapsing fevers, so called because of their continuing over a more or less definite space of time.

CONTRACEPTION is the prevention by artificial means of fertilization of the ovum ensuing from sexual intercourse. Five main groups of contraceptives are in general use: (1) The occlusive (or Dutch) cap, which covers the entrance to the womb and thereby prevents entrance of spermatozoa to the womb. (2) The sheath (or condom), which prevents spermatozoa entering the vagina. (3) Chemical pessaries or solutions, which, when placed in the vagina, destroy the spermatozoa. (4) The oral contraceptives: these are steroid hormones which are taken in the form of a pill and act by inhibiting ovulation. (See also NORETHYNODREL.) (5) The intra-uterine contraceptive devices which prevent implantation of the fertilized ovum in the uterus.

The method of *coitus interruptus*, or withdrawl of the penis from the vagina before ejaculation – one of the oldest methods of contraception – is not as universally condemned by the medical profession as it once was. Another method is the so-called *rhythm method*, whereby intercourse is restricted to the so-called 'safe period': that is the period during each monthly menstrual cycle when conception cannot take place because there is no ovum available for the spermatazoa to impregnate. Yet another method of contraception now being introduced is that of *sterilization* of the husband. Widely practised in India, where it is encouraged by the Government as a means of helping the population problem, increasing scale. (See SAFE PERIOD; STERILIZATION; and VASECTOMY.)

CONTRACTURE means the permanent shortening of a muscle or of fibrous tissue. Contraction is the name given to the temporary shortening of a muscle.

CONTRE-COUP means an injury in which a bone, generally the skull, is fractured, not at the spot where the violence is applied, but at the exactly opposite point.

CONTUSION (see BRUISES).

CONVALESCENCE means the condition through which a person passes after having suffered from some acute disease, and before complete health and strength are regained. Many diseases have special dangers during convalescence: for example, after typhoid fever the effects of overeating may be disastrous; after measles, pneumonia, and other diseases of the respiratory tract, there is a greater risk than usual of the onset of tuberculosis in susceptible individuals; and, while convalescence from scarlet fever is proceeding, there is a special risk of kidney inflammation. These are guarded against by working the body at low pressure for a time, exposing it to no strain, partaking of a moderate diet, and taking an ample allowance of rest and sleep, till all the functions have regained their usual activity and vigour. For further details see under each disease.

CONVOLUTIONS (see BRAIN).

CONVULSIONS are rapidly alternating contractions and relaxations of the muscles, causing irregular movements of the limbs or body generally, and usually accompanied by unconsciousness. They form really only a symptom of some other trouble, often, in children, of a trifling nature, but, on account of the alarm they cause and their occasional seriousness, they are treated often as a disease by themselves.

Causes – The most common cause of convulsions in adults is epilepsy (qv). As the vast majority of convulsive seizures occur in children, however, only these will be dealt with here. The relative frequency of convulsions in infants and young children is probably due to an instability of the immature nervous system. An American investigation showed that in a group of 8823 otherwise normal children, some 6 per cent had had one or more convulsions. Some children are more liable to develop convulsions than others, and this is probably due to a neurotic inheritance.

In young infants convulsions may be due to *birth injuries*, usually the result of a difficult labour. The convulsions in these cases are due to damage of the brain, either by bleeding from torn blood-vessels or concussion of the brain. In older infants convulsions may be due to the irritability of the brain often associated with *rickets*. This is the condition known as tetany, and before the introduction of the routine administration of vitamin D to infants and children, it was one of the most common causes of convulsions in older infants and young children.

A sudden *rise of temperature*, such as may occur in any infection, may induce convulsions in an infant and young child. This is most likely in pneumonia, and it would appear as if in the child a convulsion was the equivalent of the chill or rigor which occurs in adults. *Irritation* elsewhere in the body may cause convulsions in the predisposed child. This is most likely to occur with irritation in the bowels, eg. the eating of unripe or indigestible food, colic, worms or even constipation. Infection of the kidneys or bladder may also be responsible, as may be earache, particularly if of sudden onset. The role of teething as a cause of convulsions has been exaggerated, but there is no doubt that, if painful, the teething process may occasionally produce convulsions. *Diseases of the brain*, such as meningitis, encephalitis and tumours, or any disturbance of the brain due to bleeding, blockage of a blood-vessel, or irritation of the brain by a fracture of the skull, may also be responsible for convulsions.

Asphyxia, such as may occur in a young child during a paroxysm of whooping-cough, may also bring on convulsions. Breath-holding (qv), a not uncommon condition in infants and young children, may also persist long enough to bring on convulsions. These breath-holding attacks follow a severe bout of crying, at the end of which the infant holds his breath. As a rule, the worst that happens is that the infant holds his breath until he is blue in the face, and then starts breathing again. Occasionally, however, the breath-holding persists until there is a convulsion. An occasional breath-holding attack need not be taken too seriously but, if it is repeated, medical advice should be sought.

Finally, it must never be forgotten that *epilepsy* can occur in infants and young children.

Treatment – Convulsions are rarely dangerous to life unless they occur as part of a dangerous condition which is already threatening the child's life. The time-honoured custom is to put the child in a hot bath, but this is seldom necessary. On the other hand, tepid sponging may help if there is fever. If there is any possibility of the child biting his tongue, a spoon or a spatula should be put between the teeth. There is seldom any need to restrain the movements unless they are severe enough to throw the child off the bed or couch. If the convulsions persist, it may be necessary to give inhalations of chloroform. As

a rule a sedative, or an injection of one of the barbiturates, controls the convulsions. Once these are under control, the cause of the convulsions must be sought and the necessary treatment given.

COOLEY'S ANAEMIA, or THALASSAEMIA, is a condition in which there is an inherited defect in the production of normal haemoglobin, resulting in a severe degree of anaemia.

CO-ORDINATION means the governing power exercised by the brain as a whole, or by certain centres in the nervous system, to make various muscles contract in harmony, and so produce definite actions, instead of meaningless movements. It is bound up intimately with the complex sense of localization, which enables a person with his eyes shut to tell, by sensations received from the bones, joints and muscles, the position of the various parts of his body. The power is impaired in various diseases, such as locomotor ataxia. It is tested by making the patient shut his eyes, moving his hand in various directions, and then telling him to bring the point of the forefinger steadily to the tip of the nose, or by other simple movements.

COPAIBA is a mixture of oil and resin in a thick yellow fluid, obtained by cutting into the bark of *Copaifera lansdorfii*, a South American tree. It is excreted by the mucous membranes, especially of the urinary and respiratory organs, which it stimulates.

Uses – It is used in various chronic inflammations of the urinary organs, and as an expectorant in chronic bronchitis.

COPPER is an essential nutrient for man, and all tissues in the human body contain traces of it. The total amount in the adult body is 100 to 150 mg. Many essential enzyme systems are dependent on traces of copper. On the other hand, there is no evidence that dietary deficiency of copper ever occurs in man. Infants are born with an ample store, and the normal diet for an adult contains around 2 mg of copper a day. It is used in medicine as the two salts, sulphate of copper (blue stone) and nitrate of copper. The former is, in small doses, a powerful astringent, and in larger doses an irritant. Both are caustics when applied externally.

Uses – Externally, either is used to rub on unhealthy ulcers and growths, with the

(a)   (b)

117 – Eye showing corneal opacity before corneal grafting (a), and the same eye after successful corneal grafting showing clear cornea (b).

view of stimulating the granulation tissue to more rapid healing. In very small amounts copper is necessary for the formation of red blood corpuscles. It is therefore sometimes necessary to give copper as well as iron to cases of anaemia, especially in children. In a concentration of 0·5 to 1 part per million, copper sulphate is used to prevent the growth of algae in, for example, swimming pools.

COPPER POISONING is rare. Copper itself is harmless, but sulphate of copper (blue vitriol) and acetate of copper (verdigris) are now and then taken as poisons. The use of copper salts in very small quantities to colour canned peas is said to lead to occasional unpleasant symptoms, while adverse effects have also, though rarely, been reported from stewing fruit in copper-lined vessels. (See also WILSON'S DISEASE.)

Treatment – If one of the salts above named has been taken by mistake, the treatment is that for any irritant poison: milk or white of egg as an antidote, followed by washing out the stomach. Penicillamine or sodium calciumedetate should also be given.

COPROLALIA is the condition in which insane people give utterance to filthy and obscene words.

CORDOTOMY, or CHORDOTOMY, is the surgical operation of cutting the antero-lateral tracts of the spinal cord to relieve otherwise intractable pain. It is also sometimes known as TRACTOTOMY.

CORNEA is the clear membrane in front of the eye through which light passes to its interior. (See EYE.)

CORNEAL GRAFTING is the method of treating certain conditions of the cornea

by replacing the damaged cornea with a cornea which has been taken from a human body. An Act of Parliament passed in 1952 authorized the removal of the eyes from a body for the purpose of corneal grafting, unless the deceased person previous to his death, or a surviving relative, had expressed an objection. If the eye, or cornea, is removed within ten hours of death it can be kept in a corneal bank for as long as twenty days before being used. A corneal graft can be used to restore vision in many diseases of the cornea, (illustration 117), including interstitial keratitis (qv), scarring of the cornea, or damage to the cornea due to agents such as lime and ammonia.

The Department of Health and Social Security has drawn up a list of suitable eye-banks to which people can apply to bequeath their eyes, and an official form is now available for the bequest of eyes. (See also DONORS; and TRANSPLANTATION.)

CORNS and BUNIONS – A corn is a localized thickening of the cuticle or epidermis, of a conical shape, the point of the cone being directed inwards and being known as the 'eye' of the corn. A general thickening over a wider area is called a callosity. Bunion is a condition found over the joint at the base of the great toe, in which not only is there thickening of the skin, but the head of the metatarsal bone, in consequence of bending outwards of the toe by pointed or too short boots, becomes unduly prominent beneath thickened skin (illustration 118). Hammer-toe is a condition of the second toe, often caused by short boots, in which the toe becomes bent at its two joints in such a way as to resemble a hammer, while corns form over the bends.

Causes – The cause of bunions is the wearing of ill-fitting boots. Corns are due similarly to the pressure of tight or badly fitting boots, or, when on the under-surface of the foot, to unevenness in the sole. The skin grows more rapidly in consequence of the irritation, and becomes changed by the pressure into a species of horn. Where the corns are between the toes, they become moist and sodden, and are called soft corns.

Treatment – The first requisite is to wear sufficiently large and properly shaped boots. The inner side of the sole should be straight, not cut away to a point, and the width of the sole at the level of the little toe should be as great as that of the bare foot when the weight of the body is thrown on it. Relief from the pain

118 – Two foot-soles showing on left natural appearance, on right distortion of toes produced by badly fitting boot, with tendency to bunion.

of a corn may be obtained by wearing a ring of felt (corn plaster) round the corn, so as to free it from pressure and distribute the pressure of the boot over the surrounding skin. To remove the corn, the foot should be soaked in hot soapy water, and the corn then cut or scraped away with a knife or pair of scissors. After drying, the site of the corn should be covered with a small piece of soap plaster, or painted inside the felt ring with salicylic acid collodion. This consists of 12 grams of salicylic acid in 100 ml of flexible collodion. This preparation softens and breaks up the corn, which may be picked away gradually or rubbed down with pumice-stone. After the corn is removed, the skin of the foot should be hardened by daily bathing for some time in salt water or in spirit. A tendency to bunions, flat foot,

and corns can sometimes be checked by wearing shoes of which the sole is slightly thicker along the inner side than on the outer side.

Soft corns and the deformities of bunion and hammer-toe should be treated by wearing socks made like gloves with a compartment for each toe, or in slighter cases by inserting a piece of boracic lint each morning in the spaces between the toes. In bad cases of bunion the opening of the boot should run forwards to between the first and second toes, where the lace, or a peg known as a 'toe-post', is fixed to the sole in order to keep the great toe in its proper place; or a rubber pad may be worn between the toes. In old-standing cases of bunion and hammer-toe, an operation in which the protruding toe joint is excised may be necessary for cure.

Individuals who are liable to corns and bunions would be well advised to place themselves in the hands of a well-qualified and experienced chiropodist.

CORONARY is a term applied to several structures in the body encircling an organ in the manner of a crown. The coronary arteries are the arteries of supply to the heart which arise from the aorta, just beyond the aortic valve, and through which the blood is delivered with great pressure to the muscle of the heart. Disease of the coronary arteries is a very serious condition producing various abnormal forms of heart action and the disease, angina pectoris. (See also THROMBOSIS.)

CORONARY THROMBOSIS is the acute, dramatic manifestation of ischaemic heart disease, one of the major killing diseases of western civilization. In 1977, ischaemic heart disease was responsible for 145,089 deaths in England, compared with an annual average of 109,064 in England and Wales in the period 1958 to 1960. The alternative name for ischaemic heart disease is coronary artery disease. The underlying cause is disease of the coronary arteries, which carry the blood supply to the heart muscle (or myocardium). This results in narrowing of the arteries until finally they are unable to transport sufficient blood for the myocardium to function efficiently. One of three things may happen. If the narrowing of the coronary arteries occurs gradually, then either the individual concerned will develop angina pectoris (qv) or he will develop signs of a failing heart. (See HEART DISEASES.)

If the narrowing occurs suddenly or

221

leads to complete blockage, or occlusion, of a major branch of one of the coronary arteries, then the victim collapses with acute pain and distress. This is the condition commonly referred to as a coronary thrombosis because it is usually due to the affected artery suddenly becoming completely blocked by thrombosis (qv). More correctly, it should be described as coronary occlusion, because the final occluding factor need not necessarily be thrombosis. Alternatively, it is sometimes referred to as myocardial infarction, this describing the destructive changes produced in the myocardium by lack of its blood supply. (See INFARCTION.)

Causes – The precise cause is not known, but there is a wide range of factors which play a part in inducing coronary artery disease. In the first place it is commoner in men than in women. It is more common in those in sedentary occupations than in those who lead a more physically active life. There is a strong familial element, and it is more likely to occur in those with high blood-pressure than in those with normal blood-pressure. It is more common among smokers than non-smokers. It is often associated with a high level of cholesterol (qv) in the blood. This in turn has been linked with an excessive consumption of animal, as opposed to vegetable, fats. In this connection the important factors seem to be the saturated fatty acids of animal fats which would appear to be more likely to lead to a high level of cholesterol in the blood than the unsaturated fatty acids of vegetable fats. The precise practical significance of these observations is still being argued by the experts, but what all are agreed on is that obesity and coronary thrombosis go together. Equally is this the case with stress and strain, particularly that to which those in authority and with responsibility, such as business executives, are subject.

Symptoms – The presenting symptom is the sudden onset, often at rest, of acute, agonizing pain in the front of the chest. This rapidly radiates all over the front of the chest and often down over the abdomen. It is often accompanied by nausea and vomiting, so that suspicion may be aroused of some acute abdominal condition such as gall-stone colic or a perforated peptic ulcer. The victim soon becomes collapsed, with a pale, cold sweating skin, rapid pulse and difficulty in breathing. There is usually some rise in temperature.

Treatment is immediate relief of the pain by injections of morphine. Whether or not admission to hospital is necessary is an open question to be decided in each case by the medical attendant. The essentials of subsequent treatment are absolute rest, the continued administration of drugs to relieve the pain, the administration of drugs that may be necessary to deal with the heart failure that always develops and the irregular action of the heart that quite often develops, and the administration of oxygen. A recent development has been the establishment in major hospitals of what are known as intensive care units, to which patients with coronary thrombosis can be admitted for constant supervision. Such units maintain an emergency, skilled, round-the-clock staff of doctors and nurses, as well as all the necessary instruments, drugs and resuscitation apparatus that may be required. A controversial form of treatment at the moment is the administration of anticoagulant drugs. Theoretically, these should be of value to patients with thrombosis, to prevent the thrombus spreading. Carefully controlled clinical trials, however, have given no clear picture of whether or not these drugs are indicated.

The outcome varies considerably. The first few days are the critical ones from the point of view of recovery. If these are survived, then with a first coronary thrombosis the outlook is quite good provided the patient does not have a high blood-pressure and is not overweight. Following recovery, there should be a gradual return to work, care being taken to avoid any increase in weight, unnecessary stress and strain, and to observe the golden rule about moderation in all things. Cigarette smoking should be given up. At one time, patients who had had a coronary thrombosis were kept in bed for prolonged periods. Today, however, in uncomplicated cases the aim is to get them up and about as soon as possible. Thus, one heart specialist tells his patients who have had a coronary thrombosis that they will be in hospital for about ten days and that they will be back at work in three months. He has also expressed the view that 'an average patient, three months after an uncomplicated coronary thrombosis, has the capacity to do almost everything'.

CORONAVIRUSES, so called because in electron micrographs the spikes projecting from the virus resemble a crown, are a group of viruses which have been isolated from people with common colds, and have also been shown to produce common colds under experimental conditions. Their precise significance in the causation of the common cold is still undetermined.

CORPORA QUADRIGEMINA form part of the mid-brain. (See BRAIN.)

CORPULENCE, or OBESITY, is a condition of the body characterized by over-accumulation of fat under the skin and around certain of the internal organs. The extent to which obesity may proceed is illustrated by numerous well-authenticated examples, of which only a few can be here mentioned. Thus Bright, a grocer of Maldon, in Essex, who died in 1750, in his twenty-ninth year, weighed 616 pounds (280 kg). In the *Philosophical Transactions* for 1813 a case is recorded of a girl four years of age who weighed 256 pounds (116 kg). But the most celebrated case is that of Daniel Lambert of Leicester, who died in 1809 in his fortieth year. He is said to have been the heaviest man who ever lived, his weight being 739 pounds (335 kg). Lambert had publicly exhibited himself for some years before his death, which occurred suddenly at Stamford. At the inn where he died two suits of his clothes were preserved, from which some idea of his enormous dimensions may be obtained when it is stated that his waistcoat could easily enclose seven persons of ordinary size. Lambert ate moderately, drank only water, and slept less than most persons. He is said to have had an excellent tenor voice.

For some persons, and particularly among some races, a degree of corpulence is natural, and though table 16 represents the average weight for men of twenty-five years of age and over, of varying height, it must be accepted as true for health only with a wide margin. A person's weight may be one-fifth over the figures given and yet within the limit of health, while, on the other hand, if the weight is not more than one-fifth below the average weight this is not indicative of bad health. The average woman should weight rather less for her height than the average male, as a comparison of tables 16 and 17 makes clear.

The average weight of the clothing is $\frac{1}{24}$ of the male body, and the weights given in the tables include clothing. An addition of about three pounds for every four years of age over thirty must be made to these figures, as the weight tends to increase naturally until old age sets in. (See WEIGHT AND HEIGHT.)

Causes – Various causes are assigned for the production of corpulence. Thus, in

Height		Small Frame	Medium Frame	Large Frame
Feet	Inches	Pounds	Pounds	Pounds
5	2	116–125	124–133	131–142
5	3	119–128	127–136	133–144
5	4	122–132	130–140	137–149
5	5	126–136	134–144	141–153
5	6	129–139	137–147	145–157
5	7	133–143	141–151	149–162
5	8	136–147	145–156	153–166
5	9	140–151	149–160	157–170
5	10	144–155	153–164	161–175
5	11	148–159	157–168	165–180
6	0	152–164	161–173	169–185
6	1	157–169	166–178	174–190
6	2	163–175	171–184	179–196
6	3	168–180	176–189	184–202

Table 16 – Ideal weights for men of ages 25 and over. Height, with shoes on. Weight, dressed. (Metropolitan Life Insurance Company, 1943.)

Height		Small Frame	Medium Frame	Large Frame
Feet	Inches	Pounds	Pounds	Pounds
4	11	104–111	110–118	117–127
5	0	105–113	112–120	119–129
5	1	107–115	114–122	121–131
5	2	110–118	117–125	124–135
5	3	113–121	120–128	127–138
5	4	116–125	124–132	131–142
5	5	119–128	127–135	133–145
5	6	123–132	130–140	138–150
5	7	126–136	134–144	142–154
5	8	129–139	137–147	145–158
5	9	133–143	141–151	149–162
5	10	136–147	145–155	152–166
5	11	139–150	148–158	155–169

Table 17 – Ideal weights for women of ages 25 and over. Height, with shoes on. Weight, dressed. (Metropolitan Life Insurance Company, 1942.)

some instances it may be due to disturbances of some of the endocrine glands, such as the thyroid, pituitary and sex glands. In some families there appears to be a hereditary predisposition to an obese habit of body, upon which precautions in living seem to have little effect. But, beyond this, it is unquestionable that certain habits favour the occurrence of corpulence.

A luxurious, inactive or sedentary life is a well-recognized predisposing cause. The more immediate exciting causes are overfeeding and the large use of fluids of any kind, but especially alcoholic liquors. Fat persons are not always great eaters, although many of them are; while again, leanness and inordinate appetite are not infrequently associated. Still, it may be stated generally that indulgence in food beyond what is requisite to repair daily waste goes towards the increase of fat. This is more especially the case when the non-nitrogenous (the fatty, sugary and starchy) elements of the food are in excess. It is generally held that the fat of the body is mainly, if not entirely, formed from these foods, while nitrogenous foods (proteins) increase oxidation and lead to tissue waste. Alcoholic liquors, when taken to a considerable extent, also tend to the formation of fat, partly because many of them, eg. beer, contain much sugar, and partly no doubt because a portion of the body heat is derived from the alcohol and a corresponding amount of the starchy and sugary food spared and converted into fat.

Women are more prone to become corpulent than men, and appear to take on this condition more readily after having borne a child, and after the cessation of menstruation.

In young persons excessive corpulence is sometimes associated with defective action of some of the endocrine glands, especially the pituitary and thyroid glands. In slighter cases of such defect the gland usually gains its full development as life advances, and the corpulence passes off when adult age is reached.

Defective muscular exertion has been mentioned as a cause of corpulence, but it is sometimes observed that stout men, when they begin to take active exercise, become fatter still, the reason being that the appetite is sharpened and still more food is taken.

Symptoms – Health cannot be long maintained with excessive obesity, for the increase in bulk of the body, rendering exercise more difficult, leads to relaxation and defective nutrition of muscle, while the accumulations of fat in the chest and abdomen occasion embarrassment to the functions of the various organs in these cavities. In general, the mental activity of the highly corpulent becomes impaired, although there have always been notable exceptions to this rule.

The corpulent are at least as liable as the spare to be attacked by acute diseases, and they succumb much more readily to them than do the latter. Diabetes mellitus, gall-stones, gout, arterial disease, high blood-pressure and varicose veins are all more common in the obese individual. Various skin conditions, such as eczema, and particularly a chafed and painful condition of the skin at folds where two surfaces meet (see CHAFING), are also troublesome. It is therefore not surprising that the corpulent have a poor expectation of life. Life insurance statistics show that an increase of 25 pounds (11 kg) above standard weight reduces the life expectancy of a man of 45 by 25 per cent. This means that he is likely to die at 60, whereas he might have expected to live until 80 if he had not been obese.

Treatment – For the prevention of corpulence and the reduction of superfluous fat, many expedients have been resorted to, and numerous remedies recommended. These have embraced such regimens as bleeding, purging, starving, the use of different kinds of baths, and of drugs innumerable, most of which means have been found to fail in accomplishing the desired object.

The drinking of vinegar was long popularly supposed to be a remedy for obesity. It is related of the Marquis of Cortona, a noted general of the Duke of Alba, that by drinking vinegar he so reduced his body from a condition of enormous obesity that he could fold his skin around him like a garment. Such a result was only a proof of the injury done to his health, and probably to his digestive organs, by the excessive use of vinegar.

When the obesity is due to myxoedema (qv), excellent results are obtained from the administration of thyroid gland, but this form of treatment should not be used for the treatment of obesity except under careful medical supervision.

Of far greater importance than any drugs is the question of the regulation of habits as to diet, exercise and sleep. In 1863 a pamphlet appeared, entitled a *Letter on Corpulence, Addressed to the Public by William Banting*, in which was narrated the remarkable experience of the writer in accomplishing the reduction of his own weight in a short time, by the adoption of a particular kind of diet. Mr Banting described the condition of obesity in which he was in August 1862, and which, although certainly less than the examples already mentioned, appears to have been sufficient to prove a source of much discomfort and even of actual suffering. After trying almost every known remedy without effect, he placed himself upon an entirely new form of diet, which consisted chiefly in the removal as far as possible, of all sugary, starchy and fat food, the reduction of liquids, and the substitution of meat or fish and fruit in moderate quantity at each meal, together with the daily use of an antacid draught. Under this regimen his weight was reduced 35 pounds (16 kg) in the course of a few weeks, while his health underwent a marked improvement. Mr Banting's experience induced many to follow his example, and in numerous instances the effects were all that could be desired. Such a rapid loss of weight, however, is apt to be attended with serious impairment of health, and, generally speaking, it is not advisable to aim at losing weight at a greater rate than about three or four pounds (1·4 or 1·8 kg) in each week.

Various Continental spas have elaborate courses of treatment, in which rigid rules are laid down. Since a person submits himself more easily to, and obeys more implicitly, the rules in these places than he would do at home, such a 'cure' is attended with special benefit.

Unless the individual is grossly overweight it is inadvisable to reduce weight too rapidly. Provided the diet is carefully adhered to, it is seldom necessary to give a diet containing less than 1000 to 1200 Calories. Fats and carbohydrates must be reduced as much as possible. This means that sugar, sweets, jams, tinned fruit, potatoes and fried food must be banned. It is advisable to exclude all alcoholic liquors, but if the individual is so used to these that complete abstinence would be a real hardship, then a little dry wine may be allowed. Beer, sweet wines, spirits and aerated waters must not be taken. Items which can be partaken of freely, include green vegetables (salad dressings must be made with vinegar or lemon juice, not olive oil), coffee (without milk), tea and clear soups. Saccharine, of course, can be used freely for sweetening purposes.

The following is a sample diet which contains approximately 1100 Calories:

Early Morning – Glass of water.
Breakfast – Orange or $\frac{1}{2}$ grapefruit; 1 thin slice of wholemeal bread; 1 egg or 1 oz of lean ham (cold); tea or black coffee.
Mid-morning – One cup of tea.
Lunch – Lean meat, liver, kidney, chicken, white fish or tripe (small helping); potatoes (small helping) and green vegetables; stewed apple or pear with junket.
Tea – 1 thin slice of brown or wholemeal bread; tomato, cress or lettuce; tea.
Dinner – Clear soup; small helping of white fish; small helping of lean meat, chicken, or rabbit; green vegetable; fruit.

The amount of milk allowed daily is $\frac{1}{2}$ to 1 pint (280 to 560 ml), whilst not more than 1 ounce (28·3 G) of butter (or margarine) must be taken every day.

Exercise should be abundant, and clothing should be light when an attempt is made to reduce corpulence, but care must be taken that the food is not at the same time increased to satisfy the sharpened appetite, or the effect of exercise is defeated. Sleep is a matter of importance.

The person should go to bed early, and should limit the duration of rest to seven or at most eight hours, while the habit of sleeping during the day should be broken off.

In the grossly obese individual who fails to respond to any other form of treatment, a reduction in weight may be obtained by an operation in which a large section of the small intestine is by-passed, thereby reducing the amount of food that is absorbed into the body. The results, however, are far from impressive, and the procedure is not without its hazards to life and health.

In no circumstances should so-called 'slimming drugs', such as amphetamine, be taken except under medical supervision.

COR PULMONALE is another name for pulmonary heart disease, which is characterized by hypertrophy and failure of the right ventricle of the heart as a result of disease of the lungs or disorder of the pulmonary circulation.

CORPUSCLE means a small body. (See BLOOD.)

CORPUS LUTEUM is the mass of cells formed in the ruptured Graafian follicle in the ovary from which the ovum is discharged about fifteen days before the onset of the next menstrual period. When the ovum escapes the follicle fills up with blood. This is soon replaced by cells which contain a yellow fatty material. The follicle and its luteal cells constitute the corpus luteum. In the human the corpus luteum begins to disappear after ten days, unless the discharged ovum is fertilized and pregnancy ensues. In pregnancy the corpus luteum persists and grows and secretes the hormone, progesterone (qv).

CORRIGAN'S PULSE is the name applied to the throbbing pulse found with incompetence of the aortic valve. It is so called after Sir Dominic John Corrigan (1802–80), the famous Dublin physician, who first described it.

CORROSIVES are poisonous substances which corrode or eat away the mucous surfaces of mouth, gullet and stomach with which they come in contact. Examples are strong mineral acids like sulphuric, nitric and hydrochloric acids, caustic alkalis, and some salts like chlorides of mercury and zinc. (See POISONS.)

CORROSIVE SUBLIMATE, or PER-CHLORIDE OF MERCURY, is a powerful antiseptic and an irritant poison. It is not to be confounded with subchloride of mercury or calomel. (See ANTISEPTICS; DISINFECTION; MERCURY.)

CORTICOSTEROIDS is the generic term for the group of hormones with a cortisone-like action.

CORTICOTROPHIN is the *British Pharmacopoeia* name for the adrenocorticotrophic hormone of the pituitary gland, also known as ACTH. It is so called because it stimulates the functions of the cortex of the suprarenal glands. This results, among other things, in an increased output of cortisone. Although first isolated from the pituitary gland in 1933, it was not until the discovery, in 1949, of the effect of cortisone and corticotrophin in rheumatoid arthritis that it came into general use. No means of synthesis has yet been discovered, and the only available source are the pituitary glands of animals. It is only active when given by intravenous or intramuscular injection, but there are preparations available, which give a more prolonged action and which are given subcutaneously. As its action is predominantly the same as that of cortisone, the action of the two is discussed together in the section on cortisone (qv).

CORTISOL is another name for hydrocortisone (qv).

CORTISONE, originally known as Compound E, was isolated from beef adrenal glands in 1936 by workers at the Mayo Clinic. Its chemical name is 11-dehydro-17-hydroxycorticosterone. Mainly because of difficulties in obtaining adequate amounts, little interest was taken in it until, in 1949, Hench and Kendall and their colleagues demonstrated its dramatic, if transitory, effect in rheumatoid arthritis. The precise mode of action of cortisone is still not known. Among other things, it prevents (or delays) the proliferative changes in the tissues which are the normal response to infection and in allergic conditions. Among the conditions which have been shown to benefit from cortisone are rheumatoid arthritis, rheumatic fever, gout, certain eye conditions, certain skin conditions and Addison's disease.

Cortisone has two disadvantages which will always tend to restrict its use. One is that in chronic conditions such as rheumatoid arthritis the effect of cortisone is merely temporary, and tends to stop when

administration is stopped. The other is that cortisone has certain toxic effects, and therefore it must only be used under medical supervision.

For all practical purposes corticotrophin (qv) and cortisone have the same action. (See also BETAMETHASONE; DEXAMETHASONE; HYDROCORTISONE; PREDNISOLONE; PREDNISONE; and TRIAMCINOLONE.)

CORYZA is the technical name of a 'cold in the head'.

COSTAL means anything pertaining to the ribs.

COSTALGIA means pain in the ribs.

COSTIVENESS (see CONSTIPATION).

COT DEATH is the term applied to the unexpected death of an apparently healthy baby, usually during sleep. It is also known as the Sudden Infant Death Syndrome, and it is estimated that probably at least 1800 such deaths occur every year in Britain. Most babies who die in this way have been healthy, or only slightly unwell, the day before death. Death occurs silently and suddenly, the baby being found dead in his cot in the morning. Over half these deaths occur between the ages of 2 and 6 months, and boys are more affected than girls. They are more common in social classes III, IV and V (see SOCIAL CLASSES), and the incidence is highest in the winter. Most of the infants have been bottle fed.

The cause is still not really known. Smothering by a soft pillow may account for a few of the deaths, and a certain number are due to an infection of the lungs, such as broncho-pneumonia or bronchitis, usually due to a virus. One possibility is that they may be associated with allergy to milk. Another is that they may be due to a sudden upset of the fluid balance of the baby as a result of bottle feeding. Yet another is that they may be associated with a deficiency of vitamin E. Another possible cause is the spontaneous production of botulinum toxin in the gut of young babies. All that can really be said at the moment, however, is that the baby most likely to die in this way is one who was underweight when born, comes from a poor family, whose mother is young and already has several children, who has been bottle fed, has been unwell during the preceding fortnight and has signs of a cold in the head when put to bed.

CO-TRIMOXAZOLE is an antibacterial agent which is proving of value in a wide range of infections. It is a combination of two antibacterial agents: trimethoprim and sulphamethoxazole.

COTTON-WOOL is a downy material made from the hairs on cotton plant seeds (*Gossypium herbaceum*). Ordinary cottonwool is non-absorbent, owing to its containing a considerable quantity of cotton-seed oil. The absorbent form is produced by removing this oil with alkalis. It is this absorbent form that is used in medicine for a great variety of purposes, including protection to injured parts, by reason of its combined warmth and cheapness. It is highly inflammable. It may be medicated with various substances, such as capsicum, capsicum cottonwool being used as a counter-irritant (qv) for use in dressings in the treatment of painful rheumatic conditions. Cottonseed oil can be used for purposes similar to those of olive oil.

COUNTER-IRRITANTS (see BLISTERS AND COUNTER-IRRITANTS).

COWPOX is a disease affecting the udders of cows, on which it produces vesicles. It is communicable to man, and there has for centuries been a tradition that persons who have caught this cowpox from cows do not suffer afterwards from smallpox. This formed the basis for Jenner's experiments on vaccination. (See VACCINATION.)

COXALGIA means pain in the hip-joint.

COXA VARA is a condition in which the neck of the thigh-bone is bent so that the lower limbs are turned very much outwards and lameness results.

COXSACKIE VIRUSES are a group of viruses so-called because they were first isolated from two patients with a disease resembling paralytic poliomyelitis, in the village of Coxsackie in New York State. Thirty distinct types have now been identified. They constitute one of the three groups of viruses included in the family of enteroviruses (qv). They are divided into two groups: A and B. Despite the large number of types of group A virus (24) in existence, evidence of their role in causing human disease is limited. Some, however, cause aseptic meningitis, and others cause a condition known as herpangina (qv). Hand, foot and mouth disease (qv) is another disease caused by the A group. All 6 types

of group B virus have been associated with outbreaks of aseptic meningitis, and they are also the cause of Bornholm disease (qv).

CRAB-LOUSE is another name for *Pediculus pubis*, a louse that infests the pubic region. (See INSECTS IN RELATION TO DISEASE.)

CRACKED-POT SOUND is a peculiar resonance heard sometimes on percussion of the chest over a cavity in the lung, resembling the jarring sound heard on striking a cracked pot or bell.

CRADLE is the name applied to the cage which is placed over the legs of a patient in bed, in order to take the weight of the bed-clothes off the legs.

CRADLE CAP, or CRUSTA LACTEA as it is technically known, is the form of seborrhoea of the scalp which is not uncommon in nursing infants. It usually responds to an ointment containing equal parts of Salicylic Acid Ointment of the *British National Formulary*, Sulphur Ointment B P, and White Soft Paraffin B P.

CRAMP is a painful spasmodic contraction of muscles, most commonly occurring in the limbs, but also apt to affect certain internal organs. This disorder belongs to the class of diseases known as local spasms, of which other varieties exist in such affections as tetany, and colic. The cause of these painful seizures resides in the nervous system, and operates either directly from the great nerve centres, or, as is generally the case, indirectly by reflex action, as, for example, when attacks are brought on by some derangement of the digestive organs.

NIGHT CRAMP comes on suddenly, often during sleep, the patient being aroused by an agonizing feeling of pain in the calf of the leg or back of the thigh. During the paroxysm the muscular fibres affected can often be felt gathered up into a hard knot. The attack in general lasts but a few seconds and then suddenly departs, the spasmodic contraction of the muscles ceasing entirely; or, on the other hand, relief may come more gradually during a period of minutes or even hours. Even after the sharp pain has gone there is often a persisting ache. The cause is not known. It is more common in older people, but has been reported in soldiers during their preliminary period of training. It is also common in pregnancy.

Treatment – This painful disorder can

be greatly relieved and often entirely removed by firmly grasping or briskly rubbing the affected part with the hand, or by anything which makes an impression on the nerves, such as the application of some cold substance to the part, or occasionally by warmth. Even a sudden and vigorous movement of the limb, in such a direction as to stretch the affected muscle, will often succeed in terminating the attack, though this may also exacerbate the condition. If troublesome during pregnancy, the mother should restrict her milk intake to 1 pint (0·5 litre) a day and take calcium gluconate tablets with or without vitamin D. In men and non-pregnant women, in whom the condition is irritatingly recurrent, 1 to 5 grains (60 to 300 mg) of quinine bisulphate, or 10 grains (600 mg) of calcium lactate the last thing before going to bed, have a high reputation as a preventive.

CRAMP OF SWIMMERS includes usually spasm of the arteries as well as of the muscles, due to cold and exertion, so that death is apt to occur from stoppage of the heart. If treatment can be applied, friction of the limbs, warmth, and hot drinks are essential.

CRAMP OF THE STOMACH, or GASTRALGIA, is usually a symptom in connection with some form of gastric disorder (see STOMACH, DISEASES OF). For cramp affecting the muscular wall of the bowels, see COLIC.

HABIT SPASMS, or FUNCTIONAL SPASMS, are liable to occur in individuals of almost any handicraft, and are often extremely troublesome.

Writer's Cramp, or *Scrivener's Palsy*, is a spasm which affects certain muscles when engaged in the performance of acts the result of education and long usage, and which does not occur when the same muscles are employed in acts of a different kind. This disorder owes its name to the relative frequency with which it develops in persons who write much, although it is by no means confined to them.

The symptoms are in the first instance a gradually increasing difficulty experienced in conducting the movements required for executing the work in hand. At an early stage of the disease the difficulty may be overcome to a large extent by persevering efforts, but ultimately, when the attempt is persisted in, the muscles of the fingers, and occasionally also those of the forearm, are seized with spasm or cramp, so that the act of writing is rendered impossible. Sometimes the fingers, instead of being cramped, move in a disorderly manner

and the pen cannot be grasped, while in other rare instances a kind of paralysis affects the muscles of the fingers, and they are powerless to make the movements necessary for holding the pen. It is to be noted that it is only in the act of writing that these phenomena present themselves, and that, for all other movements, the fingers and arms possess their natural power. Similar symptoms are observed and similar remarks apply in the case of musicians, typists, telegraphists, artists, compositors, seamstresses, tailors, and many mechanics.

Spasmodic Wry-neck is one of the most frequent forms which the disease takes. This comes on in shoemakers, tailors, and persons generally whose employment necessitates their following, with the head, movements which the hands are making. The result is that the muscles of the neck assume the unpleasant habit of drawing the head to one side whenever the slightest attempt is made to turn and look at anything. Indeed, although actually a rare disease, no muscle or group of muscles which is specially called into action in any particular occupation is exempt from liability to this functional spasm, which is therefore ascribed to over-use of the parts concerned.

Treatment – In the treatment of habit spasms, the only effectual remedy is absolute cessation for a time (it may be a month or longer) from the work with which the attack is associated. It is sometimes recommended that the opposite hand or limb be used, so as to afford the affected part entire rest, but this may be followed by the extension of the disorder to that locality also. Special forms of penholder and other mechanical contrivances have been suggested so as to enable the occupation to be carried on, but they do not afford any relief to the disease, for the cure of which entire rest is important. There is often a strong psychological element in such cases, and psychotherapy is indicated. Where the spasmodically acting muscles are not of great importance to the bodily economy, their action can be controlled by division of their nerves of supply. For example, spasmodic wry-neck can be checked by division of the spinal accessory nerve on one side of the neck. Such a procedure is out of the question in the case of the hand.

HEAT CRAMPS are painful contractions of muscles occurring in men (eg. stokers) working in high temperatures. The cramps are due to excessive loss of salt in the sweat, and can be cured, and prevented, by giving salt water to drink. (See also HEATSTROKE.)

CRANIAL NERVES are those arising from the brain. (See BRAIN.)

CRANIUM means the part of the skull enclosing the brain as distinguished from the face.

CRASIS is the term applied to the individual temperament or constitution. (See CONSTITUTION.)

CREAM is the oily or fatty part of milk from which butter is prepared. Average cream when purchased contains about 18 per cent of fat. A food known as '20 per cent cream' consists of the upper 4 ounces (113 ml) skimmed off a quart (1·1 litres) of milk which has stood for twenty-four hours. Heavy cream or whipped cream may contain about 48 per cent of fat. (See MILK.)
Various medicinal preparations are known also as cream, eg. *cold cream*, which is a simple ointment containing rose-water, beeswax, borax, and almond oil scented with oil of rose.

CREAM OF TARTAR is another name for bitartrate of potassium.
Imperial Drink consists of a teaspoonful of cream of tartar, a squeeze of lemon, two lumps of sugar, and a pint (570 ml) of cold water.

CREATINE is a nitrogenous substance, methyl-guanidine-acetic acid. In the adult human body there are about 120 grams of it, and 98 per cent of this is present in the muscles. Much of the creatine in muscle is combined with phosphoric acid as phosphocreatine, which plays an important part in the chemistry of muscular contraction.

CREATININE is the anhydride of creatine and is derived from it. It is purely a waste product.

CREEPING ERUPTION is a skin condition caused by the invasion of the skin by the larvae of various species of nematode worms. It owes its name to the fact that as the larva moves through and along the skin it leaves behind it a long creeping thin red line.

CREMATION (see DEAD, DISPOSAL OF THE).

CREOSOTE is a clear, yellow liquid, of aromatic smell and burning taste, prepared by distillation from pine-wood or from beech-wood, the product of the latter being of better quality. It mixes readily with alcohol, ether, chloroform, glycerin, and oils.
It is a powerful antiseptic and disinfectant. It has also a soothing action upon parts with which it is brought into contact. It is unchanged after absorption into the blood, and, being excreted by the lungs and exhaled on the breath, it exercises an effect upon these organs.
Uses – Creosote is an ingredient of some disinfectant fluids. It is also used in the form of a vapour, containing creosote 5 ml, and light carbonate of magnesia 30 grains (2 G), in water 1 ounce (28·5 ml), of which a teaspoonful is added to a pint (570 ml) of hot water and inhaled in cases of suppurating throat, foetid breath, etc. In cases of sea-sickness, it is sometimes given in doses of 2 to 10 drops to check the vomiting. It has also been used for the temporary alleviation of toothache, the aching cavity being filled with cotton-wool soaked in creosote.

CREPITATIONS is the name applied to certain sounds which occur along with the breath sounds, as heard by auscultation, in various diseases of the lungs. They are signs of the presence of moist exudations in the lungs or in the bronchial tubes, are classified as fine, medium, and coarse crepitations, and resemble the sound made by bursting bubbles of various sizes.

CREPITUS means a grating sound. It is found in cases of fractured bones when the ends rub together; also in cases of severe chronic arthritis by the rubbing together of the dried internal surfaces of the joints.

CRESOL is an oily liquid obtained from coal tar. It is a powerful antiseptic and disinfectant.
Uses – It is used combined with soap to form a clear saponaceous fluid known as Cresol and Soap Solution, BP, or lysol, which can be mixed with water in any proportions. For the disinfection of linen, bed-pans, drains, or surgical instruments a convenient strength is 2 per cent (one tablespoonful to 1¼ pints (600 ml) of water); for washing the hands 1 per cent (one tablespoonful to 2½ pints (1·25 litres)) and for a douche ½ per cent (one tablespoonful to 5 pints (2·5 litres)) are commonly used.

CRETA is a Latin name for chalk.

CRETINISM is a disease which is due to defective thyroid function in foetal life or early in infancy. It can usually be recognized within a few weeks of birth. Not only is the mind feeble, but the whole body remains undeveloped, and there are deformities of the bones, changes in the thyroid gland, and a swollen condition of the skin. The defect in the thyroid gland is responsible for most of the other bodily and mental peculiarities. If untreated, the affected child rarely reaches middle age. The condition is met with particularly in Switzerland, Northern Italy, and Tyrol, but cases crop up now and then in Britain and North America.

Treatment consists in giving extract of thyroid regularly and in attending to the general health: it is important for the disease to be diagnosed at an early stage if treatment is to have effect.

CRISIS is a word used with several distinct meanings.

1. The usual meaning is that of a rapid loss of fever and return to comparative health in certain acute diseases. For example, pneumonia, if allowed to run its natural course, ends by a crisis, usually on the eighth day, the temperature falling in twenty-four hours to normal, the pulse and breathing becoming slow and regular, and the patient passing from a partly delirious state into natural sleep. The opposite mode of ending to crisis is by lysis: for example, in typhoid fever, where the patient slowly improves during a period of a week or more, without any sudden change.

2. A popular use of the word crisis, and still more frequently of critical, is to signify a dangerous state of illness in which it is uncertain whether the sufferer will recover or not.

3. The word crisis is also used to signify a paroxysm of pain in the larynx, stomach, or bowels occurring during the course of locomotor ataxia (qv).

CROHN'S DISEASE (see ILEITIS).

CROTON OIL is a powerful purgative, seldom used now, producing copious watery evacuations, and, in large quantities, acting as an irritant poison.

Externally, croton liniment is used as a counter-irritant.

CROUP is a household term for a group of diseases characterized by swelling and partial blockage of the entrance to the larynx, occurring in children and characterized by crowing inspiration. There are various causes including diphtheritic laryngitis (see DIPHTHERIA), acute laryngitis, and the condition known as spasmodic croup or laryngismus stridulosus. It is an account of this last condition which will be given here. (See also LARYNGO-TRACHEO-BRONCHITIS.)

The important thing to remember about any form of croup is that it is always potentially dangerous – particularly in the case of an infant – because of the narrowness of the entrance to the larynx and therefore the comparative ease with which it may be blocked, thereby leading to suffocation of the infant.

Symptoms – The attack usually comes on at night, when the child is in bed, and follows a chill caught during the day, or an ordinary cold that has lasted perhaps for some days. The breathing is hoarse and croaking (hence the name of the disease), the voice thin, the cough paroxysmal and metallic in tone, and the air passes in with a harsh, loud noise. The child is frightened and excited at first, but later becomes feeble and livid. Still later, pallor, sweating, and great struggling for breath come on, and may last half an hour or several hours. After this the symptoms begin to abate, gradually pass away, and the child falls asleep, but there is always a danger that the larynx may become completely blocked, in which case death ensues in a few minutes. A fatal termination is rare if the child receives proper treatment, and the alarming symptoms usually abate on the day following the attack, to return, it may be, on the succeeding night. A child who has once had croup is liable to have future attacks, and so should be specially guarded against cold and damp till he has outgrown the tendency.

Treatment – The child should be put into a hot bath to which a tablespoonful of mustard has been added, and a tent should be made with a blanket over the bath, so that he may inhale the steam. When he is put back into bed the tent should be put over the bed and the nozzle of a steam kettle brought within it. To the water in the kettle may be added a teaspoonful of compound tincture of benzoin, of creosote inhalation (see CREOSOTE), or of other soothing substance (see INHALATION). At the beginning, an attack may be checked by the administration of a teaspoonful of ipecacuanha wine every ten minutes till vomiting takes place. Sometimes, when the spasm of the laryngeal muscles seems very great, inhalation of chloroform is resorted to.

CRUCIATE LIGAMENTS are two strong ligaments in the interior of the knee-joint, which cross one another like the limbs of the letter X. They are so attached as to become taut when the lower limb is straightened, and they prevent over-extension or bending forwards at the knee.

CRURAL means something connected with the leg.

CRUSH SYNDROME is the term given to a condition in which kidney failure occurs in patients who have been the victims of severe crushing accidents. The fundamental injury is damage to muscle. The limb swells. The blood volume falls. Blood urea rises; there is also a rise in the potassium content of the blood. The patient may survive; or he dies with renal failure. Post-mortem examination shows degeneration of the tubules of the kidney, and the presence in them of pigment casts.

CRUTCH-PALSY (see DROP-WRIST).

CRYMOTHERAPY is the term applied to the treatment of disease by refrigeration. The two main forms in which it is now used are HYPOTHERMIA (qv) and REFRIGERATION ANAESTHESIA. Perhaps the best example of the latter is when a gangrenous leg in chronic diabetes mellitus or arteriosclerosis is kept by means of ice bags at a temperature of 5°C for from 1 to 5 hours. This form of anaesthesia much reduces the risks of shock and infection.

CRYOPRECIPITATE – When frozen plasma is allowed to thaw slowly at 4° C, a proportion of the plasma protein remains undissolved in the cold thawed plasma and stays in this state until the plasma is warmed. It is this cold insoluble precipitate that is known as cryoprecipitate. It can be recovered quite easily by centrifuging. Its value is that it is a rich source of Factor VIII, which is used in the treatment of haemophilia (qv).

CRYOSCOPY means the method of finding the concentration of blood, urine, etc., by observing their freezing-point.

CRYOSURGERY is the use of cold in surgery. Its advantages include little

associated pain, little or no bleeding, and excellent healing with little or no scar formation. Hence its relatively wide use in eye surgery. The coolants used include liquid nitrogen with which temperatures as low as −196°C can be obtained, carbon dioxide (−78°C) and nitrous oxide (−88°C).

CRYPTOCOCCOSIS is a rare disease due to infection with a yeast known as *Cryptococcus neoformans*. It usually involves the lungs in the first instance, but may spread to the meninges and other parts of the body. It responds well as a rule to treatment with amphotericin B, clotrimazole, and flucytosine.

CRYPTOCOCCUS is a genus of yeasts. *Cryptococcus neoformans* is widespread in nature and present in particularly large numbers in the faeces of pigeons. It occasionally infects man, causing the disease known as cryptococcosis.

CRYSTAL VIOLET (see GENTIAN VIOLET).

CUBEB is the fruit of *Piper cubeba*, used similarly to copaiba (qv).

CULDOSCOPY is the term applied to the method of examining the pelvic organs in women by means of an instrument comparable to a cystoscope (qv) inserted into the pelvic cavity through the vagina. The instrument used for this purpose is known as a culdoscope.

CUPPING is used in cases of deep-seated congestion to draw blood to the surface. It causes sudden dilatation of the superficial blood-vessels, and so probably contracts those of underlying organs. But whatever the explanation, it gives relief in difficulty of breathing due to asthma, bronchitis and pleurisy and brings relief in lumbago and various forms of rheumatic pain, though its current popularity in Britain is low. Cupping is of two kinds: *dry-cupping* and *wet-cupping*. To dry-cup, one takes a cupping-glass (or an ordinary thick glass tumbler), puts a few drops of methylated spirit upon a fragment of blotting-paper into it, ignites this, and, while it is still burning, claps the mouth of the glass tightly on the back of the patient. A vacuum is produced, and the skin swells up into the glass as blood rushes into its small blood-vessels. This is repeated four, six, or eight times in different places. Wet-cupping is rarely used these days. The skin is first dry-cupped, the swollen skin is next scarified with a lancet or a special instrument for the purpose, and then the cupping-glass is again applied, and blood drawn off into it. The vacuum for dry- or wet-cupping may also be produced by a suction bulb.

CUPRUM is the Latin word for copper.

CURARE, known also as CURARA, WOORALI, WOURARI, URARI, and TICUNAS, is a dark-coloured extract from some trees of the *Strychnos* family. It is used by the South American Indians as an arrow poison, and is extremely potent, its action depending upon a crystalline alkaloid: *d*-tubocurarine chloride. This alkaloid paralyses the nerve endings in muscle. For many years it was considered to be much too dangerous for use in man, but research has shown that the pure alkaloid can be used with safety. Its main use is in anaesthesia, where the muscular relaxation it produces is of invaluable assistance to the surgeon. With the aid of tubocurarine adequate muscular relaxation can be obtained with a lesser degree of anaesthesia than would be required were the drug not being used. It is a drug, however, that should only be used by a skilled anaesthetist. Its action is antagonized by prostigmine. It has also been used in the treatment of spastic conditions.

CURDLED MILK (see CASEIN).

CURETTE, or CURET, is a spoon-shaped instrument used in surgery for scooping out the contents of any cavity of the body: eg. the uterine cavity.

CUSHING'S SYNDROME is the term applied to the changes that take place in the body as the result of a tumour of the pituitary gland. The changes are: obesity, hairiness, curvature of the spine, impotence, and the appearance of red lines in the skin. Harvey Cushing (1869–1939) was a famous American brain surgeon.

CUSPARIA, or ANGOSTURA, is the dried bark of *Galipea officinalis*, a tree of tropical America. An infusion is used as a bitter, in doses of one, two, or more tablespoonfuls. Incidentally it should be noted that the well-known 'Angostura Bitters' contain no angostura (or cusparia). They are so named after the town where they were first produced.

CUTANEOUS means belonging to the skin. (See SKIN; and SKIN DISEASES.)

CUTICLE (see SKIN).

CUTS (see WOUNDS).

CUT-THROAT is an injury which may be due to suicide or murder, an expert being able to tell at a glance the one from the other. Death, when it occurs at once, is usually due to bleeding from the large vessels of the neck, and later may be caused by inflammation of the air passages. Another danger is that air will enter the large veins in such amount as to bring the circulation of the blood to a standstill. In a case of cut-throat, if any vessel be seen to bleed, the haemorrhage should be checked by pressure with the finger till surgical assistance can be obtained.

CYANIDES are salts of hydrocyanic or prussic acid. They are highly poisonous, and are also powerful antiseptics. (See PRUSSIC ACID; WOUNDS.) Double cyanide of mercury and zinc is specially powerful as an antiseptic used to impregnate gauze and cotton-wool for dressing wounds.

CYANOCOBALAMIN is the name given by the British Pharmacopoeia Commission to vitamin B_{12}. It is a red cobalt-containing substance, and it owes its name to the fact that it contains cyanide and cobalt. Vitamin B_{12} was first isolated in 1948 and was found to be an effective substitute for liver in the treatment of pernicious anaemia. (See ANAEMIA.) Either it or, more usually, hydroxocobalamin (qv) is now the standard treatment for this condition. (See COBALAMINS.)

CYANOSIS is a condition of blueness seen particularly about the face and extremities, accompanying states in which the blood is not properly oxygenated in the lungs. It appears earliest through the nails, on the lips, and the tips of the ears, and over the cheeks. It may be due to blockage of the air passages, or to disease in the lungs, or to a feeble circulation, as in heart disease.

CYBERNETICS is the science of communication and control in the animal and in the machine – a science which has come very much to the fore since the introduction of the modern computers.

CYCLAMATES are artificial sweetening agents which are about 30 times as sweet as cane sugar. After being in use since 1965, they were banned by Government decree in 1969 on the ground of adverse reports received from USA.

CYCLIZINE HYDROCHLORIDE, or MARZINE, is an antihistamine drug (qv) which is mainly used for the prevention of sickness, including sea-sickness.

CYCLOCOUMAROL is an anticoagulant which is active when given by mouth.

CYCLOPHOSPHAMIDE is a nitrogen mustard derivative (qv) which is proving of value in the treatment of various forms of malignant disease, including Hodgkin's disease and chronic lymphatic leukaemia.

CYCLOPLEGIA denotes paralysis of the ciliary muscle of the eye, which results in the loss of power of accommodation in the eye. (See ACCOMMODATION.)

CYCLOPROPANE is one of the most potent of the anaesthetics given by inhalation. Its advantages are that it acts quickly, causes little irritation to the lungs, and its effects pass off quickly.

CYCLOSERINE is an antibiotic derived from an actinomycete, which is of value in the treatment of certain infections of the genito-urinary tract, and of limited value in the treatment of tuberculosis.

CYCLOTHYMIA is the state characterized by extreme swings of mood from elation to depression, and vice versa.

CYCLOTRON is a machine in which positively charged particles are so accelerated that they acquire energies equivalent to those produced by millions of volts. From the medical point of view its interest is that it is a source of neutrons. (See RADIOTHERAPY.)

CYESIS is another term for pregnancy.

CYNANCHE is an old name for severe sore throat with choking. (See QUINSY.)

CYPROHEPTADINE is a drug originally introduced as an antihistamine drug (qv), but is now known to be effective in stimulating appetite and allowing underweight children and adults to gain weight.

CYRTOMETER is an instrument for measuring the shape of the chest.

CYSTEAMINE is a drug used in the prevention and treatment of radiation sickness (qv), and the treatment of paracetamol poisoning (qv).

CYSTIC FIBROSIS (see FIBROCYSTIC DISEASE OF THE PANCREAS).

CYSTITIS means inflammation of the bladder. (See BLADDER, DISEASES OF.)

CYSTOGRAM is an X-ray picture of the urinary bladder.

CYSTOMETER is an instrument for measuring the pressure in the urinary bladder.

CYSTOSCOPE is an instrument for viewing the interior of the bladder. It consists of a narrow tube carrying a small electric lamp at its end, a small mirror set obliquely opposite an opening near the end of the tube, and a telescope which is passed down the tube and by which the reflection of the brightly illuminated bladder wall in the mirror is examined. It is of great value in the diagnosis of conditions like ulcers and small tumours of the bladder.

Fine catheters can be passed along the cystoscope, and by the aid of vision can be inserted into each ureter and pushed up to the kidney, so that the urine from each kidney may be obtained and examined separately in order to diagnose which of these organs is diseased.

CYSTS are hollow tumours, containing fluid or soft material. They are almost always simple in nature.

Varieties – (*a*) RETENTION CYSTS – In these, in consequence of irritation or other cause, some cavity which ought naturally to contain a little fluid becomes distended or the natural outlet from the cavity becomes blocked. Wens (qv) are caused by the blockage of the outlet from sebaceous glands in the skin, so that an accumulation of fatty matter takes place. Ranula is a clear swelling under the tongue, due to a collection of saliva in consequence of an obstruction to a salivary duct. Cysts in the breasts are, in many cases, the result of blockage in milk ducts, due to inflammation. Cysts also form in the kidney as a result of obstruction to the free outflow of the urine.

(*b*) DEVELOPMENTAL CYSTS – Of these,

the most important are the huge cysts that originate in the ovaries. The cause is doubtful, but the cyst probably begins at a very early period of life, gradually enlarges, and buds off smaller cysts from its wall. The contents are usually a clear gelatinous fluid. Very often both ovaries are affected, and the cysts may slowly reach a great size, often, however, taking a lifetime to do so.

A similar condition sometimes occurs in the kidney, and the tumour may have reached a great size in an infant even before birth (congenital cystic kidney).

Dermoid cysts are small cavities, which also originate probably early in life, but do not reach any great size till fairly late in life. They appear about parts of the body where clefts occur in the embryo and close up before birth, such as the corner of the eyes, the side of the neck, the middle line of the body. They contain hair, fatty matter, fragments of bone, scraps of skin, even numerous teeth.

(c) HYDATID CYSTS are produced in many organs, particularly in the liver, by a parasite which is the larval stage of a tapeworm found in dogs. They occur in people who keep dogs and allow them to contaminate their food. (See PARASITES.)

CYTO- is a prefix meaning something connected with a cell or cells.

CYTODIAGNOSIS means diagnosis of disease by examining the cells found in blood effusions from cavities, etc.

CYTOGENETICS is the study of the structure and functions of the cells of the body, with particular reference to the chromosomes (qv).

CYTOLOGY is the study of cells.

CYTOMEGALOVIRUSES are a group of viruses belonging to the herpesvirus group. They are so-called from the swollen appearance of infected cells (*cytomegals*= large cell). Their importance is that they are responsible for the condition of cytomegalic disease of the newborn. The virus is transmitted from the mother either to her unborn baby while still in the uterus or to the baby during birth. In some cases the baby may show no evidence of infection, but in others it may cause a fatal disease characterized by jaundice and an enlarged liver and spleen. In those who recover from this severe form of the disease, there may be permanent mental retardation.

CYTOMETER is an instrument for counting and measuring cells.

CYTOSTATIC means the slowing, or stopping, of the growth of cells.

CYTOTOXIC means being destructive to cells.

D

DACRYOCYSTITIS means inflammation of the tear-sac at the side of the nose, near the inner angle of the eye.

DACTYLITIS means inflammation of a finger or toe.

DAMP is the name applied generally by miners to noxious gases in a mine. 'Fire damp' is an explosive mixture of gases, chiefly marsh gas. 'After damp' or 'white damp' is the term applied to carbon monoxide. 'Choke damp' and 'stink damp' are terms applied to an evil-smelling mixture of gases, following the use of explosives, containing sulphuretted hydrogen and other irritating compounds. 'Black damp' is the name applied to the stagnant air of old workings and wells from which the oxygen has disappeared, and which consists of nitrogen and carbon dioxide. (See AIR; VENTILATION; CARBON MONOXIDE; ASPHYXIA.)

DANAZOL is a synthetic derivative of ethisterone (qv) which is proving of value in the treatment of endometriosis.

DANDELION (see TARAXACUM).

DANDRUFF is the name applied to the white scales cast off from the scalp. Scurf. (See SEBORRHOEA.)

DANGEROUS DRUGS – This term is applied to certain drugs which are scheduled under the Dangerous Drugs Act, and which must be dispensed only under certain stringent regulations. These include morphine, cocaine, ecgonine, diamorphine (commonly known as heroin), extracts and tinctures of Indian hemp and opium, as well as any preparation containing one part in 500 or more of morphine or one part in 1000 or more of cocaine, ecgonine, or diamorphine. Prescriptions containing any of these drugs must be written, dated, and signed by a practitioner, and must give the name and address of the person for whom the prescription is intended, as well as the total amount of the drug to be supplied (table 18).

All other poisonous substances are scheduled in twelve classes, the important ones from the medical point of view being those included in the first and fourth schedules. The substances included in the First Schedule are those containing the more deadly poisons, which may not be sold by chemists except to persons known to the seller, and the name and address of the purchaser must be entered in a book. The Fourth Schedule includes drugs such as barbituric acid and its derivatives. A prescription for any substance in Schedule Four must contain the prescriber's name, the name and address of the seller, and the date on which the prescription was dispensed. It must not be dispensed more than once unless the prescriber directs that it be dispensed a stated number of times or at stated intervals.

In 1968, further regulations were introduced. Under the Dangerous Drugs (Notification of Addicts) Regulations, 1968, a doctor is required to pass to the chief medical officer at the Home Office full details of any person he is attending whom 'he considers or has reasonable grounds to suspect' to be addicted to any of the drugs listed in the Schedule to the 1965 Dangerous Drugs Act. These drugs include morphine, heroin, pethidine, dextromoramide. Under the Dangerous Drugs (Supply to Addicts) Regulations, 1968, it is an offence to provide cocaine or heroin or any of their derivatives to patients other than on licence issued by the Secretary of State and in accordance with the Regulations. Such licences are not issued for use in general practice, but only to individual doctors for use in a clinic, hospital or institution approved for the purpose.

On July 1, 1973, the Misuse of Drugs Act, 1971, and the regulations under it (Misuse of Drugs Regulations, 1973) came into force. The Act, which combines and extends the Dangerous Drugs Acts, 1965, and 1967, and the Drugs (Prevention of Misuse) Act, 1964, applies to the whole of the United Kingdom. The main practical changes introduced by this new legislation are: (*a*) Dangerous Drugs are now referred to as Controlled Drugs. (*b*) Nine drugs are added to the list of such Controlled Drugs, including amphetamine, codeine, dexamphetamine, methaqualone, and pholcodine. (*c*) Notification of addiction is required in respect of the following drugs: cocaine, dextromoramide, diamorphine (heroin), dipipanone, hydrocodone, hydromorphone (Dilaudid), levorphanol, methadone, morphine, omnopon, papaveretum, opium, oxycodone, pethidine, phenazocine, piritramide. (*d*) A new category of drugs has been introduced, including the hallucinogens (eg. lysergic acid diethylamide) and cannabis, which can only be prescribed under special licence.

	I	II	III
Acts	Dangerous Drugs Acts 1965 and 1967; Dangerous Drugs (No. 2) Regulations 1964; Dangerous Drugs (Notification of Addicts) Regulations 1968; Dangerous Drugs (Supply to Addicts) Regulations 1968	Drugs (Prevention of Misuse) Act 1965	Pharmacy and Poisons Act 1933; Poisons List (No. 2) Order 1968; Poisons (No. 2) Rules 1968
Drugs controlled	Opiates including Morphine Heroin* Synthetic analgesics, eg.: Pethidine Methadone Cocaine* Cannabis*	Amphetamines* and some similar substances Lysergic acid diethylamide (LSD 25)* and some similar substances, including mescaline	All those named in the Poisons List including barbiturates and the drugs named in columns I and II *Note:* Barbiturates and the drugs mentioned in columns I and II are included in Part I of the Poisons List and Schedule IV of the Rules
Main provisions	(a) Offence to possess without authority (b) Offence to import and export except under licence (c) Persons authorized to possess have to keep records of drug movements (d) Drugs to be kept under lock and key by persons authorized to possess (e) Medical practitioners must notify all cases of persons addicted† to drugs controlled under the Act of 1965 (f) Heroin and cocaine may be prescribed only for an addict, by a specially licensed medical practitioner	(a) Offence to possess without authority (b) Offence to import except under licence	(a) Offence for a poison in Part I of the Poisons List to be sold retail otherwise than by an authorized seller of poisons from registered premises (b) Offence for substances named in Schedule IV to the Poisons Rules to be sold except on a prescription given by a duly qualified practitioner (c) Records of sales of Schedule IV substances are not required, but private prescriptions must be retained for two years
Penalties	Summary – £250 fine and/or 12 months' imprisonment Indictment – £1000 fine and/or 10 years' imprisonment	Summary – £200 fine and/or 6 months' imprisonment Indictment – unlimited fine and/or two years' imprisonment	£50 fine

* Drugs commonly obtained illegally
† As defined in the Regulations

Table 18 – Summary of statutory provisions for the control of drugs in England and Wales.

(e) Some tightening up of prescribing rules for doctors of Controlled Drugs.

DANTROLENE is a muscle-relaxing drug that is proving of value in relieving the muscular spasm in some cases of multiple sclerosis (qv).

DAPSONE is one of the most effective drugs in the treatment of leprosy.

DARTOS is the thin muscle just under the skin of the scrotum which enables the scrotum to alter its shape.

DAY BLINDNESS is a condition in which the patient sees better in a dim light or by night than in daylight. It is only found in conditions in which the light is very glaring, as in the desert and on snow, and is relieved by resting the retina, for example by wearing coloured glasses for a time.

DDT is the generally used abbreviation for the compound which has been given the official name of dicophane. It was first synthesized in 1874, but it was not until 1940 that, as a result of research work in Switzerland, its remarkable toxic action on insects was discovered. This work was taken up and rapidly expanded in Great Britain and USA, and one of its first practical applications was in controlling the spread of typhus. This disease is transmitted by the louse, one of the insects for which DDT is most toxic. Its toxic action against the mosquito has also been amply proved, and it thus rapidly became one of the most effective measures in controlling malaria. DDT is toxic to a large range of insects in addition to the louse and the mosquito; these include houseflies, bed-bugs, clothes-moths, fleas, cockroaches, and ants. It is also active against many agricultural and horticultural pests, including weevils, flour beetles, pine sawfly, and most varieties of scale insect.

DDT has thus a wide use in medicine, public health, veterinary medicine, horticulture, and agriculture, both in temperate and tropical zones. Like all potent preparations, however, its indiscriminate use is not without danger. Thus, it is toxic to bees and a number of parasites of fruit pests, and may therefore do as much harm as good if used indiscriminately as a horticultural spray. Again, if used to kill fleas in animals such as cats, which lick themselves, care must be taken in using it, as it may be toxic when swallowed. It is quite safe when applied to the skin, either in man or animals, in a watery solution, but if applied in an oily solution it may be rapidly absorbed and produce toxic effects. When used for domestic purposes or on animals, it is usually applied as a 5 per cent dust. Full details concerning its use may be obtained from the many leaflets and booklets issued by the manufacturers, by government departments, and by agricultural and horticultural institutes.

Finally, there is the most worrying factor of all: the increasing number of species of insects which are becoming resistant to DDT. Fortunately, to date newer insecticides have been introduced which are toxic to DDT-resistant insects, but there is a certain amount of anxiety as to whether this supply of new insecticides can be maintained.

DEAD, DISPOSAL OF THE – Practically, only three methods have been used from the earliest times: (a) burial; (b) embalming; (c) cremation.

(a) **Burial** is perhaps the earliest and most primitive method, and, because of its practice among the Jews, and the popularly accepted idea as to the resurrection of the body, has become intimately bound up with the Christian religion. It was customary to bury the bodies of the dead in consecrated ground around the churches till the earlier half of the nineteenth century, when the utterly insanitary state of churchyards led to legislation for their better control, and now that cemeteries are supposed to be situated outside towns and in proper sites, the interment of the dead should seldom be a menace to the health of the living. Burials in Britain take place usually upon production of a certificate from a registrar of deaths, to whom notice of the death, accompanied by a medical certificate, must be given without delay by the nearest relatives.

(b) **Embalming** was practised by several races of antiquity, notably by the Egyptians, with the view of preserving from decay the bodies of dead friends. It is still used to a certain extent, particularly in the USA. The process consists in removing the internal organs by small openings and filling the body cavities with various aromatics of antiseptic power, the skin being swathed in bandages or otherwise protected from the action of the air. Bodies are also preserved by injecting the blood-vessels with strong antiseptics like perchloride of mercury. In certain circumstances bodies become naturally changed to a non-putrefying substance known as adipocere. (See PUTREFACTION.)

(c) **Cremation** was practised among the Greeks and the early Aryan races generally, and furnishes a much speedier reduction of the body to its simple components than does burial, and one devoid of any harmful tendencies to the living. Not the least of its advantages is the amount of space that is saved and can thereby be devoted to more useful and practical purposes. It is being used to an increasing extent. In 1977, there were 405,730 cremations in Britain, which accounted for 63 per cent of all burials.

In order to prevent any abuse, special certificates are required, and the necessary forms for these are obtained from the cremating authority. The law does not distinguish in England or USA between cremation and burial, but special formalities are insisted upon by the crematorium authorities. The ceremony is conducted similarly to a burial ceremony, the coffin is lowered from the mortuary chapel, through an opening, on to a trolley which bears it direct to the furnace. The process of incineration takes between one and two hours. About five to seven pounds (2·3 to 3·2 kg) of ash result from the combustion of the body, and there is no admixture with that from the fuel.

DEAD FINGERS (see RAYNAUD'S DISEASE).

DEADLY NIGHTSHADE is the popular name of *Atropa belladonna*, from which atropine is procured. Its poisonous black berries are sometimes eaten by children. (See ATROPINE; and BERRIES, POISONOUS.)

DEAFNESS is divided into three classes, according to the section of the ear at fault (illustration 119).

EXTERNAL EAR is the passage, about $1\frac{1}{2}$ inches (33 mm) in length, leading inward from the surface to the drum. When the deafness has its cause in this part, it is due simply to obstruction of the passage by a tumour, by a foreign body, such as a pea, or a polypus, or, most commonly of all, by a plug of hardened wax.

MIDDLE EAR is the tympanic cavity separated by the tympanic membrane from the outer ear, and communicating

the middle ear. Acute inflammation in the throat, for example in measles, or chronic conditions like adenoids in children, are liable to produce middle-ear disease, perforation of the drum, and deafness. Tearing of the drum in consequence of, for example, an explosion, as a rule heals and leaves no deafness; but a perforation following inflammation in the antrum or middle ear is accompanied by suppuration, discharge from the ear, and other changes, and generally attended by impairment of hearing unless effective treatment is instituted at an early stage. It is a peculiarity of deafness in middle-ear disease that the hearing is often better during a loud noise: for example, a conversation is more clearly heard while church bells are ringing, or in the noise of a railway train.

119 – The external and middle portions of the right ear from the front. *Gray's Anatomy.*

with the mastoid antrum, a hollow in the skull, behind, and with the Eustachian (or auditory) tube, which leads to the throat, beneath. These communications are important: the connection with the throat explains the deafness that accompanies a cold in the head and other forms of inflammation which spread from the nose and throat up into the middle ear; while the connection with the antrum shows why suppuration in the antrum causes great destruction of the delicate mechanism in

INTERNAL EAR AND BRAIN constitute the receptive and perceptive apparatus for sound, the outer and middle ear forming parts of the conducting and collecting apparatus. Certain fevers like typhus and typhoid, tumours of the brain, meningitis, Menière's disease, mumps, and fractures of the base of the skull may all bring on a greater or less degree of deafness by interference with the perceptive apparatus. Some drugs produce a temporary deafness, notably quinine and certain antibiotics, particularly dihydrostreptomycin and streptomycin.

The human ear, it has been said, is such a remarkable instrument that the largest sound that can be tolerated without pain and almost instantaneous permanent damage is five million times the smallest that can be heard at all. The following list gives some idea of the wide range of intensity of sound to which the ear is exposed:

	Decibels
Threshold of hearing	0
Whisper	30
Quiet bedroom in middle of night	35
Normal conversation	60–70
Fairly noisy factory	85–90
Tube train entering station	95
Jet plane at 200 metres	120
Discomfort	120
Pain	140

In spite of its versatility there is a limit to what the human ear will tolerate, and the amount of noise in our midst is causing increasing anxiety.

Boiler-maker's disease is a condition of deafness long recognized to be due to a gradual wearing out of the nervous mechanism by the constant noise of hammering, and comes on in a few years, especially in boiler-makers, but also in sawyers, threshing-mill tenders, and persons similarly subject to constant noise. The term, boiler-maker's disease, is now a misnomer as there are so many working conditions under which noise is a major hazard to hearing. The amount of deafness due to excessive noise at work is turning out to be much higher than was suspected, and at long last steps are being taken to reduce to a minimum the amount of unnecessary noise in industry. The current view is that for an eight-hour working day an acceptable upper limit of noise is around 90 decibels. Where the amount of noise cannot be reduced to a safe level, then workmen must be supplied with effective ear-protection. No ear-protector, however, is an effective substitute for a safe level of sound. In medicolegal terms, 'impairment' of hearing means hearing loss, 'handicap' implies that the loss of hearing has social consequences, whilst 'disability' is reserved for those in whom the damage leads to difficulties in employment.

The hereditary form of deafness known as otosclerosis (qv) comes on in several members of some families shortly after puberty, owing to hardening changes in the inner ear.

It is estimated that 1·75 million people, that is 3·5 per cent of the population of England and Wales, are affected by deafness. In those over the age of 75, more than half have impaired hearing.

Treatment – Deafness due to causes in the external ear is readily dealt with, and, considering the frequency of hardened wax, it is a good and safe procedure to syringe out the ear with a tumblerful of warm water containing a teaspoonful of baking soda (bicarbonate). The stream of water is directed along the upper wall of the passage and flows out below. In cases where deafness accompanies nasal catarrh, adenoids, enlarged tonsils, etc., these conditions must be remedied. (See NOSE, DISEASES OF.) In a case of perforation of the drum, accompanied by a chronic discharge, particular care must be taken to keep the ear clean; otherwise there is a danger not only of increased deafness but of retained matter infecting some neighbouring part, and causing a dangerous abscess in the brain, meningitis, or suppuration in the mastoid antrum. (See EAR, DISEASES OF.) Boilermaker's deafness generally improves if the occupation be changed; otherwise it grows steadily worse. Deaf-mutism is a condition where deafness has been complete from early life, usually from birth, and the child has never learned to speak, though the voice-producing organs are perfect. Such children can with patience, be taught to carry on a fluent conversation by means of lip-reading, or by the finger language and signs. Where adults are concerned there are wide variations in the ability to lip-read. Some are born lip-readers, the majority have a reasonable ability, some find it most difficult. What is important in the care of both adults and children is that full advantage be taken of whatever capacity they may have for hearing. Even a minimum of hearing ability makes lip-reading much more effective. (See also DUMBNESS; HEARING AIDS; and PRESBYACUSIS.)

A large range of effective hearing aids is now available, including the Medresco hearing aid supplied under the aegis of the National Health Service. These instruments are highly successful in the case of many deaf persons, though not of great use in others. Each instrument requires to be carefully tuned for the deaf person using it. Before deciding to use a hearing aid the advice of an ear specialist should be obtained. The Royal National Institute for the Deaf, 105 Gower Street, London, WC1E 6AH, provides a list of clinics where such a specialist can be consulted. It also gives reliable advice concerning the purchase and use of hearing aids.

DEAMINATION is the term applied to the process of removal of the amino group, NH_2, from amino-acids not required for building up body protein. This is carried out mainly in the liver by means of an enzyme, deaminase. The fatty acid residue is either burnt up to yield energy, or is converted into glucose.

DEATH, CAUSES OF – Although the final cause of death is usually failure of the vital centres which govern the beating of the heart and the act of breathing, the practical question is the disease or injury which leads to this failure. A general idea of the extent to which different causes operate in terminating life can be obtained from table 19.

Ischaemic heart disease	145,089
Malignant disease	117,765
Respiratory disease (excluding tuberculosis)	71,771
Cerebrovascular disease	68,291
Motor vehicle accidents	5,492
All other accidents	7,760
Suicide and self-inflicted injury	3,657
Congenital anomalies	3,134
Diabetes mellitus	4,570
Tuberculosis	898
Total	538,652

Table 19 – Some of the principal causes of death in England in 1977.

DEATH RATE – in 1977, the death rate in England was 11·6 per thousand compared with 11·96 in Scotland. In the international death stakes, based on what is known as the Standardized Mortality Ration (SMR), which is a more satisfactory method of comparison, England and Wales occupy an intermediate position. Among the thirty-one other countries available for comparison, England and Wales comes seventeenth for males (SMR 100) and fifteenth for females (SMR 100). The range of SMR's is 72 (Iceland) to 119 (Czechoslovakia) for males, and 72 (Iceland) to 125 (Romania) for females.

DEATH, SIGNS OF – There are some minor signs, such as relaxation of the facial muscles, which produces the staring eye and gaping mouth of the *Hippocratic countenance*, as well as a loss of the curves of the back, which becomes flat by contact with the bed or table; *discoloration of the skin*, which becomes of a wax-yellow hue, and loses its pink transparency at the finger-webs; *absence of blistering and redness* if the skin be burned (Christison's sign); and *failure of a ligature* tied round the finger to produce, after its removal, the

usual change of a white ring, which, after a few seconds, becomes redder than the surrounding skin in a living person.

The only certain sign of death, however, is *stoppage of the heart*, and to ensure that this is permanent it is necessary to listen over the heart, that is, over the chest at the inner side of the nipple, for five minutes. This can be done by means of a stethoscope or by listening directly with the ear on the chest. *Stoppage of breathing* should also be noted, and this can be confirmed by observing that a mirror held before the mouth shows no haze, that a feather placed on the upper lip does not flutter, or that the reflection on the ceiling from a cup of water placed on the chest of the dead person shows no movement. An important sign is that if a cut is made in the skin or a vessel be opened no bleeding takes place after death.

In the vast majority of cases there is no difficulty in ensuring that death has occurred. The introduction of organ transplantation, however, and of more effective mechanical means of resuscitation, such as respirators, whereby an individual's heart can be kept beating almost indefinitely, has raised difficulties in a minority of cases. To solve the problem in these cases the concept of 'brain death' has been introduced. In other words, if there is no evidence of brain activity, as shown by the absence of reflexes and the electro-encephalogram (qv), death is assumed to have occurred even though breathing and the beating of the heart can be maintained by artificial methods.

Four points are important in determining the time that has elapsed since death. *Hypostasis*, or congestion, begins to appear as livid spots on the back, often mistaken for bruises, three hours or more after death. It is due to the blood running into the vessels in the lowest parts. *Loss of heat* begins at once after death, and the body has become as cold as the surrounding air after 12 hours, though this is delayed by hot weather, death from asphyxia, and some other causes. *Rigidity*, or rigor mortis, begins in six hours, takes another six to become fully established, remains for twelve hours and passes off during the succeeding twelve hours. It comes on quickly when extreme exertion has been indulged in immediately before death. Conversely it is slow in onset and slight in death from wasting diseases. It is slight or absent in children. It begins in the small muscles of the eyelid and jaw and then spreads over the body. *Putrefaction* is variable in time of onset, but usually begins in 2 or 3 days, as a greenish tint over the abdomen. (See PUTREFACTION.)

DEBILITY means a state of weakness.
Treatment – The cause must, so far as possible, be removed. The essential is then rest, combined with regulated exercises, and good food. The person must be specially guarded, for the time being, from strains of all sorts and exposure to infectious diseases.

DEBRISOQUINE is one of the many new hypotensive agents being used in the treatment of high blood pressure.

DECAPSULATION is the term applied to an operation performed upon the kidney in some cases of Bright's disease. The capsule is stripped off, so that the kidney may expand.

DECIBEL is the unit of hearing. One decibel is the least intensity of sound at which a given note can be heard. The usual abbreviation for decibel is dB.

DECIDUA is the name of the soft coat which lines the interior of the womb during pregnancy and which is cast off at birth.

DECOCTION is the name for a preparation made by boiling various plants in water and straining the fluid.

DECOMPENSATION means a failing condition of the heart after compensation has been established in a case of valvular disease.

DECUBITUS is the name applied to the peculiar positions taken up in bed by patients suffering from various conditions. For example, patients with pleurisy or pneumonia prefer to lie upon the affected side; patients suffering from peritonitis, on the back; much exhausted persons, far down in the bed.
The bed sores (qv) which such patients are liable to develop are known as decubitus ulcers.

DECUSSATION is a term applied to any point in the nervous system at which nerve fibres cross from one side to the other: eg. the decussation of the pyramidal tracts in the medulla, where the motor fibres from one side of the brain cross to the other side of the spinal cord.

DEFAECATION means the act of opening the bowels. (See CONSTIPATION; DIARRHOEA.)

DEFICIENCY DISEASE is the term applied to any disease resulting from the absence from the diet of any substance essential to good health: eg. one of the vitamins.

DEFORMITIES may be present at birth, or they may be the result of injuries, or disease, or simply produced by bad habits, like the curved spine occasionally found in children. (See BURNS; CHEST, DEFORMITIES OF; CLUB-FOOT; FINGERS; FLAT-FOOT; KNOCK-KNEE; LEPROSY; PALATE, DEFECTS OF; PARALYSIS; RICKETS; SCAR; SKULL; SPINE, DISEASES OF; JOINTS, DISEASES OF.)

DEGENERATION means a change in structure or in chemical composition of a tissue or organ by which its vitality is lowered or its function interfered with. Degeneration is of various kinds, the chief being fatty, fibroid (see CIRRHOSIS), calcareous (see CONCRETIONS), waxy, colloid, and mucoid.
Causes of degeneration are, in many cases, very obscure. In some cases heredity plays a part, particular organs, for example the kidneys, tending to show fibroid changes in successive generations. Fatty, fibroid, and calcareous degenerations are part of the natural change in old age. Defective nutrition may bring them on prematurely, as may excessive and long-continued strain upon an organ like the heart. Various poisons, like alcohol, play a special part in producing the changes, and so do the poisons produced by various diseases, particularly syphilis and tuberculosis.

DEGLUTITION means the act of swallowing. (See CHOKING.)

DELHI BOIL is a form of chronic sore occurring in Eastern countries, caused by a protozoan parasite, *Leishmania tropica*. (See LEISHMANIASIS.)

DELIRIUM is a state of perverted consciousness in which an irregular discharge of nervous energy goes on, causing incoherent talk, delusions, and ill-regulated muscular action.
Varieties – There are three types.
LOW DELIRIUM is associated with exhaustion, and consists mainly of muttering or rambling talk, in which past events are jumbled together. Surrounding per-

sons and objects are not heeded, or their identity is totally mistaken. The fingers are sometimes busily employed in picking at the bed-clothes, or there is a constant twitching of the muscles, known as subsultus tendinum, in the arms, legs, and face, which is a sign of great weakness.

TREMBLING DELIRIUM (delirium tremens) is the form most commonly due to alcoholism (see ALCOHOLISM, ACUTE). In this form the mind is more active and delusions more extraordinary. Trembling is a specially marked feature, particularly in the early stages.

RAVING DELIRIUM sometimes appears in acute fevers, is often due to alcoholism, and is characterized by violent activity of the muscular system, acting in response to such wild delusions that it may result in suicide or homicide.

Treatment is, as a rule, the treatment of the causes. (See also ALCOHOLISM, ACUTE.) As the delirium in fevers is due partly to high temperature this should be lowered by tepid sponging (see COLD, USES OF). Careful nursing is one of the keystones of successful treatment, which includes ensuring that ample nutritious fluids are taken. When delirium banishes sleep and aggravates exhaustion, sleeping draughts are often necessary, such as paraldehyde or one of the barbiturates, and in severe cases even morphine and/or hyoscine.

DELIVERY means the final expulsion of the child in the act of birth. (See LABOUR.)

DELTA WAVES is the term given to abnormal electrical waves observed in the electro-encephalogram. (See ELECTRO-ENCEPHALOGRAPHY.) The frequency of the normal alpha waves is ten per second. That of the delta waves is seven or less per second. They occur in the region of tumours of the brain, and in the brains of epileptics.

DELTOID is the powerful triangular muscle attached above to the collar-bone and shoulder-blade, and below, by its point, to the humerus, nearly half-way down the outer side of the upper arm. Its action is to raise the arm from the side, and it covers and gives roundness to the shoulder.

DELUSIONS are errors in judgment, regarding simple facts, which interfere with the ordinary conduct of life. Thus a man may have the delusion that he has no stomach and refuse to take food. No amount of argument or demonstration will convince the subject of a delusion as to the error of his belief. The existence of a delusion, of such a nature as to influence conduct seriously is one of the most important signs in reaching a decision to arrange for the compulsory admission of the patient to hospital for observation. (See MENTAL ILLNESS.)

DEMENTIA is a form of insanity consisting of mental feebleness rather than derangement. It may come on acutely after some illness, but, as a rule, is chronic, and often succeeds other forms of insanity like melancholia and mania. Dementia is one of the changes almost natural in old age, and, whatever be the cause, it is one of the least hopeful forms of insanity. (See MENTAL ILLNESS.)

DEMETHYLCHLORTETRACY-CLINE, or LEDERMYCIN, is a tetracycline (qv) preparation which is effective in relatively low dosage and is said to be more stable than other tetracycline preparations.

DEMULCENTS are substances which exert a soothing or protective influence upon the surface of the alimentary canal.

Varieties – Mucilaginous substances like gum, isinglass, Iceland moss; oils like olive, linseed, and almond oils; starchy substances like arrowroot; also glycerin, borax, and mild alkalis, and fine powders like subnitrate of bismuth.

Uses – They are used in cases of inflammation, particularly of the throat and stomach, in gargles or draughts, to protect these parts from the irritation of their own secretions; and after injury, such as that due to swallowing a corrosive poison, in order to soothe the pain and encourage healing in the injured part.

DENGUE, also called BREAK-BONE FEVER, DANDY-FEVER, and THREE-DAY FEVER, is a disease of tropical and subtropical regions caused by an arbovirus (qv) transmitted to man by the mosquito, *Aëdes aegypti*. It is a sudden and short infectious fever, with an incubation period (see INCUBATION) of a few days, characterized mainly by swelling and pains in the joints, and by skin eruptions.

Symptoms – It usually begins suddenly with pain in a joint and fever. Next appears redness of the face, spreading later over the body, very much like the rash of measles. This itches intensely. There are also sore throat and running of the eyes, and the muscles and joints generally become very painful. These symptoms endure for about three days, and then gradually pass off, leaving the person very weak. After two or three days a relapse generally takes place, very similar to the first attack. There may be a third or even a fourth relapse, and recovery from the weakness and pains in the joints is often slow, often lasting over months. Death hardly ever occurs.

Treatment – Aspirin, with or without codeine, usually relieves the pains and reduces the temperature though in more severe cases pethidine may be needed to bring relief. Calamine lotion eases the itching of the rash.

DENGUE HAEMORRHAGIC FEVER is a more acute form of the disease which occurs predominantly in young children and seems to be confined largely to the indigenous population of South-east Asia.

DENTINE is the dense white material of which the greater part of the teeth is composed, and which constitutes ivory. The dentine is pierced by numberless fine tubules which communicate with the sensitive pulp in the central hollow of the tooth, hence its sensitiveness when the enamel, which covers the dentine with a thin transparent shell, is eaten away or broken. The dentine is specially liable to decay, so that when the enamel is defective in one spot, a large cavity is apt to form beneath it. (See TEETH.)

DENTITION (see TEETH).

DEODORANTS are substances which remove or lessen objectionable odours. Some, which have a powerful odour, simply cover other smells, but the most effective act by giving off oxygen, so as to convert the objectionable substances into simple and harmless ones.

Varieties – Volatile oils of plants, such as eucalyptus and turpentine, chlorine water and chlorinated lime, peroxide of hydrogen, charcoal, dry earth, sawdust, and permanganate of potassium, are among the most powerful.

Uses – The main use is to purify sewage, bilge-water, and water-closets. Many powerful deodorants act, at the same time, as disinfectants. They are also used in sick-rooms to cover the smell of discharges, and the like. For the manner of use see under the individual deodorants.

DEOXYCORTONE ACETATE is a synthetic corticosteroid (qv).

DEPILATION is the process of destroying hair; substances and processes used for this purpose being known as depilatories. The purpose may be effected in three ways: (1) by removing the hairs at the level of the skin surface; (2) by pulling the hairs out (epilation); (3) by destroying the roots and so preventing the growth of new hairs.

Shaving is the most effective way of removing superfluous hairs. Rubbing morning and night with a smooth pumice-stone is said to be helpful. The alkaline sulphides used as depilatories tend to erode the skin as well as the hairs. Electrolysis and diathermy have a limited use. In some cases of excessive hairiness in women the cortices of the suprarenal glands may be hypertrophied. Surgical correction of this is sometimes followed by a dropping out of the excessive hairs.

DEPRESSOR is the name given to a nerve by whose stimulation motion, secretion, or some other function is restrained or prevented: eg. the depressor nerve of the heart slows the beating of this organ.

DEQUALINIUM CHLORIDE is an antibacterial and antifungal compound which is of value in the treatment of infections of the mouth, gums, and throat, and in certain skin conditions.

DERBYSHIRE NECK is a name for goitre, which is fairly common in Derbyshire. (See GOITRE.)

DERMABRASION, or 'surgical planing', is a method of removing the superficial layers of the skin, which is sometimes useful in the removal of tattoos and superficial blemishes of the skin.

DERMATITIS means inflammation of the skin, though its differentiation from eczema is by no means clear. Indeed, different dermatologists (or skin specialists) use the two terms in quite different ways. Fortunately, such terminological inexactitudes, as George Robey would have described them, do no harm to the patient as the cause and treatment of the various conditions can usually be defined, no matter what the specialist may name them. For the present purpose only three forms of dermatitis will be considered here: contact dermatitis, light dermatitis, and exfoliative dermatitis. (See also DERMATITIS under OCCUPATIONAL DISEASES.)

Atropic Dermatitis (see NEURODERMTOSES).

243

Contact Dermatitis is dermatitis caused by contact between the skin and some substance to which the skin is sensitive. The skin eruption may vary from mere redness to severe inflammation of the skin. The onset may be gradual or sudden, depending upon how sensitive the individual is to the incriminating substance. A large range of substances can produce contact dermatitis, including cosmetics such as lipstick, hair dyes, shampoos, perfumes, nail varnish, face powder and rouge; nylon hair nets; rubber sponges; dyes used in clothing; nickel, chromium and rubber, as used in suspenders; contraceptives; paints and varnishes; and plants. So far as plants are concerned, the most important in Britain is the indoor primula, *Primula abconica*; next comes chrysanthemum, anthemis (the stinking mayweed) and the giant hogweed. Medicaments applied to the skin as ointments, lotions and the like are an increasing cause of contact dermatitis. For this reason antibiotics, such as penicillin, are seldom used in the form of such local applications lest they should render the patient sensitive. Not only does this expose the patient to the unnecessary discomfort of a contact dermatitis, it may also mean that the patient can no longer be given the antibiotic in question, when it may be a life-saving measure, because the patient has been rendered sensitive, or allergic, to it by what was in fact an entirely unnecessary local application of it sometime in the past. The diagnosis of the condition is usually fairly simple, one of the important factors being the localization of the dermatitis. Thus, if it occurs on the thigh in a woman it may well be due to her suspenders, whereas if it occurs in the armpit it may be due to some dye in her clothing or to some deodorant spray she has been using. In doubtful cases the diagnosis can usually be settled by what is known as a patch test. This consists of applying a small amount of the suspected sensitizing substance to an area of normal skin. If the individual is sensitive to the substance in question, an area of dermatitis appears beneath the patch in twenty-four to forty-eight hours, and the test is said to be positive.

Prevention consists in the first instance of finding the cause and then making sure the afflicted individual has no further contact with it.

Treatment varies with the severity of the condition. In relatively mild cases the application of calamine lotion is often all that is necessary. In more severe cases this is supplemented by the application of a corticosteroid (qv). The area involved should not be washed with soap, but cleaned with olive oil, or an emulsion of water and Emulsifying Ointment, B P. When the condition has become chronic, with thickening and scaliness of the skin, there is often quite intense itching, and the resultant scratching makes the condition worse. In such a case the application of Compound Zinc Paste, B P, to which coal tar has been added, brings relief and aids healing.

Dermatitis herpetiformis is a bullous, or blob-like, eruption often mistaken for eczema or scabies. It is associated with a sensitivity to gluten (qv). It responds to a gluten-free diet or to the administration of dapsone (qv).

Light Dermatitis, or LIGHT ERUPTION, is a dermatitis, with reddening and blistering of the skin, which occurs on exposure to sunlight. It is recognized by the fact that it occurs on the parts of the body normally exposed to sunlight – the face, neck and hands – and that its incidence is between April and September. It takes two main forms. One is an exaggerated form of sunburn, and this soon passes off. The other occurs in individuals who are photo-allergic. In other words, they have been rendered allergic, or sensitive, to sunlight by some substance. This may be a drug, and the drugs most likely to be responsible are the phenothiazines which include some of the antihistamine drugs and some of the tranquillizers, and the sulphonamides. Eosin in lipstick and perfume in cosmetics may also be the responsible sensitizing agent. In some individuals no sensitizing agent can be implicated, and it is assumed that this form of the condition, sometimes referred to as *polymorphic light eruption*, is due to some innate sensitivity in the individual's skin. It is this form of the condition which is most likely to be seen in children.

Treatment consists of treating the dermatitis as already outlined. To protect the skin a powder should be applied which contains some substance such as titanium dioxide that absorbs the ultra-violet rays in sunlight which cause the trouble. For the unfortunate minority for whom no remedy can be found, the only remedy is the wearing of shady hats, long sleeves and gloves.

Exfoliative Dermatitis, or ERYTHRODERMA as it is also known, is a condition which begins with patches of erythema, or reddening of the skin, followed by gradual thickening of the skin which then begins to desquamate, or peel off. It gradually spreads until practically the whole of the body is involved. It is rare before the age of 50, and is three times more common in men than in women. In over half the cases it occurs in people with some other skin condition, usually chronic eczema or psoriasis. In about a third no cause can be found, and in the remainder it develops in patients with Hodgkin's disease (qv), mycosis fungoides (qv) or chronic leukaemia (see LEUKAEMIA).

Treatment – No matter what the underlying cause, treatment consists of large doses of corticosteroids. (See also SKIN DISEASES.)

DERMATOGLYPHICS is the study of the patterns made by the ridges and crevices of the hands and the soles of the feet. It has become an important study in medicine because of the help it provides in the diagnosis of certain diseases, such as mongolism. It is also proving of value in certain other congenital diseases. Thus, a recent study showed abnormal palmar findings in 64 per cent of patients with congenital heart disease (qv) compared with only 17 per cent of patients with acquired heart disease.

DERMOGRAPHIA, also known as DERMOGRAPHISM and URTICARIA FACTITIA, is a condition in which tracings made on the skin leave a distinct swollen, reddish mark. It occurs in allergic individuals, in whom the stimulus of scratching the skin produces an excessive amount of histamine. (See ALLERGY.)

DERMATOMYOSITIS is a disease of unknown origin, characterized by erythema of the skin and wasting of the muscles.

DERMOID CYST (see CYSTS).

DERRIS is the dried root of several species of Derris, the active constituent of which is rotenone. It is used as an insecticide and larvicide, and also for the control of warble fly in cattle. A form known as Prepared Derris used to be widely used in the treatment of scabies.

DESFERRIOXAMINE is a preparation which is proving of value in the treatment of iron poisoning.

DESQUAMATION means the scaling off of the superficial layer of the epidermis.

DETERGENTS are substances which clean the skin surface. This means that, strictly speaking, any soap, or soap-like substance used in washing, is a detergent. At the present day, however, the term is largely used for the synthetic detergents which are now used on such a large scale. These are prepared by the cracking and oxidation of high petroleum waxes with sulphuric acid. The commoner ones in commercial preparations are aryl alkyl sulphate or sulphonate and secondary alkyl sulphate.

Considering their widespread use they appear to cause relatively little trouble with the skin, but more trouble has been reported with the so-called 'biological' detergents that were introduced some years ago. They are so named because they contain an enzyme (qv) which destroys protein. As a result they are claimed to remove proteins – stains such as blood, chocolate, milk or gravy, which are relatively difficult for ordinary detergents to remove. Unfortunately these 'biological' detergents may cause dermatitis of the hands. In addition, they have been reported to cause asthma in those using them, and even more so in workers engaged in manufacturing them.

DETOXICATION means reduction or removal of the toxic properties of poisons or remedies. (See VACCINES.)

DEVONSHIRE COLIC is caused by drinking cider which has been stored in contact with lead, so that colic comes on as a result of lead poisoning. (See COLIC; LEAD POISONING).

DEXAMETHASONE is a corticosteroid derivative. As an anti-inflammatory agent it is approximately 30 times as effective as cortisone and eight times as effective as prednisolone. On the other hand, it has practically none of the salt-retaining properties of cortisone.

DEXTRAN is the name given to a group of polysaccharides which was first discovered in sugar-beet preparations which had become infected with certain bacteria. Of recent years, a homogeneous preparation of it, with a consistent molecular weight and free from protein, has been introduced as a substitute for plasma for transfusion purposes.

DEXTRIN is a soluble carbohydrate substance into which starch is converted by diastatic ferment or by heat. It is thus contained in toast, the crust of bread, biscuits, and breakfast foods. It is a white or yellowish powder which, dissolved in water, forms mucilage. Animal dextrin, also known as glycogen (qv), is a carbohydrate stored in the liver after meals, often to considerable amount.

DEXTROMORAMIDE is a potent, habit-forming analgesic, or pain-reliever, which is active whether taken by mouth or given by injection.

DEXTROSE is another name for purified grape sugar or glucose.

DIA- is a prefix meaning through or thoroughly.

DIABETES INSIPIDUS is a disease characterized by excessive thirst and the passing of large volumes of urine which has a low specific gravity and contains no abnormal constituents. It is due to lack or diminution of the antidiuretic hormone normally produced by the posterior lobe of the pituitary gland. (See PITUITARY BODY.) This faulty secretion may result from a lesion involving the posterior lobe of the pituitary gland or a lesion in the base of the brain adjacent to this gland. The condition may be hereditary or due to some pathological process, such as inflammation, a tumour, or syphilis, involving the base of the brain. Treatment consists of the administration of vasopressin, the posterior pituitary extract which contains the antidiuretic hormone. This is given either by injection or by nasal insufflation. Some cases respond satisfactorily to chlorothiazide (qv) given by mouth. Promising results are also being reported from the use of a preparation known as DDAVP as a nasal spray. This condition, which is relatively rare, must be carefully differentiated from the other form of diabetes – DIABETES MELLITUS – which is an entirely different disease.

DIABETES MELLITUS is a constitutional disorder in which the power of the muscles and other tissues to utilize sugar for purposes of nutrition is greatly diminished or lost, as a result of lack of insulin, the internal secretion of the pancreas. In consequence of this, weakness and various other symptoms appear, while the sugar accumulates in the blood and is excreted in the urine and lost to the system.
Causes – In 1889 Mering and Minkowski found that diabetes frequently followed removal of the pancreas from animals. Subsequent work gradually established that, in all cases of diabetes, there is a defect in the chemistry of the body, whereby the muscles cannot absorb the sugar derived from the food, so that a gradual wastage takes place in the muscular tissue all over the body. This defect was attributed by Sharpey-Schafer, so long ago as 1909, to the failure of the pancreas to produce a hormone for which he proposed the name of 'insulin'. Despite the general acceptance of this theory, insulin was not isolated until the year 1921, when it was successfully obtained for the first time by Banting and Best taking advantage of the degeneration in the pancreas of an animal which follows ligature of the duct of the gland. Insulin, which is produced by the cells in the pancreas known as the islets of Langerhans, is obtained from the pancreas of cattle by a special process of extraction.
It is important to remember that glycosuria (ie. sugar in the urine) can occur in conditions other than diabetes mellitus. Thus, it is a common finding in thyrotoxicosis (qv) and in certain disorders of the pituitary gland. Emotional disturbance may also cause temporary glycosuria in certain individuals. Glycosuria, which is not due to diabetes, may also occur during pregnancy.
Diabetes is more prevalent during middle age in corpulent people than in persons of average physique. In adults the disease usually appears insidiously and has in most cases been present for some time before an examination of the urine reveals the condition by chance. On the other hand, in children the onset may be sudden. Exposure to wet and cold, privation, depressing mental conditions or mental overwork are predisposing causes to the onset of diabetes mellitus in susceptible individuals, but, of all predisposing causes, infection is the most important. Obesity is another important predisposing factor. There appears to be a distinct tendency for diabetes to run in families. It is most common among adults. Certain races are particularly prone to this disease, such as the Jewish race and Hindus, but this increased liability is probably in large part due to habits of life and diet. It is estimated that more than 1 per cent of the British people, that is more than half a million people, are diabetics, but half of them remain undetected.
Symptoms – The symptoms of diabetes are usually gradual in onset, and the disease is often discovered by chance before the patient complains of any definite symptoms. The first symptoms which

attract attention are usually failure of strength and loss of weight, along with great thirst and passage of an increased amount of urine. Dryness of the skin and mouth and constipation also form frequent complaints. The urine, from the normal quantity of between 2 and 3 pints (1 and 1·5 litres) in 24 hours, may be increased to 10, or even 20 pints (5 or 10 litres). It is usually clear, pale in colour, and is of high specific gravity (1030 to 1050). The quantity of sugar passed in 24 hours may vary from a few ounces to several pounds, and it is of course markedly increased after sugary or starchy food has been taken. The amount of sugar circulating in the blood rises from about 0·1 per cent, which is normal, to 0·2, 0·3, or more per cent, and it remains high for several hours after a meal instead of being rapidly absorbed.

A troublesome symptom is the intense thirst, which the patient is constantly seeking to allay, and the quantity of liquid consumed is proportional to the amount of urine passed. There is sometimes a voracious appetite. The mouth is always parched and in severe cases a faint sweetish odour can be recognized at times on the breath, owing to the escape of acetone and diacetic acid from the blood into the air in the lungs. The patient gradually becomes more and more emaciated and suffers from increasing muscular weakness; dyspepsia and constipation are commonly present. Owing to the poor vitality of the tissues, various skin eruptions appear, boils and carbuncles being especially common, and, in fact, sometimes giving the first sign of the presence of disease. The sugar deposited from the urine is liable to cause itching about the groins, and eczema of various parts of the body is set up by the presence of sugar in the sweat. The skin, as the disease advances, becomes dry and harsh, with a papery consistency. There is a special tendency to gangrene of the skin of the feet, beginning with the toes, and this forms a very serious complication of diabetes.

Diabetes, as a rule, advances comparatively slowly except in the case of young people, in whom its progress is apt to be rapid. Indeed, in a general way, it is more serious the younger the subject of the disease. Various complications arise in its course, among which may be mentioned dimness of vision due to cataract, weakness and pains in the limbs due to neuritis, inflammatory chest affections, of which pulmonary tuberculosis is the most important and may be the cause of death.

Occasionally death occurs from exhaustion or from the condition known as diabetic coma, in which acetone and similar bodies known as ketones, accumulate in the system, and in which the breathing becomes slower and slower, the person gradually more deeply unconscious, and death ensues in a few hours or days.

Cases may continue for many years without material change for the worse, especially in elderly subjects. The most unfavourable cases are those in which serious chest or other complications have arisen, and cases in which the disease has already become of severe and established character before it is recognized.

Treatment – The aim of treatment is to restore carbohydrate metabolism to as near normal as possible, and the two main guides as to how successfully this is being attained are the blood-sugar concentration and the amount of sugar and ketone bodies (eg. acetone) in the urine. The patient's general health is also of importance here, but it will usually be found that there is a direct correlation between the first two and the patient's sense of wellbeing. The one important exception to this occurs in the case of middle-aged and elderly diabetics, many of whom feel better with a rather high blood-sugar level than they do when the blood-sugar level is brought down to within normal limits. In other words, the diabetic must not become too introspective about the amount of sugar he finds on testing his urine, nor must the doctor attach all his interest to the concentration of sugar in the blood of his diabetic patients. Generally speaking, once a diabetic patient has been stabilized in his treatment, there is no need for him to test his own urine provided he is feeling well and is attending his doctor or his diabetic clinic at regular intervals. Conversely, it is equally important that the moment he begins to feel unwell, eg. develops dyspepsia, a cough, or 'a cold', he should report at once to his doctor.

The treatment of uncomplicated diabetes mellitus can be divided into two sections: (1) diet; (2) insulin. These can, again, be divided into two stages: (a) stabilization; (b) maintenance.

DIET – Of recent years the tendency has been to give the diabetic patient as liberal a diet as possible, except in the case of the obese patient in whom it is essential to obtain a reduction of weight. It has also been recognized that, as diabetes mellitus practically always persists for the rest of the patient's life, dietetic restrictions should be reduced to a minimum so that he should be able to lead as normal a life as possible. The simplest and most satisfactory way of attaining this is to control the amount of carbohydrate in the diet and not to worry (except in special cases) with the relative proportions of fat and protein in the diet. If the ordinary diabetic patient is taking an ordinary mixed diet in which the carbohydrate content is controlled, then there is seldom any need to worry about the fat and protein. If bread is used as the standard, and it is remembered that 1 ounce of bread contains 15 grams of carbohydrate, there is little difficulty in working out the daily diet from the following data (tables 20, 21), once it has been decided how much carbohydrate is to be taken each day and how this amount is to be divided between the four main meals of the day.

Butter	Green vegetables
Cheese	Asparagus
Eggs	Celery
Bacon	Marrow
Meat	Mushrooms
Fish	Leeks
Clear soup	Tomatoes
Tea	Cranberry
Coffee	Grapefruit
	Green gooseberries
	Loganberry
	Melon
	Red currants
	Rhubarb

Table 20 – Articles of food that can be taken freely.

The following amounts of some of the commoner articles of diet are equivalent in carbohydrate content to 1 ounce of bread (table 21):–

Cereals

Flour	3 dessert-spoons
Porridge	3 dessert-spoons
Rice	1 dessert-spoon
Semolina	1 dessert-spoon
Tapioca	1 dessert-spoon

Fruit

$\frac{1}{2}$ lb of: apples, figs, pears, pineapple.
1 lb of: apricots, blackberries, black currants, cherries, damsons, greengages, peaches, plums, raspberries, strawberries.
1 oz of: prunes.
2 oz of: dates.
2 oranges.
2 bananas.

Vegetables

$\frac{1}{2}$ lb of: beetroot, broad beans, carrots, onions, peas.
3 oz of: potatoes.

Miscellaneous

$\frac{1}{2}$ pint of milk.
1 dessert-spoon of jam or marmalade.

Table 21 – Carbohydrate equivalents.

When diabetes mellitus is first diagnosed, it is usual to initiate treatment by diet alone unless the condition is very severe, when the immediate use of insulin may be called for. The usual initial diet is one containing 100 grams of carbohydrate (ie. 6–7 ounces of bread or its equivalent) daily. If the diabetes improves on this diet, then it is gradually increased by 50-gram stages every two or three weeks, so long as the blood-sugar level remains satisfactory. In milder cases such dietetic control may be all that is necessary, but if it is impossible to control the diabetes in this way, then insulin is necessary.

INSULIN – Nine forms of insulin are now available: insulin injection; biphasic insulin injection; globin zinc insulin injection; isophane insulin injection; neutral insulin injection; protamine zinc insulin injection; insulin zinc suspension; insulin zinc suspension (amorphous); insulin zinc suspension (crystalline). All these have to be given by injection. The essential difference between these nine forms is their duration of action. Thus, the action of insulin injection begins in 20 to 30 minutes and reaches its maximum in 4 to 5 hours. With protamine zinc insulin the blood sugar begins to fall in 5 to 11 hours, and the maximum effect is obtained in 15 to 20 hours. With globin insulin the effect begins in 1 to 2 hours, and reaches a maximum in 8 to 16 hours. Isophane insulin begins to act in 2 hours and its action persists for 24 hours. Insulin zinc suspension has a fairly rapid onset of action which persists for 24 hours. Insulin zinc suspension (amorphous) has also a fairly rapid onset of action, but this lasts for only 12 to 16 hours. Insulin zinc suspension (crystalline) has a somewhat delayed onset of action which persists for 24 hours.

In stabilizing a new case of diabetes which requires insulin, it is advisable to use insulin injection. A usual initial dose is 10 to 20 units night and morning. This involves an alteration in the distribution of the daily allowance of carbohydrate, the greater part having to be equally divided between the two meals corresponding to the injections of insulin: ie. breakfast and supper. The amount of insulin is gradually increased every four or five days until a satisfactory blood-sugar level is attained. The subsequent course of treatment depends upon the individual response of each patient. The aim in an active patient, who is not overweight, is to allow him to take a diet containing 200 to 300 grams of carbohydrate daily. In the case of children, 300 grams of carbohydrate daily should be considered the minimum if full health and adequate growth are to be maintained. In the case of the obese patient, a diet of 1100 Calories, containing 60 grams of carbohydrate daily, is the optimum one to obtain a reduction in weight without undue discomfort to the patient.

Once the patient is stabilized on a given diet and insulin injection, a decision is then taken as to whether the maintenance insulin is to be insulin injection or one of the others. The theoretical advantage of the delayed-action insulins is that they maintain a steadier blood-sugar level throughout the 24 hours; their practical advantage is that they involve only one injection every day instead of two. The final decision in each case as to which form of insulin to use is one to be decided by the medical attendant in charge of the case.

Oral hypoglycaemic agents – Certain sulphonamide and biguanide derivatives have recently been introduced which, when taken by mouth, lower the level of the blood sugar. The available evidence indicates that, as a substitute for insulin, they are only of value in a certain proportion of mild cases of diabetes mellitus. The great majority of severe, and, the majority of moderately severe, diabetics fail to respond to these oral agents. The use of these agents should therefore be restricted to those mild, or relatively mild, diabetics in whom: (i) Diet alone fails to bring the blood sugar within or near normal limits. (ii) The dietary restriction required to control the diabetes causes progressive loss of weight or severe hunger. (iii) The withdrawal of insulin is not followed by relapse into significant acidosis. The dose of insulin that can be replaced by these oral agents seldom exceeds 30 units. (See BI-GUANIDES; CHLORPROPAMIDE; GLIBENA-CIDE; GLYMIDINE; METFORMIN; PHENETHYL-DIGUANIDE; SULPHONYLUREAS; and TOLBU-TAMIDE.)

Dangers – The danger which is always present in cases of diabetes is the occurrence of *acidosis*, which, in severe cases, proceeds to *diabetic coma*. An indication of the presence of this condition is given when a large amount of acetone along with sugar is found in the urine. This is a dangerous condition unless it is immediately treated with full doses of insulin.

This type of coma must be carefully differentiated from *hypoglycaemic coma*, which is due to an overdose of insulin resulting in an extreme fall in the blood-

sugar concentration. Milder forms of hypoglycaemia are relatively common, manifesting themselves by a sinking feeling, a sensation of hunger, a feeling of sickness, giddiness, or breaking out in a sweat. The treatment consists of the administration of sugar in some form – by mouth if the patient is conscious, by intravenous injection if the patient is unconscious. Every diabetic subject who is subject to hypoglycaemia should carry sugar about with him, in the form of lumps of sugar or barley sugar, so that he can easily avert an attack should he feel it coming on.

Another serious danger incurred by the subject of diabetes is the occurrence of *gangrene* in the skin, especially about the toes. In order to avoid this, special care must be taken to keep the feet in a healthy condition by frequent washing, treatment of corns and abrasions, and avoidance of tight shoes. Other forms of infection, such as boils, must also be treated with special care on ordinary principles. In consequence of the generally poor vitality of the tissues, diabetic patients often form bad subjects for *surgical operations*, but since the introduction of insulin the outlook has improved considerably, and, with careful preoperative care, there is seldom much need for worry. The frequency with which *chest complications* supervene in diabetes has been mentioned, and special precautions must be taken to avoid catarrhs.

People with diabetes mellitus, or their relatives, can obtain advice from the British Diabetic Association, 3–6 Alfred Place, London, WC1E 7EE.

DIACHYLON (see LEAD).

DIAGNOSIS is the art of distinguishing one disease from another, and is essential to scientific and successful treatment. The name is also given to the opinion arrived at as to the nature of a disease. It is in diagnosis more than in treatment that the highest medical skill is required, and, for a diagnosis, the past and hereditary history of a case, the symptoms complained of, and the signs of disease found upon examination are all weighed. Many methods of laboratory examination are also used at the present day in aiding diagnosis.

DIALYSIS is the process whereby crystalloid and colloid substances are separated from a solution by interposing a semipermeable membrane, such as cellophane, between the solution and pure water. The crystalloid substances pass through the membrane into the water until a state of equilibrium, so far as the crystalloid substances are concerned, is established between the two sides of the membrane. The colloid substances do not pass through the membrane.

This is the principle upon which the artificial kidney works. (See KIDNEY, ARTIFICIAL.) When, as in the artificial kidney, the patient's blood is used, the process is known as *haemodialysis* (qv). An alternative technique is to circulate the dialysing fluid through the abdominal cavity, thus using the peritoneum (qv) as the semipermeable membrane. This is the process known as *peritoneal dialysis*.

DIAMORPHINE and DIACETYLMORPHINE are other names for heroin (qv).

DIAPEDESIS (see INFLAMMATION).

DIAPHORESIS is another name for sweating. (See PERSPIRATION.)

DIAPHORETICS are remedies which promote perspiration. By imperceptible perspiration, or insenble perspiration as it is technically known, the body loses around a pint (500 ml) of moisture daily. Under exertion or in a heated atmosphere, this natural function of the skin is increased, sweating more or less profuse follows, and, evaporation going on rapidly over the whole surface, little or no rise in the temperature of the body takes place. In some forms of disease, such as fevers and inflammatory affections, the action of the skin is arrested, and the surface of the body feels harsh and dry, while the temperature is greatly elevated. The occurrence of perspiration often marks a crisis in such diseases, and is in general regarded as a favourable event. (See PERSPIRATION.)

Varieties and uses – Many means can be used to induce perspiration, among the best known being baths, either in the form of hot-vapour or hot-water baths, or the exposure of the body to a dry and hot atmosphere or to beams of electric light in a special apparatus. (See BATHS.) Such measures, particularly if followed by the drinking of hot liquids and the wrapping of the body in warm clothing, seldom fail to excite copious perspiration. Numerous medicinal substances have a similar effect, one of the oldest of these being Minidererus spirit (acetate of ammonia). Opium acts as a diaphoretic, when in combination with ipecacuanha, as in Dover's

powder, and alcohol, as well as aspirin, and similar drugs, also produces perspiration. (See under these headings.) When employed at the start of a common cold, diaphoretics sometimes check it or at least ameliorate it. In certain circumstances, diaphoretics, particularly in the form of baths, may be unsafe, especially where there is any affection of the heart or lungs attended with embarrassed respiration.

DIAPHRAGM, or MIDRIFF, is the muscular partition which separates the cavity of the abdomen from that of the chest. It is only a small fraction of an inch in thickness, and is of a dome shape, extending up on the right side to the space beneath the fourth rib, on the left to that beneath the fifth. In contact with its lower surface are, on the right side, the liver, right kidney, and suprarenal body, and to the left the stomach, pancreas, left kidney, suprarenal body, and spleen; while upon its upper surface lies the heart, with a lung on either side. The diaphragm is attached by its edge to the lower margin of the chest all round, and consists of muscular fibres meeting round a trefoil-shaped piece of fibrous tissue in the centre. It completely shuts off the above-named cavities from one another, being pierced only by openings for the gullet, the aorta, and the inferior vena cava, with a few minute openings for nerves and small vessels. The diaphragm is of great importance in respiration, playing the chief part in filling the lungs. During deep respiration its movements are responsible for 60 per cent of the total amount of air breathed.

DIAPHYSECTOMY is the term applied to the operation whereby a part of the shaft of a long bone (eg. humerus, femur) is excised.

DIARRHOEA or looseness of the bowels, is really a symptom of some disease situated in the bowels, but deserves special mention because of its potentially serious import.

Varieties and causes – Diarrhoea forms the chief symptom of several *serious diseases*, but it would be a great mistake to imagine that, by checking the diarrhoea, the disease is of necessity successfully treated. For example, the severity of an attack of cholera or dysentery is gauged mainly by the extent to which diarrhoea is present; in typhoid fever, persons fed upon ordinary diet have much diarrhoea, so that this is a usual feature in early stages of this disease; in tuberculous ulceration of the intestine diarrhoea occurs which speedily brings down the sufferer. In some diseases of the liver, kidneys, lungs, or heart, diarrhoea ensues as a result of congestion of the bowels, or through the bowels taking up in part the eliminating functions of the damaged organs. In such cases the diarrhoea may actually be a salutary thing. These special forms are considered under the headings of the respective diseases which produce them. Recurring attacks of diarrhoea occur in some cases of habitual constipation, owing to irritation caused by the presence of hard faecal masses.

Catarrhal diarrhoea is the ordinary form, and in it the intestinal mucous membrane is in much the same condition of congestion and swelling as the nasal mucous membrane during a 'cold in the head', and secretes, in great amount, clear, viscid mucus of a similar nature. This catarrhal diarrhoea may be produced in a slight degree by indigestible food, by nervous excitement, or as the result of a chill. In a severer form, it may be due to infection by micro-organisms of the food-poisoning group (see FOOD POISONING), or to drugs such as mercury and arsenic. Atmospheric conditions may also play a part, some persons developing an attack of diarrhoea upon a change of weather, just as others develop a catarrhal condition in the air-passages.

Diarrhoea in infants is such a serious condition that it requires separate consideration. One of its features is that it is usually accompanied by vomiting. Some ten per cent of the cases in this country are due to the dysentery organisms (qv) and will not be considered here. The remainder constitute the group of cases now usually referred to as infantile gastroenteritis. The condition is rare after the age of fifteen months, and the majority of cases occur between the ages of two and four months. The younger the infant, the higher the mortality rate. This is the type of diarrhoea which used to be known as 'summer diarrhoea' because of its high incidence in the late summer, but during recent years this seasonal incidence has tended to disappear. The precise cause is still obscure, but certain strains of the organism known as *Escherichia coli* (*E. coli*) are responsible for some cases, whilst in others a virus may be the cause. One important predisposing factor is artificial feeding. The condition is rare in breast-fed babies, and when it does occur in these it is usually less severe. The environment of the infant is also important. The condition

is highly infectious and, if a case occurs in a maternity home or a children's hospital, it tends to spread like wildfire. This is why such an institution is closed to all further admissions if a case of infantile gastro-enteritis occurs; and is not opened until the infection has been completely eradicated. A third factor is infection elsewhere in the body, particularly in the ear or the mastoid.

Lienteric diarrhoea is a chronic form, in which a movement of the bowels occurs shortly after every meal. The condition may become so aggravated that food passes rapidly and undigested through the body, and the sufferer becomes very thin.

Pancreatic diarrhoea is a form occasionally met in children of imperfect development, in consequence of failure by the pancreas to secrete its proper digestive fluid.

Ulcerative colitis is a serious condition characterized by the passage of frequent stools containing blood. (See COLITIS.)

Diarrhoea may also be a symptom of ulceration or gangrene of the bowels, and is then associated with the passage of *blood and mucus*, or even of shreds of membrane produced by the destruction of the inner surface of the bowels.

Treatment – The treatment of diarrhoea which is an incident of special diseases like cholera, typhoid fever, dysentery, is considered under these heads.

ACUTE DIARRHOEA, it must be remembered, is often merely a symptom either of one of the above diseases or of some local disease like intussusception, so that if the symptom be treated as if it were the real disease, the consequence may be disastrous to the sick person. Assuming that we are dealing simply with cases of uncomplicated *catarrhal diarrhoea*, we may consider the treatment of an adult and child separately. In the case of both, rest in bed is essential until the diarrhoea has subsided.

In adults, if the attack has followed the eating of some indigestible substance, a dose of a purgative may be given. To control the diarrhoea the two most effective drugs are kaolin and opium. Kaolin may be given in doses of one tablespoonful thrice daily; alternatively, in doses of 30 grains (2 G) it may be combined in a mixture with 10 minims (0·6 ml) of chlorodyne. If the diarrhoea lasts more than a couple of days, an enema consisting of starch cream (4 ounces (115 G)) with laudanum (20 drops) is useful, given every six hours. If there is much discomfort with distension of the abdomen, a turpentine stupe (qv) may be of value. During the first twenty-four hours of an acute attack, no food should be given, but the individual must be given ample water. In less acute cases barley water may be given. This, as in the case of water, should be given in small amounts at frequent intervals. Later, milk or arrowroot made with water is given. After the severer symptoms of diarrhoea have passed off, the affected person must exercise great caution for several days in respect to diet. A gradual return should be made to ordinary food, consisting at first of eggs, milk, and milk puddings, followed later by fish, and only after the lapse of several days by meat and vegetables.

In infants treatment is highly specialized, and much depends upon efficient nursing. The child or infant must be completely isolated from all other children. Drugs play little part in the treatment, which is largely dietetic. Opium and its derivatives are badly tolerated by these infants and should not be used. The evidence concerning the value of the sulphonamide drugs and antibiotics is contradictory, but recent reports suggest that when the infant is not responding to dietetic treatment and the temperature is raised, one of the sulphonamides or one of the antibiotics should be given. Severe cases should receive such therapy from the outset. If there is any evidence of infection elsewhere in the body, eg. the ear, this must be treated at once. When there is no evidence of dehydration, ie. the infant has not lost much fluid in the stools or the vomit, the infant should be starved for twelve to twenty-four hours, but during this period should be given plenty of fluid to drink in small amounts at frequent intervals. A useful guide as to how much should be given is that up to the age of 6 months the average daily requirement of a baby is $2\frac{1}{2}$ ounces per pound of body weight. A suitable drink is the Compound Sodium Chloride and Dextrose Powder of the *British Pharmacopoeia Codex*, which can be obtained from any chemist. One of these powders should be dissolved in 500 millilitres (18 ounces). An alternative is $\frac{1}{4}$-strength saline and 5 per cent glucose, either together or alternating with each other, by mouth. When feeding is re-instituted, this should consist of half-strength, half-cream National Dried Milk, alternating with the glucose-saline mixture, in frequent small feeds. After 24 hours, if progress is maintained the infant is given half-strength, half-cream milk. The strength of the milk is gradually in-

creased until, usually within a matter of five to seven days, the infant is able to take all feeds of full-strength National Dried Milk.

When dehydration is present, the outlook is much more serious, and adequate fluid must be given either subcutaneously or intravenously. The fluid is usually glucose in saline, but some prefer to use Hartman's solution (isotonic sodium lactate) instead of the saline. During the first twelve or twenty-four hours of intravenous administration, nothing is given by mouth. By the end of this time vomiting has usually stopped, and then feeding by mouth can be started very gradually.

TODDLER DIARRHOEA is a form of diarrhoea in otherwise healthy-looking infants who are growing normally, in which frequent loose stools are passed containing undigested food. The cause is not known and no treatment is needed. It usually clears up after the age of about 2 years.

CHRONIC DIARRHOEA requires, above all things, full investigation to try and determine the cause, complete rest in bed and a simple diet, such as peptonized milk, or white of egg in water, or tea and toast. Washing out of the lower bowel through a soft rubber tube, and the injection of various soothing and astringent fluids, may be of benefit. Kaolin in doses of 1 teaspoonful or more in water after meals has sometimes a beneficial effect.

DIASTASE is the name of a ferment found in germinating seeds, and is contained in large quantity in malt, which has the property of converting starch into sugar. It can be extracted as a white soluble powder. *Takadiastase* is a diastatic ferment produced by the action of a fungus, *Aspergillus oryzae*, upon wheat bran. It is used as a medicine in cases where starch is improperly digested.

DIASTASIS is a term applied to separation of the end of a growing bone from the shaft. The condition resembles a fracture, but is more serious because of the damage done to the growing cartilage through which the separation takes place, so that the future growth of the bone is considerably diminished.

DIASTOLE means the relaxation of a hollow organ. The term is applied in particular to the heart, to indicate the resting period between the beats (systoles), while blood is flowing into the organ.

DIATHERMY is a process by which electric currents can be passed into the deeper parts of the body so as to produce internal warmth and relieve pain; or, by using powerful currents, to destroy tumours and diseased parts bloodlessly. The form of electricity used consists of high-frequency oscillations, the frequency of oscillation ranging from 10 million to 25,000 million oscillations per second.

The so-called ultra-short-wave diathermy (or short-wave diathermy, as it is usually referred to) has replaced the original long-wave diathermy, as it is

By concentrating the current in a small electrode, the heating effects immediately below this are very much increased, and the method may be used to produce the effects of a cautery in surgical conditions. It differs from ordinary forms of cautery because it is cold when brought into contact with the patient, and gradually becomes heated by the current. Its surgical application has been used in treating malignant ulcers, particularly of the mouth, throat, and bladder, where ordinary surgical means are not readily available.

120 – A microwave diathermy machine. *The Practitioner.*

produced consistently at a stable wavelength (11 metres) and is easier to apply. In recent years microwave diathermy (illustration 120) has been developed, which has a still higher oscillating current (25,000 million cycles per second, compared with 500 million for short-wave (diathermy).

When the current passes, a distinct sensation of increasing warmth is experienced and the temperature of the body gradually rises; the heart's action becomes quicker; there is sweating and increased excretion of waste products. The general blood-pressure is also distinctly lowered. The method is used in painful rheumatic conditions, both of muscles and joints, and in severe cases of neuritis, such as sciatica.

DIATHESIS is another name for constitution. (See CONSTITUTION.)

DIAZEPAM is a tranquillizing drug related to chlordiazepoxide (qv), which is said to possess muscle-relaxant properties and therefore to be of value in the treatment of muscular rheumatism.

DIBUTYL PHTHALATE is an insect repellent. It is less effective than dimethyl phthalate (qv), but has the advantage of being harmless to clothing and resists washing better. When rubbed into clothing it may give protection for up to a fortnight.

DICEPHALUS is the term applied to a foetal 'monster' having two heads.

253

DICHLORALPHENAZONE is a non-barbiturate sedative, consisting of a complex of chloral hydrate (qv) and phenazone (qv).

DICHLOROPHEN is a drug for the treatment of tapeworm infestations. The dose is 70 mg per kg body weight, given as a single dose or in three divided doses eight-hourly.

DICOPHANE is the official name for DDT (qv).

DICOUMAROL is a substance isolated from spoiled sweet clover which causes a haemorrhagic disease in cattle. Dicoumarol has been synthesized and is used in clinical medicine to reduce the coagulability of blood in conditions in which this is desired: eg. in the prevention and treatment of thrombosis. It is active when given by mouth, and much cheaper than heparin. (See ANTICOAGULANTS.)

DICROTIC pulse is one in which at each heart-beat two impulses are felt by the finger. A dicrotic wave is naturally present in a tracing of any pulse as recorded by an instrument for the purpose, but in health it is imperceptible to the finger. In fevers, a dicrotic pulse indicates considerable prostration, in which the heart continues to beat violently while the small blood-vessels have lost their tone. (See PULSE.)

DIELDRIN is one of the most effective insecticides available as it combines a prolonged action with a highly lethal action on insects. In addition, it is toxic to a wide range of insects. On the other hand, it is more toxic to man than DDT, and must therefore be handled with care.

DIENOESTROL is a synthetic oestrogen closely related to stilboestrol (qv). It is not as potent as stilboestrol, but as it would appear to be less toxic, it may, for this reason, have certain advantages over stilboestrol.

DIET is a subject of the greatest importance. Information as to the change in diet necessary in special diseases will be found in the sections on these diseases, and what will be said here refers to general principles of feeding. Details regarding the diet of young children are given under INFANT FEEDING.

Dietetic principles – The body is, in many respects, comparable to an engine. Like a piece of machinery it requires fuel to supply the muscles, etc., with energizing power for the various bodily activities, and it likewise needs building materials to repair loss from wear and tear. For the latter purpose, food containing nitrogen is necessary, the protein of which the muscles and other tissues are composed being replaceable only by fresh nitrogen-containing protein. For the necessary supply of energy protein would suffice but, as its use for this purpose would throw upon the kidneys and other excretory organs the necessity of getting rid of a large residue, fats and carbohydrates (including starch and sugars), which contain only carbon, hydrogen, and oxygen, are more convenient for the purpose. In addition to these three varieties of food, water must be taken in sufficient quantity to make up for the loss by the urine, sweat, etc., and also various salts, of which, however, there is always a surplus in the food. Certain substances known as vitamins, which are present in small quantities in a variety of foods, are also essential, as are certain minerals.

The daily protein requirement of the average man lies between 70 and 100 grams a day, or a bit more than 1 gram of protein for every kilogram of body weight a day. Growing children require, in proportion to their weight, a greater allowance of protein than adults.

The scientific mode of expressing the food requirements is stated in terms of energy-producing power. Kilocalorie, or large Calorie, is the name applied to the amount of heat necessary to raise the temperature of a kilogram (2 pounds) of water from 15° to 16° C, and of these Calories of energy 4·1 are obtainable by burning a gram of protein or of carbohydrate, and 9·3 by combustion of the same amount of fat. In estimating the energy expended by an individual in climbing a mountain, doing his daily work, and the like, one expresses it as so many Calories, while the amount of food which is burned up in the body by the process may be similarly stated.

Quantity of food – The total daily amount of food necessary for a fair-sized man, doing average hard work, should provide over 3000 Calories of energy, and since about 4 ounces (110 grams) of the daily food must be protein, to supply wear and tear, this leaves 2500 Calories to be supplied by carbohydrate and fat together. The proportion of these to one another

Occupation	Energy expenditure (kCal./day)		
	Mean	Minimum	Maximum
		Men	
Elderly retired	2330	1750	2810
Office workers	2520	1820	3270
Colliery clerks	2800	2330	3290
Laboratory technicians	2840	2240	3820
Elderly industrial workers	2840	2180	3710
Building workers	3000	2440	3730
University students	2930	2270	4410
Steel workers	3280	2600	3960
Farmers	3420	2900	4000
Army cadets	3490	2990	4100
Coal miners	3660	2970	4560
Forestry workers	3670	2860	4600
		Women	
Elderly housewives	1990	1490	2410
Middle-aged housewives	2090	1760	2320
Laboratory technicians	2130	1340	2540
Assistants in department store	2250	1820	2850
University students	2290	1380	2500
Factory workers	2320	1970	2980
Bakery workers	2510	1980	3390

Table 22 – Daily rates of energy expenditure by individuals in Scotland with various occupations. *Davidson and Passmore.*

depends upon minor considerations; for example, the Eskimos make it up in fat, because, in the northern regions, sugar and cereals are unobtainable. The natives of India, and the poorer classes of the world in general, use cereal food because of its great cheapness as compared with fat, and persons of feeble digestive power consume large quantities of soft fats, because – fat being, bulk for bulk, more than double the caloric value of carbohydrate – the digestion of a sufficiency of food is rendered easier by the use of a predominance of the former. For a diet giving about 3000 Calories a day these may be suitably provided thus: carbohydrate, 400 grams; fat, 110 grams; protein, 90 grams; providing, respectively, 1640, 1020 and 370 Calories.

The degree of physical activity plays a large part in deciding how many calories an individual requires. Table 22 shows the daily rates of energy expended by individuals in various occupations in Scotland, whilst table 23 shows the recommendation of the Department of Health and Social Security for individuals undertaking varying degrees of activity. In western communities, such as the United Kingdom and the United States of America, the emphasis today must be on the number of Calories consumed by those in sedentary occupations, for it is these members of the community – directors, other office workers and the like – who are tending to consume far more Calories than are good for them, and are thereby putting on weight.

Quality of food – After the energizing

power of a substance has been ascertained, there remain several other factors which determine its suitability as a food. *Digestibility* is one of the most important, for, while petroleum, sawdust, and the like have a high energy-producing power, they are absolutely useless as foods. *Absorbability* is also of importance, for few substances are completely absorbed into the system, and some, like vegetable proteins, are even rejected if taken as food in large amounts, and passed by the bowels unchanged. Thus a considerable amount of all food eaten, and especially of the coarser kinds, remains unused. *Satisfying power* is of great importance, and depends partly upon the bulk of the food and

Age	Occupation	Calories
Men		
18–35	Sedentary	2700
	Moderately active	3000
	Very active	3600
35–65	Sedentary	2600
	Moderately active	2900
	Very active	3600
65–75	Sedentary	2350
75 and over	Sedentary	2100
Women		
18–55	Most occupations	2200
	Very active	2500
55–75	Sedentary	2050
75 and over	Sedentary	1900
Pregnancy		2400
Lactation		2700

Table 23 – Recommended average daily intake of Calories for adults in the United Kingdom. The ages are from one birthday to another. Thus 18 to 55 means from the 18th birthday up to, but not including, the 55th birthday.

partly upon its preparation. Except in certain special circumstances, such as food for invalids, food should not be capable of too rapid digestion. Hence also the value of cooking certain foods with fat, which, when it penetrates the other food, retards digestion. To a certain extent, the more satisfying a food is the less digestible it proves; and this is one of the chief reasons why different foods and different methods of cooking suit persons of diverse physique and digestive powers. *Preparation* by cooking is also important. The effect of cooking is partly to develop flavours in the food, and so make it more palatable and digestible; partly to kill organisms and animal parasites which may be present in it; and, mainly, in the case of meats, to soften the connective tissues which bind the meat proper, and, in the case of vegetables, to burst or tear the fibres and capsules of cellulose which surround the starchy and sugary material. *Cheapness* is of immense importance to the less well paid sections of the community. Animal protein, as beef, forms the dearest food, and bread is by far the cheapest, well deserving the name of 'the staff of life'. Among the cheapest and most efficient forms of protein food are skimmed milk, cheese and fish. Fat has double the energy-producing power of carbohydrates, but butter is more than four times as expensive as its equivalent in bread. Hence fatty foods are called 'rich foods'. Nevertheless margarine falls into the list of cheap foods and is quite as nutritious as butter, and, since September 1939, all margarine has had the vitamins A and D added up to the level of some butter. *Freshness* is important, since preserved foods tend to lose their vitamins, and the daily diet should include vegetables, fruit, milk, butter, cheese.

WATER	PROTEIN	FAT	CARBO-HYDRATE	ASH

122 – Bacon

Fuel value per lb = 3090 calories

	per cent
Water	18·8
Protein	9·4
Fat	67·4
Ash	4·4

123 – Cod

Fuel value per lb = 300 Calories

	per cent
Water	82·6
Protein	15·8
Fat	0·4
Ash	1·2

124 – Oyster

Fuel value per lb = 230 calories

	per cent
Water	86·9
Protein	6·2
Fat	1·2
Carbohydrate	3·7
Ash	2·0

121 – Beef Steak

Fuel value per lb = 1090 Calories

	per cent
Water	61·9
Protein	18·6
Fat	18·5
Ash	1·0

125 – White Bread

Fuel value per lb = 1180 calories

	per cent
Water	35·3
Protein	9·2
Fat	1·3
Carbohydrate	53·1
Ash	1·1

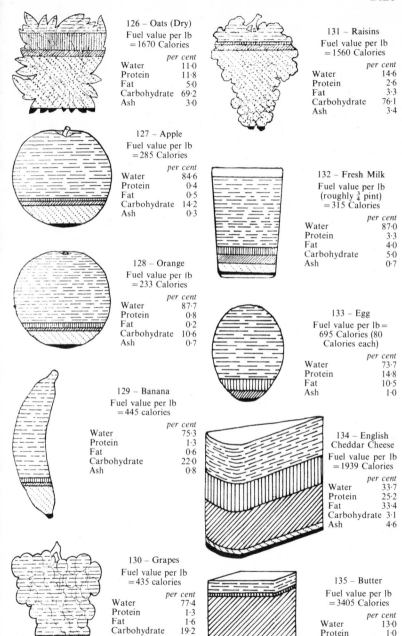

126 – Oats (Dry)

Fuel value per lb
= 1670 Calories

	per cent
Water	11·0
Protein	11·8
Fat	5·0
Carbohydrate	69·2
Ash	3·0

127 – Apple

Fuel value per lb
= 285 Calories

	per cent
Water	84·6
Protein	0·4
Fat	0·5
Carbohydrate	14·2
Ash	0·3

128 – Orange

Fuel value per lb
= 233 Calories

	per cent
Water	87·7
Protein	0·8
Fat	0·2
Carbohydrate	10·6
Ash	0·7

129 – Banana

Fuel value per lb
= 445 calories

	per cent
Water	75·3
Protein	1·3
Fat	0·6
Carbohydrate	22·0
Ash	0·8

130 – Grapes

Fuel value per lb
= 435 calories

	per cent
Water	77·4
Protein	1·3
Fat	1·6
Carbohydrate	19·2
Ash	0·5

131 – Raisins

Fuel value per lb
= 1560 Calories

	per cent
Water	14·6
Protein	2·6
Fat	3·3
Carbohydrate	76·1
Ash	3·4

132 – Fresh Milk

Fuel value per lb
(roughly $\frac{3}{4}$ pint)
= 315 Calories

	per cent
Water	87·0
Protein	3·3
Fat	4·0
Carbohydrate	5·0
Ash	0·7

133 – Egg

Fuel value per lb =
695 Calories (80
Calories each)

	per cent
Water	73·7
Protein	14·8
Fat	10·5
Ash	1·0

**134 – English
Cheddar Cheese**

Fuel value per lb
= 1939 Calories

	per cent
Water	33·7
Protein	25·2
Fat	33·4
Carbohydrate	3·1
Ash	4·6

135 – Butter

Fuel value per lb
= 3405 Calories

	per cent
Water	13·0
Protein	1·0
Fat	83·0
Ash	3·0

136 – Cabbage

Fuel value per lb
= 123 Calories

	per cent
Water	93·0
Protein	1·6
Fat	0·3
Carbohydrate	4·5
Ash	0·6

137 – String Bean

Fuel value per lb = 190 Calories

	per cent
Water	89·2
Protein	2·3
Fat	0·3
Carbohydrate	7·4
Ash	0·8

138 – Potato

Fuel value per lb
= 375 Calories

	per cent
Water	78·3
Protein	2·2
Fat	0·1
Carbohydrate	18·4
Ash	1·0

139 – Chestnut

Fuel value per lb
= 1820 calories

	per cent
Water	5·9
Protein	10·7
Fat	7·0
Carbohydrate	74·2
Ash	2·2

140 – Walnut

Fuel value per lb
= 3180 Calories

	per cent
Water	2·5
Protein	16·6
Fat	63·4
Carbohydrate	16·1
Ash	1·4

The *source* of food is not indifferent. It might be thought that a person well fed on peas would have the same powers as one fed on their equivalent in beef, but those races and individuals who feed upon a largely animal diet are characterized by the power of doing work more rapidly, by greater spirit, and by greater power of resisting disease. Although, as a general principle, this is true, and although it forms the main argument against the suitability of vegetarianism for those doing severe work, it may be carried to a very fanciful extreme, as in the case of Kean, the actor, who would choose his dinner according to the part he was to play, taking pork for a tyrant, beef for a murderer, and mutton for a lover. Probably, in such a case, ease of digestion had more to do with the effect of the food than its source.

The main objection to *vegetarianism* – at least in its extreme form – apart from that just stated, lies in the enormous bulk of vegetable food necessary, mainly in consequence of the relatively large amount of water it contains. Thus, if one were to subsist on nothing but lentil porridge, about 5 pounds (2·25 kg) of it would be necessary daily; or if one lived solely on green vegetables and succulent fruits, the impossible weight of about 30 pounds (13·5 kg) every day would be necessary to a fairly hard-working healthy man. Those vegetarians who add milk, eggs, and cheese to their food reach at once a healthy and rational diet, and one which, in those liable to gout and rheumatism – and for most people – is more salutary than a full ordinary diet.

External conditions produce great differences in the need for food. In cold climates, or in those persons unusually exposed to the weather, a special addition of fats or carbohydrates must be made to the diet in order to maintain the body heat. For the same reason a tall, spare man requires a much greater supply of these foods than a short, fat man of the same weight. Such a difference in configuration may mean the necessity for adding one-quarter or more of the amount of food.

Age and sex are important considerations. A woman requires about four-fifths of the diet of a man about the same size and build, the reduction affecting chiefly the starchy and sugary elements of her food. Children require much more protein – ie. building material – in proportion to their size than adults; whilst old people, on the other hand, if they wish to keep healthy, should be sparing eaters, particularly of animal foods.

The recommended daily intakes for children and adolescents in the United Kingdom are shown in table 24, whilst those for men and women are shown in table 23 (on page 255).

Age (years)	Calories
Boys and Girls	
0 to 1	800
1 to 2	1200
2 to 3	1400
3 to 5	1600
5 to 7	1800
7 to 9	2100
Boys	
9 to 12	2500
12 to 15	2800
15 to 18	3000
Girls	
9 to 18	2300

Table 24 – Recommended average daily intake of Calories for children and adolescents in the United Kingdom. The ages are from one birthday to another. Thus, 0 to 1 means from birth up to, but not including, the first birthday.

Articles of diet – Further details, regarding the various articles in common use as foods, are given under BREAD; CANNED FOODS; CEREAL; MILK; PROTEIN; INFANT FEEDING. Some of the substances added to foods are mentioned under ADULTERATION OF FOODS. The articles of food which may most suitably be taken in various diseased conditions are mentioned under the headings of the various diseases.

Diet for athletes and manual workers – For long it has been traditional for athletes in training to eat large amounts of meat. There is, however, no evidence to suggest that this is necessary. Carbohydrate, and not protein, is the best source of energy. Although there is still considerable difference between theory and practice, the views of dietitians and athletes are now converging, and it is now generally accepted that a simple and sufficient diet is what is required. The same holds true for manual workers. In the case of an athlete, it is probably advisable for him to go on a lighter diet for a day or two before the contest for which he is training, making certain that this contains ample carbohydrate. There is probably also much to be said in favour of taking glucose shortly before the event. There is also some evidence that the requirements of certain components of the vitamin B complex increase with exercise, so that care should be taken to ensure that there is ample vitamin B in the diet. Ample fluids should also be taken, but there is no evidence that alcohol is of any advantage.

The total daily Calories should be about 4500, and the following list gives some indication of the foods to be taken:

Foods for Calories – Dripping, suet, butter, margarine, bacon, cheese, bread, flour, sugar, jam, syrup, dried fruits, potatoes, cereals.
Foods for first-class proteins – Milk, cheese, eggs, meat, fish.
Foods for vitamins – Vitamin A: dairy foods, liver, tomatoes, green and yellow vegetables. Vitamin B: yeast, liver, kidney, whole-meal bread, bacon, ham, wheat germ. Vitamin C: citrus fruits, swedes, potatoes, green vegetables, liver. Vitamin D: fat fish, summer milk, and butter.

Invalid diet – One of the advances of recent years has been the recognition of the importance of diet in the treatment of disease. Whilst this is best exemplified in the case of diabetes mellitus, there are many other conditions in which special diets are ordered. Thus, in chronic constipation a high-roughage diet is indicated, containing whole-meal bread, bran, vegetables (particularly salads and coarse green vegetables), fruit, nuts and the drinking of plenty of water. In chronic cholecystitis a low-fat diet is necessary, whilst in jaundice a diet rich in first-class protein and carbohydrate is prescribed. Low-Calorie diets are the most effective for obesity, whilst a low-sodium diet is an essential part of the treatment of dropsy.

In febrile conditions the diet depends upon the expected duration of the fever. Thus, in a long-continued fever, such as typhoid fever, the essentials are that the diet should have a high Calorie value (3000 Calories), a large proportion of carbohydrate (380 grams), adequate protein (70–80 grams), and be given in easily digestible form in small amounts every two hours.

On the other hand, in fevers of short duration, eg. pneumonia, the amount of nourishment taken is not of such importance. If the individual is receiving ample fluid, including at least two pints (1 litre) of milk daily, there is little to worry about for several days. Again, small feeds should be given every two hours. To increase the nutritional value of the diet, and yet still impose no strain upon the digestive organs, glucose may be added to the water the patient drinks, and this can be flavoured with fruit juice, the addition of which ensures an adequate intake of vitamin C. If the patient desires more food, this may be given in the form of eggs (lightly boiled or poached), milk puddings (eg. junket, arrowroot), or jellies.

DIETHYLCARBAMAZINE CITRATE

During convalescence it is necessary to give as nourishing a diet as possible. On the other hand, digestion is sometimes not satisfactory, and the appetite is fickle. The following is a typical convalescent diet which provides approximately 2500 Calories:

Early morning – Sweetened orange juice.

Breakfast – Fruit, breakfast cereal with milk, egg, toast with butter and marmalade (or honey), weak tea (or coffee) with milk and sugar.

Mid-morning – Glass of milk, biscuit (or sandwich) and Marmite.

Lunch – Steamed white fish, or chicken, or rabbit, or sweetbreads, or tripe; potatoes (mashed with milk), vegetable purée, milk pudding or custard with stewed fruit.

Tea – Sandwiches – cress or Marmite, biscuits or sponge-cake, weak tea with milk and sugar.

Dinner (or Supper) – As for lunch. An egg-dish may be preferred to fish or meat, eg. an omelette.

Bed-time – Glass of hot milk, or Horlicks, or Ovaltine, biscuit if desired.

DIETHYLCARBAMAZINE CITRATE is a derivative of piperazine, which is proving of value in the treatment of filariasis and other parasitic diseases.

DIETL'S CRISES (see KIDNEY, DISEASES OF under MOVABLE KIDNEY).

DIGESTION, ABSORPTION, and ASSIMILATION are the three processes by which food is incorporated in the living body. In digestion, the food is softened and converted into a form which is soluble in the watery fluids of the body, or, in the case of fat, into very minute globules. In absorption, the substances formed are taken up from the bowels and carried throughout the body by the blood. In assimilation, these substances, deposited from the blood, are united with the various tissues for their growth and repair. For the maintenance of health each of these must proceed in a regular manner. Transit time through the digestive tract in young and middle-aged people in Britain averages two to four days, all but twelve hours of this being in the colon. Transit time is probably longer in the elderly.

SALIVARY DIGESTION begins as soon as the food enters the mouth. Saliva runs from the minute orifices of the salivary gland ducts, and contains a ferment named ptyalin, which actively changes the starch of bread, potatoes, and the like, into sugar. The object of chewing is not only to bruise the food, and make it more permeable for the gastric juice, but also to mix the starchy parts thoroughly with saliva. This process goes on, after swallowing, for the first twenty minutes or half-hour that the food remains in the stomach, after which the action of the saliva is checked by the acid of the gastric juice.

GASTRIC DIGESTION begins a little time after the food enters the stomach, the gastric juice exuding rapidly from the openings of the minute glands with which the interior surface of this organ is covered. The gastric juice begins to be secreted even before the food enters the stomach, at the sight and smell of food (psychic secretion). This juice contains ferments or enzymes, named pepsins, which have the power to break down the proteins of food into smaller molecules containing fewer amino-acids and to clot milk. There are also present free hydrochloric acid, which aids the action of pepsin and prevents putrefaction of the food, and acid salts, such as phosphate of soda, which have a similar action. The slow, churning movements which take place in the walls of the stomach have the effect of thoroughly mixing the food and gastric juice, and, to a slight extent, of breaking up the former. The main function of the stomach is to render the ingested food soluble, and mix it thoroughly with the gastric juice until it assumes a gruel-like consistency. This material, known as *chyme*, is then passed through the pylorus into the intestine. Very soon after soft food has been taken, waves of movement may be seen on X-ray examination, the orifice at the lower end of the stomach (pylorus) opens, and the food is squeezed quickly in small quantities into the bowel; but if any hard food comes in contact with the stomach wall near the exit the orifice at once closes. Gastric digestion of a simple meal of tea, bread, butter and jam should be complete in about an hour, a meal containing milk, eggs or light meat requires three or four hours, while a heavy dinner with soup, meat, fruit, and wine or beer is not entirely treated by the stomach till six or seven hours have elapsed. Hence the English plan of taking the heavy meal of the day (dinner) in the evening is a sound one, giving time during the night for the later stages of digestion.

INTESTINAL DIGESTION – The softened food, or chyme, which leaves the stomach is exposed in the bowels to the action of four factors: (*a*) bile, (*b*) pancreatic juice, (*c*) intestinal juice, (*d*) bacteria. Bile is collected from the liver and gall-bladder into the common bile-duct, which, together with the duct from the pancreas, opens into the duodenum a short distance from the exit of the stomach (illustration 141). The bile consists mainly of complex salts and pigments, which assist in digesting the fats of the food, and partly of waste products removed from the blood. The pancreatic juice contains four powerful ferments, which have the

141 – Diagram of alimentary canal to illustrate the organs concerned in digestion. M, Mouth; Ph, pharynx; OE, oesophagus; S, stomach; D, J, I, small intestine; into the duodenum D open P, the pancreatic duct, and DC, the common bile duct; G, gall-bladder; H, hepatic duct; C, AC, TC, DC, large intestine; R, rectum; AV, appendix.

following effects: lipase breaks down fats into glycerol and fatty acids; amylase completes the digestion of starch; and trypsin and chymotrypsin carry on the breaking down of proteins begun in the stomach. Intestinal juice contains small amounts of enzymes which (1) complete the breakdown of proteins into the constituent amino-acids; (2) act upon the disaccharides, maltose, sucrose and lactose, converting them into the monosaccharide glucose; (3) split fats into fatty acids and glycerin. Bacteria are normal inhabitants of both small and large intestine. In the former they have a fermentive, in the latter a putrefactive, action. In the former they act upon carbohydrate to produce acetic, butyric, and lactic acids. In the latter, bacteria decompose protein into such products as histamine, phenol, cresol, indole, skatole. These are no longer believed to be responsible for the ill-effects of constipation. The intestinal bacteria also play an important and valuable role in the manufacture of certain components of the vitamin B complex.

ABSORPTION – The only substance absorbed from the stomach to any extent is alcohol. Water is quickly passed from the stomach into the intestine, and considerable quantities are there absorbed in a few minutes. But it is only after subjection to digestion in the intestine for several hours that the bulk of the food is taken up into the system. The semi-solid chyme which leaves the stomach is converted into a yellowish fluid of creamy consistence called chyle by the action of bile and pancreatic fluid. From this the fats, in the form of a fine emulsion, are taken up by lymph vessels called lacteals, and ultimately reach the blood, while sugars, salts, and amino-acids formed from proteins pass directly into the small blood-vessels of the intestine. The process is facilitated by the extreme unevenness of the intestinal wall, which is folded into many ridges and pockets, while, in microscopic structure, the surface is covered by fine finger-like processes named villi (illustration 142), which are bathed in the fluids passing down the intestine. Further, absorption is probably assisted by the leucocytes, or white cells of the blood, which are increased in numbers after a meal, and which have the power of wandering out of the blood-stream and taking up particles into their substance. Food materials are absorbed almost exclusively by the small intestine. The large intestine, or colon, absorbs water and salts. The food is passed down the intestine by the contractions of its muscular coat, and, finally, the indigestible residue, together with various waste substances excreted from the liver and intestinal walls, is cast out of the body in the stools.

142 – Section of small intestine (jejunum), showing four of the villi with which the inner surface is covered. Magnified 110 times. 1, villus; 2, intestinal gland, crypt of Lieberkühn; 3, muscularis mucosae; 4, submucosa; 5, circular muscular coat; 6, longitudinal muscular coat; 7, serous coat; 8, 9, nerve plexuses. From *Hewer's Textbook of Histology*. William Heinemann Ltd.

ASSIMILATION takes place more slowly, the blood circulating through every organ, and each taking from it what is necessary for its own growth and repair. Thus the cells in the bones extract lime salts, muscles extract sugar and protein, and so forth. When the supply of food is much in excess of the immediate bodily requirements it is stored up for future use, fat being deposited in various sites, sugar

being converted into glycogen in the liver. The greater bulk of nutriment is assimilated by the muscles for heat production and work, the sugar and amino-acids being built up into a substance which forms the permanent part of the muscle. The substance so formed undergoes chemical changes, and is broken down to form carbonic acid, lactic acid and other waste products as the muscle does work. Various hormones, such as insulin, which is an internal secretion of the pancreas, circulate in the blood and are concerned in these processes. For all these processes to function satisfactorily an adequate daily intake of water is necessary; about three pints (1·5 litres) are drunk or taken with the food and absorbed daily, a similar amount being discharged from the body in the urine, perspiration, and other excretions.

DIGITALIS is the leaf of the wild foxglove, *Digitalis purpurea*, gathered when the flowers are at a certain stage, dried, and powdered. The leaf contains several active principles, which can be extracted in various ways. Its action is to strengthen involuntary muscular contraction, particularly that of the muscle fibres in the heart and blood-vessels. It is one of the most valuable remedies we have in cases of disease of the heart, associated with rapid or irregular beating of this organ, and with dropsy. Upon the heart it has the double action of increasing the strength of each beat and of lengthening each intervening pause (diastole), so that the muscle of the damaged organ obtains longer periods for rest and repair. It also lessens the conductivity of the heart muscle, so that feeble and ineffective beats tend to disappear, when the action is irregular. By thus acting on the heart, it causes the production of more urine by the kidneys and a consequent decrease of existing dropsy in cases in which the dropsy is due to heart failure.

Uses – Digitalis may be given as a powder, as tincture, as infusion and also in the form of sugar-coated 'granules' which contain the active principle of the drug. The most common form of administration is the powder given in the form of a tablet. It is the great stand-by in the treatment of heart failure accompanied by, or likely to be accompanied by, dropsy. Its action is particularly useful when the heart failure is due to atrial fibrillation, the condition in which the heart rate is wholly irregular. In such cases the digitalis slows the heart rate by abolishing many of the weak heart-beats which, although of no value in helping to maintain an efficient circulation, yet put an additional and useless strain on the heart muscle. (See also DIGOXIN.)

DIGITALIS POISONING may occur from taking medicinal doses over too long a period, or from taking a single overdose. There are nausea and vomiting, and blurring of vision may occur, with objects appearing yellow or green. The heart, which is made slower and more regular by taking small doses, becomes again quicker and more irregular as the result of excessive administration. At the same time breathing gets more difficult, and there may be convulsions or unconsciousness. The amount of urine passed gets less and less, thus causing retention in the system of the drug, which is naturally got rid of by the kidneys.

Treatment – The drug must be stopped. If a single overdose has been swallowed, the stomach should be washed out.

DIGOXIN is a crystalline glycoside obtained from *Digitalis lanata*. It is used for the same purpose as digitalis, and has the advantage that it can be given by intravenous injection as well as by mouth.

DI-IODOHYDROXYQUINOLINE is a drug used in the treatment of chronic amoebic dysentery, usually as a supplement to treatment with emetine.

DILAUDID is dihydromorphinone hydrochloride, a derivative of morphine. It is more potent than morphine, but its effect lasts for a shorter time. It is just as liable as morphine to lead to addiction.

DILUENTS are watery fluids of a non-irritating nature, which are given to increase the amount of perspiration or of urine, and carry solids with them from the system. Examples are water, milk, barley-water, and solutions of alkaline salts.

DIMENHYDRINATE, or DRAMAMINE, is a drug which is widely used, with considerable success, in the treatment of travel sickness.

DIMERCAPROL is the official name for BAL (British Anti-Lewisite), the antidote to lewisite poisoning which was discovered during the 1939–45 War. It was subsequently found to be an excellent antidote to poisoning with certain heavy metals, including arsenic, mercury and

gold, and it is now widely used for this purpose.

DIMETHYL PHTHALATE is an organic compound which was found, during the 1939–45 War, to be a most effective repellent for mosquitoes. It is also effective against flies, midges, blackflies, mites, fleas and ticks. Under the proprietary names of MYLOL and SKEETO-FAX, it is available as a cream and as a liquid. This is smeared on the face, arms, hands, legs or other exposed parts of the body. It has to be re-applied every three or four hours. Care must be taken not to allow it to get into the eyes or to come into contact with plastic spectacle-frames. It does not kill, but merely prevents the insect from alighting on the skin.

DIOCTYL SODIUM SULPHOSUC-CINATE is a faecal-softening agent that is proving useful in the treatment of constipation in old people.

DIODONE is a complex, organic, iodine-containing preparation. It is used primarily for contrast radiography of the kidney passages, but can also be used for contrast radiography of the biliary tract.

DIOPTRE is a term used in the measurement of the refractive or focusing power of lenses; one dioptre is the power of a lens with a focal distance of one metre and is the unit of refractive power. As a stronger lens has a greater refractive power, this means that the focal distance will be shorter. The strength in dioptres therefore is the reciprocal of the focal length expressed in metres.

DIPHENHDYRAMINE is a widely used antihistamine drug (qv).

DIPHENOXYLATE is a drug chemically related to pethidine that is proving of value in the treatment of travellers' diarrhoea by quietening down the gut. It has no anti-infective action.

DIPHTHERIA is the term applied to an acute infectious disease, which is accompanied by a membranous exudation on a mucous surface, generally on the tonsils and back of the throat or pharynx.

Causes – The infection is essentially a local one in the throat due to the development there of the *Corynebacterium diphtheriae*, and the general symptoms are referable to the absorption of toxins (qv) which damage the heart muscle and the nerves. Among the first signs of the disease is inflammation of the throat, where a membrane develops, composed partly of the dead surface of mucous membrane and partly of products effused from the blood and lymph. In this membrane the causative organisms swarm, along with many other varieties of organisms, particularly streptococci.

The disease is generally conveyed by direct contagion, as by kissing an affected person, using his cup or spoon, or receiving a drop of saliva or fragment of membrane upon the lips or face through incautiously approaching him when he is coughing. The organism grows freely in milk, and infection may be conveyed in this way.

Three strains of *Corynebacterium diphtheriae* are now recognized as causing clinical diphtheria: *gravis, intermedius, mitis.* *Gravis* and *intermedius* strains are almost always virulent; about 10 per cent of *mitis* strains are non-virulent.

It is predominantly a disease of the autumn and winter and, although it occurs at all ages, it is commonest in childhood. It is rare under six months of age as the young infant has a transmitted immunity from the mother.

A method known as the *Schick test* has been devised for detecting the susceptibility of individuals to diphtheria. A minute quantity of toxin filtered off from growing diphtheria bacilli is injected with a very fine needle into the skin of the arm. Individuals possessing naturally a considerable amount of antitoxic power show no reaction, but if the individual has very little resisting power to diphtheria, an area of inflammation is produced on the skin at the site of the injection.

In 1977 there were only two cases of diphtheria, with no deaths, in England, compared with over 45,000 cases and 2400 deaths in England and Wales 1940, the year in which a national immunization campaign was launched by the Minister of Health. The substance injected is diphtheria toxoid, which is diphtheria toxin so treated that it is harmless but will produce antibodies to the diphtheria bacillus and thereby give the injected individual an immunity to the disease.

Very few children are immunized solely against diphtheria at the present day. They are more usually given a combined vaccine against diphtheria, tetanus and whooping-cough. (See VACCINES.)

Symptoms – The severity of diphtheritic inflammation in general, and the fact that it is accompanied by serious constitu-tional symptoms, suffice usually to distinguish this disease from croup, which, although resembling diphtheria, differs from it in being a merely local inflammation of the larynx. There are several other diseases of the throat, such as acute suppurative quinsy, which are even more liable to be mistaken for diphtheria. The diagnosis is often difficult, even for a skilled physician.

In doubtful cases, the deciding point is the taking of a throat swab. A swab of cotton-wool mounted on a wire is rubbed against the throat, and then sent to a bacteriologist for examination. A culture of the organisms from the swab is made upon dried serum, for 16 to 24 hours at body temperature, and if the organisms found in the resulting culture be pronounced to be *Corynebacterium diphtheriae*, the case can be safely diagnosed as one in which this disease is present.

Cases of diphtheria differ as to their intensity from the mildest forms, which resemble an ordinary catarrhal sore throat, to those of the most severe character (such as the gangrenous form), in which the disease is hopelessly intractable from the first.

Following an incubation period of two to six days after infection, symptoms set in like those commonly accompanying a cold: chilliness and depression. Sometimes very severe disturbances usher in an attack, such as vomiting and diarrhoea. A slight feeling of uneasiness in the throat is experienced along with some stiffness of the back of the neck. When looked at, the throat appears reddened and somewhat swollen, particularly in the neighbourhood of the tonsils, the soft palate, and upper part of pharynx, while along with this there are tenderness and swelling of the glands at the angles of the jaw. The affection of the throat spreads rapidly, and soon the characteristic exudation appears on the inflamed surface in the form of greyish-white specks or patches, increasing in extent and thickness until a yellowish-looking membrane is formed. This deposit is firmly adherent to the mucous membrane beneath, or is incorporated with it, and, if forcibly removed, it leaves a raw, bleeding, ulcerated surface, upon which it is reproduced in a short period. The appearance of the exudation has been compared to wet parchment or washed leather, and it is dense in texture. It may cover the whole of the back of the throat, the cavity of the mouth, and the posterior nares, and may spread downwards into the air passages and into the alimentary canal, while any wound on the surface of the body is liable to become covered with it. As it loosens, it becomes decomposed, giving a most offensive and characteristic odour to the breath. There are pain and difficulty in swallowing, but, unless the disease has affected the larynx, no affection of the breathing. The voice acquires a snuffling character. When the disease invades the posterior nares, an acrid, foetid discharge, and sometimes also copious bleeding, take place from the nostrils.

Along with these local phenomena there is evidence of severe constitutional disturbance. There may not be great fever, and the temperature seldom rises above 102° or 103° F (39° to 39·5° C), but there are marked depression and loss of strength. The pulse becomes small and rapid, the countenance pale, the swelling of the glands in the neck increases, which, along with the presence of albumin in the urine, testifies to a condition of blood-poisoning. Unless favourable symptoms emerge, death takes place within three or four days or sooner, either from the rapid extension of the membrane into the air passages, giving rise to asphyxia, or from a condition of general collapse, which is sometimes remarkably sudden owing to sudden failure of the heart, for which the diphtheria toxin has a special predilection. For the same reason death occasionally takes place suddenly during convalescence, from acute dilatation of the weakened heart, if a considerable effort be made at too early a period. Death may also ensue if the temperature rises excessively.

In cases of recovery, the change for the better is marked by an arrest in the extension of the membrane, the detachment and expectoration of that already formed, and the healing of the ulcerated mucous membrane beneath. Along with this, there is a general improvement in the symptoms, the power of swallowing returns, and the strength gradually increases, while the glandular enlargement of the neck diminishes, and the albumin disappears from the urine. These favourable symptoms should appear within three or four days, but recovery is generally slow, and it may be many weeks before full convalescence is established. During this period it is particularly necessary in the case of diphtheria to guard against premature over-exertion, and for this reason patients are kept in bed for several weeks even though feeling quite well.

Even when diphtheria ends quite favourably, certain sequels may follow, generally in a period of two or three weeks after all the local evidence of the disease has disappeared. These effects, which are due to neuritis caused by the effect of the diphtheria toxin upon various nerves, may occur after mild as well as after severe attacks, and they are principally in the form of paralysis affecting the soft palate and throat, causing difficulty in swallowing, with regurgitation of fluid through the nose, and giving a peculiar nasal character to the voice. Another form of paralysis is one affecting the muscles of the eye, and producing loss of the power of accommodation and consequent difficulty in reading without glasses, which often lasts for a period of several months; another form may be paralysis of a limb, or of both legs, or even of the respiratory muscles. These symptoms, however, after continuing for a variable length of time, almost always ultimately disappear.

Treatment – The first essential of treatment is the immediate injection of *antitoxin*. (See SERUM THERAPY.) Every moment of delay increases the danger to the patient. As diphtheria antitoxin contains horse serum, the possibility of an anaphylactic reaction (see ANAPHYLAXIS) must be borne in mind. In addition to antitoxin, the patient is given penicillin daily for five days, as this antibiotic has a bactericidal action on *C. diphtheriae*.

The second essential is *complete rest in bed* for at least three weeks. Adequate nourishment should be freely administered in the form of milk, soup, etc., as long as there exists the power of swallowing, and when this fails, fluids, in the form of Hartmann's solution (qv), glucose and plasma, should be given by infusion or by nasal catheter. The strict maintenance of the recumbent position is of great importance in preserving the strength of the heart. If the infection spreads to the larynx (laryngeal diphtheria), additional antitoxin is given and the patient is kept in a steam tent. If obstruction to breathing is not relieved by this, it may be necessary to perform the operation of tracheotomy (qv).

Most cases of diphtheritic paralysis recover without special treatment. In cases in which the respiratory muscles are paralysed, it may be necessary for a time to resort to artificial respiration till the paralysis passes off, by means of some form of apparatus which rhythmically inflates and deflates the chest.

As the disease is notifiable a case of diphtheria should be notified immediately to the community physician, and arrangements made for urgent admission to a hospital for infectious diseases. Cases are isolated until cultures from three successive nose and throat swabs, taken at intervals of not less than two days, are negative.

If a case of diphtheria occurs in a closed community, such as a school, a daily examination of the throats of all contacts should be made during the incubation period, and throat swabs should be taken. Those with positive throat swabs should be given an intramuscular injection of antitoxin and also penicillin. They must also be isolated until three successive throat swabs free of virulent *C. diphtheriae* are obtained. The Schick test should also be carried out on all contacts, and those who give a positive reaction should be given a course of toxoid immunization.

DIPHYLLOBOTHRIUM LATUM is a fish tapeworm which infests man and may cause a form of megabolastic anaemia. (See ANAEMIA.)

DIPLEGIA means extensive paralysis on both sides of the body. (See PARALYSIS.)

DIPLO- is a prefix meaning twofold.

DIPLOCOCCUS is the term applied to a group of bacterial organisms which have a tendency to occur in pairs: eg. pneumococci.

DIPLOË is the layer of spongy bone which intervenes between the compact outer and inner tables of the skull.

DIPLOPIA means double vision. It is due to some irregularity in action of the muscles which move the eyeballs, in consequence of which the eyes are placed so that rays of light from one object do not fall upon corresponding parts of the two retinae, and two images are produced. It is a symptom of several nervous diseases, and often a temporary attack follows an injury to the eye, intoxication, or some febrile disease like diphtheria.

DIPROSOPUS is the term applied to a foetus which has two faces instead of one.

DIPSOMANIA is a morbid and insatiable craving for alcohol. (See ALCOHOLISM, CHRONIC.)

DIPYGUS is the term applied to a foetus which has a double pelvis.

DISABLED PERSONS now have a wide range of services available to help them to lead as normal and active a life as possible. Officially, the disabled include those with significant impairment of any kind, including impairment of sight and hearing, mental subnormality, and chronic illness as well as disablement due to accidents and the like.

Financial help is available for the disabled as follows: *Invalidity benefit* for those who have paid national insurance contributions. *Non-contributory invalidity pension* for those who have not been able to work and pay national insurance contributions. *Attendance allowance* for disabled persons who are dependent on others: for example, need frequent attention to bodily needs. *Invalid care allowance* for people who have stopped working to look after an invalid. Normally, housewives cannot draw this benefit. *Mobility allowance* is intended for people aged 5 to 65 (60 for women) who are unable or virtually unable to walk. At present it is only payable up to the age of 58, but this is being gradually extended. Full details of all these can be had from a local Department of Health and Social Security Office. If asked, someone from the local office will call to see the disabled person in his own home.

Social services are provided by Local Authority Social Services Departments. Those laid down under the Chronically Sick and Disabled Persons' Act 1970 include: (1) Practical help in the home (usually through home helps or aids to daily living). (2) Provision of, or help in obtaining, a radio, television, library or similar facilities. (3) Provision of lectures, games, outings or other recreational facilities outside the home, and assistance in taking advantage of available educational facilities. (4) Assistance in carrying out adaptations in the disabled person's house. (5) Assistance in taking holidays. (6) Provision of meals whether in the disabled person's home ('Meals on Wheels') or elsewhere (Luncheon Centres). (7) Help in obtaining a telephone. Many of these facilities involve the disabled person in some expense, but full details can be obtained from the local Social Services Department, which will, if necessary, send a social worker to discuss the matter in the disabled person's home. A warning is necessary here to the effect that, owing to lack of funds and staff, many Local Authority Social Service Departments are unable to provide the full range of services.

Aids to daily living – There is now a wide range of aids for the disabled. Full details of these can be obtained from:

Disabled Living Foundation, 346 Kensington High Street, London W14 8NS

Birmingham Disabled Living Centre, 84 Suffolk Street, Birmingham 1

Medical Aids Department, British Red Cross Society, 76 Clarendon Park Road, Leicester LE2 3AL

Merseyside Aids Centre, Youens Way, East Prescot Road, Liverpool 14

National Demonstration Centre, Pinderfield Hospital, Wakefield, Yorkshire

Newcastle upon Tyne Aids Centre, Mea House, Ellison Place, Newcastle upon Tyne NE1 8XS

Scottish Information Service for the Disabled, 18 Claremont Crescent, Edinburgh EH7 4QD

Aids cannot be bought at these centres.

Aids to mobility and transport – The Department of Health and Social Security invalid vehicles are no longer provided, having been replaced by the mobility allowance. The major car manufacturers make specially equipped or adapted cars, and some have official systems for discounts. Details can be obtained from local dealers. Help can also be obtained from Motability (Room 550, State House, High Holborn, London WC1R 4SX) which provides advice to enable the disabled to make the most of the mobility allowance, and financial assistance for buying, adapting or running a car. The disabled travelling in a car, either as a passenger or driver, may be eligible for an orange badge if they have considerable difficulty in walking or if they are blind. It allows the holder some parking concessions, and is obtainable on a doctor's certificate. A wide variety of wheelchairs is available from the Department of Health and Social Security Appliance Centres, which issue them on permanent loan and maintain them.

For help in making full use of these facilities the disabled should consult their general practitioner. Citizens' Advice Bureaux are another useful source of information. The following is a selected list of some of the more practical leaflets and pamphlets available for the disabled. All of them are free:

Help for the Handicapped. Available from local telephone sales offices.

Electric Aids for Disabled People. Available from local electricity showrooms.

How Gas Makes Life Easier for the Disabled. Available from local gas showrooms.

People in Wheelchairs – Hints for Helpers. Available from local offices of the British Red Cross Society.

Who looks after You at Heathrow Airport? Published by the British Airports Authority. Similar booklets for other airports are available from the Public Relations Office, British Airports Authority, at the airport concerned.

Care in The Air. Advice for Handicapped Passengers. Obtainable from Airline Users Committee, Space House, 43-59 Kingsway, London WC2B 6TE.

The following official leaflets published by the Department of Health and Social Security are available free from their local offices:

Help for Handicapped People. Leaflet HB1.

Aids for the Disabled. Leaflet HB2.

Family Benefits and Pensions. Leaflet FB1.

(See also REMPLOY.)

DISARTICULATION is the amputation of a bone by cutting through the joint of which the bone forms a part.

DISCHARGE is the term applied to abnormal emissions from any part of the body. It usually applies to purulent material: eg. the septic material which comes away from an infected ear, or nose.

DISCISSION is the term applied to an operation for destroying a structure by tearing it without removal: eg. the operation of needling the lens of the eye for cataract.

DISINFECTION is the process of rendering harmless any persons, articles, rooms, and the like, which are liable to communicate disease. *Disinfectants* are potent, but toxic, preparations or procedures which are able to destroy micro-organisms but not necessarily resistant spores. (See BACTERIOLOGY.) *Antiseptics* are substances which kill or prevent the growth of micro-organisms, and which can safely be applied to living tissue without harming it. *Germicides* are measures or preparations which kill germs or micro-organisms. *Deodorants* are substances which suppress foul smells, and, although many deodorants are disinfectants, they are so only on much more effective application than is necessary to subdue smell. Thus charcoal exposed in a sick-room clears away smell but does not disinfect the room, and eucalyptus

DISINFECTION

sprinkled on the floor renders the air of a room sweet, but does not destroy the germs of disease in the room.

FORMS OF DISINFECTANT – **Light and fresh air** are too apt to be neglected. There can hardly be found a more powerful disinfectant than direct sunlight, for few bacteria can survive exposure to it in the open for an hour. This applies, for example, with special force to the tubercle bacillus.

Heat is of great importance. Exposure to moist heat at 212° F or 100° C (ie. boiling in water) kills bacteria in five to ten minutes but longer exposures to higher temperatures (eg. 15 minutes at 121° C) are necessary to kill off resistant spores. (See BACTERIOLOGY). Steam under pressure, as in the autoclave (qv), is the most effective means of sterilization for materials that will withstand damp and moisture, such as clothes and dressings. For instruments, such as knives and scalpels, however, dry heat is necessary, as in a hot-air oven. A higher temperature and a longer exposure (eg. 160° C for an hour) are necessary than with moist heat.

CRUDE CARBOLIC in a dilution of 1 in 20 is used for disinfecting clothing and bedding. Although it does not harm fabrics or affect colours or metals, it is liable to stain, due to the presence of impurities.

PURE PHENOL is a satisfactory disinfectant in a dilution of 1 in 100. Although not as efficient as crude carbolic, it has the advantage of not staining.

CRESOL, in the form of a 1 per cent emulsion of saponified cresol, is an excellent disinfectant.

IZAL, CYLLIN AND LYSOL are other satisfactory coal-tar disinfectants. Izal and cyllin, which have a carbolic coefficient of 20, are used in a dilution of 0·5 per cent, whilst lysol, with a carbolic coefficient of 5 to 10, is used in a 1 per cent solution.

PERCHLORIDE OF MERCURY in a 1 in 1000 solution is a potent disinfectant, killing organisms in thirty minutes. Its use is restricted by the fact that it corrodes metals, and is not suitable for disinfecting faeces and sputum, as it forms insoluble compounds with albuminous material. Because of its extreme toxicity and the fact that it forms a colourless solution like water, it is coloured blue to prevent accidents. The following formula gives a 1 in 960 solution: mercury perchloride 0·5 ounce (14 grams), hydrochloric acid 1 ounce (28·5 ml), aniline blue 5 grains (300 mg), water 3 gallons (13·5 litres).

FORMALDEHYDE may be used either as a gaseous disinfectant or in solution as formaldehyde solution (formalin).

POTASSIUM PERMANGANATE, which is a disinfectant by virtue of being a powerful oxidizing agent, is a useful and safe disinfectant. Its use is restricted by the fact that it is rendered inert by organic matter. Five minutes in a 1 in 1000 solution of permanganate is an effective way of sterilizing drinking and eating utensils. Although it stains textiles, the stain can be removed by oxalic acid or lemon juice. Condy's fluid contains potassium permanganate.

SODIUM HYPOCHLORITE is unstable in solution and corrodes metal, but in 1 in 3000 solution it is a useful disinfectant for floors and latrines.

LIME, one of the cheapest of disinfectants, kills organisms in a few hours in a 1 per cent solution.

CHLORINATED LIME (bleaching powder) is less stable than lime. It has the further disadvantage of being destructive to fabrics. In a 0·5 to 1 per cent solution it kills most organisms in one to five minutes.

HYDROGEN CYANIDE, which, because of its intense toxicity, must only be used by experienced personnel, is used for destroying bed bugs and for fumigating ships.

SULPHUR DIOXIDE is also used for fumigating ships.

METHODS OF DISINFECTION – **The person** – The hands must always be carefully disinfected after being in contact with an individual suffering from an infectious disease, or before dressing a wound. The best method is to wash the hands thoroughly in plenty of warm water, using an antiseptic soap such as hexachlorophane soap and a sterilized nail-brush. The hands should then be carefully rinsed in one of the following: pink potassium permanganate solution; perchloride of mercury solution (1 in 2000); biniodide of mercury solution (1 in 1000 solution in water); 75 per cent isopropyl alcohol; or 1 in 500 parts of 90 per cent alcohol. An alternative measure is to apply chlorhexidine cream to the hands after drying them.

Dressings and instruments – The former are now sterilized by high-pressure steam sterilization. Surgical instruments, including syringes and needles, can be sterilized by boiling in water for ten to twenty minutes, but more usually nowadays instruments are sterilized by autoclaving and syringes by insertion in the hot-air oven at a temperature of 160° C for one hour.

Rooms – Provided reasonable precautions are taken during the illness, disinfection of the sick-room is not now considered necessary in the case of ordinary infectious diseases such as measles and diphtheria. Thorough washing with soap and water and plenty of fresh air are all that are required. At the beginning all unnecessary ornaments and hangings should be removed and the room should be kept well ventilated. During the illness dusting and sweeping must be reduced to a minimum and carried out only with damp dusters and mops. Recent work has shown that certain organisms remain alive in dust and in fluff from blankets for considerable periods. To overcome spread of infection by this means blankets and floors are now being treated by oil in hospitals. If it is considered necessary to disinfect a room after an infectious illness, the first preliminary is to burn articles of little value and to send bedding and mattresses for steam disinfection. The only satisfactory way of disinfecting a room is by a spray, and for this purpose the best is formalin: 8 ounces to the gallon of water (230 ml to 4·5 litres), and 1 gallon (4·5 litres) for every 400 square feet (111 square metres) of surface. A room sprayed in this way in the morning can be occupied again the same evening, provided all windows and doors are kept open during the spraying.

Clothes and bedding – Bed linen, blankets and similar articles should be soaked in cresol or a 5 per cent solution of carbolic acid for twelve hours before being washed. It should be remembered that if soiled linen is boiled without preliminary soaking it will be permanently stained, and that blankets do not stand repeated boiling or steam disinfection. Putting them out in the sunshine and fresh air has been described as 'one of the cheapest and most effective ways of disinfecting them'. Other articles, such as boots and leather materials, which cannot be soaked in disinfectant or destroyed, should be left in the room during disinfection, and afterwards exposed to the open air for an entire day. Where a central disinfecting station exists, arrangements should be made with the local health authoritiy to have the disinfecting done there.

Sputum, stools and other discharges – Sputum and discharges from the nose should be collected in gauze and burnt. If there is sufficient sputum to justify a sputum flask, this should contain a 5 per cent solution of carbolic acid. The bed-pan should also contain 5 per cent solution of carbolic acid, or cresol. After use, more disinfectant should be added, well mixed with the contents and allowed to stand for two hours before being emptied down the water-closet.

DISINFESTATION means the destruction of insect pests, especially lice, whether on the person or in dwelling-places.

DISLOCATIONS are injuries to joints of such a nature that the ends of the opposed bones are forced more or less out of connection with one another. Besides displacement of the bones, there is more or less bruising of the tissues around them, and tearing of the ligaments which bind the bones together.

Varieties – Dislocations, like fractures, are divided into simple and compound, the bone in the latter case being forced through the skin. This seldom occurs, since the round head of the bone has not the same power to wound as the sharp end of a broken bone. Dislocations are also divided according as they are (1) congenital, ie. present at birth in consequence of some malformation, or (2) acquired at a later period in consequence of injury, the great majority falling into the latter class.

Causes – The causes of dislocation are similar to those of fracture, the fact as to whether a bone or a joint gives way depending upon the manner in which force is applied, and still more upon the relative strength of bones and joints. Thus in very young and very old persons dislocations are rare, because the bones are relatively easily broken, and thereby the joints are saved from damage. Congenital dislocations are mainly due to some defect in development of the bones.

Signs and symptoms – The injured limb is useless, but, as a rule, there is little pain, unless the dislocated bone presses upon some nerve trunk. When the limb is compared with that of the opposite side, the joint is found to be unduly prominent in one place, and shows an abnormal hollow in another. Further, there is loss of movement at the joint in question, but no grating (crepitus) as in a case of fracture. Each joint shows further special signs dependent upon its conformation.

Treatment – So far as temporary treatment is concerned, nothing is necessary but a splint, bandage, sling or the like, to keep the injured part moderately quiet, because there is not the same danger of damage to nerves, vessels, and the like, by the rounded head of the bone as by the sharp fragments of a fracture. The greatest care is necessary in reduction, ie. putting the dislocated bone back in place, for great damage may be done by an unskilled person in the way of breaking the bone, tearing nerves and blood-vessels, or even leaving the bone dislocated in a new direction. After reduction to the natural position, the limb must be fixed for a time so as to prevent a recurrence, which will take place if it be used at once. The length of time depends upon the severity of the injury; as a rule, after about ten days, gentle movements are made to prevent the joint becoming stiff, and the bandages, and the like, left off after about three weeks. But care in using the limb is necessary for much longer.

SHOULDER – This may be reduced in one of two methods. (*a*) By *manipulation*, in which the bone is gently worked back into place by a method too complicated for description here. (*b*) By *extension*. The injured person lies on his back upon a couch or upon the floor. The operator then, sitting down by the injured side opposite the patient's hip and facing towards his shoulder, grasps the limb with one hand by the wrist, with the other above the elbow, while at the same time he places his foot, from which the shoe has been removed, in the armpit, on the edge of the shoulder-blade, to steady it, and give him something against which to pull. He then pulls on the injured arm gently, steadily, and strongly, first in a direction parallel with the injured person's body, and, if this be unsuccessful, at right angles to it, pressing all the while with his foot against the edge of the shoulder-blade. The injured person must at the same time relax all his shoulder muscles. The bone goes into place generally with a snap, and the appearance of the joint is then like that of its fellow.

ELBOW – This joint may be dislocated backwards by a fall on the hand, or forwards by a fall on the point of the elbow. In both cases it is reduced by bending steadily across the knee of the operator, who at the same time pulls on the forearm.

WRIST – This joint is seldom dislocated, and the dislocation is readily replaced by pressure, and is then kept in position by a well-padded splint on the palm and front of forearm. A fracture of the lower end of the radius (Colles's fracture) is sometimes mistaken for a dislocated wrist.

FINGERS AND TOES may be dislocated and are difficult to reduce, because the tight ligaments close round the displaced bone, and because of the difficulty in grasping the finger to pull on it. This may be overcome by winding strips of sticking-plaster round the finger, or by a device of interlacing tapes known as the 'Indian puzzle'. Dislocation of the thumb at its base is particularly hard to reduce, and may even require an operation to enlarge the opening through which the bone has passed.

HIP – This joint, being extremely strong, is seldom dislocated, and, when dislocated, is very difficult to reduce. The head of the thigh bone usually passes backwards and upwards, so that the limb appears much shortened and the toes turned inward. Reduction is effected by a special form of manipulation, or, failing this, by extension. For the latter, the injured person lying on his back, the limb is pulled straight downwards, one assistant steadying the pelvis by pressing one of his hands upon each iliac spine, and another pulling the whole thigh outwards by means of a towel passed round it as high up as possible. A very steady, powerful pull is necessary if reduction is to be effected.

CONGENITAL DISLOCATION OF THE HIP is commoner in girls than in boys. Its incidence is between 2 and 3 per 1000 births. If detected at, or soon after, birth, the results of treatment are excellent. This is why the routine examination of the newborn baby always includes a careful examination of the hips. Any undue instability of the hip, particularly if accompanied by a clicking sound on movement of the hip, indicates the probable presence of dislocation. When diagnosed within the first few days of life, treatment merely consists of the application for a few months of a simple splint maintaining the hips in abduction and flexion, and the results are excellent. If the condition is not detected at this stage it is often missed until the child starts walking, when she is seen to have a characteristic waddling gait. Treatment at this stage is more complicated and less satisfactory.

KNEE – This joint is very seldom dislocated, and such an injury to it is specially severe, being accompanied by the tearing of strong ligaments.

ANKLE – This joint is hardly ever dislocated, most severe injuries near it being fractures of the leg bones.

SPINE – Dislocation of the spine is only produced by great violence, such as that of a horse rolling over a man, and is usually combined with fracture. Very often pressure on, or tearing of, the spinal cord takes place, which may produce paralysis of the lower limbs, or even death from shock.

JAW – This joint is sometimes dislocated forwards when the mouth is very widely opened, as in yawning or singing. It can usually be replaced by a person pressing downwards with his thumbs upon the farthest back teeth and at the same time pressing up the chin. He should take care that his thumbs do not get bitten.

DISODIUM CROMOGLYCATE is a drug that is proving of value in the treatment of asthma when given as an inhalation.

DISOPYRAMIDE is a drug that is proving of value in the prevention, and treatment of disturbances of the rhythm of the heart, particularly in those which occur following a coronary thrombosis (qv).

DISORIENTATION is a term applied to a symptom in mental disease or delirium in which the patient is confused as to sense of time or place.

DISPLACEMENT is a term used in psychological medicine to describe the mental process of attaching to one object painful emotions associated with another object.

DISSEMINATED SCLEROSIS (see MULTIPLE SCLEROSIS).

DISTICHIASIS is the term applied to the condition in which there are two complete rows of eyelashes in one eyelid (or in both).

DISTOMA is a general term including various forms of trematodes, or flukeworms, parasitic in the intestine, lung and other organs.

DISULFIRAM, or ANTABUSE, the full chemical name of which is tetraethylthiuram disulphide, is used in the treatment of alcoholism. It is relatively non-toxic by itself, but when taken in conjunction with alcohol it produces most unpleasant effects: eg. flushing of the face, palpitations, a sense of oppression and distress, and ultimately sickness and vomiting. The rationale of treatment therefore is to give the alcoholic subject a course of disulfiram and then demonstrate, by letting him take some alcoholic liquor, how unpleasant are the effects. If the patient is co-operative, the results of treatment are often very satisfactory. It is a form of treatment, however, that is not without risk, and it must therefore be given under skilled medical supervision.

DIURETICS are substances which produce diuresis, that is, a copious excretion of urine by the kidneys.

Varieties – There is a host of substances which can produce diuresis, although only a small proportion of these are now used. Water, for instance, is an excellent diuretic, and if the diminished output of urine is due to inadequate intake of fluid or excessive loss of fluid through other channels, eg. sweating, diarrhoea, water is often the best diuretic to rectify matters. Salts of potassium, calcium chloride and ammonium chloride produce diuresis by temporarily altering the chemistry of the blood. Urea acts as a diuretic by stimulating the glomeruli of the kidneys. Vasodilators (qv) act as diuretics by increasing the blood supply to the kidneys. Among the vasodilators used for this purpose are caffeine, theophylline, aminophylline and theobromine. Spirit of nitrous ether, a popular constituent of fever mixtures, falls into this group, but is a much weaker diuretic than the others mentioned. Gin used to be a commonly used diuretic; here there was a twofold action – the alcohol acted as a vasodilator and the oil of juniper acted as a mild irritant of the kidney, thereby acting as a stimulant to the excretion of urine. Needless to say, gin is never used now for this purpose. The digitalis group of drugs act as diuretics in cases of dropsy due to heart failure; this they do mainly by improving the action of the heart they increase the circulation through the kidneys and thereby increase the output of urine.

For many years the most widely used diuretics were the organic mercurial diuretics, eg. mersalyl (qv), which act by diminishing the activity of the renal tubules. These, however, had certain disadvantages, including the fact that they had to be given by injection. They are now being largely replaced by a new group of diuretics, which are benzothiadiazine (qv) derivatives, and which are effective when taken by mouth. (See CHLOROTHIAZIDE; and HYDROFLUMETHIAZIDE.) Like the organic mercurial diuretics, they act on the renal tubules. The most recent additions to the list of diuretics are spironolactone (qv) and frusemide (qv).

Uses – The removal of dropsical fluid is the main function of diuretics. If the dropsy is due to heart failure the best diuretics to use are the digitalis group of drugs. These are often supplemented by the organic mercurial diuretics, or the new benzothiadiazine derivatives. In the case of dropsy due to disease of the kidneys, the choice of diuretic depends upon the condition of the kidneys. In febrile conditions, when so much fluid is being lost in the excessive sweating caused by the fever, it is often advisable to give diuretics to maintain the excretion of urine, and for this purpose a combination of the milder diuretics, such as potassium nitrate and spirit of nitrous ether, may be used.

DIVERTICULITIS is inflammation of diverticula (see DIVERTICULUM) in the large intestine. It is characterized by pain in the left lower side of the abdomen, which has been aptly described as 'left-sided appendicitis' as it resembles the pain of appendicitis but occurs in the opposite side of the abdomen. The onset is often sudden, with fever and constipation. It may, or may not, be preceded by diverticulosis (qv). Treatment consists of rest in bed, no solid food but ample fluid, and the administration of tetracycline. Complications are unusual but include abscess formation, perforation of the colon, and severe bleeding.

DIVERTICULOSIS means the presence of diverticula (see DIVERTICULUM) in the large intestine. Such diverticula are not uncommon over the age of 40, increasing with age until over the age of 70 they may be present in one-third to one-half of the population. They mostly occur in the lower part of the colon, and are predominantly due to muscular hyperactivity of the bowel forcing the lining of the bowel through weak points in the bowel wall, just as the inner tube of a pneumatic tyre bulges through a defective tyre. There is increasing evidence that the low-residue diet of western civilization is a contributory cause. The condition may or may not produce symptoms. If it does, these consist of disturbance of the normal bowel function and pain in the left side in the lower abdomen. If it is causing symptoms, treatment consists of a high-residue diet (see DIET) and an agar (qv) or methylcellulose (qv) preparation.

DIVERTICULUM means a pouch or pocket leading off a main cavity or tube. The term is especially applied to protrusions from the intestine, which may be present either at the time of birth as a developmental peculiarity, or which develop in numbers upon the large intestine during the course of life. The process of formation of these intestinal pockets is known as diverticulosis, and inflammation of them as diverticulitis.

DIZZINESS (see VERTIGO).

DOG BITES (see BITES, STINGS and POISONED WOUNDS; and RABIES).

DOLICHOCEPHALIC means long-headed and is a term applied to skulls the breadth of which is less than four-fifths of the length.

DOMETTE BANDAGE is a bandage of union fabric of plain weave, in which the warp threads are of cotton and the weft threads of wool. It is used especially when a high degree of warmth, protection and support is needed. (See also BANDAGES.)

DONORS – The inception, and increasing amount, of transplantation (qv) have created an ever-growing demand for donors of eyes, kidneys and other organs of the body. This is in addition to the already existing demand for blood donors. There is still also a demand for bodies for dissecting purposes in the anatomy departments of our medical schools.

Those who wish to bequeath their bodies for dissection purposes should get in touch with: H.M. Inspector of Anatomy, Department of Health and Social Security, Alexander Fleming House, Elephant and Castle, London, SE1, who will give full advice as to the correct procedure to be followed.

There is a steadily increasing demand for blood for transfusion (see TRANSFUSION OF BLOOD), as the present supply scarcely meets the demand. More donors are therefore required. There are fifteen blood transfusion centres in England, four in Scotland and one in Wales. Details of how to become a donor can be obtained through general practitioners, the local medical officer of health (or community physician as he is now known) at the local town hall, from any hospital, or, in the case of those in employment in large organizations, from the organization's medical officer. Alternatively, in Wales full details can be obtained from the Director of the Welsh Regional Blood Transfusion Centre, Rhyd-Lafar, St Fagans, Cardiff CF5 6XF. In Scotland such details can be obtained from the Secretary of the Scottish National Blood Transfusion Association, 5 St Colme Street, Edinburgh EH3 6AE.

In the case of organs of the body, such as the eyes, kidneys and the heart, the problem is that, to be capable of transplantation, they must be removed from the body within a matter of a few hours of the death of the donor. In practice this means that it is highly desirable that the permission of the donor for such removal be obtained in advance in writing. Otherwise, if the matter is left until after the death of the donor, there is inevitable delay in getting permission from the relatives to remove the organ in question. Not only, as in the case of a sudden death due to road accident, may this be difficult, but it may cause unnecessary distress to the relatives at a time when they are already emotionally upset.

So far as corneal grafting (qv) is concerned, the Department of Health and Social Security has drawn up a list of suitable eye-banks to which people can bequeath their eyes, and an official form is available for the bequest of eyes. Copies of this can be obtained on application to the Department at: Alexander Fleming House, Elephant and Castle, London, SE1.

In the case of kidney transplantations the Department of Health and Social Security has prepared a kidney donor card to be signed by the donor and countersigned by the donor's next of kin. Copies of this card can be obtained in any pharmacy, or from general practitioners. The card, when duly signed, should always be carried about by the donor, so that it is readily available, even though his (or her) death should occur unexpectedly – as in a road accident. Although the number of kidneys becoming available for transplantation has been increasing, there is still an urgent need for more. At present it is estimated that over 800 people are waiting for a kidney transplant in Britain.

No special arrangements have been made to date for obtaining permission for the transplantation of hearts, livers or lungs, and other organs, but anyone who is willing to become a donor of one or more of these should sign, and have countersigned, a form comparable to the kidney donor card.

DOPAMINE is a catecholamine (qv) and a precursor of noradrenaline (qv). Its highest concentration is in that portion of the brain known as the basal nuclei (see BRAIN) where its function is to convey inhibitory influences to the extrapyramidal system. There is good evidence that dopamine deficiency is one of the causative factors in Parkinsonism (qv).

DOSAGE – Many factors influence the activity with which drugs operate. Among the factors which affect the necessary quantity are age, weight, sex, idiosyncrasy, genetic disorders, habitual use, disease,

fasting, combination with other drugs, the form in which the drug is given, and the route by which it is given.

Age is but one factor. Normally, a young child requires a smaller dose than an adult. There are, however, other factors to be taken into consideration. Thus, children are more susceptible than adults to some drugs such as morphine, whilst they are less sensitive to others such as atropine. Various methods have been introduced for calculating roughly and quickly the dose generally suitable for a child of any given age. One, for instance, is:

$$\text{adult dose} \times \frac{\text{age next birthday}}{20}$$

Another formula is:

$$\text{adult dose} \times \frac{\text{weight in pounds}}{150}$$

Yet another is:

$$\frac{\text{age} \times \text{adult dose}}{\text{age in years} + 12}$$

According to *Young's Rule*, the fraction of the adult dose is measured by dividing the child's age by the child's age plus 12. Another method is to base the dosage on the surface area of the child rather than the weight.

There is, however, no simple way of calculating the dose of a drug for an infant child. The body weight is probably the best and simplest, but it must be used with discrimination, bearing in mind the other factors that have to be taken into consideration.

Old people, too, often show an increased susceptibility to drugs. This is probably due to a variety of factors, such as decreased weight in many old folk; diminished activity of the tissues and therefore diminished rate at which a drug is utilized; and diminished activity of the kidneys resulting in decreased rate of excretion of the drug.

Weight and sex have both to be taken into consideration. Women require slightly smaller doses than men, probably because they tend to be lighter in weight. The effect of weight on dosage is partly dependent on the fact that much of the extra weight of a heavy individual is made up of fatty tissue which is not as active as other tissue of the body. In practice, the question of weight seldom makes much difference unless the individual is grossly overweight or underweight.

Idiosyncrasy occasionally causes drugs

administered in the ordinary dose to produce unexpected effects. Thus, some people are but little affected by some drugs, whilst in others certain drugs, such as potassium iodide, or atropine, produce excessive symptoms in minute doses. In some cases this may be due to hypersensitiveness, or an allergic reaction, to the drug. This is a possibility that must always be borne in mind, particularly with penicillin. As a rule the individual has had the drug in question previously. Penicillin comes into this category; so much so that an individual who is known to be allergic to penicillin is strongly recommended to carry about with him wherever he goes a card to this effect. The carrying of such a card may well prevent his being given in some emergency a dose of penicillin that could possibly prove fatal.

Habitual use of a drug is perhaps the influence that causes the greatest increase in the dose necessary to produce the requisite effect. The classical example of this is opium and its derivatives, as many a drug addict knows to his or her cost. Arsenic is another example that was often encountered in the days when arsenical drugs were one of the great stand-bys in the Pharmacoepia.

Disease may modify the dose of medicines. This can occur in several ways. Thus, in serious illnesses the patient may be more susceptible to drugs, such as narcotics, that depress tissue activity, and therefore smaller doses must be given. Again, absorption of the drug from the gut may be slowed up by disease of the gut, or its effect may be enhanced if there is disease of the kidneys, interfering with the excretion of the drug.

Fasting aids the rapidity of absorption of, and also makes the body more susceptible to the action of, drugs. Partly for this reason, as well as to avoid irritation of the stomach, it is usual to prescribe drugs to be taken after meals, and diluted with water.

Combination of drugs is now frowned upon as it is often difficult to assess what their combined effect may be. In some cases they may have a mutually antagonistic effect, which means that the patient will not obtain full benefit from the prescription. In other cases the combination may have a deleterious effect, whilst in others again the combination may so enhance the effect on the patient as to produce harmful effects.

Form of administration is important in two respects. In the first instance, there is a tendency today to give a drug in the form of the active principle rather than, say, the leaf from which it is obtained as was the case at one time. This means, of course, that a smaller dose of the active principle is required than of the leaf or the tincture. In the second place, it involves the question of whether the drug is given as a tablet, a mixture or a powder. Various factors have to be taken into consideration; but today the common practice is to give a drug in tablet form, mainly because of the convenience of both patient and prescriber.

Route of administration naturally affects dosage. In Britain, medicines are given *by mouth* whenever possible, unless there is some degree of urgency, or because the drug is either destroyed in, or is not absorbed from, the gut. In these circumstances, it is given *intravenously, intramuscularly* or *subcutaneously.* In some cases, as in cases of asthma or bronchitis, the drug may be given in the form of an *inhalant* or *aerosol* (qv), in order to get the maximum concentration at the point where it is wanted: that is, in the lungs. If a local effect is wanted, as in cases of diseases of the skin, the drug is applied *topically* to the skin. On the Continent there is a tendency to give medicines in the form of a *suppository* which is inserted in the rectum. By British standards there is seldom any occasion for giving drugs in this way.

Genetic disorders are now coming to assume an increasing importance. Perhaps the classical example is the individual who suffers from a congenital deficiency of the enzyme known as glucose-6-phosphate dehydrogenase. Such individuals develop an acute haemolytic anaemia (see ANAEMIA) if they are given certain drugs, including phenacetin or a sulphonamide.

DOTHIEPIN is a drug that is being used in the treatment of depression. One of its practical advantages is that only one tablet needs to be taken daily.

DOUCHE is an application of water to the body, directly, through a pipe.

Action – Douches fall into two divisions: (*a*) those which act by virtue of some substance which they contain, such as astringent douches, cleansing douches; (*b*) those which act by virtue of their temperature, producing the effects which have been described under BATHS, and COLD, USES OF, with the distinction that douches act locally and so produce an action, upon one part only, greater than if the application were made to the whole body at one time.

Uses – (*a*) MEDICATED AND CLEANSING DOUCHES are used as a rule to wash out infected cavities. Thus, *bladder douches* are used in inflammation of this cavity, containing, for example, either half-saturated boric lotion; or oxycyanide of mercury, 1 in 10,000; or chlorhexidine, 1 in 5000 given at a temperature of 110° F (43° C). Such a douche is administered by means of a douche-can holding

permanganate, 1 in 500; boric acid, 1 in 50; or normal saline (ie. 4 G in 1 litre), at a temperature of 104° F (40° C) are used in some cases of leucorrhoea or 'whites'. A quart (1 litre) or larger douche-can is used at a height of 5 or 6 feet (1·5 or 2 metres). It leads by an india-rubber tube to a large nozzle, which should be made of glass for ready disinfection. Such a douche is sometimes used at a temperature of 115° F (46° C), or as hot as the hand can bear, in order to obtain also the soothing

143 – Apparatus for washing out the bladder.

one quart (1 litre) or more, connected by india-rubber piping with a three-way or T-shaped tube of glass, which, on its other two ends, has an outflow tube and a tube leading to a catheter introduced into the bladder (illustration 143). The douche-can, being suspended at a height of 3 feet (1 metre) or so above the bed on which the patient lies, is filled with fluid, which runs into the bladder as soon as the outflow tube is pinched. When sufficient has entered, it can be at once drawn off by pinching the inflow tube and releasing the outflow. This is repeated several times. *Vaginal douches* of chloroxylenol solution ('dettol'), 4 ml in 0·5 litre; potassium

and constricting action of a hot douche on the blood-vessels of the surrounding parts.

(*b*) TEMPERATURE DOUCHES may be hot or cold, or in general the two alternated. The action upon the circulation has been explained under the heading of BATHS, with the exception that the douche acts strongly upon a single part. Douching, combined with massage, is a useful procedure for rheumatism, neuralgia, and other pains. The Scotch douche consists of an alternate hot water or steam douche and a cold douche. It is used for similar purposes, and it is important that the hot stream should be given first, and that it should last four or five times as long as the

275

cold stream. Such a douche acts powerfully upon the skin and nerves, and can be continued for a few minutes only.

DOVER'S POWDER, also known as IPECACUANHA AND OPIUM POWDER, is made from 10 per cent each of powdered opium and ipecacuanha, with 80 per cent of lactose. (See OPIUM.) Still one of the most popular remedies in medicine, it was introduced by Captain Thomas Dover (1660–1742), one of the most romantic figures in the history of medicine. Perhaps his greatest claim to fame is that he was a member of the privateering expedition which rescued Alexander Selkirk from Juan Fernandez, an island off the coast of Chile. It was upon the story of Alexander Selkirk that Daniel Defoe based his immortal *Robinson Crusoe*.

Uses – It is widely used as a diaphoretic, analgesic and sedative in the treatment of feverish colds and influenza. It is also an excellent remedy for dry, hacking coughs. The dose is 5 to 10 grains (300 to 600 mg).

DOWN'S SYNDROME (see MONGOLISM).

DOXYCYCLINE is a wide-spectrum, long-acting antibiotic of the tetracycline group (qv), which is active against a wide range of micro-organism, including the causative organism of scrub typhus.

DRACONTIASIS is the disease caused by the guinea worm, *Dracunculus medinensis*. It has been described as the oldest known human parasite, and is believed to be the Mosaic fiery serpent that harassed the Israelites on the shores of the Red Sea. It is found in India, Arabia, Iran, the Nile valley, East and West Africa, Brazil, and the islands of the Caribbean. The female may attain a length of four feet (120 cm). It is transmitted by *Cyclops*, and man is infected by drinking contaminated water. The worm causes no trouble for about a year, when it approaches the surface of the body and causes a local painful swelling which is usually accompanied by fever. The essential treatment, ie. removal of the worm, has changed little since Biblical days. Niridazole and thiabendazole are proving of value in controlling the disease.

DRAINS (see SEWAGE AND SEWAGE DISPOSAL).

DRAMAMINE is the trade name for dimenhydrinate, a drug which is widely used, with considerable success, in the treatment of travel sickness.

DRASTICS are substances which have a violent purgative action, such as croton oil, jalap, scammony. (See PURGATIVES.)

DRAUGHT, or DRAFT, is a small mixture intended to be taken at one dose. It consists generally of two or four tablespoonfuls of fluid.

DRAW SHEET (see BED).

DREAMS (see SLEEP).

DRENCH is an old term still used in parts of England for a draught of medicine.

DREPANOCYTOSIS is another term for sickle-cell anaemia (qv), which is characterized by the presence in the blood of red blood corpuscles sickle-like in shape. The anaemia is a severe one and afflicts the Negro race.

DRESSINGS (see WOUNDS).

DROP ATTACKS are attacks, usually in a middle-aged woman, whose legs suddenly 'give way', so that she falls to the ground without any warning. There is no loss of consciousness. In some cases the loss of tone in the muscles, responsible for the fall, may persist for several hours. In such cases moving the patient or applying pressure to the soles of the feet may restore the tone to the muscles. In most cases, however, recovery is immediate. The cause is probably a temporary interference with the blood supply to the brain. In others there may be some disturbance of the vestibular apparatus which controls the balance of the body. (See EAR.)

DROP-FOOT is a condition in which there is difficulty in raising the front part of the foot from the ground, or in which, when the condition is severe, the foot hangs limp.

Causes – The commonest form is that due to neuritis of the nerve (anterior tibial) supplying the muscles on the front of the leg. It may be caused by alcohol, lead poisoning or trauma to the leg, or it may follow some infection such as typhoid fever or diphtheria. In drop-foot from these causes there are apt to be disturbances of sensation on the leg also. Drop-foot may occur in children who have had poliomyelitis, but in this condition there is no sensory disturbance. It is also liable to occur in patients who are confined to bed for any length of time. In order to prevent this occurring the weight of the bedclothes should be taken off the patient's feet by means of a cradle (qv). If the condition is not so severe as to prevent the patient from going about, he walks by lifting the foot high so as to prevent the toes from catching on objects on the ground.

Treatment – If the condition is due to neuritis, it tends gradually to become better as the neuritis passes off. (See NEURITIS.) While the condition lasts, it is usual for the patient to wear a shoe the front part of which is supported by an elastic band attached to the front of the leg, in order to prevent the weak muscles from being over-stretched and the toes from dropping. Massage and electrical treatment are also required to maintain the tone of the affected muscles.

DROPPED BEAT means the missing out of a regular beat of the heart. It can be detected either by listening to the heart or by feeling the pulse. It may be due to *heart block* (qv) or to an *extrasystole* (qv). Dropped beat due to extrasystole is of no great significance.

DROPSY, or HYDROPS, means an abnormal accumulation of fluid beneath the skin, or in one or more of the cavities of the body. The term is a general one, the accumulation in special localities having special names: eg. dropsy beneath the skin is known, when limited, as *oedema*, when widespread, as *anasarca*; dropsy in the abdomen as *ascites*, in the chest as *hydrothorax*.

Causes – Dropsy is not a disease, although this is a popular idea, supported by the fact that at one time many deaths were recorded as due to 'dropsy' without a further statement of the cause. Dropsy may be due to one of three conditions: (1) weakening of the walls of the capillary vessels, by injury of the part in which dropsy occurs, by ill-health of the body generally, by poverty of the blood circulating through and nourishing the vessels, or by poisonous materials in the blood; (2) obstruction to the blood-flow through the veins; (3) a watery condition of the blood, allowing fluid to escape through the capillary walls. Dropsy may also result from obstruction to the flow of lymph in the lymph channels.

Heart disease, which produces increased pressure in the veins, and also an impure condition of the blood, in consequence of the defective pumping action of the heart, and *Bright's disease*, in which the kidneys

fail in their functions of excreting poisonous substances and a certain amount of water from the blood, are the main causes of general dropsy. In heart disease the dropsy is more marked after exertion; in kidney disease it is found chiefly after resting. Thus one of the chief characters of dropsy due to Bright's disease is that it appears in the morning, affects loose tissues like the skin beneath the eyes, and passes off as the day advances. Dropsy due to heart disease, on the other hand, tends to appear towards evening, affects dependent parts like the feet, and diminishes during the night. When the two diseases are combined, the state of dropsy may become very grave.

In *hunger oedema*, due to diminution of the amount of protein in the blood as a result of starvation, the dropsy is generalized, but in the earlier stages is most marked in the feet and legs, especially after exertion. The swelling which sometimes follows serpent-bites, bee-stings or the eating of poisonous shell-fish, and constitutes an extreme and rapidly ensuing form of *nettle-rash*, is a special variety of dropsy. *White-leg*, which may appear after some acute disease like typhoid fever or pneumonia, or after the birth of a child, due to a thrombosis or plugging of the main vein in the affected limb, is one of the localized forms of dropsy. A similar condition may be caused by a *tumour* pressing upon a large vein of the arm or leg. Dropsy in the legs may be due to varicose veins. *Cirrhosis*, tumours, and other diseases of the liver may, by interference with the circulation through it, cause dropsy, first of the abdomen and later of the lower limbs.

Treatment – There is no general treatment which will meet every case. The particular cause has, in each case, to be removed. Dropsy due to heart or kidney disease yields as the disease producing it is alleviated. In cases of localized dropsy, elevation of the dropsical part is of great importance, and the person should adopt the recumbent position. In the case of heart disease, digitalis, which improves the action of the heart, and benzothiadiazine diuretics form the chief means employed. In acute kidney disease the treatment of the dropsy consists in the routine treatment of Bright's disease. In dropsy due to liver conditions, occasional purges with blue-pill or calomel may help the condition. When the dropsy will not yield to drugs, some of the fluid may have to be drawn off (see ASPIRATION); when this is done partially, the kidneys are sometimes enabled to cope with the remainder of the fluid.

DROP-WRIST, or wrist-drop, is a condition in which, owing to partial or complete paralysis of the muscles which extend the hand, the latter droops at the wrist.

Causes – Perhaps the commonest form

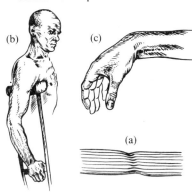

144 – Transient block of radial nerve (a) from crutch pressure (b), resulting in wrist-drop (c). From Illingworth, *A Short Textbook of Surgery*, 9th edition. Churchill Livingstone.

is that known as crutch-palsy (illustration 144), in which, owing to the constant pressure of a crutch in the armpit, the large nerve (radial) that controls the extensor muscles of the forearm becomes damaged, and hence the muscles in question are paralysed. The same effect may be produced when a person sleeps with his head resting on the upper arm, or with the arm over the back of a chair. A blow on the back of the arm may produce a similar condition. Poisoning by alcohol or by lead may also cause the condition, which may also be brought about by a chill.

Treatment – The forms due to pressure on the nerve or to chill require only rest and application of massage and electricity to the muscles to prevent their wasting, for recovery usually takes place gradually but surely. In the cases due to lead, the appropriate treatment for lead poisoning is necessary.

DROSTANOLONE PROPIONATE is an anti-cancer drug which is proving of value in the treatment of some advanced cases of cancer of the breast.

DROWNING, RECOVERY FROM – In Britain, more than a thousand people are drowned every year; two-thirds of

these are accidental and one-third suicidal. An analysis by the Royal Life Saving Society of 715 fatal drowning accidents in Great Britain in 1973 shows that 21 per cent of these occurred while swimming, bathing or paddling, 16 per cent from boats, 4·4 per cent while fishing, and 21 per cent among children playing near water. This last group included five children drowned in private swimming pools. Thirty per cent of these drowning fatalities occurred in children under 16 years of age, 14 per cent of them in the 0 to 5 years age-group. In drowning, death as a rule ensues from asphyxia (see ASPHYXIA), although, in falls from a height upon water, or in cases where the body in falling has encountered blows upon the head or abdomen, death may be due to shock. In the latter case, instead of the signs of asphyxia, the skin is pale, the face placid, and the lungs are empty of water because no attempts at breathing have taken place. In slight cases of shock the chances of resuscitation are rather more hopeful than in cases of asphyxia, because little water has been drawn into the lungs, and because there has been no struggling. Artificial respiration must be persisted in until the signs of death are unmistakable. Speed and immediate treatment on withdrawal from the water are of paramount importance. Recovery is more likely in the case of sea-water drowning than freshwater drowning.

The specific gravity of the body being slightly greater than that of water, it sinks at first; then if the person is able to struggle, his efforts bring him to the surface, only to sink again as he becomes exhausted. This may be repeated several times. In these struggles, water mixed with air is drawn into the air-passages, and the two are churned up with mucus into a froth which forms a great obstacle to the entrance of air into the lungs during subsequent attempts at resuscitation. The first step in this process should be taken *on the instant the body is drawn from the water*, without delay for any examination, removal of clothing, or the like, and consists in the attempt to restore breathing by *artificial respiration*. Before beginning the actual movements of artificial respiration a few seconds should be spent in getting rid of as much water as possible from the lungs and air-passages: for example, a child may be held up by its heels, and the water will run out of his mouth; when an adult is lying prone on the ground, the operator's arms can be linked round the patient's middle, which is then raised, and

146 – The mouth-to-mouth method of artificial respiration. *The Practitioner.*

water will flow out of the mouth. Any seaweed or other matter in the mouth should be quickly removed by the finger. According to the St John Ambulance Association, the St Andrew's Ambulance Association and the British Red Cross Society, expired air resuscitation, or the mouth-to-mouth (or -nose) method, is the method of choice.

1. **Expired-air resuscitation** consists of the old Biblical method of breathing direct into the victim's mouth. Careful investigations carried out in the United States of America, this country and Australia indicate that it is a more efficient method of artificial respiration than any of the more indirect methods.

As in all methods of artificial respiration, speed is the essence of success. Briefly, the technique is as follows:

(1) Lay the victim on his back and kneel opposite his ear. (2) Turn his head towards you and extend it to the sniffing position (illustration 145). (3) Open his mouth, and sweep a finger round the mouth and throat to remove any obvious debris. (4) Place the thumb of the right hand between the teeth and grip the lower jaw in the centre and hold it forwards so that the lower front teeth protrude (illustration 145b). (5) Close the victim's nose by pinching the nostrils with the thumb and index finger of the left hand (illustration 145b). (6) Take a deep breath and, placing your mouth over the victim's mouth (illustration 145c), sealing it, blow forcefully in adults, gently in children, and with puffs of the cheeks in infants, so that the chest is seen to rise. (7) Remove your mouth and allow passive expiration. (8) Repeat about 20 times a minute at first; later slow down to 15.

Three important points to remember are: (i) The victim's head must be extended: ie., bent backwards. (ii) The lower jaw must be kept thrust forwards. (iii) You must take a deep breath each time.

2. **Schafer's prone-posture method.** – Immediately on removal from the water, place the patient face downwards on the ground, with a folded coat under the lower part of the chest, and lose no time by removing clothing. Turn the victim's face a little to one side, so that the mouth and nose are not obstructed (illustration 146). Let the operator *kneel astride* of, or to one side of, the victim, facing his head, and let him place his hands over the lower part of the patient's back, one on each side (on the lowest ribs). Let him throw the weight of his body forward upon his hands, so as to press the air (and water if there is any)

out of the patient's lungs. Then let him immediately raise his body to take the pressure off and allow the patient's chest to expand. Repeat these movements twelve or fifteen times per minute.

146 – Artificial respiration by Schafer's method.

This method has the advantages of extreme simplicity and great effectiveness. Further, no time is lost in freeing the air passages of water and mucus, which may drain from the mouth during the whole procedure; there is no trouble caused by the tongue falling backwards into the throat, as in the face-up methods; the victim is not so liable to bruising as in the Marshall Hall method, or to injury of the ribs. The introducer of the method also claimed that, while the amount of air taken into the lungs of an average-sized healthy person is about 5850 millilitres per minute, the amount that can be drawn in by this method is about 6760 millilitres, an amount far in excess of that possible by the Marshall Hall method.

3. **Holger-Nielsen's method** – The principle is that the chest is compressed against the ground for expiration and raised by the arms for inspiration. The patient is turned face downwards, with the arms upwards and the elbows flexed, so that his head is turned to the side and rests on his hands. The operator kneels on one knee at the patient's head and facing his feet, with his opposite foot near the patient's elbow. For the inspiratory movement grasp the arms above the elbows and rock backwards, raising the arms until tension is felt. Count 1, 2, 3 while doing this (= $2\frac{1}{2}$ seconds). For expiration drop the arms and put your hands on the patient's back just below the shoulder blades, with the thumbs touching, and count 4 as you do this. Rock forwards with your elbows straight and exert steady pressure on the chest. Count 5, 6, 7 while doing this (= $2\frac{1}{2}$ seconds). Slide your hands off the back and on to the patient's arms as you count 8. This cycle should be repeated 10 to 12 times a minute. If the

arm is injured, inspiration is achieved by lifting from the shoulders rather than the upper arms.

4. **Marshall Hall's ready method** is valuable for two reasons: first, because it frees one lung thoroughly from its frothy water; and secondly, because it is an easy and simple method. A roll about 6 to 8 inches (12 to 16 cm) thick is made, for example, out of a rolled-up coat and vest, or a large stone or spar of wood may be used for the purpose. With this under his chest, the patient is placed face downwards, and firm pressure made with both hands upon the back to expel air and water. Then the body, grasped by the shoulders, is turned steadily upon one side, still lying upon the bundle or stone, so that one lung is expanded. Then the body is turned again upon the face so that the air is expelled from the chest, and so forth, each movement being repeated about fifteen times per minute. It is important always to turn the body upon the same side, otherwise water is apt to run from the lung which was previously the lower one, and again choke up the air passages of the one which has been cleared.

5. **Rocking method,** originally recommended by Dr F. C. Eve, is carried out by

147 – Artificial respiration by rocking method. from Belilios, *First Aid and Bandaging.* Baillière, Tindall.

securing the patient face-down on a stretcher. The stretcher is then rocked at the rate of 12 to 15 double rocks per minute (illustration 147). It is an excellent form of artificial respiration provided the stretcher and suitable appliances for rocking it are available.

After-treatment for drowning – As soon as the patient makes efforts at breathing, these measures are stopped. But no such effort may be made for twenty minutes, an hour, or even, in some recorded cases, for several hours, and still the person may

recover, so that artificial respiration should be persevered with so long as there is the slightest sign of life. Efforts must next be made to restore the feeble circulation, and, in cases in which the body has been long in water or much exposed during artificial respiration, to regain the body warmth. To this end the patient should be wrapped in hot blankets, with hot bottles to the sides and feet, and the arms and legs should be rubbed upwards towards the body. So soon as the power of swallowing returns, sips of hot water, and teaspoonfuls of hot brandy and water, or hot coffee, may be administered. Ammonia, nitrite of amyl, or smelling salts may for the same purpose be now and then held to the nose. Finally, if the patient shows a tendency to sleep, this should be encouraged.

Immersion hypothermia – This is responsible for a large number of unnecessary deaths every year, particularly in young people who have been involved in sailing or boating accidents. The summer sea temperature around southern Britain is about 15°C. An unprotected adult of average weight in such water will cool to dangerous levels within two hours. A thin person will reach this critical stage in an hour; a fat one, with his layers of protective insulating fat, may survive indefinitely. Children, particularly boys, who are on average thinner than girls, may be at risk within half-an-hour. Survival times are greatly increased if thick conventional clothing, as well as a lifejacket, is worn, and are shortened for those who swim about rather than float still in a lifejacket, thus retaining their heat. In practice this means that the way to prevent this potentially fatal lowering of body temperature is on abandoning ships or small craft to put on thick clothing, or special insulated clothing such as thermofloat jackets if available, as well as an efficient lifejacket, and to float still while awaiting rescue. A further precautionary measure for yachtsmen is never to take even small amounts of alcohol in exposed conditions unless a large meal is eaten at the same time.

A point to be borne in mind by rescuers, if several people are involved, is that the quietest people are most likely to be reaching a dangerously low temperature, that small boys are most at risk, and that older girls and women are the most likely to remain in good condition if all cannot be rescued on the first rescue trip. Equally important is it to remember that a small child drifting away from shore, holding a float, needs immediate rescue if he or she is not to risk cooling to a dangerous degree.

Treatment consists of getting the victim into warm surroundings as quickly as possible, preferably a bath of water as hot as the attendant can stand with his own hand – about 45° C. The temperature should be a little lower for conscious patients. The hot bath should be tried even though the victim is apparently dead. Cardiac massage (qv) should be given at half the normal rate if the heart is stopped. In most cases the hot bath will cause rapid recovery, and it is best to discontinue the bath as soon as the victim is clearly improving. Excessive rewarming may do harm, expecially in older people. Once a healthy victim of acute immersion is recovering, and has been taken from the bath and allowed to rewarm slowly, lying flat under blankets in a warm place, all is likely to be well. In the case of older people, or those in whom there has been evidence of the heart being affected, removal to hospital for further treatment and investigation is indicated. First and foremost, however, is the necessity for taking prompt action to raise the body temperature to normal limits. (See also HYPOTHERMIA.)

DRUG ADDICTION – A wide range of drugs comes into this category of drugs of addiction or dependence. Some, such as aspirin, are comparatively harmless in this respect. Others, such as the morphine-like drugs, are among the greatest social evils of the day. The characteristics of some of these drugs are shown in table 25. *Physical dependence* is the result of an adaptation of the body to a drug so that if the concentration of the drug falls below a certain level the body is unable to function properly. This produces what is known as the *abstinence syndrome*, characterized by the individual becoming ill and remaining ill until he receives a further dose of the drug. *Tolerance* means that a larger and larger dose of the drug is needed in order to produce the same effect. Drug dependence can develop without tolerance; conversely, tolerance may occur without any concurrent dependence. *Psychic dependence* is a complex factor not yet fully understood. Basically it is the state of mind induced in an individual by a certain drug. It may include what is shown in the table as '*overpowering need*', but not necessarily so. As is shown in the table, psychic dependence may occur in individuals who do not have an overpowering need to take the drug in question, as in the case of cannabis and LSD. On the other hand, over-

powering need is always accompanied by psychic dependence. *Acquired desire* is perhaps best illustrated in the case of cannabis. Devotees of cannabis have to learn to enjoy the drug. If they fail, they may give it up. If, however, they are unfortunate and acquire a desire for the drug, then psychic dependence develops and pleasure is associated with this dependence. *Psychotoxic effects* appear as disturbances in the normal behaviour pattern of the individual. They may vary with the drug being used and are influenced by the psychological make-up of the individual. *Psychotic on withdrawal* is part and parcel of the abstinence syndrome, which develops when the individual stops taking the drug. The number of notified narcotic addicts in the United Kingdom at the end of 1977 was 2033.

Morphine and heroin – Opium and all its derivatives (heroin (qv) is a derivative of morphine) are the classical example of drugs of addiction, with a history stretching back into very early times. Dangerous though they are in western civilization, it has to be borne in mind that by some Oriental peoples opium is widely used, not in an excessive and pernicious manner, but almost in the same sense as tobacco or alcohol is used in the West. Indeed, in the East opium smoking is used as an aid to contemplative serenity, and there can be no doubt that the habit in such a culture by someone brought up in its traditions can be a relatively harmless procedure. Equally, however, it should be noted that opium smoking can be grossly abused in the East as well as in the West. The two great dangers of opium in this sphere, apart from addiction – and whatever expert discussion there may be as to what is meant by addiction, opium is unquestionably accepted as a drug of addiction – are the tolerance the individual develops to it, and the appalling effects of sudden stoppage of its use. The first means that the individual has to take larger and larger doses, whilst the second means that he (or she) is unable to stop the habit alone as the moment dosage is reduced to any appreciable extent he becomes violently ill.

Until comparatively recent years the vast majority of opium addicts were what were known as 'therapeutic' addicts or professional addicts. Therapeutic addicts were individuals who had acquired the habit as a result of having been prescribed some form of the drug for quite legitimate medical reasons. Professional addicts were doctors, nurses or pharmacists who had acquired the habit through being in constant contact with it and therefore open to the temptation offered by easy access to the drug in times of depression, overwork or emotional stress and strain. Today, however, the picture is completely changed. Not only have the majority of addicts of morphine-like drugs started the habit on their own initiative, but many are taking the much more dangerous heroin. Thus, the number of heroin addicts coming to the notice of the Home Office rose from 132 in 1961 to 959 in 1971. The comparable figures for all opiate addicts were 470 and 2769.

The addict to this group of drugs degenerates steadily, physically and mentally. His face becomes sallow, his appearance prematurely aged, and his muscles wasted.

1955 and 1966 showed that 22 per cent were due to suicide or violent death, and 61 per cent were due to suicidal overdose, narcotic overdose (accidental), sudden death (related to addiction) and septic conditions. The high incidence of sepsis is due to the septic conditions under which the addict injects the drug.

Cannabis – Cannabis, or Indian hemp, is a plant which subserves the eminently practical purpose of providing fibre for the making of cord and textiles; it also provides one of the oldest drugs of addiction. Its terminology has become increasingly involved in recent years. The resin (hashish) or the dried flowers (marijuana) may be smoked in cigarettes or through a water pipe. The elixir may be drunk, marijuana

Drugs	Physical Dependence	Tolerance	Over-powering Need	Acquired Desire	Psychic Dependence	Psycho-toxic	Psychotic on With-drawal
Morphine-like	+	+	+		+	+	+
Barbiturates and other hypnotics	+	+	+		+	+	+
Cocaine			+		+	+	
Amphetamine	+	+	+	+	+	+	
Cannabis				+	+	+	
L S D and other Hallucinogens		+		+	+	+	
Inhalation Drugs		?	+ *	+	+		
Aspirin		?	+ *	+	+	+	
Caffeine		+		+	+		
Nicotine		+		+	+		
Alcohol	+	+	+	+	+	+	

* Only some of the users display this.

Table 25 – Comparison of the characteristics of drugs of dependence. *The Practitioner.*

His memory becomes bad, he suffers from insomnia, and he complains of generalized aches and pains. The appetite fails and the liver functions inefficiently. He loses interest in his work and his surroundings. His character changes, and a person who previously was honest and truthful becomes utterly untrustworthy and an inveterate liar. Delusions of various sorts develop, and under their influence criminal acts may be performed. The death-rate is high, particularly among heroin addicts. In one series it was found to be 28 times the average death-rate. In another series the mean age of death was 24·8 years. In most of the cases the causes of death are either related to use of the drug or what has been described as 'non-natural'. Thus, an analysis of the causes of death among non-therapeutic heroin addicts in the United Kingdom between

may be eaten, and the drug is also taken as snuff. Currently used slang terms are 'grass' and 'pot', and a marijuana cigarette is known as a 'stick' or a 'reefer'.

The propensities of the drug have been known for thousands of years. The Chinese were using it as an anaesthetic in surgery 2000 years ago, and it has been claimed that 'soma', a potent hallucinogenic potion referred to in Indian writings around 800 BC, contained cannabis. Herodotus, writing around 400 BC, refers to the Scythians as throwing some mysterious seeds on to red hot stones, and then inhaling the vapour, and it has been said that the seeds were probably those of cannabis. It was probably not until around the 10th century AD that the use of cannabis became widespread in Africa and Asia. How it became introduced to Britain is not quite clear, but the probability is that the habit came from the United States of America, where it was introduced from Mexico, where marijuana smoking is a long-established practice, around the 1930s. Its widespread use throughout Asia is almost part and parcel of the cultural life, the Brahmin in India using it, for example, to help him say his prayers.

When marijuana is smoked, the effects appear quickly, reach a peak in two hours and then pass off. The physical effects are quickening of the pulse, a rise in blood-pressure, congestion of the eyes, frequency of passing of urine, and often nausea and vomiting or diarrhoea. The psychological effects vary according to the individual, but by and large are dependent upon the mood of the individual when he takes the drug. If he is in an optimistic mood he will become exhilarated; if he is depressed he will become even more depressed. The ideal that the users of marijuana aim at has been described as a 'mood of pleasant euphoria, which is accompanied by a feeling that his thoughts are coming more quickly, that the world is more intensely interesting, and by a general loosening of inhibition'. This is what is meant by being 'high'. The expert regular smoker may achieve this without intoxicating or incapacitating himself, but all too often the individual becomes increasingly restless and lethargic, or dreamy and withdrawn, and there may be transient disorientation. Tremors and unsteadiness of gait may develop, and in the initiate the feeling of loss of control may evoke unpleasant anxiety. Whether or not it can produce a psychotic state is open to question. According to one expert in this field, 'marijuana releases what is latent in the individual's thoughts and emotions, but does not evoke responses which would be totally alien to him in his undrugged state'.

Although marijuana is not as vicious an addiction-forming drug as heroin, its potentialities for evil, and the risk of the user becoming dependent on it, are such as to justify steps to bring its use strictly under control or to render its use illegal in Britain. As has been pointed out over and over again, the argument that the stable personality might be able to continue using the drug without any deleterious effect, does not justify anyone, and particularly the adolescent and young adult, embarking on its use. Equally, whilst there is no logical reason why the use of marijuana need necessarily lead on to the use of heroin, all the evidence indicates that the individual – and again particularly the adolescent and young adult – who embarks on the use of marijuana sooner or later is liable to find himself (or herself) in the company where the temptation to try heroin may be so overwhelming and tempting as to brook no refusal – with dire effects.

Hallucinogens – The hallucinogenic drugs include lysergic acid diethylamide (LSD as it is popularly known), dimethyltryptamine, mescaline, psilocybin and psilocin. They are a group of compounds that since ancient days American Indians have used as intoxicants to produce ecstatic states for religious occasions. LSD is the one most widely used today in western civilization. It produces distortion of perception, visual and emotional changes, emotionally charged fantasies that may induce extreme states of panic, feelings of omnipotence or bodily and mental dissolution, panic reactions or transcendental calm and psychotic or near-psychotic reactions. Three recorded incidents may be quoted as examples of the tragic sequelae that may ensue from the use of LSD, or indeed any other member of this group of drugs: a youth of 20 who leapt from the roof of a chapel after taking LSD, thinking he could fly; a youngster who, in a state of agitation after taking a derivative of LSD, drove his car at 100 miles an hour into a house at the foot of a hill; a man, allegedly under the influence of LSD, who raped the 9-year-old daughter of his mistress in the belief that the child was his mistress.

The value of LSD in the field of treatment is still a matter of debate, but there seems little doubt that under skilled supervision, and used with the utmost caution and care, it can prove of value in the treatment of certain neuroses and phobic states. One experienced worker in this field has summed up the position as follows: 'One cannot emphasize too strongly the need for all LSD therapy to be carried out in a carefully controlled environment by trained staff working as a therapeutic team with their patients. If this is done, much can be achieved with a group of patients who often otherwise defy our therapeutic efforts: the phobic states, the sexual neuroses and some inadequate and neurotic psycopaths'.

Otherwise, *pace* Aldous Huxley, the propensities for evil in this group of drugs are such that there can be no questioning the ban on its use except by specified medical practitioners and psychiatrists. Its present use by the so-called hippie culture can do nothing but harm, apart altogether from the fact that there is more than a suspicion that they can produce genetic damage.

Amphetamines – These drugs were originally introduced as stimulants of the nervous system. It was then found that they inhibited appetite, and as a result they were used widely in the treatment of obesity. The first warning of the dangers of amphetamines was given by the finding that a disturbingly high number of housewives, who had originally been prescribed these drugs for obesity, were becoming dependent upon them as a means of keeping up their spirits and counteracting household blues. The next warning was the finding that a number of patients on amphetamines were developing a psychosis, with ideas of persecution and hallucinations. Then, somewhere in the early 1960s, youngsters started taking them for the 'kicks' they obtained. Initially this reaction takes the form of euphoria (feeling pleased with oneself and the world), a tendency to talkativeness, and diminution of inhibitions. In due course, with larger doses, and especially if the drug is taken by injection rather than by mouth, restlessness develops, rapid, often slurred speech, irritability and anxiety, unsteadiness, dilatation of the pupils and dryness of the mouth. If this last item is relieved by alcohol the results can be catastrophic. The effects are heightened if, as tends to happen, the amphetamines are taken with other drugs, such as the barbiturates.

Barbiturates and tranquillizers – For the anxiety-ridden, immature, unstable, highly wrought individual the barbiturates and tranquillizers can prove such a boon and anchor amid the emotional storms of life that it is scarcely surprising that, having once sampled their efficiency, he or she is reluctant to dispense with their aid. Whether this is a true state of addiction, in the strict sense of the term, may be arguable, but certainly these members of the community become reliant, if not dependent, on them. This may be at least a partial explanation of the fact that between 1962 and 1968, in England and Wales, the number of National Health Service prescriptions for tranquillizers rose from 6·6 million to 16 million (by 1975 in England to 20·5 million), the number of prescriptions for barbiturates remaining more or less the same (15·8 million in 1962 and 15·3 million in 1968), whilst prescriptions for non-barbiturate hypnotics rose from 2·6 million to 5·8 million. The slight fall in prescriptions for barbiturates partially represents the recognition by doctors of the dangerous potentialities of barbiturates in this field. It has been estimated that between one and two million persons regularly receive prescriptions for hypnotic drugs. The disturbing development in recent years has been the increasing use of barbiturate-like drugs by the younger generation. These are often taken by injection, and usually in conjunction with other drugs such as the amphetamines, as in the notorious 'purple hearts'. A recent survey showed that 62 of 65 heroin addicts interviewed had taken barbiturates and 52 of these had injected the drug.

The main dangers of this group of drugs are threefold. In the first place, the individual may become so dependent on them that he, or she, refuses to go to bed at night without taking one or more tablets, even though the original cause of sleeplessness has been removed. Unless the dose has been carefully worked out, the individual may well waken up in the morning with the equivalent of a 'hangover' and find it difficult to 'come to' sufficiently to do an efficient day's work. Indeed, it has been suggested that much of the current industrial discontent is due to a generation of barbiturate-, or 'tranquillized'-, workmen and workwomen. The next stage is that the individual may start taking the prescribed tablet to cope with any problem that may crop up during the day. This, in turn, may lead to experimenting with other more dangerous drugs, such as the amphetamines, or even heroin, and so the plunge is taken down one of the most slippery paths in human experience.

Inhalation drugs – These include benzenes, paint thinners, glue, amphetamines and ether. In some instances, as in the case of benzedrine inhalers, once widely prescribed for relieving the congestion in nasal catarrh, and of certain inhalers used by asthmatic subjects, the habit was acquired as a result of the inhaler being prescribed by a doctor for a perfectly legitimate purpose. The patient, however, derived so much pleasure and comfort from the inhaler that he found it increasingly difficult to dispense with it, even though there was no longer any physical need for it. Ether addiction is predominantly an occupational hazard of anaesthetists. Other anaesthetics may have the same propensity, but ether seems to be the most dangerous in this respect.

Other drugs – As shown in table 25, these include caffeine, nicotine and aspirin. They also include many hypnotics, such as chloral hydrate and bromides, which are less of a problem today in view of their diminishing use. By and large this form of dependence seldom causes much trouble and can usually be controlled, with the possible exception of My Lady Nicotine, whose charms seem to be irresistible to so many of her admirers.

Cocaine – The action of this drug is described under COCAINE. It is generally taken hypodermically by its addicts, or the leaves may be chewed. A hypodermic dose of around 1 grain (60 mg) may produce after a few minutes a feeling of suffocation, anxiety and faintness, but this rapidly passes off and is followed by mental exhilaration, rapidity of thought, and a feeling of buoyancy. After a short time, however, this passes off, and as dose after dose is taken, a reaction of deeper and deeper depression ensues upon each. At the same time, dyspepsia, loss of appetite, restlessness, sleeplessness, forgetfulness and failure of the power to apply the mind to any task appear. Finally, the person may pass into a state of melancholia or mania. Marked physical deterioration, in the form of emaciation and digestive disorders, is also found. In the United Kingdom the number of known cocaine addicts has risen from 25 in 1958 to 564 in 1968. Many of these use the drug in combination with heroin. This combination was introduced in London as a result of a mistaken belief on the part of some doctors that the combination was safer than either drug alone. In fact, the combination is much more dangerous and almost impossible to treat with any degree of success.

DRUGS – The sale and supply of medicines are controlled by part III of the Medicines Act 1968, the underlying principle of which is that medicines should normally be sold under the supervision of a pharmacist, but it also enables the Health Ministers to modify the application of this principle. Thus, the Medicines (General Sale List) Order lists the medicines which can with reasonable safety be sold or supplied at non-pharmacy premises. These are the medicines where the hazard to health, the risk of misuse, or the need to take special precautions in handling is small, and where wider sale than in pharmacies would be a convenience to the purchaser. At the other end of the scale the Medicines (Prescription Only) Order specifies the medicines which may only be supplied in accordance with the prescription of a doctor, dentist or veterinarian. These are the medicines whose use in treatment needs to be supervised by a practitioner because their use in-

volves a known or potential toxic hazard. In between these two categories are the medicines (unlisted) which can be sold only at pharmacies under the supervision of a pharmacist. Exemptions from the pharmacy sale restrictions are contained in the Medicines (Pharmacy and General Sale – Exemption) Order and the Medicines (Exemption from Restriction in the Retail Sale or Supply of Veterinary Drugs) Order. These include exemptions for particular products such as homoeopathic products; for professional groups, such as state registered chiropodists; and for agricultural merchants selling or supplying medicines to farmers. There is also an Order, the Medicines (Retail Sale or Supply of Herbal Remedies) Order, specifically relating to herbal remedies. (See also DOSAGE; and PRESCRIPTION.)

DRUNKENNESS (see ALCOHOLISM, ACUTE and CHRONIC).

DUCT is the name applied to a passage leading from a gland into some hollow organ, or on to the surface of the body, by which the secretion of the gland is discharged: eg. the pancreatic duct and the bile duct opening into the duodenum, and the sweat ducts opening on the skin surface.

DUCTLESS GLAND is the term applied to any one of certain glands in the body the secretion of which goes directly into the blood stream and so is carried to different parts of the body. These glands – the pituitary, thyroid, parathyroid, adrenal and reproductive – are also known as the ENDOCRINE GLANDS (qv). Some glands may be both duct glands and ductless glands. For example, the pancreas manufactures a digestive juice which passes by a duct into the small intestine. It also manufactures, by means of special cells, a substance called insulin which passes straight into the blood and not by way of any duct.

DUCTUS ARTERIOSUS is the bloodvessel in the foetus through which blood passes from the pulmonary artery to the aorta, thereby by-passing the lungs, which do not function during intra-uterine life. (See CIRCULATION OF THE BLOOD.) The ductus normally ceases to function soon after birth and within a few weeks is converted into a fibrous cord. Occasionally this obliteration does not occur: a condition known as patent ductus arteriosus.

This is one of the more common congenital defects of the heart, and one which responds particularly well to surgical treatment. (See HEART DISEASES.)

DUCTUS DEFERENS, or VAS DEFERENS, is the tube which carries spermatozoa from the epidydimis to the seminal vesicles. (See TESTICLE.)

DUMBNESS means an inability to pronounce the elementary sounds which make up words.

Varieties The important classification of cases of deficient power of speech is into (a) those associated with deafness and (b) those in which hearing is good. In a case associated with deafness, the person may be dumb merely because he has been born deaf, and, having no knowledge of sound, cannot understand or make intelligible sounds, although provided with good voice mechanism; or a person who has lost his hearing by some disease in childhood may be unable to speak otherwise than as a child for the same reason. It is estimated that 1 per 1000 deaf children are so deaf that natural speech is impossible. When hearing is good, on the other hand, dumbness is due generally to some mental defect or sometimes to some failure in the organs of voice production.

Causes – Deafness is the most important cause, because the one most capable of treatment. Of those due to some congenital brain-deficiency, some arise in children of persons who were themselves deaf-mutes. Another class of cases, in which there is also mental deficiency, arises from brain disease, such as that due to syphilis. Those children who are mentally bright and whose hearing is good have occasionally some structural defect, such as tongue-tie or enlarged tonsils and adenoids in the throat, which allow of attempts at speaking but prevent proper formation of words. Dumbness is sometimes a hysterical manifestation. Lisping and lalling speech are slight forms of dumbness due to inefficient control of the voice mechanism, but can generally be cured by careful training. (See STAMMERING; and VOICE.)

Treatment – A dumb child is cut off from other people and so cannot develop normally, unless carefully treated; a careful examination should be made of any child who does not speak by two years of age. Deafness is easily discovered by finding that the child pays no attention to noises made behind its back. Mental ability can be measured by special tests. Physi-

cal obstructions, like tongue-tie or large tonsils, should be removed if present.

Deaf-mutes may be trained to read the lips and throat movements of others by sight, and to use their powers of voice through a complicated process, which should begin about the age of six or seven. It is hard for adults to pick this up, and persons who are to be instructed in this method should not learn the finger language first.

The training required for this 'oral' method is long, and, if the deaf person is to gain a modulated voice and a fair command of language, the constant attention of an expert tutor is necessary all through childhood and youth. In England and Wales a local education authority can compel a parent of any child of two years of age or over to submit the child for medical examination. If this shows that special educational treatment is required, the authority must provide such treatment. In the case of deaf-mutes, attendance is compulsory between the ages of 5 and 16.

Training in lip-reading should be started as soon as possible, and special educational methods should be begun as soon as possible after the age of two years.

DUODENAL ILEUS is the term applied to dilatation of the duodenum due to chronic obstruction of the duodenum, caused by an abnormal position of arteries in the region of the duodenum pressing on it.

DUODENAL ULCER has much in common with gastric ulcer. (See STOMACH, DISEASES OF.) The two together are known as peptic ulcers, and in recent years there has been a tendency for the two forms of ulceration to be regarded as modifications of one entity known as peptic ulcer, rather than as separate disease entities. Part of the reason for this is that, as increasingly detailed statistics have become available, it has become clear that the incidence of the disease (or diseases) has been changing over the last century. Be all that as it may, it is abundantly clear that, as one authority has expressed it, 'peptic ulcer in general is still a large health problem' in Britain, probably as many 'as one in ten of the population suffering at some time or other during his or her lifetime from ulcer-type dyspepsia'.

Duodenal ulcer is ten to fifteen times more common than gastric ulcer. The age incidence of the two forms of ulcer differs. Thus, duodenal ulcer occurs at any age from 20 years onwards, whereas gastric ulcer usually occurs after the age of 40. Duodenal ulcer is three times as common in men as in women; indeed, in some series the ratio between men and women is as high as ten. In gastric ulcer, on the other hand, the sex ratio is less than two men to one woman. Gastric ulcer is rare in women until after the menopause. Here it should be interpolated that these figures, as indeed the whole of this section, is concerned with chronic peptic ulcer. It is such ulcers that are practically always referred to when mention is made of duodenal or gastric ulcer. Acute peptic ulcers are quite uncommon. Indeed, there is some evidence that they may be an entirely different disease from chronic peptic ulcers. This does not mean, however, that chronic peptic ulcers, whether duodenal or gastric, do not pass through stages when their manifestations can be justifiably described as acute. There is also a different social incidence between the two forms of ulcer. Duodenal ulcer is more common in the upper social classes, although it is to be found in all classes, but gastric ulcer is more common among the lower social classes. There is also a higher incidence of duodenal ulcer in individuals who belong to blood group O. (See BLOOD GROUPS.) Not the least interesting observation in the field of peptic ulcer is that the large increase in incidence since the turn of the century has been due to the increase in duodenal ulcers. There is some statistical evidence that this 'epidemic' is now on the wane, and that the incidence of duodenal ulcer in Britain is beginning to fall.

There is no general consensus of expert opinion as to the precise cause of peptic ulcers. What probably happens is that there is some abrasion, or break, in the lining membrane (or mucosa) of the stomach and/or duodenum, and that it is gradually eroded and deepened by the gastric juice. What is not known, however, is why this only occurs in some people. After all, the probability is that such abrasions occur in everyone of us at some time or other, but it is only in a minority that these develop into peptic ulcers. Equally puzzling is why the acid and pepsin in the gastric juice erode the stomach (or duodenum) lining downwards into the depth of the wall of the stomach (or duodenum), but does not erode, or digest, it all along the surface of the lining. Needless to say, all sorts of theories have been advanced to explain these discrepancies. None is proven, but some are probable, whilst others have practical implications. Thus, mental stress and

strain are probably provocative factors, thus explaining the increased incidence of duodenal ulcer in the managerial and executive grades of society. Smoking seems to accentuate, if not cause, duodenal ulcer, and the drinking of alcoholic liquors is probably harmful. The apparent association with a given blood group, and the fact that relatives of a patient with a peptic ulcer are unduly likely to develop such an ulcer suggest that there is some constitutional factor. Equally interesting is the suggestion that oestrogen (qv), the predominant female sex hormone, may prevent the development of a gastric ulcer. This suggestion is based upon the fact that women are much more likely to develop gastric ulcers at, or after, the menopause, when the normal output of oestrogen in the body begins to diminish.

Symptoms and signs – These are similar in some ways to those of gastric ulcer, but there are certain differences. The presenting symptom is pain in the middle of the upper part of the abdomen, or somewhat to the right. This tends to come on two or three hours after a meal, and to be relieved by taking food (eg. a glass of milk). It also tends to occur during the night. The pain varies in intensity, and, if not treated, may persist for up to an hour. The appetite is not usually affected, and, though the individual tends to remain thin, there is not usually much loss of weight. Vomiting is not common. When it does occur, it usually means that the ulcer is causing obstruction of the exit of the food from the stomach into the duodenum. The main finding on examination is tenderness over the area of pain, accompanied by stiffening, or guarding, of the overlying muscles. The diagnosis is clinched by the radiological demonstration of what is known as a 'niche' in the duodenum. This niche is the actual ulcer, and it is made visible by giving the individual some radio-opaque substance, such as barium sulphate, to swallow. This fills up the ulcer crater, which is then visible when an X-ray is taken, or when the duodenum is studied by fluoroscopy (qv). Another useful method of examination is gastric analysis. (See TEST MEAL.) In patients with duodenal ulcer this usually reveals a high gastric acidity.

As in the case of a gastric ulcer, the patient with a duodenal ulcer is liable to two complications: perforation of the ulcer, and haemorrhage (see HAEMATEMESIS). If the bleeding from the ulcer is slight, there may be no vomiting of blood (or haematemesis), the blood being passed down the gut. In the course of its passage through the gut it is chemically altered and becomes black in colour. Then, when it is finally passed in the stools, the stools are dark and shiny, or tarry, in appearance. (See MELAENA.)

Treatment consists basically of rest, a diet, and the administration of alkalis. In severe cases a period of rest in bed may be advisable. This in itself has a most beneficial effect. No complicated dietetic regime is called for nowadays. The basis of the diet is the avoidance of all condiments, a minimum of fried food, and something to eat every two hours. The rationale of this is to counteract the increased acidity of the gastric juice. In practice, two-hourly feeding means breakfast, lunch and dinner (or supper), with a glass of milk mid-morning, a snack in mid-afternoon and a snack the last thing at night on going to bed. The basis of the snacks should be milk or something milky. Strong tea and coffee should be avoided, as should smoking. Alcohol is better avoided, but a glass of wine with food will do no harm. There is a large range of alkalis to be chosen from, and the individual choice should be made in conjunction with the family doctor. Promising results are being reported from the use of cimetidine, a drug which reduces the hyperacidity of the gastric juice. If the ulcer does not respond to adequate medical treatment along these lines, or if it leads to obstruction of the pylorus (qv), then operation is called for. Operation is also indicated should perforation occur. A perforated duodenal (or gastric) ulcer is an emergency, and must be dealt with immediately. The majority of surgeons still favour immediate operation. Should a haemorrhage occur, the treatment depends upon its severity. As a rule, a blood transfusion is called for.

DUODENUM is the first part of the intestine immediately beyond the stomach, so named because its length is about twelve fingerbreadths. (See INTESTINE.)

DUPUYTREN'S CONTRACTURE is a thickening and drawing together of the skin and the underlying tissues in the palm of the hand, which cause gradual and permanent bending of the fingers. The cause of the condition is not known. It is more common among white-collar workers than among manual labourers. The ring and little fingers are most often affected. It is treated in early cases by mas-

sage and the occasional wearing of a splint, but the only cure is by means of surgery: by dividing the fibrous bands beneath the skin.

DURA MATER is the outermost and strongest of the three membranes or meninges which envelop the brain and spinal cord. In it run vessels which nourish the inner surface of the skull. (See BRAIN.)

DWARF, or DWARFISM, is a term applied to under-development of the body. The causes are either developmental or due to food insufficient in quantity or unsuitable in quality, or to defects in some of the body secretions which can be corrected. The first-named group includes pituitary dwarfism, the subjects being very small persons with normally proportioned parts, also achondroplasic dwarfs (see ACHONDROPLASIA) with large globular head and shortened limbs and stumpy fingers. It is now known that in a certain proportion of children of short stature this can be remedied by administration of the growth hormone of pituitary gland (qv), provided this is given at an early enough age. All children who by the age of 5 years are at least what is technically known as 'three standard deviations below the mean' should be referred for examination by specialists to determine whether or not their lack of height is due to lack of growth hormone and therefore likely to respond to treatment with the hormone. In the class of dwarfism which is partly curable, there are included cretins, whose want of growth in mind and body is attributable to a primary defect of the thyroid gland. (See CRETINISM.) In this class are also included various forms of defective growth associated with defects in the secretions of the digestive organs, especially the pancreas; this type of defect, often known as pancreatic infantilism, is mainly confined to a retardation of physical development, while the mental changes are little marked. Another form of dwarfism, associated with a deformity of the bones, is produced by rickets in early life, such persons showing high forehead, great bending of the leg bones, and deformity of the chest. (See RICKETS.)

DYNAMOMETER is an elliptical ring of steel to which is attached a dial and moving index. It is used to test the strength of the muscles of the forearm, being squeezed in the hand, and registering the pressure in pounds or kilograms.

DYS- is a prefix meaning difficult or painful.

DYSCHEZIA is the term applied to constipation due to retention of faeces in the rectum. This retention is the outcome of irregular habits, which damp down the normal reflex causing defaecation.

DYSCRASIA means a diseased constitution. (See CONSTITUTION.)

DYSDIADOKOKINESIA means loss of the ability to perform rapid alternate movements, such as winding up a watch. It is a sign of a lesion in the cerebellum.

DYSENTERY also called bloody flux, is an infectious disease with a local lesion in the form of inflammation and ulceration of the lower portion of the bowels. It occurs in two main forms: bacillary dysentery and amoebic dysentery, which will be discussed separately.

BACILLARY DYSENTERY is found in practically every part of the world.

Cause – The disease may occur sporadically or in epidemics. The causative organism is the dysentery bacillus, or shigella as it is now known, of which there are several strains, named after their discoverers: Shiga, Flexner and Sonne. In England, where there were 7,758 cases in 1973, the Sonne strain (*Shigella sonnei*) is responsible for the vast majority of cases. The infection is spread by flies, by direct contact, or by pollution of the water by faeces from infected patients, which contain the bacillus. Epidemics are thus encouraged by overcrowding and insanitary conditions. In the East, uncooked vegetables, especially salads, are a potent source of infection, as are cooks and other foodhandlers who are carriers of the disease. In Britain the disease is more common in the winter. The incubation period is 1 to 7 days. The severity of the disease depends partly upon the strain responsible for the infection. Thus, Shiga infections are usually severe, whilst, except in infants, Flexner and Sonne infections run a more benign course.

The dysentery bacilli affect mainly the large intestine. In mild cases there may be only a catarrh of the intestine with excessive mucoid excretion, whilst in severe cases there may be extensive ulceration involving practically the whole of the large intestine.

Symptoms – These vary from those of a mild attack of diarrhoea to those of an acute fulminating infection. The first symptoms usually consist of colicky pain in the abdomen followed by diarrhoea. There may also be nausea, aching pain in the limbs, and shivery feelings. There is always fever. The number of stools varies, but there may be as many as fifty daily in acute cases, The stools consist mainly of mucus and blood. The duration of the diarrhoea varies from a few days to a fortnight, depending upon the severity of the infection. Diagnosis is established by finding dysentery bacilli in the stools. Complications only occur in severe cases, and consist of perforation of the intestine and severe haemorrhage from the gut. At one time one of the killing diseases of the world, with mortality rates up to 50 per cent during epidemics, the outlook has been entirely altered by the introduction of the sulphonamides, but it is still a serious condition in young infants, old people and the malnourished.

Treatment – PREVENTIVE – This consists of adequate sanitation, the destruction of flies, careful disposal of all garbage, and careful protection of all food from flies. In addition no carrier of dysentery bacilli should be allowed to handle food.

CURATIVE – Complete rest in bed is essential, and precautions must be taken to ensure that the stools are disposed of without any risk of their spreading the infection. For the first twenty-four hours only water is given. In the case of acutely ill babies or young children it may be necessary to give fluids intravenously, in the form, for example, of 4·3 per cent glucose in $\frac{1}{5}$ normal saline, for the first twenty-four hours or so. This is gradually supplemented with milk, milk puddings, and chicken broth, but it is necessary for the diet to be kept light, and to contain as little residue as possible, until the diarrhoea has settled. Purgatives and laxatives are not given. The sheet-anchor of treatment is now the sulphonamides: usually phthalylsulphathiazole, succinylsulphathizole or sulphadimidine. Alternatively, neomycin may be used. If there is much abdominal pain, morphine may be given during the first day, but usually the application of heat in some form to the abdomen is sufficient.

AMOEBIC DYSENTERY is almost entirely confined to tropical and subtropical countries. Around 200 new cases occur annually in England and Wales.

Cause – The causative organism is the *Entamoeba histolytica* (illustration 148). Infection occurs as a result of food, eg. uncooked vegetables, or drinking water which has been contaminated either by a carrier of the disease or by flies. The amoebae settle in the wall of the large intestine, where they cause first of all inflammatory changes and then ulceration. These ulcers then tend to become infected with other organisms. From the ulcers the amoebae may spread through the portal vein, where they cause abscesses. An amoebic abscess of the liver is not infrequent. More rarely, the amoebae may spread elsewhere, eg. to the lungs or brain, and cause abscesses. Occasionally a mass may be formed in the colon, known as an amoeboma.

Symptoms – These may appear within a week of infection or be delayed for months or even years. The onset of the disease is usually gradual, with the passage of several stools daily, which ultimately contain blood. Occasionally there may be an

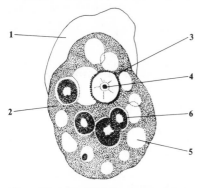

148 – *Entamoeba histolytica*, unencysted. 1, ectoplasm; 2, endoplasm; 3, nucleus; 4, karyosome; 5, vacuoles; 6, ingested red blood cells. From Blacklock and Southwell, *A Guide to Human Parasitology*. H. K. Lewis & Co. Ltd.

acute sudden onset as described for bacillary dysentery. Even in the cases with gradual onset there is loss of weight, with dyspepsia and anaemia. Complications which may occur include perforation of the intestine, haemorrhage from the gut, and abscess formation in the liver, brain, bones or testes. The condition is very liable to run a chronic course. Any individual who has been in the tropics and who complains of abdominal pain and dyspepsia should have the stools examined for the presence of *Entamoeba histolytica*, even though there is no history of dysentery.

Involvement of the liver (amoebic hepatitis) may occur months or years after the occurrence of amoebic dysentery. Such involvement is marked by the occurrence of pain and tenderness over the liver, with fever.

Treatment – PREVENTIVE – This consists of the protection of food from flies, the avoidance of contamination of water and uncooked vegetables, and steps to ensure that those handling food are not carriers of the amoeba.

CURATIVE – Emetine, one of the alkaloids of ipecacuanha, is the most effective drug for the treatment of severe cases of amoebic dysentery. It is usually given in the form of emetine hydrochloride or dehydroemetine given by injection. A recently introduced drug which is proving of value is diloxamide furoate. Metronidazole is also proving of value. Tetracycline is often used in the treatment of mild cases. Emetine hydrochloride, by intramuscular injection, is given for the treatment of amoebic hepatitis. If an amoebic abscess has formed in the liver, this is aspirated and emetine is given as in the case of amoebic hepatitis. To a certain extent emetine is being replaced by metronidazole for the treatment of amoebic abscess as well as amoebic dysentery. Chloroquine given by mouth is also of value in the treatment of amoebic hepatitis.

DYSIDROSIS means disturbance of sweat secretion.

DYSLEXIA is difficulty in reading or learning to read. It is always accompanied by difficulty in writing and particularly by difficulties in spelling correctly. It is a condition which is attracting increasing attention, particularly the form known as specific dyslexia. This is the name given to difficulties in learning to read and write which affect a minority of children exposed to normal educational processes who do not show backwardness in other school subjects.

Parents of such children would be well advised to get in touch with the British Dyslexia Association, 18 The Circus, Bath BA1 2ET.

DYSMENORRHOEA means painful menstruation. (See MENSTRUATION.)

DYSPAREUNIA means painful or difficult coitus.

DYSPEPSIA is merely another, somewhat old-fashioned, name for indigestion. In other words, it describes a condition in which the individual is complaining of pain or discomfort, usually in the upper part of the abdomen or the lower part of the front of the chest, which may, or may not, be associated with other disturbances such as heartburn (qv), flatulence (qv), or nausea (qv). It may be due to a multiplicity of causes, such as gastritis, peptic ulcer, hiatus hernia, cancer of the stomach, all of which involve the stomach, and all of which are discussed in the appropriate section. In some it may be due to disease of the gall-bladder or pancreas, or it may be due to disease in some other part of the body, such as heart failure, uraemia, and diabetes mellitus. In all of these conditions the relief of the dyspepsia is dependent upon the treatment of the underlying cause.

Nervous dyspepsia – There is one form of dyspepsia, in which the name is still retained, and that is nervous dyspepsia. This is the form of indigestion that is brought on by psychological or emotional stress. It occurs in the anxious, worrying, highly strung, 'nervous' type of individual. Whenever such individuals get worked up, become unduly tense or excitable, and find life is proving too difficult, whether this be due to difficult conditions in the home or at work, illness or death in the family, they develop rather vague, but nevertheless disturbing signs of indigestion. These may take the form of loss of appetite, pain, flatulence or heartburn. Although in some the manifestations of indigestion may be constant, in others – and these constitute the majority – they vary from time to time. Once the stress or strain is relieved or eased, the indigestion disappears, and the individual is able to eat a normal diet – and enjoy it. Among the features characteristic of this form of dyspepsia are the tendency for it to be accompanied by attacks of sweating, weakness, palpitations, a feeling of tenseness, and insomnia. The inability to sleep is not due to the indigestion, which as a rule does not tend to be troublesome at night. Rather is the insomnia due to the stress or strain that is responsible for the dyspepsia.

Treatment is based upon finding the cause of the emotional or psychological disturbance and trying to alleviate this. In some this may be difficult as it is basically the nature of the individual's make-up and cannot be changed. These are the unfortunates of this world who are quite convinced that they have a 'weak' or 'delicate' stomach. Even they, however, benefit if they can be reassured that there is no 'organic' cause for their dyspepsia. If the individual is suffering from an exceptional spell of stress or strain, a holiday may do a world of good. No dietetic restrictions are necessary, except that the diet should be nutritious, attractive and reasonably bland. Excessive smoking, often a feature of these cases, should be curtailed, and, particularly in the case of the harassed business man, a restriction on 'homework' and work at weekends should be imposed.

DYSPHAGIA is the medical term for difficulty in swallowing.

DYSPITUITARISM means disordered function of the pituitary body. (See PITUITARY BODY.)

DYSPNOEA means difficulty in breathing. Orthopnoea means breathing possible only when sitting up.

DYSTOCIA means slow or painful birth of a child.

DYSTROPHY means defective or faulty nutrition, and is a term generally applied to some developmental change in the muscles occurring independently of the nervous system. The best-known forms are those known as *progressive muscular dystrophy*, in which groups of muscles, especially those of the calves and buttocks, undergo a fatty degeneration associated with increase in size but weakness in power; and *adiposogenital dystrophy* associated with defect of the pituitary gland.

DYSURIA means difficulty or pain in urination.

E

EAR – The ear is concerned with two functions. The more evident is that of the sense of hearing, the other is the sense of equilibration and of motion. The organ is divided into three parts: (*a*) the external ear, consisting of the auricle on the surface of the head, and the tube which leads inwards to the drum; (*b*) the middle ear, separated from the former by the tympanic membrane or drum, and from the internal ear by two other membranes, but communicating with the throat by the Eustachian tube; and (*c*) the internal ear, comprising the complicated labyrinth from which runs the vestibulocochlear nerve into the brain.

149 – The auricle, with its various parts named.

External ear – The auricle or pinna, (illustration 149), shaped in man something like a crumpled-up funnel, is not essential to the sense of hearing, although in animals it appears to play an important part. It consists of a framework of elastic cartilage covered by skin, the lobule at the lower end being a small mass of fat. From the bottom of the concha the external auditory (or acoustic) meatus (illustration 150) runs inwards for 1 inch (25 mm), to end blindly at the drum. This passage is short in young children, in whom the drum is almost at the surface, and it lengthens as the skull bones develop. The outer half of the passage is surrounded by cartilage, lined by skin, on which are placed fine hairs pointing outwards, and glands secreting a small amount of wax. In the inner half, the skin is smooth and lies directly upon the temporal bone, in the substance of which the whole hearing apparatus is enclosed. The two parts meet at a slight angle, so as to give the whole passage a curve, which can be straightened by pulling the auricle upwards and backwards, when the drum can often be clearly seen by a good light.

Middle ear – The tympanic membrane, forming the drum, is stretched completely across the end of the passage, being placed rather obliquely, so that it makes an angle of about 60° with the floor (illustration 150). It is about one-third of an inch (8 mm) across, as thick as a piece of goldbeater's skin, and white or pale pink in colour, so that it is partly transparent, and some of the contents of the middle ear shine through it. From this description it can be readily understood how easily it is torn, and how dangerous are blows on the side of the head, and rough manipulations to remove wax. The cavity of the middle ear is about one-third of an inch (8 mm) wide and one-sixth of an inch (4 mm) in depth from the tympanic membrane to the inner wall of bone. Although important structures, like the facial nerve which runs down behind it, lie close around, its only important contents are three small bones, the malleus (hammer), incus (anvil), and stapes (stirrup), collectively known as the auditory ossicles, with two minute muscles which regulate their movements, and the chorda tympani nerve which runs across the cavity. The auditory ossicles are of great importance. The malleus has a long spicule of bone, the handle, embedded in the substance of the drum, while its head is in contact with the incus. The incus, suspended by one process of bone, has another affixed to the stapes, and the latter fits, by what would in a real stirrup be the footpiece, into one (fenestra vestibuli) of the two openings which lead through the inner wall of the middle ear into the internal ear. Accordingly these three bones form a chain across the middle ear, connecting the drum with the internal ear. Their function is to convert the air-waves, which strike upon the drum, into mechanical movements which can affect the fluid in the inner ear, because air-waves produce little effect upon fluid directly.

The middle ear has two connections which are of great importance as regards disease: in front, it communicates by a passage 1½ inches (37 mm) long, the Eustachian (or auditory) tube, with the upper part of the throat, behind the nose; behind and above, it opens into a cavity known as the mastoid antrum. The Eustachian tube

293

150 – The external and middle portions of the right ear. *Gray's Anatomy.*

admits air from the throat, and so keeps the pressure on both sides of the drum fairly equal. Serious deafness is produced by its closure, and it also, unfortunately, forms a channel by which acute inflammation, as in measles, can and does spread to the ear. The antrum occupies the interior of the projecting mass of bone, the mastoid process, which is felt on the surface of the head behind the ear, and this cavity, along with the middle ear, is separated from the interior of the skull only by a thin plate of bone about the thickness of a playing card.

Internal ear – This consists of a complex system of hollows in the substance of the temporal bone enclosing a membranous duplicate. Between the membrane and the bone is a fluid known as perilymph, while the membrane is distended by another collection of fluid known as endolymph. This membranous labyrinth, as it is called, consists of two parts (illustration 151). The hinder part, comprising a sac, the utricle, and three short semicircular canals opening at each end into it, is the part concerned with the balancing sense; the forward part consists of another small bag, the saccule, and of a still more important part, the cochlear duct, and is the part concerned in hearing. In the cochlear duct is placed the spiral organ of Corti, on which the sound-waves are finally received

and by which the sounds are communicated to the cochlear nerve, a branch of the vestibulocochlear nerve, which ends in filaments to this organ of Corti. The essential parts in the organ of Corti are a double row of rods and several rows of cells furnished with fine hairs of varying length. Different musical notes are perhaps appreciated by different rods and hair cells.

151 – DC, Cochlear duct; *dr*, ductus reuniens; S, saccule; U, utricle; *dv*, ductus endolymphaticus; SC, semicircular canals.

The act of hearing – When sound-waves in the air reach the ear, the drum is alternately pressed in and pulled out, in consequence of which a to-and-fro movement is communicated to the chain of ossicles. The foot of the stapes communicates these movements to the perilymph. Finally these motions reach the delicate filaments placed in the organ of Corti, and so affect the nerve of hearing, which conveys impressions to the centre in the brain. There are two theories of hearing. The first is that of Helmholtz, who compared the organ of Corti to a piano and presumed that each sound caused a vibration of a corresponding part of Corti's organ. The second and later theory assumes that the entire organ of Corti is thrown into vibration by sounds, and that the nature of the sound is analysed and perceived by the hearing-centre in the brain.

EAR, DISEASES OF – Troubles connected with the ear should be treated early. Mention has been made of the importance of the connection between throat and middle ear by way of the Eustachian tube, both as regards the maintenance of good hearing and as regards the spread of inflammation. There are several simple procedures connected with the management of the ear which demand explanation.

Examination of the external ear is carried out by placing the person's head in a good light near a window, inclining the

152 – Electric auriscope. The battery is situated in the handle.

head away from the window a little, pulling the auricle upwards and backwards, and if a conical speculum be at hand, introducing this with a gentle screwing movement. The drum and deeper part of the external ear may then be viewed. If available, an electric auriscope (illustration

152) is a much more satisfactory means of carrying out the examination.

Syringing is done with a large-sized glass or metal syringe provided with a short blunt point (not longer than 1 inch (25 mm), so that no damage to the drum can result). The auricle is pulled gently up and back, while a steady stream from the syringe is directed along the upper wall, and flows out along the lower one (illustration 153). In syringing the ear of a child the point of the syringe should not be inserted within the shallow passage at all.

153 – Method of syringing ear.

Inflation of the middle ear is performed for cases in which the Eustachian tube is partly blocked and the drum indrawn. A catheter is passed along the floor of the nose into the opening of the Eustachian tube in the throat, and forcible inflation made through this by means of an india-rubber bag (Politzer's bag). Or the bag is used to blow up one nostril, the other being closed, while the Eustachian tube is kept open by one of the following devices. The person swallows a mouthful of water, or pronounces some guttural, such as 'Huck', so as to raise the soft palate and close the opening between the nose and throat; and at this moment the bag is suddenly squeezed. The Eustachian tube may also be inflated by forcibly expelling air from the chest while the mouth and nose are closed. The fact of whether air enters the middle ear becomes plain to the person himself by a click followed by a slight ringing in the ear, and often by improved hearing, as so many people nowadays have learned from experience by clearing their ears while coming in to land in an aircraft.

Tuning-fork test is used to test the internal ear. When a vibrating fork is placed on the centre of the forehead it is heard equally in both ears, the sound being conducted through the bones of the head. If one ear be closed, it is heard better in that ear. Accordingly, if one ear be deaf, and the sound of the fork placed on the forehead is heard better in that ear, the deafness is due to middle ear disease. While if the ear be deaf to the fork when placed on the forehead, as well as when held near the ear, the internal ear or nerve mechanism is at fault.

General symptoms – The following are some of the chief symptoms of ear disease: DEAFNESS (see DEAFNESS).

EARACHE is most commonly due to acute inflammation in the middle ear, but may also be due to chronic inflammation, or to acute inflammation of the external ear, boils, eczema, wax, or neuralgia affecting the outer ear. Pain in this region may also be caused by carious teeth. The treatment varies, with the cause, but the pain may generally be relieved to some extent by applying hot flannel or a hot-water bag to the side of the head. For subsequent treatment see later in this section.

RINGING in the ear, or TINNITUS, is sometimes a very annoying symptom. It may take various forms, but is in general accompanied by catarrh of some part of the ear. Pulsating or throbbing in the ear is sometimes due to bloodlessness, or to large doses of quinine or salicylate of soda, and passes off as the bloodlessness is treated or the drugs producing it are discontinued. Blowing, hissing, and whistling noises, like those made by an escape of steam or by a boiling kettle, are the most common and most annoying forms. Usually they are associated with middle-ear catarrh, but they are often associated with high blood-pressure, and diminish as the general disease is treated. Accompanied by deafness, ringing is not infrequently due to wax. Musical tinnitus sometimes occurs, in which the sound of bells, or of short passages of music, is repeated constantly. It is due to similar causes. A high crescendo musical note, followed by giddiness, is one of the symptoms of Menière's disease (qv).

DISCHARGE from the ear may arise in the external ear as the result of eczema, boils, or the irritation caused by a plug of wax or foreign body, but, in the absence of these, comes in the great majority of cases from suppuration in the middle ear through a perforation in the drum. There are two common fallacies regarding this condition. One is that a discharge from the ear is a trifling thing. In reality the presence of suppuration is accompanied usually by increasing deafness, and is attended always by the risk of an abscess in the mastoid antrum, or even within the skull. The other fallacy is that a perforation in the drum necessarily entails great deafness. As a matter of fact, unless the perforation be so large as to interfere with the tension of the drum, it causes little interference with hearing, the real cause of deafness in suppurative middle-ear disease being adhesions which bind down the ossicles and prevent their movements. Treatment depends upon whether the cause of the discharge is in the outer or the middle ear.

OTITIS EXTERNA, or infection of the outer ear, is commonest in tropical countries with a high humidity, as many a Serviceman found to his discomfort when serving in the Far East. Hence the names of 'Singapore ear' and 'Hong Kong ear' that it has been given. It is not uncommon, however, in Britain. Many factors may cause it, including scratching or poking the ears with dirty fingers or with contaminated objects such as a matchstick or Kirby grip. Badly fitting and infrequently cleaned hearing-aid earpieces are another cause. In some it is the result of spread of infection from the middle ear, whilst quite a number of cases are allergic in origin, the allergic factor often being some ear-drops that have been prescribed in the past. It may be due to a boil, which is discussed elsewhere in this section. It manifests itself by pain in the ear accompanied by a discharge. There is usually also a considerable degree of itching. Deafness develops if the discharge from the infection blocks the meatus.

Treatment consists of careful syringing out of the meatus with normal saline (see ISOTONIC) at a temperature of 38° C, followed by careful packing of the external ear with some soothing lotion, such as 10 per cent ichthammol in glycerin, or 8 per cent aluminium acetate. Once the acute phase is over, the meatus may be painted with an alcoholic solution of gentian violet or crystal violet. For the pain in the initial stages hot packs or hot applications may be applied to the ear or, simpler and often just as effective, a rubber hot-water bottle. Ear-drops are seldom used nowadays. If the itching is particularly intense at night – which it tends to be – it may be advisable to cover the ear with a gauze bandage, or to wear cotton gloves, to prevent scratching, which may well make the condition worse.

OTITIS MEDIA, or infection of the middle ear, usually occurs as a result of infection spreading up the Eustachian tube from the nose, throat or one of the sinuses. In other words, it may occur as a complication of a cold, tonsillitis, sinusitis or adenoids. It is above all a disease of children. It is not uncommon at the beginning of the swimming season every year, due to the fact that diving and underwater swimming force infected secretions from the nose or throat up through the Eustachian tube into the middle ear. This is most likely to occur after jumping into swimming pools without holding the nose. Pain is always present and, particularly in acute cases of sudden onset, it may be intense and throbbing or sharp in character. It is accompanied by deafness and often tinnitus (qv), and the temperature rises. In infants, crying, for which there is no obvious cause, may be the only sign that something is wrong, though this is usually accompanied by some localizing manifestation such as shaking of the head or the infant putting his hand to the ear. Examination of the ear is difficult because it is so tender but when it is carried out it reveals redness, and sometimes bulging, of the ear drum. In the early stages there is no discharge, but in the later stages there may be a discharge as a result of perforation of the ear drum as a result of the pressure created in the middle ear by the accumulated pus.

Treatment consists of the immediate administration of an antibiotic, and the one of choice is usually penicillin. While it is taking effect the pain may be eased by the use of heat in the form of a rubber hot-water bottle. If the antibiotic does not quickly bring relief, then it may be necessary to perform the minor operation of myringotomy, or incising the ear drum. This gives immediate relief in those cases in which the middle ear is full of pus; the moment the ear drum is incised, the pus pours out, and the pressure in the middle ear, which has been causing the pain, is relieved. The main complication of otitis media is mastoiditis, which is discussed later in this section. It cannot be too strongly emphasized that, if otitis media is treated immediately with ample doses of the appropriate antibiotic, the chances of any permanent damage to the ear or to hearing is reduced to a negligible degree, as is the risk of any complications such as mastoiditis.

SECRETORY OTITIS MEDIA, or GLUE EAR, is a form of otitis that has come to the fore as the commonest inflammatory condition of the middle ear in children, and one of the commonest causes of the form of deafness known as conduction deafness. (See DEAFNESS.) It is due to a persisting sticky (hence the name of 'glue ear') exudation in the middle ear. It is often associated with enlarged adenoids. If removal of these does not clear the condition, further treatment is needed. If this fails, in bad cases it may be necessary to remove the ossicles and the remains of the ear drum, and so to convert the middle ear into a simple cavity, which can be easily kept clear of infection.

OTOMYCOSIS is infection of the external ear by fungi such as Aspergillus (qv) or Candida (qv). It is a common condition in tropical and subtropical countries, but is occurring more often in Britain. It is characterized by persisting irritation in the ear and rapid reaccumulation of discharged material in spite of this being repeatedly removed. Treatment consists of cleansing of the external ear by dry mopping, and the application of an antifungal agent such as nystatin (qv). Drops of 2 per cent salicylic acid in alcohol are sometimes helpful.

WAX in the ear is the commonest cause of deafness, sometimes even of several years' standing. It is removed by syringing (illustration 153) with warm water ($37°$ C) containing two teaspoonfuls of baking soda to a tumblerful of water. If the wax be very hard it should be softened by making the person lie down on his side for half an hour with the affected ear upwards, into which is poured some of this solution, or a few drops of warm olive or castor oil. At the end of half an hour the syringing is repeated. In some cases it may be necessary to insert the drops several nights running in order to soften the wax sufficiently. If there is a perforation of the drum, the removal of wax should only be carried out by a specialist.

FOREIGN BODIES, such as peas, gravel, beads or bits of india-rubber, are often pushed by children into the ear, and are extremely difficult to remove. No attempt to remove such a foreign body should be made until it is known whether it is vegetable in nature (eg. a pea) or not. The reason for this is that syringing causes a pea to swell up or to become wedged in the ear, difficult to remove and causing exquisite pain. Non-vegetable foreign bodies such as beads, can be removed by syringing or forceps. No attempt should be made by unskilful persons with hairpins, bent wires, or the like, to remove the object, which is apt by such means to be pushed through the ear-drum.

BOILS in the skin lining the outer ear give rise to intense pain. This pain is much relieved by packing the ear lightly with a piece of gauze dipped in a 10 per cent solution of ichthammol glycerin, or in 8 per cent aluminium acetate. Relief is also gained by applying heat to the ear by means of a rubber hot-water bottle. The essential of treatment, however, is a five-day course of penicillin given intramuscularly.

ECZEMA, consisting of a cracked condition of the skin in the ear, with watery discharge and intense irritation, is common, as an acute affection in infants, and as a chronic one in gouty and rheumatic adults and as a sequel to, or accompaniment of, chronic otitis externa. In children, syringing with Goulard's water affords relief. In adults, weak nitrate of mercury ointment, or tar ointment applied several times daily, does good.

TUMOURS in the ear are mostly either outgrowths from the surrounding bone or soft polypi. The former may block the passage and interfere with hearing, but have often a narrow neck, so that they can be easily removed. Polypi usually develop as a result of the irritation set up by a chronic discharge, and shrivel up as the discharge is cured, though a large one may have to be removed in order to get to the drum.

MASTOIDITIS is a serious complication of inflammation in the ear, the incidence of which has been dramatically reduced by the introduction of the sulphonamides and penicillin.

The mastoid antrum and its connection with the middle ear have been mentioned under EAR. As a rule, inflammation in this cavity arises by direct spread of a long-standing suppuration from the middle ear, sometimes in consequence of neglect to keep the ear clean and prevent discharge from accumulating. The signs of this condition include swelling and tenderness of the skin behind the ear, redness and swelling inside the ear, pain in the side of the head, feverishness, and a discharge from the ear. Current expert opinion is divided as to the best method of treatment: whether this should be by antibiotics, or by antibiotics plus operation. On the whole, the majority opinion today probably is to reserve operation for those cases which do not respond to a full course of penicillin.

EBURNATION is a process of hardening and polishing which takes place at the ends of bones, giving them an ivory-like appearance. It is caused by the wearing away, in consequence of osteoarthrosis, of the smooth plates of cartilage which in health cover the ends of the bones.

ECBOLICS are drugs which cause contraction of the womb, such as ergot.

ECCHYMOSIS means the discoloured patch resulting from escape of blood into the tissues just under the skin, often from bruising.

ECHINOCOCCUS is the immature form of a small tapeworm, *Taenia echinococcus*, found in dogs, wolves, and jackals from which human beings become infected, so that they harbour the immature parasite in the form known as hydatid cyst. (See TAENIASIS.)

ECHOCARDIOGRAPHY is the use of ultrasonics (qv) for the purpose of examining the heart. By thus recording the echo (hence the name) from the heart of ultrasound waves it is possible to study, for example, the movements of the heart valves (see HEART), as well as the state of the interior of the heart.

ECHOLALIA is a term applied to the meaningless repetition, by a person suffering from mental degeneration, of words and phrases addressed to him.

ECHOVIRUSES, of which there are more than 30 known types, are a recently discovered group of virus. Their full name is Enteric Cytopathogenic Human Orphan (hence the abbreviation, E C H O, from the first letter of each word). They owe their cumbersome full name to the fact that they were originally found in the stools of children without disease. Practically all of them, however, have now been identified with definite diseases. They are more common in children than in adults, and have been responsible for outbreaks of meningitis, common-cold-like illnesses, gastro-intestinal infections, and infections of the respiratory tract.

ECLAMPSIA is the name applied to convulsions arising in pregnancy. This condition is said to occur in around 50 out of every 100,000 cases of pregnancy. It occurs especially in the later months and at the time of delivery, but a certain proportion of cases are manifest only after delivery has taken place. The cause of the condition is not known. In practically all cases the kidneys are profoundly affected.

Symptoms – There are several warning symptoms, such as dizziness, headache, vomiting, and the secretion of urine which is found to contain albumin. These symptoms may be present for some days or weeks before the seizure takes place. The seizure consists of rigidity of the body, with unconsciousness, followed by twitching in the face and limbs lasting for one or two minutes and then passing into a state of deep unconsciousness with stertorous breathing. In mild cases there are a few fits at long intervals and the patient recovers consciousness between them, but in severer cases the fits succeed one another so rapidly that there is no appreciable interval. In cases which progress to a fatal termination, the pulse and temperature rise, and cerebral haemorrhage, uraemia or pneumonia may supervene, or the breathing may gradually cease. It accounts for one in 12 of all maternal deaths and in 1970–72 it was responsible for 12·5 deaths per million women delivered in England and Wales. Among 43 cases of eclampsia delivered in Cardiff maternity units during 1969–74, none of the mothers died, but 10 of the 47 babies were lost.

Treatment – The treatment of the seizures is that generally applicable to convulsions of any kind, morphine and chloral being especially used as sedatives. This is usually supplemented with thiopentone sodium (qv) given intravenously. Alternatively a combination of chlorpromazine (qv) and pethidine (qv) may be used. Some obstetricians recommend controlling the initial fit by the inhalation of chloroform, and then switching on to the other drugs mentioned. Magnesium sulphate given intramuscularly sometimes helps to control the fits. In severe cases oxygen should be given, and, if heart failure threatens, digoxin should be given intravenously. Some authorities recommend that the birth of the child should be hastened, but at the present day the tendency is to leave this part of the treatment to nature.

ECSTASY is a term applied to a morbid mental condition in which the mind is entirely absorbed in the contemplation of one dominant idea or object, and loses for the time its normal self-control. This condition usually presents itself as a kind of temporary religious insanity, and has frequently appeared as an epidemic.

ECTHYMA is the term applied to a pustular eruption accompanied by surrounding inflammation. The pustules burst and discharge, leaving pigmented scars.

ECTO- is a prefix meaning on the outside.

ECTOPIC means out of the usual place. For example, in congenital displacement of the heart outside the thoracic cavity it is said to be ectopic, while an 'ectopic gestation' means a pregnancy outside of the womb.

ECTROMELIA means the absence of a limb or limbs, from congenital causes.

ECTROPION is a condition of the eyelid, usually the lower, in which the skin is contracted so as to turn the inside of the lid outwards. It is caused usually by scars due to burns and the like, and is remedied by operation.

ECZEMA is a term that trips much too lightly off the tongue of doctors and patients alike. So much so that it is sometimes difficult to know what exactly a dermatologist (a skin specialist) means by the term. The confusion is not alleviated when terms such as eczematous dermatitis are used. For ease of description a relatively simplified form of classification will be used here.

Eczema is a reaction of the skin to a wide range of stimulants or irritants, some known, many unknown. In some cases, if not all, there is apparently some constitutional factor that renders the skin vulnerable, so that it responds in this abnormal manner to stimuli which have no effect upon the skin of normal individuals. The two classical criteria of the eruption in eczema are that it itches and that it causes vesication, or blistering, of the skin. Its first manifestation is erythema, or reddening of the skin. This is due to dilatation of the blood-vessels in the skin. The next stage is the formation of vesicles (qv) or papules (qv), and these gradually break down and there is then oozing from the affected area of skin. If the condition persists, the skin tends to become thickened and to start scaling off.

NUMMULAR ECZEMA, or DISCOID ECZEMA as it is sometimes known, consists of coin-shaped areas of eczema, usually on the limbs, which, like all forms of eczema, tend to itch intensely. It is not uncommon in girls when they first start doing manual work, occurring on the back of the hands and fingers, the probability being that the eczema is due to trauma to the skin at work. It also occurs in middle-aged men, usually on the shins, being often aggravated by too frequent hot baths. The outlook for cure is poor, but lotions or pastes containing coal tar are often helpful.

INFECTIVE ECZEMA is a form of eczema that appears on a burn or cut. It comes on suddenly and spreads rapidly. In some cases it is due to sensitivity to the antiseptic that has been applied to the burn or cut. In some instances the eruption may be so severe that admission to hospital may be necessary. Treatment consists of the local application of a corticosteroid (qv) combined with an antibiotic. Alternatively, the application of wet dressings of $\frac{1}{4}$-strength Dilute Hypochlorite Solution, B P C is often effective. Calamine lotion is a soothing local application.

ATOPIC ECZEMA is one of the most widespread and worrying forms of eczema. Atopy means an inherited state of hypersensitivity which may manifest itself as asthma, hay fever or eczema. Hence the name given to this form of eczema. It is also known as INFANTILE ECZEMA as it starts in infancy at about the age of 3 or 4 months. There is a family history of asthma, hay fever or eczema in about 70 per cent of these infants, and it has been estimated that 3 per cent of all infants suffer from moderate eczema, and that many more probably suffer from a mild degree of it. The condition appears first as red areas or papules on the edge of the scalp, spreading to the face, which soon erupt and start oozing or weeping. In some cases the eruption spreads all over the body and, as it is intensely itchy, the unfortunate infant or child is often worked up into a frenzy and scratches himself until he is bleeding all over. Cold, frosty weather aggravates the condition, as does exposure to heat. Fortunately, parents can console themselves that the outlook is not too gloomy. Many of the children start improving around the age of 2 years, and in one series of 500 cases, only 10 per cent had any appreciable eczema at the age of 10 years. A late appearance of the eczema tends to mean a poor outlook, as does a bad family history of atopy.

Treatment – Local treatment consists of the application of a 1 per cent hydrocortisone ointment (see HYDROCORTISONE). If crusts have formed, these are removed by the application of equal parts of lead diachylon plaster and soft paraffin, applied thickly in strips of lint, and left on for twenty-four hours. Local treatment, however, is only part of the treatment. Equally important is it that parents should not over-protect a baby or child with eczema. He or she must be allowed to lead a perfectly normal life, without any pampering or unnecessary restrictions. The vast majority of children with this form of eczema can eat a normal diet. Only occasionally does such a child prove to be allergic to some particular food. Whether or not soap should be used in washing the baby is an open question. In the more severe cases soap should probably be avoided, and the skin cleaned with Emulsifying Ointment, B P. In cold weather, if there is a tendency for the skin to become dry and crack easily, Oily Cream, B P, may be gently rubbed into the skin at bedtime. If a soap is used for washing, then one of the less alkaline soaps should be used.

People with eczema and their relatives can obtain advice from the National Eczema Society, 27 Doyle Gardens, London NW10 3DB.

EFFERENT is the term applied to vessels which convey away blood or a secretion from a part, or to nerves which carry nerve impulses outwards from the nerve-centres.

EFFERVESCING DRAUGHTS (see CITRIC ACID).

EFFLEURAGE is a form of massage by gentle stroking movements.

EFFORT SYNDROME, or DAH (Disordered Action of the Heart), also known as Da Costa's syndrome, is a condition in which symptoms occur, such as palpitations and shortness of breath, which are attributed by the patient to disorder of the heart. There is no evidence, however, of heart disease, and psychological factors are thought to be of importance.

EFFUSION means a pouring out of fluid from the vessels in which it is naturally enclosed into the substance of the organs, or into cavities of the body, as a result of inflammation or of injury: for example, pleurisy with effusion, effusions into joints, and effusion of blood.

EGG is a term applied to any animal ovum. The hen's egg forms an easily digestible article of food, and weighs on an average 2 ounces (57 grams). One egg consists of 6 grams of protein and 6 grams of fat, providing energy equivalent to 80 Calories. The yolk of the egg is of special value as a food. The best test for a stale egg is to dissolve 2 ounces (57 grams) of salt in a pint (500 ml) of water; fresh eggs placed in the solution sink; stale eggs float.

ELBOW is the joint formed between the humerus above and the radius and ulna below (see illustration 83 on page 127). The humerus has at its lower end a rounded surface, against which the head of the radius moves, and a deep groove to which a saddle-shaped surface at the upper end of the ulna fits. The head of the radius rests upon a projection of the ulna and is bound to it by a stout annular ligament, within which it can rotate. Two important movements take place at this joint: a flail-like backward and forward movement of the radius and ulna moving together upon the humerus, and a rotary movement of the radius on the ulna, by which the lower end of the radius is crossed over the ulna and again brought side by side with it, according as the hand is turned palm downwards and palm upwards. The joint is secured at the sides by strong lateral ligaments, and at the back and front is covered by powerful muscles. The ulnar nerve as it passes down to the forearm has an exposed position behind the inner edge of the humerus at its lower end; this is popularly known as the 'funny-bone'. The elbow is seldom dislocated, but a not uncommon accident consists in the chipping off, through a fall on the elbow, of the olecranon process which forms the point behind the joint.

Miner's Elbow, or *Beat Elbow,* is the term applied to an inflammatory condition of the bursa over the point of the elbow, caused by resting the weight of the body on the elbow in hewing coal. The condition corresponds to housemaid's knee in the lower limb, and occurs not only in miners but sometimes in school children and other persons who lean upon or bruise the point of the elbow. (See BURSITIS.) *Tennis Elbow* is a term applied to a pain over the elbow due to mild inflammation in the tendons of the muscles that extend, or straighten, the elbow, caused by strains and jars in playing tennis and similar games. The condition generally clears up spontaneously if games such as tennis, badminton and squash, or clothes wringing, are avoided, though this may be a somewhat slow process, taking up to a year or longer. A quicker result may be obtained by an injection of hydrocortisone (qv) into the affected area. The local appli-

cation of ultrasonics (qv) may also be helpful. *Pulled Elbow* is the name applied to a painful condition of the elbow in young children, constituting a slight dislocation of the head of the radius from beneath the ligament which should bind it to the ulna, caused by a jerk of the arm. It is most likely to occur in 1- and 2-year-olds. The condition, which is usually accompanied by loss of power of the arm, may be induced in a variety of ways; by being pulled up when sitting on the floor, when being swung between their parents when walking, when being held firmly by the arm, when in an obstreperous, recalcitrant mood. The pain may occur in the wrist or shoulder. It responds well to manipulation.

ELECTRICAL INJURIES are usually caused by the passage through the body of an electric current of high voltage owing to accidental contact with a live wire or to a discharge of lightning. The general effects produced are included under the term electric shock, but vary greatly in degree. The local effects include spasmodic contraction of muscles, fracture of bones, and in severe cases more or less widespread destruction of tissues which may amount simply to burns of the skin or may include necrosis of masses of muscle and internal organs. Fright due to unexpectedness of the shock and pain due to the sudden cramp of muscles are the commonest symptoms and in most cases pass off in a few minutes or less. In more severe cases, especially when the person has remained in contact with a live wire for some time or has been unable to let go of the electrical contact owing to spasmodic contraction of his muscles, the effects are more pronounced and may be those of concussion of the brain or of compression of the brain. (See BRAIN, DISEASES OF.) In still severer cases, death may ensue either from paralysis of the respiration or stoppage of the heart's action. In either instance, the condition may be at first one of suspended animation, and death may not ensue if prompt measures are taken for treatment.

With regard to the after-effects of an electric shock, recovery in slighter cases is almost immediate, but in cases in which the discharge of current has been prolonged the process of recovery may be prolonged. The more permanent effects depend upon the extent to which tissues have been destroyed. Fractures and splitting of bones are often caused by very powerful currents. Dislocation of a joint is sometimes produced by violent muscular spasm. Masses of muscle and areas of skin may be destroyed, and if these injuries are extensive, a long time may be required for the absorption or sloughing away of the dead tissues and for healing. Electrical injuries show little tendency to become septic as compared with similar injuries due to other causes, and while loss of a part of the body may take place, healing is in the end usually satisfactory.

With regard to the amount of current necessary to produce serious results, this varies enormously according to circumstances. Alternating current is more dangerous than direct current, the risk of death being greatest at 50 cycles per second. So far as voltage is concerned, the lowest recorded fatal shock voltage in Britain is 60; few deaths occur at voltages below 100. Contact with high-tension currents (1000 volts or more) of the alternating type is immediately fatal. Physical factors are important in regard to the effects produced by a given strength of current; after a shock is received through dry shoes or dry clothing, the effect may be negligible as compared with that of contact made with a bare part of the body, especially when the skin is damp or perspiring, or of contact through wet feet. This is why electrical apparatus should never be allowed in a bathroom unless it is out of all possible contact with individuals using the bathroom. Water is a good conductor of electricity. Therefore if an individual touches an electrical heater or fire with wet hands, he may receive a severe shock. If the contact occurs while the individual is still in his bath the result will probably be fatal. Even touching a faulty switch with dripping hands may prove fatal.

In Britain there are an average of 110 deaths a year from electrocution, half of these occurring in the home. (See ACCIDENT PREVENTION IN THE HOME.)

Treatment – No electrical apparatus or switch should be touched by anyone who is in metallic contact with the ground, such as through a metal pipe, especially, for example, from a bath. The first necessity in regard to a person through whose body a powerful electric current is passing is to break the current. This can sometimes be done by turning off a switch. If the victim is grasping or in contact with a live wire, the contact may be severed with safety only by someone wearing rubber gloves or rubber boots, but as these are not likely to be immediately available, his hands may be protected by a thick wrapping of dry cloth, or the live

wire may be hooked or pushed out of the way with a long wooden stick. If the injured person is unconscious, and especially if breathing has stopped, *artificial respiration should be applied and continued even for hours*, as described under DROWNING, RECOVERY FROM. When the patient begins to breathe again, he must be treated for shock: ie. put to bed and given hot-water bottles and hot drinks. Electrical burns are treated on the same lines as ordinary burns. If the patient shows undue excitement and restlessness, sedatives may be necessary. The local destructive effects of a powerful current, including burns, fractures, and sloughing of large masses of tissue, are treated later by ordinary surgical means, but strong and irritating antiseptics should be avoided. Bleeding from damaged blood-vessels is liable to occur a few days after a severe injury, and is treated by the ordinary means for arrest of haemorrhage.

ELECTRICITY IN MEDICINE – As electricity has proved to be a form of energy, of great usefulness and extremely convenient in application, it has become widely employed in medicine. It has, however, been credited with powers of healing far beyond those that it is capable of achieving. Electricity is generally spoken of as existing in different forms, but these differ in pressure, in amount, and in duration, rather than in any essential quality. They are named as follows: (*a*) Static, or Frictional, or Franklinic; (*b*) Galvanic or Voltaic; (*c*) Faradic or Induced; (*d*) Alternating or Sinusoidal; (*e*) High Frequency or D'Arsonvalism.

Static electricity has been recognized, by some of its simplest phenomena, from the earliest times. The name electricity is derived from the Greek word, $\eta\lambda\epsilon\kappa\tau\rho\sigma\nu$, meaning amber, because it is said that Thales of Miletus first discovered this force by noticing that a piece of amber, rubbed with a dry cloth, had the power of attracting small bodies to itself. Subsequently it was found that other bodies, such as sulphur, wax and glass, have similar properties, and a treatise, *De Magnete*, was published on the subject by William Gilbert, physician to Queen Elizabeth, in 1600. This form of electricity is often called Franklinic, after Benjamin Franklin, who, in the middle of the eighteenth century, experimented much with it in the United States. It is also interesting to note that Wesley, the famous preacher, was greatly interested in the subject of electricity, and about the same time published a treatise on its medical applications known as *The Desideratum, or Electricity made Plain and Useful, by a Lover of Mankind and Common Sense.*

When a glass rod is rubbed with a piece of dry flannel, the two gain certain properties. If the glass rod be brought near a light pith-ball or piece of paper hanging by a dry silk thread, the pith-ball is attracted towards the rod, but if the two be allowed to touch for a moment, the pith-ball is now as energetically repelled when the rod is brought near it. If, however, the piece of flannel be brought near the ball, the latter is attracted to it. To express these facts conveniently it is said that there are two 'kinds' of electricity, positive and negative, the glass rod becoming positively electrified by the rubbing, the flannel negatively electrified, and further, that like electricities repel one another. Accordingly, when the positively electrified glass rod is brought near the pith-ball, the negative electricity in the latter is supposed to separate from the positive (the ball having till now been uniformly charged with the two) and to collect on that side of the ball nearest to the rod, while the positive electricity is repelled to the point farthest off. When the rod and ball touch, the negative electricity escapes to the rod, leaving the ball positively electrified, so that it is now repelled by the positive electricity of the rod and attracted by the negative electricity of the flannel. Positive electricity is designated shortly by the sign +, and negative by the sign −, while the power possessed by the electricity of passing from pith-ball to glass rod, carrying the ball with it, is known as potential, or pressure, or electromotive force (EMF). All bodies have these properties, developing, when suddenly separated or broken, this difference of potential, the amount and nature of the force produced depending on the nature of the bodies in question. But while in the case of certain bodies called nonconductors, such as glass, porcelain, sealing-wax, india-rubber, guttapercha, dry wool, silk, and amber, the electricity remains upon the surface where it is produced, in the case of others, known as conductors, such as metals, salt solutions, and the bodies of animals and plants, it flows away through the body as soon as formed, and therefore does not show its presence. Static electricity is closely related to magnetism, a set of properties possessed only by iron, steel, nickel, cobalt, and an iron-ore called lodestone.

Static electricity may be stored up in large amounts by means of the Leyden jar. This consists of two conducting surfaces, such as tinfoil, placed one outside, the other inside, a glass jar, so that they are everywhere separated by a thin plate of glass. The outer one simply rests in contact with the earth, the inner is connected to a metal rod ending in a knob. Electrified bodies, like a rubbed glass rod, may be brought up to the knob time after time till the inner sheet of tinfoil becomes highly charged with positive electricity, which attracts negative electricity from the earth into the outside sheet. If the knob of a charged Leyden jar be connected with the outside sheet of foil the two electricities combine suddenly, and if this contact be made through the human body, a severe momentary shock is felt.

For practical medical purposes, static electricity is produced by an influence machine consisting of several pairs of circular glass or vulcanite plates, which are driven in opposite directions. Each plate carries at starting a small amount of electricity; and, as they revolve, the alternate plates generate increasing quantities of + and − electricity, which are drawn off to opposite sides of the machine by fine metal brushes. The electricity can be stored in Leyden jars, or used directly to electrify the body. For the latter purpose, the person sits upon a chair or couch, carefully insulated from the earth by glass legs, india-rubber mats, or other nonconductors, and becomes charged positively or negatively according to the manner in which he is connected with the machine. During the process of charging, a peculiar tingling over the skin is felt and the hair stands upright; the breathing becomes more rapid, and during a séance of fifteen to twenty minutes the chemical changes which accompany bodily activity are markedly increased. The electricity is discharged by bringing a metal point or ball gradually towards the charged person, when, in the former case, a spray of air or 'souffle' passes towards the point as the charge passes off, in the latter case sparks are drawn. Either form of discharge, especially the latter, has a stimulating effect. The atmosphere, both upon high wooded mountains and in the neighbourhood of breaking waves, has, as Lord Kelvin demonstrated, a different electric state from the quiet air of inland plains, so that it is quite possible that some of the advantage derived from summer change to mountain and seaside resorts may be due to stimulation from this cause.

Galvanic electricity is so named after Galvani, professor at Bologna, who published researches upon what he called 'animal electricity' in 1791. It also received the name 'voltaic', after Volta, professor at Pavia, who in 1799 published researches showing that this type of electricity is really due to chemical action. He found that dissimilar metals, moistened and brought in contact, became electrified, so that, when parts of these metals not in contact are connected by a conductor, such as copper wire, a constant current passes through the wire. As chemical action proceeds almost continuously, this current is also continuous; and for this reason, added to the fact that it is of moderate potential or pressure and is easily produced, it is the most convenient for general medical use.

The choice of metals depends upon the fact that one must be very liable to chemical action, the other as little affected as possible by an oxidizing agent. The principal metals may be arranged in a series, thus:

+ Sodium	Iron
Magnesium	Copper
Zinc	Silver
Lead	Gold
Tin	Platinum
	− Carbon

− of which each one is more oxidizable than that following it, and becomes positively electrified when brought into contact with one of those lower down in the series. Zinc and carbon, or zinc and copper, on account of their distance apart in this scale, and their comparative cheapness, are the metals usually selected. A vessel containing two metal plates, for example, zinc and copper, immersed in a fluid which maintains chemical action, for example, sulphuric acid in water, is known as a galvanic cell. A collection of such cells is called a battery. When the plates are joined by a conducting wire an electric current passes along it from the copper (+ pole) to the zinc (− pole). At the same time there is set free, on the surface of the zinc plate, oxygen, which acts upon the zinc, and also produces sulphuric acid; while hydrogen is set free at the surface of the copper plate and escapes.

It is important to bear in mind also that if the current passing along the wire be passed for some distance through a moist decomposable substance, such as the tissues of the human body, a similar chemical action is produced at the points where the wire enters and leaves the substance, which are called the electrodes. Thus oxygen is set free and acids formed at the electrode connected to the + pole (the anode), while hydrogen is set free and alkalis developed at the other, or − electrode (the cathode). This action, known as electrolysis, is much used in medicine for removing hairs, destroying naevi or birthmarks, and reducing the size of certain tumours, unsuitable for removal by the knife. There is a great difference between the action of the two electrodes, because the substances formed at the anode are caustic and germicidal in action, whilst those produced at the cathode have no such action. Accordingly, the anode (+ pole) is generally applied to the structure which it is desired to destroy.

Another important property of electric currents, the fact that a powerful current passing through a circuit heats any part which is of feeble conducting power, is utilized to heat cauteries for delicate surgical work, especially about the nose and throat, and also to light small incandescent lamps for internal examinations. The cautery consists of a piece of platinum (low conducting power), joining the ends of two large copper wires (high conducting power), so that, when the current passes, the former immediately becomes red or white hot, according to the intensity of the current.

Another method in which the galvanic current is employed is in order to carry drugs through the unbroken skin by the process known as iontophoresis (qv).

Faradic electricity dates only from 1831, when it was discovered by Faraday that if two coils of wire be placed near one another, and if a galvanic current be suddenly passed through one of them and again stopped, a current is induced in the second coil at the moments of closing and of opening the first circuit. This secondary current differs from the continuous galvanic current in two important particulars: (1) it is only momentary in duration; (2) it has a much higher potential or pressure, and is therefore much more capable of traversing poor conductors like the human body. The currents induced in the secondary coil at opening and closing the primary coil run in opposite directions; accordingly, if the primary current be very rapidly closed and opened, as, for example, by the vibration of a steel spring, an almost continuous series of alternating currents is obtained in the secondary circuit.

A faradic current sufficient for medical

purposes can be obtained from an apparatus consisting of the following: a single galvanic cell connected to a primary coil, with an appliance to make and break the circuit; a secondary coil, which is connected by wires with two electrodes provided with handles, by which the electrodes can be applied to the surface of the body; and a core of iron which fits inside the primary coil, and which, becoming magnetized as the current passes through this coil, increases the effect upon the secondary coil. Such an apparatus can be obtained in the small compass of a box 4 or 5 inches (10 or 12 cm) each way.

The faradic current can be administered to the surface of the body generally by immersion of the patient in a warm bath into which two electrodes dip.

For certain purposes, such as X-ray work, secondary coils with an enormous length of wire are used, the potential or pressure of the faradic current increasing with the number of turns taken by the wire in the secondary coil.

The potential of faradic currents is high: in medical coils it may reach 20,000 or 100,000 volts, or about five hundred times as high as that of the powerful current which supplies a town, but the amount of electricity is very small. The difference between faradic and galvanic electricity presents some resemblance to the difference between a shower of swiftly falling rain-drops, in which the total amount of water is small, and a large, sluggish river.

Alternating or sinusoidal currents – An alternating current differs from the faradic current in the fact that the latter consists of a rapid series of sudden impulses or shocks, while with the sinusoidal or alternating current the strength gradually rises from nothing to a maximum, and falls away again to be followed immediately by a current in the reverse direction, which also grows to a maximum and wanes in the same manner. These currents rapidly succeed one another, so that the effect on the body is very much the same as that produced by the faradic current. Most systems of public distribution of electrical energy are carried out by alternating currents of this type, and by means of transformers they can be very readily converted into forms of electricity more suitable for medical use. The sinusoidal current, suitably reduced by apparatus, may be used for the electric bath, or may be used for stimulating nerves or muscles, especially when the current is rhythmically cut off and restored by an instrument known as a rhythmic interrupter.

Sinusoidal currents on a small scale can be produced by bringing a magnet rapidly up to and away from a secondary coil, or making the coil move while the magnet remains fixed. The sinusoidal form of current generally has a very stinging effect on sensory nerves, and in this way is somewhat unpleasant for use.

High-frequency currents – By apparatus constructed on the principle of the induction coil, but with other complicated arrangements designed to make and break the primary current several hundred thousand times a second, currents, huge in pressure but minute as regards duration, can be produced which have an action similar to that of a discharge of static electricity. The sensation is merely one of slight tingling when sparks are drawn, and there is no stimulation of muscles or nerves. This may possibly be explained by the currents being confined to the surface, and not passing through the substance of the body at all, or more probably by the theory of D'Arsonval, that the nerve endings are incapable of perceiving such extremely short vibrations. These high-frequency currents formed at one time a very popular mode of stimulating treatment.

The apparatus by which these currents are produced consists essentially of Leyden jars, whose outer coats are united through a solenoid or spiral of thick copper wire. The jars are rapidly charged and discharged by some source of high potential electricity; and, since the discharges from a Leyden jar have the property of taking place in an oscillatory manner, they induce in the solenoid corresponding secondary currents, which are of immensely rapid frequency. A second coil of thick wire, known as a resonator, is in general connected to the solenoid with the purpose of allowing of variations in the potential of the high-frequency discharges.

The currents are applied to the patient in various ways. (a) He may be connected to the two ends of the solenoid by thin wires provided with ordinary flat electrodes, from which the currents are simply passed through his body (direct application). (b) He may lie upon a couch connected with one end of the solenoid, while the cushion of the couch isolates him from a metal plate connected with the other end; he then becomes rapidly charged and discharged (condensation). (c) He may stand or lie within a wide secondary coil, and have currents induced in his body (auto-conduction). (d) One end of the solenoid may be connected to earth, while to the other end is attached an electrode, which is cautiously approached to any desired part (local application). (*e*) The method of diathermy or thermo-penetration may be used to produce heat within the body. (See DIATHERMY.)

As already stated, the passage of high-frequency currents through the body produces no stimulation of muscles and no sensation, apart from that of heat caused by the resistance. There is a powerful effect, lasting many minutes, in diminishing the sensitiveness of the skin; the fullness of the blood-vessels in the skin, the output of body heat and of carbon dioxide by the lungs are increased, and the quantity of urine passed becomes much greater.

Applications of electricity – The galvanic and faradic currents are of value as a means of *diagnosis* in many conditions affecting nerves and muscles. In their natural condition nerves react to faradic or to interrupted galvanic currents, muscles to the latter. When excitability by faradization is lost, it shows that the nerves in question are degenerating. The sudden initiation of a weak galvanic current should produce a contraction of muscles to which the cathode is applied, but, if a much stronger current be required, or if a contraction be obtained more readily with the anode, it shows that the muscles in question are also in process of degeneration. This is expressed by the statement that when the anodal closing contraction is stronger than the cathodal closing contraction the reaction of degeneration is present, or, put briefly,

$$A C C > K C C = R D.$$

PAIN, whether headache, neuralgia, sciatica, a chronic rheumatic condition, or due to several other causes, is almost always relieved temporarily, and sometimes, after a protracted course of treatment, severe pain is entirely removed by one of the following. The static breeze may be tried, applied to the seat of pain for some minutes every day. In painful nerve conditions like neuralgia, greater benefit is often derived from the galvanic current, a strong current of 20–30 milliamperes being used, and the anode (+ electrode) being placed over the course of the affected nerve. In most cases of vague but severe pain the faradic current is the simplest of application, and very effective. A small button electrode or wire-brush is applied to the seat of pain, the other electrode, moistened with common salt solution, to

the neck, back, or other convenient part. The séance lasts, perhaps, a quarter of an hour, and is repeated several times daily.

SPASMODIC CONDITIONS of all sorts, such as writer's cramp, are relieved or lessened by the static breeze, and still more by a strong galvanic current arranged so that the anode is close to the nerve or nerves connected with the spasmodically acting muscles. The anode decreases the conducting power of nerves for motor impulses as well as for painful sensations.

PARALYSIS, such as poliomyelitis, or that following a stroke or apoplexy, or injury to a nerve, calls specially for the application of interrupted galvanic currents. The muscles in these and similar cases, where the nervous control usually exerted over them is lost, tend to waste. The application of interrupted galvanic currents of about 10 milliamperes strength, or of these combined with faradization, and assisted in every case by massage, and movements of the neighbouring joints, not only keeps up the nourishment of the paralysed muscles and prevents stiffness and wasting, but actually assists recovery. So far as possible, treatment should be daily, and must extend over very long periods.

DESTRUCTION OF HAIRS is almost painlessly accomplished by electrolysis.

BIRTH-MARKS, consisting of masses of blood-vessels beneath the skin (naevi), are successfully destroyed, without leaving a scar, by electrolysis. The electrodes consist of two needles which are pushed through the skin into the mass, and an anaesthetic is usually given during the process.

STRICTURES of the gullet, bowel, and urethra may, it is claimed, also be painlessly dilated by electrolysis, though the process must be repeated several times at intervals of a fortnight or thereabout, in séances of fifteen minutes.

REMOVAL OF STEEL PARTICLES which have penetrated the eye may often be effected by a powerful electro-magnet consisting of a soft iron core round which is wound an electric coil, through which a heavy current can be passed.

X-RAYS AND ULTRA-VIOLET RAYS are produced by the aid of electricity, and used in the treatment of many skin and other diseases. (See under LIGHT TREATMENT; and X-RAYS.)

ELECTROCARDIOGRAM is the term applied to a record of the variations in electric potential which occur in the heart as it contracts and relaxes. Any muscle in use produces an electric current, but when an individual is at rest the main muscular current in the body is that produced by the heart. This can be recorded by connecting the outside of the body by electrodes with an instrument known as an electrocardiograph. This instrument contains a galvanometer of great delicacy, consisting essentially of a silvered wire which vibrates in a magnetic field in response to these currents. While it is vibrating, an electrographic record is obtained upon a moving photographic plate or tape, and this, subsequently developed, can be studied by the physician at his convenience. The patient is con-

ELECTROCOCHLEOGRAPHY is a method of recording the activity of the cochlea, the part of the inner ear concerned with hearing. (See EAR.)

ELECTRO - ENCEPHALOGRAPHY – It has been found that in the brain there is a regular, rhythmical change of electric potential, due to the rhythmic discharge of energy by nerve cells. These changes can be recorded graphically and the 'brain waves' examined. These records – electro-encephalograms – are useful in diagnosis. For example, the abnormal electro-

154 – Normal electrocardiogram. The wave marked P represents atrial activity. The waves marked Q, R, S, and T represent ventricular activity. From Evans, *Cardiology*.

nected to the electrocardiograph by leads from either the arms and legs or different points on the chest. The normal electrocardiogram of each heart-beat shows one wave corresponding to the activity of the atria and four waves corresponding to the phases of each ventricular beat (illustration 154). Various readily recognizable changes are seen in cases in which the heart is acting in an abnormal manner, or in which one or other side of the heart is hypertrophied. This record therefore forms a useful aid in many cases of heart disease.

ELECTROCAUTERY (see CAUSTICS and CAUTERIES).

encephalogram occurring in epilepsy is characteristic of this disease. The normal waves, known as alpha waves, occur with a frequency of 10 per second. Abnormal waves, with a frequency of 7 or less per second, are known as delta waves and occur in the region of cerebral tumours and in the brains of epileptics.

ELECTRON is one of the subatomic particles. (See RADIOTHERAPY.)

ELECTRO-OCULOGRAPHY is a method of recording movements of the eyes, which is proving of value in assessing the function of the retina (qv).

307

ELECTROPHORESIS means the migration of charged particles between electrodes. Of recent years a simple method of electrophoresis, known as paper electrophoresis, has been introduced which is proving of value in examining the proteins in body fluids. This method consists in applying the protein-containing solution as a spot or a streak to a strip of filter paper which has been soaked in buffer solution and across the ends of which a potential difference is then applied for some hours.

ELECTRORETINOGRAPHY is a method of recording the activity of the retina (qv) in health and disease (illustration 155). Typical of its value is its use in the degenerative condition of the eye known as retinitis pigmentosa. (See RETINA, DISEASES OF.)

ELECTUARY, or CONFECTION, is a soft paste containing drugs mixed with sugar or honey. (See CONFECTIONS.)

ELEPHANTIASIS (synonyms, ELEPHANTIASIS ARABUM, BARBADOS LEG, BOUCNEMIA) is a term applied to a disease which is characterized by gross overgrowth of the skin and subjacent textures. This condition arises from repeated attacks of inflammation of the skin and subcutaneous tissue, and concurrent obstruction of the lymphatic vessels. The common cause in the tropics is infection with certain parasitic worms (filariae) which invade the lymphatic vessels. (See FILARIASIS.) These worms are conveyed to man by mosquitoes. They may attack any portion of the body, but most commonly the leg, which becomes so enlarged and disfigured by the great thickening of its textures as to resemble the leg of an elephant, whence the name of the disease is derived. The thickening is due to excessive increase in the connective tissue, which results from the inflammatory process, and which by pressure on the muscles of the limb causes them to undergo atrophy or degeneration. Hence the limb becomes weak. When affecting the scrotum it often produces a tumour of enormous dimensions. The health ultimately suffers, and serious constitutional disturbance is apt to arise. In elephantiasis of the leg much relief is obtained from the use of elastic bandaging, massage, rest, and elevation of the limb. Prevention must be carried out by destruction of mosquitoes. Promising results are being reported

from the use of diethylcarbazine in the early stages of the disease.

ELIXIR is a diluted tincture made pleasant to the taste by the addition of aromatic substances and sugar. The name was specially applied to several preparations greatly used in the Middle Ages, which had the effect of acting as a tonic to

155 – Electroretinograph. (Cambridge Medical Instruments. Photo: Terence Reeve)

the stomach and relieving constipation, and which were known, for example, as the elixir of Paracelsus, the elixir of long life. The main constituent of all of these was tincture of aloes. At the present day they are mainly used as a vehicle for potent and nauseous drugs.

EMACIATION means pronounced wasting, and is a common symptom of many diseases, particularly of those which are associated with a prolonged or repeated rise of temperature, such as tuberculosis. It is also associated with diseases of the alimentary system in which digestion is inefficient, or in which the food is not fully absorbed: for example, in diarrhoea of long-standing, whatever be its cause. It is also a marked feature of malignant disease.

EMBALMING (see DEAD, DISPOSAL OF THE).

EMBOLISM means the plugging of a small blood-vessel by material which has been carried through the larger vessels by the blood stream. It is due usually to fragments of a clot which has formed in some vessel, or to small portions carried off from the edge of a heart-valve when this organ is diseased; but the plug may also be a small mass of bacteria, or a fragment of a tumour, or even a mass of air bubbles sucked into the veins during operations on the neck. The result is usually more or less destruction of the organ or part of an organ supplied by the obstructed vessel. This is particularly the case in the brain, where softening of the brain, with aphasia or apoplexy, may be the result. If the plug be a fragment of malignant tumour, a new growth develops at the spot; and if it be a mass of bacteria, an abscess forms there. Air-embolism occasionally causes sudden death in the case of wounds in the neck, the air bubbles completely stopping the flow of blood. Fat-embolism is a condition which has been known to cause death, masses of fat, in consequence of such an injury as a fractured bone, finding their way into the circulation and stopping the blood in its passage through the lungs.

EMBROCATIONS are mixtures, usually of an oily nature, intended for external application in cases of rheumatism, sprains, and other painful conditions. Their action is due partly to the massage employed in rubbing in the embrocations, partly to the counter-irritant action of the drugs which they contain. (See LINIMENTS.)

EMBRYO means the foetus in the womb prior to the end of the second month. (See FOETUS.)

EMESIS means vomiting. (See VOMITING.)

EMETICS are drugs or other means which produce vomiting.
Varieties – Emetics are divided into two important classes: (1) direct emetics,

which, being taken by the mouth, irritate the stomach and so cause vomiting, and (2) indirect emetics, which will cause vomiting, even when injected into the blood, by action upon the centre in the brain controlling the act of vomiting. Examples of the first type are sulphate of zinc, mustard in water, alum, sal volatile, sulphate of copper, and even copious draughts of warm salt water. In the second class we have apomorphine, ipecacuanha, and tartar emetic; to this class also belong such means as tickling the throat, or presenting evil-smelling substances to the nose.
Uses – Emetics are now relatively seldom used except in certain cases of poisoning to remove the poisonous substance as rapidly as possible from the stomach. They must only be given if the victim is conscious, one drink of salty water, containing sodium chloride (common salt), or a dose of Ipecacuanha Syrup USP: 15 millilitres followed by 200 millilitres (a tumblerful) of water, should be given. Emetics in smaller doses than will produce vomiting, are often used in cough mixtures, as they render the secretions in the bronchial tubes more fluid and therefore more easily coughed up. Wine of ipecacuanha is used for this purpose.

EMETINE is one of the active principles of ipecacuanha. (See IPECACUANHA; and DYSENTERY.)

EMICTORY is a drug which provokes the excretion of urine.

EMMENAGOGUES are drugs which restore the flow at the menstrual periods. when this is scanty or absent. Certain substances, which are mainly dangerous irritant poisons, are credited with the power of producing this effect. Other substances act indirectly by removing the state of ill-health to which the failure is due, such as iron in anaemia. (See MENSTRUATION.)

EMMETROPIA is a term applied to the normal condition of the eye as regards refraction of light rays. In this state when the muscles in the eyeball are completely relaxed the focusing power is accurately adjusted for parallel rays, so that vision is perfect for distant objects.

EMOLLIENTS are substances which have a softening and soothing effect upon the skin. They include dusting powders such as French chalk, oils such as olive oil and almond oil, and fats such as the various pharmacopoeial preparations of paraffin, suet, and lard. Glycerin is also an excellent emollient.

Uses – They are used in various inflammatory conditions such as eczema, when the skin becomes hard, cracked, and painful. They may be used in the form of a dusting powder, an oil or an ointment.

EMPHYSEMA means an abnormal presence of air in certain parts of the body. In its restricted sense, however, it is generally employed to designate an affection of the lungs, of which there are two forms. In one of these there is over-distension of the air-cells of these organs, and in parts destruction of their walls, giving rise to the formation of large sacs, from the rupture and running together of a number of contiguous air-vesicles. This is much the more common of the two forms and is the one which is usually meant when the term 'emphysema' is used. In the other form the air is infiltrated into the connective tissue beneath the pleura and between the pulmonary air-cells, constituting what is known as *acute interstitial emphysema.*

Causes – Where a portion of the lung has become wasted, or its vesicular structure permanently obliterated by disease, without corresponding falling-in of the chest wall, the neighbouring air-vesicles, or some of them, undergo dilatation to fill the vacuum.

In cases of bronchitis, and especially of bronchial asthma, where numbers of the smaller bronchial tubes become obstructed, the air in the pulmonary vesicles remains imprisoned, the force of expiration being insufficient to expel it; on the other hand, the stronger force of inspiration being adequate to overcome the resistance, the air-cells tend to become more and more distended, and permanent alterations in their structure, including emphysema, are the result.

Emphysema also arises from exertion involving expiratory efforts, during which the glottis is constricted, as in paroxysms of coughing, in straining, and in lifting heavy weights. Whooping-cough is well known as an exciting cause of emphysema.

Symptoms – In the affected portions of the lungs there are loss of the natural elasticity of the air-cells, destruction of many of the pulmonary capillary blood-vessels, and diminution of aerating surface for the blood. As a consequence there is a strain on the heart and the venous system generally, leading to dilatation of the right side of the heart, and so to dropsy. The chief symptom in this complaint is shortness of breath, more or less constant but greatly aggravated by exertion, and by attacks of bronchitis, to which persons suffering from emphysema are specially liable. The respiration is of a wheezy character. In severe forms of the disease the patient comes to acquire a peculiar bluish and bloated appearance, and the configuration of the chest is altered, assuming character known as the *barrel-shaped chest.*

Treatment – The main element in the treatment of emphysema consists in attention to the general condition of the health, and in the avoidance of all causes likely to aggravate the disease or induce its complications. The same general plan of treatment as that recommended in asthma and bronchitis is applicable in emphysema. During attacks of urgent breathlessness anti-spasmodic remedies should be given, while inhalation of oxygen will often afford marked and speedy relief.

ACUTE INTERSTITIAL EMPHYSEMA, arising from the rupture of air-cells may occur as a complication of the vesicular form, or separately as the result of some sudden expulsive effort, such as a fit of coughing, or, as has occasionally happened, in parturition. Occasionally the air infiltrates the cellular tissue of the mediastinum, and thence comes to distend the integument of the neck and even the whole surface of the body. This air, however, is rapidly absorbed, and the condition soon subsides.

SURGICAL EMPHYSEMA is the term applied when air is present under the skin. It may get there, for example, if the lungs are wounded through the chest wall, or if the wind-pipe is pierced at any point in its path.

EMPIRICAL treatment is that school of treatment which is founded simply on experience. Because a given remedy has been successful in the treatment of a certain group of symptoms, it is assumed, by those who uphold this principle, that it will be successful in the treatment of other cases presenting similar groups of symptoms, without any inquiry as to the cause of the symptoms or reason underlying the action of the remedy. It is the contrary of 'rational' or 'scientific' treatment. Sometimes a course of treatment must perforce be empirical for want of knowledge.

EMPLASTRUM is the Latin term for a plaster.

EMPROSTHOTONOS is the term applied to the spasm of the belly muscles that occurs in tetanus, making the body arch forwards.

EMPYEMA is a term applied to an accumulation of pus within a cavity, the term being generally reserved for collections of pus within one of the pleural cavities. The condition is virtually an abscess, and therefore gives rise to the general symptoms accompanying that condition; but, on account of the thick unyielding wall of the chest, it has very little tendency to burst through the surface, and therefore it is of particular importance that the condition should be recognized early, and, as a rule, treated by surgical means.

Causes – The condition most commonly follows an attack of pneumonia. It may also occur in the advanced stage of pulmonary tuberculosis. Empyema also occurs at times through infection from some serious disease in neighbouring organs, such as cancer of the gullet, or follows upon wounds penetrating the chest wall.

Symptoms – In empyema following a case of pneumonia, symptoms of the former generally appear as the pneumonia is subsiding, and when an ordinary attack of pneumonia does not come satisfactorily to an end after the lapse of eight to ten days, it is usual for the physician to suspect and search for the signs of empyema. A certain amount of inflammation in the membrane lining the pleural cavity always accompanies pneumonia, and the fluid which is thus produced may show any stage between that of clear yellow serous fluid and thick pus of the consistence of cream. When the fluid is clear or merely turbid, absorption generally takes place naturally in course of time, and the mild type of infection which is present is readily overcome by the ordinary powers of the tissues. When, however, a severe infection, due usually either to a virulent pneumococcus or streptococcus, is present, the fluid is of the thicker purulent variety, and active measures of treatment are required. The temperature of the patient, which should revert to normal at the end of the attack of pneumonia, tends to show a daily rise to 102° or 103° F (39° to 39·5° C); there is profuse sweating and the patient presents a flushed appearance. The severity of these symptoms is proportional to the degree of virulence in the infection of the pleural membrane, the symptoms generally being less marked the clearer the fluid. On examination of the chest a dull percussion-note, faint or absent breath sounds, and other characteristic signs of the presence of fluid are found. It is usual for the physician to complete the diagnosis by puncturing the chest by means of a fine needle attached to a small aspiration syringe. A sample of the fluid is thus obtained, and its characteristics as regards the bacteria present, etc., are investigated. The collection of fluid may be very small in size and limited by adhesions to a small portion of the chest, especially in those cases due to the pneumococcus, and it may be necessary in such cases to insert the needle at various points before the purulent fluid is definitely located.

Treatment – In those cases in which the fluid is clear or only slightly turbid, the measures commonly employed for pleurisy (see PLEURISY) are often sufficient to bring about absorption. In cases in which the fluid is thick and purulent, and especially those following acute pneumonia, it is usually necessary to perform an operation for the drainage of the cavity, an incision being made through the skin and a portion of rib removed. The fluid is thus evacuated, and the lung can then expand naturally against the chest wall, a drainage tube being left in the wound so that the cavity can be irrigated and any fresh fluid which tends to collect can escape freely until the natural closure of the cavity is completed. Penicillin is also given, both intramuscularly and into the cavity. In the great majority of cases the lung ultimately reverts completely to a normal state.

EMULSIONS are mixtures containing oily substances in a state of very fine division. The division is effected and the oil kept suspended in the fluid by means of alkalis and sticky ingredients such as albumin, glycerin, or mucilage. Milk is an example of a perfect emulsion of fat globules each surrounded by an envelope of albumin. The various preparations of cod-liver oil are usually emulsified by the aid of glycerin. The oil is not only rendered more devoid of taste, but digestion and absorption are also rendered easier by emulsification.

EMUNCTORY is a term applied generally to excretory organs, such as the kidneys and bowels.

ENAMEL is a thin, hard, transparent layer which covers the surface of the teeth, at least that part of them which projects

311

above the gums. It is composed almost entirely of the earthy salts found in bone, and is the hardest tissue in the body. It is arranged in the form of long six-sided prisms, each about $\frac{1}{5000}$ inch (5 micrometres) in thickness, and set on end upon the dentine of the tooth. (See TEETH.)

ENCEPHALITIS means inflammation of the brain. It is usually a virus infection, and may occur as a complication of the common infectious diseases, including measles (in which it occurs in around 1 in 1000 cases).

ENCEPHALITIS LETHARGICA, also known as SLEEPY SICKNESS and as EPIDEMIC ENCEPHALITIS, and VON ECONOMO'S DISEASE, is a disease that appears from time to time, especially in the spring, in the form of epidemics. There has not been an epidemic in Britain since the late 1920's. It is probably a virus infection, and attacks chiefly the basal ganglia, the cerebrum, and the brain stem. These undergo dropsical swelling, haemorrhages, and ultimately destruction of areas of tissue involving both nerve-cells and fibres. The process may involve other parts of the brain, the spinal cord, and even other organs.

Symptoms – The illness begins usually with a rise of temperature and increasing drowsiness or lethargy, which may gradually proceed to a state of complete unconsciousness. In some cases, however, the patient instead of being drowsy passes at first through a stage of restlessness which may amount to maniacal excitement. As a rule the drowsiness deepens gradually over a period of a week or more, and accompanying it there appear various forms of paralysis, shown by drooping of the eyelids, squint, and weakness of one or both sides of the face. The nerves controlling the muscles of the throat are also sometimes paralysed, causing changes in the voice and difficulty in swallowing. In some cases the disease affects the spinal cord, producing severe pain in one or more of the limbs, and it is often followed by partial paralysis. Signs of inflammation are not infrequently found in other organs, and haemorrhages may be visible beneath the skin and may occur in the muscles, or blood may be vomited up or passed in the stools. The effects last usually for many months, the patient remaining easily tired and somnolent or frequently showing rigidity of muscle, mask-like facies, festinant gait (see FESTINATION), and rhythmical coarse tremors, resembling the clinical picture of Parkinsonism (qv).

Treatment – There is no specific treatment for the disease. During the acute stage the patient must be kept at rest in bed. After the acute stage is over, physiotherapy in the form of massage, passive movements and exercises should be given to control the muscular rigidity. Prolonged convalescence, ie. three months, is essential to reduce the risk of relapse.

ENCEPHALOID is the name applied to a form of cancer which, to the naked eye, resembles the tissue of the brain.

ENCEPHALOMYELITIS means inflammation of the substance of both brain and spinal cord.

ENCEPHALOPATHY is the term used to describe certain conditions in which there are signs of cerebral irritation without any localized lesion to account for them. The two best examples are *hypertensive encephalopathy* and *lead encephalopathy*. In the former, which occurs in the later stages of chronic Bright's disease, or uraemia (qv), the headache, convulsions, and delirium which constitute the main symptoms are supposed to be due to a deficient blood-supply to the brain. In the latter the symptoms are probably due to spasm of the arteries in the brain.

ENCHONDROMA means a tumour formed of cartilage. (See TUMOURS.)

ENCYSTED means enclosed within a bladder-like wall. The term is applied to parasites, collections of pus, etc., which are shut off from surrounding tissues by a membrane or by adhesions.

ENDARTERITIS means inflammation of the inner coat of an artery. (See ARTERIES, DISEASES OF.)

ENDEMIC is a term applied to diseases which exist in particular localities or among certain races. Some diseases, which are at times epidemic over wide districts, have a restricted area where they are always endemic, and from which they spread. For example, both cholera and plague are endemic in certain parts of Asia.

ENDO- is a prefix meaning situated inside.

ENDOCARDITIS means inflammation of the smooth membrane lining the heart, especially that over the heart valves. (See HEART, DISEASES OF.)

ENDOCRINE GLANDS are organs whose function is to secrete into the blood or lymph substances known as hormones which play an important part in general chemical changes or the activities of other organs at a distance. Some organs have a double function, such as the pancreas, which pours digestive secretions by a duct into the intestine, and, at the same time, has an endocrine or internal secretion (insulin) which is secreted direct into the blood. Various diseases arise as the result of defects or excess in the internal secretions of the different glands. The chief endocrine glands are the thyroid gland, adrenal bodies, pituitary body, parathyroid glands, pancreas, ovaries, and testicles. A certain amount of antagonism exists between the different endocrine glands: for example, secretion of the adrenal glands checks the action of the pancreatic secretion of insulin. Other glands have an associated action: for example, extract of pituitary gland stimulates the production of normal secretion of the thyroid. During healthy bodily activity there appears to be a constant state of balancing between the action of the different endocrine secretions. The structure of these glands is noted elsewhere under the appropriate headings, and only a short account will be given here of the action of their secretion.

THYROID GLAND – This gland, situated in front of the neck, produces a secretion which has a very important effect in regulating the general nutrition of the body. When it is defective, the conditions known as myxoedema and cretinism result; whilst excess or perversion of the secretion is associated with different types of the condition generally known as exophthalmic goitre or thyrotoxicosis. An extract is prepared from the thyroid glands of sheep and other animals, and is used in cases where the secretion is defective. The active principle of this secretion is thyroxine.

ADRENAL BODIES – These two glands, also known as SUPRARENAL GLANDS, lie immediately above the kidneys. The central or medullary portion of the glands forms the secretions known as adrenaline or epinephrine, and noradrenaline. Adrenaline acts upon structures innervated by sympathetic nerves; its action is therefore said to be sympathomimetic. Briefly, the blood-vessels of the skin and of the abdominal viscera (except the intestines) are constricted, and at the same time the arteries of the muscles and the coronary arteries are dilated; systolic blood-pressure rises; blood-sugar increases; the metabolic rate rises; muscle fatigue is di-

minished. Adrenaline can be synthetically prepared in the laboratory. This substance is widely used in medicine in 1 in 1000 solutions, for the purpose of checking bleeding, relieving congestion of mucous membranes, for the relief of asthma, and in the treatment of anaphylactic shock. The superficial or cortical part of the glands produce a series of chemical substances, the full range of which is not known. They have as their basis a complicated steroid nucleus. The best known of these are aldosterone, cortisone, hydrocortisone, and deoxycortone acetate. These substances are essential for the maintenance of life. It is the absence of these substances, due to atrophy or destruction of the suprarenal cortex, that is responsible for the condition known as Addison's disease (qv).

PITUITARY GLAND – This gland is attached to the base of the brain and rests in a hollow on the base of the skull immediately above the hinder part of the throat. The anterior, intermediate, and posterior parts of the gland produce different secretions: that from the intermediate and posterior parts has a powerful action in stimulating the contractions of unstriped muscle-fibres found, for example, in the uterus, intestine, and blood-vessels. Pituitary extract (posterior lobe) is therefore widely employed in obstetric practice for its valuable action in checking bleeding and increasing the contractions of the uterus during delivery. It is also used in the treatment of shock on account of its action in contracting blood-vessels and raising the blood-pressure.

The anterior part secretes hormones which stimulate growth, development of sex, and secretion of milk, and exert a controlling influence on most of the other endocrine glands – thyroid, adrenal, and reproductive glands.

PARATHYROID GLANDS – These are four minute glands lying at the side of, or behind, the thyroid. They have a certain effect in controlling the absorption of lime salts by the bones and other tissues. When their secretion is defective, tetany occurs.

PANCREAS – This gland is situated in the upper part of the abdomen and, in addition to the digestive ferments which it produces, a substance known as insulin is absorbed from it into the circulating blood. This has the effect of adapting sugary foods for incorporation in the muscles and other tissues that particularly require such foodstuffs. Lack of it is followed by the production of the disease known as diabetes mellitus.

OVARIES AND TESTICLES – In addition to their main function of producing reproductive cells, these organs secrete substances which have a general effect upon the other bodily tissues.

The ovary secretes at least two hormones, known, respectively, as oestradiol (follicular hormone) and progesterone (corpus luteum hormone). Oestradiol, develops (under the stimulus of the anterior pituitary lobe) each time an ovum in the ovary becomes mature, causes extensive proliferation of the endometrium lining the uterus, a stage ending with shedding of the ovum about 14 days before the onset of menstruation. The corpus luteum, which then forms, secretes both progesterone and oestradiol. Progesterone brings about great activity of the glands in the endometrium. The uterus is now ready for the nesting of the ovum if it is fertilized. If fertilization does not occur, the corpus luteum degenerates, the hormones cease acting, and menstruation takes place.

The hormone secreted by the testicles is known as testosterone. It is responsible for the growth of the male secondary sex organs.

ENDOMETRIOSIS is the condition in which the endometrium (ie. the type of cells lining the interior of the uterus) is found in other parts of the body. The most common site of such misplaced endometrium is the muscle of the uterus. The next most common site is the ovary, followed by the peritoneum (qv) lining the pelvis (qv), but it also occurs anywhere in the bowel. The cause is not known. It never occurs before puberty and seldom after the menopause. The main symptoms it produces are menorrhagia (qv), dyspareunia

156 – Endothelium. From Schafer, *Essentials of Histology*. Longman.

(qv), dysmenorrhoea and pelvic pain. Treatment is usually by removal of the affected area, but in some cases satisfactory results are obtained from the administration of progestogens (qv) such as norethisterone (qv) and norethynodrel (qv).

ENDOMETRITIS means inflammation of the mucous membrane lining the womb. (See UTERUS, DISEASES OF.)

ENDOMETRIUM is the mucous membrane which lines the interior of the uterus.

ENDOTHELIUM is the term applied to the membrane lining various vessels and cavities of the body, such as the pleura, pericardium, peritoneum, lymphatic vessels, blood-vessels, and joints. It consists of a fibrous layer covered with thin flat cells, which render the surface perfectly smooth and secrete the fluid for its lubrication (illustration 156).

ENEMA means an injection of fluid into the bowel.

Uses – PURGATIVE ENEMAS are given generally in large bulk, so as to distend the rectum; they also contain various stimulating substances. For an adult, 1 to 2 pints (450 to 900 ml) are injected, for a young child about 6 ounces (170 ml). The process of injection should be slow, and the person should retain the enema as long as he can, in order to obtain the maximum effect. The water should be tepid: about $100°$ F ($38°$ C). The usual constituent is soft green soap B P, $\frac{1}{2}$ ounce (14 G) in 1 pint (450 ml) of water. Yellow soap is also satisfactory. In some cases an olive oil enema (5 to 8 ounces (140 to 230 ml) of olive oil) is preferred, or a glycerin enema (not more than 5 ounces (140 ml) of equal parts of glycerin and water). To expel flatulence, two tablespoonfuls of turpentine may be added to each pint of warm water. The frequent use of enemas is unhealthy, as they ultimately increase the constipation.

DISPOSABLE ENEMAS are largely supplanting the traditional soap-and-water enemas – largely on account of their convenience. The ingredients, usually sodium diphosphate and sodium phosphate in the case of a purgative enema, are contained in around 100 ml of solution in a small plastic bag with tube and plug.

MINIATURE ENEMAS are in increasing use. Their great advantage is that they are of a much smaller volume – only 2 millilitres, and therefore much more comfortable for the patient. They are also prepared much more easily and are supplied ready made up in a plastic container with a soft nozzle. They may be self-administered. As a rule, a movement of the bowels occurs within fifteen minutes. A widely used formula for such a miniature enema is: 5 mg of bisacodyl; 0·5 millilitre of glycerin; made up to 2 millilitres with sulphonated castor oil BPC.

SEDATIVE ENEMAS are used to quiet spasm, and check excessive action of the bowels. There are two types. A *starch enema* is made by rubbing 120 grains (8 G) of powdered starch to a smooth paste with a little cold water, and then adding 5 ounces (140 ml) of boiling water. It is used when it has been allowed to cool. A *starch-and-opium enema* is prepared by adding 10 to 40 minims (0·5 to 2·5 ml) of tincture of opium to 2 ounces (60 ml) of starch enema.

157 – Enema syringe.

NUTRIENT ENEMAS are given when the stomach is seriously deranged and cannot retain or cannot digest food, but are not widely used today. A nutrient enema consists of dextrose, 5 per cent solution in normal saline solution, that is, ½ ounce (14 G) of dextrose and ½ teaspoonful of common salt to ½ pint (220 ml) of warm water. The enema, which is warmed to 100° F (38° C), must be administered very slowly, and preferably run in through a small funnel and catheter tube. It may be given, to the amount of 8 or 10 ounces (230 to 285 ml), every 4 hours, that is five times in 24 hours.

IRRIGATION, or CLEANSING, ENEMAS are used for healing and cleansing purposes. Several pints of warm, weak salt solution (2 teaspoonfuls of salt to every pint (450 ml) of water) or boric acid solution are introduced very slowly, by a douche, into the bowel, and then allowed to run off by lowering the tube, very much in the same way that the stomach is washed out.

Mode of administration – Nutrient enemas are administered by means of an india-rubber tube 3 or 4 feet (90 to 120 cm) in length, with a funnel at one end, and soft rubber nozzle, with rounded end, at the other. For purgative enemas, the rubber syringe with a ball in the centre (illustration 157) may be used, and for small enemas an india-rubber bag which contains the exact amount required. In all cases the old bone or metal nozzle should be replaced by a soft rubber one, because much pain and injury may be inflicted by a rigid one carelessly or forcibly introduced.

The patient lies upon his left side with the hips raised on a thick pillow, and should remain so after the enema has been given. The nozzle is oiled, introduced forwards and upwards with a screwing motion, and should be passed gently up for 3 or 4 inches (75 or 100 mm). The fluid is now pumped, or, if a tube and funnel be used, allowed to flow gently in by raising the funnel. In the case of nutrient enemas, fully fifteen or twenty minutes should be spent in letting the fluid slowly enter; otherwise the bowels may move or the whole enema be rejected.

ENOPHTHALMOS is a term applied to abnormal retraction of the eye into its socket: for example, when the sympathetic nerve in the neck is paralysed.

ENTAMOEBA (see AMOEBA).

ENTERALGIA is another name for colic.

ENTERIC FEVERS are typhoid fever and paratyphoid fever.

Until the middle of last century typhoid was not distinguished from typhus fever. The distinction between the two diseases appears to have been accurately made first in 1836 by Dr Gerhard, of Philadelphia, and still more fully demonstrated by Dr A. P. Stewart, of Glasgow, in 1840. Subsequently all doubt upon the subject was removed by the careful clinical and pathological observations made by Sir William Jenner at the London Fever Hospital (1849–51). At the end of the nineteenth century it was noticed that cases of fever resembling typhoid but of shorter duration occurred, and these were found to be due to bacilli resembling the typhoid bacillus and are known as paratyphoid fevers. This group of fevers again has a resemblance, both as regards symptoms and as regards the causal bacteria, to cases of food-poisoning and dysentery.

In 1977, there were 225 cases of typhoid fever in England, compared with 162 in 1969, and in 196 of these the infection was contracted abroad. The number of cases of paratyphoid fever in England in 1973 was 97 (188 in 1969), 68 of which were acquired abroad.

ENTERIC FEVERS

Causes – A bacillus, discovered first by Eberth in 1880, and known as *Salmonella typhi*, is the cause of typhoid fever. (See BACTERIOLOGY.) The bacilli responsible for cases of paratyphoid fever are known as *Salmonella paratyphi A* and *Salmonella paratyphi B*, the latter being the commoner. Other bacilli which do not altogether correspond to either of these are also responsible for mild attacks of fever, sometimes grouped as paratyphoid C. For the rest of this section the description will apply to typhoid fever, and paratyphoid fever will then be discussed. Where the discharges, sheets, etc., from typhoid patients are carefully disinfected, there is little risk of direct spread from person to person. In many hospitals patients with typhoid are therefore treated in the general wards, with little or no risk to the other patients, provided certain precautions be taken.

All insanitary conditions in respect of drainage of houses and localities furnish the most ready means for the spread of the contagion of typhoid fever. The most certain means of preventing its appearance or checking its spread are: the water-carriage system of sewage disposal; prevention of pollution of water-supplies, food, milk, and shell-fish with human excreta; chlorination of drinking water; pasteurization of milk; control of the house-fly; personal cleanliness; detection of carriers of enteric bacilli. The bacillus resides in the stools and urine of typhoid patients. Thus, in badly laid drains, where the contents stagnate, the bacillus may increase indefinitely, and, by the contamination of drinking-water in places where wells or cisterns are exposed to sewage pollution, convey infection to a whole community. Dust may also act as the medium which conveys the bacilli, in cases where the discharges of a typhoid patient or the sewage are allowed to dry, and so get blown into drinking-water or on to food. Milk may readily be contaminated by the bacillus and forms the cause of an epidemic, when a case of the fever has occurred in a dairy. The source of an epidemic has also been traced to the eating of oysters taken from oyster-beds near which contaminated sewage is discharged. During an epidemic it can be readily understood that flies may also form a means of contamination between uncovered stools and uncovered food. It may therefore be said that the spread of typhoid fever depends upon food or drink contaminated by a bacillus which is derived more or less directly from the discharges of previous typhoid cases.

The incubation period is usually ten to fourteen days, but may be as short as five days or as long as twenty-one days.

The chief symptoms will be better understood by a brief reference to the principal changes that take place in the body during the disease. The bowels are chiefly affected, particularly the lower end of the small intestine, where the Peyer's patches on the inner surface of the bowel (see INTESTINES) pass through changes that bear a distinct relation to the symptoms exhibited by the patient during the course of the disease. (1) During the first eight or ten days of the illness these patches, which in health are comparatively indistinct, become enlarged and prominent as the result of inflammation. (2) During the second week of the fever these enlarged patches undergo a process of sloughing, being cast off either in fragments or *en masse*. (3) From the second week onwards during the remainder of the fever, and even into the stage of convalescence, the ulcers formed by this process remain open, though slowly healing. The ulcers vary in size according to the Peyer's patches that have sloughed away, and they may be few or many in number. They are frequently, but not always, oblong in shape, with their long axis in that of the bowel, and they have somewhat thin and ragged edges. They may extend through the thickness of the bowel to the peritoneal coat, and they may perforate this, or may erode blood-vessels in their progress. (4) During convalescence the ulcers usually heal, leaving no contraction in the wall of the bowel.

The mesenteric glands associated with the intestine become enlarged, but usually subside without abscess formation as recovery takes place. The spleen becomes soft and enlarged, this enlargement being a useful guide to the physician in cases which are difficult to diagnose. As in other fevers, the muscular tissues soften and waste, and various complications affecting other organs may arise.

Symptoms – The symptoms at the *onset* of typhoid fever are much less marked than those of most other fevers, and the disease in the majority of instances sets in somewhat insidiously. Indeed, it is no uncommon thing for patients with this fever to go about for a considerable time after it has begun. The most marked of the early symptoms are headache, lassitude, and discomfort, together with sleeplessness and feverishness, particularly at night; this last symptom is that by which the disease is most readily detected in its early stages. Bleeding from the nose is also an early symptom in many cases. The course of *the temperature* is one of the important diagnostic features. During the first week it rises about 2° F in the evening and falls 1° F in the morning so that by the end of the first week it has reached a plateau of 102° to 104° F (38·8° to 40° C). Because of this feature of rising by steps, so to speak, it is known as a step-ladder temperature. During the second week the daily range of temperature is comparatively small, a slight morning remission being all that is observed. In the third week the same condition continues more or less; but frequently a slight tendency to lowering may be discerned, particularly in the morning temperature, and the fever gradually dies down as a rule between the twenty-first and twenty-eighth day, although it is liable to recur in the form of a relapse. Although during the earlier days of the fever the patient may be able to move about, he feels languid and uneasy; and usually before the first week is over he has to take to bed, and soon the effects of the attack become more apparent. He is restless, hot, and uncomfortable, particularly as the day advances, and his cheeks show a red flush, especially in the evening or after taking food. The *pulse* in an ordinary case, although more rapid than normal, is not accelerated to an extent corresponding to the height of the temperature, and, at least in the earlier stages of the fever, is rarely above 100 a minute. In severe and protracted cases, where there is evidence of extensive intestinal ulceration, the pulse becomes rapid and weak. The *tongue* has at first a thin whitish fur and is red at the tip and edges. It tends, however, to become dry, brown or glazed-looking, and fissured transversely, while sordes may be present about the lips and teeth. There is much thirst, and, in some cases, vomiting.

From an early period in the disease *abdominal symptoms* show themselves and are often of great help in diagnosis. The abdomen is somewhat distended, and pain accompanying some gurgling sounds may be elicited on light pressure about the lower part of the right side close to the groin – the region corresponding to that portion of the intestine in which the morbid changes already referred to are progressing. *Diarrhoea* is a common but by no means constant symptom. When present, it may be slight in amount, or, on the other hand, extremely profuse, and it corresponds, as a rule, to the severity of the intestinal ulceration, and to the nature of the diet which the patient has been taking. The discharges are highly characteristic, being of light-yellow colour, resembling 'pea soup' in appearance. Sometimes, especially in milder cases, constipation is found instead of diarrhoea. Should intestinal haemorrhage occur, the stools may be dark brown, or composed entirely of blood. Enlargement of the spleen and liver can usually be made out by the physician. The urine is scanty and high-coloured. When the fever is well developed from the second week onwards, the *blood* shows a well-marked feature known as the Widal reaction. (See AGGLUTINATION.)

About the beginning, or during the course, of the second week of the fever, an *eruption* often makes its appearance on the skin. It consists of small isolated spots, oval or round in shape, of a pale pink or rose colour, which are seen chiefly upon the abdomen, chest, and back, and they come out in crops, which continue for four or five days and then fade away. At first they are slightly elevated, and disappear on pressure. In some cases they are very few in number, and their presence is made out with difficulty; but in others they are numerous and sometimes show themselves upon the limbs as well as upon the body. They do not appear to have any relation to the severity of the attack, and in a large proportion of cases (particularly in children) they are entirely absent. Besides this eruption there are often numerous very faint bluish patches or blotches about half an inch in diameter, chiefly upon the body and thighs. When present, the rose-coloured spots continue to come out in crops till nearly the end of the fever, and they may reappear should a relapse subsequently occur.

These various symptoms persist throughout the third week, usually, however, increasing in intensity. The patient becomes prostrate and emaciated; the tongue is dry and brown, the pulse quickened and feeble, and the abdominal symptoms more marked; while nervous disturbance is exhibited in delirium, in tremors and jerkings of the muscles (*subsultus tendinum*), in drowsiness, and occasionally in 'coma vigil'. (See TYPHUS FEVER.) In severe cases the exhaustion reaches an extreme degree, but even in such instances the condition should not be regarded as hopeless. In favourable cases a change for the better may be expected between the twenty-first and twenty-eighth days, although it takes place by a lysis or gradual subsidence of the symptoms (the morning and evening temperatures descending, the pulse becoming stronger, the diarrhoea passing off, the tongue becoming clean, etc.), not by a crisis as in typhus fever or pneumonia. Convalescence proceeds slowly, and relapses are apt to occur (due often to errors in diet). Such relapses may prolong the fever for two or three months, though this is not common.

Abscesses sometimes arise, especially in connection with inflammation in the periosteum of the bones, found after the patient has been convalescent for some time, and these form a troublesome and prolonged complication. Stiff back, known as 'typhoid spine', is an occasional sequel to this disease, due either to inflammation in the spine or more commonly to changes in the muscles with development of fibrous tissue, causing the patient for long, it may be for years, to suffer from severe 'rheumatic' pains. Inflammation of the bile passages, with retention of the bacilli in these and their constant discharge in the stools, is also an occasional sequel; and, although this may cause no trouble to the patient, it renders him a source of danger to others as a 'carrier' of the disease. (See INFECTION.)

When death takes place, it is generally due to one of the following causes: (1) Exhaustion in the second or third week or later; (2) haemorrhage from the bowels; (3) perforation of an ulcer and the onset of peritonitis; (4) excessive rise of temperature; (5) complications, such as inflammation of the lungs.

Treatment – The preventive treatment includes all the municipal and domestic measures that aim at securing pure supplies of water and milk and well-laid drains. (See SANITATION.) Inoculation with anti-typhoid vaccine is a precaution which ought to be adopted by persons about to proceed overseas, particularly to Africa, Asia, South America, or any country around, or any island in, the Mediterranean, or in the Balkans. It should be repeated every three years. (See VACCINE.)

When an outbreak of typhoid fever occurs in a family, the source of the milk supply especially should be scrutinized. The discharges of a typhoid patient should be mixed so soon as passed with a strong disinfectant. (See DISINFECTION). Similar care should be taken to sterilize all sheets, towels, etc., soiled by the patient. Special care is necessary on the part of those in attendance upon a typhoid-fever case to cleanse the hands at once after touching the patient, and especially after they have become in any way soiled by contact with his discharges.

As an expert in this field has recently expressed it, 'the introduction of chloramphenicol has transformed a fever that lasted three to four weeks into a sharp febrile illness of three to four days'. This means that diet is not so important as it was, but milk, or milk dishes, are still the great standby. It must, however, be administered with due regard to time and to the digestive powers of the patient. The usual quantity given is from 3 to 4 ounces (85 to 110 ml) administered every two or three hours: that is $1\frac{1}{2}$ to 2 pints (850 to 1100 ml) daily. In the intervals water or bland fruit drinks may be given from time to time. When given too frequently or in too great quantity, milk may, by its imperfect digestion, prove a source of irritation to the bowels. In such a case its admixture with lime-water, or peptonizing it, may render its digestion less difficult, but sometimes its use must for a time be suspended. Barley water or simple soups, such as chicken-broth, beef-tea, are occasionally useful either as substitutes for, or in addition to, milk. In convalescence, the diet should still be largely milk and soft food, such as custards, light puddings, egg dishes, meat jellies, or one of the numerous proprietary invalids' foods; but other solid foods, with the exception of fish, should be avoided. In changing the diet it is of importance to note its effect upon the temperature, which may sometimes be considerably disturbed from this cause, even after the apparent subsidence of all fever. In serious cases, particularly in hot countries, replacement of fluid may be a matter of urgency and it may be necessary to give fluids either intravenously or intraperitoneally.

The more prominent symptoms which mark the course of typhoid fever may call for special treatment. Thus, when diarrhoea is excessive, it may be restrained by such remedies as Dover's powder or a starch-and-opium enema. (See ENEMA.) In the event of perforation of the bowel, immediate operation is called for, though the hazards of this complication have been considerably reduced since the introduction of chloramphenicol. With regard to the condition of the mouth and tongue, much comfort is gained if the patient's mouth and teeth be washed occasionally with boric lotion in tepid water, and the lips and tip of the tongue lightly smeared with boroglyceride or some emollient ointment.

The introduction of chloramphenicol

(qv) has revolutionized the outlook in typhoid fever. There is usually a dramatic improvement within 48 to 60 hours after this antibiotic is administered. Ampicillin (qv) is also proving of value, but the relative value of these two antibiotics has not been determined. Whichever is used, however, it is still necessary to keep the patient in bed for three weeks, and to keep him on a bland nutritious diet during this period. Otherwise complications may arise. The patient should be considered infective until six consecutive specimens of stools and urine are found to be negative on bacteriological examination.

In the convalescent stage, and even after apparently complete recovery, the utmost care should be observed by the patient as to diet, all hard and indigestible substances being dangerous from their tendency to irritate or reopen unhealed ulcers and bring on a relapse of the fever or cause a sudden perforation. Lastly, the general health demands careful attention for a length of time.

PARATYPHOID FEVER is a continued fever which closely resembles mild attacks of typhoid and which, like typhoid fever, is due to one or more members of the genus *Salmonella*.

Causes – Paratyphoid fever is due to infection with one of three micro-organisms: *Salmonella paratyphi A, B,* or *C.* The most common variety in Britain is *Salmonella paratyphi B.* These organisms closely resemble that of typhoid fever in appearance and some of its reactions, but inoculation against typhoid only does not afford protection against these, and a quadruple vaccine should be used for protective inoculation, prepared from all four organisms and known as TABC. The infection is usually conveyed by a 'carrier' case who has already had the disease, or it is due to contaminated food or water. In 1973, there were 97 cases in England, 68 of which were acquired abroad. In the five-year period, 1973–77) there were 509 cases in Britain, one of them a double infection with *S. paratyphi A* and *B.* Of the 158 cases of paratyphoid, 97 per cent were contracted abroad (116 in the Indian subcontinent. Of the 352 cases of paratyphoid B, 57 per cent were contracted abroad (95 in the Mediterranean).

Symptoms resemble those found in a mild case of typhoid fever. The incubation period is shorter (one to ten days), and rose spots are seen less commonly. The onset of the disease is often more sudden than in typhoid fever, but the fever tends to be less prolonged and less severe.

Treatment is the same as for typhoid fever.

ENTERITIS means inflammation of the intestines. (See DIARRHOEA; and INTESTINES, DISEASES OF.)

ENTEROBIASIS is infection with *Enterobius vermicularis,* the threadworm, or pinworm as it is known in U.S.A. It is the most common of all the intestinal parasites in Britain and the least harmful. The male is about ¼ inch (6 mm) in length and the female (illustration 158) about ½ inch (12 mm) in length. Each resembles a little piece of thread. These worms live in considerable numbers in the lower bowel, affecting children particularly. They cause great irritation round the anus, especially in the evening when the female worm emerges from the anus to lay its eggs and then die. It lays around 10,000 eggs and these may be found in dust, especially after bedmaking, in the bedclothes and pyjamas, on toys and furniture, and on the fur of cats and dogs, as well as floating in the air. Apart from this irritation around the anus, they seldom cause any symptoms, though in some cases they may cause diarrhoea and, occasionally in girls they may be responsible for a discharge from the vagina.

Treatment – The most effective form of treatment is either viprynium embonate or piperazine citrate. The former has the advantage of only one dose being necessary repeated twice at 15-day intervals, whereas a 7-day course of piperazine is necessary repeated after a week's interval. Whichever drug is used, a second course should be given after a period of three weeks. If one member of a household is infected, it is necessary to examine all other members of the household and to treat simultaneously all those found infected. During treatment steps must be taken to prevent patients reinfecting themselves or infecting others. This is done by the wearing of drawers day and night to prevent scratching of the anus, and of gloves at night, the daily washing of all infected linen, and scrupulous cleanliness. The local irritation around the anus may be relieved by the application of weak white precipitate ointment.

ENTEROCELE means a hernia of the bowel. (See HERNIA.)

ENTEROGASTRONE is a hormone derived from the mucosal lining of the small intestine which inhibits the movements and secretion of the stomach.

158 – *Enterobius vermicularis* (or Threadworm). Female. 1, cervical alae; 2, oesophagus; 3, bulb behind oesophagus; 4, intestine; 5, ovary; 6, vulva; 7, uterus; 8, anus. From Blacklock and Southwell, *Human Parasitology*. H. K. Lewis & Co. Ltd.

ENTEROGENOUS CYANOSIS is a rare condition characterized by blueness of the lips and face (cyanosis) and the presence in the blood of sulphaemoglobin and methaemoglobin, especially the former. It is usually the result of taking drugs, especially those derived from aniline (eg. phenacetin). Recovery follows discontinuance of the drug.

ENTEROKINASE is the enzyme (qv) secreted in the duodenum (qv) and jejunum (qv) which converts the enzyme, trypsinogen, secreted by the pancreas (qv) into trypsin (qv). (See also DIGESTION.)

ENTEROPTOSIS means a condition in which, owing to a lax condition of the mesenteries and ligaments which support the bowels, the latter descend into the lower part of the abdominal cavity. The condition is aggravated by tight lacing and by the lax condition of the abdominal walls which follows repeated child-bearing, and so is commoner in women.

Treatment – Massage of the abdominal muscles and viscera, and the wearing of a well-shaped abdominal belt give most relief.

ENTEROSTOMY means an operation by which an artificial opening is formed into the intestine.

ENTEROVIRUSES are a family of viruses which include the poliomyelitis, coxsackie and echo groups of viruses. Their importance lies in their tendency to invade the central nervous system. They receive their name from the fact that their mode of entry into the body is through the gut.

ENTROPION means a condition in which, as a result of disease, the edge of the eyelid is turned inwards towards the ball of the eye.

ENURESIS means the unconscious or involuntary passage of urine. (See NOCTURNAL ENURESIS.)

ENZYME is the name applied to a chemical ferment produced by living cells. Enzymes are present in the digestive fluids and in many of the tissues, and are capable of producing in small amount the transformation on a large scale of various compounds. Examples of enzymes are found in the ptyalin of saliva and diastase of pancreatic juice which split up starch into sugar, the pepsin of the gastric juice and the trypsin of pancreatic juice which break proteins into simpler molecules and eventually into the constituent amino-acids, the thrombin of the blood which causes coagulation.

EOSINOPHIL is any cell in the body with granules in its substance that stain easily with the dye eosin. About 2 per cent of the white cells of the blood are eosinophils. Eosinophil cells are also present in the pituitary gland.

EOSINOPHILIA means an abnormal increase in the number of eosinophils in the blood. It occurs in Hodgkin's disease, in asthma and hay fever, in some skin diseases, and in parasitic infestation.

EPHEDRINE is an alkaloid derived from the Chinese plant *Ma Huang*, much used for asthma and other allergic disorders, in doses of $\frac{1}{4}$ to 1 grain (15 to 60 mg). It is similar to adrenaline in pharmacological action.

EPHELIS is a freckle. *Ephelis ab igne* is the dark-brown pigmentation produced on the legs by constant exposure of them to a fire, as by sitting constantly in front of a fire. A similar discoloration of the skin of the abdomen may be produced by constant use of a hot-water bottle.

EPI- is a prefix meaning situated on or outside of.

EPIDEMIC is a term applied to a disease which affects a large number of people in a particular locality at one time. The term is, in a sense, opposed to endemic, which means a disease always found in the locality in question. A disease may, however, be endemic as a rule – for example, malaria in swampy districts, and may become at times epidemic, when a n unusually large number of people are affected.

As a rule an epidemic disease is infectious from person to person, but this is not necessarily the case, since many persons in a locality may simply be exposed to the same cause at one time; for example, outbreaks of lead-poisoning are epidemic in this sense.

The laws which govern the outbreak of epidemics are by no means fully understood. Infected food supplies, such as drinking water contaminated by the evacuations of persons sick of cholera or typhoid fever, or milk tainted by the organism of scarlet fever have been traced as the cause of outbreaks of these diseases. The migrations of certain of the lower animals, such as rats, are in some cases responsible for the spread of plague, from which these animals die in great numbers. Certain epidemics come with regularity at certain seasons. Thus scarlet fever and diphtheria are autumnal complaints, and produce their epidemics in September, October and November. Whooping-cough, on the other hand, is a spring complaint, and very few cases occur in autumn. Measles produces two epidemics, as a rule, one in winter and one in March. Influenza, the common cold, and other infections of the upper respiratory tract, such as sore throat, occur predominantly in the winter.

These seasonal variations depend largely, no doubt, upon conditions like the amount of sunshine, the rainfall, the temperature of the ground and the aggregation of susceptible individuals.

There is another variation, both as regards the number of persons affected and the number who die in successive epidemics: the severity of successive epidemics rising and falling over periods of five or ten years. Further, scourges like plague and cholera have swept over whole continents at longer periods, and then died down without apparent cause. The reason for these latter variations is still obscure.

EPIDEMIC ENCEPHALITIS is another term for ENCEPHALITIS LETHARGICA (qv).

EPIDURAL ANAESTHESIA (see ANAESTHETICS).

EPIDYDIMIS is the name applied to an oblong body attached to the upper part of each testicle, composed of convoluted vessels and ducts. It is liable to be the seat of tuberculous and other inflammation. (See TESTICLE.)

EPIGASTRIUM is the region lying in the middle of the abdomen over the stomach. (See ABDOMEN, REGIONS OF.)

EPIGLOTTIS is a leaf-like piece of elastic cartilage covered with mucous membrane, which stands upright between the back of the tongue and the glottis, or entrance to the larynx. In the act of swallowing, it prevents fluids and solids from passing off the back of the tongue into the larynx.

EPIGLOTTITIS – Acute epiglottitis is an acute inflammatory oedema of the epiglottis, due to *Haemophilus influenzae*, which causes laryngeal obstruction due to swelling and immobilization of the epiglottis. It is a disease predominantly of children, occurs usually in the winter, and may prove rapidly fatal.

EPIGNATHUS is the term used to describe a mal-development of the foetus in which the deformed remains of one twin are united to the upper jaw of the other.

EPILATION means the removal of hair by the roots. (See DEPILATION.)

EPILEPSY, or FALLING SICKNESS, is a term applied to a nervous disorder characterized by a fit of sudden loss of consciousness, attended with convulsions. There may, however, exist manifestations of epilepsy much less marked than this, yet equally characteristic of the disease. On the other hand, it is to be borne in mind that many other attacks of a convulsive nature have the term 'epileptiform' applied to them because they resemble epilepsy.

Epilepsy was well known in ancient times, and was regarded as a special infliction of the gods, hence the names *morbus sacer, morbus divus*. It was also termed *morbus Herculeus*, from Hercules being supposed to have been epileptic, and *morbus comitialis*, from the circumstances that when any one at a meeting in the forum was seized with an epileptic fit the assembly was at once broken up. Other famous epileptics are said to include Socrates, Alexander the Great, Julius Caesar, St Paul, Dante, Handel, Byron, Berlioz, Dostoevski, Edward Lear, and possibly Napoleon, though in some cases, as for example St Paul and Dante, the evidence is by no means impressive. *Morbus caducus, morbus lunaticus astralis, morbus demoniacus, morbus major* were all terms used to designate epilepsy.

There are two well-marked varieties of the epileptic seizure. To these the terms, *le grand mal* and *le petit mal*, are generally applied. The former of these is that which attracts most attention, being what is generally known as an epileptic fit. In addition to these two forms there is a type known as *Jacksonian epilepsy*, in which the seizure consists of convulsive movements starting in a single muscle or group of muscles, consciousness being in general retained. Cases of this type shade off, however, into *grand mal*, and indeed the

subjects of Jacksonian epilepsy may, at a later stage, be affected by typical seizures of severe type.

Incidence – It is estimated that in England and Wales there are around 290,000 epileptics: 190,000 adults and 100,000 children under the age of 16 years. It is also estimated that approximately 33,000 new cases occur every year. Probably one person in 20 has a fit of some sort in the course of a lifetime, but only one in 8 of those who have a fit will suffer from chronic epilepsy: that is, have a continuing liability to fits. The onset of epilepsy occurs before the age of 5 in nearly a quarter of the cases, and before school-leaving age in more than half.

Causes – The disease is commonly regarded as one of disordered function of the brain. Those cases, which begin with the Jacksonian type of seizure, appear to be due to some organic disease of the brain, such as a tumour, inflammation of the membranes of the brain, or the scar of some old injury, but this certainly does not occur in the majority of cases of epilepsy.

Practically all that can be said about the direct cause is that in the healthy brain nerve energy is capable, under control of the will, of being expended in a sudden and explosive but regulated manner, whilst, in the disease known as epilepsy, uncontrolled discharges of energy, devoid of any purposive action, take place from time to time in an unusual manner.

Although there is a hereditary disposition to epilepsy in a number of cases, quite a number of those who inherit the disposition never develop epilepsy. This means that, unless there is a strong family incidence of the disease, epilepsy *per se* is not a contraindication to marriage or having children, but there is a legal obligation for the prospective marriage partner to be informed of the position by the epileptic subject. It was found in one investigation that the risk of epilepsy for the child of an affected parent is around 4 per cent. If in doubt, the wise rule is to consult a specialist or the British Epilepsy Association. It may, however, be a ground for annulment of marriage.

Age is of importance in reference to the production of epilepsy. The disease may appear at any period of life, but it most often first manifests itself before adult life, usually during infancy or at puberty.

Among precipitating factors which are influential in the development of epilepsy in predisposed individuals may be mentioned sudden fright, prolonged mental anxiety, overwork and alcoholism. Epileptiform fits, which at a later period may develop into typical epileptic seizures, also occur in connection with injuries of the head and organic disease of the brain, as well as with a depraved state of the general health.

Epilepsy is occasionally feigned by malingerers, but an experienced medical practitioner will rarely be deceived. Although many of the phenomena of an attack, particularly the convulsive movements, can be readily simulated, that of the condition of the pupils, which are dilated during the fit, cannot be feigned, and the impostor seldom bites his tongue or injures himself in falling, choosing some soft object instead of falling headlong like the true epileptic. The electro-encephalogram (see ELECTRO-ENCEPHALOGRAPHY) in true epilepsy is characteristic.

Symptoms – Although in most instances an epileptic attack comes on suddenly, it is in some cases preceded by certain premonitory indications or warnings. These are of very varied character, and may be in the form of some temporary change in the disposition, such as unusual elevation or depression of spirits, or of some alteration in the look. Besides these general symptoms, there are often peculiar sensations which immediately precede the onset of the fit, and to such the name of *aura epileptica* is applied. The so-called aura, which occurs in over 50 per cent of cases, may be of mental character, in the form of an agonizing feeling of momentary duration; of sensory character, in the form of pain in a limb or in some internal organ, such as the stomach; or an unusual feeling connected with the special senses, such as a strange smell or extraordinary vision; or of a motor character, in the form of contractions or trembling in some of the muscles. The aura may be so distinct and of such duration as to enable the patient to lie down or seek a place of safety before the attack comes on.

The seizure is usually preceded by a loud scream or cry, which is not to be ascribed, as was at one time supposed, to terror or pain, but is due to the convulsive action of the muscles of the larynx, and the expulsion of air through the narrowed glottis. If the patient is standing he immediately falls, and often sustains serious injury. Unconsciousness is complete, and the muscles generally are in a state of stiffness or tonic contraction, which may be found to affect those on one side of the body in particular. The head is turned towards one or other shoulder, the breathing is for the moment arrested, the countenance first pale then livid, the pupils dilated, and the pulse rapid. This, the first stage of the fit, generally lasts for about half a minute, and is followed by the state of clonic (ie. tumultuous) spasm of the muscles, in which the whole body is thrown into violent agitation. The eyes roll wildly, the teeth are gnashed together, and the tongue is often severely bitten. The breathing is noisy, and foam (often tinged with blood) issues from the mouth, while even the contents of the bowels and bladder may be ejected. This stage lasts for a period varying from a few seconds to several minutes, when the convulsive movements gradually subside and relaxation of the muscles takes place, together with partial return of consciousness, the patient looking confusedly about him and attempting to speak. This, however, is soon followed by drowsiness and stupor, which may continue for several hours. When he awakes either apparently quite recovered, or fatigued and depressed, he is occasionally in a state of excitement which sometimes assumes the form of mania.

Epileptic fits of this sort succeed each other with varying degrees of frequency, and occasionally though not frequently with regular periodicity. In some persons they only occur once in a lifetime, or once in the course of many years, while in others they return every week or two, or even are of daily occurrence, and sometimes there are numerous attacks each day. Occasionally there occurs a constant succession of attacks extending over many hours, and with such rapidity that the patient appears as if he had never come out of the one fit. The term *status epilepticus* is applied to this condition, which is sometimes followed with fatal results. In many epileptics the fits occur during the night as well as during the day, but in some instances they are entirely nocturnal, and in such cases the disease may long exist and yet remain unrecognized either by the patient or by the physician, until observed and described by some other person.

The other variety of epilepsy, to which the name *le petit mal* is given, differs from that just described in the absence of the convulsive spasms. It consists essentially in the sudden arrest of consciousness, which is of but short duration, and may be accompanied with staggering or some alteration in position or motion, or may simply exhibit itself in a look of absence or confusion, and, should the patient happen to be engaged in conversation, by an

323

abrupt termination of the act. In general, it lasts but a few seconds, and the individual resumes his occupation without perhaps being aware of anything having been the matter. In some instances there is a degree of spasmodic action in certain muscles which may cause the patient to make some unexpected movement, such as turning half round, or walking abruptly aside, or may show itself by some unusual expression of countenance, such as squinting or grinning. There may be some amount of aura preceding such attacks, and also of faintness following them.

Allusion has already been made to the occasional occurrence of maniacal excitement as one of the results of the epileptic seizure. Such attacks, to which the name of *furor epilepticus* is applied, are generally accompanied with violent acts on the part of the patient, rendering him dangerous, and demanding prompt measures of restraint.

There is another sequel of an epileptic fit, particularly *petit mal*, which may have medico-legal implications. This is what is known as *post-epileptic automatism*. In this state, following an attack, an epileptic may carry out or perform some action, of which he is entirely unaware when he recovers. Thus, he may proceed to undress himself no matter where he may be, or he may pick up the first thing he lays his hands on, or he may attack someone. An interesting feature of this phenomenon is that the action performed by any one epileptic is stereotype: that is, it is always the same odd action he performs. The possible medico-legal implications of this automatism are, of course, obvious.

Treatment – During the fit, little can be done beyond preventing the patient as far as possible from injuring himself while unconsciousness continues. Tight clothing should be loosened, and a cork or pad inserted between the teeth. When the fit is over, the patient should be allowed to sleep, and have the head and shoulders well raised.

In the intervals between the attacks, the general health of the patient is one of the most important points to be attended to. The strictest hygienic rules should be observed, and all the causes which have been mentioned as favouring the development of the disease should as far as possible be avoided. Of medicinal remedies, the most commonly used is phenytoin, which is tending to replace phenobarbitone, either alone or in combination with one of the increasing number of other drugs being introduced for the treatment of epilepsy. The bromides, originally the great stand-by in the treatment of epilepsy, are seldom used for this purpose at the present day. Other drugs that have proved of value include methoin, and primidone. In severe cases which do not respond satisfactorily to one or more of these drugs, there is a further choice of drugs including carbamazepine clonazepam, and sodium valproate. One of the most effective drugs for controlling *petit mal* is troxidone. The secret of success in controlling epilepsy is to remember that every case must be considered individually, and that once a successful means of control has been established, it should not be altered unless there is some special reason for so doing. Alcohol is strictly forbidden.

As few restrictions as possible should be placed on the activities of an epileptic. Particularly does this apply to children. Unless the fits are severe and frequent, the child should be allowed to lead as normal a life as possible. At long last the position with regard to car driving has been clarified. Under regulations which came into force on June 1, 1970, from that date driving licences can now be issued in suitable cases to persons with epilepsy who, on the basis of medical evidence, have been free from attacks for at least three years, with or without treatment, or who for more than three years have had a history of attacks only during sleep.

Epileptic colonies have been established, where persons seriously afflicted in this way can carry out productive work under safe conditions. These colonies are particularly useful for the 20 per cent or so of epileptics who are mentally retarded.

Patients with epilepsy and their relatives can obtain further advice and information from the British Epilepsy Association, 3–6 Alfred Place, London, WC1E 7 E1.

EPILOIA (see TUBEROSE SCLEROSIS).

EPIPHORA means a condition in which tears, instead of passing from the eye down into the nose, run over on the cheek. It is due either to excessive production of tears or to blocking of the tearducts. (See EYE DISEASES AND INJURIES.)

EPIPHYSIS means the spongy extremity of a bone, attached to it for the purpose of forming a joint with the similar process of another bone. An epiphysis is covered on its surface by cartilage, is developed from a distinct centre of ossification, and in a young person is connected with the shaft of the bone by a plate of cartilage that disappears in the adult. Separation of an epiphysis is a form of fracture which sometimes occurs in children, and is apt to be more serious than a break through bony tissue because it involves damage to the plate of growing cartilage, so that, although union takes place readily, the subsequent growth of the bone may be interfered with and the full growth of the limb may afterwards fail to be attained.

EPISIOTOMY is the operation of cutting the outlet of the vagina in childbirth so as to facilitate the birth of the child.

EPISPASTICS are substances which produce blistering of the skin. (See BLISTERS.)

EPISTAXIS means bleeding from the nose. (See HAEMORRHAGE.)

EPITHELIOMA is a tumour of malignant nature arising in the epithelium covering the surface of the body. (See CANCER.)

EPITHELIUM means the cellular layer which forms the cuticle upon the skin, covers the inner surface of the bowels, and forms the lining of ducts and hollow organs, like the bladder. It consists of one or more layers of cells which adhere to one another, and is one of the simplest tissues of the body. It is of several forms (illustration 159): for example, the cuticle is formed of scaly epithelium, the cells being in several layers and more or less flattened. (See SKIN.) The bowels are lined by a single layer of columnar epithelium, the cells being long and narrow in shape. The air passages are lined by ciliated epithelium (illustration 160): that is to say, each cell is provided with lashes which drive the fluid upon the surface of the passages gradually upwards.

EPIZOÖTIC is a term applied to any disease in animals which diffuses itself widely. The term corresponds to the word epidemic as applied to human beings. In plague, for example, an epizoötic in rats usually precedes the epidemic in human beings.

EPSOM SALTS is the popular name for sulphate of magnesium, which is perhaps the most commonly used saline purgative. For a dose, a heaped teaspoonful or more of the salt should be mixed with as little water as will dissolve it, and

taken in the morning before breakfast, or the same quantity may be taken divided into three or four small doses, one of which is taken every quarter of an hour. (See PURGATIVES.)

Magnesium sulphate is also used for the treatment of inflammatory conditions of the bowels in order to remove by purgation the cause of the irritation. It is sometimes injected through a stomach tube direct into the duodenum in order to produce a copious flow of bile in disorders of the liver and gall-bladder. It has also

159 – Diagram of various types of epithelium. (A) Squamous epithelium seen in section. (B) Squamous epithelium seen in face view. (C) Cuboidal epithelium. (D) Columnar epithelium. (E) Cuboidal and columnar epithelium in face view. (F) Transitional epithelium. (G) Stratified, squamous non-keratinized epithelium. (H) Stratified, squamous keratinized epithelium. From *Hewer's Textbook of Histology for Students*. Heinemann.

160 – Diagram of ciliated epithelium (A) and pseudostratified columnar ciliated epithelium (B). From *Hewer's Textbook of Histology for Students*. Heinemann.

been used for injection intramuscularly or into the spinal canal in the treatment of tetanus, eclampsia, and other convulsive disorders. External fomentations of 5 to 25 per cent magnesium sulphate solution are applied in cases of rheumatic joints and other forms of inflammation, whilst a paste of magnesium sulphate in glycerin is a useful form of treatment of boils.

EPULIS is a term applied to any tumour connected with the jaws.

ERB'S PARALYSIS is a form of paralysis of the arm due to stretching or tearing of the fibres of the brachial nerve plexus. Such damage to the brachial plexus may occur during birth, and it is found that the arm lies by the side of the body with elbow extended, forearm pronated, and the fingers flexed. The infant is unable to raise the arm.

ERGOMETRINE is one of the active constituents of ergot (qv). It has a powerful action in controlling the excessive bleeding from the womb which may occur after childbirth. The official *British Pharmacopoeia* preparation is ergometrine maleate.

ERGOSTEROL is a sterol found in yeasts and fungi and in plant and animal fat. Under the action of sunlight or ultraviolet rays it produces vitamin D_2. The substance produced in this way is known as calciferol, and is used for the prevention and cure of rickets and osteomalacia. A similar change in the ergosterol of the skin is produced when the skin is freely exposed to sunlight. Calciferol is probably not so active as, and differs chemically from, the vitamin D occurring in fish-liver oils.

ERGOT is the spawn of *Claviceps purpurea*, a fungus which grows in the grain of rye. It contains several active principles, including the alkaloids, ergometrine, ergotoxine and ergotamine. Ergot causes prolonged contraction of unstriped muscle fibres all over the body, particularly the muscle fibres of the blood-vessels and of the womb. This action on the womb makes the drug of great value in midwifery, and it has been in use in midwifery since the 16th century.

Uses – Ergot is used mainly to check haemorrhage, particularly that which is apt to follow upon childbirth. It is also given in small doses for some time after childbirth to reduce the womb to its proper size in cases in which this is not taking place naturally.

ERGOTAMINE is one of the alkaloids in ergot. In the form of ergotamine tartrate it is most effective in the treatment of migraine (qv). It is usually given by injection, but is sometimes effective when given by mouth. Its continued use is not without risk, occasionally leading to gangrene of the tips of the fingers, so it should only be used under medical supervision. It has also been used for the relief of the itching of the skin which is sometimes such a troublesome feature of uraemia.

ERGOT POISONING occasionally occurs among persons who eat bread made from diseased rye. Several terrible epidemics (*St Anthony's Fire*) occurred in France and Germany during the Middle Ages. Its symptoms are the occurrence of spasmodic muscular contractions, and the gradual production of gangrene in parts like the fingers, toes and tips of the ears.

EROSION means a process of gradual wearing down of structures in the body. The term is applied to the effect of tumours, when they cause destruction of tissue in their neighbourhood without actually growing into the latter: for example, an aneurysm may erode bones in its neighbourhood. The term is also applied to minute ulcers, for example, erosions of the stomach, caused by extreme acidity of the gastric juice.

ERRHINES are drugs which cause running at the nose; eg potassium iodide.

ERUCTATION, or belching, means the sudden escape of gas or of portions of half-digested food from the stomach up into the mouth. Many nervous persons, and also persons who suffer from acid dyspepsia, have a bad habit of gulping down mouthfuls of air when digestion is uncomfortable. This air is belched up again after a little while. Some persons, especially those in whom dyspepsia occurs from time to time, have at other times the peculiarity of bringing up fragments of food an hour or two after meals.

ERUPTION or RASH, means an outbreak, in a scattered form, upon the surface of the skin, usually raised and red, or it may be covered with scales, or crusts, or vesicles containing fluid. The appearance of an eruption depends, to a certain extent, upon the nature of the disease, or other source of irritation, which causes it: for example, the eruption of measles is always distinguishable from that of chickenpox. But the same disease may also produce different eruptions in different persons, or in the same person in different states of health, or even on different parts of the body at one time.

Eruptions may be acute or chronic. Most of the acute eruptions belong to the exanthemata (qv): ie. they are bright in colour and burst out suddenly like a flower. These are the eruptions of scarlet fever, measles, German measles, smallpox and chickenpox. In general the severity of these diseases can be measured by the amount of eruption, but in cases in which the eruption is suppressed, or, as it is popularly termed, 'goes in', the disease is apt to be serious.

Some eruptions are very transitory, like nettle-rash, appearing and vanishing again in the course of a few hours.

(For chronic eruptions see SKIN, DISEASES OF.)

ERYSIPELAS – synonyms, *the Rose, St Anthony's Fire* – is a disease characterized by diffuse inflammation of the skin, or of the subcutaneous cellular tissue, attended with fever. In the Middle Ages this disease was confused with ergot poisoning.

Causes – It has long been known that the disease is of a highly infectious nature. This contagiousness of erysipelas was often illustrated in the surgical wards of hospitals, where, having once broken out, it was apt to spread with great rapidity, and to produce disastrous results, as well as in lying-in hospitals, where its occurrence gave rise to the spread of a form of puerperal fever of virulent character. The infecting organism is the *Streptococcus pyogenes*. Erysipelas is slightly commoner in women than in men, and is commonest between the ages of 50 and 60.

Symptoms – When the erysipelas is of moderate character, there is simply a redness of the skin, which feels somewhat hard and thickened, and upon which there often appear small vesicles. This redness, though at first circumscribed, tends to spread and affect the neighbouring sound skin, until an entire limb or a large area of the body may become involved in the inflammatory process. There is usually considerable pain, with heat and tingling in the affected part. As the disease advances, the portions of skin first attacked become less inflamed, and exhibit a yellowish appearance, which is followed by slight desquamation of the cuticle. Besides the

skin, the subjacent tissues may become involved in the inflammation and give rise to the formation of pus. This is termed *phlegmonous erysipelas*, and is much more apt to occur when the disease starts in a wound or ulcer. Occasionally the affected parts become gangrenous. Certain complications are apt to arise in erysipelas affecting the surface of the body, particularly inflammation of serous membranes, such as the pericardium, pleura and peritoneum.

Erysipelas of the face usually begins with symptoms of general illness, the patient feeling languid, drowsy and sick, while often there is shivering followed by fever, and the temperature may rise to 104° or 105° F (40° or 40·5° C). Sore throat is sometimes felt, but, in general, the first indication of the local affection is a red and painful spot at the side of the nose or on one of the cheeks or ears. Occasionally the inflammation begins in the throat, and reaches the face through the nasal fossae. The redness gradually spreads over the whole surface of the face, and is accompanied with swelling, which, in the lax tissues of the cheeks and eyelids, is so great that the features soon become unrecognizable and the eyes quite closed. The spreading edge of the red area is usually sharply marked and raised. Advancing over the scalp, the disease may invade the neck and pass on to the trunk, but in general the inflammation remains confined to the face and head. While the disease progresses, besides the pain, tenderness and heat of the affected parts, the constitutional symptoms may be severe, and delirium may occur. The attack in general lasts for a week or ten days, during which the inflammation subsides in the parts of the skin first attacked, while it spreads onwards in other directions, and after it has passed away there is some slight desquamation of the cuticle.

Although in general the termination is favourable, serious and occasionally fatal results follow from inflammation of the membranes of the brain, and in some rare instances sudden death has occurred from suffocation arising from oedema of the glottis, the inflammation having spread into, and extensively involved, the throat.

Erysipelas occasionally assumes from the first a violent form, under which the patient sinks rapidly. It is sometimes a complication in certain forms of exhausting disease, such as tuberculosis or typhoid fever, and is then to be regarded as of serious import. A very fatal form occasionally attacks new-born infants, particularly in the first four weeks of life (*erysipelas neonatorum*).

Treatment – The patient must be isolated, and great care must be taken to ensure that the infection is not transmitted to others by those in attendance on the patient. The outlook has changed considerably for the better since the introduction of the sulphonamides and of penicillin, and one or other of these should be given in full doses as soon as the condition is recognized. For local application the best preparations are either cold compresses of a saturated solution of magnesium sulphate or a 10 per cent solution of ichthyol in water. The patient must be kept in bed until the temperature has settled, and as nourishing a diet as possible should be given.

ERYTHEMA is a general term signifying several conditions in which areas of the skin become congested with blood, and consequently a red eruption appears. The eruption is accompanied by tingling, and often by itching and pain.

Causes – It may be due to heat, such as exposure to the sun, or the constant exposure, by cooks or iron-workers, of the face, hands or legs to a blazing fire, *Erythema ab igne* is the reddening of the skin of the leg producing a net-like pattern that is found in women who sit huddled over the fire. Another form, known as *erythema pernio*, is due to exposure to cold and wet. (See CHILBLAINS.) A variety, which appears, usually on the front of the legs, in the form of red or livid, tender swellings, often over an inch in breadth, is known as *erythema nodosum*, and is thought to be a manifestation of rheumatism, or of tuberculosis. Children and young adults, especially women, may also suffer from a severer form, which begins as red blotches on the hands, and, spreading up the arms to the body, produces lumps and vesicles, or even large blebs full of fluid. This form, on account of the diversity of the appearances in different parts, is known as *erythema multiforme*. The cause in some cases is a virus. It also occurs as a drug-rash from the use of such drugs as sulphonamides and barbiturates. *Erythema infectiosum*, or slapped cheek disease, is characterized by a fiery red rash on the cheeks: hence its alternative name. It occurs in children, in the spring. The rash which spreads to the rest of the body, lasts for up to three weeks. Although highly infectious, the causative organism, probably a virus, has not been discovered.

ERYTHRASMA is a reddish-brown macular eruption of the skin, caused by a micro-organism known as *Nocardia minutissima*.

ERYTHROBLASTOSIS FOETALIS (see HAEMOLYTIC DISEASE OF THE NEWBORN).

ERYTHROCYTE is another name for a red blood corpuscle.

ERYTHROCYTE SEDIMENTATION RATE (see SEDIMENTATION RATE).

ERYTHROEDEMA – Other terms for this condition are ACRODYNIA and PINK DISEASE. This is a disease of infants in which there are the following features: restlessness, weakness, neuritis and swelling and redness of the face, fingers and toes. In the vast majority of cases it is a manifestation of mercurial poisoning, often due to the infant having been given teething powders containing a mercurial laxative.

ERYTHROMELALGIA, or RED NEURALGIA, is a condition in which the fingers or toes, or even larger portions of the limbs, become purple, bloated in appearance, and very painful. In persons suffering from this condition, which is not a common one, the attacks come and go, being worse in summer (unlike chilblains), and worse on exertion or when the affected parts are warmed or allowed to hang down. The condition may appear without apparent cause, but is often associated with vascular diseases, such as hypertension and polycythaemia vera. It also occurs in association with certain diseases of the central nervous system, and in cases of metallic poisoning: eg. arsenic, mercury and thallium. Treatment is unsatisfactory. Residence in a moderate climate, the wearing of light-weight stockings or socks, and sandals, and the avoidance of excessive heat help to relieve the discomfort. Aspirin also gives marked relief.

ERYTHROMYCIN is an antibiotic derived from *Streptomyces erythreus*. Its antibacterial range of activity is comparable to that of penicillin, and it is effective when taken by mouth.

ESCHAR is a piece of the body killed by heat or caustics.

ESCHAROTICS are the more powerful

varieties of caustics, such as mineral acids, which produce death, to some depth, of tissues with which they come in contact. (See CAUSTICS.)

ESCHERICHIA is the generic name given to the group of gram-negative, rod-shaped bacteria found as normal inhabitants of the lower bowel: eg. *Escherichia coli.*

ESERINE is another name for physostigmine (qv).

ESMARCH'S BANDAGE is a rubber bandage which is applied to a limb from below upwards in order to drive blood from it.

ESSENCES are strong solutions of active substance. Some of these are made by solution in water, but the aromatic essences are usually solutions of volatile oils (eg. essence of peppermint), in rectified spirit of the strength 1 in 5.

ESSENTIAL HYPERTENSION is the most common form of high blood-pressure. Other causes of a high blood-pressure include kidney disease, especially Bright's disease; certain diseases of the endocrine glands; and a congenital abnormality of the aorta known as coarctation of the aorta.

Cause – In spite of its being such a common condition, the cause of essential hypertension is still obscure. It has been recognized for a long time that arteriosclerosis and hypertension often occur together, and at one time it was considered that the arteriosclerosis was the primary lesion and that the raised blood-pressure was a compensatory effort on the part of the heart to maintain an adequate circulation of blood through the thickened and narrowed arteries. This view is now considered to be wrong, and the general consensus of opinion is that the raised blood-pressure is the cause of the arteriosclerosis in these cases, although it must be remembered that arteriosclerosis can occur without hypertension. At the present moment it is generally believed that the primary lesion in essential hypertension is spasm of the smaller arteries (or arterioles). What is still undecided is what is responsible for this spasm. We know that such spasm can be produced by adrenaline and that adrenaline is produced by emotional, mental and physical strain. On the other hand, it has never been possible to demonstrate an excess of

adrenaline in the blood of people with hypertension, nor does this theory explain why only some people exposed to strain develop hypertension. Although we still do not know why this spasm of the arterioles is produced in the first instance, there is now evidence that spasm of the arteries to the kidneys results in the production of a substance called *renin* which produces a rise in the blood-pressure. It is therefore possible that the course of events in essential hypertension is as follows:

spasm of arterioles→renin→hypertension→arteriosclerosis of kidneys.

It must be realized, however, that this is a marked simplification of a most complicated problem, but it is useful as a working basis.

The following are among some of the other factors that we know about essential hypertension. It is much more common among western races than among eastern races. There is a strong hereditary factor. It is more common in males than in females, and it is rare under the age of 40 years. The highest incidence is between the ages of 50 and 60 years. It is also more common among obese individuals than among those who are normal in weight or under-weight. There is no evidence that the consumption of meat has anything to do with essential hypertension.

Symptoms – Essential hypertension may be present without any symptoms whatsoever, and the condition may be discovered accidentally during a routine medical examination. The basis for a diagnosis of hypertension is usually taken to be a systolic pressure which is persistently greater than 150 mm of mercury and a diastolic pressure which is persistently greater than 95 mm of mercury. The emphasis is upon the persistence of the raised pressure, because it is not unusual for the blood-pressure in a normal individual to be raised temporarily by excitement. From the point of view of prognosis, the height of the diastolic pressure is much more important than that of the systolic pressure.

When essential hypertension is accompanied by symptoms, these usually consist of headache, ringing in the ears (tinnitus) and giddiness. When headache is present, it is often in the back of the head and often worst on wakening in the morning, wearing off during the course of the day, and then becoming worse again towards evening.

When essential hypertension runs its natural course, it usually causes death in the end as a result of heart failure, but a proportion of its victims die of a stroke, whilst some die of failure of the kidneys. To a certain extent it is true to say that the earlier the onset of essential hypertension, the poorer the expectation of life, but many people with this condition live to a ripe old age.

Treatment – As the cause of essential hypertension is not known, there is no specific treatment. In the majority of cases, treatment consists in the individual leading a quiet life, avoiding undue effort or strain, getting off to bed early at night, and insisting upon resting at the week-ends. Unless there are signs of heart failure there is no need for the individual to take to bed. Sedatives are useful if the individual is worrying unduly, is not sleeping well, or is subject to headaches. If there is overweight, this should be treated dietetically so as to bring the weight down to within normal limits. The operation of sympathectomy has been recommended for the treatment of essential hypertension. This operation consists of cutting practically all the sympathetic nerve fibres to the abdominal organs. The rationale of the operation is that it is through these nerve fibres that are carried the impulses which are responsible for producing vasoconstriction, or spasm of the arteries, and thereby hypertension. Whilst there is no doubt that an extensive sympathectomy lowers the blood-pressure in most hypertensive subjects, it is now evident that it is only in a minority of cases that the pressure remains down.

During recent years, certain drugs have been introduced which are proving of value in the treatment of certain cases. These drugs include bretylium tosylate (qv), hydrallazine (qv), mecamylamine (qv), methonium compounds (see METHONIUM), pempidine (qv), rauwolfia (qv) and veratrum derivatives (see VERATRUM). The decision as to which, if any, of these drugs should be used in any given patient is often a difficult one, and there is no rule of thumb by which this decision can be reached. Each case must be looked upon as an individual problem. Their greatest value is in the treatment of malignant hypertension (qv).

ESTER is an organic compound formed from an alcohol and an acid by the removal of water.

ETHACRYNIC ACID is a potent diuretic (qv), which is clinically unrelated to any of the other diuretics.

ETHAMBUTOL is a synthetic drug which is proving of value in the treatment of tuberculosis.

ETHAMIVAN is chemically similar to nikethamide (qv) and has a similar action in stimulating the respiratory centre.

ETHANOL is another name for ethyl alcohol. (See ALCOHOL.)

ETHER is a colourless, volatile, highly inflammable liquid formed by the action of sulphuric acid upon alcohol, with the aid of heat. Ether boils below the body temperature, and so, when sprayed over the skin, rapidly evaporates. It dissolves many substances, such as fats, oils and resins, better than alcohol or water, and is accordingly used in the preparation of many drugs.

Uses – Externally it is used as a cleansing agent before operations. By inhalation it is used as a general anaesthetic. (See ANAESTHETICS.) Internally it is used occasionally for relieving pain such as colic. (For its use as an intoxicant, see DRUG HABITS.)

ETHINYLOESTRADIOL is a highly active oestrogen (qv), which is about twenty times as active as stillboestrol (qv). It is active when given by mouth.

ETHISTERONE is the name approved by the *British Pharmacopoeia* for the orally active analogue of progesterone. It is given in certain cases of menorrhagia and habitual abortion, where a deficient secretion of the corpus luteum is suspected. (See PROGESTERONE.)

ETHMOID is the name of a bone in the base of the skull which separates the cavity of the nose from the membranes of the brain. It is a spongy bone with numerous cavities or sinuses.

Chronic suppuration in the ethmoidal sinuses causing a nasal discharge is sometimes responsible for inflammation in neighbouring parts such as the eye.

ETHOGLUCID is an alkylating agent (qv), which is proving of value in the treatment of cancer.

ETHOSUXIMIDE is a drug that is proving of value in the treatment of the form of epilepsy known as petit mal.

ETHYL BISCOUMACETATE, is an anticoagulant which is active when taken by mouth. Its action is similar to that of dicoumarol (qv), but less prolonged. It is used in the prevention, and treatment, of thrombotic conditions. (See also ANTICO-AGULANTS.)

ETHYL CHLORIDE is a gas at ordinary temperatures and pressures, but is liquefied by slight compression. It is extremely volatile, and rapidly produces freezing of the surface, when sprayed upon it. Accordingly it is used to produce insensibility to pain for small and short operations. It is put up in graduated glass or metal tubes, with a fine nozzle. The tube is warmed by the hand and the liquid jets out in a fine spray which evaporates at once and so freezes the skin upon which it is sprayed. At one time it was used by inhalation to produce general anaesthesia for very brief operations, and to induce anaesthesia in patients in whom the anaesthesia is subsequently to be maintained by some other anaesthetic such as nitrous oxide or ether, but is seldom used now for this purpose.

ETHYLENE is a colourless inflammable gas used as an anaesthetic.

ETIOLOGY, or AETIOLOGY, means the group of conditions which form the cause of any disease.

EU- is a prefix meaning satisfactory or beneficial.

EUCALYPTUS, or BLUE-GUM (*Eucalyptus globulus*), is a tree, originally a native of Australia, and now grown all over the world. Its important constituent, oil of eucalyptus, is an oil of pleasant smell and spicy taste, which is obtained by distillation from the leaves of the tree. Similar oils are obtained in varying amount from most species of gum-trees, some of which have peculiar and fragrant odours. Groves of eucalyptus trees exert a marked influence upon the soil and air in their neighbourhood. The trees, which reach a great size, and have wide-spreading roots, remove much moisture from the soil, and have accordingly a powerful action in drying up swampy ground. The oil constantly exhaled from the leaves has the power of oxidizing and destroying large quantities of the foul gases which emanate from swamps, and of checking to some extent the growth of microbes. Accordingly these trees have a beneficial influence upon unhealthy districts in which they are planted.

Uses – The oil is used as a disinfectant and deodorant. Two ounces (57 ml) of oil of eucalyptus, placed in a porous earthenware vessel so as to impregnate its substance, will keep the air of a water-closet in which the vessel is suspended perfectly free from smell for several months. For a similar purpose, it may be mixed with eight times its weight of sawdust and used to sprinkle on floors.

It is also used as an inhalation or internally in bronchitis and in coryza.

EUGENICS is a term applied to the study and cultivation of conditions that may improve the physical and moral qualities of future generations.

EUPAD is a mixture of chlorinated lime and boric acid, 25 grams of which, dissolved in 1 litre of water, form 'eusol' (qv).

EUSOL, which stands for Edinburgh University Solution, is a solution of 12·5 G of boric acid and 12·5 G of chlorinated lime in 1 litre of water. It was introduced during the 1914–18 War as an antiseptic for the treatment of wounds, and proved to be one of the most valuable antiseptics then available. Although largely replaced by modern antiseptics, and the introduction of the sulphonamides (qv) and antibiotics, it is still a useful dressing for infected wounds. (See EUPAD; and HYPO-CHLOROUS ACID).

EUPHORIANTS are drugs which induce a state of euphoria or well-being. A typical example is amphetamine (qv).

EUSTACHIAN TUBES are the passages, one on each side, leading from the throat to the middle ear. Each is about 1½ inches (38 mm) long and is large at either end, though at its narrowest part it only admits a fine probe. The tubes open widely in the act of swallowing or yawning. The opening into the throat is situated just behind the lower part of the nose, so that a catheter can be passed through the corresponding nostril into the tube for inflation of the middle ear. (See also EAR; and NOSE.)

EUTHANASIA means the procuring of an easy and painless death. It has been advocated in some quarters that a medical man should have the power to put to death painlessly, by means of such drugs as morphine, any person suffering from a painful, distressing and incurable disease the outcome of which is inevitably fatal, the patient or his relatives consenting. Various legal safeguards have been proposed, but there are obvious moral and religious – not to mention medical – objections to the recognition of such a procedure.

EVACUANT is a name for a purgative medicine.

EXANTHEMATA is an old name used to classify the acute infectious diseases distinguished by a characteristic eruption. (See ERUPTION.)

EXCIPIENT means any more or less inert substance added to a prescription in order to make the remedy as prescribed more suitable in bulk, consistence, or form for administration.

EXCISION means literally a cutting out, and is a term applied to the removal of any structure from the body, when such removal necessitates a certain amount of separation from surrounding parts. For example, one speaks of the excision of a tumour, of a gland, of a joint. When an opening is simply made into the body the term incision is used. When a limb, or part of one, is removed, the term amputation is employed.

EXCITEMENT (see DELIRIUM; HYSTERIA; and MENTAL ILLNESS).

EXCITING CAUSE of a disease is the name given to the direct or immediate cause, as opposed to predisposing causes, which merely render the body more liable to the disease in question. For example, poor expansion of the chest may be a predisposing cause of tuberculosis, but the exciting cause is infection with the tubercle bacillus, or *Mycobacterium tuberculosis* as it is now known.

EXCORIATION means the destruction of small pieces of the surface of skin or mucous membrane. (See CHAFING OF THE SKIN.)

EXERCISE is a matter of great importance in the maintenance of health at all ages, but particularly for those who are normally engaged in sedentary occupations. (See also CHEST DEVELOPMENT.)
Effects of exercise – The right amount of the right type of exercise results in all parts of the body working at their best. The muscles are firm in tone, strong and

working at maximum efficiency, so that the onset of fatigue, with its accompanying aching and soreness, is postponed. The heart, too, works more efficiently, pumping more blood round the body. For instance, when an individual is resting, the output of the heart per minute is 5 litres. When running at $7\frac{1}{2}$ miles (12 km) per hour, this shoots up to around 25 litres: a five-fold increase. This increased volume of blood dealt with by the heart per minute is achieved with increasing efficiency, as is shown by the fact that at each contraction the heart expels 150 millilitres, compared with 70 millilitres at rest. The lungs also function more efficiently. Again taking the example of the individual running at $7\frac{1}{2}$ miles an hour, the amount of oxygen used up increases twelvefold, although the output of the heart has only increased five-fold. The digestive tract, including the liver, also functions better, partly because it is not being overloaded by unnecessary food. The increased expenditure of energy involved in exercise ensures that the food eaten is metabolized, or used up, immediately to cope with the increased energy demands. The nervous system also works more efficiently, reflexes becoming brisker and the muscles thereby being able to respond more promptly and more effectively to any special stress or strain. Finally, possibly more imponderable but nevertheless of great practical importance, there is considerable emotional benefit. The individual feels more satisfied with life, is less affected by the normal worries of life in so far as he can forget them in exercising himself – whether this be in some form of athletics or games, or merely tramping the countryside – and when he falls into bed at night his physical tiredness, combined with his emotional peace of mind, allows him to fall asleep – and sleep soundly.
Want of exercise – Failure to take adequate exercise affects the body adversely at all ages. In children it leads to slouching, faulty posture and flabbiness of the muscles. This leads to the typical round-shouldered child who, in addition, may develop scoliosis (qv), or curvature of the spine. As often as not this physical flabbiness is accompanied by mental lethargy and emotional instability. As these children seldom use their lungs to the full in breathing, not only is inadequate oxygen brought to the blood, and therefore to all the cells of the body, which at this period of rapid growth are demanding in their call for oxygen and nutriment, but they render themselves

 (*continued on page 336*)

161 – *Position of attention*, which forms commencement for most exercises. Heels together, feet turned out at an angle of 45°, knees straight, trunk erect, arms hanging naturally from the shoulders, with palms turned towards thighs, neck erect, and eyes looking forwards.

NECK EXERCISES

162 – *Head bending backward.* In the position of attention, the head is bent slowly backward as far as possible, and then raised slowly to its former position.

163 – *Head turning.* The head is turned slowly but strongly to the left as far as possible, then turned to its former position; then to the right as far as possible, and, finally, the position of attention resumed.

164 – *Position of hips firm.* The hands are raised quickly to grasp the waist with fingers in front and thumbs behind. This is the starting position for most arm exercises.

DORSAL EXERCISE

165 – *Trunk downward bending.* Assume the position of illustration 161. Bend the body as far downward as possible from the hips without rounding the back; slowly resume original position.

JUMPING EXERCISE

166 – *Upward jumping.* Assume position of illustration 164. Suddenly extend the knees and ankles and place the arms straight at the sides, springing from the ground vertically upward; drop to the ground on the toes with the knees practically straight, but allowing the ankles and knees to give, so that the position of illustration 163 is resumed after landing. Repeat the movement.

333

EXERCISE

167 – *Arms bending.* Keeping the elbows to the sides, the arms are quickly and sharply bent by carrying the hands up in front of the body and clenching the fists; the arms are then sharply stretched downward to the side.

168 – *Arms stretching upward.* The arms are stretched sharply upwards to their fullest extent, palms inwards and fingers fully extended.

169 – *Arms stretching sideways.* The arms are stretched sharply in line with the shoulders, palms downward and fingers fully stretched. The last three exercises strengthen the muscles of the arms and shoulders.

170 – *Rising on tiptoe.* The heels are raised from the ground as high as possible and slowly lowered to the ground again. This develops the calf muscles.

171 – *Full knee bending.* Keeping the heels together, these are raised from the ground as high as possible; the knees are then bent as much as possible, so that the buttocks are lowered to touch the heels; the original standing position is then slowly resumed. This strengthens the leg and thigh muscles and keeps the ankle, knee and hip joints supple.

172 – *Foot placing sideways with knee bending.* Each foot is carried one foot sideways; the heels are raised from the ground; the knees are bent till thigh and leg form a right angle; the knees are then straightened; the heels are slowly lowered and the original position of attention resumed. This exercises the adductor muscles of the thigh.

LATERAL EXERCISES

173 – *Trunk turning*. Each foot is carried one foot outward, the hands are placed behind the neck, and, with the feet firm on the ground, the trunk is turned steadily as far as possible to the left; the original position is resumed, and the movement repeated to the right.

174 – *Trunk bending sideways*. The arms are stretched upward, each foot is carried one foot outward, and, with the feet firm on the ground, the trunk is then bent steadily as far as possible to the left; the original position is resumed, the trunk is then bent to the right, and the original position again resumed.

175 – *Lunging with arms stretched*. With the left foot carried three feet to the left, lunge outward stretch upward the arm corresponding to the forward foot and stretch downward, one hand's-breadth from the thigh, the arm corresponding to the rear foot, the movement of the arms being completed as the forward foot reaches the ground. Resume the position of attention, repeat towards opposite side.

ABDOMINAL EXERCISES

176 – *On the hands*. Keeping the heels together, these are raised from the ground and the knees bent; at the same time the palms of the hands are placed on the ground rather more than the width of the shoulders apart, with arms straight. Keeping the arms straight, the feet are shot backward till the body and legs are straight, and fully stretched, the weight supported on the toes and hands.

177 – *Turning on the hand and leg-raising*. From position of illustration 169 raise the right hand from the ground and place it on the waist, at the same time turning the body to the right and placing the right foot immediately over the left; keeping left arm straight, raise right leg slowly as high as possible and slowly resume original position. Repeat by turning on the right hand.

178 – *Trunk backward bending*. Keeping the knees straight, raise the arms above the head and bend the upper part of the trunk slowly backwards as far as possible. Slowly resume the original position.

179 – *Trunk backward bending with foot support.* Sitting on the ground with feet supported above and arms stretched upwards, bend slowly backward to touch the ground. Slowly resume original position.

180 – *Leg-raising – on the hands.* Assume the position of illustration 169; keeping the right leg straight, raise it as high as possible with toe pointed. Resume starting position and repeat with left leg.

181 – *Leg-raising – on the back.* Assume the position of illustration 164; place both hands on the ground to the rear and lower the body quickly backward to the ground, shooting the legs to the front. The body is then stretched flat on the back, feet together, and arms to the sides; stretch arms upward, keeping the knees straight, raise the right leg steadily without arching the back, lower the leg, and repeat with left leg. Repeat with both legs at one time.

more liable to lung disease. The appetite is poor or capricious, and the skin fails to acquire that healthy, glossy appearance of ebullient childhood, which is the envy of adults – and particularly the ladies. In adolescence these features all become enhanced, associated often with a cigarette hanging out of the corner of the flabby mouth. In adult life, and particularly in middle age, lack of exercise leads to the putting on of weight, with all the hazards to life that this involves (see CORPULENCE), constipation, not to mention dyspepsia as often as not due to overeating. What is of even more serious import is that there is

an increased tendency to atherosclerosis (qv) and coronary thrombosis (qv). The motor car is a lethal weapon, not only because of the accidents it causes, but also because it is the means whereby hundreds of thousands of middle-aged men (and women) are deprived of the useful form of exercise provided by walking to work – or at least part of the way. Cycling to health was the motto of a well-known heart specialist in the United States of America who lived to a ripe old age. It is one which might well be adopted in the United Kingdom.

Over-exercise seldom does any permanent harm except in the rapidly growing adolescent and in the old, provided the individual is healthy. For instance, there is no evidence that a healthy heart can be damaged by exercise. The circulatory system is so adaptable that, if there is any possibility of undue strain being placed upon the heart, certain mechanisms come into play which cause giddiness or fainting, so that the exercise in question is automatically stopped before any real harm is done. On the other hand, should there be any undetected disease of the heart, then undue exercise may produce permanent harm. This is why a careful medical examination is an essential preliminary to any severe form of exercise. This is particularly important, indeed essential, in the case of school children.

The secret of success here, as in most spheres of life, is moderation in all things. The man in his fifties or sixties must realize that he can no longer do many of the things that he did when he was thirty years younger. If he bears this in mind, there is little chance of his damaging himself by exercise. For instance, if he finds that an afternoon's tennis begins to make him uncomfortably breathless, then he should give up the game for a less exacting one, or alternatively be satisfied with one or two sets instead of several.

In the case of adolescents and young adults, the wise rule is to ensure that the individual, and particularly his heart, is sound, and then to insist upon his undergoing a careful course of training before embarking upon any severe form of exercise such as racing or rugger.

Training involves a certain regimen and practice prior to engaging in special athletic efforts. The objects of training, generally speaking, are:

(1) To accustom certain muscles to perform certain movements with the maximum efficiency as, for example, the thigh and leg muscles to contract sharply and in

a particular order for jumping; (2) to strengthen the heart and deepen the breathing for prolonged efforts; and (3) to bring the whole body, and especially the nervous system, to a state of perfect health. For these objects, a course of special practice, combined with various general exercises, lasting usually over three weeks before the event for which the training is intended, is combined with a healthy form of diet. (See DIET.) Different trainers have, in addition, special

182–184 – Three examples of remedial exercises for helping the disabled.

182 – (*right*) A Harris belt. *The Practitioner*.

183 – (*below*) A form of balancing exercise. *The Practitioner*.

184 – (*below right*) Resisted shoulder exercise. *The Practitioner*.

rules of their own, usually founded on experience.

Training exercises – The exercises shown in illustrations 161 to 181 include groups of exercises for the different parts of the body. If ten or twelve of these exercises be chosen, and if each movement be carried out ten or twelve times slowly and methodically, this is sufficient to provide fifteen minutes of exercise. If these are carried out during dressing in the morning by business men and others whose duties prevent them from obtaining outdoor exercise by games, sufficient exercise is obtained to maintain a reasonable standard of physical fitness, but, if at all possible, they should be supplemented by a modicum of exercise in the open air at, say, the weekends or a stroll 'round the square' at bedtime.

Remedial gymnastics – Equally important is the value of exercises in restoring the physically disabled to health. (See also FRENKEL'S EXERCISES.) Illustrations 182–184 show some typical forms of remedial exercises. (Illustration 182 shows a Harris belt which is a useful aid when giving walking exercises. Illustration 183 shows one form of balancing exercise, in which a patient with loss of joint sense is walking along a bench, balancing a bean bag on her head, whilst illustration 184 shows a patient performing resisted shoulder exercises.

EXFOLIATION means the separation, in layers, of pieces of dead bone or skin.

EXOMPHALOS is the term applied to a hernia formed by the projection of abdominal organs through the umbilicus.

EXOPHTHALMIC GOITRE is a disease in which there is an enlargement of the thyroid gland, protrusion of the eyes, and other symptoms. (See GOITRE.)

EXOPHTHALMOS is abnormal protrusion of the eyeball. The commonest cause is hyperthyroidism (see GOITRE). It may also occur as a result of a tumour at the back of the eye pushing the eyeball forwards.

EXOSTOSIS means an outgrowth from a bone; it may be due to chronic inflammation, constant pressure or tension on the bone, or tumour-formation. (See BONE, DISEASES OF.)

EXPECTANT is a term applied to a form of treatment in which the cure of the patient is left mainly to nature, while the physician simply watches for any unsatisfactory developments or symptoms, and relieves them if they occur.

EXPECTATION OF LIFE at 1 year of age in England and Wales, based on the figures for 1974, was 69·7 years for men and 75·7 years for women. The comparable figures for Scotland were 67·8 and 74, whilst for Northern Ireland they were 67·2 and 74·3. These are all slightly below the best figures recorded in other countries, which are 73·5 for men in Greece and 78·7 for women in Iceland. In USA the comparable figures are 68 for men and 76·2 for women. In all countries for which statistics are available, the expectation of life for women is greater than that for men. There is also a certain variation within socio-economic groups. Thus in England in 1970–72 the expectation of life for men at age 45 was 22 for those in the Armed Forces, 29·3 for farmers on their own account, 28·9 for self-employed professional workers and 26·1 for unskilled manual workers. With the steady rise in the expectation of life, the number of centenarians in our midst is rising. Thus, a Londonderry general practitioner, in 1978, reported that he had three centenarians in his practice, the oldest (a woman) being 104. The eastern states of the USSR, however, seem to specialize in centenarians. In 1978 it was reported that the oldest man in the Soviet Union had celebrated his 143rd birthday in Azerbaijan. (See also AGE, NATURAL CHANGES IN.)

EXPECTORANTS are drugs which assist the removal of secretions from the air passages.

Varieties – Most drugs used as expectorants have a complicated mode of action. (1) Some act chiefly by making the secretion in the bronchial tubes more watery, and therefore less sticky; (2) others have exactly the opposite action, drying up the secretion where it is very copious; (3) a third group assists the act of coughing in feeble persons, and so helps the removal of secretion; (4) those in a fourth group soothe the lining membrane of the air passages and quiet ineffectual coughing. Some of the chief drugs, arranged as far as possible in the order of these groups, though several have a double action, are as follows: (1) steam inhalations, draughts of hot milk or water, chloride of ammonium, iodide of potassium, and, generally speaking, all alkalis; (2) volatile oils like anise, eucalyptus, and turpentine, menthol, balsam of tolu and Friars' balsam, syrup of squills and infusion of senega, inhalation of creosote or tar, and, generally speaking, all acids; (3) ipecacuanha, carbonate of ammonia and sal volatile, and tincture of nux vomica; (4) linctuses and codeine.

Uses – These drugs are combined in various ways in bronchitis and other chest conditions. For example, those in the first group are used in the early stages of acute and in chronic bronchitis, those in the next group are better for later stages of acute bronchitis, those of the third group are necessary for aged persons with pneumonia and bronchitis, and the members of the fourth group are applicable to a constant hacking cough.

EXPECTORATION means either material brought up from the chest by the air passages, or the act by which it is brought up. The term is also used in place of sputum for anything spat out. Expectoration varies considerably in character according to the site in which it is produced, and the disease with which it is associated.

Characters of expectoration – There may be much cough productive of a very small amount of sputum at the start of acute bronchitis or inflammation of the throat, but it must be remembered that young children and some older persons swallow their expectoration as soon as they have brought it up instead of spitting it out.

The sputum from the throat in catarrh of this region is usually thick and sticky, speckled with black owing to dust and smoke inhaled and deposited on the throat.

Watery, frothy expectoration is brought up in considerable quantities during the greater part of an attack of acute bronchitis, particularly in old people. A similar fluid is spat up when the lungs are oedematous or dropsical, as occurs sometimes in the course of heart or kidney disease. At a later stage of an acute bronchitis the sputum becomes more yellow and thicker in consistence.

When cavities are present in the lungs their contents are often expectorated as thick, yellow, oily-looking material, with few air-bubbles in it; and expectoration from this source, when spat into water, flattens out into a round disc resembling a coin, and hence gets the name of nummular sputum (Lat. *nummulus*, money).

Sputum with a 'rusty' tinge, and so sticky that it adheres to the dish into which it is expectorated, when the latter is turned upside down, is characteristic of pneumonia.

Bright red blood in large quantities may be brought up from the lungs. This is the condition known as *haemoptysis* (qv) and usually indicates the presence of pulmonary tuberculosis, carcinoma of the lung or certain forms of heart disease. On the other hand, it must be remembered that spitting of blood may be due merely to bleeding in the nose from which the blood has run backward down the throat: or to the rupture of a small vessel on the wall of the throat in cases in which this part of the air passages is inflamed. Bleeding from the stomach has totally different characteristics from those of lung bleeding. That brought up from the lungs is bright red, frothy and usually comes up with a hawk or with a few suppressed coughs, it may be by mouthfuls. Blood from the stomach is usually dark brown and granular from the action of the gastric juice, and is brought up by a definite act of vomiting. It results generally from some ulcerated or congested state of the stomach.

Expectoration of a 'prune juice' colour occurring in the course of pneumonia is an ominous sign, and indicates usually that softening of parts of the lungs is setting in.

In some diseases the sputum possesses a very foul smell, particularly in gangrene of the lung and in the condition known as bronchiectasis. (See LUNGS, DISEASES OF.)

Microscopic examination of the sputum is of importance in diagnosing the cause of an infection of the lung. Thus the presence of tubercle bacilli, or *Mycobacteria tuberculosis* as they are now known, denotes that the individual is suffering from pulmonary tuberculosis. It is also of importance in determining to which antibiotic the causative micro-organisms are sensitive. In cancer of the lung the microscope may disclose malignant cells in the sputum.

Disposal of expectoration is a matter demanding public attention. The habit of spitting on the ground in public places is one which, in view of the dangerous nature of diseased sputum, should never be tolerated. Where spittoons are provided, these should be washed and disinfected every day.

Most tuberculous patients are supplied with a sputum flask containing a small quantity of some strong antiseptic (eg. carbolic acid solution 1 in 5 or 1 in 20) into which the expectoration is received and by which it is disinfected before it is poured down the drains.

EXTENSION is the term applied to the process of straightening or stretching a limb. In cases of fractured limbs, extension is employed during the application of splints, in order to reduce the displacement caused by the fracture, and prevent movement of the broken ends of bone. It is effected by gently and steadily pulling upon the part of the limb beyond the fracture. Extension of a more permanent type is used in the after-treatment of some fractures, as well as in diseases of the spine, by placing the patient upon an inclined bed and affixing weights to his lower limbs or to his head by means of adhesive plaster or of straps. A similar procedure is often adopted in tuberculous disease of the knee or hip, to prevent the starting pains, which are apt to occur as the affected person is dropping off to sleep.

EXTRA – is the Latin prefix meaning outside of, or in addition, such as extra-capsular, meaning outside the capsule of a joint, and extrasystole, meaning an additional contraction of the heart.

EXTRACTS are preparations, usually of a semi-solid consistence, containing the active parts of various plants extracted in one of several ways. In the case of some extracts the juice of the fresh plant is simply pressed out and purified; in the case of others the active principles are dissolved out in water, which is then to a great extent driven off by evaporation; other extracts are similarly made by the help of alcohol, and in some cases ether is the solvent.

EXTRASYSTOLE is a term applied to premature contraction of one or more of the chambers of the heart. A beat of the heart occurs sooner than it should do in the ordinary rhythm and is followed by a longer rest than usual before the next beat. In an extrasystole the stimulus to contraction arises in a part of the heart other than the usual. Extrasystoles often give rise to an unpleasant sensation as of the heart stumbling over a beat, but their occurrence is not usually of serious import.

EXTRAVASATION means an escape of fluid from the vessels or passages which ought to contain it. Extravasation of blood due to tearing of vessel walls is found in apoplexy, and in the commoner condition known as a bruise. Extravasation of urine takes place when the bladder or the urethra is ruptured by a blow on the abdomen or on the crutch (or perineum), or torn in a fracture of the pelvis.

EXUDATION means the process in which some of the constituents of the blood pass slowly through the walls of the small vessels in the course of inflammation, and also means the accumulation resulting from this process. For example, in pleurisy the solid, rough material deposited on the surface of the lung is an exudation.

EYE – The eyes are set, one on each side, in a deep four-sided cavity in the skull, called the orbit. The edges of this are so prominent, especially above and to the inner side, that a flat object resting on them does not touch the eyeball, and therefore the eye is seldom injured by a blow. The prominence of the eyebrow is largely due to air-spaces known as the frontal sinuses, lying in the substance of the frontal bone, and connected with the interior of the nose. The space behind the eyeball, and between it and the bone, is filled up by loose fat, which supports the eye as on an elastic cushion. The walls of the orbit almost meet in a point behind, leaving only two small gaps, through which pass nerves and vessels. The most prominent point of each eyeball is about $1\frac{1}{4}$ inches (30 mm) from the middle line of the face, so that the two are $2\frac{1}{2}$ inches (60 mm) apart. The eye is protected by two lids, upper and lower, which cover a varying amount of the globe, leaving usually an almond-shaped opening between their edges, which widens slightly as the eyes are turned up and down. The points where the lids join are known as the outer canthus and inner canthus, respectively. The inner canthus is tightly bound to the side of the nose, as may be seen by drawing the lids outwards, when a band stands out beneath the skin, between the nose and inner canthus; but the outer angle is freely movable up and down. Just within the inner canthus lies a small red swelling, the caruncle, which is merely a soft piece of skin, and often bears a few hairs. Within this, again, is a small fold, the semilunar fold, in the membrane covering the eyeball which in some persons is fairly large, and represents the third eyelid found in birds and some other animals.

Eyelids – Each of these consists of four layers. On the surface is skin, similar to the skin elsewhere on the body, but specially thin, loose and pliant. Behind this comes a layer of muscle, the orbicular muscle, the fibres of which run round and round from one lid to the other, and serve to shut the eye. Next comes a stiff, fibrous layer, the tarsus, or tarsal plate, which gives stiffness to the lids, but which does not extend upwards and downwards the whole height of the lids, reaching, in the upper lid, only about one-third of an inch (8 mm) from the margin, in the lower one about half that distance. In the substance of this plate is embedded a row of straight glands, the Meibomian, or tarsal, glands, the openings of which can be seen on the edge of the lid as a row of minute punctures. Small cysts often form as a result of obstruction to these glands, and produce small, round, painless swellings upon the surface of the lid. Farthest back of all is a moist, red layer of mucous membrane, known as the conjunctiva. This rubs over the surface of conjunctiva covering the eyeball, with which that on the lids is in fact continuous, at the upper margin of the upper lid and the lower margin of the lower lid. The conjunctiva, in passing from the lid to the surface of the eyeball, forms a pocket above and below. From the free margin of the lid projects a row of long, curved, elastic hairs, the eyelashes, which protect the eyes from dust insects and the like. About one-fifth of the length of each lid away from the inner canthus one sees, on turning the lid a little outward, a small puncture on the margin of the lid. This puncture, the lacrimal puncture, leads off the tears from the surface of the eye.

Front of the eye – When one separates the lids widely, a large part of the white of the eye comes into view. The white appearance is due to the sclera, or sclerotic coat, composed of dense, white, fibrous tissue, shining through the translucent conjunctiva. In the centre of the sclerotic is set the clear transparent cornea, through which light passes into the eye. Behind the cornea, again, is the beautifully coloured iris, with a hole in its centre, the pupil, which looks black against the dark interior of the eye. A space is seen to exist between the cornea and iris, particularly if the eye be looked at from a little to one side, this space being filled with a clear transparent fluid. The colour of the iris depends upon the way in which the pigment is arranged in it: blue or grey eyes owe their colour to the presence of pigment at the back of the iris (in the posterior epithelial layer); in brown eyes pigment is present also in the pigment cells in the middle layer (the stroma). If one attempts to look in through the pupil, one sees nothing, because, just as in looking into a camera, one obscures the entering light by placing one's head in front of it, and very little of the light which enters from the sides is reflected out again. If, however, one holds a mirror in front of the eye into which one wishes to look, in this way reflecting a bright beam of light into the eye, and if one then looks from behind the mirror through a small hole in its centre, the interior of the eye can be seen brightly lit up. The ophthalmoscope (qv) is an instrument constructed on this principle. By its help, the interior is seen as a general red ground. At one point is a round, pale area, the end of the optic nerve, and from the centre of it arteries and veins spread out over the inner surface of the eyeball. The signs of various diseases, not only of diseases of the eye, but also of various constitutional maladies which to some extent affect the structure of this organ, can be minutely studied with the help of the ophthalmoscope, which often therefore is of inestimable value to the physician.

Coats of the eyeball – The eyeball rests upon a pad of fat in the cavity of the orbit, where it is held in place by the pressure of the eyelids; by the attachment of the

185 – A diagram of the eye. *Hewer's Textbook of Histology for Medical Students.* Heinemann.

conjunctiva; by the orbital fascia and an envelope of fibrous tissue known as the capsule of Tenon; by six small muscles, which move it in different directions; and finally by the optic nerve, which enters from behind. The eyeball has three distinct coats (illustration 185):

(*a*) THE SCLERA, or sclerotic coat, is composed of dense white, fibrous tissue, which gives its appearance to the white of the eye. This coat completely encloses the eyeball, except behind, where the optic nerve pierces it, while in front it is

341

modified so as to form the transparent cornea. It maintains the shape of, and gives its strength to, the ball of the eye, being very hard to cut or tear. The *cornea*, which has a greater curvature than the rest of the eye ball, is the front, or anterior, part of this outer fibrous coat and is quite transparent. In front of and behind these layers is a thin protective membrane, and both surfaces, back and front, are covered by a layer of cells. All these are transparent, and the cornea forms, as it were, a window let into the front of the sclera.

(*b*) THE UVEAL TRACT, or vascular coat, lies within the sclerotic coat, and consists of three parts. The *choroid*, which forms its greatest part, and lines more than two-thirds of the sclera, consists mainly of a network of vessels which nourish the sclerotic coat and the interior of the eyeball. It is formed by the endings of a few ciliary vessels which pierce the sclerotic coat on the front and back of the ball. The choroid is prolonged forward into the *ciliary body*, a very complex structure, which forms a thickened ring opposite the line where the sclerotic passes into the cornea. To this line of junction between the sclerotic and cornea the ciliary body is firmly attached by the ciliary muscle, and, from the line of junction as a fixed point, the ciliary muscle takes its bearing, and, in contracting, slackens the suspensory ligament of the lens, so as to allow the lens of the eye which is suspended from, or, as it were, 'set' in, the ciliary body, to grow thicker and thinner in the act of accommodation for near and distant vision. (See ACCOMMODATION.) The iris and ciliary body are easily infected, and injuries to them are more dangerous for the whole eye than injuries to the cornea or to the eyeball farther outwards. The farthest forward part of the choroid coat is known as the *iris*, and, as already stated, it is seen lying behind the cornea and separated from the latter by a slight space. The iris consists partly of fibrous tissue, partly of muscle fibres, interspersed with pigment cells, some of the fibres being arranged in a circular manner, others running from the edge of the pupil to the outer margin of the iris. These fibres, by their contraction, serve to narrow or dilate the pupil, according as the light entering the eye is strong or weak, and according as the eye gazes at a near or distant object. In the sharp angle formed by the meeting of the cornea and iris round their edges the fluids which keep the eyeball naturally tense filter out and in, to and from the neighbouring vessels. In the disease known as glaucoma the angle through which this process takes place is blocked up, and the eyeball becomes very tense, painful and hard till sight is lost. The iris and ciliary muscle are powerfully acted on by certain drugs. Thus when atropine is put in the eye or taken internally the pupil becomes widely dilated, whilst under the influence of moderate doses of opium or morphine, or of physostigmine locally applied, it contracts. This action is a valuable sign of poisoning by these drugs.

(*c*) THE RETINA, or nervous coat, is the innermost of the three coats of the eyeball. The optic nerve ends, after piercing the sclerotic and choroid coats, by a sudden spreading out of its fibres in all directions to form this coat, which also contains blood-vessels and nerve and pigment cells. The retina in microscopic section can be seen to consist of no fewer than ten layers (illustration 186). Of these, the outermost is a layer of pigment cells preventing the diffusion of light inside the eye, and the layer next to this is that of the rods and cones upon which light is received, and from which impressions are conveyed by the optic nerve to the brain, where the

186 – Diagrammatic section of the retina showing its various layers. A, pigment cells; B, cones; C, rods; D, F, felt-work of dendrons; E, axon of one of the cells which lie between the rods and cones and G, the ganglion cells; H, axons passing from ganglion cells to optic nerve. From Hill, *Manual of Human Physiology*. Edward Arnold & Co.

sensations to which the various forms of light give rise are perceived. The rods are coloured a purple hue, visual purple, which fades for a time on exposure to bright light. They are excessively minute, less than $\frac{1}{400}$ inch (0·06 mm) long and about $\frac{1}{1000}$ inch (25 micrometres) in thickness. The cones are still shorter. The total number of cones in the human retina is about 6,500,000, and there are many more rods – about 115,000,000. It is probable that in order that two points of light may be seen as separate they must be sufficiently far apart for the rays proceeding from them to the eye to affect at least two cones. In the middle of the retina, at the very back of the eye, is a yellow spot, known as the macula lutea, in the centre of which a central pit (the fovea centralis) marks the point of clear vision. Here the retina is very thin, and consists entirely of cones. Rods and cones stand closely side by side over the whole retina, except over the area where the optic nerve enters. As there is none over the ending of the nerve, no light is perceived at this point, which is therefore called the blind spot. The presence of the blind spot in each eye can easily be proved by taking a clean sheet of paper, making an X in the middle of it, and then, while one eye is closed, following with the other eye the point of a pencil which is slowly moved to the right in the case of the left eye and to the left for the right eye. When the pencil is about 3 or 4 inches (75 to 100 mm) from the X the latter suddenly disappears, reappearing as the pencil is followed farther on.

The contents of the eyeball – The clear fluid separating the cornea from the iris is known as the aqueous humour of the eye. Immediately behind the iris and opposite the ciliary body, to which it is attached round its edge by a ligament, known as the ciliary zonule, lies the lens, a clear elastic body about $\frac{1}{3}$ inch (8 mm) in diameter and convex on both surfaces. If the lens becomes opaque, as it sometimes does in later life, the condition is known as cataract. Behind the lens and filling up the greater part of the interior of the eyeball is a soft, transparent, jelly-like mass known as the vitreous body. The lens and vitreous body are both of an albuminoid nature in chemical composition. The vitreous body usually contains small specks and filaments, which cast shadows upon the retina when the eye looks at a bright cloud or whitened wall. They appear as floating blots or strings and often cause alarm, but are of no importance and occur in almost every eye.

The lacrimal apparatus (illustration 187) is an attachment to the eye designed to keep its surface clean. In the upper and outer part of the orbit, between the eyeball and the bone, lies the lacrimal gland, which secretes a saltish, clear, watery fluid, which is constantly conveyed, drop by drop, through several fine ducts to the upper part of the sac formed by the conjunctiva, between the upper lid and the eyeball. From here the fluid spreads out over the front of the eye, and is removed partly by evaporation (25 per cent) and partly through the minute lacrimal punctures (puncta lacrimalia) which can be seen, one on the margin of each eyelid, about one-fifth of its length from its inner end. When the fluid runs over the margin of the lid it forms tears. From the lacrimal punctures the fluid runs, carrying with it specks of dust, etc., through two small canals into the lacrimal sac and duct, which lie alongside the nose, and thence into the lower part of the nose.

A negligible amount of tears is formed during sleep. In babies the secretion of tears does not begin until a few weeks after birth. It has been estimated that during the waking daily period 0·5 to 1·25 grams are produced daily, but there is a considerable range of individual variation. In addition to inorganic salts (mainly sodium chloride) and a small amount of protein, tears have an antibacterial enzyme, known as lysozyme, which plays an important part in protecting the eyes from infection.

Effect of light – When rays of light from an object fall upon the eye, they are strongly refracted at the front surface of the cornea; next, they pass through the aqueous humour and then the lens, by which they should be so much refracted as to be brought to an accurate focus on the retina, producing upon the rods and cones a small inverted image of the object viewed (illustration 188). If a bright light falls upon the eye, the pupil is narrowed by muscular action of the iris, causing, if the light continues very bright, considerable eye-strain. Therefore, in reading, one should not let a bright light shine full into the eyes, but should set it above one's head, behind one's back, or carefully shade it from the eyes. If the gaze turns to an object close at hand, the eyes look inwards, the pupils narrow, and the lenses become more convex by the automatic action of the muscles outside the eyeball, and of the muscle fibres in the iris and ciliary body. (See ACCOMMODATION.) As the eyes look at a distant object again, they take up the position of rest, the pupils

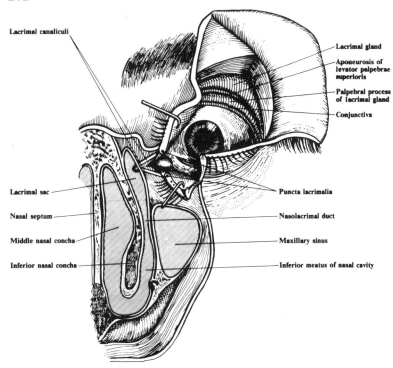

Lacrimal canaliculi

Lacrimal gland

Aponeurosis of
levator palpebrae
superioris

Palpebral process
of lacrimal gland

Conjunctiva

Lacrimal sac

Nasal septum

Middle nasal concha

Inferior nasal concha

Puncta lacrimalia

Nasolacrimal duct

Maxillary sinus

Inferior meatus of nasal cavity

187 – Dissection to show lacrimal apparatus. From *Gray's Anatomy*. Longman.

widening, the ciliary muscle relaxing, and both eyes looking straight forwards. Hence the sensation of restfulness derived from looking in moderate light at a distant scene or even at a landscape picture. The images formed upon the retina are reversed in every way; thus rays from points towards the right hand fall upon the left side of both retinae, and vice versa, while rays from the ground affect the upper part, and those from above the lower part of both retinae. The different colours corresponding to rays of various wave length produce different effects upon the retina, and these, being converted into

188 – Diagram showing the inverted image on the retina produced by the lens.

nerve impulses, are carried along the optic nerves to the hinder part of the brain, where they produce the varied sensations of light and colour, very much in the same way, probably, as the voice is received by a telephone, transmitted along wires in an altered form, and again reproduced in the receiver with all its original tones and modulations.

The sense of distance, solidity and form implies an act of judgment based upon experience. To an infant the universe is a mass of colour spread before his eyes, but gradually he learns, with the help of other senses, that objects which appear large and distinct are close at hand and may be grasped, those which seem small and indistinct are far off. The impression of solidity is gained by the image of any object upon one retina being slightly different from the image of it upon the other which can, so to speak, see a little way round the side of the object. This principle is utilized in making and viewing stereoscopic photographs. These, being taken from two different points, form, when viewed side by side, different images upon the two retinae. The two images are combined by the mind into the sensations derived from a single scene which has depth as well as breadth and height. (For further information, see VISION.)

EYE DISEASES AND INJURIES –
The delicacy of structure of the eye renders any disorder of this organ highly important. Many of its disorders cannot be cured or can be remedied only to a small extent, such as, for example, as loss of transparency in the cornea; whilst, in the case of others, such as cataract and high errors of refraction, the skill of the specialist may restore the eye from a state of almost complete uselessness to that of good vision. Most of the diseases are intricate in their course and treatment, requiring the highest degree of skill in handling. In the following account, some of the simpler and commoner diseases are dealt with. The subjects of CATARACT; CHEMOSIS; CHOROIDITIS; GLAUCOMA; IRITIS; RETINA, DISEASES OF; SQUINTING; SPECTACLES; TRACHOMA; and VISION, DISORDERS OF, are dealt with under these headings.

STYE consists of an inflammation situated round an eyelash, which occurs especially in young people. It begins as a general swelling of the lid accompanied by pain, and gradually suppurates. As one stye subsides another often appears. Styes are most likely to occur in debilitated individuals. Treatment consists of hot compresses or hot spooning (illustration 189). Once the stye has burst, neomycin ointment may be of value.

Wooden spoon

Bowl of boiling water

189 – Eye bathing by means of hot spooning. A piece of flannel or flannelette is wrapped round an ordinary kitchen wooden spoon. This is then soaked in a bowl of boiling water, the excess of water is squeezed out against the side of the bowl, and the hot spoon then applied gently to the closed eye. This procedure is repeated for around five minutes several times a day.

BLEPHARITIS, or chronic inflammation of the margin of the lids, occurs in weakly children. It is known by a variety of names, and, if not treated, it may prod-

uce, a red, watery condition of the eyelids, with loss of the eyelashes, known as 'blear eyes', which persists throughout life. It begins with swelling near the edge of the eyelid, usually the upper one, redness and the constant formation of a crust round the roots of the eyelashes. The onset often follows one of the acute diseases of childhood, especially measles. The lower lid becomes infected later.

Treatment consists in removing the crusts from the lids twice a day with warm solution of bicarbonate of soda (a teaspoonful to a tumblerful of water), drying carefully, and at once applying some astringent and antiseptic, of which the favourite is ammoniated mercury ointment or yellow oxide of mercury ointment. Neomycin ointment has proved of value in the treatment of this condition.

190 – Meibomian cysts. From Parsons and Duke-Elder, *Diseases of the Eye*. Churchill Livingstone Ltd.

CYSTS of the lids often arise in connection with the Meibomian glands (illustration 190). They may last for many years, and give no trouble beyond that of irritation and disfigurement caused by their size, if they be large. They may be removed, when desired, by an opening on the hinder surface of the lid, which is turned outward for the purpose. The contents being scraped out, the cyst does not tend to refill. This small operation is done under local anaesthesia.

PARALYSIS of the lids may occur from many causes, producing a drooping of the upper lid known as ptosis when the 3rd cranial nerve is affected, or a turning outward of the lower lid, together with inability to close the eye, when the 7th (facial) nerve is injured. (See PARALYSIS.) Paralysis of the muscles that move the eyeballs, causing double vision and an appearance of squinting, is a frequent symptom of chronic nervous diseases, such as multiple sclerosis. It may also be caused by injuries to, and various morbid conditions within, the skull, causing interference with the 3rd, 4th and 6th cranial nerves, which regulate these muscles.

345

SPASM of the lid is sometimes a troublesome condition. It may occur either in the form of frequent fluttering of the lid, popularly called 'life' in the eyelid, or there may be a partial closure of the eye, which will not relax. Fluttering of the lid is common and usually has no obvious cause, the person being simply tired or 'run down'. Small doses of quinine are worth trying if the condition persists.

NYSTAGMUS – involuntary, rapid, rhythmical, usually fine, up-and-down or side-to-side flickering movements of the eyeball – is a symptom of many nervous disorders, but, being due to a want of control of the nervous system over the action of the muscles which move the eyeball, is not really an eye disorder. It is observed also in persons who have had bad eyesight from childhood, and in miners.

WATERY EYE, or EPIPHORA, in which the tears overflow on to the face, is a slight but very annoying trouble. It results either from some irritation which causes over-secretion of tears, such as exposure to cold wind, bright light, smoke, irritating vapours, a foreign body in the eye, or some disease of the eye such as a corneal ulcer, or from some interference with the ducts which should convey the tears away to the lower part of the nose. This last cause is particularly common in older people, particularly women. Sometimes in old people with flabby eyelids, or in cases in which there is a contracting scar on the face, the lower eyelid turns outwards so that the lacrimal puncture is drawn away from the eye and the tears cannot enter it, but collect in the hollow of the lid, and then run over the face. Usually there is a blockage, it may be of the canaliculus by an eyelash or other small object, or, more often, of the duct upon the side of the nose as a result of inflammation. In the latter case a small swelling forms upon the side of the nose, and, if one presses upon this with the finger, tears and mucus ooze back on to the eyeball. If this condition be permitted to continue, not only is there the annoyance of tears constantly trickling down the cheek, but suppuration is apt to occur in the obstructed duct and to produce a small but unsightly sinus on the side of the nose, which can be closed only with difficulty. The presence of a suppurating tear sac is a source of danger to the eye, because, after any accident to or operation on the eye, virulent organisms are apt to spread from the sac and set up ulceration of the cornea.

Treatment of epiphora – Where the cause is due to conjunctival irritation, a mild astringent lotion, eg. tannic acid in the strength of 2 to 5 grains (125 to 300 mg) to the ounce (28·5 ml) of water, may be employed. Foreign bodies blocking the lacrimal punctures or canaliculi must be removed. When the lacrimal sac is distended with mucus and pus the canaliculus should be dilated, and a probe passed down the nasal duct into the nose, so as to remove any obstruction and allow free drainage into the nose. Gentle washing out of the sac with a small syringe often helps to restore the parts to a more healthy state. In very bad cases many surgeons advocate removal of the lacrimal sac by operation.

CONJUNCTIVITIS, or inflammation of the conjunctiva, is a very common eye affection. Not in itself a serious condition, it may yet give rise to grave complications, as, for instance, ulceration of the cornea.

A chronic state of redness or congestion of the eye, hardly amounting to conjunctivitis, is common in people whose eyes are much exposed to irritation from, for example, dust, smoke, cold winds. In gouty or plethoric people a similar congested state of the conjunctivae is often met with. Even the strain upon the eyesight due to errors of refraction may cause the eyes to appear reddened and tender. A cold in the head is often associated with congestion of the conjunctiva, or even with a conjunctivitis more or less severe. In some infectious diseases, notably in measles, conjunctivitis is a well-recognized symptom. Micro-organisms are the cause of nearly all cases of acute and subacute conjunctivitis. This explains why epidemics of conjunctivitis often occur in schools, orphanages and similar institutions, the infection being readily conveyed on towels, sponges, and the like, from one person to another.

Signs of conjunctivitis – The most characteristic sign of conjunctivitis is that the affected eye becomes red or *bloodshot*. This is due to the dilatation of the numerous vessels which ramify over the conjunctival surface. The colour is often described as brick red, and it is specially to be noted that the redness is general, and not most marked round the cornea, as is the case in iritis. The *swelling* of the conjunctiva in severe cases may be marked, and a thickened fold may form round the edge of the cornea. Haemorrhages in the conjunctiva from rupture of small blood-vessels are often seen in acute cases, but their presence does not afford any special cause for anxiety. Subjective symptoms vary greatly in severity. In mild cases there may be merely an annoying feeling of roughness or sand in the eyes, while in severe cases there may be great *pain. Photophobia* (dread of light) is a constant symptom. but is not usually so intense as in iritis and keratitis.

The *discharge* from the eyes in the early stages is thin and serous, but assumes more or less the character of pus after a few days. The sticky secretions tend to keep the lids gummed together, so that there may be great difficulty in opening the eyes, especially in the morning. Both eyes are usually affected, but often the disease begins in one eye some days before it attacks the other; the second eye in such cases becoming infected by accidental contamination with discharges from the inflamed eye. An attack of acute conjunctivitis lasts for one to two weeks.

Varieties of conjunctivitis – In addition to the type of *simple acute conjunctivitis* just described, there are various more severe forms.

A very severe type of conjunctivitis, *ophthalmia of the newborn* or *ophthalmia neonatorum*, may attack children a few days after birth. It is due to infection with discharges, usually gonorrhoeal, from the maternal passages, and may be attended with very severe corneal ulceration, thereby destroying or doing great permanent harm to the eyesight. At one time responsible for practically 50 per cent of cases of blindness in children, it is now gradually disappearing. In 1970, there were 59 cases in England. Infection from the genital passages in cases of gonorrhoea may in the adult cause a *gonorrhoeal conjunctivitis* of the most severe type.

Follicular conjunctivitis is characterized by the presence of numerous small reddish elevations about the size of a pin's head, often arranged in rows on the conjunctiva lining the eyelids. It is often seen in children and young adults, but its effects are not serious, and it must not be confused with trachoma (qv), which it may closely simulate.

Phlyctenular conjunctivitis is a form seen usually in weakly, ill-nourished children. At one time very common, it has now almost disappeared in Britain. Little, elevated, yellowish-red, flattened nodules (phlyctenules) are seen on the conjunctiva near the corneal margin. The disease may involve the cornea, producing ulceration and great irritation and photophobia. It is then known as keratoconjunctivitis.

Treatment of conjunctivitis – In *simple cases* all that is needed is to keep the eyes clean by frequent bathing with a mild antiseptic lotion: eg. boric lotion. The bathing is best done by pledgets of cotton-wool which can be burned after use. A special small flask known as an undine (illustration 191) with a long nozzle may be used to direct a stream of lotion over the eyeball. A mild antiseptic ointment, eg. boric or zinc ointment, or one containing an antibiotic, should be smeared on the lid margins to prevent gumming of the lids. Bandaging the eye is not good treatment, as it prevents the escape of discharges from the eye, and thus encourages the growth of organisms. Similarly, poultices of bread, porridge, etc., so often employed as a household remedy for inflamed eyes, may do great harm. The eyes may,

191 – Undine, used for irrigating the eye with fluid.

however, be protected from light and draught by an eye-shade, which at the same time allows access of air. Alternatively, dark glasses may be worn.

In *severe cases* of conjunctivitis, and especially in the stage when the secretion is becoming purulent, sulphacetamide or chloramphenicol eye-drops are of the greatest value. Silver salts are also used on account of their astringent and antiseptic actions. Silver nitrate (1 per cent) may be applied gently on a camel-hair brush once or twice. Its application is very painful, and, on this account, an organic salt of silver, eg. Protargol, 5 or 10 per cent, or Argyrol, 20 per cent, applied twice daily, may be substituted. Thorough and frequent bathing of the eye is of primary importance.

The severe *ophthalmia of infants* can also be treated by these silver salts. These, however, have been almost entirely replaced by penicillin eye-drops, supplemented sometimes in severe cases by sulphonamides given by mouth. In some maternity hospitals a few drops of weak nitrate of silver solution ($\frac{1}{2}$ per cent) are instilled into the eyes of every child at birth, but this practice has now been largely given up in Britain.

Many cases of *subacute conjunctivitis*, accompanied by inflammation of the lid margins, will yield readily to the use of zinc salts. Zinc sulphate lotion (1 to 2 grains (60 to 120 mg) to the ounce (28·5 ml) of water) may be instilled thrice daily, and an ointment of zinc oxide rubbed into the lid margins at bedtime.

In *phlyctenular conjunctivitis* the best treatment is the daily application of a 1 per cent ointment of yellow oxide of mercury. In using the ointment a piece about as large as a small grain of barley should be laid gently within the lower-lid margin, and then the eye, being closed, the lid should be gently massaged so as to rub the ointment over the whole eye. (Similarly, when drops are applied to the eye, the lower lid is pulled down, so as to form a sort of pocket into which the drops are allowed to fall.) Should the cornea be affected, the addition of atropine ($\frac{1}{2}$ to 1 per cent) to the ointment will greatly relieve photophobia and promote healing. Corticosteroids in the form of eye-drops or eye-ointment are also of value but must only be used under skilled medical supervision.

General treatment is important in these cases. The diet should be plain and simple, but nourishing, including especially milk, butter and eggs. Fresh air, sunlight and the strictest attention to cleanliness are of the greatest importance. Children with this affection tend to suffer from nasal catarrh and overgrowth of the tonsils and adenoid tissue of the nasopharynx. Proper treatment of these affections will do much to improve the general health and expedite the cure of the ocular troubles. (See NOSE, DISEASES OF.)

KERATITIS, or INFLAMMATION OF THE CORNEA, is due to several causes, including the herpes virus. In these herpetic cases an eye ointment containing the anti-viral agent, adenine arabinoside, is proving of value. It may be caused by an abrasion of the cornea, or it may be caused by a burn from molten metal, acids or alkalis. Such burning accidents are not uncommon in certain industries, such as the heavy metal industries and the chemical industry. If the eye is injured by acids, alkalis or irritant gases it must be irrigated immediately with a copious gentle stream of water or by blinking under water. This must be continued for up to 20 minutes depending on the severity of the injury. If the eye is still painful after irrigation, a few drops of castor oil may be put into the outer corner of the eye, which is then covered lightly with a sterile pad or bandage. The patient is then sent for immediate further medical attention.

Acute infection of the cornea tends to lead to corneal ulcer (qv). Chronic keratitis occurs in association with tuberculosis, syphilis and leprosy. Syphilitic interstitial keratitis is nearly always a manifestation of inherited syphilis, and comes on between the ages of seven and twenty years. The cornea gets dull and hazy, the sight being a good deal interfered with, and at the same time there are pain and intolerance of light. This disorder lasts usually four to six months, or longer, both eyes being affected, and it is almost always accompanied by iritis, which renders it still more serious. The treatment generally adopted is the use of atropine drops and the wearing of dark glasses. If the condition is syphilitic the appropriate anti-syphilitic treatment must be given. The chief danger of the disorder is that it leaves behind it opaque patches in the cornea, or changes in the choroid membrane, which interfere with vision or even obscure it altogether.

One dramatic advance in treatment has been the grafting of a new cornea (illustration 192) in place of one that is so opaque by disease as to hinder vision. (See CORNEAL GRAFTING.)

ULCER of the cornea arises from various causes, several of which have been mentioned. Two chief dangers attend an ulcer here, one being the fact that a white scar, which interferes with vision, especially if the ulcer has been severe, is certain to follow the ulcer; the other danger being that of perforation of the cornea (which is only about one millimetre in thickness), followed by more or less destruction of the eye.

Treatment of corneal ulcer – The great essential is to keep the eye clean. Hence bandages, poultices and such applications are in most cases likely to be harmful. Antibiotics are used in full dosage to overcome the infection. Weak corrosive sublimate lotion (1-6000), or boric or Argyrol lotion, may be used to bathe the eye. Atropine is used to combat the iritis which always attends severe ulceration of the cornea. In severe cases not apparently responding to treatment, corticosteroids

(a)   (b)

192 – Eye showing corneal opacity before corneal grafting (a); same eye after successful corneal grafting showing clear cornea (b).

may be used. If the ulcer is spreading, various methods are adopted to check it, such as application of a cautery to the spreading margin, the division of the ulcer and opening up of the anterior chamber by a fine knife. A corneal ulcer of the severe spreading kind may, if not checked, destroy the cornea in a few days, and with it all hope of useful vision in that eye. Hence the necessity for prompt and efficient treatment.

XEROPHTHALMIA is the term given to a condition in children characterized by inflammation of the cornea and eyelids, which leads to blindness unless treated in time. It is due to a deficiency of vitamin A in the diet, and is cured, not by local applications, but by giving vitamin A concentrates or food rich in this vitamin: eg. milk, eggs, butter, carrots.

ARCUS SENILIS is the name given to a white ring which forms round the edge of the cornea with advancing years. (See AGE, NATURAL CHANGES IN.)

EPISCLERITIS, at one time thought to be associated with rheumatism and gout, is now considered to be an allergic reaction to some toxin such as that of tuberculosis or streptococci. It consists of an inflammation of the sclera accompanied by patches of dusky redness over the white of the eye, pain and watering of the eye. The condition subsides when protective glasses are worn, and the constitutional condition is treated; but it is very obstinate to cure and liable to recur.

SCLERITIS involves a deeper inflammation of the sclera than episcleritis, and is not so common. Treatment is as for episcleritis.

BLACK-EYE is an effusion of blood under the loose skin over and round the lids, due to a blow. Within the first few hours of a blow on the eye, much may be done to diminish the blackness by a pad of linen wrung out of cold water, or of Goulard's water, and tightly bound on by a handkerchief passing round the head. A time-honoured pad is a raw beef-steak, which is moist and cold. After the first day absorption may be hastened by gentle massage and the bruise may be made less apparent by the application of flesh-coloured grease paint.

WOUNDS OF THE EYE – The eyebrow, cheek, nose and even the eyelids are often wounded, but seldom the eye itself, on account of the efficient protection afforded to it by these parts. The danger of a wound to the eye consists, not so much in the wounding of any important structure, which will heal with great rapidity, as in the introduction of organisms which may set up inflammation. The most dangerous position for a wound is in the ciliary region or iris, that is, just outside the margin of the cornea (see EYE), from whence a destructive inflammation not only of the wounded eye but also of the other, causing total blindness, is apt to be set up. (See IRITIS.) Metallic particles which penetrate the eye should always, if possible, be removed, because the fluids of the eye act upon them to form irritating chemical compounds. Most eye hospitals are provided with a powerful electromagnet, which will draw small particles of iron or steel from the deeper part of the eye into the anterior chamber, where they can be seen by the operator and successfully removed.

Cinders or dust may lodge behind one of the lids or may be embedded in the cornea and cause much pain. In this case the eye should not be rubbed, but a handkerchief may be gently pressed against it. The lids should be drawn gently apart, and if the body be seen it should be wiped

193 – Method of turning out the upper eyelid in order to examine its inner surface and the upper part of the eyeball.

off the eye with a wet camel-hair brush or clean wet rag. If it cannot be seen, the eyelids should be turned outwards and the inner surface of each lid examined. The lower lid is simply pulled downwards. To examine the upper lid, the person is told to look steadily downwards, a flat pencil, or penholder, or a match is laid horizontally along the centre of the lid, and the lid, being grasped by the eyelashes between the finger and thumb of the person who is looking for the foreign body, is gently and quite painlessly folded upwards over the pencil, etc. (illustration 193). The irritating body is then brushed away, and the lid turned down again. If a piece of lime has got upon the eye it should be sponged with vinegar and water, and if acid has got into the eye it should be copiously bathed with baking-soda in water. The first-aid treatment for cement powder in the eye is to wash it out with copious amounts of water. The patient should then be taken to hospital for examination by an eye specialist, whether the cause of the eye injury be lime, acid or cement. In the case of lime burns of the eye promising results are being obtained from the use of disodium edetate eye lotion (0·4 per cent).

EYE STRAIN (see VISION).

F

FACE is that part of the head extending from the forehead to the chin (illustration 194). It is supported by 14 bones: 2 nasal bones. 2 superior maxillae which carry the upper teeth. 2 lacrimal bones, 2 zygomatic bones, 2 palatine bones, 2 nasal bones at the sides of the nose, the vomer, forming a partition between

direction instead of being sloped backwards as in animals. This facial angle has formed one means of classifying different races. The angle, which is measured by drawing one line from the centre of the forehead to the projecting part of the upper jaw and another line from the lower margin of the ear to the base of the nasal

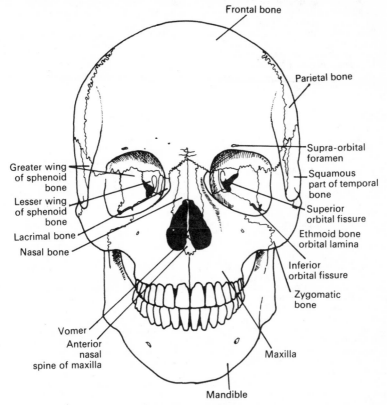

194 – The skull seen from the front.

the nostrils, and the mandible carrying the lower teeth. The lower jaw forms a joint of hinge-shape with the temporal bones of the skull, whilst the other bones of the face are firmly fixed together by sutures. The face in man is relatively small, as compared with that in lower animals, on account of the development of the cranium containing the brain. For the same reason, the face has an almost vertical

opening, is in Negroid races an acute angle, in most European races almost a right angle, while in the ancient Greek statues the face has an overhanging character.

The general character of the features depends chiefly upon the presence of air spaces in the frontal bone, situated immediately behind the eyebrows and in the upper jaw-bones. The varying expressions

351

which are connected with the emotions and the general expression denoting character are chiefly due to the action of numerous thin muscles situated around the openings of the eyes, nose, and mouth. (See MUSCLE.) These are controlled by the 7th cranial nerve, which springs from the hinder part of the brain, passes through the skull to the ear, and, emerging immediately below the latter, passes forward on to the face round the edge of the lower jaw. In this position it is liable to be wounded or injured by such conditions as cold, then giving rise to a flat and expressionless appearance of one side of the face, known as *Bell's palsy* (or *paralysis*) or *facial paralysis*. (See BELL'S PARALYSIS.) The sensory nerve of the face is the 5th cranial nerve, which originates from the neighbouring part of the brain and within the skull divides into three portions called, respectively, ophthalmic, maxillary, and mandibular divisions. Each of these sends branches on to the face through a notch that can be felt near the inner end of the eyebrow, through an opening immediately beneath the eye, and through another opening near the middle of the chin. On their way to the face these nerves supply the parts about the eye, the teeth, and the muscles which move the lower jaw in chewing. The various parts of this nerve are subject to a particularly painful form of neuralgia, known sometimes as 'tic-douloureux'. (See NEURALGIA.)

The face is liable to certain deformities, of which hare-lip and cleft palate are the principal. (See PALATE, MALFORMATIONS OF.) The skin of the face, which has an unusually free blood supply, bleeds with great freedom when wounded, but, for the same reason, wounds heal with special rapidity and freedom from suppuration. The contraction of scars after severe injuries, such as burns, sometimes leads to marked deformity of the eyelids, mouth, and nose. The skin condition known as acne (see ACNE) is very common in young persons about the chin and brow, disappearing as age advances. Boils, carbuncles, and other infectious conditions often occur on the face, and, when situated about the upper lip, present a considerable degree of danger from the liability of the infection to spread to the interior of the head. The tuberculous disease known as lupus is more frequent on the face than in any other situation and may lead to unsightly ulceration and scarring. Certain simple tumours, particularly sebaceous cysts and naevi or birth marks, commonly affect the skin in this region, and cancer, in the form of epithelioma, is not uncommon in the later stages of life about the margins of the lip, nostril, or eyelid. This is also one of the commonest sites of the slow-growing form of cancer known as rodent ulcer.

FACIAL NERVE is the seventh cranial nerve, and supplies the muscles of expression in the face, being purely a motor nerve. It enters the face immediately below the ear after splitting up into several branches. (See BELL'S PARALYSIS.)

FACIES is a term applied to the expression or appearance of the face, which often gives indications of the presence of disease in other parts of the body. Thus the *abdominal facies* is a pinched, anxious expression associated with severe disease in the abdomen. The *cardiac facies* is a condition present in some valvular defects of the heart, showing bright purplish cheeks and lips, with a sallow hue of the rest of the face. The *typhoid facies* is a vacant, bewildered, and apathetic expression seen in typhoid fever and other debilitating diseases. The *Hippocratic facies* is a cast of countenance originally described by Hippocrates, in which the face is drawn, pinched, and livid, indicating approaching death.

FAECES is another name for the stools. (See CONSTIPATION; DIARRHOEA; STOOLS.)

FAINTING, or SYNCOPE, is a temporary loss of consciousness.

Causes – The manner in which the loss of consciousness is produced appears to be that temporarily there is an inadequate supply of blood to the brain. If the person who threatens to faint lies down, or, still better, if she sits and then bends forward so as to bring the head below the knees, the faint is averted. Fainting may occur as part of the general muscular relaxation which takes place in a hot bath. Powerful emotion, generally of a sorrowful nature, but sometimes even great joy, is a cause. Extreme pain, such as that due to the crushing of a limb, and shocks to the nervous system, such as a blow on the head or on the abdomen, are apt to cause fainting, or even the more serious condition known as shock. It is liable to occur on first getting up after a prolonged period of illness with confinement to bed. Another not uncommon cause, particularly in adolescents and young adults, is prolonged standing: eg. on the parade ground. Disgusting smells and sights, breathing of bad air, and general exhaustion are also causes. As a rule, a combination of these causes is necessary, except in hysterical persons, and persons weak from some illness, who are specially liable to faints. Certain drugs, such as tobacco or alcohol, when taken in excess, produce syncope. Occasionally it may be due to heart disease.

Symptoms are well known. There are certain warning symptoms, such as pallor, feebleness of the pulse, a sinking feeling, and a dullness of sight and hearing. When the faint has occurred, the person lies still, breathing very faintly, with feeble pulse, pallid complexion, and often perspiration standing in drops on the face.

The faint, as a rule, lasts only a few seconds or minutes, but it may last for hours, and hysterical persons may pass from one faint, only to fall into another several times.

Treatment – The faint may often be prevented by attending to the cause, as already noted. Sitting down and bending forwards so as to bring the head on a level with the knees, or taking rapid gulps of cold water, is often enough to prevent a threatened faint. The person in a faint should be laid flat on the back, and care should be taken that breathing is unimpeded. If care is not taken to leave the fainting person lying flat, death may ensue, but if this be attended to, nothing more is usually necessary. Stimulants may be applied to the skin in the form of cold compresses on the head, slapping of the hands, pinching of the cheeks; or to the nose in the form of smelling-salts or eau-de-Cologne, or the pungent fumes of burnt feathers. After recovery has taken place from the faint the tendency to its recurrence may be prevented by administration of some stimulant such as sal volatile or brandy.

FALLING SICKNESS is an old name for epilepsy. (See EPILEPSY.)

FALLOPIAN TUBES, or UTERINE TUBES, are tubes, one on each side, which are attached at one end to the womb, and have the other unattached but lying close to the ovary. Each is between 4 and 5 inches (10 and 12·5 cm) long, large at the end next the ovary, but communicating with the womb by an opening which admits only a bristle. These tubes conduct the ova from the ovaries to the interior of the womb. Blockage of them by a chronic inflammatory process resulting from infection is a not uncommon cause of infertility in women.

FALSE MEMBRANE is the name given to the deposit which forms upon the walls of the air passages in cases of diphtheria. It consists partly of fibrin derived from the blood, partly of the destroyed surface of the mucous membrane upon which it rests, and it contains bacteria in enormous numbers. If it be removed, it leaves a raw and bleeding surface upon which new membrane quickly forms.

FANGO is the name of a kind of mud, derived from thermal springs at Battaglio in Italy, which is applied warm to gouty and rheumatic joints.

FANSIDAR is a combination of pyrimethamine (qv) and sulfadoxine (qv) which is being used for the prevention of malaria (qv). It has the advantage of only needing to be taken once a week, or even only once a fortnight.

FARADISM (see ELECTRICITY IN MEDICINE).

FARCY is another name for glanders. (See GLANDERS.)

FARMER'S LUNG is a form of external allergic alveolitis (see ALVEOLITIS) caused by the inhalation of dust from mouldy hay or straw.

FASCIA is the name applied to sheets or bands of fibrous tissue which enclose and connect the muscles.

FASCIOLIASIS is the disease caused by the liver fluke, *Fasciola hepatica* (illustration 195). This is found in sheep, cattle and other herbivorous animals, in which it is the cause of the condition known as liver rot. It measures about 35 × 13 mm, and is transmitted to man from the infected animals by snails. In Britain it is the commonest disease found in animal slaughterhouses. The danger to man is in eating vegetables, particularly wild watercress, that has been infected by snails. There have been several outbreaks of fascioliasis, the disease caused by the fluke, in Britain due to eating contaminated wild watercress. Much larger outbreaks of fascioliasis due to eating wild watercress have also been reported in France. The disease is characterized by fever, dyspepsia, heavy sweating, loss of appetite, abdominal pain, urticaria, and a troublesome cough. In the more serious cases there may be severe damage to the liver with or without jaundice. The diagnosis is clinched by the finding of the eggs of the fluke in the stools. The two drugs used in treatment are bithionol and chloroquine. Even though many cases are quite mild and recover spontaneously, prevention is particularly important. This consists primarily of never eating wild watercress, as this is the main cause of infestation. Lettuces have also been found to be infested.

195 – Adult fluke of *Fasciola hepatica*.

FASTIGIUM means the highest temperature reached in a feverish state.

FASTING means the abstention from, or deprivation of, food and drink.

The practice, which some persons carry out, of fasting one day a week or even of changing to a light diet at stated intervals, in the interests of health or of religion, has much to commend it in certain cases, because it gives the digestive organs a periodic rest.

If food and drink be entirely suspended, two results quickly follow: the body becomes thinner and lighter as it draws upon its stored-up nourishment, and also the temperature gradually falls. If water be taken, the process of using up the fat and muscles in order to maintain the activity of the heart, lungs, and other vital organs, proceeds to an extreme extent, and the body becomes very emaciated before

death. If water be withheld, death results much sooner, and the sufferings are great. If the body be well protected by clothes and blankets, the loss of heat is slower, and life is prolonged beyond the time that it lasts if the fasting person be poorly clad or exposed to severe cold, as in the case of Arctic explorers. It follows, too, that a person fasting and doing no work can survive very much better than one who is compelled at the same time to put forth great exertions, and so use up more of the bodily store of food. Persons are subjected to the worst combination then, when they are not only deprived of food, but have also a poor supply of water, are exposed to severe cold, and must make great muscular efforts.

Under the last-named conditions life could not be prolonged more than two or three days. But in the case of miners imprisoned by a fall of earth or flooding in a mine, and well supplied with water, life and health may be prolonged without any food for over a week. In the case of five miners imprisoned in Redding Pit, Scotland, in September 1923, they were brought up little the worse after being deprived of food for 214 hours. Whilst it is most unusual to survive for more than four or five days without water a case was recorded in the 1977 Bucharest earthquake who survived under the rubble for 252 hours without food or water.

Dogs may be kept alive with nothing but drinking-water for considerable periods. One case is on record of a dog which was starved for 117 days. At the end of this period it had lost 63 per cent of its weight but was fairly active. Human beings can also survive long fasts. The longest period for which anyone has gone without food, according to *The Guinness Book of Records*, is 382 days. This was achieved by a patient in Maryfield Hospital, Dundee, who lived on tea, coffee, water and soda water from June 1965 to July 1966. His weight in this period fell from 214 to 81 kilograms. One of the most historic fasts of modern times is that of Terence McSweeney, the Mayor of Cork, who in 1920 went on hunger strike and died 74 days later.

The professional fasters who profess to subsist entirely without food for a month or six weeks probably have small supplies administered to them in their drinking-water, or by other surreptitious means.

After prolonged fasting the return to food should be gradual, and no heavy meal should be taken for a day or two.

FAT as a food has more energy-producing power weight for weight than any other food. Animal fat is a mixture in varying proportions of stearic, palmitic, and oleic acids combined with glycerin. Butter contains about 80 per cent of fat, ordinary cream contains 20 per cent fat, and rich cream 40 per cent, whilst olive oil is practically a pure form of fat. Fat requires, when taken to a large extent in the diet, to be combined with a certain proportion of either carbohydrate or protein in order that it may be completely consumed, otherwise harmful products, known as ketones, are apt to be formed in the blood. Each gram of fat has an energy-producing equivalent of 9·3 Calories.

From the medical point of view, fats are divided into saturated fats, that is, animal fats and dairy produce, and unsaturated fats which include vegetable oils from soya bean, maize and sunflower, and marine oils from fish (eg. cod-liver oil). (See ADIPOSE TISSUE; CORPULENCE; LIPID.)

FATIGUE – Fatigue is brought about in two ways. In the first place muscles become fatigued by the lactic acid accumulating in them as the result of their activity. For the removal of lactic acid in the recovery phase of muscular contraction oxygen is needed. If the supply of oxygen is not plentiful enough, or cannot keep pace with the work the muscle is doing, then lactic acid accumulates and fatigue results. There is also a nervous element in muscular fatigue: it is diminished by stimulation of the sympathetic nervous system.

Industrial workers – Many factors enter into the maintenance of efficiency and the avoidance of fatigue, mental and physical. Intensity and direction of illumination, ventilation, temperature and humidity of the air, adequate diet, posture at work, rest pauses, monotony, and, above all, hours of work are among some of these factors. There is a level beyond which the human machine can no longer produce work satisfactorily. If this is exceeded it is shown by a reduction in the quantity and quality of the work done. If work is done under conditions of fatigue, damage to health results and accidents may occur. The shortening of unduly long hours of labour under improved hygienic conditions is followed by increased productive efficiency.

Children are especially liable to suffer from over-pressure at work. This applies especially to children of nervous temperament, those who are anaemic or badly fed, those who are rapidly growing, and those who have too little sleep and recreation or have various physical defects: eg. in sight, hearing. The time devoted to a lesson in any particular subject should not exceed three-quarters of an hour, and there should be an appropriate variation of subjects, sufficient intervals for rest, recreation, physical exercise and food. Fresh air and quiet in the classroom diminish fatigue. Home work should not be given to children under the age of nine years, and for several years after that age it should not take longer than one hour. The teachers should be carefully on the look-out for imperfections of vision and hearing which cause strain and brain fatigue. (See CHILDREN, PECULIARITIES OF; and SCHOOL CHILDREN.)

FAT NECROSIS – In injury to, or inflammation of, the pancreas the fat-splitting enzyme in it may escape into the abdominal cavity, causing death of fat-containing cells.

FATTY DEGENERATION – As a result of anaemia, interference with blood or nerve supply, or because of the action of various poisons, body cells may undergo abnormal changes accompanied by the appearance in their substance of fat droplets.

FAUCES is the name given to the somewhat narrowed opening between the mouth and throat. It is bounded above by the soft palate, below by the tongue, and on either side by the tonsil. In front of, and behind, the tonsil are two ridges of mucous membrane, the anterior and posterior pillars of the fauces.

FAVISM is a fulminating haemolytic anaemia, attacks of which occur within an hour or two of eating broad beans (*Vicia faba*) or inhaling their pollen. It is a hereditary disease due to lack of an essential enzyme which is largely confined to inhabitants of the Mediterranean littoral.

FAVUS is another name for honeycomb ringworm. (See RINGWORM.)

FEBRICULA means a little fever. The term – at one time popular in medical parlance – is seldom used now.

FEBRIFUGES, or antipyretics, are remedies employed to reduce the temperature of the body when it has been raised above that found in health (see BATHS;

COLD, USES OF; and FEVER). In addition to the application of cold, some of the chief febrifuges are aspirin, quinine, and salicylate of soda. (See also under each of these headings.)

FEEBLE-MINDEDNESS (see MENTAL SUBNORMALITY).

FEEDING (see CEREAL; DIET; DIGESTION; INFANT FEEDING; and PROTEIN) – The manner and times of administering food are matters of considerable importance in illness. In health appetite forms the usual guide to the amount of food and to meal-times. Most persons in health take four meals in the course of the day, one meal being much larger than any of the others and taken either in the middle of the day or in the evening. During the course of a disease or in convalescence, when the digestive powers are weak and a large meal cannot be borne, it is usually found more suitable to feed the patient in small amounts given at frequent intervals. The nature of the food must be such that it is readily digested and the food is usually fluid. Except in certain special cases, milk is the ideal food for this purpose, supplemented by drinks containing glucose. The quantity of milk given at one time is 6 to 8 ounces (170 to 230 ml). If milk tends to produce nausea or vomiting, it may be diluted with equal parts of water and given warm. The total amount of milk given in twenty-four hours should be 2 to 3 pints (1 to 2 litres). Glucose is given in preference to ordinary sugar (ie. sucrose) because it is not so sweet, and therefore it is possible to give larger amounts without making the dish too sweet. In order to produce variety, and at the same time to ensure an adequate amount of vitamin C, the glucose drinks should be flavoured with fresh fruit juice: eg. orange or lemon. Milk puddings and eggs should be added to the diet as soon as possible. Beef tea, although it has no energy value, adds variety to the invalid diet, as do jellies. Small feeds should be given: two-hourly during the day, and during the night if the patient is awake.

It is sometimes convenient to feed the patient by means of a spoon, but, as a rule, the patient's head being raised by the nurse's arm passed beneath the pillow, the spout of a feeding-cup (illustration 196) is introduced into his mouth and the patient is thus able to drink without spilling the fluid. A form of glass from which the patient can drink more naturally con-

sists of a tumbler with an elongated lip on one side, and this is often preferable. Still another method in which the patient may be fed with thin fluids is through a straw

196 – Two forms of feeding-cup. The cup on the left is used for patients who are further advanced in convalescence, and who are partly raised in bed.

or piece of narrow india-rubber tubing. In this case the straw must be thrown away after use and the rubber tubing carefully boiled before being used again.

Food may be peptonized for administration to invalids. (See PEPTONIZED FOODS; see also MILK, and for preparation of fluid foods for invalids, see ALBUMIN WATER; BARLEY WATER; BEEF-TEA; GRUEL; RICE WATER; TOAST WATER.)

FEHLING'S TEST for glycosuria (see URINE).

FEMUR is the bone of the thigh (illustration 83), and is the longest and strongest bone in the body. As the upper end of the femur is set at an angle of about 120 degrees to the rest of the bone, and since the weight of the body is entirely borne by the two femora, fracture of one of these bones close to its upper end is a common accident in old people, whose bones are becoming brittle. The femur fits, at its upper end, into the acetabulum of the pelvis, forming the hip-joint and, at its lower end, meets the tibia and patella in the knee-joint.

FENESTRATION is the operation whereby a new opening is made into the labyrinth of the ear. It has proved most valuable in restoring hearing to patients with otosclerosis (qv), particularly in young people with this disease.

FENFLURAMINE is one of the more recent anorexiant drugs (qv), introduced to aid the slimming process by suppressing or reducing appetite. Although less likely to become a drug of addiction than some of the other anorexiant drugs, it is not without its risks and must only be used under skilled medical supervision. One of its disadvantages is that in some people it induces an increased frequency of dreaming or even nightmares.

FENNEL is the seed-like fruit of *Foeniculum vulgare* used as a carminative: ie. to relieve griping, flatulence, and distension of the stomach. Fennel water used to be a popular remedy for griping.

FENOTEROL is a drug that is proving useful by inhalation in the treatment of asthma.

FERMENTS are substances which produce chemical changes in other bodies while remaining unchanged themselves.

FERRUM is the Latin name for iron.

FESTER is a popular term used to mean any collection or formation of pus. It is applied to both abscesses and ulcers. (See ABSCESS; ULCER; WHITLOW.)

FESTINATION is the term applied to the involuntary quickening of gait seen in some nervous diseases, especially in PARALYSIS AGITANS, or PARKINSONISM (qv).

FEVER is the condition of the body characterized by a rise in temperature. It is one of the most common accompaniments of diseases in general, and serves to make the distinction between *febrile* and *non-febrile* ailments.

Causes – In many cases the fever must be regarded as only secondary to, and symptomatic of, the disordered state with which it is found associated. For example, a certain amount of fever may arise in consequence of some nervous shock. But there is a large class of diseases in which fever is the predominant factor, and which arise from the formation in the system of something of the nature of a poison (toxin), upon which all the symptoms depend. To such diseases, the term primary or specific fevers is applied, and, as examples, may be mentioned typhoid fever, scarlet fever, diphtheria. These diseases depend on the growth of bacteria in the blood or tissues of the body, the toxins being formed by the activity of these organisms.

In considering the general subject of fever, regard must be had in particular to the two main features of the febrile process: the abnormal elevation of temperature, and the changes affecting the tissues of the body in reference thereto.

The average temperature of the body in health ranges between 98·4° and 99·5° F (36·9° and 37·5° C). It is liable to slight variations from such causes as the ingestion of food, the amount of exercise, the menstrual cycle, and the temperature of the surrounding atmosphere. There are, moreover, certain appreciable daily variations, the lowest temperature being between the hours of 1 am and 7 am. (01.00 and 07.00 hours), and the highest between 4 pm. and 9 pm. (16.00 and 21.00 hours), with trifling fluctuations during these periods. (See TEMPERATURE.)

The development and maintenance of heat within the body are generally regarded as depending on the destructive oxidation of all its tissues, consequent on the changes continually taking place in the processes of nutrition. In health this constant tissue disintegration is exactly counterbalanced by the introduction of food, whilst the uniform normal temperature is maintained by the due adjustment of the heat thus developed, and of the processes of exhalation and cooling which take place, especially from the lungs and skin. In the febrile state this relationship is no longer preserved, the tissue waste being greatly in excess of the food supply, while the so-called 'law of temperature' is in abeyance. In this condition the body wastes rapidly, the loss to the system being chiefly in the form of nitrogen compounds (eg. urea). In the early stage of fever a patient excretes about three times the amount of urea that he would excrete on the same diet if he were in health – the difference being that in the latter condition he discharges a quantity of nitrogen equal to that taken in with the food, whilst in the fevered state he wastes the store of nitrogen contained in the tissues and the blood. The amount of fever is estimated by the degree of elevation of the temperature above the normal standard. When it reaches as high a point as 106° F (41·1° C) the term hyperpyrexia (excessive fever), is applied, and is regarded as indicating a condition of danger; while, if it exceeds 107° or 108° F (41·7° or 42·2° C) for any length of time, death almost always results. Occasionally the temperature may reach 110° to 112° F (43·3° to 44·4° C) prior to the fatal issue.

Symptoms – The onset of a fever is usually marked by a rigor or shivering, which may exist only as a slight but persistent feeling of chilliness, or, on the other hand, be of a violent character, and, as occasionally happens with children, find expression in the form of well-marked

197 – Temperature chart from a case of pneumonia, showing a high degree of fever with increased pulse and respiration. The heavy line at 98·4 shows the level of the normal temperature. Note the rapid fall in temperature: ie. by crisis.

convulsions. Although termed the *cold stage* of fever, in this condition the temperature of the body is really increased. There are, besides, various accompanying feelings of illness, such as pain in the back, headache, sickness, thirst, and great lassitude. In all cases of febrile complaints it is of importance for the physician to note the first occurrence of shivering, which in general fixes the beginning of the attack. This stage is soon followed by the full development of the febrile condition, the *hot stage*. The skin now feels hot and dry, and the temperature, always elevated above the normal standard, will often be found to show daily variations corresponding to those observed in health – namely, a rise toward evening, and a fall in the morning. There is a relative increase in the rate of the pulse and quickness of breathing. The tongue is dry and furred; the thirst is intense, while the appetite is gone; the urine is scanty, of high specific gravity, containing a large quantity of solid matter, particularly urea, the excretion of which, as already stated, is increased in fever; while, on the other hand, certain of the saline ingredients, such as chlorides, are often diminished. The bowels are in general constipated, but they may be relaxed, especially if the gut is the primary site of infection, as in typhoid fever. The nervous system participates in the general disturbance, and sleeplessness and disquietude are common accompaniments,

and there may be delirium. The wasting of the muscles, and corresponding loss of strength, may be marked, and continue even although considerable quantities of nutriment may be taken.

The decline of the fever takes place either by the occurrence of a *crisis* (illustration 197), ie. a sudden termination of the symptoms, often accompanied with some discharge from the body, such as profuse perspiration, copious flow of thick urine, and occasionally diarrhoea, or by a more gradual subsidence of the temperature, technically termed a *lysis*. If death ensues, this is due to failure of the vital centres in the brain or of the heart, as a result of either the infection or hyperpyrexia. Such terminal failure may be gradual, the patient passing into what is sometimes known as the *typhoid state* (a condition of extreme prostration, associated with low delirium or coma). In other cases death occurs suddenly after slight exertion, as a result of the additional strain on the heart.

Certain well-marked types of fever are recognized. The term *continued fever* is applied to those forms in which the febrile temperature persists for a more or less definite period, uninterrupted by any distinct intermission till the crisis is reached. To this type belong typhus and typhoid fevers, and the eruptive fevers or exanthemata: eg. smallpox, measles, and scarlet fever. *Relapsing fever* is a form of continued fever, the chief characteristic of which is the occurrence in about a week after the crisis of a distinct relapse and repetition of all the symptoms. Occasionally second and third relapses take place.

The term *remittent* is applied to those forms of fever the course of which is interrupted by a short, usually daily, diminution of the fever, followed by a recurrence of all the symptoms. Such fevers are chiefly met in tropical climates, but occasionally continued fevers assume this form, particularly in children. The condition known as *hectic fever*, which occurs in the course of wasting diseases, is markedly remittent in its course.

In *intermittent fever* there is a distinct periodic subsidence of the symptoms, which, according to its duration, characterizes the variety as *quotidian* (where the paroxysm recurs in twenty-four hours), *tertian* (in forty-eight hours), *quartan* (in seventy-two hours). Hectic fever is also not infrequently of the intermittent type.

The term *malignant* is employed to describe forms of fever in which the blood appears to undergo rapid deteriorating changes. Yellow fever may be said to belong to this category, and the continued fevers, more especially typhus and the exanthemata, occasionally assume a malignant form from the beginning.

Treatment – Fever is a symptom, and the correct treatment is therefore that of the underlying condition. Occasionally, however, it is also necessary to try and reduce the temperature by more direct methods. For this latter purpose it will be sufficient to refer to two methods: namely, the external application of cold and the administration of antipyretic remedies or febrifuges. The former of these methods is accomplished by means of baths, in which the patient is placed, the water being somewhat below the febrile temperature and gradually cooled down by the addition of cold water till a temperature of from 60° to 70° F (15·5° to 21° C) is reached. This process, when continued for only a short time and frequently repeated, yields most valuable results in many instances of high temperature. The relief to the patient is remarkable, the body rapidly parting with its heat, and the effect usually continues for hours. The cooler the bath the longer the effect lasts. Sponging with cold water and the wet pack are other methods used to reduce temperature and exert a soothing influence. (See COLD, USES OF.)

Certain drugs possess the power of reducing the temperature by their action on the heat-regulating centres in the brain, thereby causing an increased loss of heat through dilatation of the blood-vessels in the skin. These drugs include sodium salicylate, aspirin, quinine, and Dover's powder.

FIBRILLATION is a term applied to rapid contraction or tremor of muscles, especially to a form of abnormal action of the heart muscle in which individual bundles of fibres take up independent action. It is believed to be due to a state of excessive excitability in the muscle associated with the stretching which occurs in dilatation of the heart. Fibrillation is distinguished as atrial or ventricular, according as the muscle of the atria or of the ventricles is affected. As a result, the heart-beats and the pulse become extremely irregular both as regards time and force. The condition of atrial fibrillation is responsible for more than half of all marked and persistent cases of irregular pulse.

FIBRIN is a substance formed in the blood as it clots. Its formation indeed causes clotting. The substance is produced in threads. After the threads have formed a close meshwork through the blood, they contract, and produce a dense felted mass. The substance is formed not only from shed blood but also from lymph which exudes from the lymph-vessels. Thus fibrin is found in all inflammatory conditions within serous cavities like the pleura, peritoneum, and pericardium, and forms a thick coat upon the surface of the inflamed membranes. It is also found in inflamed joints, and in the lung as a result of pneumonia. (See COAGULATION.) (illustration 198.)

FIBRIN FOAM is one of a series of absorbable haemostatics introduced into surgical use. A haemostatic is a preparation which arrests bleeding, and the great advantage of an absorbable haemostatic is that it produces no irritation in the tissues into which it is introduced and that it does not need to be removed after the bleeding is arrested, but is gradually absorbed by the tissues. Fibrin foam is a spongy material which is soaked in a solution of thrombin immediately before use. Other absorbable haemostatics now in use include oxidized cellulose (oxycellulose) which is prepared as a gauze, and calcium alginate (derived from seaweed) which is prepared as a gauze and as wool. These absorbable haemostatics, which constitute

198 – Section of blood clot, showing network of strings of fibrin. Magnified 400 times. From Schafer's *Histology*. Longman.

a great advance in surgery, are of particular value in operations on the brain and in operations on blood-vessels and nerves.

FIBRINOGEN is the soluble protein in the blood which is the precursor of fibrin (qv), the substance in blood-clot.

FIBROCYSTIC DISEASE OF THE PANCREAS, or MUCOVISCIDOSIS, which is also known as cystic fibrosis, is the commonest serious genetic disease in Caucasian children, with an incidence of about 1 per 2500 births. It is a disorder of the mucus-secreting glands of the lungs, the pancreas, the mouth, and the gastro-intestinal tract, as well as the sweat glands of the skin. It is characterized by failure to gain weight in spite of a good appetite, repeated attacks of bronchitis, and the passage of loose, foul-smelling and slimy stools. A simple, cheap, reliable test for detecting the disease by examination of the stools has now been evolved, which permits the early diagnosis of the disease. The earlier treatment is started, the better the results. Parents of children with cystic fibrosis, seeking help and advice, can obtain this from the Cystic Fibrosis Research Trust, 5 Blyth Road, Bromley, Kent BR1 3RS.

FIBROID is a term sometimes applied to tumours of the womb consisting partly of muscular and partly of fibrous tissue. (See UTERUS, DISEASES OF.)

FIBROMA is a tumour consisting of fibrous tissue. (See TUMOURS.)

FIBROSIS means the formation of fibrous or scar tissue, which is usually due to either infection or deficient blood supply.

FIBROSITIS is another name for muscular rheumatism. (See RHEUMATISM.)

FIBROUS DYSPLASIA is a rare disease in which areas of bone are replaced by fibrous tissue (qv). This renders the bone fragile and liable to fracture. It may involve only one bone, usually the thigh bone, or femur (qv), or several bones. This latter form of the disease may be accompanied by pigmentation of the skin and the early onset of puberty. There is another form of the disease known as cherubism because of the appearance it gives to the face, in which the abnormality of bone is confined to the upper and lower jaw-bones (the maxilla and mandible). The cause of the disease is not known.

FIBROUS TISSUE is one of the most abundant tissues throughout the body. White fibrous tissue consists of fibres of a substance known as collagen, which yields gelatine on being boiled. Between these fibres lie flattened or star-shaped cells, by which the fibres are produced. The fibres, like the cells, are of microscopic size, and are grouped into bundles which are held together by other fibres running round them. Yellow fibrous tissue is a rarer form, and consists of bundles of long yellow fibres, formed from a substance known as elastin. White fibrous tissue is very unyielding and forms sinews, ligaments, the material which binds muscle fibres together, the substance of the true skin. It is also the tissue which is laid down in the repair of wounds, or as a result of inflam-

199   *Wuchereria bancrofti* (*Filaria bancrofti*). From Manson's *Tropical Diseases*. Baillière Tindall.

mation, and so forms the tissue composing a scar. It has the property of contracting and becoming denser as time goes on, and hence the puckering seen in scars, and the contraction resulting from burns and inflammation. Yellow fibrous tissue is highly elastic, and so is found in the walls of arteries, and in ligaments, like that on the back of the neck, which are often put upon the stretch. (See also ADHESIONS; SCAR; WOUNDS.)

FIBULA is the slender bone upon the outer side of the leg (illustration 83).

FILARIASIS is the name given to a group of tropical diseases in which minute Nematode worms, called filariae, are found in the blood (illustration 199). The most widespread of these is Bancroftian filariasis, so called after Dr. Joseph Bancroft. The causative worm is *Wuchereria bancrofti*, also known as *Filaria Bancrofti*. This is a threadlike worm (illustration 199) which is transmitted by certain mosquitoes. It is named after Wucherer, who discovered microfilariae in the urine of a filarial patient in Brazil in 1866 and Bancroft, who first described the adult worms in Australia in 1876. The adult female worm measures up to 100 millimetres in length. One of the striking features of these worms is that they are found in the circulating blood in large numbers in the evening, whilst during the day they disappear from the blood-stream. Its geographical distribution is widespread in warm countries, but it is most prevalent in India, South China, South Japan, the Dutch East Indies, and the Pacific islands.

The form of filariasis produced by *W. bancrofti* is characterized by inflammation and blockage of the lymphatics. In the early stages this leads to enlargement of the lymphatic glands. There is also involvement of the testicles, which become painful and enlarged, and this is accompanied by the formation of a hydrocele. Repeated inflammation of the lymphatic vessels ultimately leads to their blockage and this is responsible for the most characteristic of the later stages of the disease – elephantiasis, ie. gross enlargement of the lower limbs and the scrotum. This may be so marked that the leg may attain a circumference of several feet, whilst the scrotum may weigh 50 pounds (23 kg). Elephantiasis may occur elsewhere in the body, eg. the arms, but not very commonly. (See ELEPHANTIASIS.)

Treatment – Encouraging results are being obtained, particularly in early cases, from the use of the piperazine derivative, diethylcarbamazine. Surgery is required for the treatment of elephantiasis. Prevention consists primarily of (*a*) destroying the mosquitoes which transmit the worm, and (*b*) protection of the individual against mosquito bites by the use of mosquito nets and repellents.

FINGERS consist of three bones called phalanges united by hinge-joints and strong ligaments. The thumb, like the great toe, differs from the others in having only two bones. These are bent or flexed, and straightened or extended by powerful sinews, two in front and two behind, which are brought into action by the contraction of muscles in the forearm. The sinews are enveloped in complicated synovial sheaths, through which they slide without friction, and are attached to the bases of the middle and end phalanges, back and front.

Running up each side of each finger are two small arteries and two small nerves, which supply the various structures and especially the overlying skin. The skin of the fingers is specially strong and particularly sensitive, and the end of the finger has a highly specialized part, the nail (see

361

SKIN). Each finger is set upon a bone, the metacarpal, which lies in the substance of the hand between the finger and the carpus or wrist.

FINSEN LIGHT (see LIGHT TREATMENT).

FIRST AID – Courses of instruction in first aid comprise six to twelve sessions, each of about two hours' duration. Syllabuses of instruction are published by various organizations, the principal ones being the British Red Cross Society, the St John Ambulance Association, and the St Andrew's Ambulance Association. For full details reference should be made to the secretary of one of these associations: British Red Cross Society, 9 Grosvenor Crescent, London, S.W.1; St John Ambulance Association, 1 Grosvenor Crescent, London, S.W.1; St Andrew's Ambulance Association 36 Palmerston Place, Edinburgh, 12.

(For subjects connected with first-aid, see under INJURED, REMOVAL OF; BANDAGES; BURNS; CONVULSIONS; DROWNING; FAINTING; FRACTURES; HAEMORRHAGE; NURSING; POISONING; WOUNDS.)

FISH (see DIET; PROTEIN).

FISSURE is a term applied both to clefts of normal anatomical structure and also to small narrow ulcers occurring in skin and mucous membrane. The latter type of fissure occurs especially at the corners of the mouth and at the anus. (See LIPS; and RECTUM, DISEASES OF.)

FISTULA is an unnatural, narrow channel, leading from some natural cavity, such as the duct of a gland, or the interior of the bowels, to the surface. Or it may be a communication between two such cavities, where none should exist, as, for example, a direct communication between the bladder and bowel.

Causes – Sometimes a child is born with a fistula, as a result of some defect in development, for example, a fistula from the thyroid gland to the surface; but, as a rule, the cause of the formation is either disease or injury. Often, the blockage of the duct of a gland leads to a fistula and the escape of the secretion from the gland on to the surface. Thus a salivary fistula may form on the face as a result of blockage by a concretion of the salivary duct in the cheek, and saliva then runs out on the cheek instead of into the mouth. Injury may also be the cause. For example, if the pelvis be fractured, the urethra may be torn across, so that urine, instead of being properly voided, passes among the tissues, and, by a process of suppuration, gradually bursts its way out through the skin, forming a permanent urinary fistula. A fistula from the bowel or bladder occasionally arises in women as a result of injury during protracted child-birth. Disease is another cause; thus an abscess may form at the side of the lower end of the bowel, and, bursting into the bowel on one side, and through the skin on the other, forms a fistula. This fistula in ano forms the best known and most important variety of fistula. The abscess which produces the fistula may be tuberculous or an acute abscess due to other micro-organisms. (See ABSCESS, ACUTE.) Sometimes a fish-bone or pin, which has been swallowed, travels through the whole digestive canal without doing damage, till it reaches this point, where it lodges and produces a fistula.

Treatment – As a rule, a fistula is extremely hard to close, especially after it has persisted for some time. The treatment consists in an operation to restore the natural channel, be it salivary duct, or urethra, or bowel. This is effected by appropriate means in each locality, and when it is attained the fistula heals quickly under simple dressings.

Fistula in ano is a very troublesome condition, and is kept from healing by the constant entrance into it of material from the bowel. It is only to be cured by dividing the tissues which separate it from the bowel, and, each day, after the bowels move, packing the wound in such a way as to compel it to heal gradually from its deepest part. The process of healing is therefore a tedious one.

FIT is a popular name for a sudden convulsive seizure, although the term is also extended to include sudden seizure of every sort. During the occurrence of a fit of any sort the chief object should be to prevent the patient from doing any harm to himself by the convulsive movements, so that the person should be laid flat, and the head supported on a pillow or other soft material. To prevent the tongue from being bitten, some object of moderate hardness may be placed between the teeth. (See APOPLEXY; CONVULSIONS; ECLAMPSIA; EPILEPSY; FAINTING; HYSTERIA; URAEMIA.)

FLAT-FOOT or PES PLANUS, is a deformity of the foot in which its arch sinks down so that the inner edge of the foot comes to rest upon the ground (illustration 200). Flat-foot seldom occurs in active, energetic people, and its presence debars persons from the public services, or even from engagement in positions where physical activity is needed, for example, as sailors.

Causes – Most cases occur in growing and undernourished young men and young women who have much standing on the feet. The ligaments which support the arch are in these persons still soft, the four muscles (two tibial muscles on the inner side, and two peroneal muscles on the outer side) which sling it up become weak or tired, and hence the arch gradually subsides. It also tends to develop in obese middle-aged individuals who have to stand about a great deal without actually exercising the muscles: eg. fat housewives.

200 – Flat-foot showing complete loss of the arch.

Symptoms – There is pain both along the instep and beneath the outer ankle, the foot is stiff and broad, walking is tiresome, and the toes turn far out. The footprints of a flat-foot are broad all the way from toe to heel, instead of being a mere line at the instep. The extent to which the flatness has proceeded may be tested by wetting the bare feet with inky water and causing the person to stand on a piece of clean white paper.

Treatment – Change of occupation to one which allows of sitting is sometimes necessary. In early cases the leg muscles may be strengthened by tiptoe exercises performed for ten minutes night and morning, the legs being thereafter bathed with cold salt water and massaged. This may be enough, or a steel sole, with instep to support the arch, may have to be worn inside the boot. Sponge rubber pads also make an effective, and resilient, support for the arch. In other cases providing the boot with a sole, which is thicker on the inner side of the foot by $\frac{1}{4}$ to $\frac{1}{2}$ an inch (5 to 10 mm) than it is on the outer side, may both relieve discomfort in walking and

help to remedy the flat-foot by throwing the weight of the body on to the outer edge of the foot. The toes should be habitually turned inwards in walking. In very bad cases of long standing it may be necessary either to wrench the foot into position, under a general anaesthetic, and put it in plaster of Paris for a month, or even to remove part of the bone from its inner side, so as to shorter the instep and make a new arch.

FLATULENCE means a collection of gas in the stomach or bowels. In the former case the gas is expelled from time to time in noisy eructations by the mouth; in the latter case it may produce unpleasant rumblings in the bowels, or be expelled from the anus.

Causes – The presence of gas in the stomach has been explained under the heading of ERUCTATION. When gas is found in large amount in the bowels its production is usually due to fermentation set up by bacteria. Marsh gas and hydrogen are formed from the cellulose of vegetables, sulphuretted hydrogen and carbon disulphide from eggs, peas, and other articles of diet containing much sulphur. Many cases of flatulence are much aggravated by a bad habit of gulping mouthfuls of air.

Treatment – Flatulence in the stomach is treated by relieving the dyspepsia which causes it. It may also be relieved, or eased, by the administration of carminatives (qv). In many cases the flatulence is aggravated by a nervous condition which must receive appropriate treatment. If the flatulence is due to, or aggravated by, the habit of swallowing air, the patient must, by taking a careful note of the occasions when he does this almost unconsciously, break himself of this bad habit. When this is done the flatulence often passes off. In cases of intestinal flatulence, articles of diet which tend to decompose, eg. green vegetables and starchy foods, should be avoided, and the food should be light and quickly digestible.

FLAVINE (see ANTISEPTICS).

FLEAS (see INSECTS IN RELATION TO DISEASE).

FLEXIBILITAS CEREA is the term applied to an abnormal state in which the limbs remain in any position into which they are moved.

FLEXION means bending, and is a term applied either to the bending of joints or to an abnormal shape of organs.

FLIES (see INSECTS IN RELATION TO DISEASE).

FLOATING KIDNEY (see KIDNEY, DISEASES OF).

FLOCCITATION means the fitful picking at the bed-clothes by a delirious patient, as, for example, in typhoid fever.

FLOODING is a popular name for an excessive blood-stained discharge from the womb. (See MENSTRUATION.) In the majority of cases flooding is the sign of a miscarriage. (See MISCARRIAGE.)

FLOUR (see BREAD).

FLUCLOXACILLIN (see PENICILLIN).

FLUCTUATION is a sign obtained from collections of fluid by laying the fingers of one hand upon one side of the swelling, and, with those of the other, tapping or pressing suddenly on a distant point of the swelling. The thrill communicated from one hand to the other through the fluid is one of the most important signs of the presence of an abscess, or of effusion of fluid into joints or into the peritoneal cavity.

FLUCYTOSINE is a drug that is proving of value in the treatment of certain fungal infections such as candidiasis (qv) and cryptococcosis (qv).

FLUFENAMIC ACID is a drug with analgesic, anti-inflammatory and anti-pyretic actions which is proving of value in the treatment of osteoarthrosis and rheumatoid arthritis.

FLUKES are a variety of parasitic worms. (See FASCIOLIASIS.)

FLUOCINOLONE is a corticosteroid for application to the skin as a cream, lotion or ointment. It is more potent than hydrocortisone. It must not be given by mouth.

FLUORESCIN is an orange-coloured powder which, dissolved in water, is dropped into the eye in order to detect scratches or ulcers of the cornea.

FLUORINE, one of the halogen series of elements, is one of the constituents of bone and teeth. During recent years evidence has accumulated that supplementing the daily intake of fluorine

diminishes the incidence of dental caries. American and British evidence indicates that people who, throughout their lives, have drunk water with a natural fluorine content of 1 part per million, have less dental caries than those whose drinking-water is fluorine free. All the available evidence indicates that this is the most satisfactory way of giving fluorine, and that if the concentration of fluorine in drinking-water does not exceed 1 part per million, there are no toxic effects.

FLUOROSCOPE is an apparatus for rendering X-rays visible after they have passed through the body by projecting them on a screen of calcium tungstate. The technique of using it is known as FLUORO-SCOPY. It provides a method of being able to watch, for instance, the beating of the heart, or the movements of the intestine after the administration of a barium meal. (See X-RAYS.)

FLUOROURACIL is a drug that is proving of value when given intravenously, in the treatment of recurrent and inoperable carcinoma of the colon and rectum, as well as secondaries from cancer of the breast.

FLUPENTHIXOL is a tranquillizer that is proving of value in the treatment of schizophrenia (qv).

FLUPHENAZINE is one of the phenothiazine derivatives which is proving of value as an anti-psychotic drug.

FLURBIPROFEN is a drug that is proving of value in the treatment of rheumatoid arthritis and ankylosing spondylitis.

FLUSPIRILENE is a tranquillizer that is proving of value in the treatment of schizophrenia (qv). It is given by intramuscular injection, and the effect of one injection lasts for six to fifteen days.

FLUTTER, or ATRIAL FLUTTER, is the term applied to a form of abnormal cardiac rhythm, in which the atria contract at a rate of between 200 and 400 beats a minute, and the ventricles more slowly. The abnormal rhythm is the result of a diseased heart.

FLUX means an excessive discharge from any of the natural openings of the body. 'Bloody flux' is a popular name for dysentery, 'white flux' or 'whites' for leucorrhoea.

FOETOR OF THE BREATH (see
BREATH, DISORDERS OF).

FOETUS, or EMBRYO, is the name given
to the child while still within the womb.
The human being, like the young of all
animals, begins as a single cell, the *ovum*,
in the ovary. After fertilization with a spermatozoon the ovum becomes embedded
in the mucous membrane of the uterus, its
covering being known as the decidua. Increase in size is rapid, and development of
complexity is still more marked. The original cell divides again and again to form
new cells, and these become arranged in
three layers, known as the ectoderm,
mesoderm, and endoderm. From the first
are produced the skin, the brain and
spinal cord, and the nerves; from the
second the bones, muscles, blood-vessels,
and connective tissues; while the third
develops into the lining of the digestive
system and the various glands attached
to it.

The ovum produces not only the foetus
but several membranes and appendages
which serve it till birth, and are then cast
away. The embryo develops upon one side
of the ovum, its first appearance consisting
of a groove, the edges of which grow up
and join to form a tube, which in turn
develops into the brain and spinal cord. At
the same time, a part of the ovum beneath
this is becoming pinched off to form the
body, and within this the endoderm forms
a second tube, which in time is changed in
shape and lengthened to form the digestive canal. From the gut there grows
out very early a process called the allantois, which attaches itself to the wall of the
womb, forming later on the navel-string
and afterbirth, by which nourishment is
gained for growth. (See AFTERBIRTH.)

The remainder of the ovum, which
within two weeks of conception has increased to about $\frac{1}{12}$ inch (2 mm) in size,
splits into an outer and inner shell, from
the outer of which are developed two
covering membranes, the chorion and
amnion, while the inner constitutes the
yolk sac, attached by a pedicle to the
developing gut of the foetus. From two
weeks after conception onward, the various organs and limbs appear and grow,
the name of *embryo* being now applied to
the developing being, while it is almost
indistinguishable in appearance from the
embryo of other animals, till the middle of
the second month, when it begins to show
a distinctly human form. After this stage it
is called the *foetus*. The property of 'life' is
present from the very beginning, although

the movements of the foetus are not felt by
the mother till the fifth month.

During the first few days after conception the eye begins to be formed, beginning as a cup-shaped outgrowth from the
mid-brain, its lens being formed as a thickening in the skin. It is very soon followed
by the beginnings of the nose and ear,
both of which arise as pits on the surface,
which increase in complexity, and are
joined by nerves that grow outward from
the brain. These three organs of sense
have practically their final appearance
as early as the beginning of the second
month.

As already stated, the body closes in
from behind forward, the sides growing
forward from the spinal region. In the
neck, the growth takes the form of five
arches, similar to those which bear gills in
fishes. From the first of these the lower jaw
is formed, from the second the hyoid bone,
all the arches uniting, and the gaps
between them closing up by the end of the
second month. At this time the head and
neck have assumed quite a human
appearance.

The digestive canal, as already stated,
begins as a simple tube running from end
to end of the embryo, but it grows in
length and becomes twisted in various directions to form the stomach and bowels.
From this tube also the lungs and the liver
arise as two little buds, which quickly increase in size and complexity. The kidneys
also appear very early, but go through
several changes before their final form is
reached.

The genital organs appear late. The
swellings, which form the ovary in the
female and the testicle (or testis) in the
male, are produced in the region of the
loins, and gradually descend to their final
positions. The outward organs are exactly
similar in the two sexes till the end of
the third month, and the sex is not clearly
distinguishable till late in the fourth
month.

The blood-vessels appear in the ovum
even before the embryo. The heart, originally double, forms as a dilatation upon
the arteries which later produce the aorta.
These two hearts later fuse into one. (For
the circulation in the foetus, see CIRCULA-
TION OF BLOOD.)

The limbs appear about the end of the
third week as buds which increase quickly
in length and split at their ends into five
parts, for fingers or toes. The bones at first
are formed of cartilage, in which true bone
begins to appear during the third month.

The following table gives the average

365

size and weight of the foetus at different periods:

Age	Length	Weight
4 weeks	5 mm	1·3 grams
3 months	8 to 9 cm	30 to 60 grams
5 months	15 to 25 cm	170 to 340 grams
7 months	32 to 35 cm	1360 to 1820 grams
Birth	45 to 60 cm	3200 grams

Table 26 – Approximate length and weight of the foetus at different periods.

The foetus is legally viable after the end of the 28th week of pregnancy (see BIRTH), when it weighs around 3 pounds (1400 grams), but the number of babies who survive such premature birth is small. Thus, in England in 1977, of the 2471 babies born with a weight of under $3\frac{1}{4}$ pounds (1500) grams), 833 died within 28 days of birth. On the other hand, modern methods of dealing with premature infants are so efficient that babies weighing as little as $1\frac{1}{2}$ pounds (680 grams) have survived.

FOLIC ACID, one of the constituents of the vitamin B complex, derives its name from the fact that it is found in many green leaves, including spinach and grass. It has also been obtained from liver, kidney, and yeasts. In 1945 it was synthesized by American workers, who proposed that the chemical name should be pteroylglutamic acid. It has proved of value in the treatment of macrocytic anaemias, particularly those associated with sprue and nutritional deficiencies. It also relieves pernicious anaemia but does not prevent the onset of the nervous complications of this disease, namely, subacute combined degeneration of the cord. It should therefore never be used in the treatment of pernicious anaemia.

FOLIUM is the latin term for leaf: eg. digitalis folium is digitalis leaf. (Plural: folia.)

FOLLICLE is the term applied to a very small sac or gland: eg. small collections of adenoid tissue in the throat and the small digestive glands on the mucous membrane of the intestine.

FOLLICULAR HORMONE (see OESTRADIOL).

FOMENTATION (see also POULTICES) is the term applied to any warm application to the surface of the body in the form of a cloth. Usually the fomentation cloth is heated by being wrung out of hot water, but the term is also applied to dry applications and to hot cloths upon which various drugs are sprinkled. A fomentation dilates the blood-vessels of the part to which it is applied and has a soothing effect upon the endings of the nerves, so that it both aids the absorption of effusions and relieves pain. In the case of superficial abscesses it softens the skin and helps the abscess to 'point'.

Method of preparation – HOT MOIST FOMENTATIONS are made as follows. The requisites are a piece of flannel sufficiently large when folded double to cover the part to which it is desired to apply heat, a towel, a basin, a kettle of boiling water, a piece of jaconet slightly larger than the fomentation, a layer of cotton-wool to cover the fomentation, and a binder with safety pins (illustration 201). The towel is placed open across the basin; the fomentation flannel is laid upon the towel and pressed down into the basin; boiling water is then poured from the kettle upon the fomentation cloth until it is well soaked (illustration 202); the ends of the towel are then twisted firmly in opposite directions by the hands holding its dry ends; and the hot water is thus squeezed out of the fomentation cloth (illustrations 203, 204). The towel is now untwisted, the fomentation cloth is shaken out flat, so as to admit air between its folds (illustration 205), and laid upon the jaconet, which in turn is laid on the layer of cotton-wool (illustration 206). The whole is now laid upon the body with the fomentation cloth against the skin, and is fixed in place with the binder and safety pins. The preparation of the fomentation should be carried out at the bedside, so that it does not cool unduly before being applied. If the fomentation is large, it may be found more convenient to use a roller towel and to twist it up by passing a couple of sticks through each end. Instead of the cotton-wool and binder a large bath towel may be used to keep the fomentation in contact with the body. The fomentation retains its heat only a short time, and, if it is to be renewed, this should be done about every twenty minutes.

TURPENTINE FOMENTATION – This is also known as a stupe. It is prepared in the same way as the hot fomentation, but, in addition, after the boiling water is poured on the cloth and before it is wrung out, a few teaspoonfuls of turpentine are sprinkled on the cloth.

LAUDANUM FOMENTATION – This may be prepared in the same way as the hot fomentation, with the addition that, after

201 – Requisites for a hot fomentation.

205 – Shaking the fomentation cloth to admit air between folds.

206 – Fomentation cloth laid on jaconet (or mackintosh), which is laid on cotton-wool. Ready to apply and fix with flannel binder.

202 – Fomentation cloth laid on towel in bottom of basin; boiling water poured on fomentation cloth.

203 – Towel twisted round fomentation cloth.

204 – Wringing out the hot water.

the cloth is wrung out and just before the fomentation is applied, two or three teaspoonfuls of laudanum are sprinkled over its surface. Another method of preparing this soothing fomentation is to take half a dozen dried poppy heads, break them up and boil them with $1\frac{1}{2}$ pints (850 ml) of water in a saucepan for twenty minutes, and then, proceeding as before, to pour the water from the saucepan through a strainer on to the fomentation cloth as it lies on the towel in the basin.

COLD-WATER DRESSINGS are sometimes also known as fomentations because they become gradually warmed by the heat of the body. They are prepared by dipping a piece of lint in saturated boric acid lotion or other weak antiseptic, applying to the part, and then covering with a piece of gutta-percha tissue or oiled silk which is larger than the piece of lint and projects at least half an inch beyond it all round.

DRY FOMENTATION – This is made by toasting a piece of thick flannel in front of the fire and laying it on the part to be fomented, covering with a thick layer of cotton-wool and on the outside a hot-water bag. This does not retain its heat for long, but the heat is longer retained by a flannel bag containing salt or bran which is warmed and applied in a similar manner. Flat india-rubber bags, 'thermophores', which retain their heat for many hours, contain a mixture of salts which

367

liquefies when the bag is boiled. The bag is boiled for a few minutes in a kettle each time it is required, and then applied and covered with cotton-wool. These dry applications are very useful for relieving the pain of colic, neuralgia, and the like. An ordinary rubber hot-water bottle, of course, is often as effective a method of applying heat as any.

FOMITES is a term used to include all articles which have been brought into sufficiently close contact with a person sick of some infectious disease to retain the infective material and spread the disease. For example, clothes, bedding, carpets, toys, books, may all be fomites till disinfected.

FONTANELLE is the term applied to areas on the head on which bone has not yet formed. The chief of these is the anterior fontanelle, situated on the top of the head between the frontal and two parietal bones. In shape it is four-sided, about an inch square (25 mm) in size at the time of birth, gradually diminishing until it is completely covered by bone, which should happen by the age of 18 months. The pulsations of the brain can be readily felt through it. Delay in its closure is particularly found in cases of rickets, as well as in other states of defective development. The fontanelle becomes more tense than usual in acute fevers, whooping-cough, and bronchitis, and tends to bulge in cases of hydrocephalus. It becomes unusually depressed in all cases of diminished vitality, such as that due to diarrhoea or wasting from any cause.

FOOD (see ADULTERATION OF FOODS; BREAD; CANNED FOODS; CEREAL; DIET; DIGESTION; FAT; FEEDING; INFANT-FEEDING; MILK; PROTEIN; FRUIT; VITAMIN).

FOOD POISONING is characterized as a rule by vomiting, diarrhoea, and abdominal pain, the result of eating food contaminated with metallic or chemical poisons, or with bacteria, or with the toxins of bacteria; or as a result of eating poisonous 'foods', such as poisonous mushrooms. (See FUNGUS-POISONING.) One of the characteristics of food poisoning due to chemical or metallic causes is its relatively quick onset – within ten minutes to ten hours of eating the food.

Bacterial food poisoning is now what is commonly meant by the term 'food poisoning'. It comprises those conditions formerly and erroneously described as 'ptomaine poisoning'. The gravest, and fortunately the rarest, form of food poisoning is botulism (qv).

In staphylococcal food poisoning, certain staphylococci produce in the food they contaminate an enterotoxin which after ingestion makes the consumer suddenly ill within a matter of one to six hours, with vomiting, diarrhoea, and abdominal pain. The staphylococci themselves do not act thus on ingestion; it is the preformed toxin which is noxious. Contamination of food with staphylococci can usually be traced to faulty handling and is usually human in origin. Foods, such as meat products (often cold meat served as sandwiches), milk, custard, and egg products, can be contaminated either before or after cooking. As the toxin produced by the *Staphylococcus aureus* is heat resistant, subsequent cooking will not make the toxin-contaminated food safe.

Many cases of food poisoning are caused by infection with one of a group of bacteria belonging to the genus *Salmonella*. *Salmonella typhimurium* is responsible for 65 to 70 per cent of all outbreaks of food poisoning due to salmonellae. Other salmonellae commonly involved are *Salmonella bredeny*, *Salmonella enteritidis*, *Salmonella heidelberg*, *Salmonella newport*, *Salmonella stanley*, and *Salmonella thompson*. Salmonellae are found in all foods of animal origin: meats, meat products (such as pies), soups, milk, eggs and foods such as custards and cream cakes in which the egg products are only partially cooked. The onset of food poisoning due to salmonellae occurs twelve to forty-eight hours after eating the contaminated food.

Salmonella infections are common in pigs, sheep, rabbits, cattle, rats, mice, dogs, and cats. If a cow is infected with a *Salmonella* – eg. *S. enteritidis* – the organism may get into the milk, and the consumer of the milk suffer from food poisoning. Food may become infected by the excreta of rats or mice. Ducks are susceptible to *Salmonella* infections, especially *S. typhimurium*, and the organism may get into the duck's egg – an occasional source of human infection. Most types of salmonella are killed by heating to 60°C for fifteen minutes, but a much higher temperature is required for much longer to ensure that the temperature is raised throughout the whole of the food being cooked. Thus, a sausage taken from the deep freeze and gently fried on all sides may still show spicules of ice in the centre. It is therefore essential to ensure that frozen food is well thawed before being cooked. In practice this means that a frozen chicken needs twelve hours to thaw out, and a large turkey twice as long, while roasting requires a temperature of 375° to 400°C in the oven and twenty minutes per pound of bird.

In recent years an increasing number of outbreaks of food poisoning have been due to *Clostridium welchii*. This is a common cause of food poisoning in communal feeding establishments, and is usually associated with meat dishes, soups or gravy, which have been cooked the day before consumption. To reduce the incidence of this form of food poisoning, the pre-cooked dish must be rapidly cooled, kept in a refrigerator overnight, and when reheated it must be cooked as thoroughly as if it were raw meat. This type of food poisoning comes on eight to twenty-four hours after eating the contaminated food.

Food poisoning is now a notifiable disease. In 1976, 11,912 cases were notified in England, but this is only a fraction of the total number of cases that must occur. Of these, 69 per cent were due to *Salmonellae*, 15 per cent to *C. welchii* and 3 per cent to staphylococci. Regulations are also now in force that lay down requirements relating to the construction of, and equipment used in, food premises, the transport of certain foods, the temperature at which food must be stored, and regulations relating to food handlers in food businesses. Thus, food handlers who are suffering from, or are carriers of, a salmonella infection including typhoid and paratyphoid), or who have a staphylococcal infection likely to cause food poisoning must be reported to the local district community physician. Such individuals can be suspended from work as food handlers and in certain circumstances they can be allowed compensation for loss of wages.

FOOT is that portion of the lower limb situated below the ankle-joint. Its structure (illustration 207) is very similar to that of the hand. There are seven tarsal bones, of which the talus, supporting the leg bones, and the calcaneus, forming the heel, are the largest. The others are the navicular, three cuneiform, and the cuboid bones. Then comes a row of five metatarsal bones (known together as the metatarsus), and finally fourteen phalanges contained in the toes, the great toe having two only, while each of the others has three. The arrangement of the arteries (illustration 208) and nerves is similar to that found in the hand and fingers.

The arch of the foot is a most important structure. The bones are so arranged that

207 – Bones of the foot as seen from above ie. superior aspect.

208 – Arteries of the foot. From Passmore and Robson. *A Companion to Medical Studies.* Backwell Scientific Publications.

the sole is hollow both from before back and from side to side. In walking, the outer edge only, at the middle of the sole, should touch the ground. The arch is further supported by a short plantar ligament situated in the hollow of the arch, running from the calcaneus to the cuboid bone, and by a long plantar ligament situated nearer the surface. It is also slung up by two sinews on either side, coming from muscles in the leg, the two tibial muscles on the inner side, and the two peroneal muscles on the outer side. When this arch gives way, flat-foot is the result. (See FLAT-FOOT.)

For diseases of the foot see BONES, DISEASES OF; CHAFING OF THE SKIN; CHILBLAINS; CLAW-FOOT; CLEFT-FOOT; CLUB-FOOT; CORNS AND BUNIONS; DROP-FOOT;

FLAT-FOOT; GOUT; HALLUX RIGIDUS; HALLUX VALGUS; MALLET TOE; METATARSUS VARUS; METATARSALGIA; NAIL.

FORAMEN is the Latin term for a hole. It is especially applied to natural openings in bones, such as the foramen magnum, the large opening in the base of the skull through which the brain and spinal cord are continuous.

FORCED FEEDING (see GAVAGE).

FOREHEAD (see FRONTAL BONE).

FORGETFULNESS in many people is an inborn misfortune, in others it arises as the result of some disease. Memory is defined by William James as 'the knowledge of an event or fact, of which meantime we have not been thinking, with the additional consciousness that we have thought or experienced it before'. This process necessitates two things: the retention of an event and the reproduction of it, both depending upon the same process in the nervous system. In this system there are, according to Meynert, some 600,000,000 nerve-cells. These are united together by numberless nerve-fibres into countless combinations. When a sensation affects the brain it influences certain of these groups, and if the sensation be very powerful or very often repeated the groups of associated nerve-cells develop a habit of acting in concert and tend, upon future stimulation by any means, to reproduce this sensation in its entirety. This process is known as association, and the multitudinous fibres which connect cell with cell and group with group, forming the chief bulk of the brain, are known as association fibres.

Sound memory depends upon the rational grouping of ideas of things in the mind, so that one may call up the other, and the man who thinks most over the occurrences of his daily life will, other things being equal, have the best memory. No training will make up for a deficiency of nerve-cells or association fibres, which are inborn characters.

For good memory of important facts, a certain amount of forgetfulness is necessary. Facts in the past should become 'foreshortened', so to speak, and the inability to recount an incident without going over all its petty details forms a type of mental weakness. For this purpose, mental relaxation and change of employment are just as necessary as the quiet pondering over past events that leads to their classification and orderly retention.

According to modern psychological theory, forgetting is often an active process. Painful memories may be repressed out of consciousness, and, buried in the 'unconscious mind', may be the source of anxiety and neurotic behaviour.

There are certain changes in which memory becomes impaired. Chief among these is old age. (See AGE, NATURAL CHANGES IN.) In the old man's memory the events of yesterday are a blank, and only the events of youth, and later of childhood, forgotten in busy middle age, are again brought to light, all, however, crumbling and half rubbed away. When this defect is extreme it is due to degenerative changes in the old man's arteries and brain. Apoplexy is another cause either of permanent impairment (see APHASIA) or, in slighter cases, of frequent losses of memory which occur in old people, and last a few hours or a few days. In hypnotism and various mental diseases, especially dementia, curious vagaries occur. Concussion of the brain, too, may produce at first total unconsciousness, followed by partial loss of memory, lasting for some time. (See BRAIN, DISEASES AND INJURIES OF.)

Treatment – For improving the memory there are three methods.

Judicious methods are those of classification, repeated presentation of facts to be remembered in different guises, and the formation of numerous connecting links between these facts and facts already in the mind. This method is exemplified in all the sciences, and lies at the root of present-day school-teaching.

Mechanical methods are sometimes useful in remembering new facts. For example, little children are taught to read in unison words or figures clearly written on the blackboard, so that ideas of these entering by the channels of eye, ear, and muscular sense may form on the brain deep impressions upon which future memories can be built. Similarly, a person, hearing a new name, repeats it several times, so that it may make a lasting impression upon his brain-cells.

Artificial memories (*memoriae technicae*) are often constructed by persons who have either very few facts in mind with which to form new associations, or who wish in a short time, and for a special purpose, such as an examination, to remember certain facts, and then blot out the whole as a useless encumbrance of memory.

FORMALDEHYDE – The *British Pharmacopoeia* preparation, Formaldehyde Solution, also known as FORMALIN, contains 34 to 38 per cent formaldehyde in water. It is a powerful antiseptic, and has also the power of hardening the tissues. The vapour is very irritating to the eyes and nose.

Uses – For disinfection it is largely used in the form of a spray. It can also be vaporized by heat. One of its advantages for this purpose is that it does not damage metals or fabrics. In 3 per cent solution in water it is used for the treatment of warts on the palms of the hands and the soles of the feet.

FOSSA is a term applied to various depressions or holes, both on the surface of the body and in internal parts, such as the iliac fossa in each lower corner of the abdomen, and the fossae within the skull which lodge the different parts of the brain.

FOWLER'S SOLUTION is another name for ARSENICAL SOLUTION which contains arsenic and is a colourless, odourless fluid. The dose is 2 to 8 minims (0·12 to 0·47 ml).

FOXGLOVE (see DIGITALIS).

FRACTURES are breaches in the structure of bones produced by violence.

Varieties – The great division of fractures is into those which are simple and those which are compound. (See also MARCH FRACTURE.)

SIMPLE FRACTURES form the commonest variety, consisting of those in which the bone is broken, with or without much laceration of the surrounding parts, but in which there is no wound leading from the fracture through the skin.

COMPOUND or OPEN FRACTURES are those in which the skin is injured, so that a wound leads from the outer air to the broken bone, which may indeed protrude through this wound. The fact that a fracture is compound renders it very much more serious, even though there be little splintering of the bone or laceration of the soft tissues. The special dangers attending compound fractures are as follows. The injury is apt to be much more serious than in simple fracture, and a large quantity of blood may be lost. The union of the bone is delayed, repair taking place by a much slower process when there is an open wound, and a lengthy illness is the result. The greatest danger, however, is

that the wound may become infected with virulent micro-organisms, so that suppuration or blood-poisoning may ensue, and amputation of the limb may even become necessary. For all these reasons the greatest care is necessary in handling a fractured limb, so that a simple fracture may not be converted into a compound one.

COMPLETE FRACTURES are those in which the bone is broken completely across, and no connection left between the pieces.

INCOMPLETE FRACTURES are those in which the bone is broken only partly across, or in which the periosteum, the tough membrane surrounding the bone, is not torn. This variety occurs in children, whose bones contain more fibrous material and less bone earth than those of old people, a fact which renders them tougher and more pliant in earlier life. A child's bone may, like a twig, crack half-way across and then split some distance up its length, suffering in this way what is called a 'greenstick' fracture.

FISSURED FRACTURES are mere cracks in the bone, and are found commonly in the skull.

DEPRESSED FRACTURES occur generally on the skull, and consist of fractures in which a fragment of bone is forced inwards below the general level. This may give rise to interference with the brain, either when the fracture is produced or at a later date from thickening consequent on repair of the bone.

COMPLICATED FRACTURES are those in which, in addition to the fracture, some other serious injury is produced: eg. a dislocation, or tearing of a nerve.

COMMINUTED FRACTURES are those in which there is much splintering.

IMPACTED FRACTURES are those in which, after the break has occurred, one fragment is jammed inside the other, usually at an angle.

UNUNITED FRACTURES are those in which, after the time has elapsed in which the fracture usually mends, it is found that union has not taken place. The failure to unite may be simply due to delayed union, in which the process of repair is proceeding slowly on account of ill-health, or of damage to the chief artery which supplies the bone with blood, or usually in consequence of the fact that the fractured limb is not kept sufficiently at rest. Or there may be actual failure of the healing process to take place. In the latter case the ends of the bone are thoroughly rubbed together under a general anaesthetic, and the fracture again set. If this produces no good effect, an operation is usually performed in order to remove any piece of muscle which may have got between the ends, or to fasten the ends with wire or with metal plates.

MALUNITED FRACTURES are those which have not been properly set, or in which displacement occurs after setting, so that the bone is twisted, or united with a neighbouring bone, as sometimes happens after fracture of the forearm, or is enlarged and shortened, or does not unite by bone, but forms what is known as a 'false-joint'. Sometimes malunion is unavoidable, owing to spasm of muscles or to production of an excessive amount of new bone.

Causes – Certain causes render some persons more liable than others to fracture of bones. Of these, far the most important is old age. The bones decrease in thickness after middle age, the fibrous tissue composing them becomes less resilient, and there is an increase of the merely earthy part - facts which all tend to produce increasing brittleness. In old age, a fall upon a hard surface, even a moderate strain like that of jumping off a moving vehicle, is apt to be followed by a fracture. Rickets, tuberculosis of bones, osteomalacia, and malignant disease all render the bones more easily broken. Apart from these causes, fractures are due to force, which may be applied in three ways.

DIRECT VIOLENCE, as, for example, the blow of a hammer or crush of a wheel, may cause a fracture, and in such a case the fracture is apt to be a compound one, or attended by serious complications, such as damage to the brain where the skull is fractured, or to the lungs in fracture of the ribs.

INDIRECT VIOLENCE is the most common cause. In this case the violence is applied at some distance from the seat of the fracture, and whether a fracture or a dislocation occurs depends upon the point which in the circumstances is weakest and exposed to most stress. Thus a fall on the palm of the hand may cause a Colles's fracture at the wrist, or dislocation of the shoulder, or fracture of the collar-bone, according to the position of the arm. Similarly, a twist of the foot may cause fracture of the leg, as well as other injuries.

MUSCULAR ACTION in rare cases produces fracture. The most common example is fracture of the knee-cap, which may be snapped across the end of the thigh-bone in the sudden pull given to recover the balance after missing a step on a flight of stairs. Throwing a cricket ball has also been known to fracture the arm.

Symptoms and signs – *Uselessness of the part* is the main symptom, if the fracture affects a limb. If the lower limb be affected, it is useless for support; if the upper limb, the part beyond the fracture cannot be raised. *Pain* is a variable sign. So long as the affected part remains at rest, it is generally slight; movement, however, is apt to be painful. In fracture of the ribs, the moderate movements of tranquil respiration are free from pain, whilst a deep breath or squeezing of the chest causes considerable pain. *The sound of a crack* is sometimes heard, or the sensation of something giving way may be experienced by the injured person at the moment of the accident, but this is not a reliable symptom, because it occurs also when a muscle or sinew is torn. *Deformity* is found at the site of fracture. There is *shortening* of' the limb in consequence of contraction of the muscles which pass over the fracture. There is also *swelling*, partly owing to the overlapping of the ends of the bone, partly in consequence of the blood and lymph which are at once poured out from the torn vessels around the injury. *Unnatural mobility* is also found, the limb giving way at a point where it should be rigid. *Crepitus* or grating is the final and only certain sign of fracture, experienced when the ends are rubbed together. It should never be felt for except by skilled hands, since much damage can be done by the sharp broken ends of bone to surrounding structures.

Healing of fractures – When the bone breaks, many vessels both in its substance and in the periosteum are torn, and accordingly a large clot of blood forms around the ends, between them, and for some distance up the inside of the bone. Later, great numbers of white corpuscles find their way into this clot, which becomes organized, blood-vessels and, later, fibrous tissue being formed in it (soft callus). Next lime-salts are gradually deposited in this fibrous tissue, which thus develops into bone (hard callus). In this process a thick ring of new bone forms round the broken ends, filling up all crevices, and when union is complete this thickening is again gradually absorbed, leaving the bone as it was before the injury. When the fragments have not been properly set, but allowed to remain overlapping, considerable thickening remains, the ring of new bone being permanent for the sake of strength.

Treatment – After the fracture has been

recognized, a certain amount of temporary treatment is advisable till the broken bone can be properly fixed in place by a surgeon, and in the following descriptions the temporary treatment will be given, short reference being made to the permanent treatment where it differs from the temporary.

A compound fracture is treated first of all as a wound (see WOUNDS) by cleansing and by dressings, and then as a simple fracture. It is particularly necessary that the skin around should be well cleansed, and the wound itself is often very dirty. A thorough washing and scrubbing of the wound, under an anaesthetic, is usually

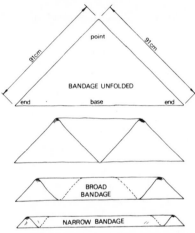

209 – Triangular bandage. The narrow cravat is the form into which it is folded for fixing splints.

necessary, and some surgeons fasten the fragments with silver wire or plates.

For temporary treatment the splints, etc., may be applied above the clothes in the case of simple fractures, and little padding is then necessary. But, for a compound fracture, the limb must be exposed, the wound dressed, and then the splints have to be carefully padded.

For permanent treatment, the fracture must first of all be 'reduced': ie. the broken ends must be brought accurately together; then it must be 'set': ie. the ends firmly fixed in good position; and finally it must be kept at rest, with attention to the patient's general health, till union has taken place. Reduction is effected usually by one person, who pulls gently and steadily upon that part of the limb beyond the fracture (extension), so as to overcome the shortening and bring the ends a little

apart from one another, in order to prevent grating, and so avoid pain. At the same time, a second person should steady the limb above the seat of fracture (counter-extension). This he maintains while a third person applies the necessary splints, bandages, etc. For keeping the bone in position, various devices, such as bandages, plaster, cradles, splints of wood, leather, or poroplastic felt, sandbags, and extension by weight and pulley are adopted in different cases. Splints are generally made from strips of wood, about $\frac{1}{4}$ inch (6 mm) thick, but they may be improvised from bundles of twigs, broomhandles, rifles, folded-up newspapers, and many other rigid articles. Care must be taken, especially in old people confined to bed for a fracture, that no bed sores form. In the case of fracture of the lower limbs it is a general practice to keep the person in bed with the limb fixed by ordinary splints for two or three weeks, and then to apply a case of plaster of Paris to the whole limb, and allow the patient to get up and go about with crutches.

For bandages to fix splints, one uses either a strip of calico bandage 3 inches (7·5 cm) wide or an Esmarch's triangular bandage folded narrow. The latter (illustration 209) is a triangle made by cutting a yard of calico across from corner to corner (so as to form two pieces), and then doubling in the point of the triangle three times, so as to form a sort of flat cravat. (See BANDAGES.)

COLLAR-BONE – This bone is apt to be fractured by falls on the hand, or by blows or falls on the point of the shoulder. As it supports the weight of the arm to a large extent, and gives squareness to the shoulder, when it is broken the shoulder droops downwards, forwards, and inwards towards the chest. On account of the shortness of the bone, splints are useless, and the deformity is remedied by bandages. These are applied in many different ways, of which the following is one of the simplest (illustration 210a, b). A pad of cloth or wool, the size of the fist, is first placed high up in the armpit, and the elbow is bent so that the arm lies across the chest. An unfolded triangular bandage is then placed on the chest with one end over the sound shoulder, the base running down over the elbow of the injured arm, and the point of the bandage lying on the front of the chest. The other end, which is hanging down, is brought up behind the elbow of the injured arm, carried up across the back, and tied as tightly as possible to the first-mentioned end behind the neck. The point

211 – Alternative method of treatment of fractured collar-bone, with two triangles folded narrow.

210 – Treatment of fractured collar-bone. *a*, Sling applied; *b*, finished.

212 – Treatment of fractured humerus, with two splints, two ties, and narrow sling.

of the bandage hanging loose beneath the wrist is folded up round the wrist and pinned to the bandage above it. Finally a triangular bandage, folded narrow, is carried round the chest and elbow of the injured arm and tied tightly, thus levering the shoulder outwards round the pad in the armpit. After this bandage is applied, there is a special necessity to feel that the pulse is not stopped by its tightness. Instead of this sling and narrow-folded bandage, one may use a couple of narrow-folded bandages similarly applied with a pad (illustration 211).

The permanent treatment is usually carried out by a roller bandage applied in somewhat the same way, or by broad strips of plaster, or by a figure-of-eight bandage passing in front of the shoulders and crossing between the shoulder-blades, the arm then being supported by a triangular sling tied over the opposite shoulder.

The fractured bone is fairly strong in three weeks, and the bandage can then be

374

discarded. During this three-week period the fingers, wrist and elbow must be exercised regularly every day.

UPPER ARM – This fracture is usually due to a direct blow, and is easily recognized. For setting, two splints, 2 to 3 inches (5 to 7·5 cm) wide, and long enough to reach, the one from the armpit, the other from the shoulder, to beneath the elbow, are taken and well padded (illustration 212). The forearm being laid across the chest, one splint is applied to the front of, the other behind, the upper arm, and fixed by two ties, the first above, the second below, the site of fracture. A narrow sling is then applied to support the wrist.

This fracture takes up to ten weeks to

mend. The permanent treatment is similar, with the arm splinterd by Gooch splintering or a plaster of Paris splint which fixes the elbow. The wrist is supported by a collar and cuff sling.

FRACTURES NEAR ELBOW – These all cause great swelling as they implicate the joint more or less, and it is usually very difficult to recognize the precise nature of the injury. The temporary treatment of all is the same. An L-shaped, or rectangular, splint 3 inches (7·5 cm) wide, and resembling a mason's 'square', is used, one limb being long enough to reach from the tips

213 – Treatment of injuries near elbow, with L-shaped splint and two ties.

of the fingers to the elbow, the other from the elbow to the armpit (illustration 213). It is fastened to the inside of the arm and forearm by one tie round the hand and round the forearm, and one round the upper arm. A broad sling is applied to support the forearm.

For permanent treatment, the same plan is very satisfactory and is often adopted, though it is more common to fix the arm in plaster of Paris. Sometimes the elbow is bent as far up as possible and tightly bandaged in this position. When the fracture consists in the chipping off of the olecranon process of the ulna, ie. the point of the elbow, as tends to happen in a fall on the bent elbow, the fragment may be drawn upwards by the triceps muscle, leaving a distinct gap behind the elbow. To correct this an operation is necessary to fix the fragment to the ulna by means of a silver wire or screw. If there is no such displacement, then all that is necessary is a bandage and a sling.

All fractures round the joint are apt to cause some permanent stiffness, and in order to lessen the risk of this the patient is encouraged to move the joint after three or four weeks, in order to prevent adhesions forming.

FOREARM – One or both bones may be broken by a blow or fall, and the condition is easily recognized. For treatment the forearm is laid across the chest with the thumb upwards (illustration 214). Two splints, at least 4 inches (10 cm) wide, and long enough to reach from the elbow to beyond the tips of the fingers, are well padded (especially down the centre) and placed one behind and one in front of the forearm. The splints are fixed by one tie round the hand and wrist, and another above the fracture.

214 – Treatment of fractured forearm, with two splints, two ties, and broad forearm sling.

A rectangular splint, similar to that used for fractures about the elbow, is applied to prevent movement at this joint, though not absolutely essential in the temporary treatment, and finally a broad sling to support the forearm.

This fracture is put up for permanent treatment in precisely the same way in plaster of Paris. It takes about the same time to heal as a fracture in the upper arm. There is a danger that the movements of turning the hand palm up and palm down (pronation and supination) may be permanently interfered with by malposition of the bones, unless the fracture be very carefully set.

WRIST – Fracture of the radius close to the wrist, known as Colles's fracture, is a common result of a fall on the palm of the hand. The forearm and hand present a peculiar 'dinner-fork' bend, in consequence of the lower fragment turning upwards and backwards. The temporary treatment is similar to that for fractures of the forearm higher up. For permanent treatment, the

375

forearm is fixed in plaster of Paris with the wrist flexed and the fingers and thumb free.

The danger of stiffness, after union has taken place, is even greater here than in fractures near the elbow, and is prevented by similar means.

HAND AND FINGERS – A splint is laid along the palm, reaching from the tips of the fingers to the elbow, and the hand and forearm are bandaged to it, or the fist is closed on a thick pad and tightly bandaged in this position. A sling is then applied. The fingers mend quickly.

THIGH – In all fractures of the upper limb the person is usually allowed to go about while he is wearing the splints, but in all fractures of the lower limb he lies in bed. Fracture of the neck of the thigh-bone, or femur, is a specially common accident in old people, following upon falls on stairs or ice, but in the young this strong bone is broken only by great violence. There are complete inability to move the limb, shortening amounting to 2 or 3 inches (5 to 7·5 cm) on comparison with the other limb, and rotation outwards of the foot. For treatment a long splint, reaching from the armpit down to below the foot, is laid along the side (illustration 215), and three shorter splints reaching from the groin to the knee may be laid, one in front, one on the inner side, and one behind the thigh, but are not essential for treatment. The long splint, if no regular splint be procurable, may be easily improvised from a broom-handle (illustration 216), plank, or rifle. These splints are fixed by the following ties. One broad band, for example a bolster case, round the chest, with or without a narrow-folded bandage round the hips; two ties round the thigh, one above and one below the fracture, fixing the short splints; two narrow ties round the leg below the knee. Finally, the feet are tied together.

The permanent treatment varies with the site of the fracture. If it is in what is known as the neck of the fracture – ie. at the very upper end of the femur – the usual procedure is to fix the fragments internally by a metallic device. After operation the patient is allowed to move about freely in bed for a few days, and then allowed up on a couch. Walking with a crutch is allowed in a few weeks, but weight-bearing is not allowed for three months. If the fracture is in the shaft of the femur the usual form of treatment is to reduce the fracture – ie. get the two pieces of bone into alignment – and then hold them there by fixing the leg in a Thomas's splint and applying traction

215 – Treatment of fractured thigh with Liston's long splint: (1) shows ties by which extension is effected, the foot being secured first and the upper tie gradually tightened through two holes in the upper end of the splint; (2) shows arrangement complete.

216 – Fractured thigh secured by means of a broom, and tying of legs together.

217 – Treatment of injuries about the knee, with splint and three ties.

to the lower part. Firm union of the fracture takes twelve to sixteen weeks.

KNEE-CAP – This bone is seldom fractured. A long splint is laid along the back of the limb and fixed by ties to thigh and leg. The fragments of the knee-cap may be fixed together by a bandage passing round above the knee-cap, crossing behind the joint, and then passing round below the knee-cap (illustration 217).

It is extremely difficult to get good bony union, and for the permanent treatment most surgeons prefer to cut in to the fracture and unite the fragments with silver wire.

LEG – There is particular need for care in the handling of this fracture, because the tibia, or shin-bone, which lies in its whole length just beneath the skin, usually breaks with a sharp-pointed end, like a pen-nib, that is very readily pushed through the skin, thus making the fracture compound. Two splints, about 4 inches (10 cm) wide, and long enough to reach from a few inches above the knee to beyond the foot, are carefully padded, above and below the

218 – Treatment of fracture of the leg, with two splints and three ties; the two limbs are afterwards tied together, as in illustration 216. *a* shows the method of pushing through the ties so as not to jerk the limb. A second pair of hands should be shown applying extension to the foot, but for clearness are omitted. *b* shows setting finished.

knee-joint, and above and below the ankle-joint, so as to prevent them from pressing upon the skin where the bone lies just beneath (illustration 218). They are applied one along the outer, one along the inner side of the leg, and fixed with two ties, one above and one below the fracture. A third tie is applied above the knee to fix this joint, and the feet are finally tied together.

For permanent treatment the leg is encased in plaster of Paris after reduction of the fracture, with the plaster extending half-way up the thigh. Care must be taken to ensure that the foot is fixed in the position of dorsiflexion: ie. bent upwards. The plaster is kept on for eight to twelve weeks but, if all goes well, walking is encouraged after two or three weeks. A careful watch must be kept of the foot, to ensure that the plaster is not interfering with the circulation to the foot.

Fracture of the fibula, the slender bone on the outer side of the leg, may take place in consequence of a kick or twist of the foot, while the tibia is uninjured. If the fracture occurs in the middle or upper part of the fibula the person may be quite able to walk, though with considerable pain. If, however, the fracture occurs at the lower end of the fibula, it is more likely to be due to indirect violence to the foot as a result of severe strains. This injury, which is one of those included under the term, 'Pott's fracture' is accompanied by considerable tearing of the ligaments on the inner side of the ankle-joint. The temporary

treatment is as for fracture of both bones. Permanent treatment consists of applying plaster of Paris – from below the knee downwards. In the case of a fracture of the fibula alone this is worn for three weeks. In the case of a Pott's fracture it is worn for six to ten weeks.

PELVIS – The bones of the pelvis are broken only by excessive violence, such as a crush from the wheel of a heavily laden cart, a fall of coal in a mine, and the like. For temporary treatment the injured person should have a broad binder fastened round the hips and be lifted on a rug or shutter. The seriousness depends upon the extent of damage done to internal organs.

RIBS are commonly fractured by a blow or kick on the side. If only one or two be broken and the fracture be simple and uncomplicated, the accident is comparatively trivial but painful. The traditional treatment of restricting movement of the chest by a broad bandage or strips of sticking plaster has largely been given up, and all that is considered necessary is the taking of pain-relieving drugs such as aspirin. If this does not suffice, a local anaesthetic may be injected by a doctor. The ribs usually heal fairly quickly, those above and below the broken ribs acting as splints If the injured person spits up blood after the injury the condition is serious, this being a sign that the broken ribs have pierced the pleura and wounded the lung.

SPINAL COLUMN – Mere damage to the bone, as in the case of the so-called com-

Compression Fracture

219 – Injury to the spine: compression fracture with no involvement of spinal cord. Dotted lines indicate outline of undamaged spinal cord. From Illingworth, *A Short Textbook of Surgery*, 9th edition. Churchill Livingstone.

Fracture Dislocation

220 – Injury to the spine: fracture-dislocation with cord involvement. Dotted lines indicate outline of damaged spinal cord. From Illingworth, *A Short Textbook of Surgery*, 9th edition. Churchill Livingstone.

pression fracture (illustration 219), in which there is no damage to the spinal cord, is not necessarily serious. If, however, the spinal cord is damaged, as in the so-called fracture dislocation (illustration 220), the accident may be a very serious one, the usual result being paralysis of the parts of the body below the level of the injury. Therefore the higher up the spine is fractured, the more serious the consequences. The injured person should not be moved till medical assistance is at hand, or, if he must be removed, this should be done on a rigid shutter or door, not on a canvas stretcher or rug, and there should be no lifting which necessitates bending of the back. In such an injury an operation designed to remove a displaced piece of bone and free the spinal cord from pressure is often necessary and successful in relieving the paralysis.

SKULL – Simple fissured fractures and depressed fractures of the skull often follow blows or falls on the head, and are not at all serious, as a rule, apart from the damage which may have been done to the brain at the same time.

Compound fractures are attended by risk of suppuration which may spread within the skull, and if the skull be extensively broken and depressed the operation of trephining (see TREPHINING) is often done in order to cleanse the wound thoroughly. Another risk of fracture is that some of the small arteries on the inner surface of the skull may be torn and may

bleed, thus causing compression of the brain. For this reason also the skull is often trephined. Thorough cleansing of the wound, and confinement to bed in a darkened room constitute the treatment.

JAW – The lower jaw is often fractured by a blow on the face. There is generally bleeding from the mouth, the gum being torn. Also there are pain and grating sensations on chewing, and unevenness in the line of the teeth. The treatment is simple (illustration 221), the line of teeth in the upper jaw forming a splint, against which the lower jaw is bound, with the mouth closed. One bandage is passed below the chin and tied on the top of the head;

221 – Treatment of fractured jaw, with two triangular bandages folded narrow.

222 – Two forms of feeding-cup. The cup on the left is used for patients who are further advanced in convalescence, and who are partly raised in bed.

another passes in front of the chin, and is tied on the back of the neck. The two are then prevented from slipping forward and backward, respectively, by tying the one to the other on the crown of the head. It is essential that the victim be seen as soon as possible by a specialist surgeon to ensure that the jaw heals properly with the teeth in correct alignment. The patient must be fed for two or three weeks with liquid food, eg. eggs and milk, poured into the corner of the mouth from a feeding-cup with a spout (illustration 222).

NOSE – The bridge of the nose may be fractured by a fall. The bleeding is copious, and should be arrested by the usual means. (See HAEMORRHAGE.) An operation may later be performed to restore the shape of the nose.

FRAMBOESIA is another name for YAWS (qv).

FRAMYCETIN is an antibiotic derived from *Streptomyces decaris*. It is active against a wide range of organisms, when taken by mouth or applied locally to infections of the skin.

FRECKLES, or SUMMER-SPOTS, are small yellow or brown spots which appear on the exposed parts of the body, ie. face, neck, and hands, during hot or windy weather. They appear especially in people with fair skin and red hair. They consist of small pigmented areas in the deeper part of the cuticle, which are stimulated to increased development by exposure.

FREMITUS is the name given to a sensation which is communicated to the hand of an observer when it is laid upon the chest in certain diseases of the lungs and heart. Friction fremitus is a grating feeling communicated to the hand by the movements of lungs or heart when the membrane covering them is roughened, as in pleurisy or pericarditis. Vocal fremitus means the sensation felt by the hand when a person speaks; it is increased when the lung is more solid than usual. The 'thrills' felt over a heart affected by valvular disease are also varieties of fremitus.

FRENKEL'S EXERCISES are a series of movements of precision intended to be performed by patients suffering from difficulty of control of the muscles, with a view to regaining lost power of co-ordination. The exercises for the lower limbs of a patient confined to bed begin with such movements as those of raising the foot and carefully bringing it down upon a particular part of the edge of a padded board. At a later stage, the patient, supported if necessary under the armpits, practises walking along a broad strip painted on the floor, later still on a narrow strip, and afterwards tracing out marked patterns with the toes and placing the feet carefully as he walks on marked positions. Similar exercises are devised for re-establishing co-ordination of the muscles in the arms: eg. carefully inserting pegs into small holes in a board, picking up pins from a smooth surface, and similar movements.

FREUD'S THEORY is the term applied to a theory that emotional and allied diseases are due to a psychic injury or trauma, generally of a sexual nature, which did not produce an adequate reaction when it was received and therefore remains as a subconscious or 'affect memory' to trouble the patient's mind. As an extension of this theory Freud's treatment consists in encouraging the patient to tell everything that happens to be associated with trains of thought which lead up to this memory, thus securing a 'purging' of the mind from the original 'affect memory' which is the cause of the symptoms. This form of treatment is also called psychocatharsis or abreaction. The general term, psychoanalysis, is applied, in the first place, to the *method* of helping the patient to recover buried memories by free association of thoughts. In the second place, the term is applied to the body of psychological knowledge and theory accumulated and devised by Freud and his followers. The term 'psychoanalyst' should be applied only to those who have had a strict Freudian training, not to anyone who happens to practise psychotherapy.

FRIARS' BALSAM (see BALSAM).

FRICTION is the name given either to the fremitus felt, or to the grating noise heard, when two rough surfaces of the body move over one another. It is characteristically obtained over the chest in cases of dry pleurisy.

FRIEDREICH'S ATAXIA is a hereditary disease resembling locomotor ataxia, and due to degenerative changes in nerve tracts and nerve cells of the spinal cord and the brain. It occurs usually in children, or at any rate before the twentieth year of life, and affects often several brothers and sisters. Its chief symptoms are unsteadiness of gait, with loss of the knee jerks, followed later by difficulties of speech, tremors of the hands, head, and eyes, deformity of the feet, and curvature of the spine. There is often associated heart disease. The sufferer gets gradually worse, but may live, more or less helpless, for twenty or thirty years.

FRÖHLICH'S SYNDROME is the name given to a condition in children characterized by obesity, physical sluggishness, and retarded sexual development. It is the result of disturbed pituitary function.

379

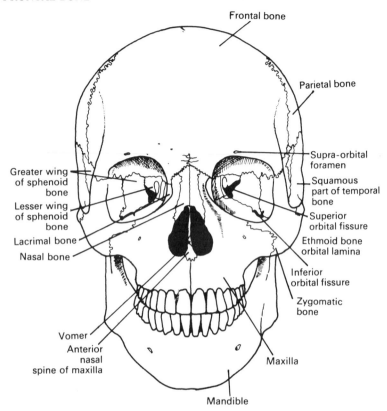

Frontal bone

Parietal bone

Supra-orbital foramen

Squamous part of temporal bone

Superior orbital fissure

Ethmoid bone orbital lamina

Inferior orbital fissure

Zygomatic bone

Maxilla

Mandible

Greater wing of sphenoid bone

Lesser wing of sphenoid bone

Lacrimal bone

Nasal bone

Vomer

Anterior nasal spine of maxilla

223 – The skull seen from the front.

FRONTAL BONE is the bone which forms the forehead (illustration 223) and protects the frontal lobes of the brain. Before birth, the frontal bone consists of two halves, and this division may persist throughout life, a deep groove remaining down the centre of the forehead. Above each eye is a heavy ridge in the bone, most marked in men, and, behind this, in the substance of the bone, is a cavity on each side, the frontal sinus, which communicates with the nose. Catarrh in these cavities produces the frontal headache characteristic of a 'cold in the head', and suppuration may occur in them, producing discharge from the nose. (See NOSE, DISEASES OF.)

FROSTBITE results from the action of extreme cold. In mild cases, the condition sometimes known as frostnip, the skin on exposed parts of the body, such as the cheeks or nose, becomes white and numb with a sudden and complete cessation of cold and discomfort. In more severe cases blisters develop on the frozen part, and the skin then gradually hardens and turns black until the frozen part, such as a finger, is covered with a black shell of dead tissue. Swelling of the underlying tissue occurs and this is accompanied by throbbing and aching. If, as is often the case, only the skin and the tissues immediately under it are frozen, then in a matter of months the dead tissue peels off, leaving behind it shiny red babyskin, as it is known, which at first is exquisitely tender. In the most severe cases of all, muscles, bone and tendon are also frozen, and the affected part becomes cold, swollen, mottled and blue or grey. There may be no blistering in these severe cases. At first there is no pain, but in time shooting and throbbing pains usually develop.

Prevention – This consists of wearing the

right clothing and never venturing on even quite short expeditions in cold weather, particularly on mountains, without taking expert advice as to what should be worn. Recent experience in the Scottish Highlands has shown how careless people can be in such matters.

Treatment – Frostnip is the only form of frostbite that should be treated on the spot. As it usually occurs on exposed parts, such as the face, each member of the party should be on the lookout for it in the other. The moment whitening of the skin is seen, the individual should seek a place sheltered from the wind, or turn his back on the wind, and warm the affected part by covering it with his warm hand or a glove until the normal colour and consistency of the affected part are restored. In more severe cases treatment should only be given in hospital or a well-equipped camp. In essentials this consists of warming the affected part, preferably in a container filled with water at 44° C. This temperature must not be exceeded. If there is no thermometer available, the alternative is a normal unfrostbitten finger. If the water is too hot for comfort, then cold water should be added. If no container is available, the alternative is hot water poured over towels or a cloth wrapped round the affected part. Rewarming should be done for spells of twenty minutes at a time. If facilities are not available for warming in this way, the alternative is to place the affected part in contact with a warm abdomen or armpit, or held in warm air. It should never be placed near an open fire. Generalized warming of the whole body may also be necessary, and this is achieved by giving hot drinks, and putting the victim in a sleeping bag. Extra heat may be supplied by his companions lying alongside him – either in their own sleeping bags, or by one getting into the same sleeping bag. After rewarming, the part should be very gently cleaned. Blisters should not be pricked. Antibiotics may be given to reduce the risk of infection. An important point to bear in mind is that no-one should be allowed to walk on a thawed, or partly thawed, foot, as this will almost certainly do irreparable damage. On the other hand, walking on frostbitten feet for a period does not appear to increase the liability to further damage.

The treatment of frostbite which has resulted in gangrene is given under GANGRENE.

FROZEN SHOULDER is the name given to a painful condition of the shoulder accompanied by stiffness and considerable limitation of movement. The usual age-incidence is between 40 and 50. The cause is not known. There is no specific treatment, but there is always complete recovery, even though this may take twelve to eighteen months. A course of deep X-ray therapy is sometimes beneficial.

FRUCTOSE is another name for laevulose, or fruit sugar, which is found along with glucose in most sweet fruits.

FRUIT – Almost all fresh fruits contain about 80 per cent of water, and the nutritive material, consisting chiefly of starch and sugar, does not exceed one-fifth of the fruit. The banana is the most nutritious of the fresh fruits, followed by grapes, plums, and apples. In addition to their food value, fruits contain vegetable acids, such as tartaric, citric, and malic acids, which have an agreeable flavour, a mildly laxative action, and are beneficial to the kidneys. Oranges, lemons, and grapefruit are specially useful in this way. The importance of fruits lies in the fact that they are the chief source of vitamin C, especially the citrus fruits and black-currants. The odour and flavour of fruits, which depend upon volatile oils and ethereal bodies, render them an agreeable article of food and improve appetite and digestion.

Dried fruits, such as apples, figs, dates, prunes, and grapes (raisins), form a highly nutritious form of diet, containing 60 or 70 per cent of starch, gum, and sugar; thus dried dates, figs, or raisins are more nourishing than an equal weight of bread. They are also a relatively rich source of iron and calcium, but a poor source of vitamin C.

FRUSEMIDE is a recently introduced potent diuretic.

FUGUE literally means flight and it is used to describe the mental condition in which an individual is suddenly seized with an unconscious motiviation to flee from some intolerable reality of everyday existence. This usually involves some agonizing interpersonal relationship. As a rule, it lasts for a matter of hours or days, but may go on for weeks or even months. During the fugue the individual seldom behaves in a particularly odd manner though he may be considered somewhat eccentric. When it is over there is no remembrance of events during the fugue.

FULLER'S EARTH is a grey powder free from all grittiness. It consists mainly of aluminium silicate, but differs from kaolin in containing traces of iron. It is a valuable dusting powder for tender, moist skins, such as those of infants.

FUMIGATION is a means of disinfection by the vapour of powerful antiseptics. (See DISINFECTION.)

FUNCTIONAL DISEASES (see PSYCHOSOMATIC DISEASE).

FUNGOID TUMOURS are ulcerating growths which sprout rapidly and have therefore a mushroom-like appearance.

FUNGUS-POISONING – Several diseases are due to the growth of minute fungi in the tissues of the body; for example, actinomycosis (caused by the ray-fungus), ringworm, and Madura foot of India. As to the large fungi, or mushrooms as they are often called, although they grow in dead and decaying material, they do not infest the living body, but many of them contain a poisonous alkaloid known as muscarine, others a body called phallin, both of which are poisons when swallowed. About 2000 of these larger fungi grow in England, of which 200 are edible. There are about a dozen which are classified as poisonous, but several of these cause no more than indigestion. The most poisonous of all is the 'death cap' or *Amanita phalloides* (illustration 224). The distinguishing features of this fungus are that it has a yellowish green cup, the gills

are white and at the base of the stem, or stalk, there is a cup, or volva. These features distinguish it from the common edible mushroom (*Psalliota campestris*), which has brownish purple gills and no cup at the base of the stem (illustration 225). Other poisonous mushrooms include *Amanita virosa, Amanita vernu*, and *Amanita muscaria* (illustration 226). Deaths from mushroom poisoning are relatively rare in England: between 1920 and 1940

225 – Edible Mushroom (*Psalliota campestris*), Gills brownish purple. Base of stem clubbed. No volva. (Height 3¾ inches (9·5 cm); width of cap 5 inches (12·5 cm); width of stem 1 inch (2·5 cm).) *The Practitioner.*

224 – The Death Cap (*Amanita phalloides*). Gills white. Volva at base of stem. Cap yellowish green. (Height 4½ inches (11·25 cm); width of cap 3½ inches (8·75 cm); width of stem ⅝ inch (1·5 cm).) *The Practitioner.*

226 – Fly Agaric (*Amanita muscaria*). Cap red with white patches. (Height 10 inches (25 cm); width of cap 7 inches (17·5 cm); width of stem 1 inch (2·5 cm).) *The Practitioner.*

only 39 cases were recorded in England and Wales.

Symptoms – Apart from indigestion, actual deadly poisoning is attended by three symptoms. There are, first of all, vomiting and purging from irritation of the stomach and bowels; then feebleness of the heart's action, due to the muscarine, producing pallor and faintness; and, finally, unconsciousness or delirium, which may, in a few hours, end in death. Fungi therefore act as narcotico-irritant poisons.

Treatment – The first thing is to give an emetic in order to remove the fragments of fungus from the stomach (see EMETICS) or, preferably, wash out the stomach (see STOMACH TUBE), and then leave in the stomach 2 fluid ounces (60 millilitres) of White Mixture of Magnesium Sulphate BPC. Stimulants, such as nikethamide (qv), should be given if the pulse be weak and the person collapsed. If the fungi have been eaten several hours before, a powerful purgative, such as a large dose of castor oil or Epsom salts, should be given as well as an emetic. Finally, in all serious cases atropine should be administered, since it forms a direct antidote to muscarine. There is also an antiphallinic serum which is sometimes of value. Another form of treatment which is sometimes used is to give five uncooked rabbits' stomachs and brains daily. This line of treatment is based upon the observation that rabbits do not die after eating *Amanita phalloides*.

FURAZOLIDONE is a drug used in the treatment of bacterial diarrhoea, bacterial food-poisoning and typhoid fever.

FURFURACEOUS is a term applied to skin diseases which produce scaliness of the surface, resembling bran.

FURUNCLE is another name for a boil. (See BOILS.)

FUSIDIC ACID is an antibiotic derived from the fermentation products of the fungus, *Fusidium coccineum*. It is particularly active against staphylococci, including those which are resistant to penicillin.

G

GAIT is an important sign of health and disease. Children, as a rule, begin to walk between the ages of twelve and eighteen months, having learned to stand before the end of the first year. If a good-sized child shows no ability to make movements by this time the possibility of his being mentally retarded must be borne in mind, and if the power of walking is not gained by the time the child is a year and a half old, he is probably the subject either of rickets, cerebral palsy, or a malformation of the hip-joint. (See RICKETS; PARALYSIS.)

Lameness in later life may be due to flat-foot (qv), when the spring of the foot is lost and the person walks with his toes turned out at right angles; or to the stiffness following disease of the knee-joint (see JOINTS, DISEASES OF), when the limb is carried forward like a rigid bar; or to the stiffness following hip-joint disease, when the person walks in a lop-sided manner, alternately taking a long step with the sound limb and swinging the whole pelvis round with the lame leg, as well as bending over to one side.

In **hemiplegia,** or paralysis down one side of the body following apoplexy (qv), the person drags the paralysed leg, and carries the paralysed side as if it were, so to speak, hung upon the healthy one. There is a tendency for this walk to improve gradually, the paralysed leg regaining power almost completely even when the arm remains helpless and bent stiffly across the body.

Steppage, or heather-step, gait occurs in certain cases of alcoholic neuritis, lead palsy, and other conditions where the muscles that raise the foot are weak and the toes in consequence droop. The person bends the knee and lifts the foot high, so that the toes may clear obstacles on the ground, much as a person steps in going through heather or long grass. (See DROP-FOOT.)

In **locomotor ataxia** (qv) the sensations derived from the lower limbs are blunted, and consequently the movements of the legs are uncertain and the heels planted on the ground with unnecessary force. When the person tries to turn or stands with the eyes shut he is apt to fall over. When he walks he feels for the ground with a stick or keeps his eyes constantly fixed upon it.

In **spastic paralysis** the limbs are moved with jerks. The foot first of all clings to the ground (the person being very apt to trip over small objects), and then leaves it with a spasmodic movement, being raised much higher than necessary.

In **trembling palsy,** paralysis agitans, or Parkinsonism (qv) as it is now known, the movements are tremulous, and as the person takes very short steps, he has the peculiarity of appearing constantly to fall forward, being, in advanced cases, unable to stop himself till he brings up against some object of which he can lay hold.

In **St. Vitus's dance (chorea)** (qv) the walk is bizarre and jerky, the affected child often seeming to leave one leg a step behind him, and then, with a screwing movement on the other heel, go on again.

GALACTAGOGUES are drugs which increase the flow of milk in nursing women. The normal stimulus of an infant's lips is the most powerful agent in producing milk, and a mother who has little or no milk should nevertheless hold her infant to the breast. Good food and the hormone, prolactin, from the pituitary gland increase the quantity and improve the quality of milk.

GALACTOCELE is the term applied to a cyst-like swelling in the breast which forms as a result of obstruction in the milk-duct draining the swollen area.

GALACTOPHORITIS means inflammation of the milk-ducts of the breast.

GALACTORRHOEA is a recurrent or persisting discharge of milk from the breast.

GALACTOSAEMIA is a hereditary disease due to the lack of the enzyme which normally converts galactose, the sugar derived from lactose, or sugar-milk, into glucose. The incidence is around 1 in 75,000 births. Soon after birth the affected baby becomes jaundiced and lethargic. If he survives and is not treated, he becomes mentally retarded. Treatment consists basically of a diet free of lactose. Special lactose-free milks are now available.

GALENICAL PREPARATIONS are preparations of drugs sanctioned by the pharmocopoeia, the list of drugs and remedies published under government regulations. The term, official, is more commonly used in the same sense; offi-

GALL-BLADDER, DISEASES OF

cinal means drugs procurable in the ordinary shops.

GALL is another name for bile. (See BILE.)

GALL-BLADDER, DISEASES OF –

The bile ductules begin as minute passages scattered throughout the liver, and lying between its rows of cells, from which they collect the bile secreted by the latter. They unite into larger and larger vessels just as do the tributaries of a river, and finally a single, large hepatic duct emerges from the right lobe and another from the left lobe of the liver. (See LIVER.) The connection of these with the gall-bladder is somewhat complicated (illustration 227). The right and left ducts unite first into one vessel,

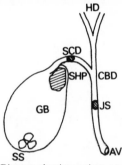

227 – Diagram showing various positions of gall-stones. GB, the gall-bladder; CBD, the bile duct; HD, hepatic ducts; SS silent stones; SHP, stone in Hartmann's pouch; SCD, stone in cystic duct; JS, stone in common bile duct; so-called jaundice stone; AV, ampulla of Vater. From Handfield-Jones and Porritt, *The Essentials of Modern Surgery.* E. & S. Livingstone, Ltd.

the common hepatic duct, which meets the cystic duct coming from the gall-bladder, and the two unite to form the bile duct, which opens into the small intestine a few inches below the outlet of the stomach. The importance of this arrangement lies in two facts: first, the entrance to the gall-bladder is a cul-de-sac, bile in entering it from the liver running down the hepatic and up the cystic duct; and, secondly, if the gall-bladder or its cystic duct becomes blocked, the bile can still escape from the liver down the common hepatic and bile ducts, into the bowel. The size and condition of the gall-bladder can be determined in many cases by X-ray examination. A substance which is opaque to X-rays, such as iopanoic acid, when taken by mouth is

excreted in the bile and passed into the gall-bladder. If an X-ray photograph be taken some sixteen hours afterwards, the gall-bladder and any stones that it may contain are seen outlined as a shadow in the plate. Inflammation of the gall-bladder is known as cholecystitis. The condition characterized by the presence of gall-stones is known as cholelithiasis.

CHOLECYSTITIS – Catarrh, or inflammation, may occur in the gall-bladder and bile passages as in other cavities lined by mucous membrane. It may either arise in the bile-ducts themselves, or may follow upon a catarrhal condition in the bowels, spreading up from the point where the bile duct opens into the small intestine. Cholecystitis may be either acute or chronic. Both forms are more common in women than in men, and are more liable to occur in the obese than in the thin. The condition is more liable to occur in middle age. Hence the description of the individual subject to cholecystitis as 'fair, fat, and forty'. Since the bile is expelled from the liver largely by the movements of breathing, any condition which impedes this causes stagnation of the bile, and favours catarrh. Pigments are deposited from the bile in the finer vessels, producing 'bile-sand', and thick, stringy mucus collects in these passages and in the gall-bladder, the irritation caused by these deposits still further aggravating the catarrh. Finally, this bile-sand may collect into small masses in the larger ducts or gall-bladder, and, chemical changes in the mucus taking place, a crystalline substance incorporating cholesterol encrusts them in a gradually thickening layer, so that finally large gall-stones may be produced.

Symptoms – An acute attack of cholecystitis causes, in general, pain and tenderness to touch beneath the margin of the ribs on the right side: ie. over the edge of the liver and the gall-bladder. This may be followed by a certain degree of jaundice. (See JAUNDICE.) In chronic catarrh there is general ill-health and indigestion, associated with a dark, sallow skin, and occasional attacks of 'biliousness'. There is often, too, a vague, uneasy feeling in the region mentioned above, and in advanced cases there may be recurring attacks of gall-stone colic.

Treatment – The treatment of acute cholecystitis consists of rest in bed, the administration of antibiotics and pain-relieving drugs and a diet containing ample carbohydrate and protein but a minimum of fat. The patient should be encouraged to drink as much bland fluid as possible: eg. glucose drinks flavoured with fruit juice. If the condition does not settle quickly. operation may be necessary.

Even in cases which settle satisfactorily, the possibility of operation at a later date must be considered. Such elective operation, as it is known, is recommended by most surgeons today. Removal of the gall-

that it helps to drain the biliary passages. To cleanse the bile passages, large quantities of water should be taken with meals, and one or two tumblerfuls of warm water an hour before each meal are specially beneficial. The bowels must be carefully regulated.

SUPPURATION is a rarer but much

228 – Gall-stones. Reproduced by permission of the President and Council of the Royal College of Surgeons of England.

bladder, the operation known as cholecystectomy, is the only satisfactory treatment for chronic cholecystitis. If, however, surgical treatment is not carried out for any reason, the regime followed should be based upon a simple life, with not more than three meals daily, the avoidance of alcoholic beverages and highly spiced food, and the taking of more exercise together with the practice of deep breathing. The administration by mouth of a concentrated solution of magnesium sulphate one hour before breakfast is sometimes of value by virtue of the fact

more serious condition which occasionally appears in the course of a chronic cholecystitis. It may also arise as the result of an infective fever like typhoid, and sometimes results from the irritation of a growing gall-stone. Its symptoms are an exaggeration of those of catarrh along with shivering, high fever, and often delirium. The treatment is an operation to drain the gall-bladder of its suppurating contents, after which recovery often ensues, though the outlook is serious.

GALL-STONES – The manner of formation of these has been already described. The smaller stones consist of a combination of bile-pigment with lime (bilirubin-calcium), and are deep brown in colour; the larger ones have a core of this surrounded by cholesterol, and are lighter or even white in colour. The size varies from that of small gravel, in which case several hundred stones may be present, to the size of a goose egg, when the stone is single. When there are several stones they are faceted so as to fit against one another (illustration 228). Gall-stone disease is a major affliction in modern society, and operations on the gall-bladder are now the commonest form of major abdominal surgery in the United Kingdom. They are equally common in U.S.A., where approximately 16 million of the inhabitants are said to have gall-stones.

Symptoms – To begin with, there are the symptoms described under the heading of cholecystitis, which causes the formation of the stones. Apart from these, stones may lie for years in the gall-bladder and give no trouble, being found accidentally at an operation or after death. But as a rule they produce symptoms in one of three ways (illustration 227).

(1) The mere presence of stones in the gall-bladder may give rise to much irritation, and the tenderness and pain over the region of the gall-bladder then become very marked. These symptoms are specially liable to become aggravated during digestion, so that the condition is taken for a form of dyspepsia, although the pain is at the right side of the body. When bacteria find an entrance from the bowel, high temperature, shiverings, and sweatings develop, and suppuration may come on.

(2) The usual way in which gall-stones show their presence is by passing out of the gall-bladder along with the bile. If the stone be small, it reaches the bowel and is voided, without attracting attention beyond perhaps passing discomfort in the upper part of the abdomen, after a meal. If the stone be large enough to stick in the cystic or bile-duct, and particularly if it be angular, it sets up great spasm of the muscle fibres in the wall of the duct, causing the most agonizing pain shooting up to the right shoulder. It comes on, as a rule, very quickly, and is accompanied by collapse, cold sweat, and vomiting. It lasts usually several hours, and often ceases quite suddenly as the stone passes into the bowel or back to the gall-bladder. Next day there is usually some jaundice, which may last for a week or two.

(3) Sometimes the stone remains jammed or impacted in one of the ducts, passing neither up nor down. In this case, the pain passes slowly off as the muscle fibres of the ducts become tired out, only to return again and again, till, in a milder degree, it becomes almost constant. Gradually increasing jaundice may develop till the skin becomes even a dark olive brown. At the same time loss of weight and strength, and often dropsy, progress so far that the case may be very difficult to diagnose from cancer. In this case, too, suppuration may come on.

Treatment – To prevent gall-stones, what has been said in the section on cholecystitis holds good, and if the accompanying cholecystitis be cured, even after large gall-stones have been formed, they may be comparatively harmless. Many substances, which will dissolve gall-stones outside the body, have been recommended in the hope that, taken into the system for long periods, they may gradually dissolve the stones in the gall-bladder – for example, ether, turpentine, and olive oil, but they are of no practical value. The one exception to this is chenodeoxycholic acid which will dissolve gall-stones in about one in five patients, but it must be given for a relatively long period – even up to a year. Fortunately it is a relatively safe drug. It is taken by mouth.

When an attack of gall-stone colic occurs, hot fomentations should be at once applied to the abdomen. Morphine sulphate, $\frac{1}{4}$ grain (15 mg), with or without atropine, $\frac{1}{150}$ grain (0·6 mg), should be given hypodermically. Inhalations of amyl nitrite are also useful. If the pain is excessive, chloroform or ether may have to be given for the fifteen or twenty minutes that elapse before the morphine can take effect. A hot bath sometimes gives great relief.

As to a surgical operation, if a person suffers from constant catarrh and repeated attacks of gall-stone colic, it is well that he should undergo the comparatively simple operation of having the gall-bladder removed (cholecystectomy), which may relieve both conditions. In cases in which a gall-stone is impacted, operation is practically always essential. Sometimes, as when the duct is permanently closed, a fistula follows upon operation, and the bile drains away permanently through a wound in the abdomen. In this case, the jaundice and colic at least are alleviated, and the fistula can be closed at a later operation by the surgeon, who makes an opening between the gall-bladder and adjacent bowel.

GALLS, or NUTGALL, is the name of an excrescence growing upon oaks and containing a large quantity of tannic acid which gives the galls a strongly astringent action. Galls are chiefly used in the form of ointment of galls, and ointment of galls with opium, for application to bleeding piles.

GALL-STONES (see GALL-BLADDER, DISEASES OF.)

GALTON'S WHISTLE is a metallic whistle producing extremely high notes which is used in testing the sense of hearing.

GALVANISM (see ELECTRICITY IN MEDICINE).

GALVANOCAUTERY means a cautery (see CAUSTICS and CAUTERIES) made by a wire heated by a galvanic current.

GAMETE is a sexual or germ cell: for example, an ovum (qv) or spermatozoon (qv).

GAMGEE TISSUE is a surgical dressing composed of a thick layer of cotton-wool between two layers of absorbent gauze, introduced by the Birmingham surgeon, Sampson Gamgee.

GAMMA BENZENE HEXA-CHLORIDE is a drug that is used in the treatment of pediculosis (qv) and scabies (qv).

GAMMA-GLOBULIN – It has been known for a long time that the protective antibodies of the body are closely associated with the proteins of the blood. Gamma-globulin is a concentrated solution of the antibody fraction of human blood which has proved of great value in providing immunity against certain infectious diseases, particularly measles. It is of little value once the disease is begun but, if given before the disease manifests itself, it either prevents its onset or modifies its severity very considerably.

GAMMEXANE is the proprietary name for a synthetic insecticide which is a formulation of benzene hexachloride. It is active against a large range of insects and pests, including mosquitoes, fleas, lice, cockroaches, house-flies, clothes moths, bed-bugs, ants, and grain pests.

GANGLION is a term used in two senses. In anatomy, it means an aggregation of nerve-cells found in the course of certain nerves. In surgery, it means an enlargement of the sheath of a tendon, containing fluid. The latter occurs particularly in connection with the sinews in front of, and behind, the wrist.

Causes – The cause of these dilatations on the tendon-sheaths is either some irregular growth of the synovial membrane which lines them and secretes the fluid that lubricates their movements, or the forcing out of a small pouch of this membrane through the sheath in consequence of a strain. In either case a bag-like swelling forms, whose connection with the synovial sheath becomes cut off, so that synovial fluid collects in it and distends it more and more.

Symptoms – A soft, elastic, movable swelling forms, most often on the back of the wrist. When noticed first it is perhaps the size of a pea, and its connection with a tendon can easily be made out. It may remain of this size for many years and occasion no trouble at all, but generally a ganglion gives a peculiar feeling of weakness to the wrist, and on account of its size or position it may be very inconvenient. A ganglion which forms in connection with the flexor tendons in front of the wrist sometimes attains a large size, and extends down the sinews to form another swelling in the palm of the hand.

Treatment – Sudden pressure with the thumbs may often burst a ganglion and disperse its contents beneath the skin, after which it should be prevented from refilling by bandaging the part tightly, a very efficient pad being made by wrapping up a large coin in a piece of lint. If it cannot be burst, there only remains the opening of the ganglion, with scraping of its interior. As the ganglion may disappear spontaneously there should be no rush to remove it unless it is causing inconvenience or pain.

GANGRENE, or MORTIFICATION, means the death of a part of the body sufficiently large to be seen. When the process is slow and superficial, only microscopic parts dying in succession, the process is called ulceration, whilst the term necrosis is usually restricted to the death of internal parts, particularly of bones. There are two varieties of gangrene, dry and moist, dry gangrene being a process of mummification, in which, as a rule, the circulation simply stops, and the part, so to speak, withers up, whilst in moist gangrene there is inflammation accompanied by putrefactive changes. The dead part, when formed of soft tissues, is known as a slough, and, when part of a bone, is called a sequestrum.

Causes – Certain diseases which lessen the strength and vitality of the tissues throughout the body render them more liable to die when subjected to injury. Chief among these are Bright's disease and diabetes mellitus. The nervous system, too, exerts an important influence over the nutrition and repair of the body, so that where it is diseased a quite trifling injury may produce gangrene of the injured part: for example, in paralysis bed sores are apt to form, owing to the mere pressure of the body on the bed.

Direct injury is perhaps the commonest cause. If a limb be badly crushed, or frozen, or burned by heat or powerful chemicals, it may not recover.

Interference with the nutrition of a part by the gradual closure of the arteries, which may occur in old age; by their sudden closure in Raynaud's disease; or after the eating of diseased rye (see ERGOT POISONING); or by prolonged mechanical compression, may also cause it.

Infection by bacteria is another, and the most serious, cause, although fortunately it is rare and seldom occurs save in people of very low vitality. The hospital gangrene, so much dreaded by surgeons last century, belonged to this type, but is now practically unknown, thanks to aseptic surgery.

Symptoms – DRY GANGRENE usually comes on in old people with diseased arteries, and is preceded by pain in the affected limb, which gradually becomes a dusky red colour and later brown and black. The line between the dead and living tissues is quite sharp (line of demarcation), and marked by a red ring, where a slight degree of inflammation is going on. There is some smell, especially if care be not taken to keep the foot or other affected part absolutely dry. There is little or no pain after gangrene has occurred, nor any fever, and the red ring gradually deepens till the gangrenous part drops off in the course of some months.

MOIST GANGRENE is the more common form, and is accompanied by putrefaction. The part becomes swollen, livid, and covered with blebs; later it turns bluish-green and black in places. The smell is very offensive, and much fluid is effused from the decaying tissues, speedily soaking the dressings applied. There is not much pain, but the general symptoms are apt to be very serious, and there is then high fever. In the latter case the person may die of blood-poisoning, and in any case the line of demarcation is not definite, and the gangrene is apt to extend up the limb.

GAS GANGRENE is a form which may occur when wounds are infected with soil from highly cultivated fields like those of Belgium. Gas-producing bacilli (eg. *Clostridium welchii*) from the soil then grow with great rapidity in the wound, and the gas spreads along the spaces in the muscles and connective tissues. Some of these bacilli grow only in the absence of oxygen, so that incisions to admit the air, together with application of oxidizing agents, and use of gas-gangrene antitoxin, check their spread. In this form speedy amputation may be necessary. Experience gained in the 1939–45 War clearly demonstrated the value of penicillin, in conjunction with surgery, in the treatment of this condition.

Treatment – The dry form must be kept dry by wrapping in cotton-wool, and, when the line of demarcation has distinctly formed, amputation may be performed close above it. In the moist form, which is not spreading quickly, the surgeon also waits till he can see clearly how much is to become gangrenous, and an attempt is made to control any infection by means of antibiotics. The gangrenous area is left dry. When small parts, like the fingers, become gangrenous after frost-bite, they may be treated by applying on lint some simple antiseptic ointment, such as boric acid ointment, containing a small amount of eucalyptus or other volatile oil, to subdue the smell. (See also FROST-BITE.)

GARGLES – Gargling is a process by which various substances in solution are brought in contact with the throat without being swallowed. The watery solutions used for the purpose are called gargles.

Gargles are used in the treatment of infections of the throat: ie. 'sore throat', pharyngitis, and tonsillitis. They are also of value in the treatment of the condition known as 'relaxed throat' or 'clergyman's sore throat' (qv). A gargle consists of either (*a*) a solution (in warm water) of an antiseptic, eg. potassium permanganate; or (*b*) a concentrated solution of common salt or glycerin in warm water. It exerts its beneficial action in throat infections by virtue of one or more of the following properties: (1) the mechanical effort of gargling induces a hyperaemia in the throat which has a beneficial effect on the infection. (2) The heat of the gargle has the same effect and is also soothing to the inflamed tissues. (3) A strong solution of common salt, or glycerin, induces a hyperaemia. (4) If the gargle contains an antiseptic, this may help to control the infection.

One of the simplest and most effective gargles is common salt: sufficient should be added to a tumblerful of warm water to give it a strong salty flavour. Potassium chlorate is also a satisfactory gargle: 12 grains (800 mg) to a tumblerful of warm water. Another simple and effective gargle is one containing sufficient potassium permanganate to give it a faint pink colour. A more elegant gargle consists of: sodium bicarbonate, 60 grains (4 grams); compound thymol solution, 2 ounces (57 ml); glycerin, 2 ounces (57 ml). A tablespoonful of this mixture is added to a cup of warm water. Another useful glycerin gargle is: boric acid, borax, glycerin (60 grains (4 grams) of each); water, 6 ounces (170 ml).

For 'relaxed throats' a gargle containing alum (5 to 10 grains (300 to 600 mg) per ounce (28·5 ml) of water) is usually most effective, because of its astringent action.

An aspirin gargle (10 grains (600 mg) to a cupful of warm water) is sometimes useful in relieving local discomfort, especially following tonsillectomy.

Mode of use – About a tablespoonful of the warm solution is taken into the mouth after the person has drawn a deep breath. The head is then tilted far back and a constant stream of bubbles is blown up through the fluid, so as to serve the double purpose of preventing it from running down the larynx and of sending fine drops in every direction about the throat. When the throat is much inflamed gargling is painful. The gargle is then allowed to pass back as far as possible into the throat and kept there as long as the breath can be held.

GARGOYLISM is a rare condition in childhood, characterized by abnormalities of growth of the skeleton which result in a large head with coarse, ugly features.

GAS (see ANAESTHETICS; NITROUS OXIDE GAS; DAMP).

GAS GANGRENE (see GANGRENE).

GAS-POISONING may be the result of working at some dangerous trade, as in the case of miners, or may result from accident as in escapes of coal-gas. (See CARBON MONOXIDE; DAMP.)

GASTRALGIA means pain in the stomach. (See DYSPEPSIA.)

GASTRECTOMY means an operation for removal of the whole or part of the stomach.

GASTRIC means anything connected with the stomach, such as gastric ulcer.

GASTRIC FEVER is an old name for typhoid fever.

GASTRIC ULCER (see STOMACH, DISEASES OF).

GASTRITIS means inflammation of the stomach. (See DYSPEPSIA.)

GASTROCNEMIUS is the large double muscle which forms the chief bulk of the calf, and ends below in the tendo calcaneus.

GASTROENTERITIS means inflammation of the stomach and intestines. Its main symptoms are vomiting and diarrhoea. (See DIARRHOEA.)

GASTROENTEROSTOMY is an operation performed usually in order to relieve some obstruction to the outlet from the stomach, and consists in making one opening in the lower part of the stomach, another in a neighbouring loop of the small intestine, and stitching the two together.

GASTROPTOSIS is the condition in which the stomach occupies an abnormally low position in the abdomen. (See STOMACH, DISEASES OF.)

GASTROSCOPE is an instrument for viewing the interior of the stomach, by means of a special arrangement of light and mirrors attached to a hollow tube, which is introduced into the stomach via the mouth and gullet. A special camera attachment makes it possible to photograph the interior of the stomach.

GASTROSTOMY means an operation on the stomach by which, when the gullet is blocked by a tumour or other cause, an opening is made from the front of the abdomen into the stomach, so that fluid food can be passed into the organ.

GATHERING is a popular term applied to an abscess.

GAUCHER'S DISEASE is a disease characterized by abnormal storage of lipoids, particularly in the spleen, bone marrow, and liver. This results in enlargement of the spleen and the liver, particularly the former, and anaemia. It runs a chronic course. There is no curative treatment, but splenectomy (removal of the spleen) is often helpful.

GAULTHERIA, or WINTERGREEN, is an American evergreen plant (*Gaultheria procumbens*) containing an oil with peculiar smell and aromatic taste. The oil consists almost entirely of methyl salicylate. Externally, oil of wintergreen is applied by rubbing on painful joints, in cases of acute and chronic rheumatism, often giving great relief.

GAVAGE means forced feeding by a soft rubber tube in cases when a person cannot swallow owing to weakness or other cause, or when an insane person refuses food. The tube, in the former case, is passed through the mouth into the stomach, and in the latter case a small tube is often simply passed through one nostril into the back of the throat, from which the person must automatically swallow food. By this means only liquid food, like strong soup, whipped eggs, or milk, can be administered.

GEL is the term applied to a colloid substance which is firm in consistence although it contains much water: eg. ordinary gelatin.

GELATIN is derived from collagen (qv), the chief constituent of connective tissue. It is a colourless transparent substance which dissolves in boiling water, and on cooling sets into a jelly. Such a jelly is a pleasant addition to the invalid diet, especially when suitably flavoured, but it is of relatively little nutritive value as not more than 1 ounce can be taken in the day: ie. the amount required to make one pint of jelly. Although it is a protein, it is lacking in several of the vital amino-acids. The ordinary household 'stock' made from boiling bones contains gelatin. Mixed with about two and a half times its weight of glycerin, gelatin forms a soft substance used as the basis for many pastilles and suppositories.

GELSEMIUM is the root of the yellow jasmine, *Gelsemium sempervirens*, a climbing plant of the Southern United States. Its action upon the body is to dull the central nervous system. It must be used with caution, because in larger doses it is a dangerous poison. Its main use is in the relief of migraine, when it is given in the form of tincture of gelsemium combined with other drugs. (See GOWERS'S MIXTURE.)

GENERAL PARALYSIS OF THE INSANE, also known as GPI, GENERAL PARALYSIS, DEMENTIA PARALYTICA, is a disease in which both bodily and mental powers degenerate; though in some cases the bodily symptoms are for a time most marked, whilst in others the mental change appears first.

Causes – The disease is a late manifestation of syphilis, usually beginning eight to twenty years after infection: ie. it usually begins between the ages of 30 and 50 years. It is much commoner among males than among females. Occasionally it is found in adolescents, when it is due to congenital syphilis.

When a person dies in an advanced stage of the disease, certain very marked changes are found in the brain and its membranes. There is inflammatory thickening of the latter, and they are more or less adherent to the brain, in the superficial part of which the blood-vessels show various signs of chronic inflammation, while the brain tissue of nerve cells and fibres has to a great extent disappeared. The cells of the neuroglia or supporting tissue of the brain are found increased in size ('spider cells') and numbers, on microscopic examination.

Symptoms come on very insidiously, as a rule, and the disease is often far advanced before it is recognized, although, on the other hand, it may now and then be ushered in by convulsive seizures, by a sudden maniacal attack, or by a rapid nervous breakdown.

The first stage is characterized by slight physical symptoms, which generally escape the notice of the affected person's friends. These are tremors of the tongue and facial muscles in speaking, transient paralysis of eye muscles producing slight squint and double vision for a time, stammering over difficult words like 'British Constitution' or 'hippopotamus', and, later on, increasing feebleness in walking and disinclination for exertion of all sorts. Furthermore, the handwriting degenerates greatly, and this is often the first symptom that excites remark. All these physical signs are apt to be masked by the peculiar state of mental exaltation which sometimes ushers in the disease. The person often feels himself to be stronger and better than usual, and is never tired of stating that he is 'all right', or 'as strong as an elephant', or that he 'could jump over a house'. But these are delusions, and, if he be actually put to the proof, his weakness is discovered. Often these delusions go further and he believes himself to be very rich, or embarks upon great commercial schemes, or identifies himself with some well-known personality; but however grand his dreams be, there is in them an element of foolishness. Sometimes the first sign of the malady is a squandering of money on useless trifles; or foolish and criminal actions may be done which bring the incipient general paralytic into conflict with the law. In other cases the first mental symptoms consist of depression with delusions of poverty or of personal unfitness, the type of delusion being largely a matter of temperament. Great emotionalism is another feature, and the affected person is excited to tears by very little pathos, or to laughter with equal facility, while the memory at the same time fails and the patient gets notably absent-minded. Important early signs, in addition to the mental excitement or mental enfeeblement, are diminished reaction of the pupil of the eye to light, and alteration of the knee-jerks and other reflexes.

In the second stage the physical weakness becomes more and more marked. The sight grows bad, and the affected person loses his power to feel pleasure or sorrow. Gradually, too, he loses feeling for actual physical pain, so that he is liable to get bruised and cut. The mind, too, becomes quite clouded, and unfit to sustain the simplest exercise.

In the third stage the mental failure is profound, and the sufferer cannot recognize even his nearest relatives. Speech degenerates to a series of meaningless noises. The paralysis becomes complete, and the person lies oblivious to all around him, and unable even to control his bladder and bowels. In this stage he becomes a ready prey to any infectious disease, and large bed sores.

The whole course of the disease lasts usually only two to three years, and, though occasional remissions take place, which may prolong life to ten years or more, a genuine case of general paralysis must be regarded as affording little ground for hope, unless effective treatment is instituted at as early a stage as possible.

Treatment – Recognition of general paralysis at a very early stage is of the greatest importance for two reasons. In the first place, treatment at this stage affords considerable prospect of stopping the progress of the disease. In the second place, the person suffering from an early stage of this disease is liable through mental weakness to transact his business affairs badly and lose his means, although still regarded by his friends as merely slightly peculiar or eccentric. The most effective form of treatment is penicillin, particularly if given early enough.

In the late stages of GPI the patient's mental condition is such that admission to a mental hospital is either desirable or necessary.

GENES are the biological units of heredity. They are arranged along the length of the chromosomes (qv). (See HEREDITY.)

GENETIC COUNSELLING is the procedure whereby advice is given to married couples, or to people proposing to marry, as to the likelihood of their having congenitally abnormal children. It is a procedure which is assuming enhanced value now that by means of antenatal diagnosis it is possible in certain cases to foretell in the early stages of pregnancy whether or not the unborn child is abnormal: for example, whether or not he or she is a mongol. There are now over twenty genetic advisory centres in the United Kingdom, to which patients can be referred by their family doctors.

GENETICS is the science which deals with the origin of the characteristics of an individual or the study of heredity.

GENITALIA are the organs of reproduction.

GENITO-URINARY TRACT consists of the kidneys, ureters, bladder, and urethra and, in the male, the genital organs.

GENTAMICIN is an antibiotic derived from a species of micro-organisms, *Micromonospora purpurea*. Its main value is that it is active against certain micro-organisms such as *Pseudomonas pyocyanea*, *E. coli* and *Aerobacter aerogenes* which are not affected by other antibiotics, as well as staphylococci which have become resistant to penicillin.

GENTIAN is the root of the yellow gentian (*Gentiana lutea*), a European plant. Preparations made from it are very bitter, and it is one of the most commonly used bitters (qv) in dyspepsia and loss of appetite.

GENTIAN VIOLET, or CRYSTAL VIOLET, is a dye belonging to the rosaniline group. Gentian violet is a good superficial antiseptic. It is used in the treatment of burns, either alone or in conjunction with brilliant green and proflavine. Applied to a burn, gentian violet forms a tough pliable film.

GENU VALGUM is the medical term for knock-knee (qv).

GENU VARUM is the medical term for bow leg (qv).

GERIATRICS is that branch of medicine which treats of the disorders and diseases associated with old age.

GERMAN MEASLES, or RUBELLA, is an acute infectious disease of a mild type, which may sometimes be difficult to differentiate from mild forms of measles and scarlet fever. It is also known by the name of rötheln.

Cause – The cause of infection is a virus. It is spread by close contact with infected individuals, and is infectious for a week before the rash appears and at least four days afterwards. It occurs predominantly in the winter and spring, and is more likely to occur in young adults than measles. The incubation period is usually 14 to 21 days.

Symptoms are very mild, and the disease is not at all serious. On the day of onset there may be shivering, headache, slight catarrh with sneezing, coughing and sore throat, very slight fever, not above 100° F (37·8° C), and at the same time the glands of the neck become enlarged. These symptoms are usually slight. Within 24 hours of the onset a pink, slightly raised eruption appears, first on the face or neck, then on the chest, and the second day spreads all over the body. The appearance of the rash is intermediate between that of measles and scarlet fever, being less blotchy, and remaining more as minute pink spots than the rash of measles, and the spots being more definite than the fairly uniform redness of scarlet fever. The rash is very bright on some parts of the body, while other parts are almost entirely free. The duration of the rash is variable. It may last for the greater part of a week, and, as it disappears, fine bran-like scales separate from the surface. The most distinguishing feature of this disorder is a well-marked but transient enlargement of the glands in the neck.

An attack of German measles during the early months of pregnancy may be responsible for congenital defects in the foetus, and it is for this reason that the disease has assumed such great importance in recent years. The incidence of such defects is not precisely known, but probably around 20 per cent of children, whose mothers have had German measles in the first three months of the pregnancy, are born with congenital defects. These defects take a variety of forms, but the most important ones are: low birth weight with retarded physical development; malformations of the heart; cataract, and deafness. Parents of such handicapped children can obtain help and advice from the National Association for Deaf, Blind and Rubella Handicapped, 164 Cromwell Lane, Coventry CV4 8AP.

Treatment – The only treatment necessary is confinement to bed so long as there are any symptoms. Infectivity ceases within 4 days provided there are no symptoms. Children who develop the disease should not return to school until they have recovered, and in any case not before four days have passed from the onset of the rash. In view of the mildness of the disease, contacts are seldom kept in quarantine, but they should be carefully watched from the tenth to the twenty-first day from exposure to infection.

In view of the possible effect of the disease upon the foetus, particular care should be taken to isolate pregnant mothers from contact with infected subjects. As the risk to the foetus is particularly high during the first sixteen weeks of pregnancy, any pregnant mother exposed to infection during this period should be given an intramuscular injection of gamma-globulin (qv). Female members of the school staff who have not had the disease or been vaccinated against it, who might probably become pregnant should be recommended not to attend the school until the risk of infection is over. A vaccine is now available which should make it possible to give a girl an immunity to the disease before she attains adult life, and it is now officially recommended that such vaccination should be offered to all girls between 11 and 14 years of age. It is also recommended that all women of childbearing age, who have been shown by a simple laboratory test not to have had the disease, should be vaccinated, always provided the woman is not pregnant at the time and has not been exposed to the risk of pregnancy during the previous eight weeks.

GERMS (see BACTERIOLOGY).

GESTATION is another name for pregnancy.

GIARDIASIS is a condition caused by a parasitic organism known as *Giardia lamblia*, which is found in the duodenum (qv) and the upper part of the small intestine. This organism is usually harmless, but is sometimes responsible for causing diarrhoea. This responds well to metronidazole or mepacrine.

GIDDINESS (see VERTIGO).

GIGANTISM (see ACROMEGALY).

GIN is an alcoholic beverage made from rye or barley with the addition of juniper berries and hops. In the days when there were few satisfactory diuretics, it used to be given as a diuretic, but it is now seldom used for this purpose. (See ALCOHOL.)

GINGER is the root of *Zingiber officinale*, a plant which grows in India, Jamaica, and other tropical countries. In the case of black ginger the bark is left on, whilst white ginger is the root minus bark. Its properties are due to a hot volatile oil and an aromatic resin. The tincture and syrup of ginger act like preparations of other volatile oils, and are given in doses of about a teaspoonful. They are used in cases of flatulence to stop griping, and are added to purgatives for the same purpose.

GINGIVITIS means inflammation of the gums. (See TEETH, DISEASES OF.)

GLANDERS, or EQUINIA, is a specific infectious disease to which certain animals, chiefly those possessing an undivided hoof – such as horses, asses, and mules – are liable, and communicable by them to man. The term farcy is also used to designate a variety of the disease in which the lymphatic glands are first and chiefly affected. Glanders is happily a rare form of disease in man. It occurs chiefly among those who from their occupation are in contact with horses, such as grooms, farmers, cavalry soldiers, veterinary surgeons, and seems to be produced either by direct inoculation of the organism from

a diseased animal into the broken skin or by inspiration. The cause of glanders is a short rod-shaped organism, known as the *Loefflerella mallei* or *Acinetobacter mallei*. It has been eradicated from Britain, but still occurs in Eastern Europe and Asia.

In the untreated acute form of the disease, the case generally terminates fatally in a period varying from two or three days to as many weeks. A chronic form of glanders and farcy is more common, in which the symptoms advance much more slowly, and are attended with relatively less constitutional disturbance. Around 30 to 50 per cent of patients with chronic glanders survive without treatment. Promising results have been reported from the use of sulphonamides, penicillin and streptomycin.

GLANDS are divisible into several classes. In the first place, the term is applied to organs like the liver, pancreas, and kidneys, which produce a secretion; but in general the term is limited to smaller structures concerned in the production of some excretion from the body, or of some substance needful to its working. These latter are divided into two quite distinct groups: (1) glands which produce some form of secretion or excretion; (2) lymphatic glands.

(1) SECRETING AND EXCRETING GLANDS comprise glands in almost all parts of the body, which vary much in appearance, in size, and in the character of the substances they produce. The skin, for example, is richly supplied with sebaceous glands, which secrete an oily material, and with sweat glands, which are placed in rows whose openings can be seen with a weak magnifying lens upon the ridges of the palms and soles. The lining membrane of the stomach is made up of long tubular glands set closely side by side, and in these the gastric juice is formed. The structure of the mucous membrane in the intestine is much the same. In all these mucous membranes there are situated other glands, generally formed each of a small mass of twisted tubes, which secrete a clear shining fluid known as mucus, that gives to these membranes their soft, smooth appearance and their name (illustration 229). The glands so far mentioned are all of microscopic size, but there are many of large dimensions. The parotid gland, situated just in front of the ear, the submaxillary gland, which can be easily felt, of the size of a chestnut beneath the jaw, and the sublingual gland, which can be seen beneath the tongue, are occupied in producing

229 – Diagram of various types of glands. 1, simple tubular (eg. intestinal glands); 2, simple coiled tubular (eg. sweat glands); 3, 4, simple branched tubular (eg. gastric glands); 5, simple alveolar; 6, simple branched alveolar (eg. sebaceous glands); 7, compound (eg. salivary and mammary glands). The secretory part of the gland is black. From *Hewer's Textbook of Histology*. William Heinemann, Ltd.

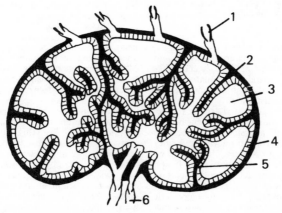

230 – Diagram of structure of a lymph gland. 1, afferent lymphatic; 2, capsule; 3, cortical lymph follicle; 4, lymph sinus; 5, trabecula; 6, efferent lymphatic. From *Hewer's Textbook of Histology*. William Heinemann, Ltd.

saliva, and known as salivary glands. The breasts or mammary glands are a pair of large glands situated in the skin over the front of the chest, and secrete milk. The thyroid gland, situated in front of the neck, has no outlet to the exterior, but produces a very important secretion which is absorbed by the blood and carried throughout the body. The suprarenal glands situated immediately above the kidneys act under similar conditions. Many of the glands which have an outlet through which one secretion comes, such as the pancreas and testes, also produce what is called an internal secretion that is absorbed by the blood, and exerts a profound effect upon general nutrition.

Glands which produce an internal secretion are known as endocrine glands. (See ENDOCRINE GLANDS.)

(2) LYMPHATIC GLANDS are scattered all through the body in connection with the system of lymphatic vessels. They vary much in size, from that of microscopic masses to that of large beans, but they have essentially the same structure everywhere (illustration 230). Round each gland is a fibrous tissue capsule, from which partitions and bands run into the gland to join one another and give it cohesion. In the meshes of these lie enormous numbers of lymph corpuscles in the circulating blood. These corpuscles are arranged in masses round which the lymph circulates freely. Numbers of lymph-vessels (afferent vessels) pierce the capsule of the gland, and the lymph, after passing from them, percolates through the gland and leaves its central part, carrying with it many corpuscles, by a few larger lymph-vessels (efferent vessels). The vessels leaving one gland pass on to enter another, the glands being, as a rule, arranged in chains.

In the limbs the lymph-vessels pass from the foot and hand up to the knee and elbow, respectively, before they encounter glands. A few glands are situated in the bend of each of these joints, and the vessels passing from these reach large chains of glands in the groin and armpit, respectively. The chains of glands beneath the jaw and down each side of the neck are known to everyone from the frequency with which they become inflamed and swollen. Inside the abdomen small lymph vessels known as lacteals collect certain parts of the food from the intestine, and pass their contents through mesenteric glands, situated deep in the abdominal cavity. Deep in the chest, too, lie many large bronchial glands, receiving lymphatics from the lungs. The lymph-vessels from the lower limbs and abdomen, after passing through numerous glands, unite into a single trunk, about the size of a quill, called the thoracic duct, which passes upwards through the chest, collecting the lymphatics of the chest, left arm, and left side of the neck, to open into the veins on the left side of the neck. A shorter lymphatic vessel collects the lymphatics from the right side of the chest, right arm, and right side of the neck, opening into the veins of the right side. The point where the lymphatic system on each side opens into the venous system is at or close to the point of union of the subclavian vein with the internal jugular vein. By means of these connections the lymph corpuscles formed in the glands may reach the blood. Beyond forming these corpuscles, the glands have another function, acting as a species of filters upon the lymph circulation, and keeping back micro-organisms and other dangerous impurities from entering the blood circulation.

GLANDS, DISEASES OF – The diseases of the chief secreting glands are described under various headings, and reference is made here only to diseases of the lymphatic glands. Most of the diseases which affect these glands are of an inflammatory nature, various poisonous substances lodging in them in the attempt to pass through the system by way of the lymphatic vessels. (See also ENDOCRINE GLANDS.)

SIMPLE ENLARGEMENT AND SUPPURATION OF A GLAND is the commonest condition. This is generally the result of a wound or other source of infection in the area drained by the lymphatic vessels going to the gland. For example, any source of irritation about the head, such as lice or eczema, is apt to produce swelling of the glands behind the ear and down the neck; or a wound of the foot or hand to cause inflammation of the glands in the groin or armpit, respectively.

Treatment – The object at first is to prevent suppuration of the enlarged and inflamed gland. For this purpose the source of irritation must be removed by opening the gumboil, cleaning the head, dressing the wound of the foot, etc. If the infection is due to a penicillin-sensitive organism, penicillin should also be given unless the infection is very mild. The gland itself is best left entirely alone, or at most kept supported and at rest by a pad and flannel bandage. If the swelling becomes soft and the skin over it reddened, suppuration is taking place, and the condition must be treated as an acute abscess. (See ABSCESS, ACUTE.)

TUBERCULOUS GLANDS. or SCRO-FULA, is a disease of childhood, especially in the neck. In many cases the glands become infected by the tubercle bacillus, *Mycobacterium tuberculosis*, through the tonsils. The chain of glands under the jaw and that running up and down the neck become affected in most cases, whilst in others the glands inside the abdomen are diseased, producing the condition of wasting known as tabes mesenterica. The condition progresses very slowly, as a rule, the glands enlarging for some months, then becoming matted together, to form an irregular mass, which softens, reddens here and there, and finally bursts through the skin to produce sinuses, which may go on discharging for years, healing finally with red, puckered, unsightly scars.

Treatment – Tuberculous glands are often the result of infection with the bovine tubercle bacillus. Therefore, one of the most important preventive measures is to see that no child drinks raw milk but only milk that has been pasteurized. In the first stage, while the glands are simply enlarging, general treatment to improve the constitution is required, as well as the administration of anti-tuberculous drugs. The diet should be constructed upon the same principle as that for other tuberculous conditions. (See TUBERCULOSIS.)

The introduction of the anti-tuberculous drugs has meant that in many cases the infection can be brought under control without any of the procedures about to be described, but there is still a certain number of cases in which they are necessary. A bandage or other appliance is often used in order to keep the part where the enlarged glands are situated more effectually at rest. This form of treatment may be persevered with so long as the glands are not becoming matted together. When the latter change takes place it is usually best to have the whole mass removed by operation, after which healing is, usually, immediate, and a narrow, barely visible scar is left. When a chronic abscess has formed but has not burst, it is treated like a chronic abscess in other sites. (See ABSCESS, CHRONIC.) If suppuration be allowed to take place, and the abscess to burst of itself, it is almost impossible to avoid a unsightly scar. When this accident has occurred, and a discharging sinus is present, the best that can be done, in general, is for the surgeon to aid healing by scraping the sinus out and dressing it

frequently in such a way that it may heal from the bottom.

CANCER, when it is present in any organ, sooner or later affects the neighbouring lymphatic glands. It is by way of the lymphatic system, indeed, that cancer usually spreads to parts at a distance, and glands in a part of the body far removed from the original cancer may become affected, while the intervening tissues remain healthy. This is the chief reason for the recurrence of cancer after apparently complete removal. As an example of this, it may be noted that the glands on the left side of the neck are prone to be diseased as a result of cancer in the stomach; those in the armpit become affected early in cancer of the breast.

OTHER CONDITIONS which produce enlargement of glands are the venereal diseases, leukaemia, and the disease known as lymphadenoma, or Hodgkin's disease. (See also BUBO.)

GLANDULAR FEVER, or INFECTIOUS MONONUCLEOSIS, is an acute virus infection which occurs predominantly among older children, adolescents and young adults. The incubation period is variable and may be as long as seven weeks. The glands of the neck become, in the course of a day or two, much enlarged and tender. This is accompanied by fever and a sore throat, and the patient loses all appetite for food. Jaundice may occur in a few cases. One of the characteristics of the disease is the presence in the blood of a large number of mononuclear, non-granular white cells. There is also a specific test for the disease known as the Paul-Bunnell Test (qv). Children recover fairly quickly but in adults convalescence may be prolonged.

Treatment – The patient should be confined to bed until the temperature has settled or the patient feels fit to get up. Analgesics, such as aspirin or paracetamol, should be given to relieve pain and discomfort, and the neck should be kept warm and still by a flannel bandage and cotton-wool.

GLAUBER'S SALT, or SULPHATE OF SODA, is used as a saline purgative in doses of a quarter of an ounce to half an ounce (5 to 15 grams), dissolved in a wine-glassful of water.

GLAUCOMA is a disease of the eye, occurring most commonly after the age of 50 years, in which the pressure within the eye rises and destroys the visual nerve fibres. It is responsible for over a quarter of all blindness after the age of 45. Certain families seem to be prone to it.

Causes – The manner in which it arises is as follows. It has been explained (see EYE) that a sharp angle exists all round the ring of junction between the iris and cornea, and in this angle the fluids of the eye filter out and into the blood-vessels situated in the neighbouring ciliary body. Sometimes in later life, owing to increasing size of the lens or to some inflammatory change in the eye, the iris becomes pushed forward at its outer margin against the cornea, and thus the angle where filtration occurs is shut up. Accordingly fluid collects in the hinder part of the ball, and the pressure inside the eyeball rises, causing damage, especially to the optic nerve fibres.

Symptoms – Quite often glaucoma appears so slowly, and with so little pain, that the condition is far advanced before it attracts special attention, but sometimes a series of well-marked acute attacks gives warning that a serious condition is present, and allows it to be averted or lessened by early treatment. An acute attack usually begins at night with great pain in one eye, shooting through one side of the head, and this pain may be so severe as to produce sickness and vomiting at first. In more prolonged cases coloured haloes are seen round lamps and candles, and there are various other peculiarities of vision. The veins on the surface of the eye are distended, giving it a bloodshot appearance, and the pupil is often wide and oval in shape instead of small and round like that of the sound eye. The peculiar grey-green haze which gives the disease its name may or may not take the place of the absolute blackness shown by the healthy pupil. When the eye is closely examined by a specialist, the tension of the ball is found to be increased, so that the eye is harder than usual; the anterior chamber lying between iris and cornea is shallow, and both the latter appear hazy; the field of vision is much restricted; and on examination with the ophthalmoscope the optic disc is found to be deeply indented, or cupped, if the disease has been present any length of time. The severe pain may last for two or three days, gradually decreasing, but if the condition be not recognized and treated, it reappears in a few weeks. Attacks become more and more frequent as time goes on, and the vision gets steadily worse. In chronic glaucoma the eye becomes gradually blind without these acute attacks.

Treatment – Prior to 1857 the disease was incurable, but in this year von Graefe introduced the operation of iridectomy for glaucoma. This operation is performed by making an incision into the anterior chamber of the eye along the line where the cornea merges into the sclerotic, grasping the iris, and partly by cutting, partly by pulling, removing a segment of it, so as to free the angle of filtration at one point. A more modern operation is that of sclerotomy, in which a wide incision is made in the same situation as for iridectomy, or a small circle bored out of the sclerotic coat (trephining) but no part of the iris removed. The fluids in the eye can then filter out through the scar, and thus the pressure within the eyeball is lessened.

When the condition is progressing very slowly, or when, for any reason, operation is inadvisable, a solution containing 0·25 to 5 per cent of pilocarpine nitrate is dropped into the eye night and morning, and since this drug powerfully contracts the pupil the iris is drawn away from the cornea and the angle between them opened up for filtration. This treatment may be continued daily for months or years.

GLEET means a chronic form of gonorrhoea.

GLENOID is the term applied to the shallow socket on the shoulder-blade into which the humerus fits, forming the shoulder-joint.

GLIBENACIDE is a drug which stimulates the beta cells of the pancreas to liberate insulin, and is thereby proving of value in some cases of diabetes mellitus (qv).

GLIOMA is the name given to a tumour which forms in the brain or spinal cord, composed of neuroglia, which is the special connective tissue that in these organs supports the nerve-cells and nerve-fibres.

GLOBULIN is the term applied to a class of proteins which are insoluble in water and alcohol and soluble in weak salt solution. (See also GAMMA-GLOBULIN.)

GLOBUS is a term applied generally to any structures of ball shape, but especially to the sensation of a ball in the throat causing choking, which forms a common symptom of hysteria.

GLOMERULONEPHRITIS is the term applied to inflammation of the kidney that chiefly affects the glomeruli. (See BRIGHT'S DISEASE.)

GLOMERULUS is the term applied to a small knot of blood-vessels (illustration 277) about the size of a sand grain, of which around 1,000,000 are found in each kidney, and from which the excretion of fluid out of the blood into the tubules of the kidney takes place.

GLOSSITIS means inflammation of the tongue.

GLOSSOPHARYNGEAL nerve is the ninth cranial nerve, which in the main is a sensory nerve, being the nerve of taste in the posterior third of the tongue and the nerve of general sensation for the whole upper part of the throat and middle ear. It also supplies the parotid gland and one of the muscles on the side of the throat.

GLOTTIS is the narrow opening at the upper end of the larynx. (See AIR PASSAGES; CHOKING; LARYNX.)

GLUCAGON is a hormone secreted by the alpha cells of the islets of Langerhans in the pancreas, which increases the amount of glucose in the blood.

GLUCOCORTICOIDS is the group of steroid hormones produced by the adrenal cortex, which includes cortisol and cortisone (qv), and which particularly affect protein, fat and carbohydrate metabolism.

GLUCONEOGENESIS means the formation of sugar from amino-acids in the liver.

GLUCOSE (DEXTROSE; GRAPE SUGAR) is the form of sugar found in honey and in grapes and some other fruits. It is also the form of sugar circulating in the blood stream and the form into which all sugars and starches are converted in the small intestine before being absorbed. Glucose is a yellowish-white crystalline substance soluble in water and having the property of turning the ray of polarized light to the right. It is often given to patients as an easily assimilated form of carbohydrate. It has the further practical advantage in this context of not being nearly as sweet-tasting as cane sugar and therefore relatively large amounts can be consumed without sickening the patient. For patients unable to take food by the mouth, glucose is sometimes administered in the form of an enema consisting of 5 per cent of glucose in normal saline fluid, or one ounce (28·5 grams) of glucose to the pint (570 ml) of water. The same fluid, when carefully sterilized, may be injected by a hollow needle beneath the skin or directly into the veins, and is quickly absorbed. (See SUGAR; URINE.)

GLUCOSIDE is a glycoside (qv) formed from glucose.

GLUE EAR is another name for secretory otitis media. (See EAR, DISEASES OF.)

GLUTAMIC ACID is an amino-acid with the formula $C_3H_5(NH_2)(COOH)_2$. It has been used in the treatment of epilepsy.

GLUTEAL is the name applied to the region of the buttock and the structures situated in it, such as the gluteal muscles, arteries, and nerves.

GLUTEN is the constituent of wheat-flour which forms an adhesive substance on addition of water, and therefore permits of the 'raising' of bread. It can be separated from the starch of flour, and being of a protein nature is used to make bread for those diabetics who are debarred from starchy and sugary foods.

It is also responsible for certain forms of what is now known as the malabsorption syndrome (qv). In these cases an essential part of treatment is a gluten-free diet.

GLUTETHIMIDE is a non-barbiturate hypnotic, which induces sleep fairly rapidly, and whose effects last about six hours.

GLYCERIN, or GLYCEROL, is an alcohol, $C_3H_8O_3$, which occurs naturally in combination with organic acids in the form of fats or triglycerides. It is a clear, colourless, thick liquid of sweet taste. It dissolves many substances, and it has a great power of absorbing water, in consequence of which, in the pure state, it diminishes congestion in surfaces with which it is brought in contact.

Uses – Glycerin has many varied uses. Numerous substances, such as carbolic acid, tannic acid, alum, borax, boric acid, starch, are dissolved in it for application to the body. It is frequently applied along with other remedies to inflamed areas for its action in extracting fluid and thus diminishing inflammation.

Mixed with an equal quantity of water it forms a useful mouth-wash when the tongue and gums are furred or dry, and, as a spray, is one of the best ways of relieving the discomfort of laryngitis. It is also useful for application to the skin in order to prevent chapping in cold weather, and to protect and heal all sorts of small abrasions.

Internally, pure glycerin, in doses of 1 or 2 teaspoonfuls, acts as a laxative, administered either by the mouth or as an enema. For its pleasant taste it is added to various medicines. It is mixed with gelatin to form a basis for pastilles. (See GELATIN.)

GLYCERITE is a mixture of glycerin with a medicinal substance. The principal glycerites are those of alum, borax, boric acid (known as boroglycerin), gallic acid, subacetate of lead, carbolic acid, starch, and tannic acid. These are used as applications, especially to the mucous membrane of the mouth and throat, for the action of the various medicinal substances contained.

GLYCEROL is another name for glycerin (qv).

GLYCEROPHOSPHATES are compounds of glycerin and phosphates, supposed by some to be beneficial as tonics in debility, because glycerophosphoric acid is a constituent of nerve tissue.

GLYCERYL TRINITRATE, or TRINITRIN, is a dilator of arterioles (qv), which is used in the treatment of angina pectoris (qv). Also known as TRINITRIN and NITROGLYCERIN, it is a thick oily liquid of sweet taste and explosive properties. When a small quantity is taken internally it produces marked effects in about two minutes, relaxing the smaller arteries, capillaries (qv) and veins so as to cause the skin to flush visibly, quickening the pulse, and causing a sense of fullness all over the body and throbbing in the head. It greatly lessens the blood pressure and temporarily relaxes all muscle, whether striped or unstriped.

Uses – This sudden action in relaxing muscle fibres and lessening blood-pressure proves very valuable in conditions where serious effects are produced by spasm, particularly in angina pectoris, but also in bronchial asthma (due in part to spasm of the small bronchial tubes), in gall-stone and renal colic, and in the vomiting of sea-sickness. In these it diminishes the spasmodic condition and gives relief.

It is used in the form of glyceryl trinitrate tablets B.P., each containing 500 micrograms made up with chocolate. These should not be swallowed intact, but allowed to melt in the mouth before being swallowed. (See ANGINA PECTORIS.)

Other substances have a similar action. Nitrite of sodium and nitrite of potassium are used in doses of 3 to 5 grains (200 to 500 mg), and have the advantage of producing their effect more slowly and more permanently. Erythrol tetranitrate has a similarly prolonged effect. Nitrite of amyl, on the other hand, produces its effect in a few seconds, and, being volatile, may be inhaled as well as swallowed. For this purpose small thin glass perles are prepared, and are carried in the pocket by those liable to angina pectoris or other sudden convulsive seizure. Immediately the spasm comes on, one of these perles is crushed between the finger and thumb and held to the nostrils.

GLYCO- is a prefix meaning of the nature of, or containing, sugar.

GLYCOGEN, or ANIMAL STARCH, is a carbohydrate substance found specially in the liver, as well as in other tissues. It is the form in which carbohydrates taken in the food are stored in the liver and muscles before they are converted into glucose as the needs of the body require.

GLYCOPYRRONIUM BROMIDE is an anticholinergic, or atropine-like, agent which is used in the treatment of duodenal ulcer.

GLYCOSIDE is a compound of a sugar and a non-sugar unit. Glycosides are widespread throughout nature and include many important drugs such as digoxin.

GLYCOSURIA means the presence of sugar in the urine. By far the most common cause of glycosuria is diabetes mellitus, but it may also occur in exophthalmic goitre, certain other glandular disturbances, following a general anaesthetic, and occasionally following great emotional stress.

GLYCYRRHETINIC ACID is the active principle of liquorice (qv) and has been shown to have an anti-inflammatory action resembling, though much weaker than, that of cortisone. (See CARBENOXOLONE.)

GLYMIDINE is one of the oral hypoglycaemic agents: that is, a drug which, when taken by mouth, is able to control certain milder cases of diabetes mellitus without the help of insulin.

GOA POWDER (see CHRYSAROBIN).

GOITRE, also known as BRONCHOCELE or DERBYSHIRE NECK, is a term applied to a swelling on the front of the neck caused by an enlargement of the thyroid gland. This structure, which lies between the skin and the front of the windpipe, and which in health is not large enough to give rise to any external prominence, is liable to occasional variations in size, more especially in females, a temporary enlargement of the gland being not uncommon at the menstrual periods, as well as during pregnancy. The gland is liable to fluctuations in function as well as in size. When its functions are lessened, either by wasting of the gland (atrophy) or by failure of secretion in a gland either of ordinary size or in an enlarged state, the general name of hypothyroidism is applied; when the functions are increased, which may happen in a gland of ordinary size or more commonly accompanies certain types of enlargement, the name hyperthyroidism is given. Atrophic conditions of the gland are considered under the heading MYXOEDEMA. Here we shall consider conditions in which the gland is enlarged, although it must be noted that the symptoms depend not so much upon enlargement as upon the fact of whether the gland is acting sluggishly or in excess. Two main forms of enlargement are recognized: (*a*) *Simple goitre*, and (*b*) *Exophthalmic goitre*.

SIMPLE GOITRE occasions a swelling which is well marked, and is not only unsightly, but by its growth may occasion much discomfort, and even give rise to serious symptoms from its pressure on the windpipe and other important parts in the neck.

Causes – Simple goitre is an excellent example of an endemic disease. There are few parts of the world where it is not found prevailing in certain localities, these being for the most part deep valleys in mountainous districts. For example, in Germany it occurs in the Black Forest; it is also found in Styria, in the Italian Alps, and, above all, is common in parts of Switzerland. In India it is common among the Himalayas, in China it affects the dwellers in various hill districts, and in England it was so frequent in the Peak district that the disease has received for one of its titles the name of Derbyshire neck. It is also very common in certain places far removed from the sea and supposed to have a deficiency of iodine in the soil: eg. in the Middle States of America, especially Michigan. The widespread nature of the disease has naturally led to inquiry and speculation as to its origin. The most generally accepted view is that which ascribes the malady to the use of drinking water deficient in iodine. Although this view is supported by the fact that goitre has been much decreased in whole districts by the expedients of either obtaining a new water supply or giving iodized salt to the entire population, there is evidence which suggests that other factors may occasionally come into play. For instance, certain wells in some areas are known to be goitre-producing, whilst neighbouring wells with apparently the same water are safe; the goitre-producing water may be rendered innocuous by boiling. It has been suggested that it may be due to a micro-organism or other parasite infesting particular waters. It has also been suggested that want of sunlight, etc., combine with the effect of the drinking water in developing the disease. Certain foods, especially the Brassica family (eg. cabbage) are also known to be goitrogenic: ie. induce goitre. Goitre can often be cured by removal from the district where it prevails, and it may be acquired by previously healthy persons who settle in goitrous localities. It is only in such places that the disease shows any hereditary tendencies. Women are far more often affected than men.

Symptoms – In districts where the disease prevails, the goitre usually appears in early life, often from the eighth to the twelfth year. Its growth is at first slow, but, after several years of comparative quiescence, a somewhat sudden increase occasionally occurs. In the earlier stages of the disease, the condition of the thyroid gland is simply an enlargement of the gland, which retains its normal, soft consistence, and is distended by colloid material. But in the course of time other changes supervene, and the gland may become the seat of cystic formations, or acquire hardness from increase of fibrous tissue or calcareous deposits. Occasionally the enlargement of the gland is uniform, but more commonly one of the lobes, generally the right, is the larger. The growth is unattended by pain, and is compatible with ordinary health. Sometimes, when the goitre becomes large, the voice grows hoarse and toneless, but only when the gland becomes very large is there any interference with breathing or swallowing.

Treatment – In endemic areas the incidence of simple goitre has been reduced to a very low figure by the routine administration of iodine. This is usually given in the form of iodized table salt, the concentration of iodine in the salt varying between 1 part in 5000 to 1 part in 250,000. Another method used in some areas is to give iodine to school children for ten days in the spring and in the autumn, and to women during pregnancy. The usual dose in these cases is 0·2 gram of potassium iodide daily.

When a goitre is already present, treatment consists of the administration of iodine, usually in the form of Lugol's solution (qv), 15 to 30 minims (1 to 2 millilitres) daily. If this fails to control the condition, thyroid extract is usually tried. Surgery is resorted to in those cases in which the goitre is unduly large or unsightly or is causing unpleasant symptoms by pressing on the windpipe. When the goitre is removed in this way, care must be taken to leave sufficient of the gland to ensure an adequate supply of thyroid secretion. Otherwise signs of hypothyroidism, or myxoedema (qv), will develop.

EXOPHTHALMIC GOITRE is the name applied to another form of enlargement of the thyroid gland, in which marked constitutional changes occur. In this disease, the goitre is one of several symptoms which form the most noticeable features of the disease: ie. extreme nervousness, muscular tremors, palpitation of the heart and throbbing of the great vessels, enlargement of the thyroid gland, and protrusion of the eyeballs. This group of symptoms is often known also by the names of Graves' disease, Parry's disease, and von Basedow's disease, in reference to the physicians by whom the disease was first recognized and described. It is also known as thyrotoxicosis.

Causes – The exact nature of exophthalmic goitre is still uncertain, but its symptoms are due either to an increase of the normal secretion of the thyroid gland, or, in other cases, to perversion in quality of this secretion. Many of the symptoms produced are due to the action of this secretion on the sympathetic nervous system, and a number of the symptoms are also caused by changes in the other endocrine glands related to the thyroid.

This type of goitre is not more common in the districts where simple goitre occurs than it is elsewhere. Women are more often affected than men, in the proportion of 8 to 1, or even higher. The age of onset is usually between sixteen and forty years.

The predisposition to the disease seems to occur in certain families, and cases which previously were slight are often greatly aggravated by fright or anxiety or mental strain. The general appearance of the disease, apart from the goitre, shows a great similarity to the characters of intense fear. Sometimes the disease first attracts attention after the patient has suffered from some infectious disease, or it may be preceded by anaemia, or by various nervous or emotional manifestations.

Symptoms – The first of the symptoms to appear are generally the nervousness and the palpitation of the heart, which is aggravated by the slightest exertion and may be very severe. The rate of the pulse is much increased, commonly to 120 per minute or more. An uncomfortable sensation of throbbing is felt throughout the body, and many of the larger blood-vessels are seen to pulsate strongly. There are marked tremors of the muscles and limbs, especially after any exertion. The enlargement of the thyroid gland generally comes on gradually; it rarely increases to any great size, thus differing from simple goitre.

Accompanying the goitre a change is observed in the appearance of the eyes, which attract attention by their prominence and by the fact that a space of the white of the eye is left exposed all round the iris (exophthalmos). A startled or frightened expression is thus given to the countenance. In extreme cases the eyes protrude from the sockets to such a degree that the eyelids cannot be closed, and injury may thus arise to the constantly exposed eyeballs. Apart from such risk, however, the vision is rarely affected in this disease. Much difference of opinion prevails as to the immediate cause of the protrusion of the eyes, but it is generally ascribed to the increase of the fatty tissue and distension of the blood-vessels of the orbits. The eyelids show a characteristic sign (von Graefe's sign) by failing to descend along with the eyeball as the person glances downwards. It occasionally happens that in undoubted cases of the disease one or other of the above-named characteristic phenomena is absent, generally either the goitre or the exophthalmos. The palpitation of the heart is the most constant symptom. Sleeplessness, irritability, disorders of digestion, diarrhoea, uterine derangements, muscular tremors, and an unusual readiness to perspire freely are common accompaniments. All the bodily activities are carried on at high pressure, and there is consequent wasting of the fatty and muscular tissues, with increasing thinness. The basal metabolism is much higher than it is in the normal individual.

Exophthalmic goitre is not often a directly fatal malady, but the nervousness, palpitation, and muscular weakness may render the patient unfit for even the slightest exertion. Heart failure and atrial fibrillation are grave risks. Partial improvement and relapses occur from time to time, especially after periods of rest. In some cases, the patient in old age passes into the opposite condition of myxoedema, the thyroid gland appearing to be completely worn out.

THYROTOXIC ADENOMA is a variety of exophthalmic goitre, in which a simple goitre containing one or more large hard nodules, which may have been present for some time, suddenly takes on the characters of exophthalmic goitre, with the symptoms of this condition. The symptoms in such a case are, however, not so marked, except that there is a marked tendency for atrial fibrillation and heart failure to develop. A simple goitre occasionally develops gradually into a case of exophthalmic goitre.

Treatment – Three lines of treatment are now available: drugs, surgery, and radioactive iodine. Drugs are usually the first line of attack, and the two most widely used are carbimazole and propylthiouracil. Surgery, which consists of removing around seven-eighths of the gland, is usually resorted to if the condition fails to respond to drugs, if the condition is severe or of long standing, or if the goitre is particularly big. The patient is usually prepared for operation by drugs and then by a course of potassium iodide. Radioactive iodine (see ISOTOPES) is usually reserved for middle-aged or elderly patients.

GOLD SALTS have been used in the treatment of tuberculosis and of chronic rheumatic disorders. They have now been given up for the treatment of tuberculosis, but are still used in the treatment of rheumatoid arthritis. Gold may be administered in various forms, such as sodium aurothiomalate. It is injected in very small doses intramuscularly and produces a reaction in the affected tissues which leads to their scarring and healing. If gold is administered in too large quantities skin eruptions, albuminuria, metallic taste in the mouth, jaundice, and feverishness may be produced, so that it is necessary to prolong a course of this remedy over many months in minute doses.

GOLDEN OINTMENT is another name for yellow oxide of mercury ointment, which is used for inflammation of the eyelids.

GONAD is a gland which produces a gamete: an ovary or a testis.

GONADOTROPHINS, or GONADOTROPHIC HORMONES, are hormones that control the activity of the gonads (ie. the testes and ovaries). In the male they stimulate the secretion of testosterone and the production of spermatozoa. In the female they stimulate the production of ova and the secretion of oestrogen (qv) and progesterone (qv). There are three gonadotrophins produced by the pituitary gland. *Chorionic gonadotrophin* is produced in the placenta and excreted in the urine.

GONAGRA means an attack of gout affecting the knee. (See GOUT.)

GONORRHOEA is an inflammatory disease affecting especially the mucous membrane of the urethra in the male and that of the vagina in the female, but spreading also to other parts. It is the most common of the venereal diseases (qv).

Causes – The disease is directly contagious from another person already suffering in this manner, usually by sexual intercourse, but occasionally it is conveyed by the discharge on sponges, towels, or clothing as well as by actual contact. The infecting agent is the gonococcus or *Neisseria gonorrhoeae*. This is found in the discharge expressed from the urethra, which may be spread as a film on a glass slide, suitably stained, and examined under the microscope; or a culture from the discharge may be made on certain bacteriological media and films from this, similarly examined under the microscope. Since discharges resembling that of gonorrhoea accompany other forms of inflammation, the identification of the organism is of great importance.

Symptoms – These differ considerably, according to whether the disease is in an acute or a chronic stage. In *men*, after an incubation period of between two and ten days, irritation in the urethra, scalding pain on passing water, and a viscid yellowish-white discharge appear; the glands in the groin often enlarge and may suppurate. The urine when passed is hazy and is often found to contain yellowish threads of pus visible to the eye. After some weeks, if the condition has become chronic, the discharge is clear and viscid, there may be irritation in passing urine, and various forms of inflammation in neighbouring organs may appear, the testicle, prostate gland, and bladder becoming affected. At a still later stage the inflammation of the urethra is apt to lead to gradual formation of fibrous tissue around this channel. This contracts and produces narrowing, so that the passage of water becomes difficult or may be stopped for a time altogether (the condition known as stricture). Inflammation of some of the joints is a common complication at this or an earlier stage, the knee, ankle, wrist, and elbow being the joints most frequently affected, and this form of 'rheumatism' is very intractable and liable to lead to permanent stiffness. The fibrous tissues elsewhere may also develop inflammatory changes, causing lumbago, pain in the foot, etc. In occasional cases, during the acute stage, a general blood-poisoning results, with inflammation of the heart-valves (endocarditis) and abscesses in various parts of the body. The infective matter occasionally is inoculated accidentally into the eye producing a very severe form of conjunctivitis. In the newly born child this is known as *ophthalmia neonatorum* and until recently was one of the chief causes of blindness. (See EYE DISEASES.)

In *women* the course and complications of the disease are somewhat different. It begins with a yellow vaginal discharge, pain on passing water, and very often inflammation or abscess of the Bartholin's glands, situated close to the vulva or opening of the vagina. The chief seriousness, however, of the disease is due to the spread of inflammation to neighbouring organs, the uterus, Fallopian tubes, and ovaries, causing permanent destructive changes in these, and leading occasionally to peritonitis through the Fallopian tube, with a fatal result. Many cases of prolonged ill-health and sterility or recurring miscarriages are due to these changes.

Treatment – Prevention is always better than cure, and this applies *par exellence* in the case of gonorrhoea, as in the case of all forms of venereal disease. If, however, risks have been run and the infection acquired, the chances of cure are better the earlier treatment is instituted. The treatment of gonorrhoea was revolutionized by the introduction of the sulphonamides. These, in turn, have now been replaced by the antibiotics. Penicillin is now the antibiotic of choice: a single injection of 2·4 or 4·8 mega units of procaine penicillin. Unfortunately, the gonococcus is liable to become resistant to penicillin. In patients who are infected with penicillin-resistant organisms, one of the other antibiotics is used, usually either oxytetracycline (qv) or tetracycline (qv). In all cases it is essential that bacteriological investigation should be carried out at weekly intervals for three or four weeks, to make sure that the patient is cured.

GOSSYPIUM is the Latin word for cotton.

GOULARD'S WATER is the popular name for the dilute solution of subacetate of lead, which is employed in the treatment of sprains, bruises, and localized inflammations. It is commonly mixed with laudanum in the proportion of 60 minims (4 ml) of laudanum to 1 ounce (28·5 ml) of the Goulard's water, and the mixture, known as lead and opium lotion, is applied on a piece of moist warm flannel, and covered with waterproof cloth.

GOUT is a constitutional disorder connected with excess of uric acid in the blood, and manifesting itself by inflammation of joints usually therein of urate of soda, and also by morbid changes in various important organs.

The term, gout, which was first used about the end of the thirteenth century, is derived through the French *goutte* from the Latin *gutta*, a drop, in allusion to the old pathological doctrine (which in the present case seems to be essentially the correct one) of the dropping of a morbid material from the blood within the joints. The disease was known and described by the ancient Greek physicians under various terms, which, however, appear to have been applied by them alike to rheumatism and gout. The general term, *arthritis*, was employed when many joints were the seat of inflammation; whilst in those instances where the disease was limited to one part the name referred to such locality; hence *podagra* when the foot was involved, *chiragra* when the hand was involved and *gonagra* when the knee was involved.

Chalk-stones have been found in the feet of Egyptian mummies. Hippocrates (460–375 BC) in his *Aphorisms* speaks of gout as occurring most commonly in spring and autumn, and mentions the fact that women are less liable to it than men.

Galen regarded gout as an unnatural accumulation of humours in a part, and the chalk-stones as the concretions of these; and he attributed the disease to over-indulgence and luxury. Gout is alluded to in the works of Ovid and Pliny, and Seneca, in his ninety-fifth epistle, mentions the prevalence of gout among the Roman ladies of his day as one of the results of their high living and debauchery. Lucian, in his *Tragopodagra*, gives an amusing account of the remedies used for the cure of gout.

Sydenham, the famous English physician of the seventeenth century, wrote an important treatise on the subject, and his

passing off in the urine being 0·1 to 2 grams daily. In the healthy human subject the blood contains 3 to 6 mg per 100 millilitres, but in gout it is increased, both before and during the acute attack, while in chronic gout the amount in the blood and elsewhere in the body is always above the normal level. The gouty paroxysm appears to rid the system to a certain extent of the accumulated uric acid, although such relief is generally of but temporary duration.

Gout is in a marked degree hereditary. A family history of the disease is obtained in from 50 to 80 per cent of cases. Gout is said to affect the sedentary more readily

231 – Urate crystals (magnified × 400) from a tophus. From Copeman, Textbook of Rheumatic Diseases. E. & S. Livingstone.

description of the gouty paroxysm, all the more vivid from his having himself been afflicted with the disease for thirty-four years, is still quoted by writers as the most graphic and exhaustive account of the symptoms of gout. William Cullen, in his time Professor of Medicine in both Edinburgh and Glasgow Universities, was among the first, in 1778, to contend that gout afflicted the wise. The tradition still persists and, whether or not statistically valid, there are certainly quite a number of the sages of this world, such as William Harvey, Sir Isaac Newton and Charles Darwin, who have suffered from the disease.

Causes – The cardinal feature of gout is the presence of an excessive amount of uric acid, and its deposition in the joints in the form of sodium monourate (illustration 231). The cause of this excess of uric acid is not known. Uric acid is formed in the system in the processes of nutrition, and is excreted by the kidneys, the amount

than the active, but this cannot be taken as a constant rule. On the other hand, inadequate exercise, a luxurious manner of living, habitual over-indulgence in animal food and rich dishes, and especially in alcoholic beverages, are undoubtedly important precipitating factors in the production of the disease. These, however, are no more than precipitating factors, and the disease can occur in vegetarians and teetotallers.

Gout is more common in mature age than in the earlier years of life, being infrequent before the age of 40, but it may occasionally affect very young persons in whom there is a strong family history. About 95 per cent of patients are males. In women it most often appears after the cessation of the menses. Persons exposed to the influence of lead-poisoning, such as plumbers and painters, are apt to suffer from gout; and it would seem that impregnation of the system with this metal

405

markedly interferes with the uric acid excreting function of the kidneys.

Attacks of gout are readily excited in those predisposed to the disease. Exposure to cold, disorders of digestion, fatigue, and irritation or injuries of particular joints will often precipitate the gouty paroxysm.

Symptoms – An attack of gout may appear without warning, or there may be premonitory symptoms. Among the more common of these are disorders of the digestive organs, with a feeble and capricious appetite, flatulence, uneasiness in the right side in the region of the liver, and irritation in the urinary organs. Various forms

takes place, and the patient may fall asleep. The pain, however, returns next night, and these nocturnal exacerbations occur with greater or less severity during the continuance of the attack, which generally lasts for a week or ten days. As the symptoms decline, the swelling and tenderness of the affected joint abate, but the skin over it pits on pressure for a time, and with this there is often associated slight desquamation of the cuticle. During the attacks the patient is restless and extremely irritable, and suffers from cramp in the limbs, and from dyspepsia, thirst, and constipation. The urine is scanty and

232 – The hands in a case of classical gout. Professor E. G. L. Bywater.

of nervous disturbance also present themselves in the form of extreme irritability of temper, and numbness and coldness in the limbs. On the night of the attack, the patient retires to rest apparently quite well, but about two or three o'clock in the morning is awakened by a painful feeling in the foot, most commonly in the ball of the great toe, but it may be in the instep or heel, or in the thumb. With the pain there often occurs a distinct shivering, followed by feverishness. The pain soon becomes of an agonizing character.

When the affected part is examined it is found to be swollen and of a deep red hue. The skin is tense and glistening, and the surrounding veins are more or less distended. After a few hours there is a remission of the pain, slight perspiration

high-coloured, with a copious deposit, consisting chiefly of urates. It is rare that the first is the only attack of gout, although by care and treatment recurrences may be warded off. In the earlier recurrences the same joints as were the original seat of the gouty inflammation suffer again, but in the course of time others become implicated, until in advanced cases scarcely any joint escapes, and the disease becomes chronic. When gout assumes this form, the frequently recurring attacks are usually attended with less pain, but chalk-stones, or tophi, are gradually formed round the affected joints. These deposits, which are highly characteristic of gout, at first occur in the form of a semi-fluid material, consisting for the most part of bi-urate of soda, which gradually becomes more dense, and ultimately quite hard. In some cases of chronic gout the deposit is so slight as to be barely appreciable externally, but on the other hand it occasionally causes great enlargement of the joints, and fixes them in a flexed or extended position which renders them entirely useless. Any of the joints may be thus affected, but most commonly those of the hands (illustration 232) and feet. The deposits occur in other structures besides those of joints, such as along the course of tendons, underneath the skin and periosteum, in the sclerotic coat of the eye, and especially on the cartilages of the external ear. When bi-urate of soda is largely deposited in joints the skin sometimes gives way, and the concretion is exposed.

Gout, when of long standing, is often found associated with degenerative changes in the heart and large arteries, the liver, and especially the kidneys, which are apt to assume the granular contracted condition already alluded to as one of the forms of Bright's disease (see BRIGHT'S DISEASE). A variety of urinary calculus – the uric acid – formed by concretions of this substance in the kidneys is a not infrequent occurrence in connection with gout; hence the well-known association of this disease and gravel.

Treatment – The usual plan of treatment is somewhat as follows. During the acute attack the affected part should be kept at perfect rest, and be enveloped in cotton-wool covered with oil-silk. The diet should be light, and the use of a laxative is of service, as well as the free administration of fluids. The medicinal agent upon which most reliance is placed is colchicum. The first known record of the use of this drug, which is said to derive its name from Colchis in Asia Minor, is in the Eber papyrus of around 1500 BC. The mode of action of colchicum is uncertain, but it is probable that it has simply a special sedative action upon the gouty inflammation without affecting the excretion of uric acid. It is usually administered as colchicine, which is the active principle of the drug and was first isolated in 1820. In cases which do not respond satisfactorily to colchicine, phenylbutazone may be used, or indomethacin or allopurinol, or corticotrophin or cortisone (or one of its derivatives).

In chronic gout the most commonly used drugs are allopurinol, phenylbutazone, sulphinpyrazone (a derivative of phenylbutazone), probenecid, sodium salicylate, or aspirin.

The diet and regimen to be employed in the intervals of the gouty attacks are of importance. Restriction must be laid upon the amount and quality of the food, and still more upon alcoholic stimulants. Regular but moderate exercise in the form of walking or riding, in the case of those who lead sedentary lives, is of great advantage, and all overwork, either physical or mental, should be avoided. The effect upon the gouty constitution of certain mineral waters and baths is well known, the alkaline waters being the favourite.

GOWERS'S MIXTURE was introduced, in 1888, by Sir William Gowers for the treatment of migraine. It contains sodium bromide, solution of glyceryl trinitrate, dilute hydrobromic acid, tincture of nux vomica, tincture of gelsemium, and syrup of lemon. It is still widely and successfully used for the purpose for which it was introduced.

GRAFT is the term applied to a small piece of skin or other tissue removed from one person or animal and implanted in another or the same in order by its growth to remedy some defect. Skin grafts are the tissues most commonly used. If a large piece of skin is required for covering an old ulcer or wound, the operation of grafting is usually done in two stages, the piece of skin to be grafted being first raised from its bed but allowed to remain attached at one end so that it may be nourished by its own blood-vessels while it is establishing connections with the tissues of the gap which it is desired to fill. After one or two weeks the graft is cut away from its original position and firmly fixed in the new one. Bone grafts are also used to replace bone which has been lost by disease: for example, a portion of rib is sometimes removed in order to furnish support for a spine weakened by disease, after the disease has been removed. Also, the bone of young animals is used to afford additional growth and strength to a limb bone which it has been necessary to remove in part on account of disease or injury. (See SKIN GRAFTING.)

GRAM, or GRAMME, is the unit of weight in the metric system and is equal to a little over 15·4 grains. For purposes of weighing food, 30 grams are usually taken as approximately equal to 1 ounce.

GRAM'S STAIN, named after the bacteriologist, H. C. J. Gram, who first described it in 1884, is one of the most valuable methods of differentiating certain micro-organisms. The principle involved depends upon the fact that certain bacteria, when treated with a dye such as gentian violet and then with iodine, fix the dye, whereas other bacteria do not do so. Those bacteria, such as the pneumococcus, that fix the dye are known as Gram-positive, whilst those that do not fix it, eg. the gonococcus, are said to be Gram-negative.

GRAND MAL is the name applied to a convulsive epileptic attack, in contrast to petit mal, which includes the milder forms of epilepsy (qv).

GRANULAR KIDNEY is the name given to the state of the kidney in chronic Bright's disease (see BRIGHT'S DISEASE), which often occurs in association with chronic arterial disease.

GRANULATIONS are small masses of formative cells containing loops of newly formed blood-vessels which spring up over any raw surface, as the first step in the process of healing of wounds. (See ULCER; WOUNDS.)

GRANULOMA is a term applied to a tumour or new growth made up of granulation tissue. This is caused by various forms of chronic inflammation, such as syphilis and tuberculosis.

GRAVEL is the name applied to any sediment which falls down in the urine, but particularly to small masses of uric acid. It produces various unpleasant symptoms. (See BLADDER, DISEASES OF; GOUT; URINE.)

GRAVES' DISEASE is another name for exophthalmic goitre. (See GOITRE.)

GRAVID means pregnant.

GREEN SICKNESS is a popular name for chlorosis. (See ANAEMIA.)

GREENSTICK FRACTURE is the term applied to an incomplete fracture, in which the bone is not completely broken across. It occurs in the long bones of children and is usually due to indirect violence. (See FRACTURES.)

GREGORY'S MIXTURE or POWDER is a powder of light-yellow colour containing rhubarb, magnesia, and ginger. In doses of 10 to 60 grains (0·6 to 4 grams) it is used as an antacid and purgative.

GRENZ RAYS are very soft, poor penetrating X-rays which are used in the treatment of certain skin diseases. (See X-RAYS.)

GREY POWDER is a powder composed of mercury and chalk. It was at one time much used as an ingredient of powders intended to check infantile diarrhoea, but is not used now for this, or any other, purpose in children because of the risk of inducing mercurial poisoning. (See ERYTHROEDEMA.)

GRINDELIA is an American plant used as an asthma remedy. The leaves are generally used soaked in nitre, dried, and then either burned on a plate, from which the fumes are inhaled, or rolled in a cigarette and smoked.

GRINDER'S ROT is the term applied to a disease of the lung in steel-grinders caused by inhaling particles of the metal.

GRIPES is a popular name for the colic of infants, generally due to irregular feeding. (See COLIC.)

GRIPPE is a popular name for influenza. (See INFLUENZA.)

GRISEOFULVIN is an antibiotic obtained from *Penicillium griseofulvum Dierckse*, which is proving of value in the treatment of various forms of ringworm.

GROIN is the name applied to the region which includes the upper part of the front of the thigh and lower part of the abdomen. A deep groove runs obliquely across it, which corresponds to the inguinal ligament, and divides the thigh from the abdomen. The principal diseased conditions in this region are enlarged glands (see GLANDS), and hernia (qv).

GROMMET is a small bobbin-shaped tube (illustration 233) used to keep open the incision made in the ear-drum in the treatment of secretory otitis media. (See EAR, DISEASES OF.) It acts as an artificial Eustachian tube (qv) and aids healing.

GROWING PAINS occur in children during the course of development. They occur most commonly in the legs and back. As often as not they are of no significance, but they must not be entirely ignored because they may on occasion be the first manifestation of rheumatic fever. Severe pains in young children are occasionally due to actual disease in a bone, either of tuberculous nature or caused by acute inflammation (osteomyelitis), and special attention is required in such cases.

GROWTH is a popular term applied to any new formation in any part of the body. (See CANCER; CYST; GANGLION; TUMOUR.) For growth of children, see WEIGHT AND HEIGHT.

GRUEL is the name given to a thin paste or thick fluid made of oatmeal or maize meal and milk or water. Gruel is made by mixing 3 tablespoonfuls of meal with 1 pint (570 ml) of cold milk or water, allowing to stand for 15 minutes, then straining and boiling for 15 minutes, and finally flavouring with salt and, if desired, with sugar.

GUAIAC is a resin obtained from the wood of *Guaiacum officinale* or *Lignum vitae*, a West Indian tree. It is seldom used now, except in the form of guaiac lozenges, which are sometimes of value in the treatment of sore throats.

GUANETHIDINE is one of the hypotensive drugs which act by inhibiting the action of the sympathetic nervous system (qv).

GUANOCLOR is another of the hypotensive drugs which act by blocking the action of the sympathetic nervous system.

GUANOXAN has a similar action to guanoclor.

GUINEA-WORM (see DRACONTIASIS).

233 – A grommet (Downs Surgical Ltd.)

GULLET, or OESOPHAGUS, is the tube down which food passes on its way from the throat to the stomach. (See OESOPHAGUS.)

GUM is a complex viscid substance which exudes from the stems and branches of various trees, and consists principally of arabin or bassorin. The two best-known gums are gum acacia and gum tragacanth. Gum-resins such as asafoetida, galbanum, and myrrh also contain resin. For gum-saline, see ACACIA.

GUMBOIL is a condition of inflammation, ending generally as an abscess, situated about the root of a carious tooth.

Symptoms – One tooth becomes a little painful and seems a little raised above the others, but the pain is at first relieved by clenching the teeth tightly, although after a day or more the affected tooth becomes extremely tender. A thickening forms at the side of the tooth, which is also at first relieved by pressure, as by holding a pad of cotton-wool, or similar soft mass between gum and cheek. After some days the pain lessens, and either the swelling gradually subsides, or an abscess forms and bursts, generally between gum and cheek, but it may be on the cheek.

Treatment – If there be any cavity in the tooth it should be stopped with cotton-wool soaked in a volatile oil, such as oil of cloves, or with a mixture of zinc oxide and oil of cloves, and if the pain and swelling do not speedily abate, the tooth should be pulled. Relief of the inflammation in the early stages is often gained by painting the gum freely with tincture of iodine. These, however, are only first-aid remedies, and expert dental advice should always be sought as soon as possible.

GUMMA means a hard swelling situated usually in connective tissue, although it may be in internal organs, muscle, or brain, and resulting from syphilis. The swelling is usually painless, but it may produce very marked symptoms by interference with the organ in which it is situated. A gumma generally disappears speedily when the treatment appropriate to syphilis is administered.

GUMS, DISEASES OF (see MOUTH, DISEASES OF; and TEETH, DISEASES OF).

GUTTA PERCHA is used in the preparation of some varieties of sticking-plaster, but its main use is, rolled out in

409

thin films, known as gutta-percha tissue, to keep surgical dressings moist by preventing evaporation.

GYMNASTICS (see EXERCISE; and CHEST DEVELOPMENT).

GYNAECOLOGY means that branch of medical science which deals with diseases peculiar to women.

GYNAECOMASTIA is the term used for describing an abnormal increase in size of the male breast.

GYRUS is the term applied to a convolution of the brain.

H

HABITS (see DRUG HABITS; also CHILDREN, PECULIARITIES OF).

HAEMARTHROSIS is the term used to denote bleeding into, or the presence of blood in, a joint.

HAEMATEMESIS means vomiting of blood. Blood brought up from the stomach is generally dark in colour, and is often so far digested as to form small brown granules resembling coffee grounds. Vomiting of blood is one of the chief symptoms of ulcer of the stomach, but it may also occur in gastritis, especially when this is due to the action of irritant poisons or alcohol. It should always be remembered that the blood may come from the nose or throat, and, after being swallowed, provoke vomiting. (See HAEMORRHAGE.)

HAEMATOCELE means a cavity containing blood. Generally as the result of an injury which ruptures blood-vessels, blood is effused into one of the natural cavities of the body, or among loose cellular tissue, producing a haematocele.

HAEMATOCOLPOS is the term applied to the condition in which menstrual blood is held up in the vagina as a result of an imperforate hymen.

HAEMATOCRIT is a graduated capillary tube for estimating the concentration of red corpuscles in the blood. The blood, made non-coagulable, is drawn into the tube; this is placed in a centrifuge and revolved at a speed of 3000 revolutions per minute for 30 minutes. The red corpuscles will then congregate at the end of the tube. Above this will be a clear layer of plasma. Normally, plasma occupies 55 divisions of the tube, and the red corpuscles 45 divisions.

HAEMATOIDIN and HAEMIN are crystalline bodies derived from the blood when it is allowed to clot and dry up. The former is produced where blood is effused in internal haemorrhages and then partly absorbed, for example, in cases of apoplexy. Chemical analysis proves it to be the same substance as bilirubin, the chief colouring matter of the bile. It produces the yellow colour noticed in a bruise as the blood is being absorbed and the bruise fading away. *Haemin* is of great medico-legal importance, because it can be obtained from long-dried stains on clothing, knives, etc., its discovery proving such stains to be due to blood. To obtain it, one scrapes off a few particles of the stain upon a microscopic slide, adds a drop of strong acetic acid, and a small crystal of common salt. One then heats the drop till it dries up, and examines it under the microscope. Haemin appears as minute, dark brown plates and prisms.

HAEMATOLOGY is the term applied to that branch of medical science devoted to the study of diseases of the blood.

HAEMATOMA means a collection of blood forming a definite swelling. It is found often upon the head of new-born children after a protracted and difficult labour. It may occur as the result of any injury or operation.

HAEMATOXYLON, or LOGWOOD, is the wood of *Haematoxylon campechianum*, which is used as a dye in staining tissues in histology. As it has a mildly astringent action, it is used for checking diarrhoea.

HAEMATURIA means the condition of blood in the urine. (See URINE.) The blood may come from any part of the urinary tract. When the blood comes from the kidney or upper part of the urinary tract, it is usually mixed throughout the urine, giving the latter a brownish or smoky tinge. This condition is usually the result of acute or subacute Bright's disease, or it may be present in persons suffering from high blood pressure or pyelitis (qv). Blood may also appear in the urine from time to time in considerable quantities when a stone or gravel is present in the pelvis of the kidney setting up irritation, especially when the person undergoes unwonted exercise. The blood may also originate from the bladder in cases in which this is inflamed, and is then present in smaller quantities as a rule. The presence of a stone in the bladder is also productive of blood, and in either of the latter cases the urine is generally turbid from admixture with pus. A condition which leads to the passage of bright red blood at occasional intervals is the presence of a species of warty growth (papilloma) on the wall of the bladder. Blood may also be derived from the urethra following some inflammatory condition in this passage, or injury

411

to it as by a fracture of the pelvic bones. Occasionally the bleeding may be due to purpura.

The recognition of the site of the haemorrhage is important in relation to the measures to be adopted for its treatment. This can often be made out by the character of the blood, whether intimately mixed with the urine or in the form of clots, also by the shape of the clots, and by the presence of other abnormal constituents in the urine. For the final diagnosis, examination of the interior of the bladder by the cystoscope and the passage of fine catheters up the ureters to the kidneys is often of importance. (See CYSTOSCOPE.)

HAEMIC MURMUR is a term applied to unusual sounds heard over the heart and large blood-vessels in severe cases of anaemia. They disappear as the condition is recovered from. Murmurs of this type are to be distinguished from 'organic murmurs', which are due to some disease of the heart-valves or vessel walls.

HAEMOCHROMATOSIS, or BRONZED DIABETES, is the name of a disease in which cirrhosis of the liver, enlargement of the spleen, pigmentation of the skin, and diabetes mellitus are associated with the abnormal and excessive deposit in the organs of the body of the iron-containing pigment, haemosiderin.

HAEMOCYTOMETER is an instrument for counting corpuscles in the blood.

HAEMODIALYSIS is the principle used in the artificial kidney (see KIDNEY, ARTIFICIAL), whereby the patient's blood is circulated through a cellophane tube, on the other side of which is a dialysing solution containing electrolytes in the concentration they should be in normal blood, but no urea. In this way the patient's blood is restored to its normal state as it would were it passing through normally functioning kidneys. (See also DIALYSIS.)

HAEMOGLOBIN is the colouring material which produces the red colour of blood. It is a chromoprotein, made up of a protein called globin and the iron-containing pigment, haemin. When separated from the red blood corpuscles, each of which contains about 600 million haemoglobin molecules, it is crystalline in form. It exists in two forms: simple haemoglobin, found in venous blood, and oxyhaemoglobin, which is a loose compound with oxygen, found in arterial blood after the

blood has come in contact with the air in the lungs. This oxyhaemoglobin is again broken down as the blood passes through the tissues, which take up the oxygen for their own use. This is the main function of haemoglobin: to act as a carrier of oxygen from the lungs to all the tissues of the body. When the haemoglobin leaves the lungs it is 97 per cent saturated with oxygen. When it comes back to the lungs in the venous blood it is 70 per cent saturated. The oxygen content of 100 millilitres of blood leaving the lungs is 19·5 millilitres, and that of venous blood recturning to the lungs is 14·5 millilitres. Thus each 100 millilitres of blood delivers 5 millilitres of oxygen to the tissues of the body. Human male blood contains 13 to 18 grams of haemoglobin per 100 millilitres. In women, there are 12 to 16 grams per 100 millilitres. A man weighing 70 kilograms (154 pounds) has around 770 grams of haemoglobin circulating in his red blood corpuscles.

HAEMOGLOBINURIA means the presence of blood pigment in the urine caused by the destruction of blood corpuscles in the blood-vessels or in the urinary passages. It produces in the urine a dark red colour or a brown colour resembling porter. In some persons this condition, known as intermittent haemoglobinuria, occurs from time to time, especially on exposure to cold. It is also produced by various poisonous substances taken in the food. It occurs in malarious districts in the form of one of the most fatal forms of malaria: blackwater fever (qv).

HAEMOLYSIS means the breaking up of blood corpuscles by the action of poisonous substances, usually of a protein nature, circulating in the blood, or by certain chemicals. It occurs, for example, gradually in some forms of anaemia and occurs rapidly in poisoning by snake venom.

HAEMOLYTIC DISEASE OF THE NEWBORN (also known as ERYTHROBLASTOSIS FOETALIS and ICTERUS GRAVIS NEONATORUM) is a severe disease of the newborn characterized by severe haemolytic anaemia and jaundice. There is also some oedema, and when this is severe, with excess fluid in the pericardial, pleural, and peritoneal cavities, the condition is known as HYDROPS FOETALIS. The fundamental cause is the haemolysis (or breakdown) of the red blood cells, and this is due to a Rhesus-negative mother bearing a Rhesus-positive child. Such a mother becomes sensitized to the Rhesus-positive factor in her unborn child, thereby producing agglutinins (or antibodies) to it, and these pass through the placenta into the foetus and destroy its red blood cells. (See BLOOD GROUPS.)

Treatment consists of blood transfusion: either a simple transfusion or an exchange transfusion. (See TRANSFUSION OF BLOOD.) The efficacy of treatment is largely dependent upon the awareness of

done by giving her gamma-globulin (qv) which contains antibodies, or anti-D immunoglobulin as it is known, that will destroy the Rhesus-positive cells from the foetus. Thus these cells are destroyed before they can induce the production of antibodies in the mother's tissues. The injection of gamma-globulin is given within forty-eight hours of delivery as it is usually during delivery that most of the child's cells pass into the mother's bloodstream.

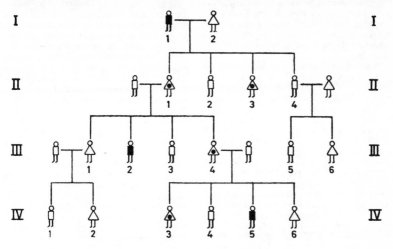

Transmission through an affected male (I, 1) and carrier females (II, 1 and III, 4).

234 – Mode of inheritance of haemophilia. *The Practitioner.*

the fact that the baby may be born with haemolytic disease, and that all the necessary steps have been taken to start treatment immediately after birth. This is the reason why so much importance is attached nowadays to the careful blood-grouping of all mothers early in pregnancy. As a result of modern treatment the mortality for this condition has dropped from around 75 per cent to around 5 per cent.

Two recent advances have gone far towards reducing the incidence of this disease. One is the method whereby the Rhesus-negative mother can be prevented from developing antibodies should the child she bears be Rhesus-positive. This is

The other preventive measure is to give the Rhesus-positive foetus an intra-uterine transfusion of Rhesus-negative blood. In skilled hands this is a perfectly feasible procedure, the blood being injected directly into the peritoneal cavity of the foetus any time from the 20th week onwards.

HAEMOPHILIA is a hereditary disease, confined almost entirely to members of the male sex, and characterized by a tendency to uncontrollable haemorrhage even after quite slight wounds. The victims are popularly known as 'bleeders'.

Causes – The defect is in the blood and is one of clotting, or coagulation. The coagulation time may be prolonged up to 12 hours or even longer, compared with a normal of 4 to 10 minutes. The cause of the prolonged coagulation time is deficiency of the antihaemophiliac factor, or Factor VIII as it is known, which is part of the globulin fraction of plasma. The most characteristic feature of the disease is its manner of hereditary transmission, this being through the mother, who is not a bleeder, although her brother may be. In other words as shown in illustration 234 the males of the affected family are bleeders but do not transmit the disease to their male offspring, whilst the females are not bleeders but their male children may be.

The disease occurs predominantly in white races, and it has been estimated that the over-all incidence of the disease is 8 per 10,000 of the population, the incidence of severe cases being 3 to 4 per 100,000. Correlated with births, the incidence is thought to be 1 haemophiliac in every 3000 to 4000 live births. There are around 3000 haemophiliacs in Britain. At one time probably only around 10 per cent of bleeders survived beyond puberty. Today advances in treatment have so altered the outlook that few bleeders die of the disease. As a result of this longer survival, the number of bleeders, or haemophiliacs, in the community will steadily rise.

Symptoms – The characteristic feature of haemophilia is the slow, persistent oozing of blood from any wound or injury that, untreated, may go on for hours or even days despite all attempts to stop it by local pressure or by the application of haemostatics (qv). Even when the bleeding does stop, it is liable to start again some days later. On the other hand, contrary to popular belief, superficial cuts and scratches do not cause much trouble with bleeding unless they involve mucous membranes, such as that of the mouth, for instance. Neither do haemophiliacs bleed rapidly to death from deep cuts unless, of course, as in the case of non-bleeders, they involve a major artery or vein. One of the major risks a haemophiliac runs is a large haemorrhage into a muscle or joint. Recurrent bleeding into the joints is one of the commonest features of the disease, the symptoms starting as soon as the child begins to walk. By the age of 10 years, 80 per cent of severe haemophiliacs have abnormal joints. This is why it is so important to try and reduce such bleeding into the joints as much as possible and so reduce the amount of crippling. Bleeding from the kidney is quite common, manifest-

ing itself by the passage of blood in the urine. (See HAEMATURIA.)

Treatment – The fundamental treatment of bleeding in a haemophiliac is the intravenous administration of Factor VIII. This is now available in various forms, including fresh frozen plasma, freeze-dried human antihaemophiliac globulin concentrate (AHG), and cryoprecipitate (qv). Cryoprecipitate, which is prepared from human plasma, can be prepared by most blood transfusion centres, and is proving a most useful source of Factor VIII. If any operation has to be performed on a haemophiliac, even such a minor one as the extraction of a tooth, the patient must be carefully prepared by having adequate amounts of Factor VIII. As always, of course, prevention is better than cure, and, in the case of the teeth, this means that every care should be taken with the teeth of a haemophiliac, whether child or adult, by ensuring that he should see a dentist at regular intervals so that preventive action can be taken that will reduce the possibility of dental extraction to a minimum. To facilitate treatment and ensure that the best possible care is available to every haemophiliac, a National Haemophilia Register has been established in Great Britain, and some thirty Haemophilia Centres have been set up throughout the country where expert treatment can be obtained at any time. Every haemophiliac whose name is on this Register is provided with a card which gives full details about his condition.

It is now realized that the general management of the haemophiliac is just as important as the actual treatment of the bleeding episode. He must be allowed to lead as normal a life as possible, going to an ordinary school and participating in sport. In this last respect, body-contact games such as rugby should be avoided, but there is no reason why a haemophiliac should not go in for cycling, running, or swimming, for instance. In planning such a social life parents and relatives can obtain advice, not only from the Haemophilia Centres, but also from The Haemophilia Society, 16 Trinity Street, London, SE1 DE1.

HAEMOPTYSIS means the spitting up of blood from the lower air passages. The blood is usually coughed or gently hawked up, it may be in mouthfuls at a time, and is bright red and frothy, thus differing from the blood brought up from the stomach. Generally the condition results from some disease of the heart or lungs. It should be remembered, however, that in elderly people haemoptysis may be due to a varicose condition of the small veins in the throat, not to haemorrhage in the lungs; while in young people this condition is often due to bleeding from the nose, in which, owing to the position of the head, the blood happens to run backwards instead of forwards through the nostrils. (See HAEMORRHAGE; TUBERCULOSIS.)

HAEMORRHAGE means any escape of blood from the vessels which naturally contain it. It may occur from a wound of the skin, in which case it escapes externally, or into some internal cavity such as the stomach or bowels, or may simply be poured out into the tissues in consequence of a blow or similar injury; but, in all cases alike, the blood escaping from the vessels is lost to the circulation. Haemorrhage is classified according to the vessels from which it occurs, as (a) *arterial*, in which case the blood is bright and appears in jets or spurts, corresponding to the heart-beats; (b) *venous*, when it comes from veins, is dark, and wells up gradually into the wound; (c) *capillary*, when it flows merely from torn capillaries, and comes in a gentle ooze out of the general surface of the wound. The immediate result of a severe haemorrhage is great anaemia, so that in extreme cases the bodily organs may be unable to continue their functions, and the person dies in consequence, with symptoms of shock.

In general, arterial haemorrhage is the most serious, and if a large artery, such as the femoral, be wounded, the person concerned may bleed to death in a few minutes. Venous haemorrhage is so easily checked by slight pressure, and the valves in the veins so effectively prevent blood from running backwards in these vessels, that this form is not dangerous to life except in the case of ruptured varicose veins of the leg, or when a serious internal injury is received. Capillary haemorrhage stops so quickly, that only in the case of the disease known as haemophilia (qv) is it of serious import. The following terms are applied to haemorrhage from special sites: *haematemesis*, bleeding from the stomach; *haemoptysis*, bleeding from the lungs; *epistaxis*, bleeding from the nose; and *haematuria*, bleeding from the kidney or urinary passages. (See these headings.) Haemorrhage is also classed as primary, reactionary, and secondary. (See WOUNDS.)

Natural arrest – When an artery of small size is cut across, the bleeding stops in consequence of changes in the wall of the artery on the one hand, and in the constitution of the blood upon the other. Every artery is surrounded by a fibrous sheath, and, when cut, the vessel retracts some little distance within this sheath, in consequence of the shortening of its muscle fibres; and further, by the same process the end contracts so as to form an opening of smaller size than the rest of the vessel. In the space between the end of the vessel and its sheath, and afterwards for some distance up the interior of the narrowed artery, blood-clot quickly forms by the following process, and rapidly blocks the open end of the vessel. When blood is shed so as to come in contact with any surface other than the smooth lining of blood-vessels, the fibrinogen which is dissolved in its fluid becomes converted into threads of fibrin through combination with the lime salts of the blood, and the action of a ferment given off probably by the blood platelets. These threads of fibrin slowly contract and develop into a dense felt-work, in the meshes of which the corpuscles are held, and in this way a blood-clot of increasing hardness is produced, within and round the ends of the injured vessels. When an artery is only partially severed it is evident that contraction and retraction within the sheath cannot take place, and accordingly bleeding is apt to be more serious than when the vessel is completely cut across. Again, if an artery be torn across or twisted instead of cut, the opening at its end is still more narrowed, and the blood clots more rapidly on the ragged surface than it would do upon a clean cut, so that haemorrhage from a torn or bruised wound is in general much smaller in amount than from a stab or cut. The natural arrest of bleeding is usually described therefore as depending upon four factors: (a) the retraction, and (b) the contraction

235 – Artery forceps, with jaws shown enlarged.

of the cut artery: (c) the external, and (d) the internal clot formed by the blood. For the means by which circulation is subsequently carried on after an artery is cut, see ANASTOMOSIS.

Control of external haemorrhage – Four main principles are applicable in the control of a severe external haemorrhage: (a) direct pressure on the bleeding point or points; (b) elevation of the wounded part; (c) pressure on the main artery of supply to the part; and (d) application of substances known as styptics, which contract the vessels or aid the coagulation of the blood.

(a) DIRECT PRESSURE may be made with the finger, which is the best method, when a definite bleeding point is seen in a gaping wound. This is the method adopted at an operation by the surgeon, who places his finger at once upon any bleeding point, afterwards seizing the cut artery with forceps (illustration 235) and tying a piece of silk or catgut tightly round its end. If the artery lie between the skin and a hard surface, as in the case of scalp wounds, a wedge-shaped pad and tight bandage (known as a graduated compress) may be substituted for pressure with the finger, the edges of the wound being compressed between the pad and skull.

236 – Compression of arteries about the head and face. a, temporal artery, for bleeding from front of scalp; b, occipital artery, for back of scalp; c, facial artery, for face.

237 – Compression of arteries in the neck. a, carotid artery, for bleeding from head or neck; b, subclavian artery, for bleeding from upper limb. The arrow in each case shows the direction in which pressure should be exerted.

(*b*) ELEVATION of the bleeding member is an important method, the blood running off more readily by the veins, and a smaller quantity being driven into the limb the higher it is raised. This method is applicable, of course, only in cases of bleeding from the hand or foot.

(*c*) PRESSURE UPON THE MAIN ARTERY of supply to the injured limb is a certain method of stopping the circulation and consequently all bleeding, much after the manner of stopping the water supply of a district by closing the main pipe. At certain points where the arteries lie close to bones and near the surface, the pulsation of the vessel may be felt, and *pressure with the finger* over the artery serves to obliterate it against the bone, the points where this may be adopted being as follows. In cases of bleeding from the upper part of the scalp, the temporal artery may be felt and compressed immediately in front of the upper part of the ear (illustration 236a), while for wounds at the back of the head the occipital artery can be felt and compressed a short distance behind the mastoid process, the bony prominence at the back of the ear (illustration 236b).

Bleeding from the face may be checked by pressure on the facial artery, which passes on to the face about an inch in front of the angle of the jaw, across the jawbone, against which it is to be pressed (illustration 236c).

All bleeding from the head and neck may be lessened by pressure upon the common carotid artery in the neck a short distance below the prominent Adam's apple, and between it and the edge of the large sternocleidomastoid muscle (illustration 237a). In this groove the artery is pressed straight back against the transverse processes of the spinal column.

Bleeding from the region of the shoulder and armpit is checked by pressure on the subclavian artery, the pressure being applied with the thumb directly downwards in the hollow behind the middle part of the collar-bone, so as to press the artery down upon the first rib (illustration 237b).

Bleeding from the region of the elbow or forearm may be controlled by feeling for the brachial artery on the inner side of the upper arm, behind the biceps muscle, and pressing it against the humerus (illustration 238a).

Bleeding from the hand is checked by pressure on the radial artery, where it lies between the skin and radius in front of the wrist, and on the ulnar artery just before it

238 – Compression of arteries for bleeding from forearm or hand. *a*, brachial artery; *b*, radial and ulnar arteries.

239 – Compression of femoral artery, for bleeding in lower limb.

417

240 – Compression of posterior tibial artery, for bleeding in sole of foot.

enters the hand near its inner margin (illustration 238b).

In the lower limb the arteries lie deeply among the muscles, but bleeding from any part of the limb may be checked by pressure backwards on the femoral artery, which is to be felt pulsating in the centre of the groin, and which is compressed backwards against the head of the thigh-bone (illustration 239).

Bleeding from the sole of the foot may be controlled by pressure on the posterior tibial artery, which lies about half an inch behind the inner ankle (illustration 240).

A second method for applying pressure on the main artery consists in *forced flexion* at the elbow, hip, or knee, as the case may be. A pad is placed in the bend of the joint, which is then flexed as completely as possible and firmly bound in this position, the artery being thus sharply bent upon itself (illustration 241).

A third method for control of the main blood supply is by the *tourniquet*, which consists of an elastic band or ligature passed round a fleshy part of any of the limbs, and pulled or twisted tight. A surgical tourniquet consists of an india-rubber cord or band with an arrangement for

241 – Method of stopping bleeding from the forearm or hand by forced flexion at the elbow, the limb being firmly flexed over a pad placed in the bend of the elbow. The same method may be applied to compress the femoral artery at the groin or the popliteal artery behind the knee, by forced flexion with a pad at hip or knee.

fixing the ends together, or of a strap with buckle and a screw appliance for tightening it up. A tourniquet may, however, be improvised from a piece of rope, or a handkerchief folded cravatwise, tied round the limb and then twisted up tight by a piece of wood, large key, or similar object introduced beneath it. The handle of such a tourniquet is prevented from untwisting by passing a second band round the limb and including the end of the handle within it before tying. A tourniquet may be applied to the fleshy part of the thigh, leg, upper arm, or forearm. It is most important to note on a label the time of application of a tourniquet. No tourniquet should ever be left on longer than an hour. It must be loosened every fifteen minutes, to be tightened again if bleeding restarts. (See TOURNIQUET.)

Occasionally, when bleeding is continuous or when it occurs from a deep-seated wound like a stab, or injury to the root of the tongue, it is impossible to get at the bleeding point, and permanent control of the bleeding is only to be achieved by the surgeon, who cuts down upon the main artery of supply and ties a ligature round it.

(*d*) STYPTICS are applied when the bleeding is a general ooze from a wound, or when the bleeding comes from an inaccessible position, such as the interior of the nose or a wound in the side. The most important styptics are heat and cold. Although moderate warmth greatly increases bleeding, ice-cold water and also water between 115° and 120° F (46° and 49° C) (ie. a temperature which the hand can hardly bear) both favour clotting and contract the blood-vessels. Heat is much more effectual than cold, if applied directly to the wound. Various drugs, such as perchloride of iron (steel drops) and hazeline, act similarly. Adrenaline has a powerful local action in contracting vessels and stopping bleeding. Russell-viper venom is most effective as a local application in cases such as bleeding from a tooth socket. Other styptics include oxidized cellulose, gelatin by-products, calcium alginate, and thrombin powder.

Control of internal haemorrhage is not to be so certainly achieved as in the case of bleeding from the vessels of the limbs. There are certain general principles to which it is most important to adhere. Chief among these is the maintenance of the recumbent position, since the heart beats less forcibly and the blood-pressure is consequently lowered as soon as the injured person lies down. For the same reason, all excitement must be avoided, and the mind of the sufferer quieted as far as possible. The patient must also be kept warm. Stimulants must be avoided. Ice-bags or compresses wrung out of cold water may be laid over the chest or stomach, according to the origin of the haemorrhage. The most valuable drug in the treatment of internal haemorrhage is morphine given hypodermically. In the haemorrhage which sometimes follows child-birth, the source of bleeding is usually the uterus. This is controlled by the injection of ergometrine, the removal of the placenta if this has not already come away, and then compression of the uterus. This may need to be supplemented by plugging of the vagina with sterile gauze.

It should be mentioned that in operations on internal organs or other highly vascular tissue, in the case of which bleeding would be very hard to stop, the cautery is often used instead of the knife, and not only removes the part desired, but, by its heat, prevents all bleeding.

Treatment of bleeding from special sites:
NOSE – Keep quiet, lying or sitting; loosen collar; no blowing of nose; cold key or sponge to neck; if these are not successful, plugging of nostrils with lint soaked in tincture of perchloride of iron or adrenaline.

TONGUE – Ice to suck; pressure with the fingers; if serious, compression of carotid artery.

FACE OR SCALP – Direct pressure with fingers or bandage and pad on wound; if bleeding be severe, pressure in addition on facial, temporal, or occipital artery.

NECK – Pressure on carotid artery.

ARMPIT OR SHOULDER – Pressure on sub-clavian artery.

FOREARM – Pressure on brachial artery by fingers, tourniquet, or forced flexion at elbow.

HAND – Elevation and direct pressure with pad and bandage; if bleeding severe, pressure on radial and ulnar arteries, or tourniquet to forearm.

THIGH – Pressure on femoral artery at groin; tourniquet, if low down.

LEG – Tourniquet to thigh, or forced flexion at knee. In the case of ruptured varicose veins, a pad and bandage round leg extending above and below wound with elevation of limb suffice.

FOOT – Direct pressure and elevation; if bleeding severe, forced flexion at knee, or pressure on posterior tibial artery.

HAEMORRHOIDS (see PILES).

HAEMOSTATICS are any means, whether of the nature of mechanical appliances or drugs, used to control bleeding. (See FIBRIN FOAM; HAEMORRHAGE.)

HAEMOTHORAX means an effusion of blood into the pleural cavity.

HAIR DISEASES (see BALDNESS).

HAIR (see SKIN).

HAIR, REMOVAL OF (see DEPILATION).

HALIBUT-LIVER OIL is the oil expressed from fresh, or suitably preserved, halibut liver. It is a particularly rich source of vitamin A (30,000 international units per gram), and also contains vitamin D (2300 to 2500 units per gram). Because of the relatively small volume required, it is often used as a means of giving vitamin D: either as drops of the oil or in capsules. As mentioned in the section on cod-liver oil. care must be taken to ensure that the child is receiving at least 700 international units of vitamin D daily.

HALISTERESIS is the term applied to softening of a bone resulting from the disappearance of lime salts from it.

HALITOSIS is another term for offensive breath. (See BREATH, DISORDERS OF.)

HALLUCINATIONS are errors in perception, affecting some sense organ to such an extent that a person imagines he perceives something for which there is no foundation. For example, a person may fancy he hears himself called during perfect stillness, or may see lights in pitch darkness. *Illusions* are misinterpreted sensations: for example, a person may constantly mistake an article of furniture for the figure of some friend, or of an animal. Both these errors occur in sane people, and may indicate some slight brain derangement, due to sleeplessness, overwork, feverishness, or other cause. They are usually, however, a symptom of insanity. (See MENTAL ILLNESS.)

HALLUCINOGENS are compounds characterized by their ability to produce distortions of perception, emotional changes, depersonalization, and a variety of effects on memory and learned behaviour. They include lysergic acid diethylamide (qv) and mescaline (qv). (See also DRUG ADDICTION.)

HALLUX is the anatomical name of the great toe.

HALLUX RIGIDUS is stiffness of the joint between the great toe and the foot which induces pain on walking. It is usually due to a crush injury or stubbing of the toe. Such stubbing is liable to occur in adolescents with a congenitally long toe. If troublesome it is treated by an operation to create a false joint.

HALLUX VALGUS is outward displacement of the great toe and is always associated with a bunion (illustration 242).

242 – *Hallux valgus* and bunion. (*A Short Textbook of Surgery*, Charles Illingworth, Churchill Livingstone)

It is due to the pressure of footwear on an unduly broad foot. In adolescents this broad foot is inherited; in adults it is due to splaying of the foot as a result of loss of muscle tone. The bunion is produced by pressure of the footwear on the protruding base of the toe. In mild cases the wearing of comfortable shoes may be all that is needed. In more severe cases the bunion may need to be removed, while in the most severe the operation of arthroplasty (qv) may be needed. (See also CORNS AND BUNIONS.)

HALO is a coloured circle seen round a bright light in some eye conditions. When accompanied by headache it is specially likely to be caused by glaucoma. (See GLAUCOMA.)

HALOPERIDOL is one of the butyrophenone group of drugs that is proving useful in the treatment of mania and schizophrenic excitement.

HALOTHANE is a non-inflammable anaesthetic, the chemical formula of which is $CF_3CHClBr$. One of its advantages is that patients recover rapidly from its effects.

HAMAMELIS (see WITCH-HAZEL).

HAMMER-TOE is the deformity in which there is permanent flexion, or bending of the middle joint of the toe (illustration 243). The condition may affect all the

243 – Hammer toe with infected *bursa*. (*A Short Textbook of Surgery*, Charles Illingworth. Churchill Livingstone)

toes as in claw-foot (qv). More commonly it affects one toe, usually the second. It is due to a relatively long toe and the pressure on it of the footwear. A painful bunion usually develops on it. In mild cases relief is obtained by protecting the toe with adhesive pads. If this does not suffice operation is necessary. (See CORNS AND BUNIONS.)

HAMSTRINGS is the name given to the tendons at the back of the knee, two on the inner side and one on the outer side, which bend this joint. They are attached to the tibia below.

HAND is the section of the upper limb below the wrist. The hand of man is more highly developed in its structure and in its nervous connections than the corresponding part in any other animal. Indeed the possession of a thumb which can be 'opposed' to the other fingers for grasping objects is one of the distinguishing features of the human race. Of all the parts of the body, the hand, which is cconnected with a large area on the surface of the brain, is capable of the highest degree of education, and in cases in which the brain degenerates, as in general paralysis, the uses of the hand deteriorate particularly early; while in those cases in which part of

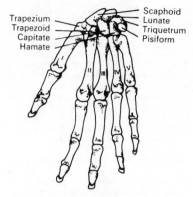

Trapezium
Trapezoid
Capitate
Hamate

Scaphoid
Lunate
Triquetrum
Pisiform

244 – The bones of the hand and wrist, anterior (or palmar) view.

the brain is destroyed by apoplexy, the hand is apt to suffer more permanently than either face or leg.

In structure, the hand has a bony basis of eight small carpal bones in the wrist, five metacarpal bones in the fleshy part of the hand, and three phalanges in each finger, two only in the thumb (illustration 244). From the muscles of the forearm twelve strong tendons or sinews run in front of the wrist. Of these, nine go to the fingers and thumb and are bound down by a strong band, the flexor retinaculum, in front of the wrist. They are enclosed in a complicated synovial sheath, and pass through the palm and down the fingers. (See FINGER.) Behind the wrist twelve tendons likewise cross from forearm to hand.

Forming the ball of the thumb and that of the little finger, and filling up the gaps between the metacarpal bones, are other muscles, which act to separate and bring together the fingers, and to bend them at their first joints (knuckles).

Deep in the palm the ulnar artery makes an arch across the hand, giving off branches which run down the sides of the fingers; while the radial artery makes an arch across at a still deeper level, lying in close contact with the bones (illustration 245).

The skin of the hand is richly supplied with nerve filaments, in accordance with its highly specialized sense of touch, the outer three and a half digits being supplied in front by the median, behind by the radial nerve, whilst the inner one and a half fingers have their nerve supply both back and front from the ulnar nerve.

In addition to the diseases mentioned above, certain nervous diseases affect the hand early. Thus in multiple sclerosis and in chorea there are tremors; in alcoholic neuritis and in lead-poisoning, drop-wrist; in progressive muscular atrophy one of the first signs is wasting of the small muscles belonging to the thumb and little finger; in syringomyelia there is loss of sensation for pain and for change of temperature in the fingers.

Deformities of the hand, in the shape of chalk-stones, may occur in gout; rheumatoid arthritis always affects the joints of the hand and all too often causes crippling disabilities; and acromegaly is characterized by great enlargement of the hands. Swellings on the back or front of the wrist are usually due to collection of fluid in the tendon sheaths (see GANGLION). Deep abscesses on the front of the fingers are serious, because of the ease with which the infection spreads up the synovial sheaths of the tendons into the palm of the hand. (See WHITLOW.) A condition in which the fingers, especially the ring and little fingers, are gradually flexed up into the palm follows sometimes on a severe

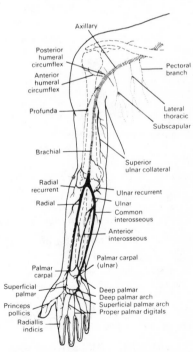

Axillary

Posterior
humeral
circumflex

Anterior
humeral
circumflex

Profunda

Brachial

Radial
recurrent
Radial

Palmar
carpal

Superficial
palmar
Princeps
pollicis
Radiallis
indicis

Pectoral
branch

Lateral
thoracic
Subscapular

Superior
ulnar collateral

Ulnar recurrent

Ulnar
Common
interosseous
Anterior
interosseous

Palmar carpal
(ulnar)

Deep palmar
Deep palmar arch
Superficial palmar arch
Proper palmar digitals

245 – Arteries of the upper limb, anterior view.

421

strain of the palm or long-continued pressure of a tool. (See DUPUYTREN'S CONTRACTURE.)

Several special terms are applied to deformities of the hand. Claw hand or *main en griffe* is applied to a condition in which the hand is atrophied and the fingers bent in paralysis of the ulnar nerve; cleft hand, or *lobster hand*, is a rare congenital defect characterized by the absence of one or more fingers and a deep central cleft that divides the hand into two; monkey hand or *main en singe* is applied to a condition in which the muscles of the thumb are wasted; obstetrician's hand is a condition in which the thumb and fingers are held together in a kind of cone in tetany and other conditions; and skeleton hand is a condition in which the muscles of the hand are generally wasted, as in progressive muscular atrophy. (See also DROP-WRIST.)

HAND, FOOT AND MOUTH DISEASE is a disease characterized by an eruption of blisters on the palms of the hands, on the feet (often the toes) and in the mouth. It is most common in children and is due to infection with coxsackie A16 virus. The incubation period is three to five days.

HANGING is a form of death due to suspension of the body from the neck, either suddenly, as in judicial hanging, so as to damage the spinal column and cord, or in such a way as to constrict the air passages and the blood-vessels to the brain. Death is, in any case, speedy, resulting in two or three minutes, if not instantaneous, although in bygone days criminals who were shored-up, or supported by their friends, have come round after half-an-hour's suspension. The mark of the noose on the neck is oblique in hanging, which serves to distinguish this form of death from strangling, in which the mark is circular. Apart from judicial hanging, and in the absence of any signs of a struggle, hanging is usually due to suicide. The resuscitation of persons found hanging is similar to that for drowning. (See DROWNING.)

HANG-NAIL means a splitting of the skin at the side of the finger-nail. It is often a painful condition and difficult to heal. This is best effected by wearing constantly for several days a wet boric dressing covered by a rubber finger-stall.

HARD METAL DISEASE is a disease that occurs in those involved in tungsten carbide grinding. Tungsten carbide is a hard metal (hence the name of the disease) that has revolutionized metal machining and metal working. It is made from tungsten and carbon with cobalt as a binder. The disease is characterized by cough, expectoration (spitting), shortness of breath and tightness in the chest. In most cases the manifestations of the disease are mild and disappear on withdrawal from exposure to the risk. In some they may be severe enough to involve giving up working with tungsten.

HARDNESS is a term applied to water that contains a large amount of calcium and magnesium salts (lime salts) which form an insoluble curd with soap and thus interfere with the use of the water for purposes of washing. Hard water is especially found in districts where the soil is chalky. Temporary hardness, which is due mainly to the presence of bicarbonates of lime, can be remedied by boiling, when the lime is precipitated as carbonate of lime. Permanent hardness is not remedied by boiling, and is due to the presence of a large amount of sulphate of lime. It may be removed by the addition of sodium carbonate (washing soda) or by the permutit process which involves the use of various combinations of silicate of alumina and soda. In the past hard water was often blamed for many of the ills to which man is heir – without any convincing evidence. Today the medical statisticians are suggesting that the drinking of soft water may lead to heart disease.

HARE-LIP (see PALATE, MALFORMATIONS OF).

HARTMANN'S SOLUTION is a solution which is commonly used as a means of fluid replacement in dehydrated patients. Each litre contains 3·1 grams of sodium lactate, 6 grams of sodium chloride, 0·3 gram of potassium chloride, and 0·2 gram of calcium chloride.

HARTSHORN is a popular name for ammonia. (See AMMONIA.)

HARVEST MITE, or HARVEST BUG (see BITES AND STINGS).

HASHIMOTO'S DISEASE is a condition in which the whole of the thyroid gland is diffusely enlarged and firm. It is one of the diseases produced by autoimmunity (qv). The enlargement is due, not to increase of colloid, but to diffuse infiltration of lymphocytes and increase of fibrous tissue. This form of goitre appears in middle-aged women, does not give rise to symptoms of thyrotoxicosis, and tends to produce myxoedema.

HAUNCH-BONE is the name of the bone which encloses the lower part of the abdomen on each side. (See PELVIS.)

HAUSTUS is the Latin word for a draught.

HAVERSIAN CANALS are the fine canals in bone which carry the blood-vessels, lymphatics, and nerves necessary for the maintenance and repair of bone. (See BONE.)

HAY FEVER, otherwise known as SUMMER CATARRH, and in America as AUTUMN CATARRH, means an allergic condition of the mucous membranes of the eyes, nose, and air passages, which year after year affects certain individuals during the summer and early autumn. It is estimated that around 3,000,000 people in Britain suffer from it, and that 500,000 of these are so severely affected as to need medical treatment.

Causes – Hay fever is an allergic reaction in individuals who are hypersensitive to the pollens of grasses, weeds or trees. This explains the seasonal distribution of the disease. In Britain, where grass pollens are the commonest cause, it occurs from the middle of May to the end of July. In North America it occurs over a longer period: in April and May, due to tree pollens; in June and July, due to grass pollens; in August and September, due to weed pollens. The inhalation of such a pollen to which the individual is hypersensitive results in the production of an excessive amount of histamine (qv) and it is the histamine which is responsible for the manifestations of hay fever.

The tendency to develop hay fever runs in certain families. What is inherited in these families is what might be described as an allergic constitution. Only some members of these families will develop hay fever, whilst others may develop other allergic manifestations, such as asthma, eczema, or food allergy.

Symptoms – The malady recurs with regularity during the summer months in those susceptible to it. It begins with an itching of the eyes and nose, followed by symptoms of a severe cold or influenza, such as headache, violent sneezing, and profuse watery discharge from the eyes and nose, together with dry, hard cough, and occasionally severe asthmatic paroxysms. The attack usually runs a course of several weeks. During rainy weather the symptoms may subside. Susceptible persons who move to the seaside early in May, or to a place where vegetation is scanty, rarely suffer.

Treatment – The most effectual method of treatment in hay fever is to avoid the exciting cause, namely, the neighbourhood of grass fields, during the summer season. Removal to the seaside often succeeds in putting an end to an attack. A course of vaccines either immediately before the hay-fever season, or spread out over the preceding winter, sometimes provides relief. Of recent years a number of antihistamine preparations (qv) have been produced which practically always bring relief. In cases in which there is some nasal defect, cauterization of the turbinate process or an operation to straighten a distorted nasal septum sometimes helps. If the watering of the eyes is particularly severe, relief may be obtained from the use of eye-drops containing 1 per cent of ephedrine in saline.

Susceptible persons living in the country should sleep with their bedroom windows shut. Ionization of the nasal mucosa with zinc sulphate may help.

HAZELINE, or HAMAMELIS WATER, is an extract made from the leaves or bark of *Hamamelis virginiana*, the witch-hazel. It is a useful astringent in checking bleeding and excessive mucous discharges. (See WITCH-HAZEL.)

HEAD (see BRAIN; FACE; SKULL; and SCALP).

HEADACHE is one of the commonest ills to which man is heir. Its significance varies tremendously. Thus, at one extreme it may denote the presence of a tumour of the brain or meningitis, whilst at the other extreme it may only be a sign of tiredness in an over-worked executive or professional man. In spite of being such a common finding, the precise mechanism whereby it is produced is still somewhat obscure. The brain itself is insensitive to pain, but the arteries supplying it and the membranes of the brain in relationship to these arteries are sensitive to pain. The general view at the moment is that headache is usually due to dilatation of these arteries or pressure (or traction) on them. This dilatation of the intracranial arteries may be due either to a lesion in the brain

423

or it may be caused reflexly: ie. by a stimulus somewhere else in the body which through the nervous system (often the vagus nerve) causes such dilatation. In other cases the headache arises in the scalp or in the muscles of the back of the neck. The following are some of the more important, or more common, conditions in which headache is present.

ANXIETY – One of the most common forms of headache is that which occurs in individuals when they are worried, anxious, or overworked. In some cases it may be a manifestation of what is known as the anxiety state or of emotional instability, but quite often it occurs in individuals who are emotionally stable. On the other hand, it seldom occurs in the phlegmatic type of person. Manual workers and those who live an out-of-door life seldom complain of headache, and there can be little doubt that the stress and strain under which the modern town-dweller lives have much to do with its incidence. Aggravating factors are inadequate ventilation of offices and excessive smoking. In women it is liable to occur during or shortly before menstruation.

MIGRAINE – This is one of the most characteristic forms of headache. For further details the section on migraine should be consulted.

REFRACTIVE ERRORS OF THE EYE are not as common a cause of headache as is sometimes thought. It occurs in the region of the brow and tends to be worse in the evening, particularly if much reading or close work has been done during the course of the day. It is sometimes accompanied by a sensation of grittiness in the eye. The remedy in such cases is the wearing of spectacles which correct the faulty vision.

INFECTION OF THE SINUSES is a common cause of headache. The location of the pain depends upon which sinus is involved. If the maxillary antrum, which lies in the cheek-bone, is infected, the pain is usually over the cheek, although it may be referred elsewhere in the head. In the case of involvement of the frontal sinuses the pain is over the eyes, whilst in the case of the deeper-lying ethmoidal sinuses the pain appears to be deep-seated behind the eyes. In such cases there is usually a history of a cold in the head followed by a discharge from the nose. The pain is usually worse about midday and tends to wear off towards evening. It is usually made worse by coughing and even sometimes by change of position.

DENTAL SEPSIS – Septic teeth may sometimes be responsible for headache. Usually, of course, there is also the classical toothache, but occasionally the pain of septic teeth is referred to the head.

INDIGESTION AND CONSTIPATION – Any form of dyspepsia due to disordered function of the stomach and which is liable to be accompanied by nausea (ie. a feeling of sickness), may be responsible for headache. On the other hand, individuals with a duodenal ulcer are not particularly liable to headache. Constipation is quite a common cause of headache, especially in children, but the old theory that the headache is due to absorption of toxic material from the gut has now been discarded. The headache is relieved so rapidly by the passing of a stool that it must be due to distension of the lower part of the bowel. Disturbances of the liver are also characterized by headache.

FEVER – Any infection, such as pneumonia or measles, causing a rise in temperature is liable to be accompanied by headache. This is probably due to dilatation of the blood-vessels in the brain resulting from the fever itself and from the infecting organism or its toxins.

URAEMIA – This is the terminal stage of Bright's disease (qv) and it is often accompanied by severe headache, which is due partly to the high blood-pressure which is always present and partly to the toxic substances which are retained in the body as a result of the failure of the kidneys.

HIGH BLOOD-PRESSURE – Although many people with a high blood-pressure are not unduly troubled with headache, the headache when it does occur is characteristic. It tends to occur at the back of the head and to be worse in the morning, wearing off during the course of the day.

RHEUMATIC CONDITIONS – Many rheumatic subjects are subject to aches and pains about the head. These are due to rheumatic changes in the muscles of the head and the back of the neck, and can usually be easily recognized by the fact that they are accompanied by tender spots elicited by pressure on the affected parts.

SUNSTROKE AND HEATSTROKE – Headache is the prominent feature in these conditions, and its occurrence after undue exposure to the sun or to exceptionally hot conditions renders easy its recognition.

DISEASES OF THE BRAIN – Finally, there are the conditions in which a headache indicates the presence of some disturbance or disease of the brain. This may take the form of infections of the brain or its membranes: eg. encephalitis, brain abscess, meningitis. There is seldom any difficulty in determining the presence of these conditions, as there are practically always other signs of involvement of the brain: eg. rigidity of the neck and squint in meningitis. In young children meningitis must always be considered when a febrile illness is accompanied by severe headache. In tumours of the brain severe headache develops sooner or later, but here again there are other manifestations, such as giddiness and apparently causeless vomiting, which indicate the cause of the headache. In middle-aged or elderly persons headache may be due to arteriosclerosis or thrombosis of the arteries in the brain. A relatively uncommon, but very acute, type of headache, usually in the back of the head, is caused by rupture of a small aneurysm (qv) in the circle of Willis, a network of arteries at the base of the brain. Headache is one of the main manifestations of concussion, whether or not this is accompanied by a fractured skull. The persistence of this headache after the individual has otherwise recovered from the concussion is sometimes most troublesome. If the concussion is due to an accident for which the victim considers he should receive compensation, this post-concussion, or post-traumatic, headache is one of the manifestations of a compensation neurosis. Once the case is settled, whether favourably or unfavourably to the claimant matters little, the headache usually clears up.

Treatment – It will be clear from this outline that in the majority of cases the treatment of headache is the treatment of the underlying cause. The main exception to this is migraine (qv). When the headache is associated with anxiety, worry or overwork, the same principle holds true. In these cases there may be an associated general debility, and for this the best remedy is a holiday with complete change of environment, adequate rest, and plenty of good food. If the headache is associated with sleeplessness, the administration of a mild sedative, eg. a small dose of a barbiturate, is helpful provided it is not continued indefinitely. Similarly with aspirin; this will relieve many a headache, but its continued use by an increasing number of the population is not in the interest of the health of the community. Used sensibly for short periods of time aspirin has its uses, but its repeated and continued use is

to be deprecated. Local soothing applications to the forehead are often of value in relieving headache. For this purpose there is much to be said for eau-de-Cologne. If the individual is lying down, a moist handkerchief on the forehead is sometimes just as effective.

HEALING (see WOUNDS).

HEALTH – The state of health implies much more than freedom from disease, and good health may be defined as the attainment and maintenance of the highest state of mental and bodily vigour of which any given individual is capable. People vary in the degree of strength and activity to which they are capable of attaining, and some persons must be content with leading a life on a lower plane of physical or mental activity than others. For the maintenance of this individual standard it is essential that each person should recognize his capabilities and limitations, and also that he should be aware of any defects of body or mind to which he is liable, either as the result of heredity or of previous disease. The recognition of, and allowance for, these in the conduct of daily life is of immense importance in maintaining health in other respects. Many persons have some inborn hereditary defect or tendency, eg. a neurotic temperament or a liability to disease of some special organ of the body, such as the heart or lungs, and the maintenance of health in such persons should be particularly directed towards avoiding conditions which lead to disorders common in their family. (See, for example, HEREDITY; HEART DISEASES; LUNG DISEASES.)

Environment is another matter with an important bearing upon health. This involves such considerations as the choice of an occupation suited to the individual's capabilities and temperament and the avoidance in dangerous occupations of the influences which are specially deleterious to health. (See OCCUPATIONAL DISEASES.) The social surroundings also involved in environment play an important part with many persons in the development of nervous affections. (See NEURASTHENIA.) Speaking generally, it may be said that the majority of persons, long before middle life is reached, have contracted some defect of body or constitution arising from their surroundings, and the maintenance of health depends largely upon making appropriate allowance for this.

The preservation of health should begin very early in life, and as infants are more prejudicially affected by improper feeding than by any other physical influence, the care of the child in this respect is of the greatest importance. (See INFANT FEEDING.) Equally important is it to nurture the child's emotional development by providing a home in which security and mutual trust and loving kindness are the keynotes. Children display at an early age peculiarities and tendencies which, if unchecked, sometimes develop into undesirable habits, and these form a matter for careful education. (See CHILDREN, PECULIARITIES OF; SCHOOL CHILDREN; and MENTAL SUBNORMALITY.)

At a later stage the most important factor in the due care of body and mind consists in attention to the natural functions of the body. Of these, the question of food that is proper in quality and in amount is one of the most important. (See DIET.) Careful attention to the functions of the bowels (see CONSTIPATION) and proper care of the teeth (see TEETH, DISEASES OF) are subjects of the utmost importance, in which children especially should be carefully instructed. In regard to the care of the skin and the maintenance of its functions, see SKIN; BATHS; and CLOTHING. A due maintenance of the relation between the exercise of the body and the amount of rest is of great importance (see EXERCISE; FATIGUE; and SLEEP), whilst the correction of bad habits in regard to the posture of the body, especially while at work, is also of importance in maintaining good health. (See CHEST DEVELOPMENT; and SPINE, DISEASES OF.) Various habits in regard to eating and drinking, and the practice of smoking, which has become almost universal, require to be carefully studied in order that due moderation may be exercised in regard to them. (See CORPULENCE; ALCOHOL; TOBACCO.)

Despite all the ordinary precautions that may be taken in regard to matters of everyday life, such as those already mentioned, people become, especially in the earlier years of life, exposed to accidents and diseases, which may, however, with care be avoided to a large extent. (See INFECTION; and SANITATION.) Certain diseases and influences are particularly liable to affect the health in different parts of the world. (For the influences exerted by climate upon health, see CLIMATE IN RELATION TO DISEASE, and for reference to the diseases which are liable to be contracted by persons in tropical countries, see references under TROPICAL DISEASES.)

HEARING (see DEAFNESS; EAR).

HEARING AIDS have been in use for many years. In the pre-electronic era they took the form of horns, ear trumpets, speaking tubes and the like. These acted by collecting the sound waves and reflecting them along a conducting tube to the ear. In other words, they were the equivalent of bringing the speaking voice close to the listener's ear. Such aids had much to be said for them, but today they would be socially unacceptable to the vast majority of the deaf.

Their place has been taken by electronic amplifiers, an adaptation which became a practical proposition when radio valves were developed, though these in turn have been superseded by transistors. Basically an electronic hearing aid consists of three elements: (1) a microphone, (2) an amplifier, (3) a miniature earphone (receiver). From the practical point of view there are three basic types of hearing aids. (1) *Body-worn aid* – In this type of aid the microphone and amplifier are housed in a small case worn on the body (eg. in a breast pocket), and the sound receiver is attached to the amplifier by a cord and situated at or near the ear. (2) *Ear-level aid* – This is a very small aid mounted in the vicinity of the ear; often behind the ear, but sometimes mounted in spectacle frames. (3) *Within-the-ear aid* – This is a very small, low-powered aid mounted, together with the receiver, directly at the outer entrance to the ear. Attractive though it may be to some, it has limited application on account of its low power.

From the point of view of hearing aids there are two types of hearing loss, or deafness. (1) *Conductive loss* is due to a defect in the conducting mechanism of the ear, usually in the middle ear. This is the type of deafness that responds particularly well to hearing aids, as the actual hearing part of the ear in the inner ear is functioning well, and the amplification produced by the hearing aid compensates almost completely for the defect. (2) *Sensorineural loss* is due to a defect in the mechanism of the inner ear, either the cochlea (see EAR) or the cochlear nerve, and the conducting mechanism is quite satisfactory. This is the type of hearing loss, or deafness, that occurs in old age. The response to hearing aids is not as satisfactory as in the case of conductive hearing loss, but in many it is satisfactory enough to justify the use of hearing aids. Part of the trouble is that the use of a hearing aid does not actually increase the ability of the affected ear to discriminate, but it may improve hearing by bringing the sound into an intensity range where a degree of discrimination is possible. Thus, the deafness sometimes takes the form of inability to recognize the sounds spoken by a very quiet speaker. By amplifying the quiet speaker's voice a hearing aid allows the deaf person to discriminate more words, and thus much of his deaf disability is overcome.

In the planning, and choice, of hearing aids it is too often forgotten that they are needed for old people who, in addition to being deaf, are also suffering from short-sightedness and are not as nimble-fingered as they were in their younger days. This means that the switches and controls on the aid must be easily managed by the elderly, and not too small. The same applies to children. So-called automatic volume control can also be an advantage in these cases as it helps to maintain a steady level without the need to make manual adjustments. With body-worn aids a polished metal case to diminish clothes rustle is helpful. An important practical point is the contact between the ear-piece and the ear. The ear-piece usually consists of a moulded insert made of special plastic resins and moulded for the individual wearer. The insert is drilled and the earphone (receiver) is fitted to it. A snugly fitting insert is essential; otherwise the aid will oscillate, producing an all too familiar howling or whistling sound. This can be a very difficult problem in the case of young children.

One final word of warning is necessary. Modern hearing aids are little master-pieces of modern technology, including, as they do, transistors, miniature circuitry and lightweight batteries; and variations of output and response characteristics, as well as automatic volume control, are provided in many of them. Fundamentally, however, these requirements are relatively marginal benefits, which are only of real value to a minority of more sophisticated individuals. To the general-ity of elderly who provide so many of the deaf people in our midst, what is required, as has already been noted, is the less sophisticated, more robust, easily managed hearing aid, an essential element of which is ample power output. In making a choice therefore from the large range of effective hearing aids now avail-able, including the Medresco hearing aid supplied under the National Health Service, the expert advice of an ear special-ist must be obtained. The Royal National Institute for the Deaf, 105 Gower Street, London, WC1E 6AH, provides a list of clinics where such a specialist can be con-sulted. It also gives reliable advice concern-ing the purchase and use of hearing aids.

A behind-the-ear hearing aid weighing 7·65 grams (about ¼ ounce) is now available under the National Health Service for all who will benefit from it.

HEART is a hollow muscular pump with four cavities, each provided at its outlet with a valve, whose function is to maintain the circulation of the blood. The two upper cavities are known as atria, the two lower ones as ventricles. The term auricle is applied to the ear-shaped tip of the atrium on each side. Owing to the fact that the heart has important connections with the nervous system, and that its action is liable to be increased or di-minished by influences which powerfully affect the latter, the heart was regarded in olden times, and is still metaphorically spoken of, as the seat of the emotions.

Position – The heart lies in the chest between the two lungs, but projecting more to the left side than to the right (illustrations 246, 247, 248). On the left

246 – Chest with the skin and muscles removed from the front, showing the position of heart and lungs. *H*, heart; *LL*, left lung; *RL*, right lung; *W*, windpipe; *L*, liver; *S*, stomach.

side its apex reaches out in the adult between $3\frac{1}{2}$ and 4 inches (8 and 9 cm), almost to the nipple, and lies beneath the fifth rib, while its right border extends only a short distance, at most an inch, beyond the margin of the breast-bone. Its lower border rests upon the diaphragm, by which it is separated from the liver and stomach, and this close connection has an important influence upon the heart in several disorders of the stomach. Above, the heart extends to the level of the second rib, where the great vessels, the aorta on the right side and the pulmonary artery on the left, lie behind the breast-bone.

Structure – The heart lies within a strong fibrous bag, known as the pericardium, and since the inner surface of this bag and the outer surface of the heart are both covered with a smooth, glistening membrane faced with flat cells and lubricated by a little serous fluid, the movements of the heart are accomplished almost without friction. The main thickness of the heart wall consists of bundles of muscle fibres, which run, some in circles right round the heart, others in loops, first round one cavity, then round the corresponding cavity of the other side. Within all the cavities is a smooth lining

1 Aorta.
2 Pulmonary artery.
3 Left ventricle.
4 Superior vena cava.
5 Right atrium.
6 Inferior vena cava.

247 – X-ray of healthy heart. From Evans, *Diseases of the Heart and Arteries*. E. & S. Livingstone.

Shape and size – The heart of any individual was described by Laennec as, roughly, of the size and shape of the clenched fist. Its weight in the male varies from 280 to 340 grams, and in the female from 230 to 280 grams. It continues to increase in weight and size up to a ripe old age, more so in men than in women. One end of the heart is pointed (apex), the other is broad (base), and is deeply cleft at the division between the two atria. One groove running down the front and up the back shows the division between the two ventricles; a circular, deeper groove marks off the atria above from the ventricles below. The capacity of each cavity is somewhere between 3 and 6 ounces (90 and 180 ml).

membrane, continous with that lining the vessels which open into the heart. The investing smooth membrane is known as epicardium, the muscular substance as myocardium, and the smooth lining membrane as endocardium.

For the regulation of the heart's action there are important nervous connections, especially with the vagus nerve and with the sympathetic system. In the hinder part of the atria lies a collection of nerve cells and connecting fibres, known as the sinu-atrial node, which forms the starting-point for the impulses that initiate the beats of the heart. Hence its alternative name of the pacemaker of the heart. In the groove between the ventricles and the atria lies

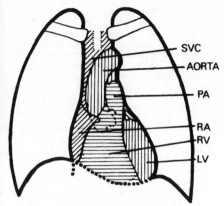

248 – Diagrammatic representation of the heart as seen by X-rays. *SVC*, superior vena cava; *PA*, pulmonary artery; *RA*, right atrium; *RV*, right ventricle; *LV*, left ventricle. From Evans, *Diseases of the Heart and Arteries*. E. & S. Livingstone.

another collection of similar nerve tissue, known as the atrioventricular node. From it there runs downwards into the septum between the two ventricles a band of special muscle fibres, known as the atrioventricular bundle, or the bundle of His. This splits up into a right and a left branch for the two ventricles, and the fibres of these distribute themselves throughout the muscular wall of the ventricles and control their contraction.

Openings – There is no direct communication between the cavities on the right side and those on the left; but the right atrium opens into the right ventricle by a large circular opening, and similarly the left atrium into the left ventricle. Into the right atrium open two large veins,

249 – Interior of the left ventricle, showing structure of mitral valve. *LA*, left atrium; *LV*, left ventricle. From Passmore and Robson, *A Companion to Medical Studies*. Blackwell Scientific Publications.

the superior and inferior venae cavae, with some smaller veins from the wall of the heart itself, and into the left atrium open two pulmonary veins from each lung. One opening leads out of each ventricle, to the aorta in the case of the left ventricle, to the pulmonary artery from the right.

Prior to birth there is an opening (*foramen ovale*) from the right into the left atrium through which the blood passes; but when the child first draws air into his lungs this opening closes and is represented in the adult only by a depression (*fossa ovalis*).

Valves – As stated above, there are four valves (illustrations 249, 250). The mitral valve consists of two triangular cusps, the tricuspid valve of three smaller cusps. The aortic and pulmonary valves each consist of three semilunar-shaped segments. The structure of a valve is a double layer of the lining membrane of the heart (endocardium) strengthened by fibrous tissue between. Two valves are placed at

250 – The aortic valve. (*a*), open; (*b*) closed. From Passmore and Robson, *A Companion to Medical Studies*, Blackwell Scientific Publications.

the openings leading from atrium into ventricle, the tricuspid valve on the right side, the mitral valve on the left, so as completely to prevent blood from running back into the atrium when the ventricle contracts. Two more, the pulmonary valve and the aortic valve, are placed at the entrance to these arteries, and prevent regurgitation into the ventricles of blood which has been driven from them into the arteries. The noises made by these valves in closing constitute the greater part of what are known as the heart sounds, and can be heard by anyone who applies his ear to the front of a person's chest. Murmurs heard accompanying these sounds indicate defects in the valves, and form one of the chief signs of heart disease.

Action – At each heart-beat the two atria contract and expel their contents into the ventricles, which at the same time they stimulate to contract together, so that the blood is driven into the arteries, to be returned again to the atria after having completed a circuit in about fifteen seconds through the body or lungs as the case may be. The heart beats from sixty to ninety times a minute, the rate in any given healthy person being about four times that of the respirations. The heart is to some extent regulated by a nerve centre in the medulla, closely connected with those centres which govern the lungs and stomach, and nerve fibres pass to it in the vagus nerve. By some of these fibres its rate and force can be diminished, by others increased, according to the needs of the various organs of the body. If this nerve centre be injured or poisoned, for example, by want of oxygen, the heart stops beating in human beings, although in some of the lower animals – eg. frogs, fishes, and reptiles – the heart may under favourable conditions go on beating for hours even after its entire removal from the body.

HEARTBURN means a burning sensation experienced in the region of the heart and up the back to the throat. It is caused by an excessive acidity of the gastric juice, and is relieved temporarily by taking alkaline substances, such as 20 grains (1·2 grams) of bicarbonate of soda or a similar amount of bismuth carbonate or carbonate of magnesia in water.

HEART DISEASES belong to that class of diseases which can be recognized only by the trained observer, although their presence may occasion severe symptoms and evident signs of general illness perceptible to every one. Their treatment, and a true appreciation of their slightness or gravity, belong still more to the department of the specialist.

Varieties – Many general diseases affect the heart; but, considering the arduous work which this organ constantly performs (see EXERCISE), and the fact that it never rests completely from the time of its formation till death ensues, it is subject to wonderfully few disorders. Its diseases are classified according to the part of the heart affected, or the nature of the changes produced. *Inflammatory affections* are divided into pericarditis, myocarditis, and endocarditis, according as the pericardium or enveloping membrane, the myocardium or muscular substance, and the endocardium or lining membrane is affected. *Valvular diseases* form one of the most important groups; any of the four valves may be stenosed: ie. the aperture between its flaps narrowed, or a valve may be incompetent, so that some blood leaks back through the opening in the wrong direction. *Hypertrophy*, in which the heart is enlarged and its wall thickened, and *dilatation*, in which one or more of the cavities is dilated, form another group often associated with the valvular diseases. *Degeneration* of the muscular tissue, producing enfeeblement of the heart's action, may occur usually as a result of inadequate blood supply to the heart muscle. Then there is a class of disorders characterized by *disturbances of rhythm*, such as palpitation, irregularity, rapidity, or slowness, of the heart action. Finally, there is *congenital heart disease*, in which a child is born with a damaged heart. (See also CARDIOMYOPATHY.)

Causes – In 1977, what are officially known as 'circulatory diseases' accounted for one-half of the 538,652 deaths in England. Circulatory diseases include diseases of the heart and of the blood-vessels. In this group, by far the commonest cause of death was ischaemic heart disease, or coronary artery heart disease, which was responsible for 145,089 deaths – or more than one-quarter of all deaths in that year.

The main causes of heart disease are disease of the coronary arteries, the arteries which nourish the heart muscle (see CORONARY THROMBOSIS), high blood-pressure, acute rheumatism, and syphilis. Acute rheumatism is predominantly a disease of childhood, and most cases of heart disease occurring between the ages of 5 and 45 years of age are of rheumatic origin. High blood-pressure and coronary-artery disease are predominantly diseases of middle age, and their incidence has increased markedly during the last fifty years. Syphilitic heart disease also occurs in later life as a result of infection acquired during early adult life.

Other causes of heart disease include diphtheria, disease of the thyroid gland (thyrotoxicosis), and certain chronic forms of disease of the lungs. A small, but important group of cases of heart disease are those due to congenital abnormalities of the heart: ie. developmental errors in the heart which occur before the birth of the child. These account for 1 to 2 per cent of all cases of organic heart disease. Bright's disease involves the heart when it is accompanied by high blood-pressure. Certain deficiency diseases involve the heart, particularly gross deficiency of vitamin B_1, which causes the condition known as beri-beri (qv).

General symptoms – The heart possesses a remarkable power, known as compensation, by which it adapts itself to new conditions. Thus if a person takes up some more arduous employment than usual the heart beats more powerfully and becomes larger, in order to overtake the extra strain; and, in a similar way, disease in one part of the organ, such as a valve, may be so compensated that not only do no symptoms arise, but the person may pass through a long life without suspecting the existence of any such defect. The establishment of this compensation is one of the chief objects of the gradual training which is necessary before undertaking any strenuous athletic exercise. It is a common mistake to suppose that disease of the heart ends always in sudden death, for only disease of the aortic valve and coronary-artery disease are associated with this accident, which even in these conditions is infrequent. If, however, the defect be so great that it cannot be remedied by compensation, or if general ill-health or the debility of age come on, the pumping power of the heart weakens and symptoms appear, some of which are referable to the organs in which the circulation is defective, others, like pain and palpitation, to the heart itself. For example, breathlessness and lividity are due to bad circulation in the lungs; faintness and giddiness to want of blood in the brain; dyspepsia, swelling of the abdomen, and dropsy of the feet, to impeded circulation in the veins of the lower part of the body.

PERICARDITIS is an inflammation of the membrane covering the exterior of the heart. It may be dry, in which case the two opposing surfaces of the membrane are covered by a layer of fibrin worked up by the movements of the heart into ridges, very like those upon the surface of two slices of bread and butter forcibly separated from one another; or effusion may accompany this condition, when the pericardial bag becomes much distended by fluid. The causes include a virus infection (the condition known as acute benign pericarditis); rheumatic fever; uraemia; tuberculosis; spread of infection from the lungs, as in pneumonia, though this is remarkably rare considering the close relationship between the lungs and the heart; injury to the chest; any acute infection in the body, such as septicaemia; neoplasm. Pericarditis with effusion generally follows the dry form, unless the latter be very slight in extent, and the amount of fluid may reach as much as two pints (one litre). The fibrin upon the surface of the membrane increases with the amount of fluid, and may form a coating like thick leather round the heart, which very greatly embarrasses its action. Pain over the heart, high fever, rapid and feeble pulse, restlessness, difficulty in breathing, and even delirium, mark the presence of this serious condition.

Recovery often takes place, but the heart is apt to be left weak and dilated, in consequence of permanent roughening and adhesions between the two surfaces of the pericardium, and in long-standing cases this resistance to its action produces great increase in the size of the heart. This condition is known as adhesive pericarditis or adherent pericardium; it leads to great hypertrophy of the heart, and it is apt to be associated with recurring attacks of rapid cardiac action accompanied by breathlessness (paroxysmal tachycardia). Treatment during the acute stage, apart from treatment of the underlying infection by penicillin or the sulphonamides, is usually effected either by the application of an ice-bag or of blisters to the front of the chest, while various stimulants are given to maintain the action of the heart. Occasionally it becomes necessary to tap the pericardial cavity and draw off some of the fluid which is embarrassing the heart's action.

ENDOCARDITIS is an inflammatory condition of the membrane lining the heart, and since the part most subjected to friction and strain is that covering the valves, so these valves are the most commonly affected parts, those on the left side of the heart being affected much more often than those on the right side. The inflammatory process consists in the appearance of small groups of nodules upon the valves. These unite to form wart-like growths, upon which fibrin is deposited from the blood to form pendants, often of some length. The condition just described is known as simple endocarditis, and occurs most commonly in connection with rheumatic fever in childhood. Tonsillitis and scarlet fever may also be complicated by simple endocarditis. Simple endocarditis arises especially in those cases of rheumatic fever which are not allowed to rest during the attack, and although the endocarditis may give no symptom of its presence, it may leave the heart with serious valvular disease. Palpitation and a slight increase of temperature may often form the only warning of the onset of endocarditis during an attack of rheumatic fever.

Another form of endocarditis is known as bacterial endocarditis. In 80 per cent of

431

cases there is a previous history of rheumatism or chorea, whilst in 10 per cent of cases it is superimposed on a congenitally deformed valve. The essential feature is a progressive microbic infection of the heart valves or the endocardium of the heart wall. It is of much more serious import than the simple type, since fragments of the ulcerating valves may be carried by the blood-stream all over the body and set up abscesses in diverse organs, this form at one time resulting almost always in death. There is, however, no hard and fast dividing line between simple and ulcerative endocarditis, and various grades of intermediate severity are found. Little could be done for the condition beyond rest and careful nursing until the introduction of penicillin, which has now been shown to be a life-saving measure in this condition.

CHRONIC VALVULAR DISEASES form the most common and most important group of heart disorders. Although, in consequence of the power of compensation already mentioned, the heart may become more powerful and so neutralize the ill-effects of a narrowed or leaking valve, it is not possible to predict how far this change will be affected by ill-health or the strain of a laborious life, and consequently the detection of valvular disease unfits a person for entrance upon any public service, and renders him subject, if he becomes a candidate for life assurance, either to refusal or to a heavily increased premium. The commonest cause of valvular disease is rheumatic endocarditis, which, instead of passing off with the disease that produced it, has become chronic, leading ultimately either to thickening and contraction of the valves, so that they become unable to close their respective openings, or to adhesion of the segments of the valves to one another at their margins, so that the opening is very much narrowed. The former condition is known as incompetence, the latter as stenosis, and the two are found either separately, or together affecting the same valve. The valves on the left side of the heart are more often affected than those on the right side, in the proportion of about 18 to 1.

AORTIC DISEASE – Of all the valvular defects, incompetence of the aortic valve is the most serious, and next to it in importance comes stenosis of the mitral opening. Aortic incompetence leads to great dilatation and hypertrophy of the heart, which in well-marked cases becomes so large as to receive the name of cor bovinum or ox-heart. Although aortic disease in young

persons follows upon rheumatic endocarditis, and may produce a rapidly fatal issue, on the other hand it may give rise to few symptoms directly referable to the heart until later in life. If the incompetence develops in childhood it may result in the child being more or less stunted in body, and feeble or capricious in mind and temper. Stenosis at the aortic valve is much rarer than incompetence and is due either to rheumatic endocarditis or a congenital lesion. Syphilis is especially apt to lead to a degenerative and hardened condition of the aortic valve, which renders it incompetent. Angina pectoris is not infrequently associated with this condition, in consequence of the spread of the degenerative process to the coronary arteries which supply the muscle of the heart itself with blood. (See ANGINA PECTORIS.) When compensation begins to fail, throbbing of the arteries becomes very noticeable, and headache, giddiness, faintness on rising quickly, and dull pain about the heart appear. Later, shortness of breath causing inability to lie down, and dropsy of the feet and legs appear. Sudden death may occur in a case of aortic stenosis, but death may also come on gradually, ushered in by increasing dropsy, great difficulty of breathing, and mental excitability.

MITRAL DISEASE is of two types. In one case the valve itself is at fault, owing almost always to endocarditis, which produces incompetence, or stenosis, or both. In the other, the left ventricle is dilated so that the two segments of the valve are held apart by their attachments to its walls, and consequently a state of temporary, secondary, or relative incompetence is produced. It is of great importance to recognize this distinction, because, whilst the former is permanent and organic, the latter, which is due to weakness of the heart muscle, as a result, for instance, of an acute infection such as diphtheria, or anaemia, may end in complete recovery. Mitral incompetence unaccompanied by stenosis may be of relatively little importance, and persons with this defect sometimes live to an advanced period of age. In defects of this valve, the symptoms relate chiefly to the lungs, breathlessness on exertion being one of the most common, and the lips and ears becoming of a bluish tint, in consequence of the slow passage of blood through the lungs. Bronchitis and spitting of blood are common, particularly in cases in which stenosis is present. When compensation is failing, these symptoms become more marked, the liver and stomach get congested, producing a jaundiced tint of the skin, together with dyspepsia, and congestion of the kidneys develops, shown by the presence of albumin in the urine. One of the most unpleasant symptoms is the sleep-start, which catches the person as he is dropping off to sleep, making him start up gasping, and feeling as if his heart were stopping. All these symptoms pass off under treatment, to be renewed again and again at intervals. When the valve is stenosed, there is a tendency to the formation of small clots in the atrium; these may be carried away and lodged in various organs: eg. in the brain, causing apoplexy. Sudden death in mitral disease is rare. Cases of mitral disease, and especially cases in which marked stenosis is present, are often, as time goes on, associated with a state of dilatation of the atria, and the condition of disordered action in these cavities is known as atrial fibrillation. This leads to great irregularity in the time and force of the heart-beats, with corresponding irregularity felt in the pulse.

DISEASE OF THE VALVES ON THE RIGHT SIDE is relatively rare. The tricuspid valve may be incompetent in consequence of far advanced mitral disease, which increases the difficulty of circulation through the lungs and so leads to dilatation of the right side of the heart. Stenosis of the pulmonary valve sometimes forms a congenital condition in children.

Treatment of valvular diseases – When a valvular defect is accidentally discovered, even though it be perfectly compensated and give rise to no symptoms, it is well that the person should take certain precautions in his daily life, and he should therefore, unless of a particularly nervous and highly strung temperament, be informed by his medical adviser of the condition found in his heart. The subject of such disease must lead a quiet and well-regulated life, avoiding, as far as may be, excitement, worry, and sudden strains, although methodical attention to business, and even hard, steady work, are quite well borne. The question of marriage is an important one, and, speaking generally, it is unwise for the subjects of aortic disease to marry, for insurance companies decline the risk in this condition. In mitral disease marriage is not attended with the same risk, although in a woman the condition of a heart with defective mitral valve tends to become progressively worse with each confinement. The excessive use of tobacco, prolonged hot baths, and excursions up mountains are bad for most cases

of valvular disease. A simple, wholesome diet is necessary.

When compensation begins to fail – and often this does not take place until middle age – the symptoms already mentioned appear, but, in early stages, rest may be the only remedy required. In the later stages the great standby is digitalis (qv). Many persons, by taking digitalis and living a carefully regulated life, manage to keep in abeyance all the symptoms of a serious valve defect, and to live a busy, useful life. Congestion of the liver, lungs, and kidneys is treated by rest in bed, digitalis, and diuretics. For dropsy in advanced cases, tapping of the legs, abdomen, or chest may be necessary, although less so since the introduction of efficient diuretics. (See ASPIRATION.) For breathlessness, the patient must often remain in the sitting posture night and day, and it is important that a comfortable bed-rest should be provided. Pain about the heart is not common, but, when it occurs, is often relieved by careful attention to the diet, so as to prevent dyspepsia. Spitting of blood, when it occurs, is not very copious, and is rather salutary than otherwise, so that it does not call for treatment.

Most satisfactory results are now being obtained from surgical treatment in selected cases of mitral stenosis, and to a lesser extent in the treatment of aortic valvular disease.

ENLARGEMENT OF THE HEART is of two types: dilatation of the cavities with HYPERTROPHY of the walls, and DILATATION with thinning of the walls. The first takes place as the result of simple, constant strain, as in professional runners and other athletes. It also arises in consequence of the increased difficulty in the circulation that results from a diseased valve, and it produces compensation of the valvular disease. It also occurs in consequence of high blood-pressure. To this extent, and while general health lasts, hypertrophy is an altogether good thing, the only sign of its presence being a large heart with an extra-powerful beat. But in the later years of life there is a special tendency for the muscle of these hypertrophied hearts to degenerate; and further, if the vessels throughout the body be weak, as in Bright's disease, the powerful beating of the heart may tear them, particularly in the brain, with apoplexy as a result. DILATATION of the heart, with thinning of its walls, is always a bad thing, leading to feeble action of the organ. It occurs also as the result of strain when the heart has not sufficient reserve force to hypertrophy. It takes place, too, in persons who are bloodless and it often occurs to a slight extent after a severe fever. Sometimes it occurs suddenly, the heart becomes unable to contract upon the blood which accumulates in it, and death results in a few minutes or hours, in consequence of some extraordinary effort by a feeble person, or in consequence of injudicious exercise too soon during convalescence from a fever.

Treatment is much the same as for valvular heart disease where compensation is failing. For a dilated heart, rest combined with regulated exercise is the special treatment. At certain spas and watering-places these exercises have been brought to great finesse. (See also TRANSPLANTATION.)

DEGENERATION OF THE HEART occurs principally in elderly people, the most common form being a change of the muscle fibres, in scattered patches, into fat. In another form of degeneration a deposition of fibrous tissue gradually takes place between the muscle fibres, which at the same time waste away. Less common forms of degeneration consist in a granular change in the fibres, producing great softening in the course of some fatal fevers; and a condition known as brown atrophy, in which the heart-muscle wastes as old age advances, and contains much brown pigment.

FATTY DEGENERATION – In stout people a deposit of fat takes place upon the heart (fatty infiltration), interfering with its action and causing shortness of breath upon slight exertion, but this is not so serious as true degeneration, in which the change involves a gradual destruction of the actual muscle. Fatty degeneration arises as a senile change, most commonly in persons addicted to alcohol, in whom it may appear early in middle life; and also as a sequence to hypertrophy of the heart. In general devitalizing diseases like pernicious anaemia, or when the coronary arteries, which supply the heart itself with blood, are narrowed by disease, fatty degeneration of the heart-muscle is common. It may come on acutely in infective diseases like pneumonia or influenza. If it comes on gradually, it causes attacks of pain in the centre of the chest and left arm, with great irregularity and palpitation of the heart on exertion. Unusual torpor in the early part of the day following on very slight exertion, is also a sign of its presence. Other symptoms are occasional fainting fits and great loss of mental activity, and there is a special danger of

sudden death in persons affected by this degenerative process.

FIBROID DEGENERATION of the muscular wall of the heart is usually a result of gradual and extensive blocking in branches of the coronary arteries, due to patches of atheromatous thickening in their walls. The muscle fibres waste or die in patches as a result of defective nourishment, and are replaced by useless fibrous tissue. Dilatation of the cavities, clotting of the blood on the fibroid patches, followed, it may be, by angina pectoris or by sudden death, take place. This condition of the heart is often associated with advanced disease in the kidneys. The symptoms are much the same as those due to fatty degeneration. In the treatment, the same drugs are used as for valvular disease, though more sparingly. Careful regulation of daily life with simple diet is of great importance. The person should beware of any excessive physical strain.

CORONARY ARTERY DISEASE, or *ISCHAEMIC HEART DISEASE* – This is the most important form of heart disease at the present day because it is the most killing. (See CORONARY THROMBOSIS; and ANGINA PECTORIS.)

DISTURBANCES OF RHYTHM – Several varieties of abnormal action of the heart are recognized. Some of these are due to a definite organic disease of the heart, but in many there is no discoverable disease, and the abnormal action is then described as of functional nature. Some of these conditions are due to disease affecting the mechanism in the heart which controls the regular sequence of contraction of the different cavities, but such disease is only recognizable during life by the abnormal action which it sets up.

Many troublesome irregularities of the heart are now known to be caused by defective action of the muscular connections. The site of these defects can be analysed by means of elaborate modern instruments. Of these the chief is the *electrocardiograph* (qv), which by means of a galvanometer registers photographically the electrical changes that take place in the body as the heart beats.

The heart-muscle has in itself, independently of nervous control, the power of contracting rhythmically when excited to do so, of conducting the impulse to contract from one part of the muscle to another, and of maintaining itself in a moderate state of tension or tone. When any of these properties is affected by disease some change in the force or rhythm of the heartbeat is apt to appear.

PALPITATION is a condition in which the heart beats fast and the person becomes conscious of its beating. (See PALPITATION.)

SINUS ARRHYTHMIA is a condition of irregular action in which the heart speeds up during inspiration and slows again during expiration. It is a normal phenomenon, but may occasionally be so accentuated that the individual becomes aware of it, when it may give rise to anxiety.

ATRIAL (or AURICULAR) FIBRILLATION is the commonest form of persistent irregularity of the heart's action, accounting for about one-half of all the cases of irregular pulse. It usually accompanies disease of the mitral valve, and is recognized by great irregularity in time and force of the pulse (what has been described as an 'irregular irregularity'), visible pulsations in the veins of the neck, and various signs which are made out by the use of the electrocardiograph and by auscultation. In this type of irregularity the atria do not empty themselves by the normal regular waves but contract partially in a rapid series of twitches, and in consequence the ventricles do not receive the normal rhythmic stimulus to contract, and they accordingly contract irregularly. This is a serious irregularity.

EXTRASYSTOLES form a common cause of irregular action in irritable states of the heart; the extrasystole is a premature beat followed by a pause of the heart for rest. This is not a serious form of disorder, and it may come and go for many years in certain individuals.

HEART-BLOCK is a serious condition in which the conducting mechanism between atrium and ventricle is impaired (incomplete heart-block), or destroyed (complete heart-block) so that the atrium and ventricle beat at different rates independently of one another. During the incomplete stage the pulse is irregular, but when the heart-block becomes complete and the ventricles contract independently of the atria, the pulse becomes regular and very slow, and the individual is liable to fainting or convulsive attacks (Stokes-Adams attacks). (See also CARDIAC PACEMAKER.)

PULSUS ALTERNANS, or ALTERNATING PULSE, is a condition in which there are regularly alternating strong and weak beats of the heart, forming a persistent type of irregularity, which is caused by degeneration of the heart-muscle. It is of serious import.

RAPID HEART (*tachycardia*) with a pulse considerably above 100 per minute is found in a large variety of conditions. In its most benign form it may be due to emotional disturbance, whether excitement, fear, or pleasure. In other cases it may be due to overactivity of the thyroid gland as in thyrotoxicosis (qv). A more common cause is fever. A rise in temperature is always accompanied by a rise in heart rate. The most common cause of all is a failing heart.

SLOW HEART (*bradycardia*) is a natural phenomenon in some individuals, the heart beating only forty, fifty, or sixty times per minute instead of the normal seventy or eighty times. Such individuals are usually of a generally lethargic temperament. Slowness of the heart-beat is also a character of complete heart-block.

CONGENITAL HEART DISEASE accounts for 1 to 2 per cent of all cases of organic heart disease. Its incidence is 6 to 7 per 1000 live births. The cause is variable. In a small minority of cases it is hereditary, but in the majority it is due to some illness of the mother, such as German measles, or some other adverse factor, such as certain drugs, affecting her during the early period of pregnancy. The abnormality may take almost an infinite variety of forms, such as an abnormality of the valves of the heart, the heart lying on the right side of the chest instead of the left, a patent ductus arteriosus (see DUCTUS ARTERIOSUS), a defect in the septum separating the chambers of the heart, or coarctation of the aorta (qv). These last three have become of great interest in recent years, in view of the satisfactory results which have been obtained with surgical treatment.

HEAT – (See also BURNS; HEAT-STROKE.) The curative uses of heat as applied by hot water and hot air are mentioned under BATHS. Hot-air applications are much used in the treatment of rheumatic conditions in the joints and muscles, and a more powerful application of heat for the same purpose is obtained by the use of high frequency electricity. (See DIATHERMY.) Excessive heat, in the form of the cautery, is also used in order to destroy diseased tissues. (See CAUSTICS AND CAUTERIES.)

HEAT-CRAMPS are painful cramps in the muscles occurring in workers, such as stokers, who labour in hot conditions. The cramps are the result of loss of salt in the sweat, and can be cured by giving salty water to drink. (See HEAT-STROKE.)

HEATING – People vary tremendously in their opinion as to what they consider to be a comfortable temperature in which to sit or do sedentary work, and this individual reaction is partly dependent upon other factors such as the efficiency of the ventilation of the room. Thus, by and large, a stuffy room will tend to feel uncomfortably hot to many people even though the temperature may be within the recognized limits of comfort. These levels are usually taken to be 60° to 65° F (15·5° to 19·8° C). In nurseries, sick-rooms and rooms for old people a higher range of 65° to 70° F (18·3° to 21° C) is usually aimed at.

The choice of domestic heating today is dependent upon three main considerations: cost, air pollution, and personal preference. Coal is gradually disappearing as a source of heat, though coke and various forms of so-called smokeless coal derivatives are still used. Gas, electricity and oil are gradually assuming the dominant position in this field.

Open fires, which warm chiefly by radiation, afford a traditionally pleasing, but wasteful and dirty, source of warmth. An open fire sends about five-eighths of its heat up the chimney, about two-eighths are used to heat the walls, leaving only one-eighth to warm the air of the room. As the open fire, burning coal, is one of the major sources of air pollution in urban areas, the use of ordinary coal is forbidden in those progressive towns that implement the enactments of the Clean Air Acts, and only smokeless fuels such as coke or the products of low-temperature carbonization such as 'coalite' can be used. Not the least of the advantages of an open fire is the contribution it makes to the ventilation of a room.

Stoves warm by radiation and convection, causing a current of warmed air to pass through the room, thereby helping to maintain a uniform temperature. They burn anthracite or coke, and are more efficient than the open fire, but care must be taken to ensure that the ventilation flue is of sufficient size to allow escape of all fumes even when the damper is in the closed position. Their main use is for heating halls or large rooms when central heating is not available.

Gas fires are efficient and share with open fires the facility of adding ventilation.

Electricity has the advantage of cleanliness, efficiency and adaptability. It may be used in the form of a fire which heats by radiation, or a convector heater in which a non-luminous element warms the air as it passes through a metal cabinet. Alterna-

tively, it can be used in radiator form, in which oil is circulated by means of an immersion heater. Electric floor heating is also used, as well as so-called storage heaters which can be heated at off-peak periods or during the night at a lower tariff.

Central heating is gradually becoming the most popular form of heating in houses, as it has been in schools and offices for a long time. Hot water is more widely used in Britain than in the United States of America where steam heating is more widely used. The three sources of heat are oil, gas, or solid fuel. The temperature of the radiator surface ranges from room temperature to 190° F (80° C). For domestic purposes the usual installation is what is known as the indirect hot-water system, in which one boiler heats the water for both radiators and the hot-water taps. Concealed pipes in the ceiling may be used as an alternative to radiators, but have the disadvantage of difficulty of access if anything goes wrong.

HEAT SPOTS is a vague term applied to small inflamed and congested areas which appear especially upon the skin of the face, neck, and chest or other parts of the body in warm weather.

HEAT-STROKE is the term applied to the effects produced on the body by exposure to excessive heat. Although most commonly observed in tropical regions, it may occur also in temperate climates during hot weather. A moist condition of the atmosphere, which interferes with cooling of the overheated body, greatly increases the liability to suffer from this ailment.

Causes – The fundamental cause of the condition is exposure of the body to amounts of radiant energy for which it cannot compensate. This inability to compensate for excessive exposure to heat results in overheating of the body and loss of fluid. In any given case one or other of these factors, or both, may come into play (table 27). In the more acute cases the condition is characterized by failure of the sweating mechanism: these are the cases which are rapidly fatal unless treatment is instituted immediately. When excessive sweating occurs, in the early stages this loss of fluid is accompanied by a corresponding loss of salt (sodium chloride), resulting in a disturbance of the electrolyte balance of the body fluids. Unless this loss of water and sodium chloride is compensated for, one of three things may occur: (i) the individual may be seized with severe cramp in the muscles: ie. heat cramps; (ii) the blood volume is diminished and the circulation of the body is seriously disturbed, resulting in a condition analogous to surgical shock; (iii) the sweating mechanism may break down, with resultant further rise in the temperature of the body, leading to a fatal termination.

Predisposing factors are bad living or working conditions, lack of acclimatization to tropical conditions, unsuitable clothing, poor health, and dietetic and alcoholic indiscretions.

Dilatation of blood-vessels of skin
Sweating
Dilution of blood
Decreased muscle tone
Inclination to reduced activity
Stretching, or extension, of body to increase loss of heat
Decrease in volume of urine
Thirst
Loss of chloride leading to heat-cramps
Difficulty in maintaining blood supply to brain, leading to dizziness, nausea and heat-exhaustion
Rising body temperature
Impairment of heat-regulating centre in brain
Cessation of breathing

Table 27 – Effects of exposure to high temperatures.

Symptoms – The symptoms, which obviously depend upon the disorganization of the normal heat-regulating mechanism as well as of the functions of circulation and respiration, vary in their intensity and likewise to some extent in their form. Four chief types of the disease are usually described.

(1) HEAT COLLAPSE – This is the mildest form of the condition. It is characterized by fatigue, giddiness, and temporary loss of consciousness. The blood-pressure is low and the pulse is slow. In the more severe cases there is a state of collapse, with cold, clammy skin and a subnormal temperature. Vomiting is not uncommon and there may be muscular cramps. The urine is much diminished in volume, is highly coloured and has a high specific gravity: eg. over 1020. This type of case practically always recovers.

(2) HEAT EXHAUSTION – The mild case of heat exhaustion is similar to one of heat collapse. The more severe case tends to occur towards the end of the hot season in the tropics. The onset is characterized by increasing weakness, dizziness, and insomnia, and this is accompanied by defective sweating in the majority of cases. Cramps and vomiting seldom occur, but large volumes of urine are voided. The temperature is usually about $100°–101°$ F $(37·8°–38·3°$

C), the pulse rate is within normal limits, and there are seldom signs of dehydration, the skin usually having quite a good colour.

(3) HEAT CRAMPS – These have been recognized for many years and occur in individuals who perform hard physical work in high temperatures. Hence the many different names by which they have been known: eg. miners' cramps, stokers' cramps, bakers' cramps. The characteristic feature is agonizing cramp, usually in the legs, arms, or back. Occasionally the abdominal muscles are involved, and in these cases the intensity of the pain may suggest some acute condition of the stomach or gut. The cramps are accompanied by sweating, pallor of the skin, and a feeling of intense anxiety. There may be headache and giddiness. The temperature is seldom raised very much.

(4) HEAT HYPERPYREXIA – This is the most serious type of all. The initial manifestations are loss of energy and irritability. Then follow mental confusion and diminution or cessation of sweating. Gradually, or sometimes with startling suddenness, this passes into restlessness and then coma and the temperature rises rapidly to $107°$ F $(41·7°$ C) or even higher. Unless treatment is instituted immediately, there is soon a fatal termination.

Prevention – Careful selection of personnel who have to perform hard physical work under tropical conditions or in high temperatures such as pertain in stokeholds, is essential. Even in the case of such selected individuals acclimatization is necessary and they should not be allowed to perform severe physical exertion at high temperatures until a period of several weeks' training has elapsed. In the tropics elderly people should move to a cool area, eg. the hills in India, during the hot season. Personal hygiene is important. Only light clothing should be worn, with a minimum of constrictions such as tight belts.

Diet should be light and nourishing and ample fluids should be taken. Salads and fruit should constitute an important part of the diet, and fluids should be bland: eg. fruit drinks, tea, iced coffee. Alcoholic drinks should be taken in moderation, and only after sundown. In the case of individuals performing hard physical exertion at high temperatures, water containing salt (ie. sodium chloride) should be drunk freely. Unless the water contains a certain amount of salt, there is an increased tendency to develop cramps. In industries where men work under such conditions, they are now provided with salt and water flavoured with lemon to disguise the salty flavour. Attention to ventilation and air-conditioning is also essential. In the tropics, when air-conditioning is not available, houses should be closed up in the early morning and opened up again at sundown. This reduces the amount of hot air entering the house during the day and allows of free circulation of the cool night air. Fans are also of value, and, in hot, dry conditions, sprinkling the compound with water during the afternoon sometimes helps to keep the house cool.

Treatment – In the case of *heat cramps, heat collapse,* and *heat exhaustion,* treatment consists of removal of the affected individual to a cool place and the administration of normal saline (see ISOTONIC). In severe cases this can be given intravenously, but it can usually be given by mouth. *Heat hyperpyrexia* is an emergency which requires immediate attention with a view to reducing the temperature. The individual should be placed in the shade, stripped, and drenched with water. To increase the cooling property of the water the surface of the body should be fanned. The patient is then wrapped in a sheet soaked in as cool water as possible (see WET PACKS), and the fanning is continued. This treatment must be stopped when the rectal temperature falls to 102° F (38.9° C) and the patient then be wrapped in a dry blanket. The reason for stopping at this temperature is that the temperature continues to fall after treatment is stopped and therefore if treatment was continued until the temperature became normal, the further fall in temperature might have serious consequences. As soon as the patient is conscious he should be given normal saline to drink, and this usually provokes sweating – a favourable sign. Whenever possible, further treatment should be carried out in hospital, as there is always a risk of circulatory collapse occurring. Convalescence may be prolonged, and the advisability of the affected individual returning permanently to a cooler climate must always be given careful consideration.

HEBEPHRENIA is a form of mental disorder coming on in youth and marked by depression and gradual failure of mental faculties with egotistic and self-centred delusions. It is one of the forms of schizophrenia.

HEBERDEN'S NODES are little hard knobs which appear at the sides of the last phalanges of the fingers in persons who are the subject of osteoarthrosis.

HEBETUDE is mental dullness, especially the temporary dullness which arises in the course of fevers.

HECTIC is a type of fever which may occur in certain severe forms of tuberculosis or septic poisoning. The temperature rises during the day to 102° or 104° F (39° to 40° C), and falls during the night almost to normal or even to below normal, 96° or 97° F (35·6° to 36·1° C), with profuse sweating. (See TUBERCULOSIS.)

HEEL is the hinder part of the foot formed by the calcaneus and the specially thick skin covering it. It is not subject to many diseases. Severe pain in the heel is sometimes a sign of gout or rheumatism.

HEIGHT (see WEIGHT AND HEIGHT).

HELIOTHERAPY is a term applied to treatment of disease by exposing the body to the sun's rays. This form of treatment by sun bath has been widely used in the treatment of tuberculosis of the bones and joints. (See LIGHT TREATMENT.)

HELIUM is the lightest gas known, with the exception of hydrogen. This property renders it of value in anaesthesia (qv), as its addition to the anaesthetic being inhaled means that it can be inhaled with less effort by the patient. Thus it can be used in the presence of any obstruction to the entry of air to the lungs.

HELLEBORE (see VERATRUM).

HELMINTHS is a name for worms. (See PARASITES.)

HEMERALOPIA is the term for describing the condition of day-blindness, in which the patient can see better in a dull light than in bright daylight.

HEMIANAESTHESIA means loss of touch-sense down one side of the body.

HEMIANOPIA, HEMIANOPSIA, and HEMIOPIA are terms meaning loss of half the usual area of vision. The affected person may see everything clearly to the left or to the right, the field of vision stopping abruptly at the middle line, or he may see things only when straight in front of him, or thirdly, he may see objects far out on both sides, although there is a wide area straight in front for which he is quite blind. The position of the blind area is important in localizing the position in the brain of the disease responsible for the condition.

HEMIATROPHY is atrophy of one side of the body, or of part of the body on one side: for example, facial hemiatrophy, in which one-half of the face is smaller than the other either in the course of development or as a result of some nervous disorder.

HEMIBALLISM is a condition characterized by a violent form of restlessness involving one side of the body. It is usually most marked in the arm. It is due to a lesion in the mid-brain.

HEMICRANIA means a headache limited to one side of the head. (See MIGRAINE.)

HEMIPLEGIA means paralysis limited to one side of the body. (See PARALYSIS.)

HEMLOCK, or CONIUM, is used in the form both of the leaves and fruit of *Conium maculatum.* Its action depends upon the property which it possesses of paralysing the endings of the motor nerves. It therefore diminishes spasmodic conditions of all sorts, producing at the same time muscular weakness and confusion of vision. In large amount it causes complete paralysis and acts as a narcotic, and was the poison by which Socrates died. The action depends upon an alkaloid, coniine.
Uses – It is seldom used in medicine now. At one time it was considered to be of value in the treatment of spasmodic or convulsive conditions such as chorea, whooping-cough, and epilepsy.

HENBANE (see HYOSCYAMUS).

HEPARIN is a substance, first obtained from the liver, which prevents coagulation of the blood. It is present chiefly in liver, muscle, and lung. It is thought to act by neutralizing thrombin. (See FIBRIN.) Heparin has a complicated chemical structure and has been prepared in crystalline form. It is carbohydrate in nature, and contains amino and sulphuric acid groups. It is used for the prevention of clot formation in the blood or to prevent the spreading of this process once it has occurred. It is not active when given by mouth and must therefore be given by injection – usually intravenously. (See also ANTICOAGULANTS.)

HEPATECTOMY is the operation for removal of the liver, or part of it.

HEPATITIS means inflammation of the liver. (See LIVER.)

HEPATITIS, ACUTE INFECTIOUS, is an acute infection of the liver, caused by a virus. The disease is an intestinal infection, the virus passing from the stools of one patient to the mouth of the next. In temperate climes it tends to occur in late summer, with a peak in winter or early spring. In the tropics and sub-tropics there is no seasonal incidence. The incubation periods varies from 15 to 50 days (commonly 28). The disease may come on suddenly or gradually. In many patients, there is no jaundice, the patient merely feeling 'liverish', off his food and complaining of some abdominal discomfort. When jaundice does occur it usually appears about the 7th or 9th day, and may persist for 2 or 3 weeks. As already noted, it is spread by the stools of the infected individual. The duration of infectivity of the patient is uncertain, but is probably from 7 to 14 days before, to 7 days after the onset of jaundice. Those who have had the disease should not return to work until at least seven days following the disappearance of jaundice or until complete clinical recovery. The disease is notifiable in Britain.

HEPATITIS, SERUM, is a closely allied disease, which differs in three respects. It has a longer incubation period (up to 100 days or even longer). It is transmitted by the transfusion of contaminated blood or by the use of contaminated syringes or needles. It is a more fatal disease, the mortality ranging from 6 to 20 per cent, compared with 1 to 2 per 1000 for acute infectious hepatatis.

HEPATIZATION means the solidified state of the lung which appears in lobar pneumonia, giving it a consistence like that of the liver.

HEPTABARBITONE is a short-acting barbiturate which induces sedation, hypnosis or anaesthesia, according to the dose given.

HEREDITY is a term indicating the principle on which various peculiarities of bodily form or structure, or of physical or mental activity are transmitted from parents to offspring, and so handed down through a family stock.

Every individual begins life as two cells, derived one from each parent. These germinal cells are in a sense half-cells, because in preparation for union the nucleus of each has extruded from the cell one-half of the rod-shaped bodies (chromosomes) by which the characters of the individual are supposed to be determined. Each germinal cell thus supplies 23 chromosomes, carrying certain characters from one of the parents, to form, with those of the other, the 46 chromosomes in the new cell from which all the other cells of the human body are derived by a process of growth and repeated division. (See FOETUS.) In the process of extrusion of chromosomes certain 'genes' or characters possessed by either parent may be lost to the offspring.

According to Weissmann's germ plasm theory, a fragment of the new cell is at once set apart for the formation of the germ cells in the new individual and thus conformity of succeeding generations with their predecessors is secured. Galton stated a rule that the total heritage of an offspring is derived, on the average, one-half from the parents, one-quarter from the grandparents, one-eighth from the greatgrandparents, and so on. This, while doubtless true in a general way, does not account for the evident differences among brothers and sisters. Mendel's theory to explain this supposes that simple or unit characters, such as height or colour of hair, are segregated or transmitted alternatively to the offspring (according to which chromosomes have been lost or retained) instead of being an average of these characters as shown in the two parents. Each unit character has a variation, which is, in a sense, its opposite, like tallness and shortness. The one of these which tends to give the appearance to the individual is called the dominant character (in this example, tallness), the other variation is called recessive, although both have an equal tendency to be transmitted.

For example, if two persons of a pure-tall stock are mated, their children will all be tall, whilst the children of a pure-short race union will all be short. If, however, a pure-tall stock person be mated with a pure-short stock person, all their children, though tending to be tall in appearance, may transmit either tallness or shortness to the next generation, and the final average result will be: out of every four children, one true tall who will transmit tallness, one true short who will transmit shortness, and two of tall appearance who

will transmit with an equal chance tallness or shortness to their children. The last is the general formula on which in modern human communities hereditary characters are likely to be transmitted.

In plants or animals the breeding of single desirable unit characters like colour or length of limb or quality of hair is a comparatively simple affair of selection in mating. In human eugenics, however, desirable qualities are complicated matters of character or intellect or general physique, which depend for their development as much upon environment and personal influence during childhood as upon heredity. It is noteworthy also that persons who appear unfit in one aspect are often well endowed in others.

The transmission of characters which predispose to certain diseases is a matter of some importance, although many serious defects tend to die out through difficulties to procreation. Disorders caused by a dominant gene are rare. The clinical example is Huntington's chorea (qv). All those born with a dominant gene such as this will develop the condition, and there is a 50 per cent chance of their children being affected. Diseases may also be caused by recessive genes, but anyone with such a disorder must have got the genes from both parents. If the recessive gene is transmitted by only one parent, the offspring will not show the disorder but will be a 'carrier': that is, he could pass it on to his children. If he marries someone with the same gene, their children could be affected. There are almost certainly many recessive genes in the population at any one time, but there are so many different ones that the chance of two carriers of the same genetic condition having children is small, though the risk is increased by marriages between close relatives – which is one of the arguments against marriages between first cousins. Thus, if the condition in question is carried by $0 \cdot 1$ per cent of the population, a particular male carrier has only a 1 in 1000 chance of marrying a female carrier unless he marries a close relative. On the other hand, a child of two carriers of the same condition has a 1 in 4 chance of inheriting the disorder and 2 in 4 of being a carrier.

Yet another way in which abnormalities of chromosomes may arise is by an accidental fault during division of the germ cells. Such abnormalities are not inherited beyond one generation.

The shape of the eye is largely a hereditary character, so that short-sight, astigmatism, etc., tend to run in families;

cataract is also largely familial; colour-blindness is handed down as a sex-linked character affecting males but transmitted by females who do not suffer from it; a rare form of blindness due to atrophy of the optic nerve is similarly transmitted. As to ear defects, the condition of otosclerosis, causing deafness, runs in families, while among deaf-mutes one in four owes this condition to defects in the nervous system which may be transmitted.

A tendency to rheumatism, or to tuberculosis or to certain skin diseases is due to defective power to resist the effective causes of these diseases, which may be a hereditary defect. Similarly, faults in the structure of certain organs, which may be inherited peculiarities, produce a liability in some families or races to goitre, diabetes, gastric ulcer, asthma, for example.

HERMAPHRODITE is the name applied to a person in whom the sexual organs are so defectively formed that it is difficult to decide the sex, or in whom there appear to be parts belonging to both sexes.

HERNIA means the protrusion of any organ, or part of an organ, into or through the wall of the cavity which contains it. Thus hernia of the brain may occur in consequence of a severe injury to the skull, hernia of the lung in consequence of a wound of the chest wall, but these are uncommon, and the most common form is hernia of the bowel, the popular term for which is rupture.

Varieties – Although far the commonest organ found in a hernia is part of the bowel, yet any of the abdominal structures, such as stomach, kidney, ovary, womb, bladder, or omentum, may be found projecting through an opening in the wall of the abdomen and lying close beneath the skin. Probably the only two organs exempt are the liver and pancreas, by reason of their position and connections. The projecting organ carries in front of it, and is enveloped by, a sac of peritoneum, the smooth membrane lining the interior of the abdomen. It is separated from the surface at least by this sac and by the skin. A hernia is usually described according to the position at which it protrudes. There are certain natural openings in the region of the groin on either side: one, known as the inguinal canal, through which the testicle descends in early life, and which the spermatic cord keeps always more or less open; the other, known as the femoral canal, which lies to

the inner side of the large femoral vessels that pass from the abdomen to the thigh. The inguinal canal ends just above the pubic bone, its exit, known as the external abdominal ring, being large enough to admit the tip of the finger. The femoral canal is less in size and is separated from the former only by the inner end of the inguinal ligament, a strong band which lies beneath the oblique groove that can be seen on the surface to separate the abdomen from the thigh. A hernia emerging from the former is known as an *inguinal hernia*, and tends to descend along the spermatic cord into the scrotum. A hernia emerging through the femoral canal comes forwards on the front of the thigh, and is called a *femoral hernia*. A weak spot exists in the centre of the abdomen at the navel, and here, not infrequently in young children of poor development, a hernia may appear, which is then known as an *umbilical hernia*. A hernia which protrudes at some accidental opening on the abdomen, as, for example, through the scar of an operation wound, is known as a *ventral hernia*. A rare form of hernia is one which passes through the gap in front of the pelvis between the ischial and pubic bones; it is known as an *obturator hernia*. Finally, there are various forms of *internal hernia*, the protruded organ passing up into the chest, or into some other region where it does not show itself on the surface. (See HIATUS HERNIA.)

A hernia may also be considered as *congenital*, that is, existing at birth, or *acquired* later on in life. The only positions in which congenital hernia is found are in the umbilical and inguinal regions. In the latter case the hernia descends along with the testicle towards the scrotum, the hernia being inside the tubular process of peritoneum which descends with the testicle in order to provide it with a smooth tunic.

An important classification of hernia is made according to the condition of the protruding organ. A *reducible hernia* is one which is so freely movable that it may be pressed back into the abdomen, although it comes down again by the same opening unless this be blocked up. An *irreducible hernia*, on the other hand, is one which cannot be returned, either because it has become adherent to its new surroundings, because it has enlarged after emerging, because much fat has been deposited inside the abdomen, or for some similar reason. An *obstructed hernia* is one in which, a part of the bowel being protruded, some of its contents become caught inside, and cannot for a time pass on, a state of costiveness arising in fact inside the hernia. A *strangulated hernia* is by far the most important variety, because of its immediate danger to life. In this form, the circulation of blood in the protruded bowel becomes cut off by the margin of the opening through which the loop of bowel has passed; and, if an operation be not immediately performed for its relief, the bowel will become gangrenous, and the patient may die within a few days. The great danger attending all forms of hernia is that they may at any time become strangulated.

Causes – Two factors come into play in causing hernia. First, some defect or injury of the abdominal wall; and, secondly, some increase of pressure within the cavity. With regard to the hernia at the umbilicus of young children, there is usually some defect in the closure of the opening through which the navel-string passes before birth, and through this opening a loop of bowel is forced by excessive crying or the like. In inguinal hernia, which, it may be noted, is far commoner in men than in women, the defect consists in some failure of the inguinal canal through which the testicle descends before birth – to close completely. There may, in congenital hernia, be a completely open passage leading out of the abdomen, or there may be simply a small pocket in the peritoneum which, by a sudden strain or by long-continued pressure, such as coughing, gets torn or stretched in front of a protruded organ. Femoral hernia is commoner in women than in men, probably on account of the special shape and inclination of the pelvic bones, and arises in a manner similar to that just stated for inguinal hernia. Both in these and in ventral hernia, the occurrence of marked changes in size of the abdomen, such as great increase in stoutness, great loss of fat, and repeated child-bearing, has the effect of greatly weakening the abdominal wall and predisposing to the formation of hernia. All laborious occupations involving great efforts, and bodily conditions involving frequently repeated strains, such as chronic cough or constipation, conduce to hernia of all sorts. Accordingly hernia is much more common in the male sex – who lead a more strenuous physical life – than among females.

Symptoms – The symptoms vary considerably, depending upon the particular organ which is protruded, upon the size of the opening, which may or may not compress the hernia, and upon the condition of the latter. In the great majority of cases the hernia consists of one or more loops of the small intestine, and, if the hernia be of small size and readily reducible, the symptoms are somewhat as follows. If the hernia be produced quite suddenly, as during the lifting of a heavy weight, the person affected may hear or feel a distant crack, and be conscious that something has given way, but, as a rule, suffers no sharp pain. More usually the hernia develops gradually, and the symptoms have then no definite onset, but simply increase till they attract attention. An undefinable sense of weakness, and occasionally pain, are felt in the region of the hernia. When any great effort is made, such as coughing, or straining at stool, or lifting a weight, a swelling appears with a gurgling feeling at the seat of the hernia, although this can be made to disappear by pressure when the person lies down. Even if the hernia does not come far down, a distinct impulse on coughing is communicated to the hand laid upon the swelling, which is situated usually at the inner end of the groin. When the hernia has become irreducible, the swelling does not vary in size, but the impulse on coughing is still to be felt. The presence, even of a small hernia, may occasion some interference with digestion, and constipation is a common accompaniment. A dragging sensation in the back is another frequent symptom.

When a hernia becomes strangulated, as the result of stoppage of its circulation by the pressure of the margin of the ring through which it comes, a marked set of symptoms ensues. The hernia first becomes inflamed, acutely painful, and then in a few hours turns gangrenous, producing general peritonitis and death if not relieved. At the same time, all passage of contents through the bowel is stopped, and as a result the bowels do not move, although some of their contents pass in the reverse direction, up to the stomach, whence they are vomited. Accordingly the onset of abdominal pain, accompanied by stoppage of the bowels and vomiting in a person possessed of a hernia, forms an ominous sign, and, even if no hernia be known to exist, the appearance of these three symptoms calls for immediate examination of the region of the groin by a medical practitioner.

Treatment – When a hernia is present, it may be treated in a palliative manner, so as to relieve unpleasant symptoms and diminish the risk of strangulation, or an attempt may be made to cure it.

PALLIATIVE TREATMENT – If the hernia be reducible, it is pushed back through the opening in the abdomen by manipulation known as taxis, and is then retained by an artificial support known as a truss. (See TRUSS.) The truss in its simplest form may consist merely of a pad of lint or folded handkerchief kept in position by a spica bandage. In infants, a very simple truss may be improvised from a skein of worsted, which is carried round the waist, one end passed through the other end over the site of the hernia, and the loose end carried down between the legs, and pinned to the circular part behind the back. For adults, the usual truss consists of a pad which fits over the opening, a spring to run round the pelvis and a strap to pass between the legs and prevent the truss from sliding upwards. The pad for an inguinal hernia is differently shaped from, and should be much larger than, that for femoral hernia. In getting a truss the particulars required are: (a) the girth round the pelvis below the crests of the haunch-bones; (b) the variety of hernia; (c) the side on which it is situated; (d) the age and sex of the patient; (e) the strength desired in the spring. No pains should be spared to get a correctly fitting truss. (See TRUSS.)

If the hernia be irreducible, a different type of truss designed merely to protect the hernia must be used.

CURATIVE TREATMENT – The danger of strangulation, involving an immediate operation with great risk to life, is present as long as a hernia exists, and, except in old people with a very wide opening, the chance of radical cure and removal of the danger offered by an operation deserve to be carefully considered. The operation, known as the radical cure, is not in itself a dangerous one, and the period of enforced idleness consequent on it amounts only to a few weeks. Many operations are performed by different surgeons, but all consist briefly in this, that an opening is made over the hernia and, after the hernia has been returned into the abdomen, the sac is cut off, bunched up, turned aside, or otherwise disposed of, and the margins of the opening united by strong sutures. Almost all cases operated upon in this way result in complete cure.

When a hernia is irreducible, some special diet or other treatment is often required before the operation, in order to diminish the amount of fat in the abdomen, reduce the size of the hernia, and so forth.

When a hernia becomes strangulated, an operation becomes urgently necessary.

The first object of this operation is to set free the hernia from the margin of the opening, tight band, or other cause that is impeding the circulation in it. This having been achieved, if the bowel is not too much damaged by the pressure it has received, it is returned to the abdomen, and the radical cure performed. Sometimes, however, the bowel has been so much damaged by several hours of pressure, that it would be too dangerous to replace it, and then, the compression having been relieved, either the damaged portion is completely cut out and the ends united by stitching, or the bowel is simply left in the wound for a few days, and the operation completed at a subsequent stage, if the bowel recovers its vitality. If the damaged loop of bowel does not recover, but sloughs away, then either the patient dies, or a fistula is left, from which the contents of the bowel escape to the exterior. This can, however, be closed by subsequent operation.

HEROIN, also known as DIAMORPHINE HYDROCHLORIDE, is a white crystalline powder of slightly bitter taste derived from morphine. It is a much more potent pain killer, or analgesic, than morphine but also a much more dangerous drug from the point of view of addiction. (See DRUG ADDICTION.)

HERPANGINA is a short febrile illness in childhood, in which minute vesicles or punched-out ulcers develop in the posterior parts of the mouth. It is due to infection with group A Coxsackie viruses (qv).

HERPES SIMPLEX is an acute infectious disease, characterized by the development of groups of superficial vesicles, or blebs, in the skin and mucous membrane. It is due to a virus, and infection can occur at any time from birth onwards, but the usual time for primary infection is between the second and fifteenth year. Once infected, the virus persists in the body for the rest of the patient's life.

Symptoms – The symptoms vary with the age of infection. In young infants it may cause a generalized infection which may prove fatal. In young children the infection is usually in the mouth, and this may be associated with enlargement of the glands in the neck, general irritability and fever. The condition usually settles in seven to ten days. In adults the vesicles may occur anywhere in the skin or mucous membranes. The more common sites are the lips, mouth and face, but the vesicles may also appear on the genitalia, or in the conjunctiva or cornea and the brain may be infected, causing encephalitis (qv) or meningitis. The first sign is the appearance of small painful swellings. These quickly develop into vesicles, containing clear fluid, and surrounded by a reddened area of skin. Some people are particularly liable to recurrent attacks of herpes simplex, and these often tend to be associated with some debilitating condition or infection, such as pneumonia.

Except in the case of herpes of the cornea, the eruption clears completely unless it becomes contaminated with some other organism. In the case of the cornea, there may be residual scarring, which may impair vision.

Treatment – The most effective local treatment, if the skin is involved, is idoxuridine. Grenz rays and soft X-rays are also used. Should the eye be involved, the patient must be referred immediately to an eye specialist. In those cases in which the eye or the brain is involved, the anti-viral agent, adenine arabinoside, is proving of value. The only preventive measure that is worth consideration is the administration of gamma-globulin (qv) in the case of infants under the age of 3 months who are in close contact with a case. This is particularly applicable if the infant suffers from eczema.

HERPES ZOSTER, or SHINGLES, is a skin eruption of acute nature, closely related to chickenpox, consisting in the appearance of small yellow vesicles, which spread over an area, dry up, and heal by scabbing. It receives its name from the Greek word, $\zeta\omega\sigma\tau\eta\rho$, a 'circingle', or girdle, because it spreads in a zone-like manner round half the chest. Herpes of the face also occurs, particularly on the brow and round the eye.

Causes – It is due to a virus identical with that of chickenpox. This invades the ganglia of the nerves, particularly the spinal nerves of the chest and the fifth cranial nerve which supplies the face. In spite of its being due to the same virus as chickenpox, it is rare for herpes zoster to occur as a result of contact with a case of chickenpox. On the other hand, it is not unusual for a patient with herpes zoster to infect a child with chickenpox. It is a disease of adults rather than children, and the older the person the more likely is he to develop the disease. Thus in adults under 50 the incidence is around 2·5 per 1000 people a year. Between 50 and 60 it is around 5 per 1000, whilst in octo-

genarians it is 10 per 1000. Most adults who acquire the disease have had chickenpox in childhood. Occasionally it may be associated with some serious underlying disease such as leukaemia, lymphadenoma, or multiple myeloma.

Symptoms – The first symptoms of herpes are much like those of any feverish attack. The person feels unwell for some days, has a slight rise of temperature, and vague pain in the side or in various other parts. The pain finally settles at a point in the side, and, two or three days after the first symptoms, the rash appears. Minute yellow blebs are seen on the skin of the back, of the side, or of the front of the chest, or simultaneously on all three, the points corresponding to the space between one pair of ribs right round. These blebs increase in number for some days, and spread till there is often a complete half girdle round one side of the chest. The pain in this stage is severe, but it appears to vary a good deal with age, being slight in children and very severe in old people, in whom indeed herpes sometimes forms a serious malady. After one or two weeks, most of the vesicles have dried up and formed scabs, which finally drop off, leaving the skin just as it was before, or covered with small scars. Occasionally the little vesicles run together into large blebs, which leave ulcers difficult to heal, and followed by marked scars. The skin is generally healed completely in two or three weeks, but a distressing peculiarity about the pain is that, in old people especially, it may not pass off when the eruption disappears, but may remain for weeks or even months: a condition known as post-herpetic neuralgia.

Treatment – In the very early stage, before the vesicles have formed, cocaine or atropine ointment rubbed into the side eases the pain and seems to prevent to some extent the outbreak of the eruption. Later, when the vesicles have formed and are discharging, a dusting-powder of starch, zinc oxide, and bismuth subnitrate gives much relief, or the side may be painted with glycerin jelly containing menthol or with a mixture of chloral, camphor, and menthol in equal parts. Alternatively, the lesions may be dabbed with calamine lotion. In any case, the part should be kept warm by a dressing of cotton-wool. Analgesics may be required for relief of the pain.

Should post-herpetic neuralgia persist, the administration of analgesics is essential. Occasionally the pain of post-herpetic neuralgia may be so persistent that radiotherapy may be required.

HERTZ is the SI (International System of Units) unit of frequency. It indicates the number of cycles per second (c/s). The abbreviation for hertz is Hz.

HESPERIDIN is a glycoside (qv) derived from the rind of citrus fruit, which is believed to control the permeability of capillaries.

HETEROGRAFT is a transplant from one animal to another of a different species. It is also known as a xenograft.

HEXACHLOROPHANE is a widely used antiseptic which is active against a range of micro-organisms, including Gram-positive and Gram-negative organisms, *Shigella dysenteriae*, and *Salmonella typhi*. One of its advantages is that it retains its activity in the presence of soap, and it is therefore often used in soaps and creams in a concentration of 1 to 2 per cent. It must be used with caution in babies as it can be absorbed through the skin and prove harmful.

HEXAMINE is a substance which when excreted by the kidneys, sets free formaldehyde, which has an antiseptic action. It is given in cases of cystitis when the urine decomposes within the bladder, and it exerts its beneficial action very speedily. It acts only in urine with an acid reaction, and, if the urine be alkaline, acid phosphate of soda is usually taken along with the hexamine. The dose of each of these is 10 to 30 grains (0·6 to 2 grams) several times daily.

HEXOBARBITONE is a short-acting barbiturate. The sodium salt injected into a vein makes the patient unconscious: this is known as intravenous anaesthesia.

HEXYLRESORCINOL is a drug used in the treatment of roundworms and threadworms.

HIATUS HERNIA is a displacement of a portion of the stomach through the opening in the diaphragm through which the oesophagus passes from the chest to the abdominal cavity.

HICCUP is a spasmodic indrawing of air to the lungs, ending with a click, due to sudden closure of the vocal cords. The cause is some irritation of the nerves which go to the diaphragm, producing sudden contractions of the latter. Most cases, especially those recurring habitually about the same hour of the day, are due to indigestion. The symptom also occurs in some serious general diseases, like the uraemia of Bright's disease and typhoid fever, being in such cases a grave sign. Hiccup lasting over some days or weeks is in some cases a symptom of mild encephalitis lethargica.

Treatment – If the condition be due to dyspepsia, it is often relieved by a copious draught of cold water or by some aromatic like a few drops of spirit of chloroform, a teaspoonful of Hoffmann's anodyne, or a tablespoonful of peppermint water or cinnamon water. When continuous and excessive it is usually controlled by the inhalation of carbon dioxide. The popular remedy of breathing in and out of a paper bag is probably successful because of the accumulation of carbon dioxide in the bag. If persistent, and resisting all these traditional measures, more potent drugs may need to be resorted to. In this respect, chlorpromazine (qv) has achieved a certain reputation for efficacy in bringing it under control.

HIERA PICRA, popularly known as 'hickory pickory', is a powder composed of aloes and canella, used as an aperient and emmenagogue.

HIGH FREQUENCY (see ELECTRICITY IN MEDICINE).

HILUM is a term applied to the depression on organs such as the lung, kidney, and spleen, at which the vessels and nerves enter it and round which the lymphatic glands cluster. The hilum of the lung is also known as its root.

HIP-JOINT is the joint formed by the head of the thigh-bone and the deep cup-shaped hollow on the side of the pelvis which receives it (acetabulum). The joint is of the ball-and-socket variety, is dislocated only by very great violence, and is correspondingly difficult to reduce to its natural state after dislocation. The joint is enclosed by a capsule of fibrous tissue, strengthened by several bands, of which the principal is the ilio-femoral or Y-shaped ligament placed in front of the joint. A round ligament also unites the head of the thigh-bone to the margin of the acetabulum.

For Hip-joint Disease see under JOINTS, DISEASES OF; and DISLOCATIONS.

HIPPUS is the term applied to a tremor of the iris which produces alternating contraction and dilatation of the pupil. This is often a sign of hysteria.

HIRSCHSPRUNG'S DISEASE, or MEGACOLON, is the term given to a condition in childhood which is characterized by great hypertrophy and dilatation of the colon.

HIRSUTIES, or HYPERTRICHOSIS, is a growth of hair of the male type and distribution in women. It is most marked in cases of certain tumours of the suprarenal glands.

HISTAMINE is an amine (qv) derived from histidine (qv). It is widely distributed in the tissues of plants and animals, including man. It is a powerful stimulant of gastric juice, a constrictor of smooth muscle including that of the bronchi, and a dilator of arterioles and capillaries. It is this last action which is responsible for the eruption of nettlerash (qv).

HISTIDINE is an amino-acid from which histamine is derived by decomposition.

HISTOLOGY is the study of the minute structure of the tissues.

HISTOPLASMOSIS is a disease due to a yeast-like fungus known as *Histoplasma capsulatum*. Most cases have been reported from USA. In infants it is characterized by fever, anaemia, enlargement of the liver and spleen, and involvement of the lungs and gastro-intestinal tract. In older children it may resemble pulmonary tuberculosis, whilst in adults it may be confined to involvement of the skin.

HIVES is a popular term applied to eruptions of the nature of nettle-rash.

HLA ANTIGENS are antigens (qv) which we inherit on the surfaces of cells throughout the body. They are known as Human Leucocyte Antigens (HLA) because they were first identified on leucocytes (qv). It is these HLA antigens which are responsible for the body rejecting a transplanted organ such as a kidney. This is because the body into which the organ is transplanted recognizes the organ as a 'foreign body' and immediately starts producing antibodies to destroy it. In some ways they are comparable to the ABO blood groups (qv). They are, however, far more complicated. Over fifty of them have already been recognized, and most people have four of them. (See also TRANSPLANTATION.)

HODGKIN'S DISEASE, so called after Thomas Hodgkin (1798–1866), the Guy's Hospital pathologist who first described it, or LYMPHADENOMA, is a condition in which the lymphatic glands all over the body undergo a gradually progressive enlargement. The cause is not known. The glands affected may reach a great size. The patient often runs a characteristic form of fever (Pel-Ebstein fever), in which bouts of fever alternate with several days with no fever. Along with these changes a considerable degree of anaemia arises, and the affected person becomes gradually weaker. Treatment consists of radiotherapy when the disease is relatively localized. When it is more widespread, however, chemotherapy is the treatment of choice. This is now given in the form of a combination of drugs, rather than one single drug. The most commonly used combination at the moment is: mustine, vinblastine, procarbazine and prednisone. The results of treatment are now such that over 80 per cent treated by radiotherapy, and 78 per cent of those treated by combined chemotherapy, are still alive after five years.

HOGBEN TEST is a pregnancy diagnosis test. (See PREGNANCY TESTS.)

HOMATROPINE is an alkaloid derived from atropine, which is used to produce dilatation of the pupil and to paralyse accommodation temporarily for the purpose of examining the interior of the eye. It is used in 1 per cent solution, and its effects pass away in the course of a few hours.

HOMOCYSTINURIA is a congenital disease due to the inability of the affected individual to metabolize, or utilize properly one of the essential amino-acids (qv) known as methionine. The main features of the condition are abnormality of the lens of the eye, mental retardation, fair complexion and fair hair and a high cheek colour.

HOMOEOPATHY is a system of medicine founded by Hahnemann at the end of the eighteenth century. It is based upon the theory that diseases are curable by those drugs which produce effects on the body similar to symptoms caused by the disease (*similia similibus curantur*). In administering drugs, the theory is also held that their effect is increased by giving them in minute doses obtained by diluting them to an extreme degree.

HOMOGRAFT is a piece of tissue or an organ, such as a kidney, transplanted from one animal to another of the same species: eg, from man to man. It is also known as an allograft.

HOOKWORM (see ANCYLOSTOMIASIS).

HOPS have been used in medicine as the powder obtained from the dried fruit of *Humulus lupulus*. The plant contains an alkaloid, lupuline, which is possessed of a weak sedative action. A poultice made from crushed hops is a household sedative in cases of localized pains, and hop pillows have been used for nervous insomnia.

HORDEOLUM is another name for a stye.

HOREHOUND is the name for the dried leaves and tops of *Marrubium vulgare*, which are used for coughs, either mixed with sugar as a syrup in doses of 2 to 4 ml or as fluid extract in doses of 4 to 8 ml.

HORMONES are substances which, on absorption into the blood, influence the action of tissues and organs other than those in which they are produced. The internal secretions of the ovary, pancreas, thyroid, pituitary and suprarenal bodies afford examples of this action.

HORNER'S SYNDROME is the description given to a combination of changes resulting from paralysis of the sympathetic nerve in the neck. They are: small pupil, sunken eye, and a drooping upper eyelid.

HORNETS (see BITES).

HORRIPILATION is another term for goose-flesh, due to contraction of the small muscles in the skin which make the hairs erect.

HORSESHOE KIDNEY (see KIDNEYS, DISEASES OF).

HOSPITAL is a building intended for receiving sick or injured persons. The introduction of the National Health Service Act in 1948 completely changed the organization of the hospitals in Great

Britain, but for the sake of historical interest the following description of the pre-1948 position has been retained. It is followed by a brief summary of the organization now in force.

In Great Britain hospitals were divided into four chief classes according to their manner of administration:

(1) VOLUNTARY HOSPITALS were supported by public subscription and administered by a board of managers chosen by the subscribers. The total number of voluntary hospitals in Great Britain was over 950, providing in all nearly 53,000 beds. The voluntary hospital was introduced into Europe from the East at the beginning of the thirteenth century, chiefly owing to the exertions and influence of Louis IX of France and Pope Innocent III. Although originally supported as a charity by the wealthier members of the community for the benefit of the poor, the voluntary hospital latterly derived the greater part of its annual revenue from the subscriptions of those who had been or were likely to be treated in it. These subscriptions in many instances were collected by small weekly payments, for example, by deduction of a few pence from weekly wages. Hospital maintenance therefore had become a kind of informal insurance against serious illness or accident.

In USA most of the large voluntary hospitals have private blocks or private wards attached, where patients pay the full cost of both maintenance and of medical or surgical treatment as required. For the same reason, the small private nursing homes, which at one time formed the main provision for private patients in Great Britain, and in which the general expenses are spread over a small number only of patients, were and are necessarily very expensive.

(2) COUNCIL HOSPITALS were supported by town and county councils, and administered by their local health authority, under the general supervision of the Ministry of Health (England) and Department of Health (Scotland). Prior to the Local Government Acts (1929), many of these were devoted to the treatment of infectious diseases and tuberculosis, but after 1929 municipal hospitals were provided in many localities for treating general medical and surgical ailments. These were supported from local rates, and the Council could recover the cost of treatment from patients. These hospitals usually had whole-time resident medical officers and salaried visiting consultants.

(3) STATE HOSPITALS were supported out

of Parliamentary grants and administered by Military, Naval, Pension, or Prison authorities; these hospitals were relatively few in number. They had a medical staff composed of officers of the service to which they belonged.

(4) PRIVATE HOSPITALS are owned and managed by private individuals or companies for profit; most of these are of small size, taking ten or twenty patients, and are then known as Nursing Homes.

As has already been mentioned, this was all changed by the National Health Service Act. Under this Act all hospitals in the country, with the exception of a few which insisted on remaining outside the National Health Service, passed under the control of the Minister of Health. With the exception of the teaching hospitals, these hospitals in the National Health Service passed to the control of Regional Boards appointed by the Minister of Health. These Regional Boards further subdivided the hospitals in their areas into units under the control of Hospital Management Committees. The endowments of the voluntary hospitals were transferred to a Hospital Endowments Fund, and the income from this is used for purposes outside the official budget. Hospitals are no longer allowed to appeal for funds. No charge is made for admission to, or treatment in, hospital, but hospitals are allowed to have special blocks of private wards for patients who wish to pay for the additional comforts of such private wards. Teaching hospitals were given a larger measure of independence. They were allowed to keep their own Boards of Governors and they retained control over their endowments.

Hospitals are also classified according to the type of case with which they deal, as follows: (a) GENERAL HOSPITALS admit both cases of disease requiring treatment by diet, drugs and other non-operative procedures (medical cases), and cases of disease and injury requiring operation (surgical cases). Most of the larger general hospitals also possess special departments (for eye diseases, diseases of ear, nose and throat, diseases peculiar to women, etc.). *Teaching Hospitals* form a special subdivision of the general hospitals, which are connected with a medical school, and are attended by medical students. (b) SPECIAL HOSPITALS are reserved for one special kind of case. Of these, the best known types are *Children's Hospitals, Eye Hospitals, Maternity Hospitals,* and *Mental Hospitals.* (c) CONVALESCENT HOSPITALS are usually situated in a rural or seaside district where light and fresh air are abundant. They receive patients, usually from general or special hospitals, who require little in the shape of treatment, but whose bodily powers are still enfeebled after serious illness or operation.

Under the National Health Service Reorganization Act 1973, a complete overhaul of the Service came into effect on April 1, 1974, bringing into a single administrative structure the hospital services previously administered by Regional Hospital Boards, Boards of Governors and Hospital Management Committees, the local authority health services and the family practitioner services. This took the form of the establishment of 14 Regional Health Authorities responsible to the Secretary of State for Health and Social Security, (formerly the Minister of Health) and 90 Area Health Authorities responsible to the Regional Health Authorities. Under the Area Health Authorities are Family Practitioner Committees which administer the family practitioner services. The boundaries of the Area Health Authorities are coterminous with the boundaries of local government authorities responsible for the social services. Under the Health Services Act 1976, private wards, or pay beds, are gradually being withdrawn from National Health Service hospitals.

HOUR-GLASS STOMACH is the term given to the X-ray appearance of a stomach which is constricted in its middle part because of either spasm of the stomach muscle or contraction of scar tissue from a gastric ulcer.

HOUSEMAID'S KNEE is an inflammation of the bursa in front of the knee-cap, often mistaken for some disease in the joint itself (see BURSITIS).

HOUSES and BUILDING SITES (see SANITATION).

HUMERUS is the bone of the upper arm (illustration 83). It has a rounded head, which helps to form the shoulder joint, and at its lower end presents a wide pulley-like surface for union with the radius and ulna. Its epicondyles form the prominences at the sides of the elbow.

HUMIDIFICATION of the air we breathe is essential for the efficient working of the lungs. (See RESPIRATION.) This is achieved largely by the nose (qv) which acts as an air-conditioner, warming, moistening, and filtering the 10,000 litres of air which we inhale daily, in the process of which, incidentally, it produces around 1·5 litres of secretion daily. Humidity is expressed as relative humidity (RH). This is the amount of moisture in the air expressed as a percentage of the maximum possible at that temperature. If the temperature of a room is raised without increasing the moisture content, the RH falls. The average outdoor RH in Britain is around 70 to 80 per cent. With central heating it may drop to 25 per cent or lower.

This is why humidification, as it is known, of the air is essential in buildings heated by modern heating systems. The aim should be to keep the RH around 30 to 50 per cent. In houses this may be achieved quite satisfactorily by having a jug or basin of water in the room, or some receptacle that can be attached to the heater. In offices and the like, some more elaborate form of humidifier is necessary. A point to be borne in mind is that those suffering from chronic bronchitis are particularly susceptible to dry air. (See also VENTILATION.)

HUMIDIFIER FEVER is a form of alveolitis (qv) caused by contamination of the water used to humidify, or moisten, the air in air-conditioning plants. The breathing of the contaminated air results in infection of the lung, which is characterized by fever, cough, shortness of breath and malaise, worse on Monday and tending to improve during the course of the week.

HUMOUR is a term applied to any fluid or semi-fluid tissue of the body: eg. the aqueous and vitreous humours in the eye. The term, humour, is also associated with a theory regarding the causation of disease, which originated with Pythagoras and lasted in a modified form until the early part of the nineteenth century. According to this theory diseases are due to an improper mixture in the body of blood, bile, phlegm and black bile.

HUNGER is the term applied to a craving for food or other substance necessary to bodily activity. Hunger for food is supposed to be directly produced by strong contractions of the stomach which occur when it is empty or nearly so. (See also THIRST.) AIR HUNGER is an instinctive craving for oxygen resulting in breathlessness, either when a person ascends to great heights where the pressure of air is low, or in some diseases such as pneumonia and diabetes mellitus.

HUNTINGTON'S CHOREA is a hereditary disease characterized by involuntary movements and dementia. Each child of a parent with the disease has a 50:50 chance of developing it. The usual time of onset is between 35 and 45, but 10 per cent of cases occur under the age of 20. Some patients show more severe mental disturbance, others more severe disturbances of movement, but in all it pursues an inexorable downward course over a period of ten to twenty years to a terminal state of physical and mental helplessness. It is estimated that there are around 6000 cases in Britain. The cause is not known and there is no effective treatment. People with Huntington's chorea and their relatives can obtain help and guidance from The Association to Combat Huntington's Chorea, Lyndhurst, Lower Hampton Road, Sunbury-on-Thames, Middlesex, TW16 5PR.

HUTCHINSON'S TEETH is the term applied to the narrowed and notched permanent incisor teeth which occur in congenital syphilis. They are so named after Sir Jonathan Hutchinson (1828–1913), the famous London physician who first described them.

HYALINE MEMBRANE DISEASE is a condition found in premature infants and infants born by Caesarean section, characterized by the onset of difficulty in breathing a few hours after birth. It is also known as the respiratory distress syndrome. About half the affected babies die, death usually occurring before the third day. At post-mortem examination the alveoli and the finer bronchioles of the lungs are found to be lined with a dense membrane. The cause of the condition is obscure.

HYALURONIDASE is an enzyme (qv) which hydrolyzes hyaluronic acid. The latter is a gel-like substance which is widely distributed throughout the body and which helps to bind together the tissue cells and also acts as a lubricant in joints. By virtue of its action in hydrolyzing hyaluronic acid, hyaluronidase is now used in subcutaneous injections of fluid as it facilitates the spread of the injected fluid and therefore its absorption.

HYDATID is a cyst produced by the growth of immature forms of a tapeworm. (See TAENIASIS.)

HYDATIDIFORM MOLE, or VESICULAR MOLE as it is sometimes known, is a rare complication of pregnancy, in which there is tremendous proliferation of the epithelium of the chorion (the outer of the two foetal membranes). It seldom occurs during a first pregnancy. Treatment consists of immediate evacuation of the womb.

HYDNOCARPUS OIL, or CHAULMOOGRA OIL, is an oil pressed from the seeds of *Hydnocarpus wightiana*, once used in the treatment of leprosy. It has now been replaced by other drugs. (See LEPROSY.)

HYDRADENITIS SUPPURATIVA is a chronic inflammatory disease of the apocrine sweat glands (see PERSPIRATION). It is more common in women, in whom it usually occurs in the armpit, than in men in whom it is most common in the perineum of the drivers of lorries and taxis. It occurs in the form of painful, tender lumps underneath the skin, which burst often in a week or so. Treatment consists of removal by operation.

HYDRAEMIA is a condition in which the blood contains an excess of water. It is found in certain forms of Bright's disease, leading to dropsy.

HYDRAGOGUE is a drug that produces a watery stool. (See PURGATIVES.)

HYDRALLAZINE is a hypotensive drug. (See ESSENTIAL HYPERTENSION.)

HYDRAMNIOS is the condition characterized by excess of fluid in the amniotic cavity. (See AMNION.)

HYDRARGYRUM is another name for mercury.

HYDROCELE is a collection of fluid connected with the testicle or spermatic cord. It is sometimes due to inflammation of the sac in which these structures are enclosed, but in many cases the cause cannot be discovered. It develops usually in middle life, although it may appear at any time, increases gradually in size, and is usually devoid of pain. The condition presents some resemblance to hernia, and there is occasionally some doubt in distinguishing between them, particularly when the hydrocele communicates with the abdominal cavity. In infants and young children the hydrocele disappears spontaneously. When treatment is required it takes one of three forms. It may take the form of aspirating, or withdrawing, the fluid with a needle and syringe. The fluid is

liable to recur and further aspirations have to be carried out. In these cases it is more satisfactory to remove the fluid and replace it with sclerosing agent that seals off the cavity. Some surgeons prefer to operate and remove the sac.

HYDROCEPHALUS is the term applied to the condition in which there is abnormal accumulation of cerebrospinal fluid within the skull. It is due to one or more of three main causes: (i) excessive production of spinal fluid (qv); (ii) defective absorption of cerebrospinal fluid; (iii) blockage to the circulation of cerebrospinal fluid. The causes of these disturbances of circulation of cerebrospinal fluid may be congenital (most commonly associated with spina bifida (qv)), meningitis, or a tumour.

Symptoms – In children the chief symptoms observed are the gradual increase in size of the upper part of the head, out of all proportion to the face or the rest of the body. The head is globular in shape, with a wide anterior fontanelle and separation of the bones at the sutures. The veins in the scalp are prominent, and there is a 'crackpot' note on percussion. The normal infant's head should not grow more than 1 inch (2·5 cm) in each of the first two months of life and much more slowly subsequently. Growth beyond this rate should arouse suspicions of hydrocephalus. Another useful rule is that the circumference of the head should not exceed that of the chest. In chronic hydrocephalus, the head of an infant 3 months old has been known to measure 29 inches (72·5 cm); and in the well-known case of the man, Cardinal, who died in Guy's Hospital, the head measured 33 inches (82·5 cm). In the museum of the faculty of medicine in Paris there is a hydrocephalic skull measuring 39 inches (97·5 cm).

The cerebral ventricles are widely distended, and the convolutions of the brain flattened, while occasionally the fluid escapes into the cavity of the cranium, which it fills, pressing down the brain to the base of the skull. As a consequence of such changes, the functions of the brain are interfered with, and in general the mental condition of the patient is impaired. The child is dull and listless, irritable and sometimes suffers from severe mental subnormality. The special senses become affected as the disease advances, especially vision, and sight is often lost, as is also hearing. Towards the end paralysis is apt to occur.

The outlook for children with hydrocephalus is not as gloomy as was at one time thought to be the case. Such a child has a 50 per cent chance of survival with the disease arrested. He then has a 75 per cent chance of being educable. Almost one-third of arrested cases can be expected to enjoy normal intelligence with little or no physical disability.

Treatment – Numerous ingenious operations have been devised for the treatment of hydrocephalus. The most satisfactory of these utilize the Holter or Pudenz unidirectional valves, whereby the cerebrospinal fluid is by-passed into the right atrium of the heart or the peritoneal cavity.

HYDROCHLORIC ACID is a colourless, pungent, fuming liquid. It is present in the gastric juice to the extent of 2 parts in 1000. (See DIGESTION.) In large quantities it is a corrosive poison.

Uses – Its chief use is in cases in which the gastric juice is deficient: ie. in cases of achlorhydria (qv). The Dilute Hydrochloric Acid of the *British Pharmacopoeia* is given in doses of 0·5 to 4 millilitres, or in some such mixture as Acid Gentian Mixture BPC, Acid Gentian Mixture with Nux Vomica BPC, or Acid Nux Vomica Mixture BPC in doses of 10 to 20 millilitres.

HYDROCORTISONE, or compound F, has the chemical formula, 17-hydroxy-corticosterone. It is closely allied to cortisone (qv) both in its structure (cortisone is an oxidation product of hydrocortisone) and in its action. Its anti-rheumatic potency is said to be 50 per cent greater than that of cortisone. Its main use to date in rheumatoid arthritis has been for local injection into affected joints. It is also used as a local application to the skin in the form of a cream or lotion in the treatment of certain skin diseases.

HYDROCYANIC ACID (see PRUSSIC ACID).

HYDROFLUMETHIAZIDE is a derivative of chlorothiazide (qv). It is a powerful diuretic which acts by causing an increased urinary excretion of sodium and chloride. On a weight for weight basis it is about ten times as potent a diuretic as chlorothiazide.

HYDROGEN PEROXIDE is a syrupy, colourless, odourless liquid which differs in chemical composition from water, by containing two atoms of oxygen (H_2O_2) to every one in water (H_2O). It has the property of readily giving up its extra oxygen

and being reduced to water, and this renders it of great value in medicine for antiseptic, deodorant, and other purposes. It is most commonly employed as a solution in water of such a strength that any quantity will give off twenty times its bulk of oxygen gas; this is known as 20-volume strength, or as Hydrogen Peroxide Solution BP. It is also prepared as Strong Hydrogen Peroxide Solution BP, also known as 100-volume strength as it gives off one hundred times its volume of oxygen. This strong solution must never be used undiluted. When added to ether the mixture is known as ozonic ether. Volatile oils which have become oxidized contain a considerable quantity of peroxide of hydrogen, and to this substance the power they possess of destroying foul odours is largely due.

Uses – The solution of hydrogen peroxide is applied externally to ulcers, and by sprays or swabs to cavities like the nose and throat, in order to act as an antiseptic, and also for the valuable property possessed by the little bubbles of oxygen that it gives off in breaking up and causing the separation of discharges. It is used to remove surgical dressings that are very adherent. Internally, it is sometimes used to wash out the stomach in cases of chronic gastritis, in a strength of $\frac{1}{2}$ ounce to the pint (14 ml to 570 ml). It is also used to bleach hair and to remove superficial stains from teeth; for this purpose it is mixed with an equal volume of water.

HYDROGEN SULPHIDE, or SULPHURETTED HYDROGEN, is a potential hazard in petroleum refining, the gas industry, tanning and the chemical industry. It is found in sewers and coalmines (stink damp), and can be given off during the vulcanization of rubber containing sulphur. It is also a fishing hazard as it is given off in trawlers' holds containing what is known as 'trash' fish, the fish used for making fishmeal. Its well-known 'rotten egg' smell is detectable at as low a concentration as 0·025 part per million (p.p.m.), and by the time the concentration attains 30 p.p.m. it is intolerably unpleasant. Unfortunately, in prolonged exposure to it the smell rapidly disappears, which explains why it can be such a dangerous poison as the exposed individual has no idea that he is breathing it. Exposure to 150 to 300 p.p.m. leads to headache, spasm of the eyelids, with pain and redness of the eyes, blurred vision and coloured haloes round lights (gas eye). It may be several hours before these effects appear and they usually take several days to go. Serious effects appear above concentrations of 500 p.p.m.: mental confusion, convulsions, and oedema of the lungs with cyanosis (qv).

There is no specific antidote, and treatment consists of the usual first-aid measures for asphyxia (qv), the patient having first been removed well away from the contaminated area. If artificial respiration (qv) is started as soon as breathing stops, recovery is usually complete.

HYDROLYZED PROTEIN is protein (qv) which has been broken down into its constituent amino-acids. (Hydrolysis means the reaction of a large molecule with one or more molecules of water, with the production of two or more smaller molecules.) This is the process which normally occurs in the course of digestion of protein, but in certain conditions, such as marasmus and severe liver disease, where the process of digestion is badly upset, it is sometimes of value to give the patient protein that has already been hydrolyzed.

HYDRONEPHROSIS is a chronic disease in which the kidney becomes greatly distended with fluid. It is due to incomplete or intermittent blockage of the ureter connecting the kidney with the bladder. The chief causes of this are stricture of the ureter as a result of infection or a new growth, and spasm of the ureter where it enters the kidney.

HYDROPHOBIA is another name for RABIES (qv).

HYDROPS is another name for dropsy.

HYDROPS FOETALIS (see HAEMOLYTIC DISEASE OF THE NEWBORN).

HYDROTHERAPY, OR HYDROPATHY, is the name for all those curative measures in which water is the agent employed. (See BATHS; COLD DOUCHES; FOMENTATIONS; WET PACK.)

HYDROTHORAX means a collection of dropsical fluid in the pleural cavities.

HYDROXOCOBALAMIN, or vitamin B_{12a}, has now replaced cyanocobalamin (qv) in the treatment of pernicious anaemia. (See ANAEMIA.) It has the practical advantage that fewer injections are required than in the case of cyanocobalamin. Like cyanocobalamin it belongs to the group of substances known as cobalamins

which have an enzyme (qv) action in practically every metabolic system in the body and are essential for normal growth and nutrition.

HYDROXYUREA is a drug that is proving of value in the treatment of chronic myeloid leukaemia.

HYDROXYZINE PAMOATE is a tranquillizer that is proving of value in the treatment of anxiety states.

HYGIENE means the science of preserving health. (See BATHS; CLOTHING; DIET; EXERCISE; HEALTH; SANITATION; VENTILATION; WATER SUPPLY; WATER-CLOSETS.)

HYMEN is the thin membranous fold partially closing the lower end of the virginal vagina.

HYOID is the name of a U-shaped bone at the root of the tongue. It can be felt from the front of the neck, lying about an inch above the prominence of the thyroid cartilage.

HYOSCYAMUS, or HENBANE, is a plant that grows commonly in the United States and in Europe. The preparations are made from the leaves, and have an effect in quieting pain and relieving spasm. In large quantities it is a narcotic poison.

Uses – In spasmodic and painful conditions, particularly in colic and in irritable states of the bladder, the tincture of hyoscyamus is used with good effect. Hyoscine, an alkaloid obtained from hyoscyamus, is used in very small doses to quiet raving mania and in some nervous diseases, eg. Parkinsonism. It is also used for the production of 'twilight sleep', and for the prevention of travel sickness.

HYPERACUSIS means an abnormally acute sense of hearing.

HYPERAEMIA means congestion or presence of an excessive amount of blood in a part.

HYPERAESTHESIA means oversensitiveness of a part, as found, for example, in certain nervous diseases. (See TOUCH.)

HYPERALGESIA means excessive sensitiveness to pain. (See PAIN; TOUCH.)

HYPERCALCIURIA means an abnormally large amount of calcium in the urine. It is the most common single cause of stones in the kidneys in Britain.

HYPERCAPNIA means an abnormal increase in the amount of carbon dioxide in the blood or in the lungs.

HYPERCHLORHYDRIA is the condition in which there is an excessive production of hydrochloric acid in the stomach. It is a characteristic finding in certain forms of dyspepsia, particularly that associated with a duodenal ulcer. It causes heartburn (qv) and waterbrash (qv). (See DUODENAL ULCER; DYSPEPSIA; and STOMACH, DISEASES OF.)

HYPEREMESIS is a term applied to excessive vomiting, especially that which occurs in pregnancy.

HYPERGLYCAEMIA means excess of sugar in the blood, the condition accompanying diabetes mellitus. The amount of sugar normally present in the blood is dependent upon how much sugar has been consumed, but in the fasting state it runs around 80 to 120 milligrams per 100 millilitres of blood. A fasting blood level of sugar above this is regarded as hyperglycaemia; in diabetes mellitus (qv) the sugar may rise to four or five times that amount. Hyperglycaemia may occur in conditions other than diabetes mellitus, though this is by far the commonest cause.

HYPERIDROSIS, or HYPERHIDROSIS, means excessive sweating. (See PERSPIRATION.)

HYPERMETROPIA or HYPEROPIA, is a term applied to long-sightedness, in which the eye is too flat from before back and rays of light are brought to a focus behind the retina. (See VISION; and SPECTACLES.)

HYPERNEPHROMA is a term applied to a tumour resembling the tissue of the suprarenal gland and occurring usually in the kidney.

HYPERPIESIS is another term for high blood-pressure. HYPERPIESIA is another term for ESSENTIAL HYPERTENSION (qv).

HYPERPLASIA means an abnormal increase in the number of cells in a tissue.

HYPERPYREXIA means an excessive degree of fever. (See FEVER; TEMPERATURE.)

HYPERTELORISM is a rare congenital deformity of the head and face. The forehead is broad and low and the orbits are large and set widely apart. The divergence of the eyes is such that focusing on near objects is impossible. The abnormal shape of the skull is thought to be due primarily to a disproportion in the growth of the brain.

HYPERTENSION is another term for high blood-pressure. (See ESSENTIAL HYPERTENSION; MALIGNANT HYPERTENSION.)

HYPERTHERMIA means abnormally high body temperature. It is also the name given to the treatment of disease by the artificial production of fever. This may be done by the intravenous injection of certain vaccines, the artificial production of malaria, or by placing the individual in a machine known as a hypertherm, in which the patient's temperature can be safely raised to 105° to 106° F (40° to 41° C).

HYPERTHYROIDISM is a term applied to excessive activity of the thyroid gland: eg. in exophthalmic goitre. (See GOITRE.)

HYPERTROPHY means the increase in size which takes place in an organ as the result of an increased amount of work demanded of it by the bodily economy. For example, when valvular disease of the heart is present and the heart is in process of dilating, compensation occurs by an increase in thickness of the heart-muscle, and the organ, by beating more powerfully, is able to overtake the strain thrown upon it. Similarly, if one kidney be removed, the other hypertrophies or grows larger to overtake the double work.

HYPNO-ANALYSIS is a method of treating certain neuroses by first releasing the patient's repressed fear under hypnosis, and then helping the patient to the necessary adjustment by suggestion.

HYPNOTICS are measures, including drugs, which produce sleep.
Varieties – As certain conditions are necessary for the onset of sleep, even a slight departure from these may be sufficient to keep persons who are not in good health awake. Thus a diminution of the circulation in the brain, and freedom from pain or irritation in any bodily organ are essential, whilst quiet and darkness are desirable, though many people can adapt

themselves to noise and there are not a few who can sleep equally well whether it be light or dark. Often some trivial alteration of the daily life or diet is enough to relieve habitual insomnia; in other cases the quieting of pain is alone necessary; in other cases drugs must be used which have a light dulling effect upon the brain itself. For the relief of pain the drugs known as anodynes (see ANODYNES) are used. Of the hypnotics, which dull the brain without much other effect, there is a large variety.

Uses – Simple remedies should always receive a fair trial first of all. Thus a person may be kept awake by severe mental labour or worry just before retiring to rest. The activity of the brain continues and sleeplessness results. Some quiet employment for the latter part of the evening, or a light meal, may relieve this. In other cases sleeplessness is often due to difficulty of digestion through a meal having been taken shortly before retiring to rest, and this may be relieved by abstaining from the last meal at night. In old people insomnia may be due to cold feet, and in such cases the best hypnotic is a pair of warm sleeping socks. A condition of anaemia of the brain occurs in old men whose arteries are unhealthy, and this also debars sleep, unless the head be kept warm or a small quantity of alcohol be taken at bedtime: ie. a night cap literally or metaphorically. Occasionally sleep can be obtained by purely external applications. Massage of the head, the wet pack, and electrical (especially high frequency) applications are all used in different cases. Should these measures fail, and a hypnotic be required, the choice of which to use can only be made satisfactorily by the family doctor. Because of the tendency for drug addiction to develop with the continued use of the barbiturates, the tendency today is to try one of the non-barbiturate drugs in the first instance.

HYPNOTISM is the process of producing a state of mind known as hypnosis. Although a process which has been known for hundreds of years, its precise nature is still unknown. One modern writer has defined hypnosis as 'a temporary condition of altered attention, the most striking feature of which is greatly increased suggestibility' (Mason). There is no evidence, as has been claimed, that women can be more easily hypnotized than men. Children and young adults are the more easily hypnotized, middle-aged people being more resistant. There are various methods of induction of hypnosis, but the basis of

them is some rhythmic stimulus accompanied by the repetition of carefully worded suggestions. The most commonly used method is to ask the patient to fix his eye on a given spot, or light, and then keep on repeating to him, in a quiet soothing voice, that his eyes will gradually become tired and that he will want to close them. There are various levels of hypnosis, usually classified as light, medium, and deep, and it has been estimated that 10 per cent of people cannot be hypnotized, 35 per cent can be taken into light hypnosis, 35 per cent into medium hypnosis, and 20 per cent into deep hypnosis.

Although in the past, hypnotism has often been frowned upon by orthodox medicine, largely because of its prostitution by charlatans, at the present day it is recognized to be a most useful method of therapy. Like all effective forms of therapy, however, it is not without its dangers, and this is why it should only be practised by those who have been adequately trained. Thus, under deep hypnosis suggestion can induce the person concerned to perform some prescribed automatic action when he awakes from the hypnotic state. Although there is good evidence that no-one can be hypnotized to perform acts which are fundamentally contrary to his moral or ethical principles and which he does not want to do, this is only reassuring if one has sound evidence that the hypnotized subject has conventional moral or ethical principles.

Apart from its use in psychiatry, it is of value in the treatment of many psychosomatic conditions: that is, conditions in which physical manifestations, such as skin lesions, headaches and other forms of pain, are primarily due to some psychological or emotional disturbance. It is also being used to an increasing extent in obstetrics for the relief of pain during labour, and for the relief of pain in dentistry. Asthma is another condition that sometimes responds well to it. Another condition in which it is proving most valuable is as part of the treatment of alcoholism.

HYPOCALCAEMIA is the condition of the blood in which its content of calcium is below normal. (Normally there are between 9 mg and 11 mg of calcium in 100 ml of serum.)

HYPOCHLORHYDRIA means an insufficient secretion of hydrochloric acid from the digestive cells of the stomach lining.

HYPOCHLOROUS ACID is a powerful antiseptic which both kills organisms and neutralizes the poisons they produce. It forms the active principle of the powder known as eupad and of its solution eusol. The powder is produced by mixing equal weights of boric acid and bleaching powder. The solution is prepared by adding 25 grams of this powder to 1 litre of water, and filtering. The clear solution so produced is eusol, and should contain 0·5 per cent of hypochlorous acid.

Uses – Popularized during the 1914–1918 War, eusol has now been displaced to a great extent by the newer antiseptics, such as the acridine derivatives, the sulphonamides and penicillin, but it is still of value in the treatment of septic wounds.

HYPOCHONDRIASIS is a chronic mental condition in which the affected person's mind is constantly occupied with a delusion that he is seriously ill. As a rule, the ailments are referred to the stomach or the liver, and very often some trivial derangement of these exists to give colour to the person's views. Along with these complaints, there is a self-centred and gloomy turn of mind that prevents the patient from doing much of his proper work. Not uncommonly this mental trouble is hereditary, and passes gradually at a later stage into melancholia. The condition, apart from the affected person making a strong effort of will and taking up some active work which may distract his thoughts, is very difficult to treat.

HYPODERMIC means: of, or pertaining to, the region immediately under the skin. Thus, a hypodermic injection means an injection given underneath the skin. A hypodermic syringe is a small syringe which, fitted with a fine needle, is used to

251 – Hypodermic syringe, with needle-holder and needle.

give such injections (illustration 251). A hypodermic injection is given for one of three main reasons: (1) because the substance administered cannot be given by mouth on account of its being destroyed in the stomach before it can be absorbed, eg. insulin; (2) because it is not possible or it is inadvisable to give anything by mouth to the patient, eg. because of vomiting; (3) because a quick action is necessary, eg. morphine in cases of severe haemorrhage.

HYPODERMOCLYSIS is injection of a fluid under the skin: for example, of a solution of glucose or of saline as a method of restoring fluids to the circulation of a person who is dehydrated.

HYPOGASTRIC means pertaining to the lower middle part of the abdomen just above the pubis.

HYPOGLOSSAL NERVE is ˉ the twelfth cranial nerve, and supplies the muscles of the tongue, together with some others lying near it.

HYPOGLYCAEMIA is the term applied to a deficiency of sugar in the blood. It may occur in states of starvation, or after the administration of insulin in too large doses, causing symptoms of weakness, tremors, nervousness, breathlessness and excitement, followed sometimes by unconsciousness. These symptoms are relieved by taking sugar or by an injection of adrenaline, which checks the action of insulin.

HYPOGONADISM is the condition characterized by deficient production of the hormones secreted by the gonads: that is, the ovaries and testes.

HYPOMANIA is a slight degree of mania.

HYPOPHOSPHITES of lime, iron etc., are administered in combination as 'a tonic'.

HYPOPHYSECTOMY means surgical excision of the pituitary gland.

HYPOPHYSIS is another name for the pituitary gland.

HYPOPIESIS means abnormally low blood-pressure.

HYPOPLASIA means excessive smallness of an organ or part, arising from imperfect development.

HYPOPYON is the term for describing an accumulation of pus between the iris and the cornea: ie. in the anterior chamber of the eye.

455

HYPOSPADIAS

HYPOSPADIAS is a developmental abnormality in the male, in which the urethra opens on the under-surface of the penis or in the perineum (qv).

HYPOSTASIS is the term applied to the condition in which blood accumulates in a dependent part as a result of a feeble circulation. Congestion of the base of the lungs in old people from this cause, and infection, is called hypostatic pneumonia.

HYPOTHALAMUS is that part of the forebrain situated beneath the thalamus on each side and forming the floor of the third ventricle. The hypothalamus contains collections of nerve cells believed to form the controlling centres of (1) the sympathetic and (2) the parasympathetic nervous systems. The hypothalamus is the nervous centre for primitive physical and emotional behaviour. It contains nerve centres for the regulation of certain vital processes: the metabolism of fat, carbohydrate and water; sleep; body temperature and genital functions.

HYPOTHERMIA means low temperature. This is a term that is used in three different contexts.

It is being widely used in conjunction with operations on the heart and on the brain. The rationale of its use is that it lowers the requirements of the tissues for oxygen. This means that the cells of the brain, which are particularly susceptible to lack of oxygen, can be safely deprived of their blood supply for a longer period than at normal temperature. In practice this means that in operations on the heart, for instance, the action of the heart can be arrested for a few minutes while the surgeon actually operates on the heart.

Two methods are used to produce hypothermia. In one the blood of the patient is circulated through a special cooling machine. In the other the body temperature is lowered by the use of ice packs, iced water or a special cooling mattress. (See also CRYMOTHERAPY.)

The term is also used to describe the condition which may develop, especially in old people and in infants, if they are exposed to abnormally low temperatures. The effects of exposure to low temperatures are as follows:

Constriction of the blood-vessels of the skin leading in extreme cases to frostbite (qv).
Increased muscle tone

Shivering
Curling up of the body to reduce exposure to the cold
Concentration of blood
Inclination to increased body activity
Increased output of urine
Increased appetite
Falling body temperature
Drowsiness
Cessation of breathing and beating of heart.

Each winter in the British Isles old people die at home as the result of cold. Accidental hypothermia occurs in apparently fit old people and has been described as 'a common domestic disorder of the elderly'. It is defined as a deep body temperature (that is, a temperature recorded in the rectum or by a thermistor (qv) in the ear) below 95° F (35° C), and it has been estimated that around half a million old people in Britain are at risk of hypothermia. One of the main causes is that old people cannot maintain their body temperature because they lose heat through the skin. Normally on exposure to cold the blood-vessels of the skin are reflexly constricted through the autonomic nervous system (qv). This is a powerful mechanism for conserving heat as it reduces the heat conductivity of the skin to that of cork, once used to plug vacuum flasks for this reason.

As many old folk cannot conserve the heat they make because they lose it through the skin, the obvious treatment is that they should wear adequate insulating clothing indoors as well as outdoors. As half the heat loss from a clothed adult is from the head, there is much to be said for the elderly reviving the old fashion of wearing nightcaps, smoking caps and mutches. They should wear long underwear, or combinations, and gloves or mittens by day, and bed socks and extra warm blankets at night. In this last respect the metallized 'space blankets' on sale for mountaineers are light and efficient. Basic to all these measures, however, is an adequately heated house. For those who cannot afford to keep their homes adequately heated, additional supplementary benefits are available for extra heating. Details of these benefits can be obtained from local offices of the Department of Health and Social Security.

There is a third important context in which hypothermia may occur: on immersion in water, usually the sea. This is the form known as immersion hypothermia. (See DROWNING, RECOVERY FROM.)

HYPOTHYROIDISM means the condition produced by defective action of the thyroid gland. (See MYXOEDEMA.)

HYSTERECTOMY means the operation of removing the uterus. HYSTERO-OOPHORECTOMY is the term applied to removal of the uterus and ovaries.

HYSTERIA is a condition or set of conditions which it is difficult to define. The condition is also known as PITHIATISM because many of its symptoms appear to be due to auto-suggestion and are readily relieved by suggestion from another person. Hysteria manifests itself by overaction of some parts of the nervous system, or by failure of other parts to perform their necessary work. In consequence, there follow mental changes, convulsive seizures, spasms and contractions of limbs, paralyses, loss of sensation over areas of the body, affections of various internal organs, derangements of joints and combinations of these which closely mimic various organic diseases. Hysterical manifestations are among the most difficult affections upon which the specialist is called to give an opinion.

Causes – The condition is far more common in women than in men. It used to be supposed that the origin of the disease, as its name indicates, lay in trouble of the womb, but, though sexual disturbances often occur in the condition, they should more probably be classed as symptoms. Heredity is of importance, the disease being most common in the Latin races, and running to a great extent in families. Faulty upbringing in childhood predisposes to hysteria, which in young women of unequally developed mind and pampered habits, may be produced by sudden fright, family worry, grief, or a love affair.

Symptoms – MENTAL CHANGES are almost always observable in hysterical cases, although the other symptoms in different cases may differ widely from one another. The affected person becomes whimsical, dominated by ideas, and incapable of the same work and concentration as before. She becomes easily excitable, and is either morbidly sensitive, feeling slight rebuffs keenly, or unusually demonstrative, bursting into fits of laughter or paroxysms of weeping upon slight provocation. In marked cases, hysterical subjects become morally unhinged, deceiving every one around them, so that little credence can be given to their statements.

CONVULSIVE HYSTERIA is the most marked form. An attack may begin upon some excitement, with laughter or weeping, or may give no warning sign. The person falls in an unconscious or half-conscious condition, but whereas the fall in epilepsy is downright, the hysterical person subsides gently in general upon a couch or chair, and rarely or never so as to hurt herself, and seldom without an audience. She may then lie still, or more generally moans or talks incoherently, rolls the head from side to side, and tosses the hands and feet about. In serious attacks, known as hystero-epilepsy, the onset resembles epilepsy and may be followed by curious posturing, the sufferer placing herself in attitudes which suggest powerful emotions of fear, ecstasy or joy. In this state visions are seen, voices heard, and conversations held with imaginary persons. This forms one of the most perverted types of hysteria and one of the least hopeful as regards a cure.

LOSS OF SENSATION over some part of the body is one of the commonest symptoms. This loss may affect a limb, or may be irregularly distributed in patches, or may affect some special sense organ, causing, for example, failure of taste, blindness for all objects to one side of the field of vision, or for objects of some special type repugnant to the patient, or deafness in one ear. Sometimes there is complete loss of the sense of pain, so that pricks, pinches, and other painful stimuli are borne without wincing.

SPASMS AND CONTRACTIONS of muscles also form a common manifestation of hysteria without any other sign save mental hebetude. If this contraction exist in the muscles of the body wall, it may, and often does, give rise to the idea that the person is the subject of a tumour. Such spasms may also lead to the drawing up of an arm or foot, so that the limb in time becomes permanently deformed. Or when the mind becomes powerfully impressed by some person or idea, the spasm may pass off, and gradual or sudden recovery takes place.

PARALYSIS is perhaps the most troublesome symptom of all to overcome. It may extend over one-half of the body, and is then very hard to differentiate from the effects of apoplexy. Most commonly the foot is affected and the person declares herself unable to walk. As the paralysis sometimes lasts for years unimproved, and then suddenly vanishes, these cases are eminently suited for successful ministration by the faith-healer or by wonder-working shrines. Such persons, when the

457

paralysis affects both legs, and is accompanied by pain in the back, have again and again been confined for years to bed or couch as cases of spinal disease, only to recover suddenly when some new interest has come into their lives, or force of circumstances has rendered an active life imperative. The muscles of the larynx are often affected, and the person may be deprived of speech for years, till some powerful influence forces her to exert her will and the organ of voice again comes into play.

CHANGES IN INTERNAL ORGANS take place in some cases and produce such signs as constant hiccup, barking noises, excessive vomiting. diarrhoea, absolute loss of appetite, and profound changes in the circulation. Among the features of the last-named may be mentioned the appearance of swollen and congested areas in the skin, and, showing the power which the mind may exert over bodily functions, there is recorded the case of Louise Lateau, who, after meditating for many days upon the Crucifixion, developed on hands and feet 'stigmata' or bleedings beneath the skin.

JOINT AFFECTIONS are among the most remarkable physical changes. A joint, especially the hip or knee, becomes swollen, stiff, and painful, and may remain so for months. (See PAIN.)

Treatment – Special care should be taken in the upbringing of children who come of hysterical stock. They should not, on the one hand, be allowed to work too hard at lessons to the neglect of healthy exercise, nor, on the other hand, should they be pampered and allowed to gratify every passing whim. No hysterical young woman should remain unoccupied, but should be provided with, and forced to do, some congenial work. Needless to say, all the bodily functions should be maintained in the best possible order. In acute hysterical attacks rest and quiet are chiefly necessary. For symptoms such as vomiting, joint affections, loss of sensation, and spasms, removal from home and from the attention of sympathetic friends to strict isolation, where the patient sees nobody but a nurse and eats only the simplest of food, is a good form of treatment. For the severest forms of hysteria isolation and absolute rest in bed are employed. Further, massage takes the place of exercise, and the patient is encouraged to eat large amounts of readily digestible food. In all cases of hysteria psychotherapy forms an important element in treatment. This is carried out especially by suggestion, but in other cases it may take the form of persuasion, psycho-analysis, or education and employment.

IATRIC is a term meaning anything pertaining to a physician.

IATROGENIC DISEASE is disease induced by a physician: eg. a neurosis resulting from a physician's diagnosis of a physical disease.

IBUPROFEN is a drug which is proving of value as an anti-inflammatory agent and as an analgesic in the treatment of rheumatoid arthritis and other forms of rheumatism.

ICE is used as a convenient form of applying cold, both externally and internally. For external application the most convenient form of application is by placing chopped ice in an india-rubber bag, known as an ice-bag. The bag is closed by a screw cap and is laid upon the head, abdomen, or other part to which it is desired to make the cold application, a layer of flannel or a garment being placed between the bag and the skin to prevent a direct freezing action on the surface. When an ice-bag is not available, ice may similarly be applied to a small area by taking a large piece of gutta-percha tissue, laying the ice upon its centre, and bunching up the corners, which are tied together with a string. Iced water is sometimes applied by means of a coiled tube, especially in cases of inflammation of the head. The iced water is allowed slowly to percolate from a jug placed a few feet above the bed through the coiled tube laid on the affected part.

For internal application ice is seldom used now. (See also COLD, USES OF; and CRYMOTHERAPY.)

ICELANDIC DISEASE is another name for epidemic neuromyasthenia. (See NEUROMYASTHENIA.)

ICHOR is the term given to the thin fluid, yellowish or bloody, which issues from a sore or a wound.

ICHTHAMMOL, ICHTHYOL, is ammonium ichthosulphonate, an almost black, thick liquid of fishy smell, prepared from a bituminous shale. It is used in several chronic skin diseases.

ICHTHYOSIS is a skin disease in which the surface is very rough and presents a dry, cracked appearance, resembling fish-scales. The peculiarity is generally hereditary, and persists through life, the skin being permanently hard, and deficient in oily material. The appearances differ considerably according to the part affected and the surrounding conditions. Thus the knees and elbows when affected become black from the collection of dirt in the deep crevices, and in winter the skin becomes specially hard and the condition still more marked.

Treatment – There is no specific internal treatment, but improvement sometimes follows the administration of vitamin A. Those who suffer from the disease should live, if possible, in a warm sunny climate. External treatment is most important and consists of daily warm baths with bran or starch, followed by the application of 20 to 50 per cent glycerin in water, olive oil, or equal parts of salicylic acid ointment (2 per cent) and glycerin. An alternative form of treatment is to add the *British Pharmacopoeia* Emulsifying Ointment to the bath: 1 ounce (28·5 grams) is added after preliminary creaming in a jug of hot water. This is followed by the application to the skin of the *British Pharmacopoeia* Hydrous Ointment as often as is required. Another promising line of treatment is the use of a urea cream. (See UREA.)

ICTERUS is another name for jaundice (qv).

ICTERUS GRAVIS NEONATORUM (see HAEMOLYTIC DISEASE OF THE NEWBORN).

ICTUS is another term for a stroke.

IDIOCY is a term no longer used. Those who were described as idiots are now included in the category of 'severe subnormality' as defined in the Mental Health Act, 1959. (See MENTAL SUBNORMALITY.)

IDIOGLOSSIA means the continued utterance of meaningless sounds, the afflicted person 'speaking' a language intelligible to no-one.

IDIOPATHIC is a term applied to diseases to indicate that their cause is unknown.

IDIOSYNCRASY means an unusual effect produced by certain drugs or other agencies in certain persons. For example, some persons are poisoned by very small doses of opium or belladonna, whilst, on the other hand, others can take large doses of these or other drugs without any effect. The same applies to alcohol, arsenic, iodides and many other drugs. Idiosyncrasies exist also for foods, some persons having an acute attack of dyspepsia, or even becoming dangerously ill, when they take milk, or fish, or eggs, or oatmeal, as the case may be. Others may be powerfully affected by smells, such as that of roses, or of particular animals, as of cats. This peculiarity as applied to sensitiveness to substances, such as foods and the pollen of plants, is known as allergy (qv).

IDOXURIDINE is a preparation that is proving of value in the treatment of some cases of herpes of the eye.

ILEITIS means inflammation of the ileum. REGIONAL ILEITIS, or CROHN'S DISEASE, is the term applied to a condition in which there is an (apparent) inflammation of an area of the small intestine. This is accompanied by colicky abdominal pain, irregularity of the bowels, loss of weight and slight fever. The abdomen is distended and the thickened intestine may be felt. The narrowed intestinal canal may become obstructed, necessitating immediate operation. The cause is unknown. The primary lesion is hyperplasia (qv) of the lymph tissue in the submucosa of the intestine and in the lymph glands.

As the cause is not known, there is no specific treatment. In the early stages, treatment is medical, including a high-vitamin, low-residue diet, sulphonamides and antibiotics. Promising results have been reported from the use of corticosteroids in some cases. Operation, consisting of removal of the damaged section of gut, is reserved for cases which do not respond to medical treatment. Even in cases apparently successfully operated on, recurrence tends to occur in 15 per cent or more of cases.

ILEO-CAECAL is the term applied to the region of the junction between the small and large intestines in the right lower corner of the abdomen. The ileocaecal valve is a structure which allows the contents of the intestine to pass onwards from the small to the large intestine, but, in the great majority of cases, prevents their passage in the opposite direction.

ILEOSTOMY is the operation by which an artificial opening is made into the ileum.

ILEUM is the lower part of the small intestine. (See INTESTINE.)

ILEUS is another name for severe colic due to obstruction of the bowels. (See INTESTINE, DISEASES OF.)

ILIUM is another name for the haunch-bone, the uppermost of the three bones forming each side of the pelvis. (See BONE; PELVIS.)

ILLUSIONS (see HALLUCINATIONS).

IMBECILITY is a term no longer used. What used to be known as imbecility is now included in the category of 'severe subnormality', as defined in the Mental Health Act, 1959. (See MENTAL SUBNORMALITY.)

IMIPRAMINE is one of the so-called tricyclic antidepressants which is proving of value in the treatment of depression.

IMMERSION FOOT is the term applied to a condition which develops as a result of prolonged immersion of the feet in cold or cool water. It was a condition commonly seen during the 1939–45 War in shipwrecked sailors and airmen who had crashed in the sea and spent long periods before being rescued. Such prolonged exposure results in vasoconstriction of the smaller arteries in the feet, leading to coldness and blueness of the feet, and finally, in severe cases, to ulceration and gangrene.

IMMUNITY is a principle by virtue of which the bodies of certain animals or human beings are protected from the invasion of certain diseases, or the action of certain poisons. It is a well-recognized fact that some persons expose themselves again and again to the risk of infection and are not affected, whilst others seem prone to contract any disease with which they are brought into contact. The immunity so enjoyed is of several types. Natural immunity is one which is inborn; but immunity may also be acquired in the course of life, or it may be produced artificially by inoculation, or by injection of the blood serum of immune animals.

Natural immunity – Certain animals seem to be little affected by poisons which to others are very deadly. Thus the snake-killing mongoose of India is said to be highly immune to cobra poison. Pigeons are little affected by large doses of morphine; rabbits and other animals eat freely the leaves of the deadly nightshade plant. (See IDIOSYNCRASY.) The rat is little affected by tuberculosis, to which other creatures, including particularly man and the guinea-pig, are very susceptible. Man, on the other hand, is unaffected by swine fever, and some other diseases which are very infectious and fatal among the lower animals, while no animal, so far as is known, contracts cholera, a disease which is so disastrous to man. Other examples are found in the fowl and the alligator, which are peculiar in being exempt from lockjaw, and white rats, which are not affected by anthrax. There is probably no such thing as absolute immunity, however, since animals are affected by any poison if their health be very low or if the amount of poison be very great.

administering by the mouth in some cases, a small dose of some particular poison insufficient to produce death. This has the effect of stimulating the animal's powers of resistance, so that next time it can withstand a larger dose. The process is repeated over and over, the dose each time increasing, till finally the animal is unaffected by many times the dose which would have originally killed it. This applies to snake poisons also, and the snake-charmers of India appear to render themselves indifferent to cobra-bites by a similar process.

With regard to disease-producing bacteria and the toxins or poisons which they form, immunity is reached by injecting small quantities of bacteria, or of their toxins, which have been weakened by

Vaccine	Age at which to give
BCG	Within first week of life if any contact likely with anyone with tuberculosis
Diphtheria, tetanus and whooping-cough (one injection of Triple vaccine) and poliomyelitis vaccine by mouth	3 months Repeated 6 weeks later and again after a further 6 months
Measles	During 2nd year
Diphtheria and tetanus (one injection) and poliomyelitis vaccine by mouth	On going to school
BCG if child is Mantoux-negative	10 to 13 years
German measles (girls only)	11 to 13 years
Diphtheria and tetanus (one injection), poliomyelitis vaccine by mouth	On leaving school

Table 28 – Timetable for routine immunization of children. – *The Practitioner.*

Acquired immunity is that which is gained by passing through an attack of some disease. Protection is probably given by all infectious diseases for a longer or shorter period against a second attack of the same disease. In the case of some, such as smallpox, typhoid fever, scarlet fever, the protection appears to last throughout life, or, at all events, for many years. Recovery from a disease is in fact a process of immunity, the poison of the disease being destroyed by antagonizing substances, known as antibodies, produced in the tissues of the body, so that the disease comes to an end after a definite period. Some individuals acquire these antibodies by coming in contact with the infecting organisms without ever actually showing signs of the disease or possibly by having it in such a mild form that it is not recognized.

Artificial immunity is of two kinds, known as active and passive immunity.

(*a*) ACTIVE IMMUNITY is produced by injecting beneath an animal's skin, or

mixing with antiseptics, by drying in air, by passing through the bodies of partially immune animals, or by other highly technical processes. The best-known practical example of this treatment is vaccination against smallpox, in which cowpox, a modified form of the disease, is produced in persons so as to render them immune to the far severer smallpox. Another is Pasteur's preventive treatment for rabies, in which, during the long incubation period before the disease has had time to appear, the person is treated by increasing doses of the poison, taken from rabbits that have been killed by the disease. (See RABIES.)

The principle of this method, then, consists in stimulating the power of the body to resist the action of poisons. Great success in preventing diphtheria has been achieved by injecting one to three doses of diphtheria toxoid (inactivated toxin). This is quite harmless, and hundreds of thousands of children the world over have now been protected against this serious disease. Other common diseases against which

461

protection can be provided in this way include typhoid fever, whooping-cough, tetanus, measles, German measles and poliomyelitis. A summary of current practice of immunization for children is shown in table 28. (See also VACCINE.)

(b) PASSIVE IMMUNITY is that form of artificial immunity obtained by injecting into the body of one animal or person, whom it is desired to render immune, blood serum drawn from an animal already rendered immune by the active method. The best-known example of this method is the treatment of diphtheria by antitoxic serum. This serum is obtained from horses already protected from diphtheria, as explained above, by a course of several months' treatment. This serum temporarily protects a person against contracting diphtheria, and after the onset of the disease, it will, if injected, neutralize the poison and bring about a milder type of disease and speedier recovery. The theory of action is, that the antitoxic serum contains certain chemical substances (antitoxins) which have been produced by the cells of the horse's blood or other tissues, and which combine with the poisons (toxins) produced by the diphtheria bacilli so as to neutralize the latter. Antitetanus serum immediately given to those injured under such conditions as to render them liable to an attack of lockjaw will prevent the onset of tetanus. (See SERUM THERAPY.)

IMMUNOGLOBULINS are the proteins in the blood which carry the antibody activity of the blood against infectious micro-organisms. The most important of them is immunoglobulin G and this is available to be given by injection to provide immediate protection against diseases such as infectious hepatitis and measles.

IMPACTION is a term applied to a condition in which two things are firmly lodged together. For example, when after a fracture one piece of bone is driven within the other, this is known as an impacted fracture; when a tooth is firmly lodged in its socket so that its eruption is prevented, this is known as dental impaction.

IMPERIAL DRINK (for composition see under CREAM OF TARTAR).

IMPERSEX is another name for infantalism (qv) or imperfect sexual development.

IMPETIGO is a skin disease of an infectious nature often found in schools and caused usually by the *Staphylococcus aureus*. It consists of vesicles which appear here and there, on the face particularly, and dry up, leaving yellowish-brown scabs from which the discharge is infectious. These scabs fall off, leaving no scars, but the disease spreads from place to place over the skin, and may last for months if untreated. When it occurs in very young children, it is liable to run a severe course unless treatment is initiated immediately. This form of the disease is known as pemphigus neonatorum (see PEMPHIGUS) because of the marked blistering of the skin that tends to occur.

Treatment – Affected children should be off school and use separate washing and eating utensils. Infected crusts are removed by washing with saline or cetrimide lotion. Starch poultices may be necessary where the crusts are extensive. Some antibiotic ointment, such as chlortetracycline bacitracin, framycetin or polymyxin, is applied night and morning, and covered by a bandage.

Penicillin is not usually used partly because of its tendency to produce sensitization of the skin, but particularly because the causative *Staphylococcus aureus* is so often penicillin resistant.

When nits are present on the hair, treatment is ineffective until these have been removed. (See PARASITES.)

IMPOTENCE is the inability to perform the sexual act. It may be partial or complete, temporary or permanent. Of the many classifications of this not uncommon condition, the most satisfactory is probably that which divides it into two main groups: *organic* and *psychological*. Among organic causes are lesions of the external genitalia, eg. a tight foreskin; disturbances of the endocrine glands, such as diminished activity of the gonads, thyroid gland or pituitary gland; diseases of the central nervous system, eg. tabes dorsalis; any severe disturbance of health, such as diabetes mellitus, addiction to alcohol and the like. Among the psychological factors are ignorance, fear, weakness of sexual desire or abnormality of such desire.

INCISION means a cut or wound and is a term specially applied to surgical openings.

INCISOR is the name applied to the four front teeth of each jaw. (See TEETH.)

INCOMPATIBILITY is a term applied to unsuitability in a prescription owing to the fact that its different contents either cannot be mixed, or that when mixed they undergo chemical changes, or that their actions are opposed to one another.

INCOMPETENCE is a term applied to the valves of the heart when, as a result of disease in the valves or alterations in size of the chambers of the heart, the valves become unable to close the orifices which they should protect. (See HEART DISEASES.)

INCONTINENCE is a term applied to the inability to retain the evacuations of the bowels and bladder. It occurs in diseases of these organs, injuries and diseases of the spinal cord, etc.

INCO-ORDINATION is a term applied to irregularity of movements produced either by loss of the sensations by which they are governed or by defects in the muscles themselves or their nerves.

INCUBATION means the period elapsing between the time when a person becomes infected by some agent and the first appearance of the symptoms of the disease. Most acute infectious diseases have fairly definite periods of incubation (table 29), and it is of great importance that people who have run the risk of infection should know the length of time which

	days
Chickenpox	14–21
Diphtheria	2–5
German measles	14–21
Measles	10–15
Mumps	18–21
Poliomyelitis	3–21
Smallpox	10–16
Typhoid fever	7–21
Whooping-cough	7–10

Table 29 – Incubation periods of the commoner infectious diseases.

must elapse before they can be sure whether or not they are to contract the disease in question. A person who has been exposed to infection is, during the incubation period, technically known as a contact. By isolating and watching contact cases in a boarding-school, barrack, or other public institution, medical officers can often successfully check a threatened epidemic. It must be noted that diseases are not communicated to others by a person while passing through the stage of incubation. Some diseases, however, such as measles, become infectious as soon as the first symptoms set in after the incubation period is over; others, like scarlet fever and smallpox, are not so infectious then as in their later stages. The incubation period for any given disease is remarkably constant, although in the case of a severe attack the incubation is usually slightly shortened, and if the oncoming attack be a mild one, the period may be

Disease	Patients	Contacts
Chickenpox	6 days from the date of the appearance of the rash.	None.
Diphtheria	Until 3 consecutive throat and nose swabs are negative.	Until nose and throat swabs are bacteriologically clear.
German measles	5 days from the appearance of the rash.	None.
Measles	7 days after the appearance of the rash if the child appears well.	Infants who have not had the disease should be excluded for 14 days from the date of appearance of the rash in the last case in the house. Other contacts can attend school. Any contact suffering from a cold, chill or red eyes should be immediately excluded.
Mumps	9 days from the onset of the disease or 7 days from the subsidence of all swelling.	None.
Smallpox	Until the patient is pronounced free from infection.	21 days, unless recently vaccinated, when exclusion is unnecessary.
Whooping-cough	21 days from the beginning of the characteristic cough.	Infants who have not had the disease should be excluded for 21 days from the date of onset of the disease in the last case in the house.

Table 30 – Quarantine periods for the commoner infectious diseases.

lengthened. So far as schools are concerned, children who have been contacts should not be allowed to return to school till several days beyond the maximum incubation period has elapsed since exposure to infection. All of these may, however, take a few days longer than the time stated to show themselves. (See INFECTION.) Several also, and especially whooping-cough, are very difficult to recognize in their early stages. For practical purposes, therefore, as regards the length of time that should be allowed to elapse after a child has been in contact with a case of infectious disease, and before he is permitted to return to school, table 30 should be followed.

INDIAN HEMP (see CANNABIS INDICA).

INDICATION is the term applied to any sign which points to the cause or particularly the treatment of a disease. The term, contraindication, is applied to some circumstance which debars a particular line of treatment.

INDIGESTION (see DYSPEPSIA).

INDOMETHACIN is a drug that is proving of value in the treatment of gout and rheumatoid arthritis.

INDUSTRIAL DISEASES (see OCCUPATIONAL DISEASES).

INFANT FEEDING – An infant may either be breast-fed or bottle-fed.
Breast feeding – Unless there is some definite contraindication, every new-born child should be breast-fed. As has been well said, 'to take in human milk and mother love at the breast and to continue to do so for several months is the best start in life for a human baby'. The advantages are clear cut and definite. The milk is specially prepared in composition for the human baby. It is at the right temperature and therefore there is no need to worry about hotting it up or cooling it down. It is available at any time no matter where the mother may be. It is most unlikely to be infected or contaminated, and it provides protection against infection at an age when the baby is particularly vulnerable in this respect. Further, breast feeding helps the womb to return to its normal shape more quickly and helps to prevent the mother from putting on weight. It also reduces the risk of the baby becoming too fat, and there is growing evidence that fat babies are more likely to have chest infections and to grow up into fat adults. Finally – but by no means least – breast feeding offers the most intimate contact between a mother and her new-born baby. A point to be borne in mind, however, is that many drugs taken by a nursing mother are excreted in her milk and may therefore affect her babe. These include antibiotics, tranquillizers, corticosteroids, vitamins, alcohol and nicotine.

The baby should be put to the breast six to eight hours after birth, and thereafter every three or four hours. Whether the baby is fed three-hourly or four-hourly depends upon how he progresses, but in the majority of healthy babies who weigh 7 pounds (3·2 kg) or more at birth, four-hourly feeding is sufficient. Five feeds are usually sufficient in the twenty-four hours, a useful time-table being feeds at 6 am., 10 am., 2 pm., 6 pm. and 10 pm. There is no reason why a healthy infant should not go through the night without a feed, although it may sometimes be found more convenient to give the first feed in the morning somewhat earlier. This undisturbed night is invaluable to the nursing mother. Both breasts should be used at each feed, and it is an advantage to start each feed on alternate breasts. For the first feed of all, one minute at each breast is sufficient, and this

	Height				Weight			
Age	Boys		Girls		Boys		Girls	
	Inches	Centi-metres	Inches	Centi-metres	Pounds	Kilo-grams	Pounds	Kilo-grams
Birth	20·0	50·9	19·5	49·5	7·5	3·4	7·3	3·3
2 weeks	20·3	51·7	20·1	51·0	7·5	3·4	7·3	3·3
3 months	23·7	60·2	23·2	58·8	12·9	5·8	12·0	5·5
6 months	26·2	66·7	25·6	65·0	17·4	7·9	16·4	7·4
9 months	28·0	71·2	27·4	69·6	20·4	9·2	19·2	8·7
1 year	29·6	75·1	29·1	73·9	22·8	10·3	21·7	9·8
2 years	34·0	86·4	33·7	85·5	27·0	12·2	25·7	11·6
3 years	37·8	95·9	36·9	93·8	31·5	14·3	30·4	13·8
4 years	40·6	103·0	40·0	101·6	35·6	16·2	34·5	15·7
5 years	43·1	109·5	42·9	108·9	40·2	18·3	39·4	17·9

Table 31 – Mean height and weight of infants and young children. Thomson.

time should be gradually increased until by the end of the first week the baby is having seven to ten minutes at each breast every feed.

The main guide as to whether an infant is being adequately fed is the weight (table 31). During the first few days of life a healthy infant loses weight, but this he should have regained by the tenth day of life. Thereafter he should gain 1 ounce (28 grams) daily. The only supplement which is required to satisfactory breast feeding until weaning takes place is vitamin C and vitamins A and D. Vitamin C is

	Protein per cent	Fat per cent	Sugar per cent	Calories per cent
Human milk	1·5	4·0	6·8	68
Cow's milk	3·5	3·5	5·0	66

Table 32 – Composition of human and cow's milk.

given in the form of orange juice: a few teaspoonfuls of equal parts of orange juice and water suitably sweetened at the age of one month, and gradually increased

aperient action on the bowels than any other form of liquid food.

Artificial feeding – If breast feeding is not possible, then some substitute for human milk must be used, and the most satisfactory is cow's milk. As will be seen from tables 32 and 33, cow's milk differs in certain important aspects from human milk: it contains less sugar, more protein, and about the same amount of fat. In addition, however, there are important qualitative differences. Milk contains two types of protein – casein and albumin. The albumin in milk is known as lactalbumin; it forms a finer clot and is more digestible than casein. In addition it contains larger amounts of two amino-acids, cystine and lysine, which are of special importance for growth. The fat in cow's milk also differs from that in human milk in that its globules are larger and coarser.

The other drawback to cow's milk is that in the liquid form it is a potentially dangerous food for infants unless it is boiled. Dangerous diseases such as tuberculosis can be conveyed by milk, and the only safe rule for infants is to boil all milk. Even the more expensive forms of graded

	Human Milk per 100 millilitres	Cow's Milk per 100 millilitres
Vitamin A	170 international units	
Summer		150 international units
Winter		100 international units
Vitamin D	1 international unit	
Summer		1·5 international units
Winter		0·5 international unit
Thiamine	17 micrograms	40 micrograms
Ascorbic Acid (Vitamin C)	3·5 milligrams	2 milligrams

Table 33 – Vitamin content of human and unboiled cow's milk.

until at the age of six months the infant is taking the juice of one orange undiluted. Tomato juice may occasionally be given instead of orange juice. Vitamins A and D are given in the form of cod-liver oil, starting with a quarter of a teaspoonful daily at about the age of 6 weeks, or the equivalent amount of any special form of cod-liver oil that may be used.

The fluid secreted by the breasts during the first few days of lactation is known as colostrum. It has a high content of protein, but only a small amount of sugar and fat. The precise function of colostrum is not known, but it may be of value in helping to establish the immunity to certain infectious diseases which the breast-fed baby so often possesses. In addition, it has of course a certain nutritional value, but it is doubtful whether it has any more

milk, such as 'TT' or 'accredited', are not safe in the unboiled state for infants. The results of infection in infants can be so disastrous that up to the age of two years all milk should be boiled. After the age of two years pasteurization is reliable and therefore above this age children should be given pasteurized milk. The simplest way of boiling milk is in a double saucepan, and it is only necessary to bring the milk up to the boil. Prolonged boiling is not necessary. Statements are sometimes made that boiling adversely affects the nutritious qualities of milk. There is no evidence in favour of this, except in the case of the vitamin C content, and this deficiency can readily be overcome by giving orange juice. What has been said here, of course, only applies to liquid milk. The processes whereby dried and condensed milks are made ensure that these are safe from all infection. Liquid, dried or condensed milk may be used for infant feeding.

GENERAL PRINCIPLES – Before dealing with details of how to prepare the milk, certain general principles will be outlined. Feeding times depend upon the weight of the infant. If the weight is over 7 to 8 pounds (3·2 to 3·6 kg), feeds are given every four hours from the tenth day, ie. at 6 am., 10 am., 2 pm., 6 pm., and 10 pm. If the weight is less than this, three-hourly feeds should be instituted, ie. 6 am., 9 am., 12 noon, 3 pm., 6 pm., and 10 pm. In all cases four-hourly feeds are sufficient after the age of three months or after the weight is 10 pounds (4.5 kg).

Absolute cleanliness is essential, This is achieved by effective sterilization of the bottle and teat – either by boiling or the use of sodium hypochlorite (qv). With both methods, the bottle and teat must first be thoroughly cleaned. Immediately after a feed, before the film of milk hardens, they are rinsed under running water. They are then thoroughly washed in warm water and detergent, using a bottle brush. The teat must be turned inside out, sprinkled inside and out with salt, rubbed with the fingers and then washed again with warm water and detergent. The bottle brush must be used for no other purpose and must be regularly washed and boiled. Having been cleaned, the bottle and teat are ready for sterilization. If this is done by boiling, they must be completely submerged in a closed pot or pan and boiled for ten minutes. If sodium hypochlorite is used, a fresh solution is made up every 24 hours, and bottle and teat soaked in this for at least three hours. After sterilization the bottle and teat are left in the boiled water or sterilizing solution covered with a lid until needed again. If chemical sterilization has been used, the excess fluid should be drained from bottle and teat before use but there is no need to rinse off the remaining drops of fluid. The hands of the mother or nurse must be carefully washed before handling the bottle, teat or feed. The teat must be as big as the baby can cope with, and the hole in it must be so adjusted that the feed drips freely through it (about 1 drop per second). This ensures that the baby is able to take each feed in ten to fifteen minutes.

The amount of each feed depends upon the daily caloric requirements of the infant, which can be taken to be 2½ fluid ounces (75 ml) of human milk or its equivalent per pound (455 grams) of body weight. Thus an infant weighing 8 pounds (3.6 kg) would require 20 fluid ounces (560 ml) of milk daily, and on the basis of five four-hourly feeds, this would mean 4 fluid ounces (140 ml) per feed. Two essential additions to all artificial feeding are vitamins C and D. The former is given in the form of diluted orange juice as already described under breast feeding. Vitamin D is given either as quarter to half a teaspoonful of cod-liver oil daily, or three drops of hali-but-liver oil daily.

DRIED MILK – Amidst the brands on the market, are three main types of dried milk: (1) 'Full cream' variety which, when reconstituted 1 in 8 (ie. 1 teaspoon or measure to 1 fluid ounce (28·5 ml) of water), gives milk of the same composition as un-diluted liquid milk. (2) 'Half-cream milk' from which some of the fat has been re-moved in the preparation, so that, when reconstituted 1 in 8, 1 fluid ounce (28·5 ml) is equivalent to about ¾ fluid ounce (22·5 ml) of human milk. To improve the feed value, some manufacturers add sugar to half-cream milk, but as this may not suit the baby, the plain varieties should be tried in the first instance. (3) 'Humanized dried milk' is so modified that reconstituted 1 in 8, 1 fluid ounce (28·5 ml) is equivalent to 1 fluid ounce (28·5 ml) of human milk. From the tenth day for a month or two, either the 'half-cream' or the 'humanized' milk should be used. The latter is the easier to use, as dilution 1 in 8 is all that is required. Thus, for a ten-day-old baby requiring 3 fluid ounces (85 ml) per feed, all that is required is to take 3 measures of the dried milk and add 3 fluid ounces (85 ml) of boiled (*not* boiling) water. The equivalent with half-cream milk would be 3 measures of dried milk, 4 fluid ounces (115 ml) of water, 1½ teaspoonfuls of sugar, and give 3 to 3½ fluid ounces (85 to 105 ml) per feed. Not later than three months, or a weight of 10 pounds (4·5 kg), a change-over is made to the full-cream variety. For an infant weighing 10 pounds (4·5 kg), 22½ fluid ounces (635 ml) of breast milk or its equivalent is necessary every day. On the basis of five feeds daily, this means that each feed would consist of 3 measures of the dried milk, 4½ fluid ounces (125 ml) of water, and 1½ teaspoonfuls of sugar. This is gradually increased until, by the age of six months (15 pounds (6·8 kg) weight), each feed is made up of 5 measures, 6 fluid ounces (170 ml) of water, and 1½ teaspoon-fuls of sugar. In order to avoid any diges-tive disturbance the switch-over from one variety of dried milk to another should always be made gradually. A further point to be borne in mind is that the scoops from different packs of food vary in size. Only the scoop supplied with the preparation in use should therefore be used. Equally important is that only level, not heaped, scoopfuls should be used. In all cases cod-liver oil and orange juice should be given daily from the age of one month.

Weaning – It is usual to start weaning about the fifth month or when the infant weighs about 17 pounds (7·8 kg), though the modern tendency is to start even earlier than this. Provided the process is carried out gradually, there is seldom any difficulty in having the child completely off the breast by the end of the ninth month. It is essential to remember that all cow's milk given to the baby must be boiled. The amount of milk, including that used for cooking, should be about $1\frac{1}{2}$ pints (850 ml) daily. From the age of six months the baby should be given a crust to chew every day. Cod-liver oil and orange juice are, of course, continued.

No hard and fast rules can be laid down for the process of weaning. If the baby has been breast-fed, then it is usually a mistake to switch on to an intermediate stage of bottle feeding. It is better, and usually not difficult, to teach baby to drink from a teaspoon or a feeding cup. The consistency of the food is important in the early stages of weaning. In the initial stage it should be semi-fluid, and for quite a long time it must be pulpy in consistency without any lumps. The large variety of powdered cereals and purées of vegetable and meat now available make the weaning process much simpler than it used to be – and much more pleasant for the baby. From a very early stage of weaning the aim should be to get baby on to a programme of three meals a day, with the meat, fish and vegetables given at the mid-day meal.

Digestive disturbances – These are much more likely to occur with artificial feeding than with breast feeding. Only mild digestive upsets associated with feeding will be mentioned here. Any serious digestive disturbance in an infant should be referred immediately to a medical practitioner. (See also DIARRHOEA.) In the case of breast feeding, overfeeding may cause vomiting, colic and diarrhoea, whilst underfeeding is accompanied by constipation. Sometimes, however, underfeeding may be accompanied by a special type of diarrhoea characterized by the passage of small, dark-green stools containing an excess of mucus – usually during or just after a feed. In the case of artificial feeding the most common digestive disturbances are colic

and diarrhoea. These may be due to either dirty feeding utensils or an unsuitable feeding mixture.

Treatment – It is important to remember that in a breast-fed baby vomiting, occurring immediately or soon after a feed, is usually of no significance provided there is no loss of weight. Should it be due to overfeeding (and this can be checked by test feeding) and should it persist, it can often be remedied by reducing the time at each breast and also by giving the infant a little boiled water before each feed. If underfeeding on the breast is confirmed by test feeding, the first essential is to reassure the mother and to ensure that she is taking sufficient diet, adequate fluid, and adequate rest. Other measures which help are to institute three-hourly feeding instead of four-hourly and to give an extra feed at night. If these fail, then complementary feeding may be used: ie. a bottle feed after one or more breast-feeds. In the case of artificial feeding, the first essential is to ensure that the feeding utensils are all being adequately sterilized by boiling and that there is no contamination of the feed. The next step is to change to some other food. Should all these measures fail, it may then be necessary to treat the milk in some special way. This may be done by adding 1 grain (60 mg) of sodium citrate to each fluid ounce (28·5 ml) of milk mixture, or peptonized milk may be used. If all else fails, it must never be forgotten that human milk is the best food for human infants and that it is sometimes possible to obtain supplies from maternity hospitals.

General rules for feeding young children – The proper routine of feeding, sleeping, and exercise forms the beginning of a child's education, and the following general rules should be observed:

1. Give food at regular hours only.

2. Take ample time; do not hurry the child in sucking or chewing.

3. If a child is disinclined to eat he should not be coaxed or forced to do so. If a child is losing weight, or off his food, he should be examined for signs of disease; otherwise the regulation of the amount of food should be left to his appetite.

4. Fancy dishes should not be given to tempt the appetite if simple food is refused; nor should food refused at meals be allowed at other times.

5. Although all food given to a child should be simple, it ought to be varied from day to day, well cooked, and attractively served.

6. Highly seasoned food, much dressed

467

food, and food with a large indigestible residue should not be given to children.

7. If a child habitually refuses some important article of diet, like milk, egg, or cereals, this should be given first and the more popular food withheld till the simpler one is taken. The refusal of some special food tends readily to become a habit with some children.

8. If a child is feverish, food should be reduced in strength and quantity. In very hot weather a young child often eats less food than usual and drinks more water.

9. The basis of a child's diet should be pasteurized milk (up to 2 pints (1 litre) a day); brown, wholemeal, or wheatmeal bread; butter or vitaminized margarine; eggs; cheese; fruit; salad vegetables; green leafy vegetables; potatoes and other root vegetables; meat; fish; sugar (but not too much); and water to drink. In the winter months a child should take one to two teaspoonfuls of cod-liver oil, or drops of halibut-liver oil, and 50 mg of ascorbic acid (vitamin C), daily.

INFANT MORTALITY is the number of deaths of infants under one year of age. The infant mortality rate in any given year is calculated as the number of deaths in the first year of life in proportion to every 1000 registered live births in that year. Along with perinatal mortality (qv), it is accepted as one of the most important criteria for assessing the health of the community and the standard of the social conditions of a country. The striking fall in the rate is well shown in the following figures:

1838–39	146	1941–45	49·8
1841–50	153	1946–50	36·4
1851–60	154	1951–55	26·9
1861–70	154	1956–60	22·6
1871–80	149	1961–65	20·6
1881–90	142	1968	18·3
1891–1900	153	1970	18·2
1901–05	138	1971	17·5
1906–10	117·1	1972	17·2
1911–15	108·1	1973	16·9
1916–20	90·9	1974	16·3
1921–25	74·9	1975	15·7
1926–30	67·9	1976	14·3
1931–35	62·2	1977	13·6
1936–40	55·3		

Table 34 – Infant mortality rate in England and Wales, 1838–1977.

On the other hand, that there is still room for improvement in this country is shown by the fact that the rate in England and Wales is still higher than that in some other countries. For instance, in 1976 the infant mortality rate was only 7·7 in Iceland, and 8·3 in Sweden, compared with 14·3 in England and Wales. In Scotland, it was 14·8.

This striking improvement in the infant mortality rate has occurred mainly in the period from the second month of life. There has been much less improvement in the neonatal mortality rate: ie. the number of infants dying during the first four weeks of life, expressed as a proportion of every 1000 live births. During the first week of life the main causes of death are asphyxia, prematurity, birth injuries and congenital abnormalities. After the first week the main cause of death is infection. The causes of death during the first year of life in England and Wales in 1911–20, 1931–39 and 1970 are shown in the following table. For 1970 the figures for the two sexes are combined.

Cause		1911–1920	1931–1939	1970
Whooping-cough	M	3·31	1·35	0·0166
	F	3·85	1·64	
Tuberculosis	M	2·88	0·80	0·0013
	F	2·26	0·65	
Measles	M	2·57	0·78	0·0115
	F	2·21	0·66	
Bronchitis and pneumonia	M	21·33	13·62	2·95
	F	16·43	10·28	
Gastro-enteritis	M		6·22	0·0013
	F		4·31	
Congenital malformations	M	4·29	6·03	3·72
	F	3·56	5·22	
Immaturity	M	21·48	16·40	2·01
	F	17·48	13·32	
All causes	M	111·70	66·17	18·19
	F	88·66	51·03	

Table 35 – Infant mortality rates per 1000 live births in England and Wales in 1911–20, 1931–1939, and 1970. M = Male. F = Female.

Social conditions also play an important rôle in infant mortality. For statistical purposes the Registrar-General divides the community into five social classes. In England and Wales the infant mortality rate in these classes in 1930–32 was: Class I (professional), 32·7; Class III (skilled workers), 57·6; Class V (unskilled workers), 77·1. The comparable figures for Scotland for 1939–45 were: Class I, 30·9; Class III, 53·4; Class V, 78·6. Many factors come into play in producing these social variations, but overcrowding is undoubtedly one of the most important. For instance, in 1936 the infant mortality rate in Bournemouth, where only 0·3 per cent of working-class families were overcrowded, was 78 per cent of that for the entire country, compared with 145 per cent in Newcastle-upon-Tyne where 10·7 per cent of working-class families were overcrowded. The same thing is evident in more recent figures available for Scotland. In 1945 the infant mortality rate in Scotland was 56, but in Port Glasgow it was 78, whilst in the county of Sutherland it was only 11.

It is thus evident that for a reduction of the infant mortality rate to the minimum figure the following conditions must be met. The mothers and potential mothers of the country must be housed adequately amid surroundings which permit of adequate fresh air and healthy exercise. The pregnant and nursing mother must be ensured an adequate diet. Effective antenatal supervision must be available to every mother, as well as skilled supervision during labour. The new-born infant must be adequately nursed and adequately fed. This means that all possible steps must be taken to encourage breast feeding. Mothers must be instructed in the proper care and feeding of their children, particularly during the first year of life. This in itself would reduce the mortality rate, but in addition adequate public-health measures must be taken to ensure a clean milk supply and full availability of such protective measures as immunization against diphtheria, measles, poliomyelitis and whooping-cough. (See also PERINATAL MORTALITY.)

INFANTILE PARALYSIS is an old name for POLIOMYELITIS (qv).

INFANTILISM is the condition characterized by imperfect sexual development at puberty. It may or may not be associated with small stature. It may be due to lack of development of certain of the endocrine glands: ie. the gonads (qv), pituitary gland or the adrenal glands. In other cases it may be associated with some generalized disease such as diabetes mellitus, asthma, ulcerative colitis, and rheumatoid arthritis.

INFARCTION means the changes which take place in an organ when an artery is suddenly blocked, leading to the formation of a dense, wedge-shaped mass in the part of the organ supplied by the artery. It occurs as the result of embolism or of thrombosis. (See EMBOLISM.)

INFECTION is the name given to the process by which a disease is communicated from one person to another. All diseases so communicable are called infectious. There is, in the case of all such diseases, some micro-organism produced in the body of the diseased person which, on being transmitted to a second person, is capable of reproducing itself in larger quantity and causing a particular disease.

This micro-organism may be a bacterium, a Rickettsia, a virus, a protozoon, or a metazoon. Invasion of the body by a metazoon (eg. by an intestinal worm) is more often known as an infestation.

The germs of disease may be grouped into those which will not flourish except about the temperature of the body, and those which are capable of maintaining their existence in decaying animal or vegetable matter, making only occasional migrations into the body and setting up disease. Speaking generally, bacteria of the first group are consistently much more deadly in their action, whilst those in the second group vary much in the severity of the disease they produce, causing a severer type if they have come direct from an infected person than if they have been germinating in drains, in the soil or floating on dust particles in the air. This principle is of immense practical importance. In the course of a surgical operation many bacteria must fall from the air into the wound, but this does not appear to be any drawback, unless the bacteria be derived direct from suppurating wounds or like virulent source. Similarly diphtheria or pneumonia bacteria of a mild type may be found in the mouth of people who are, nevertheless, quite healthy, if certain conditions, necessary to render the bacterium virulent, be not present.

The same bacterium may produce very different types of disease, not only on account of its previous life-history, but even according to the channel by which it enters the body. The *Mycobacterium tuberculosis*, for instance, produces a very different picture, depending upon whether it invades the lungs, the intestines, the joints, the glands or the skin. A certain amount of protection against the entrance of infective matter into the tissues of the body is afforded by the horny layer of the skin, by the acid of the gastric juice, and by the movements of the intestine, and a still greater measure of protection is afforded by the factors which ensure immunity against diseases. (See IMMUNITY; and SERUM THERAPY.)

Modes of infection – The infective material may be transmitted to the person by direct contact with a sick person, when the disease is said to be contagious, although such a distinction is purely artificial. Different diseases are specially infectious at different periods of their course; and the practical question of guarding against infection is rendered much more difficult by the fact that some diseases are infectious at a stage even before they are clearly recognizable. This applies particularly to the early stage of measles before the rash appears, when the infected child is showing symptoms merely resembling those of catarrh or a cold in the head.

Infection may be conveyed on dust driven by the wind, in drinking-water, food, particularly milk, evacuations with which the healthy person's hands have become contaminated, crusts and scabs from the infected person's body, or even clothes and linen which have been in contact with him.

In this connection what are termed carriers are of great importance. Some persons who have suffered from a disease, or who have simply been in contact with an infectious case, harbour the germ of the disease. This is particularly the case in regard to typhoid fever, the bacillus continuing to develop in the gall-bladder of persons who have had the disease maybe for years after the symptoms have passed away; it is estimated that 2 to 5 per cent of patients with typhoid fever become permanent typhoid carriers and where a cook or food purveyor is affected, he is apt to start an epidemic unless he exercises the most scrupulous cleanliness. In the case of cholera, which is endemic in some localities of the East, 80 per cent or more of the population may harbour the bacillus and spread infection when other circumstances favour this. Similarly in the case of dysentery, persons who have completely recovered may still be capable of infecting dust and drinking-water by their stools. Diphtheria is similarly liable to be carried by persons in whose throat the germ remains after recovery from the disease. Cerebrospinal meningitis, which is particularly liable to infect children, appears to be transmitted through the germ being carried in the nose of persons who may not develop any symptoms.

Flies pass from garbage heaps to unprotected food, and are especially dangerous as regards the infection of milk and other food with the organisms causing typhoid fever and food poisoning. Mosquitoes convey from sick to healthy the germs of malaria and yellow fever, these undergoing part of their development in the body of the mosquito. Fleas convey the germ of plague from rat to man, lice

are responsible for inoculating typhus fever and one form of relapsing fever by their bite. A tick is responsible for spreading another form of relapsing fever, and kala-azar (or leishmaniasis) is spread by the bites of sandflies.

Notifiable diseases – Certain of the common and most serious infectious diseases were scheduled in the Infectious Diseases Act of 1889 as notifiable in Great Britain. That is to say that any medical practitioner, attending or called in to visit a person suffering from one of these, must immediately, on becoming aware that the patient is suffering from it, send a notice to the local medical officer of health. The current list of notifiable infectious diseases in England and Wales is:

Acute encephalitis
Acute meningitis
Anthrax
Chlorea
Diphtheria
Dysentery
Infective jaundice
Lassa fever
Leprosy
Leptospirosis
Malaria
Marburg disease
Measles
Ophthalmia neonatorum
Paratyphoid fever
Plague
Rabies
Relapsing fever
Scarlet fever
Smallpox
Tuberculosis
Typhoid fever
Typhus
Viral haemorrhagic fever
Whooping-cough
Yellow fever

Food poisoning and suspected food poisoning are also notifiable.

In Scotland the following diseases are also notifiable in addition to the above list:

Cerebrospinal fever
Encephalitis lethargica
Erysipelas
Pneumonia (influenzal and acute primary)
Puerperal fever
Puerperal pyrexia

In Northern Ireland gastroenteritis (under 2 years of age) is notifiable.

Anthrax and toxic jaundice are notifiable as industrial diseases. Similar regulations are found in other countries.

Prevention of infection – The various channels of infection are mentioned under the heading of the different infectious diseases, and also briefly under SANITATION. As children are much more liable to contract infectious diseases than grown-up people, attempts to prevent the spread of these diseases are specially directed towards separating affected persons from healthy children. The measures taken apply particularly to schools, which form the places of dissemination in a large proportion of cases, but the rules applicable to children may well be practised with regard to persons of any age and in respect of any public institution. (See also IMMUNITY; INCUBATION.)

INFECTIOUS MONONUCLEOSIS
(see GLANDULAR FEVER).

INFERTILITY – The inability of a married couple to have children may be the fault of the husband, or the wife, or both. As one or more of many factors may be involved, it is essential, if success is to be achieved, that the problem should be approached in an unemotional and systematic manner. Nothing is more likely to lead to failure than mutual recrimination.

In the first place it must be remembered that the fertility, or ability to have children, of married couples varies considerably. This means that many a couple must have patience. Some couples may find that the wife becomes pregnant almost immediately, whilst others may have to wait months – or even years. Speaking generally, there is no need to become worried until at least a year has elapsed. Among the first factors to be looked into are the frequency and timing of intercourse and the technique. The main point about timing is its relationship to menstruation, taking this as a guide to the time of ovulation: that is, the release of the ovum from the ovary. It is in the early days of marriage that psychological factors can play a strong inhibitory part, particularly if there is inadequate mutual trust and understanding. Few things are more likely to render a husband temporarily impotent than the accusation by his wife that he is responsible for the fact that she is not pregnant. If, after a year, there is still no evidence of pregnancy, or earlier if undue anxiety is being aroused, then advice should be sought from some reliable source, such as the family doctor, or the Marriage Guidance Council (qv).

If further investigations are called for, then it is essential that these should include both partners unless it is initially clear which is responsible. The husband is usually examined first, as male infertility is probably the main factor in infertile marriages in 45 per cent of cases. Both husband and wife must have a general medical examination to make sure that it is not their general health that is at fault. If there is no such fault, the frequency, timing and technique of intercourse are investigated, and corrected if necessary. If the husband is impotent, this is investigated and can often be corrected provided full cooperation of both partners is obtained. A careful examination of the husband's semen is then carried out to decide whether or not he is sterile. Many factors can be responsible for absolute or relative sterility of the husband, and for some of these nothing can be done. Great care and experience are required in the interpretation of sperm counts obtained from an examination of the husband's semen but, if there is absolute sterility (that is, total and permanent absence of sperms), then there is nothing left that can be done to render the marriage fertile – except artificial insemination from a donor. (See ARTIFICIAL INSEMINATION.)

In the case of the wife, infertility may be due to some obstruction to the sperm reaching the ovum or to the ovum reaching the uterus. Alternatively, it may be due to some disturbance of the woman's hormones so that she is unable to produce ova or to release them into the uterus at regular monthly intervals. Modern methods of investigation can usually reveal which of these factors is responsible. If there is some physical obstruction, say, in the Fallopian tubes (qv), it may be possible to remove this. Alternatively, if there is some factor that is destroying the sperm before it can reach the uterus, this may be counteracted. If the defect is in the hormonal make-up of the wife, the so-called fertility drugs may right the matter.

If after full investigation it appears that the wife should be capable of becoming pregnant, and her husband is capable of producing healthy semen, but the marriage remains childless, artificial insemination by the husband (AIH) may be considered. If artificial insemination is not congenial to both partners – and it is certainly a practice that should not be embarked upon except after very careful thought and the obtaining of the best possible advice – and both partners are anxious to have children, there is always the well-established practice of adoption. It may not completely satisfy the woman's craving to perform her natural function of giving birth to a child, but many a couple have found it a satisfying alternative and one that has brought adopters and adopted much joy and happiness.

INFESTATION is a term applied to the occurrence of animal parasites in the intestine, hair or clothing. (See INSECTS IN RELATION TO DISEASE.)

INFLAMMATION may be defined as the reaction of the tissues to any injury, short of one sufficiently severe to cause their immediate death. The term is limited sometimes to the changes which take place when bacteria enter the body, but the changes in the latter case, though specially severe, are essentially the same as those produced by any other source of irritation. There are four cardinal symptoms of inflammation: redness, heat, pain and swelling, all of which, and particularly the last, are present in greater or less degree, so that these are also made a basis for defining the condition.

The first sign of inflammation consists in a dilatation of the arteries and veins of the affected part, so that the blood circulates in it more quickly and in larger quantity than before, thus causing heat and redness. Very soon, however, and apparently as the result of some change in the walls of the smaller blood-vessels, the circulation becomes gradually slower, and the white corpuscles of the blood are seen to adhere to the inner surface of these vessels. Later, these corpuscles push their way in great numbers through the walls of the smaller veins and capillaries, migrating into the surrounding tissues along with large quantities of the fluid material of the blood and a few red corpuscles, a process known as DIAPEDESIS. Hence the swelling, which is the most characteristic sign of inflammation. These white corpuscles subserve many functions. In the first place, they have been shown, originally by Metchnikoff, and later by other observers, to attack the bacteria which have invaded the tissues, to envelop them in their own substance, and, apparently by a process of digestion, to break them up. They also remove tissues which are dead or useless. Other corpuscles, at a later stage, when the source of irritation has been removed, play a part in producing the new tissues to repair the damage done, although the greater part of this repair is effected by cells from the surrounding tissues.

One of two results may follow inflammation. Either *resolution* may take place, when the white corpuscles, having played their part, find their way back into the circulation after the process of repair has been started at the site of injury, and the circulation proceeds as before, or *abscess-formation* results, the circulation comes to a complete standstill in the affected part, an excessive number of white corpuscles migrate from the vessels, an area of tissue becomes destroyed, and the process ends by a discharge of pus through the surface of the body, after which repair proceeds. (See ABSCESS, ACUTE.)

Symptoms – As already mentioned, redness, heat, pain and swelling are the classical symptoms of inflammation, and there are usually general symptoms of feverishness, varying with the severity of the inflammation. Various special symptoms are set up in special localities: for example, inflammation of the mucous membranes of the stomach and bowels leads to a copious excretion of mucus; inflammations of outlying parts, if they are very severe, may cause death of these parts, and are then called gangrenous inflammation; intense inflammation limited to a surface may destroy patches of the surface and convert them into a leather-like membrane, such types being known as croupous inflammations. Inflammation may become chronic, and in this case not only does the process described proceed in a minor degree, but there is an exaggerated process of repair leading to the formation of much fibrous or scar tissue, which may come to replace almost entirely the organ in which the chronic inflammation is proceeding, thus rendering the organ small, hard and irregular in outline.

Treatment – This depends upon different factors, such as the type of organism responsible, the site of infection and the severity of the infection. Thus, if the inflammation is due to tuberculosis, treatment will be by means of a combination of two or more, of streptomycin, isoniazid and para-aminosalicylic acid. If, on the other hand, it is in the appendix, immediate removal of the appendix is called for, whilst in the case of superficial inflammation of the skin, all that may be required is careful cleansing of the skin and the application of some antiseptic preparation.

Two general principles, however, apply to the treatment of all forms of inflammation: rest and the maintenance of the general health of the patient.

INFLUENZA, also known as LA GRIPPE, is an acute infectious disease, characterized by a sudden onset, fever and generalized aches and pains, which usually occurs in epidemics and pandemics.

History – The term influenza was first introduced into England in 1743 by John Huxham, a practitioner in Plymouth, and is said to be derived from *influsso*, which is the Italian form of *influxio* which means 'catarrh'. The origin of the disease is wrapped in the mists of antiquity. It has been suggested, for instance, that the epidemic of 412 BC described by Hippocrates was influenza, and that this was also the cause of the epidemic that swept across Europe in 839 AD, causing heavy losses in Charlemagne's army. To come to more modern times, there were five widespread epidemics during the nineteenth century in 1830, 1833, 1836, 1897 and 1889–90. The greatest pandemic of all, however, was that of 1918–19, which swept across the world and is estimated to have caused 15 to 20 million deaths within two years.

Cause – The disease is caused by a virus of the influenza group (illustration 252). There are at least three types of influenza virus, known respectively as A, B and C. One of their most characteristic features is that infection with one type provides no protection against another type. Equally important is the ease with which the influenza virus can change its character. It is these two characteristics which explain why one attack of influenza provides little, if any, protection against a subsequent attack, and why it is so difficult to prepare an effective vaccine against the disease.

Epidemics of influenza due to virus A occur in Britain at two- to four-year intervals, and outbreaks of virus B influenza in less frequent cycles. Virus A influenza, for instance, was the prevalent infection in 1949, 1951, 1955 and 1956, whilst virus B influenza was epidemic in 1946, 1950, 1954 and, along with virus A, in 1958–59. The pandemic of 1957, which swept most of the world, though fortunately not in a severe form, was due to a new variant of virus A – the so-called Asian virus – and it has been suggested that it was this variant that was responsible for the pandemics of 1889 and 1918. Since 1957, variants of virus A have been the predominating causes of influenza accompanied on occasions by virus B.

Symptoms – The incubation period of influenza A and B is two to three days and the disease is characterized by a sudden onset. In most cases this is followed by a short, sharp febrile illness of two to four days' duration, associated with headache, prostration, generalized aching and respiratory symptoms. In many cases the respiratory symptoms are restricted to the upper respiratory tract, and consist of signs of irritation of the nose, pharynx and larynx. There may be nose-bleeds, and a dry hacking cough is often a prominent and troublesome symptom. The fever is usually remittent and the temperature seldom exceeds 103° F (39·4° C), tending to fluctuate between 101° and 103° F (38·3° and 39·4° C).

The most serious complication is infection of the lungs. This infection is usually due to organisms other than the influenza virus. It is a complication which can have serious results in elderly people.

The very severe form which tends to occur during pandemics – and which was so common during the 1918–19 pandemic

252 – Model showing the structure of influenza virus, by J. J. Skehel. (Medical Research Council)

– is characterized by the rapid onset of broncho-pneumonia and severe prostration. Because of the toxic effect on the heart there is a particularly marked form of cyanosis, known as heliotrope cyanosis.

Convalescence following influenza tends to be prolonged. Even after an attack of average severity there tends to be a period of weakness and depression.

Treatment – Expert opinion is still divided as to the real value of influenza vaccine in preventing the disease. Part of the trouble is that, as already pointed out, there is no value in giving any vaccine until it is known which particular virus is causing the infection. As this varies from winter to winter, and as the protection given by vaccine does not exceed one year, it is obviously not worth while attempting to vaccinate the whole community. The general rule therefore is that, unless there is any evidence that a particularly virulent type of virus is responsible, only those should be vaccinated who are particularly vulnerable, such as children in boarding schools, elderly people, pregnant women, and people who suffer from chronic bronchitis. In the face of an epidemic, people in key positions, such as doctors, nurses and those concerned with public safety, transport and other public utilities should be vaccinated.

For an uncomplicated attack of influenza, treatment is symptomatic: that is, rest in bed, analgesics to relieve the pain, sedatives, and a light diet. A linctus, such as Gee's linctus, is useful to sooth a troublesome cough. The best analgesic is aspirin – either alone, or combined with paracetamol and codeine. None of the sulphonamides or the known antibiotics has any effect on the influenza virus. On the other hand should the lungs become infected, antibiotics should be given immediately, because, as has already been pointed out, such an infection is usually due to other organisms. Usually one of the tetracycline group of antibiotics is best, or chloramphenicol, but in others penicillin is the antibiotic of choice. If possible, a sample of sputum should be examined to determine which organisms are responsible for the lung infection. The choice of antibiotic then depends upon which antibiotic the organism is most sensitive to. At the moment promising results are being reported from the use of a drug known as amantadine, particularly if taken early in the illness.

INFUSIONS are preparations of vegetable drugs made by steeping them for some time in water and straining. In order that an infusion may keep well it is usually concentrated and mixed with spirit, being diluted just before it is dispensed. Among the better-known infusions are those of gentian, quassia, senega and senna. The dose of most infusions is from one to several tablespoonfuls.

Infusion is also the term applied to the injection into blood-vessels or subcutaneous tissues of warm normal salt solution, glucose solution or gum acacia solution, in the case of persons who are in a feeble state from loss of blood, loss of fluid by diarrhoea, etc. The infusion is sometimes administered in an amount of about one pint (570 ml) at a time, or is often used by a drip method in which the warm fluid is suspended at a height and allowed to pass drop by drop for several hours into a vein.

INGUINAL REGION (see ABDOMEN, REGIONS OF).

INHALATION means a method of applying drugs in a finely divided or gaseous state, so that, on being breathed in, they may come in contact with the nose, throat and lungs. There are five chief means by which drugs are mingled with the air and so taken in by breathing. These are as follows:

(a) Volatile drugs, which become gaseous at the ordinary temperature. Examples of these are chloroform, ether, nitrous oxide gas and amyl nitrite. Most drugs so administered act as general anaesthetics.

(b) Respirators are worn in front of the mouth and nose when it is desired to admit small quantities of some slowly volatile drug constantly into the air passages. The simpler and lighter such respirators are, the better. Perhaps the best variety is one consisting of a thin piece of bent, perforated metal, padded round the edge, having a small piece of sponge in its interior upon which the drug may be dropped, and pieces of elastic at its sides to pass behind the ears and keep the respirator in position.

(c) Drugs which give off volatile substances on burning are mixed with some combustible substance, and the fumes they give off inhaled. Thus asthmatic persons sometimes obtain relief during an attack from the smoke given off by smouldering blotting-paper which has been previously soaked in a strong solution of nitre and dried. (See NITRE.) Similarly, lobelia, stramonium and belladonna leaves are made into powders or rolled up in cigarettes, of which the fumes are inhaled.

(d) Steam inhalations. Steam itself, or hot moist air, has a soothing effect upon the mucous membrane of the air passages, and the steam may be impregnated with many moderately volatile drugs. This type of inhalation is used especially in bronchitis and inflammatory conditions of the throat and larynx. If it be desired to surround the patient constantly with a steamy atmosphere, the most convenient mode of doing so is by a kettle placed over a spirit lamp or electric heater, from which a long funnel leads in beneath a tent formed by a blanket over the upper half of the patient's bed (illustration 253). In cases of chronic bronchitis, one teaspoonful of the following mixture is now and then added to the hot water: pinewood oil 1 ounce (28·5 ml), eucalyptus oil 1 ounce (28·5 ml), creosote $\frac{1}{2}$ ounce (14 ml). Or in acute cases, where a soothing effect is specially necessary, a teaspoonful of the following: compound tincture of benzoin 1 ounce (28·5 ml), menthol 10 grains (600 mg), spirit of chloroform ½ ounce (14 ml). Either of these formulae may be used by simply adding it to a jug half full of boiling water, over which the mouth is held, the head being enveloped in a towel that falls down round the sides of the jug. The same remedies may be added in similar quantity to a Nelson's inhaler with mouthpiece, and the mouth directly applied to the tube leading from it.

253 – Bronchitis tent and steam kettle.

(e) The most recent form of inhalation consists of a fine spray or cloud driven off from a fluid by a stream of compressed air. By this means, various medicaments can be made to reach the farthest recesses of the lungs. The smaller of these nebulizers or atomizers are worked by a hand-ball of india-rubber, which drives a strong stream of air across the mouth of another tube dipping into the liquid. In various spas, larger nebulizers worked by force pumps are employed to fill whole rooms with medicated vapour, which patients sit and inhale for hours.

INHIBITION means arrest or restraint of some process effected by nervous influence. The term is applied to the action of certain inhibitory nerves: eg. the vagus nerve which contains fibres that inhibit or control the action of the heart. It is also applied generally to the mental processes by which instinctive but undesirable actions are checked by a process of self-control.

INJECTIONS (see ENEMA; and HYPODERMIC INJECTIONS).

INJURED, REMOVAL OF – A knowledge of the manner in which injured persons may best be removed from the spot where they have sustained the injury is of great importance, because careless or unskilful handling or moving may produce much pain and in some cases is liable to aggravate the bodily damage already done.

Precautions before removal – In the case of some injuries, such as that of the brain in apoplexy, or the perforation of the bowels caused by a bullet-wound of the abdomen, the less movement of the patient that takes place at first the better are his chances of recovery, and it is sometimes advisable that treatment should be carried out for some time near the spot where the injury has been sustained. When a bone has been broken it is essential that the fragments should be temporarily supported and made rigid by suitable devices before any attempt is made to change the patient's position (see FRACTURES). In other cases, as, for example, those of faintness, shock, immersion in water, some other form of first-aid treatment or the administration of stimulants is urgently necessary prior to removal. (See COLLAPSE; FAINTING; DROWNING; RECOVERY FROM; HAEMORRHAGE.) During removal an attendant must be constantly with the injured person, or at least the latter must be carried in such a way that one of the bearers constantly sees his face.

Position in removal – Severely injured persons, or those with any tendency to faintness, bleeding, shock or other general symptoms, should be carried lying at full length with the head slightly supported on a low pillow; a similar position should be adopted in the case of persons who have sustained any injury to the bones or joints of the lower limb, or of the shoulder-joint, or severe wounds of the head, chest or abdomen. On the other hand, injuries of the hand or forearm when properly supported, no matter how severe they may be, slight injuries of the foot, and uncomplicated wounds to the body, face or upper part of the body, permit generally of the patient either walking or being removed in the sitting posture, as by one of the forms of hand seat.

In wounds of the head care should be taken that the injured part does not press upon the stretcher.

In severe injuries to the back the greatest care must be exercised in lifting the patient, and some rigid though well-covered form of stretcher is to be preferred, upon which the patient is placed face downwards.

In fractures of the leg or thigh the

475

patient should lie upon his back inclined slightly towards the injured side and supported thus by a pillow, folded coat, or the like; in this position there is least jarring of the injured part.

In fractures of the upper limb, if the patient has to lie down, which is not usual, he should incline slightly towards the sound side, so that there is no risk of the body pressing the injured part.

In wounds or diseases of the chest there is often difficulty in breathing, which is relieved by propping the patient half up and turning him towards the affected side.

In painful conditions of the abdomen, or in the case of transverse or punctured wounds of this region, the patient should lie upon his back with the knees drawn well up and supported. In the case of a vertical wound of the abdomen the legs are kept straight.

The patient is usually carried feet first, but in going uphill or upstairs this position is reversed; in all cases, however, in which there is a fracture of the lower limb, the patient's head is kept lowest on a hill or stair so that the weight of the body may not press down upon the helpless and motionless part of the limb below the fracture. The taller bearer should be the farther down on the hill or stair.

No attempt should be made by inexperienced bearers to carry a stretcher over a wall or ditch, and on no account should a stretcher be carried upon the bearers' shoulders, because a fall may do very serious injury to the patient.

The stretcher should be carried at the full length of the bearers' arms, as horizontal as possible, and the bearers, though walking at an equal rate, must be careful not to keep in step, which causes the stretcher to swing painfully.

Care of unconscious patient – The unconscious patient must not be allowed to lie on his back. In this position he may suffocate. Particularly is this likely to occur if he should vomit or if there is any bleeding into the mouth or throat. The unconscious patient is unable to swallow properly and any blood or vomited material in the mouth drains into the lungs and interferes with breathing. Even if the patient does not actually suffocate, if such material as blood gets into the lungs it may have serious results. This means that the patient who is bleeding into the mouth or throat, as a result, for example, of a blow to the head or neck, should be treated in this respect as an unconscious patient.

Once the unconscious patient has been

removed from danger he should be placed in what is known as the semi-prone, or recovery, position (illustration 254). In this position the body lies on its side with the face turned towards the ground. To prevent the body rolling right over, both arms are bent at the elbows, and the upper, or top, leg is bent slightly at the hip and knees so that it falls forward over the lower, or under, leg.

Before rolling the patient into the semi-prone position it is essential to make sure that there are no fractures, especially of the spine. If there are, then the fractured part must be carefully supported as the patient is rolled over gently but firmly. In the case of the patient suspected of having a fractured spine, the whole body should be rolled over in one piece, without bending or twisting. If the unconscious patient has to be removed he should be placed on the stretcher in the semi-prone position.

There are certain other important rules to be observed in the management of the unconscious patient. No attempt should be

254 – Recovery position.

made to move him in the first instance if he is in no danger. If he wears false teeth, these should be removed, and any tight clothing, especially round the neck or waist, should be loosened. Under no circumstances should he be given any fluid by mouth, as he cannot swallow, and any fluid forced into his mouth will probably be breathed into the lungs, with serious consequences.

Method of removal depends upon (1) how many persons are available as bearers, and (2) the degree of assistance required by the patient, as already stated.

I. BY ONE BEARER – When an arm is injured the patient is usually quite able to walk, and, the arm being suitably supported, the bearer draws the patient's sound arm *over his shoulders* and places his own arm round the patient's waist (illustration 255).

If the bearer be strong and the patient seriously incapacitated, the latter may be carried *in the bearer's arms*, the right one passing beneath the patient's shoulder-blades, the left beneath the upper part of

255 – Removal of slightly injured person by one bearer.

farther; then stooping and pushing his head between the patient's right arm and his body, he allows the patient's body to fall over his right shoulder upon his back, while the patient's right arm comes round the bearer's neck and is steadied temporarily by his left hand (illustration 256). Finally, the bearer, passing his right arm round one or both thighs of the patient, grasps the patient's right wrist with his right hand, and bringing the weight of the body well on to the centre of his own back, rises to the erect position (illustration 256).

257 – Two-handed seat.

the thighs; in this case the patient should be carried high and supported as much upon the bearer's chest as by his arms. In other cases the patient may be carried *upon the bearer's back*, his arms round the bearer's neck and his legs under the bearer's arms.

In cases of complete unconsciousness, where the dead-weight of the patient's body must be raised and borne by one bearer, the method known as the *Fireman's Lift* is applicable. The patient is turned on his face, arms by the sides; the bearer stands at the patient's head, and, passing his hands beneath the latter's shoulders, raises him to a kneeling posture. The bearer next slides his hands under the patient's armpits and raises him still

256 – The fireman's lift.

II. BY TWO BEARERS WITH HAND SEATS – If the patient is suffering from such a condition as an injured foot and is able to give some assistance, and if there are two bearers, the bearers divide his weight by means of one of the forms of hand seats, of which the two-handed seat is the most useful. If the patient be more seriously injured, some form of stretcher must be obtained or improvised as described below.

For the *two-handed seat* (illustration 257) the bearers face one another, the one on the right interlocking the fingers of his right hand with those of the left hand of the other bearer; each places his disengaged hand behind the patient or on the other bearer's hip or shoulder. In lifting the patient, they kneel at his sides, each upon the knee nearest to his feet, and, forming the seat beneath his thighs, they rise together supporting him, while he assists if possible by putting his arms round their necks.

477

258 – Three-handed seat.

For the *three-handed seat* (illustration 258), the right-hand bearer grasps his own left forearm. The left-hand bearer places his right hand upon the shoulder of the other, and grasps the right forearm of the other with his left hand, his left forearm at the same time being grasped by the left hand of the other bearer.

For the *four-handed seat* (illustration 259), each bearer grasps his own left wrist with his right hand; each then clasps the disengaged right wrist of the other with his left hand. To carry a patient by the three-handed or four-handed seat the patient must stand up, and the bearers, stooping, form the seat behind him.

If a patient be absolutely helpless and it is urgently necessary to carry him quickly for a short distance only, the *fore-and-aft carry* may be used. One bearer stands at the patient's head and passes his hands

259 – Four-handed seat. (1) Method of formation; (2) seat ready.

behind the shoulders into the armpits, while the other bearer stands between the patient's legs facing towards his feet and takes one leg under each arm.

III. BY HELP OF A STRETCHER – If the patient be unable to walk or to sit upright in the conditions described, a stretcher must be obtained. If no regular canvas stretcher be at hand, a satisfactory one may be improvised from a pair of poles 6 or 7 feet (185 or 215 cm) in length and a couple of coats with the sleeves turned outside in. The coats are buttoned over the sleeves, through which the poles are

260 – Stretcher improvised from poles and two coats.

261 – Stretcher improvised from poles and a blanket. The edges are turned over in the order marked.

then passed (illustration 260). Or a blanket may be used, two poles, rifles or similar objects being laid upon it about 20 inches (50 cm) apart, and the ends and sides of the blanket being then successively folded over them (illustration 261). Various other articles, such as a light sofa or a window-shutter, or a blanket supported by four people, one at each corner, may also be used.

The patient having received suitable first-aid treatment is lifted on to the stretcher as follows:

(*a*) *When there are four bearers*, which is the ideal, one acts as leader. The others place themselves on one side of the

262 – The three-man lift.

patient, kneeling on the knee farthest from the head of the patient. They then place their hands and forearms under the patient as shown in illustration 262. When all are ready, at the word of command they simultaneously and carefully lift the patient on to their bent knees, taking care not to jolt the patient and to keep him absolutely straight. The leader then slips the stretcher under the patient and gives the order for the patient to be lowered on to it.

(*b*) *If only three bearers are available*, the same technique is used but, when the three bearers are all set with their arms under the patient, they then lift him directly – but just as carefully – on to the stretcher.

(*c*) *When only two bearers are available* the stretcher is placed close to the patient's head and in line with his body (illustration 263). The bearers then straddle the patient facing his head. One passes his arms under the shoulders, at the same time supporting the head. The other passes one arm under the buttocks and the other under the legs. When both are ready they gently lift the patient, walk over the stretcher and then gently lower the patient on to it.

IV. REMOVAL BY TRAILERS OR CARTS – If an ambulance in which the patient lies

263 – The two-man lift.

upon the stretcher is not obtainable, a trailer or cart, or lorry well furnished with springs in order to diminish jolting, forms a good substitute. If the patient cannot sit, the floor of the trailer or cart should be deeply covered with straw or with a mattress. To place the stretcher in the trailer or cart, it should be raised by four bearers, one taking an end of each pole. The head end of the stretcher is then rested upon the floor of the trailer or cart, and two of the bearers get in and assist the others in lifting the stretcher in. The patient may then either be lifted off on to the straw, or may be left on the stretcher.

INOCULATION is the process by which infective material is brought into the system through a small wound in the skin or in a mucous membrane. Many infectious diseases and blood-poisoning are contracted by accidental inoculation of microbes. Inoculation is now used as a preventive measure against many infectious diseases. (See VACCINE.)

INOSITOL is one of the components of the vitamin B complex. Deficiency in mice produces baldness, but little is known yet about its rôle in human nutrition.

INSANITY (see MENTAL ILLNESS).

INSECT REPELLENTS are substances which repel insects and prevent their landing on the skin. (See DIBUTYL PHTHALATE; DIMETHYL PHTHALATE.)

INSECTICIDES are substances which are fatal to insects. Since the discovery of the insecticidal properties of DDT in 1940, a steady stream of new ones has been introduced, and their combined use has played an outstanding part in international public health campaigns, such as that of the World Health Organization for the eradication of malaria.

Unfortunately, insects are liable to become resistant to insecticides, just as bacteria are liable to become resistant to antibiotics, and it is for this reason that so much research work is being devoted to the discovery of new ones.

It is against this beneficial background that must be viewed the increasing evidence that the indiscriminate use of some of these potent preparations is having an adverse effect, not only upon human beings, but also upon the balance of nature. The solution to this problem, as

479

to so many other comparable problems, is to be found in a closer observation of the old rule about the golden mean. Without such insecticides, herbicides and the like mankind would be in imminent danger from starvation or disease, but they must be used with discrimination and only under skilled supervision.

The following are some of the more common insecticides now in use, brief notes on which will be found under the name of the substance: benzene hexachloride, chlordane, DDT, dieldrin, parathion, malathion.

INSECTS IN RELATION TO DISEASE – Many insects play an important part in the transmission of infectious diseases. Thus, flies by their feet and their feeding habits carry the organisms which cause typhoid fever, the tsetse fly spreads sleeping sickness, mosquitoes transmit the germs of malaria and yellow fever, fleas convey plague germs and lice convey typhus fever and one form of relapsing fever. In addition, these creatures are nuisances as well as dangers.

HOUSE-FLY (*Musca domestica*) – This fly lays its eggs in manure, or in moist, fermenting vegetable matter. The maggot is hatched in eight hours to two days, feeds on the manure, passes through the pupa stage in anything from a few days to four weeks, and, becoming a fly, is capable of egg-laying about three weeks from its own appearance as an egg. As 120 to 150 eggs are laid in a batch by each female fly, this fly is capable, under the most favourable conditions, of producing over half-a-million progeny within her life of three months. The fly gorges on fluid food which it sucks up by means of its proboscis, and it has the habit of repeatedly vomiting and re-swallowing the contents of its crop as it feeds. It walks in filth habitually, and being provided with hairy legs and body it is apt to carry off portions of this, in which are entangled numbers of bacteria. The fly has been well described as a 'winged sponge', and its immense power to distribute disease germs over the surface of uncovered food is evident.

BLOW-FLY or *BLUE-BOTTLE* (*Calliphora erythrocephala*) lays its eggs (450 to 600 in number) on meat, fish or decaying animal matter. The maggot hatches out within a day, passes through the pupa stage and becomes a full-grown fly in about three weeks. Its habits are similar to those of the house-fly, though in numbers it is much less plentiful.

Treatment of flies – The most important measure is to destroy their breeding grounds near human dwellings. All kitchen refuse must be burned, and none should be left exposed so that flies may deposit their eggs in it. Stable litter and manure must be disposed of, or kept covered and shut up in outhouses, not allowed to accumulate in the open air and sunshine near houses. Adult flies may be destroyed to a great extent by proper protection and storage of all food. DDT (qv), which may be used as a powder, a spray or a paint, has established itself as a most efficient means of treatment, but care must be exercised that it does not come in contact with food.

LICE – There are three lice which infest man: the body louse (*Pediculus corporis*), the head louse (*Pediculus capitis*) and the crab louse (*Phthirus pubis*). The head louse is by far the most common in Britain and adults. Infestation is most common in children under school age, but it is not unusual in adults. In schoolchildren it seems to be ineradicable: a recent survey in England showed that 2·44 per cent (193,806) of the secondary and primary school population were infested. In some areas the incidence is as high as 10 per cent. It used to be much commoner in girls than boys, but this sex difference is disappearing – presumably because of the current fashion for longer hair among boys. Incidentally, a very good argument for discouraging this fashion. Head lice spread by close human contact. (See also under PARASITES.)

Treatment of lice – In individuals infested with the body louse the clothing should be dusted with 10 per cent DDT, packed in a bag and then sent for washing or storing. A temperature of 129° F (54° C) is rapidly lethal to both lice and their eggs. At a temperature of −4° F (−20° C) lice are killed in half-an-hour and eggs are killed in five hours. As the lice tend to congregate into the seams, hot ironing these is a useful measure.

For body lice a hot bath followed by thorough powdering with 10 per cent DDT powder in the form of Dicophane Dusting-Powder BPC, is effective: three dustings at weekly intervals. Calamine lotion containing 1 per cent phenol eases the itching. For crab lice, the affected area is rubbed with either Dicophane Application BPC, or Gamma Benzene Hexachloride Application BPC which is left on for two days, and the process then repeated. For head lice, one tablespoonful of Gamma Benzene Hexachloride Application BPC should be rubbed with the fingers into the hair and its roots and left for twenty-four hours. The hair is then washed. This may need to be repeated twice or three times. The hair is then carefully combed with a fine comb to remove the nits. Removal may be easier if the hairs are rubbed previously with a swab soaked in vinegar. Unfortunately the head louse is becoming resistant to Gamma Benzene Hexachloride, which is therefore being replaced by Malathion (qv). This is applied in a 0·5 per cent solution in spirit until the scalp is thoroughly moist. The hair is then allowed to dry naturally without the use of any heat. After twelve hours the hair is shampooed and combed with a fine metal comb while wet to remove the dead nits. Only one such treatment is usually necessary, but all close contacts including the mother of the infested child should be examined and treated forthwith with malathion if infested. Only in this way can the infestation be eradicated from the family.

FLEAS – *Pulex irritans* is the common flea that afflicts mankind. *Xenopsylla cheopis* is the rat flea that conveys *Pasteurella pestis*, the causative organism of plague, from rat to man. The flea lays its eggs singly. They take two to four days in summer, two weeks in winter, to hatch into larvae which are fully grown in a fortnight. The larva then becomes a pupa from which the adult emerges two weeks later. The flea can survive alive for a long time without food.

Treatment of fleas – Human beings vary tremendously in their susceptibility to flea bites. For those who are susceptible the best preventive is dimethyl phthallate sprayed on the trousers or socks where it is effective for several days. In the absence of dimethyl phthallate, alternative methods of prevention are the smearing of the skin with oil of pennyroyal, or oil of lavender, or dusting the socks and underclothing with pyrethrum powder, menthol or camphor. For disinfestation of buildings, a 5 per cent solution of DDT in kerosene is effective: 2 quarts (2·25 litres) per 1000 square feet (82 square metres). For bedding a powder containing 10 per cent DDT, or 0·5 per cent gamma benzene hexachloride, is effective.

BED BUGS (*Cimex lectulatius*) are best got rid of by a 5 per cent solution of DDT in kerosene, with or without the addition of pyrethrum. The amount required is 100 mg of DDT per square foot (9·3 square decimetres). (See BED BUG.)

MOSQUITOES – One of these (*Anopheles gambiae*) is responsible for conveying the parasite of malaria (illustration

264 – *Anopheles gambiae*. The most dangerous malaria-carrier in Africa. From Manson's *Tropical Diseases*. Cassell & Co. Ltd.

265 – *Aedes aegypti* (female). The transmitter of yellow fever and dengue. From Manson's *Tropical Diseases*, Cassell & Co. Ltd.

264), another (*Aedes aegypti*) for distributing the infection of yellow fever (illustration 265).

Treatment of mosquitoes – See under MALARIA; and YELLOW FEVER.

INSOLATION is a term applied both to treatment by exposure to the sun's rays (see LIGHT TREATMENT) and to fever caused by excessive heat (see SUNSTROKE).

INSOMNIA (see SLEEP; HYPNOTICS).

INSPISSATION is a term applied to the process of the drying or thickening fluids or excretions by evaporation.

481

INSUFFLATION means the blowing of powder or vapour into a cavity, especially through the air passages, for the treatment of disease.

INSULIN is the name applied to the internal secretion of the pancreas formed by groups of cells called the islands of Langerhans in this organ. Its existence was indicated by Schafer in 1909, and it was successfully isolated in a pure form by McLeod, Banting and Best in 1921. It acts by enabling the muscles and other tissues which require sugar for their activity to take up this substance from the blood. When it is deficient, the sugar derived from the food accumulates in the blood and is wastefully excreted in the urine. Insulin prepared from the pancreas of pigs and oxen is administered by hypodermic injection in cases of diabetes mellitus (qv), and thus enables the sugar in the circulation to be utilized so that its excretion in the urine ceases. Each unit of insulin administered to a diabetic patient enables him to utilize somewhere between one and two grams of additional carbohydrate material. The appropriate dose of insulin in any given case depends upon its severity.

Ten forms of insulin are included in the *British Pharmacopoeia* 1973. *Addendum* 1978: insulin injection; biphasic insulin injection; globin zinc insulin injection; isophane insulin injection; isophane propionate insulin injection; neutral insulin injection; protamine zinc insulin injection; insulin zinc suspension; insulin zinc suspension (amorphous); insulin zinc suspension (crystalline). The essential difference between them lies in the duration of their action.

There are two preparations of Neutral insulin injection: Nuso made from beef insulin and Actrapid made from pig insulin. In addition there are three very highly purified pork insulin preparations. Actrapid MC which is neutral insulin injection (monocomponent insulin); Semitard MC which is insulin zinc suspension amorphous (monocomponent insulin); and Monotard MC which is insulin zinc suspension (monocomponent insulin). These pure monospecies insulin are of value in that small minority of diabetics who develop hypersensitivity to beef or pig insulin, or who develop resistance to neutral insulin injection. Around 70 per cent of the raw material for insulin production is of bovine origin. It is a *British Pharmacopoeia* requirement that the species of origin shall be shown in the packaging of all insulin preparations.

INTELLIGENCE QUOTIENT, or IQ as it is usually known, is the ratio between the mental age and chronological age multiplied by 100. Thus, if a boy of 10 years of age is found to have a mental age of 12 years, his IQ will be:

$$\frac{12}{10} \times 100 = 120.$$

On the other hand, if he is found to have a mental age of 8 years his IQ will be:

$$\frac{8}{10} \times 100 = 80.$$

The mental age is established by various tests, the most widely used of which are the Stanford-Binet Scale, the Wechseer Adult Intelligence Scale, and the Mill Hill Vocabulary Test.

Average intelligence is represented by an IQ of 100, with a range of 85 to 115. For practical purposes it is taken that the intellectual level reached by the average 15-year-old is indistinguishable from that of an adult.

INTERCOSTAL is the term applied to the nerves, vessels and muscles that lie between the ribs, as well as to diseases affecting these structures.

INTERCURRENT is a term applied to one disease which occurs during the course of another disease already present, and modifies its course or increases its severity.

INTERFERON – It has been known for many years that one virus will interfere with the growth of another. In 1957, workers at the National Institute for Medical Research, in London, isolated the factor that was responsible for this interfering of one virus with another. They gave it the name of interferon. The precise nature of interferon is not yet known, but it is known to be a protein. Its practical interest lies in the possibility that it may prove to be a useful method of treating diseases caused by viruses.

INTERMITTENT is a term applied to fevers which continue for a time, subside completely and then return again. The name is also used in connection with a pulse in which occasional heart-beats are not felt, in consequence of irregular action of the heart.

INTERMITTENT CLAUDICATION is a condition occurring in middle-aged and elderly people, which is characterized by pain in the legs after walking a certain distance. The pain is relieved by resting for a short time. It is due to arteriosclerosis (see ARTERIES, DISEASES OF) of the arteries to the leg, which results in inadequate blood supply to the muscles.

INTERSEXUALITY is the condition resulting from faulty sex differentiation during the development of the foetus. Although not a common condition, it is one that is now recognized should be diagnosed as early as possible in life in order that an early decision may be reached as to the sex of the child, or at least the sex he (or she) is to be brought up as. Equally important is it that any treatment that may be possible should be instituted at the optimum moment.

INTERSTITIAL is a term applied to indifferent tissue set among the proper active tissue of an organ. It is generally of a supporting character and formed of fibrous tissue. The term is also applied to diseases which specially affect this tissue, such as interstitial keratitis. (See EYE, DISEASES OF.)

INTERTRIGO is a term applied to a chafed or abraded condition between two surfaces of skin that rub together: eg. under the breast or between the toes, in the armpit. (See ATHLETE'S FOOT; CHAFING OF THE SKIN.)

INTESTINAL STASIS (see STASIS; and CONSTIPATION).

INTESTINE is the whole of the alimentary canal situated below the stomach. In it the chief part of digestion is carried on, and through its walls all the food material is absorbed into the blood and lymph streams. (See DIGESTION.) The length of the intestine in man is about 28 to 30 feet (8·5 to 9 metres), and it takes the form of one continuous tube suspended in loops in the abdominal cavity.
Divisions – The intestine is divided into small intestine and large intestine (illustration 266). The former comprises that part of the tube which extends from the stomach onwards for 22 feet (6·5 metres) or thereabout, and at its broadest point is about 1½ inches (35 mm) in width. The large intestine is the second part of the tube, and though shorter (about 6 feet (1·8 metres) in length) is much wider than

the small intestine, reaching in places a width of 2½ inches (65 mm). The *small intestine* is divided rather arbitrarily into three parts: the *duodenum*, consisting of the first 10 or 12 inches (25 or 30 cm), into which the ducts of the liver and pancreas open; the *jejunum*, which is generally found empty after death, and comprises

266 – Diagram of the stomach and intestines. S, stomach; D, duodenum, J, jejunum, and I, ileum, together forming the small intestine; AV, appendix, C, caecum, AC, ascending colon, HF, hepatic flexure, TC, transverse colon, SF, splenic flexure, DC, descending colon, Sg, sigmoid flexure, R, rectum, together forming the large intestine; G, gall-bladder; H, hepatic ducts; DC, common bile-duct; P, pancreatic duct.

Lips of
ileocaecal valve

Frenulum of
valve

Orifice of
vermiform
appendix

Ileum

Vermiform
appendix

267 – The interior of the caecum and lower end of the ascending colon showing the appendix. From *Gray's Anatomy*. Longman.

the next 8 or 9 feet (2·4 or 2·7 metres); and finally the *ileum*, which at its lower end opens into the large intestine.

The *large intestine* begins in the lower part of the abdomen on the right side. The first part is known as the caecum, and into this opens the *appendix vermiformis* (illustration 267). The appendix is a small tube, about the thickness of a quill, from 2 to 20 cm (average 9 cm) in length, which has much the same structure as the rest of the intestine. At one end it is closed, at the other it opens into the caecum, and although it appears to play little or no part in digestion, it is of great importance because of the frequency with which serious inflammation takes place in it. (See APPENDICITIS.) The caecum is continued into the colon. This is subdivided into: the *ascending colon* which ascends through the right flank to beneath the liver; the *transverse colon* which crosses the upper part of

the abdomen transversely to the left side; the *descending colon* which bends downwards and descends through the left flank into the pelvis where it becomes the *sigmoid* colon. The last part of the large intestine is known as the *rectum*, which passes straight down through the back part of the pelvis, to open to the exterior through the *anus*.

Structure – The intestine, both small and large, consists of four coats, which vary slightly in structure and arrangement at different points, but are of the same general nature throughout the entire length of the bowel. On the inner surface there is a mucous membrane; outside this is a loose submucous coat, in which blood-vessels run; next comes a muscular coat in two layers; and finally a tough, thin peritoneal membrane. The total thickness of all four coats amounts to about one-eighth of an inch (3 mm).

MUCOUS COAT – The interior of the bowel is completely lined by a single layer of pillar-like cells placed side by side. These rest upon a smooth, fine membrane, beneath which is a loose network of connective tissue and muscular fibres, richly supplied with blood-vessels and lymphatic-vessels. There are two arrangements by which the surface in the small intestine is much increased for the purposes of digestion and absorption. Countless ridges with deep furrows between them run across the upper part, and the whole surface is thickly studded with short hair-like processes called villi (illustration 268). As blood- and lymph-vessels run up to the end of these villi, the digested food passing

268 – Diagrammatic representation of intestine. A, small intestine (magnified 15 times), B, duodenum (magnified 12 times); 1, intestinal glands; 2, muscularis mucosae; 3, submucous coat; 4, circular muscles; 5, longitudinal muscles; 6, peritoneum; 7, lymph follicles; 8, villi; 9, duodenal gland. From Blacklock and Southwell, *A Guide to Human Parasitology*. H. K. Lewis & Co. Ltd.

slowly down the intestine is brought into very close relation with the circulation. Between the bases of the villi are set little openings, each of which leads into a simple, tubular gland lined by cells, which are similar to those covering the surface, and which produce a fluid with digestive powers. In the small intestine, cells here and there produce mucus, and, in the large intestine, a great number of cells are devoted to the production of this substance for lubricating the passage of the food through the bowel. A large number of minute masses, called lymph follicles, similar in structure to the tonsils and lymphatic glands, are scattered over the inner surface of the intestine. In the lower part of the small intestine these are grouped into patches of a square inch or thereabout in size, known as Peyer's patches, which are of special interest, because the inflammation and ulceration of the bowels that occur in typhoid fever is limited to them and to the scattered follicles. The large intestine is bare both of ridges and of villi, and, as already stated, its mucous membrane produces mucus in large amount.

SUBMUCOUS COAT – This consists of a loose connective tissue which allows the mucous membrane to play freely over the muscular coat. The blood-vessels and lymphatic-vessels which absorb the food in the villi pour their contents into a network of large vessels lying in this coat.

MUSCULAR COAT – The muscle in the small intestine is arranged in two definite layers, in the outer of which all the fibres run lengthwise with the bowel, whilst in the inner they pass circularly round it. The muscular coat is of immense importance, because by its contraction and relaxation, somewhat after the mode of progression of a worm, the food is slowly squeezed down the bowel, the process being known as peristalsis. In the large intestine the only departure from this arrangement is that the fibres which are placed lengthwise are collected into three thick bands upon the outward surface of the bowel, and these bands, being slightly shorter than the other coats of the bowel, cause it to present a puckered appearance.

PERITONEAL COAT forms the outer covering for almost the whole intestine except parts of the duodenum and of the large intestine. It is a tough, fibrous membrane, covered upon its outer surface with a smooth layer of cells, which in the movements of the bowel rub against a similar surface upon the peritoneum lining the general cavity of the abdomen, and so cause a minimum of friction. From the peritoneal coat of the intestine of animals catgut is prepared.

Support – The duodenum and greater part of the large intestine are covered only in front by the peritoneum which lines the abdominal cavity, and this tough membrane serves to bind these parts of the intestine firmly against the back wall of the abdomen. The jejunum and ileum, the transverse colon, and the first part of the rectum are not only completely surrounded by peritoneum, but a double layer of this membrane suspends these parts of the bowel at a distance of several inches from the lines on the back of the abdomen, where the two layers become continuous with the rest of the peritoneum. In this way freedom is given to the movements of these parts of the bowels. These suspending structures are known as mesenteries. That of the small intestine is the largest, being shaped like a fan, 8 inches (200 mm) long at its attached margin, and spreading out to 22 feet (6·5 metres) at its frilled border, where it meets the intestine. The vessels and nerves which supply the intestine run between the two layers of the mesentery.

INTESTINE, DISEASES OF – The principal signs of trouble which has its origin in the intestines consist of pain somewhere about the abdomen, sometimes vomiting, and irregularity in movement of the bowels in the direction either of stoppage or of excessive action.

Several diseases are treated under separate headings. See APPENDICITIS; CHOLERA; COLITIS; CONCRETIONS; CONSTIPATION; DIARRHOEA; DYSENTERY; ENTERIC FEVER; HERNIA; ILEITIS; INTUSSUSCEPTION; IRRITABLE COLON; PARASITES; PERITONITIS; PILES; RECTUM, DISEASES OF.

INFLAMMATION of the bowel may affect either its outer or its inner surface. The outer surface is covered by peritoneum, and peritonitis is a serious disease. (See PERITONITIS.) Inflammation of the inner surface is known generally as enteritis, inflammations of special parts receiving the names of colitis, appendicitis, and the like. Enteritis may form the chief symptom of certain infective diseases due to special organisms: for example in typhoid fever, cholera, dysentery. Again, it may be acute, though not connected with any definite organism, when, if severe, it is a very serious condition, particularly in young children. Or it may be chronic, especially as the result of dysentery, and then constitutes a less serious though very troublesome complaint. Indiscretions in diet, such as the eating of unripe fruit, are a not uncommon cause. A very serious type results from the action of irritant poisons. In some persons inflammation of the stomach and bowels is liable to result from exposure to cold and damp.

Symptoms – Diarrhoea is the most common and most marked symptom, and in chronic cases usually the only symptom, although, when the small intestine alone is affected, constipation is a more usual result than diarrhoea. Pain, particularly of a griping nature, which comes and goes, is also common. The temperature in acute cases is raised, and there is restlessness, even delirium. If the diarrhoea is very profuse, collapse speedily comes on.

Treatment – Each case requires special handling, according to the cause and the severity. Where diarrhoea is very severe this requires special treatment. (See DIARRHOEA.) There are a few general principles which are applicable to all cases. The diet should be light, bland, non-irritating and containing a minimum of roughage. In more acute cases only milk and glucose drinks should be given for the first twenty-four hours. If there is much diarrhoea ample fluids should be given to prevent dehydration. Rest in bed is essential. Considerable quantities of warm water, containing bicarbonate of soda, have a beneficial action by flushing out the bowel and removing irritating substances. In general, water is given by the mouth, but in some cases it is introduced by an enema to irrigate the lower bowel. Various drugs which have a mildly astringent and soothing action, of which the chief are bismuth carbonate and kaolin, are given by the mouth. When the inflammation is not the result of a chemical or physical irritant, but the result of an infection, as in dysentery, treatment with a sulphonamide drug absorbed only slowly from the intestine is indicated. Phthalylsulphathiazole, succinylsulphathiazole and sulphadimidine have proved particularly useful in the treatment of dysentery.

ULCERATION of the bowels arises in a manner similar to the production of ulcers on the skin surface, although, probably these internal ulcers heal much more rapidly than others. Typhoid fever regularly produces ulcers in the lower part of the small intestine, this variety arising in the patches of lymphatic tissue found in this region. Tuberculous ulcers arise late in the course of tuberculosis, and produce a diarrhoea which is always a serious sign.

Ulceration also occurs in amoebic dysentery.

Symptoms of ulceration are much the same as those of enteritis, and the formation of ulcers is simply an advanced stage of this condition. In addition, the ulcerated surface is apt to bleed, and, if the ulcer be situated high up in the bowel, this blood is voided as black or brown material; if it comes from near the lower end of the bowel the blood is red and unchanged. The healing of these ulcers leads, in the case of all save those of typhoid fever, to the formation of scars, and, as these scars contract there is a tendency to narrowing of the bowel and obstruction. This is particularly apt to follow tuberculous ulcers, if these should heal, because they often run circularly round the inside of the bowel.

Treatment in cases of ulceration is similar to that for inflammation.

PERFORATION of the bowel may take place as the result either of injury or of disease. Stabs and other wounds which penetrate the abdomen may damage the bowel, and severe blows or crushes may tear it without any external wound. Ulceration, as in typhoid fever, or, more rarely, in tuberculosis, may cause an opening in the bowel-wall also. Again, when the bowel is greatly distended above an obstruction, faecal material may accumulate and produce ulcers, which rupture with the ordinary movements of the bowels. Whatever be the cause, the symptoms are much the same.

Symptoms – The contents of the bowel pass out through the perforation into the peritoneal cavity, and, making their way between the coils of intestine, set up a general peritonitis. In consequence, the abdomen is painful, and after a few hours becomes extremely tender to the touch, as a result of the peritonitis. The abdomen swells, particularly in its upper part, owing to gas having passed also into the cavity. Vomiting is a symptom, and the person passes into a state of collapse. Such a condition is almost invariably fatal in two, or at most three, days, if not promptly treated. Occasionally, however, the perforation is preceded by a certain amount of peritonitis, which forms adhesions in the neighbourhood of the ulcerated part, so that when perforation finally takes place a localized abscess, instead of general peritonitis, may result, and the person may recover.

Treatment – All food should be withheld, because whatever is taken into the stomach is either vomited or is liable to pass out of the perforation into the peritoneal cavity. An operation is urgently necessary, the abdomen being opened in the middle line, the perforated portion of bowel found, and the perforation stitched up. If the bowel be damaged badly, a part is often cut out and the divided ends joined together. Finally, the peritoneal cavity is thoroughly washed out, and a drainage tube left for some days in the abdominal wound. The local application of penicillin or sulphonamides to the peritoneum during operation has effected a marked reduction in the mortality rate.

OBSTRUCTION of the bowels means a stoppage to the passage down the intestine of the partially digested food. Obstruction may be due either to some cause within the abdomen or to the thrusting of a loop of bowel through an opening in the wall of this cavity. The latter class of cases has been referred to under HERNIA. Obstruction may be acute when it comes on suddenly with intense symptoms, or it may be chronic, when the obstructing cause gradually increases and the bowel becomes slowly more narrow till it closes altogether, or when slight obstruction comes and goes till it ends in an acute attack. In chronic cases the symptoms are much the same as those of the acute variety, although they are milder in degree and more prolonged.

Causes – Obstruction may be due to causes outside the bowel altogether, for example, the pressure of tumours in neighbouring organs, the twisting round the bowel of bands produced by former peritonitis, or even the twisting of a coil of intestine round itself so as to cause a kink in its wall. Chronic and partial forms of obstruction are sometimes due to such kinks near the end of the small intestine, sometimes to the pressure of the mesentery on the upper end of the small intestine. Chronic causes of the obstruction may exist in the wall of the bowel itself: for example, a tumour, or the contracting scar of an old ulcer. The condition of intussusception (qv), where part of the bowel passes inside of the part beneath it, in the same way as one turns the finger of a glove outside in, causes obstruction and other symptoms. Finally some body, such as a concretion, or the stone of some large fruit, or even a mass of hardened faeces, may become jammed within the bowel and stop up its passage.

Symptoms – There are four chief symptoms of this condition, and any case in which these are combined demands immediate treatment. These are pain, vomiting, constipation and swelling of the abdomen. The *pain* is of a griping character, and may be very severe although it comes and goes, getting now stronger and again for a time less marked. When the small intestine is the seat of obstruction the pain is almost always referred to the region round the navel; when the large intestine is affected the pain may be more accurately referred to the part from which it arises. In addition to this, acute cases are marked by great tenderness of the abdomen to touch. The *vomiting* is peculiar in character. It begins with the first onset of pain, and consists of the contents of the stomach. Later it is yellow or green, bitter, and contains much bile, while, after several hours have elapsed, it becomes brown and ill-smelling, and is then known as faecal vomiting. The *constipation* in acute cases comes on suddenly, whilst in chronic cases it may be preceded by a state in which constipation and diarrhoea alternate, or by one in which the stools gradually get smaller and smaller in size, possibly over a period lasting for several months. In chronic cases of obstruction to the large intestine, it is not uncommon for the sufferer to possess a constant desire to go to stool with straining pain, although he can pass nothing (tenesmus). In some conditions, particularly that due to intussusception, though there is constipation in the ordinary sense, the excessive straining produces a copious discharge of blood-stained mucus. The *swelling of the abdomen* varies in different cases. In acute cases the whole belly is blown up with gas, much increasing the pain of the condition. The constipation is so complete as to prevent even flatus from being passed – a very important sign of its gravity. Another grave sign is the absence of the sounds of intestinal movement which can be heard on auscultation over the normal abdomen. In chronic cases, in which the wall of the intestine is thickened, individual loops stand out now and then and become visible on the surface in their attempts to force their contents past the obstruction. When the small intestine is affected, its loops stand out one over the other, resembling the rungs of a ladder; whilst obstruction low down in the large intestine causes a bulging in the flanks and across the upper part of the abdomen.

In addition to these abdominal symptoms, in the later stages there is generally collapse, although consciousness is retained till the end. If the condition be not relieved by operation, death almost always results: in acute cases, in the course of three to six days.

Treatment – As a rule the surgeon opens the abdomen, finds the obstruction and relieves it or if possible removes it altogether. The task of the surgeon is rendered specially hard by the difficulty of determining, before he opens the abdomen, where the obstruction is, by the fact that the intestine is inflamed, and by its distension with gas and faeces. He has generally to open the abdomen in the middle line, examine the usual sites of obstruction, and, failing to find any cause at these points, to pass the whole length of intestine carefully through his hands till he finds the obstruction. Even after this is found, if it be of the nature of a tumour, it may be impossible of removal. If the obstruction be successfully removed, something must next be done, by puncturing the bowel or other means, to relieve the collection of gas and faeces, and this adds to the operation the great risk of sepsis. The introduction of the sulphonamides and antibiotics, however, has diminished this risk considerably. In all these manipulations care must be taken, by warm towels and the like, to prevent unnecessary exposure and chilling of the bowel.

TUMOURS are relatively uncommon in the small intestine and, when they do occur, they are usually benign. Conversely, they are relatively common in the large intestine where they are usually cancerous. In 1976, in England there were 16,246 deaths from cancer of the intestine, 5892 of these growths being in the rectum. The most common site for cancer of the large intestine is the rectum, with the sigmoid, caecum and ascending colon next in order of frequency. It is a disease of the older age-groups, and occurs with equal frequency in men and women. A history of altered bowel habit, in the form of increasing constipation or diarrhoea, or an alternation of these, or of bleeding from the anus, in a middle-aged person is an indication for taking medical advice. If the condition is cancer, then the sooner it is operated on, the better the result.

INTIMA is the innermost coat lining the arteries and the veins.

INTOXICATION is a term applied to states of poisoning. The poison may be some chemical substance introduced from outside, eg. alcohol (see ALCOHOLISM), or it may be due to the products of bacterial action, the bacteria either being introduced from outside or developing within the body. The term, auto-intoxication, is applied in the latter case.

INTRACRANIAL is the term applied to structures, diseases, and the like, contained in or rising within the head.

INTRATHECAL means within the membranes or meninges which envelop the spinal cord. The intrathecal space, between the arachnoid and the pia mater, contains the cerebrospinal fluid.

INTRA-UTERINE DEVICES (see CONTRACEPTION).

INTROSPECTION is a term applied to observation of one's own thoughts or feelings. It is generally applied to this process when it occurs to an abnormal extent in association with melancholia.

INTUBATION is a simple operation, consisting in the introduction, through the mouth into the larynx, of a tube designed to keep the air passage open at this point.

INTUSSUSCEPTION is a form of obstruction of the bowels in which part of the intestine enters within that part immediately beneath it. This can best be understood by observing what takes place in the fingers of a tightly fitting glove as they turn outside in when the glove is pulled off the hand. The persons affected are almost always infants. The cause is not known. The point at which it most often occurs is the junction between the small and the large intestines, the former passing within the latter. The symptoms are those of intestinal obstruction in general, and in addition there is often a discharge of blood-stained mucus from the bowel. The treatment consists – unless the symptoms rapidly subside, when it may be assumed that the bowel has righted itself – of either hydrostatic reduction by means of a barium enema, or an operation. At operation the intussusception is either reduced or if this not possible, the obstructed part is cut out and the ends of the intestine then stitched together. If treated adequately and in time, the mortality is now reduced to around 1 per cent.

INUNCTION is a method of administering drugs by rubbing them into the skin mixed with oil or fat. The method is not often used now.

IN VITRO is a term commonly used in medical research and experimental biology. Literally 'in a glass', it refers to observations made outside the body: eg. on the action of drugs on bacteria. The opposite term is IN VIVO, which refers to observations of processes in the body.

INVOLUCRUM is the term applied to the sheath of new bone which is formed round a piece of dead bone in, for example, osteomyelitis.

INVOLUTION is the term which describes the process of change whereby the uterus returns to its resting size after parturition. The term is also applied to any retrograde biological change, as in senility.

IODIDES are salts of iodine; those which are especially used in medicine being the iodide of potassium and iodide of sodium.

Action – Iodides have a threefold action. They are excreted in the mucus secretions, as well as in the urine, saliva and sweat, and have an action in liquefying the mucus secretion of the bronchial tree. They are therefore used in expectorant mixtures. Their second action is in assisting to absorb diseased tissue, particularly in syphilis. Finally, they are used to assist in providing a supply of iodine in patients with goitre, or in individuals who live in an area where goitre is liable to occur because of a deficiency of iodine in the drinking water. (See GOITRE.)

Over-dosage of iodides results in iodism (qv).

Uses – At one time the chief use of the drug was to cause absorption of the unhealthy tissues in syphilis, upon which it acted with great rapidity when taken into the system. It is used for a similar reason in chronic forms of rheumatism. Iodides are given in chronic lead-poisoning, because they dissolve the lead deposited in the tissues and so permit of its excretion from the body. They are also a common constituent of expectorant mixtures. Iodide is administered over long periods in small doses to children living in districts where goitre is common, with the object of preventing the onset of this disease.

IODINE is a non-metallic element which is found largely in seaweed. It is prepared in the form of dark violet-brown scales. It has a pleasantly pungent smell and a burning taste. It has a highly irritating action and when applied to the skin, stains the latter dark brown and causes it to peel off in flakes, while internally it is a violent irritant poison in large doses.

Uses – Externally iodine is used as an antiseptic. Its only drawback in this respect is that it is fixed by protein, which reduces its antiseptic efficiency in open wounds. Its main use in this sphere therefore is for sterilizing the unbroken skin, as before an operation. For this the Weak Iodine Solution BP, which contains 2·5 per cent iodine, is used. This solution is also used as a preventive of chilblains, applied while the hands are still red before the skin has begun to crack.

In the form of Mandl's paint (ie. dissolved with potassium iodide in glycerin) iodine is a useful remedy in inflammatory conditions of the throat and tonsils. Small doses of the weak iodine solution (2 to 5 drops) often control vomiting when other measures fail; for this purpose it is usually given in milk. Iodine – often as Aqueous Iodine Solution BP, or Lugol's solution as it is sometimes known (5 per cent iodine and 10 per cent potassium iodide in water) – is given internally in the treatment of goitre, especially before the operation of thyroidectomy for Graves' disease.

IODISM is the condition which is produced by an over-dose of iodides, but in some susceptible individuals iodism may be produced by very small amounts of iodides. It is characterized by running of the eyes and nose, sore throat, a heavy, dull feeling over the eyes, increased secretion of saliva and a typical skin eruption. These manifestations usually disappear rapidly upon the drug being withdrawn.

IODOFORM is a mild antiseptic made by the action of iodine upon a mixture of alcohol and potash. It has a most penetrating, not unpleasant odour and strong taste. It relieves pain when applied to a raw or mucous surface, and has the property of preventing putrefaction when brought in contact with discharges. When applied in large quantities to a raw surface it is apt to be absorbed and to cause symptoms of poisoning, consisting of a red rash over the body, fever, loss of appetite and, it may be, delirium.

Uses – Because of its combined analgesic and antiseptic properties, it is a useful application for ulcers and granulating wounds. In the form of Bipp (qv) it was a popular wound dressing in the 1914–18 War. It is also sometimes used as an insufflation in the treatment of ozaena and ulcers of the mouth.

ION EXCHANGE RESINS are synthetic organic substances which have the power of exchanging ions. Chemically, they are closely related to plastics. They are divided into two groups: *cation exchange resins*, which take up and liberate cations, eg. sodium, potassium, hydrogen ions; *anion exchange resins*, which take up and liberate anions, eg. chloride, hydroxyl ions. The former are used in the treatment of oedema, and the latter in the treatment of peptic ulcers.

IONIZATION means the breaking up of a substance in solution into its constituent ions.

IONTOPHORESIS is the process by which various substances are made to pass through the skin into the underlying tissues by means of the electric current. This. is also called iontherapy, galvanoionization and medical ionization. Only those drugs can be used for ionization which are soluble in water and can be dissociated when dissolved. They include inorganic salts and similar organic compounds such as salts of the alkaloids and salts of organic acids like salicylate of soda. The form of electricity used for ionization is the continuous current. Iontophoresis is largely restricted nowadays to its use as a means of alleviating rheumatic pains. Among the substances used for this purpose are sodium chloride, sodium salicylate and histamine. Zinc ionization is sometimes used for the treatment of nasal allergy.

IOPANOIC ACID is an organic iodine preparation which is radio-opaque and is used to visualize the gall-bladder on X-rays, as it is excreted in the bile. It is given by mouth.

IPECACUANHA, IPECAC, or HIPPO, is the root of *Cephaëlis ipecacuanha*, a Brazilian shrub. It contains an alkaloid, emetine, which acts as an irritant when brought in contact with the interior of the stomach, producing vomiting. This effect is also brought about after its absorption into the blood by its action on the vomiting centre in the brain. In small doses it acts, not as an irritant, but as a gentle stimulant to the mucous membrane of the stomach, bowels and respiratory passages. Emetine is also a specific for amoebic dysentery.

Uses – Ipecacuanha is a constituent of many expectorant mixtures given in the treatment of bronchitis. It is of value in this connection because of its action in liquefying the thick mucous secretion which occurs in bronchitis. It is also a con-stituent of Dover's Powder (qv), which is one of the most efficient diaphoretics for use in febrile conditions, such as the common cold.

In the treatment of amoebic dysentery ipecacuanha is now largely replaced by emetine, as a more certain action can be obtained with emetine.

IPRINDOLE is a drug that is proving useful in the treatment of depressive illness.

IPRONIAZID is a drug which inhibits monoamine oxidase (qv), an enzyme which plays an important part in the metabolism of the brain. It was originally introduced into medicine for the treatment of tuberculosis. It proved too toxic for this purpose, however. It is now being used in the treatment of depressive states.

IPROTROPIUM is a drug that is proving of value in the treatment of asthma.

IRIDECTOMY is the operation by which a piece is removed from the iris, and the pupil of the eye is thereby increased in size, as, for example, in the treatment of glaucoma (qv), or as part of the operation for the removal of a cataract (qv).

IRIDENCLEISIS is the term for describing the condition in which the iris is caught in a small gaping wound of the cornea.

IRIS is the muscular and fibrous curtain which hangs behind the cornea and serves, by alteration of the size of the pupil (the round hole in its centre), to regulate the amount of light entering into the eye. (See EYE.)

IRISH MOSS (see CARRAGEEN).

IRITIS means inflammation of the iris. Inflammation of the iris is closely associated both in cause and in symptoms with inflammation in the ciliary body and choroid membrane, which, together with the iris, make up the middle coat of the eyeball.

Causes – In the majority of cases the cause is not known, and it is generally assumed that the condition is an allergic type of reaction. In other cases it is due to syphilis, gonorrhoea, tuberculosis, infection of the iris through a wound or injury. In other cases again it is associated with diabetes mellitus, ankylosing spondylitis, rheumatism or focal sepsis elsewhere in the body.

Symptoms – The most marked symptom is pain situated either in the eye itself or more commonly in the forehead above it. There may be much watering of the eye, and bright light always occasions more or less distress. The eye is red around the margin of the iris, and for this reason the condition is often mistaken for inflammation of the conjunctiva covering the eye – a much less serious condition. (See EYE DISEASES AND INJURIES.) Dimness of vision is present, and, particularly in chronic cases, may for long be the only sign. When one looks at the eye closely, one notices that the iris has lost its lustre, and the pupil is generally narrow. If the affected person has suffered previously from iritis, the iris may be adherent behind to the lens of the eye, so that the pupil loses its usual circular outline, and ceases to vary in size in different lights. An acute attack of iritis generally lasts some weeks even when treated, and, if the condition be not carefully treated, the sight may be much impaired or lost as the result of opacities in the lens or cornea, deposit of inflammatory matter in the pupil, and the like.

Treatment – Rest of the eye is of the highest importance. To effect this, all reading and other near work, even with the unaffected eye, must be given up. To prevent the eye from being used, atropine, which paralyses the muscles of accommodation, is dropped into the eye, usually in a 1 per cent solution. This is accompanied by the administration of corticosteroids (qv) in the form of eye-drops or eye-ointment or sometimes injected under the conjunctiva. As a further protection, dark glasses are worn. The application of warmth to the eye, the administration of aspirin, and confinement to bed are also helpful. The disease which is responsible for the iritis is at the same time treated by suitable remedies whether this be an infection due to injury to the eye, syphilis, gonorrhoea or tuberculosis.

IRON is a metal which is an essential constituent of the red blood corpuscles, where it is present in the form of haemoglobin. It is also present in muscle, myoglobin, and in certain respiratory pigments which are essential to the life of many tissues in the body. Iron is absorbed principally in the upper part of the small intestine. It is then stored: mainly in the liver; to a lesser extent in the spleen and kidneys, where it is available, when required, for use in the bone marrow to form the haemoglobin in red blood corpuscles. The daily iron requirement of an adult is 15 to 20 milligrams. This requirement is increased during pregnancy. Iron salts also have an astringent action, especially the chloride, and this property is sometimes made use of when it is used as a styptic to check bleeding.

Uses – The main use of iron is in the treatment of iron-deficiency anaemias. (See ANAEMIA.) The main form in which it is used is ferrous sulphate. Iron preparations sometimes cause irritation of the gastro-intestinal tract, and should therefore always be taken after meals. They sometimes produce a tendency towards constipation. Whenever possible, iron preparations should be given by mouth. It is a very small proportion indeed of cases of iron-deficiency anaemia which will not respond satisfactorily to iron given by mouth. For the occasional cases in which oral administration is not suitable, a preparation of iron is now available which can be given intravenously.

Springs of iron-containing water are known as chalybeate springs, and in England are to be found at Tunbridge Wells and Harrogate. Such iron-containing waters have no advantage over the administration of iron. Indeed, they have the great disadvantage that they can never supply sufficient iron for a patient who is suffering from a definite degree of iron-deficiency anaemia.

IRRADIATION is the term applied to treatment by various forms of light and radiant activity.

IRRIGATION is the name given to the method of washing out wounds, or cavities of the body, like the bladder and bowels. (See DOUCHES; ENEMA.)

IRRITABLE COLON, or SPASTIC COLON, is the condition characterized by painful spasm of the colon, which tends to occur in nervous people when under stress or strain. It may be accompanied by constipation or by the passage of frequent small stools. Treatment consists of dealing with the underlying nervous condition, the avoidance of all aperients and a full diet. Whether or not roughage, or 'fibre' as it is popularly known at the moment, should be added to the diet is still an open question. It suits some patients, but not others. A useful practical compromise is to try the effect of wholemeal bread.

ISCHAEMIA means bloodlessness of a part of the body, due to contraction, spasm, constriction or blocking (by embolus or by thrombus) of the arteries: for example, of the heart.

ISCHAEMIC HEART DISEASE (see CORONARY THROMBOSIS).

ISCHIO-RECTAL ABSCESS is the name of an abscess arising in the space between the rectum and ischial bone and often resulting in a fistula.

ISCHIUM is the bone which forms the lower and hinder part of the pelvis. It bears the weight of the body in sitting.

ISCHURIA means insufficiency in the amount of urine passed, due either to suppression of excretion or retention in the bladder.

ISHIHARA TEST is used in testing for colour-blindness. It consists of a series of variously coloured charts. Some of these charts, when viewed by individuals with normal colour vision, appear to present figures and pathways which are not apparent to colour-blind individuals, whilst other charts appear to the colour-blind to have figures which are not apparent to the individual with normal colour vision. This test has been accepted as the standard by the fighting forces, including the Royal Navy.

ISO-IMMUNIZATION is the immunization of one member of a species by an antigen lacking in himself but present naturally in other members of the species, as, for example, the immunization of an Rh-negative mother by an Rh-positive foetus, the mother as a result producing anti-Rh agglutinins which injure the foetus. (See also HAEMOLYTIC DISEASE OF THE NEWBORN; and RH FACTOR.)

ISOLATION in infectious diseases is an important procedure, applied both to persons who are themselves sick and to persons who have come in contact with them, technically known as contacts or suspects, and who may later develop the disease. (See INCUBATION; INFECTION; QUARANTINE.)

ISONIAZID is one of the most potent anti-tuberculous drugs which we possess. It has the further advantages of being relatively non-toxic and of being active when taken by mouth. Unfortunately, like streptomycin, it may render the *Mycobacterium tuberculosis* resistant to its action. This tendency to produce resistance is con-

siderably reduced if it is given in conjunction with streptomycin and/or para-aminosalicylic acid.

ISOPRENALINE is a bronchodilator drug that is widely and successfully used in the treatment of asthma, mainly as an aerosol for inhalation. In view of its action on the heart it must be used with caution.

ISOTONIC is a term applied to solutions which have the same power of diffusion as one another. An isotonic solution used in medicine is one which can be mixed with body fluids without causing any disturbance. An isotonic *saline solution* for injection into the blood, so that it may possess the same osmotic pressure as the blood serum, is one of 0·9 per cent strength or containing 9 grams of sodium chloride to 1 litre of water. This is also known as *normal* or *physiological salt solution*. An isotonic solution of *bicarbonate of soda* for injection into the blood is one of 1·35 per cent strength in water. An isotonic solution of *glucose* for injection into the blood is one of 5 per cent strength in water.

Solutions which are weaker, or stronger than, the fluids of the body with which they are intended to be mixed are known as hypotonic and hypertonic, respectively.

ISOTOPE is each of two or more chemical elements or atoms which have the same chemical properties but differ in atomic weight. Isotopes have become of great interest and importance in medicine because of the developments in nuclear physics which have rendered it possible to make all the common elements radio-active. These radioactive isotopes have a twofold value in medicine: (1) as a means of studying some of the more abstruse processes of the body, of which we are still ignorant; (2) as a means of treating certain malignant conditions. For instance, radioactive iodine is proving of value in the diagnosis of diseases of the thyroid gland and in the treatment of cancer of the thyroid gland. (See RADIOTHERAPY.)

ISSUE is an old term for a suppurating sore.

ITCH is a popular name for scabies (qv).

ITCHING or PRURITUS, is an unpleasant condition of the skin surface which in some cases is so constant as to become unbearable.

Causes – It is due to many different conditions, some of which are local and can be easily removed. Some are general, while occasionally the condition becomes so chronic and the skin so changed by scratching, that it is incurable. Itching is produced by slight mechanical irritation, such as contact with rough woollen underclothing, also by parasites such as lice, or scabies ('the itch'), and these mechanical causes being removed the itching speedily vanishes. There is often a large psychological factor and this must always be borne in mind. (See NEURODERMATITIS.)

Various skin diseases, of which eczema is the chief, have itchiness as one of their main symptoms. In old age, when the skin is becoming thin and inelastic, itching sometimes becomes a troublesome complaint. In these and other conditions, a habit of scratching, which in course of time renders the skin rough and thickened, is apt to be contracted, and this of itself aggravates and keeps up the itchiness. Among the general diseases which set up itchiness, the chief is diabetes mellitus. In fact, any one who is much troubled by itchiness, especially if this be situated about the genital organs, should have his urine examined for the presence of sugar. Jaundice caused by various liver derangements, and Bright's disease, are often accompanied by itchiness in a milder degree. Dyspepsia is not uncommonly the cause of nettle-rash, which may be of an itching type and appear soon after indigestible food has been taken. Some persons are much troubled by itching of the body when changes in size of the blood-vessels in the skin take place, as occur upon getting warm in bed or upon the advent of spring and autumn. A similar condition, which affects persons on going to the tropics, is known as prickly heat (qv).

A special and often very aggravated form of itching occurs sometimes at the anus, known as *pruritus ani*. In all cases of irritation in or around the anus, a careful search should be made for threadworms. (See RECTUM, DISEASES OF.) An equally troublesome form of itching occurs round the vagina, known as *pruritus vulvae*. It may be associated with excessive vaginal discharge. (See WHITES.)

Treatment – The use of detergents should be avoided, and as little soap as possible should be used for cleansing purposes. Warm baths, alkaline or containing bran, are among the most soothing applications for general itching. (See BATHS.) The addition of an ounce or two (30 to 60 grams) of the *British Pharmacopoeia* Emulsifying Ointment is often beneficial. Calamine lotion is the most efficient local application, but talcum powder is often useful. It is essential that a proper examination should be made as to the functions of the internal organs in cases in which itching is a chronic complaint. In diabetic cases the surest remedy to prevent the itching is to treat the diabetes. In pruritus ani attention to anal hygiene is important, and the anal region should be washed twice a day, using a soft sponge, and, if possible, every time the bowels move. Talcum powder should be applied after the washing and careful drying. In persistent cases of pruritus ani and pruritus vulvae the application of a corticosteroid (qv) ointment is often helpful. If there is a psychological cause, this must always be dealt with.

-ITIS is a suffix added to the name of an organ to signify any diseased condition of that organ.

IVORY, or DENTINE, is the hard material which forms the chief bulk of the teeth. (See TEETH.)

J

JABORANDI, or PILOCARPUS, is the leaf of a South American plant, *Pilocarpus microphyllus*. It contains an alkaloid, pilocarpine, upon which its action depends. (See PILOCARPINE.)

JACKSONIAN EPILEPSY (see EPILEPSY).

JACONET is a waterproofed lightweight cotton fabric.

JAIL FEVER is another term for typhus fever.

JALAP is the tuber of *Iopmoea purga*, a Mexican plant, which contains two resins of irritating properties.

Uses – Jalap is a potent purgative which is seldom used now except in combination with milder purgatives in certain pills. On the relatively few occasions on which a powerful purgative action is required, compound jalap powder may be used, in a dose of 40 to 60 grains (2·4 to 4 grams).

JANICEPS is a foetal monstrosity characterized by one combined head and two faces.

JAUNDICE is a yellow discoloration of the skin due to the deposition of bile pigment in its deeper layers. (See also HEPATITIS, ACUTE INFECTIOUS.)

Causes – Jaundice is divided into two main classes: *hepatogenous jaundice*, arising from the absorption of bile formed by the liver, and *haemolytic jaundice*, arising from the formation of a yellow pigment in the blood, derived from the breaking down of red blood corpuscles. The former is the usual type, and is described below; the latter is found in such conditions as pernicious anaemia, haemolytic anaemia, acholuric jaundice and snake poisoning.

When the bile cannot escape into the intestine in the usual way, it is absorbed by the blood- and lymph-vessels, and some of its constituents are deposited in the various tissues throughout the body. Some obstruction to the outflow of bile is therefore a necessary condition, and this obstruction may either exist in the bile-ducts, which convey the bile from liver to intestine, or it may be caused by some disorganization in the liver (eg. hepatitis) which prevents the bile, formed by the liver-cells, from finding its way to the bile-ducts at all. The tint of the jaundice has not necessarily any direct relation to the severity of the cause. Obstruction may be due to gall-stones, and the resulting jaundice is then a symptom of this condition. (See GALL-STONES.) Obstruction may be due to some cause quite outside the liver and bile-ducts, for example, enlarged glands lying near the liver or cancer of the pancreas, the seriousness of the jaundice depending then upon the seriousness of the disease responsible for the pressure. In elderly persons, who are likely to be the subject of cancer, long-continued jaundice is for this reason a serious symptom. Cirrhosis of the liver, in which the small branches of the bile-duct become compressed by the formation of fibrous tissue, may also be a cause of chronic jaundice. (See CIRRHOSIS.)

Among the causes which disorganize the liver, one finds many poisons which are carried to it in the blood: for example, phosphorus, mercury, chloroform and snake poison. Much more common as a cause of jaundice are two inflammatory conditions of the liver, known as infectious hepatitis and serum hepatitis (qv). They are both due to viruses but they differ in that the former has a shorter incubation period. Infectious hepatitis, which is much the more common of the two, is the condition which used to be known as catarrhal jaundice. Certain infective diseases are also prone to produce this effect, of which may be mentioned yellow fever, malaria, typhoid fever and pyaemia. A serious but uncommon condition, accompanied by rapid and often fatal jaundice, is that known as acute yellow atrophy of the liver. Another form of jaundice is known as spirochaetal jaundice or *spirochaetosis icterohaemorrhagica* (qv). These conditions cause such changes in the liver that the bile is unable to escape save by reabsorption into the blood.

Symptoms – Yellowness, appearing first in the whites of the eyes and later over the whole skin, is the symptom that attracts notice. This tint varies from a pale sulphur-yellow through all gradations to a deep olive or bronze colour, according to the completeness of the obstruction and the length of time the jaundice has lasted. The urine passed during the time the jaundice lasts is of a dark greenish-brown colour, owing to the excretion of bile by the kidneys. Various digestive disturbances are present: the tongue is furred, the appetite poor, and a feeling of sickness is often felt, and is aggravated by eating fats. The stools are of a grey or white colour, owing to the want of bile in the intestine, and for the same reason constipation, relieved occasionally by diarrhoea, is present, and the stools have an excessively offensive smell. A bitter taste in the mouth is generally felt by the jaundiced person, due, as it is supposed, to the presence in the saliva of salts of the bile-acids, and the same or other substances in the sweat lead to itching of the skin. Slowness of the pulse, and, in long-continued cases, mental confusion and dullness, are other less evident accompaniments of jaundice.

Treatment – The first essential is to treat the underlying cause if possible: for instance, gall-stones, if these be the cause of the jaundice. For the actual treatment of the jaundice the patient must be kept in bed. The diet should contain as much protein and carbohydrate as possible and a minimum of fat. The diet to be aimed at should contain 3000 Calories daily, including 100 to 120 grams of protein and supplemented with vitamins. Such a diet should not be forced in its entirety in the early days of treatment when the appetite is poor and the mere thought of food nauseating. For the pruritus, or itching, which may be very severe, cala-

mine lotion containing 2 per cent phenol should be used. This may need to be supplemented with analgesics: eg. aspirin or a tablet containing aspirin, paracetamol and codeine. Sedatives may also be required.

As the jaundice clears, the amount of protein may be reduced, and if there is much residual indigestion this is best treated by a modified peptic ulcer diet.

JAW is the name applied to the bones that carry the teeth. The upper jaw-bones, the maxillae, are two in number, and are firmly fixed to the other bones of the face (illustration 269). The lower jaw, the mandible, is shaped somewhat like a horseshoe, and, after the first year of life, consists of a single bone. It forms a hinge-joint with the squamous part of the temporal bone, immediately in front of the ear. Both upper and lower jawbones possess deep sockets, known as alveoli, which contain the roots of the teeth. (See DISLOCATIONS; FRACTURES; GUMBOIL; MOUTH; TEETH.)

JEJUNUM is the name given to part of the small intestine. (See INTESTINE.)

JELLY (see GELATIN).

JIGGER is a popular term used to denote a parasite also known as the sand-

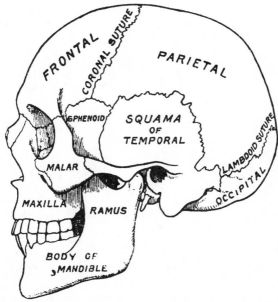

269 – Side view of skull. From Hill, *Manual of Human Physiology*. Edward Arnold & Co.

flea. The term is also used to denote the small worm-like masses of fatty material which can be squeezed out of the sebaceous glands on the face of those suffering from acne (qv).

JOINT-MOUSE is a popular term for a loose body in a joint. It is found especially in the knee. (See JOINTS, DISEASES OF.)

JOINTS – A joint or articulation is the meeting-place between different parts of the skeleton, whether bones or cartilages.

Superior pubic ligament

Interpubic disc of fibrocartilage

Hyaline cartilage

Body of pubis

Arcuate ligament

270 – The symphysis pubis (a cartilaginous joint).

Structure – The great division of joints is into those which are fixed or relatively fixed (*fibrous* and *cartilaginous joints*), and

those at which free movement can take place (*synovial joints*). In the former (illustration 270), a layer of cartilage or of fibrous tissue intervenes between the bones and binds them firmly together. This type of joint is exemplified by the sutures between the bones that make up the skull. Among these fixed joints, some have a thick disc of fibro-cartilage between the bones, so that, although the individual joint is really capable of very little movement, a series of these, like the joints between the bodies of the vertebrae, gives to the spinal column, as a whole, a flexible character (amphiarthrodial joint).

Into the formation of every *movable joint* four structures enter. These are the bones whose junction forms the joint; a layer of cartilage covering the end of each of these and rendering the ends smooth (illustration 271); a sheath of fibrous tissue known as the capsule, thickened at various points into bands or ligaments, which hold the bones together; and, finally, a membrane known as synovial membrane, which lines this capsule and produces a synovial fluid to lubricate the movements of the joint. Further, the bones are kept in position at the joints by the various muscles passing over them and by atmospheric pressure. This type of joint is known as a synovial joint (illustration 272).

271 – Vertical section of articular cartilage covering end of tibia. Magnified 30 times. *a,b,c*, groups of cartilage cells embedded in matrix; *d*, layer of calcified cartilage; *e*, bone. From Schafer, *Essentials of Histology*. Longman.

Some joints possess subsidiary structures, such as discs of fibro-cartilage, which adapt the ends of the bones more perfectly to one another in places where these do not quite correspond. In others, movable pads of fat under the synovial membrane fill up larger cavities and afford additional protection to the joint.

272 – (A) Diagrammatic representation of a simple synovial joint. (B) Diagrammatic representation of a synovial joint with an articular disc.

Varieties – Apart from the main division of joints into those which are fixed and those which are movable, the movable joints fall into several groups. Gliding joints are those in which, like the wrist and ankle, the bones have flat surfaces capable of only a limited amount of movement. In hinge-joints, like the elbow and knee, the chief movement takes place round one axis. The ball-and-socket type is exemplified by the shoulder and hip, in which free movement is possible in any direction. There are other subsidiary varieties, named according to the shape of the bones which enter into the joint.

JOINTS, DISEASES OF – The larger

joints, on account of their exposed position, are subject to constant injuries, and this, together with the wear they suffer and the richness of their blood supply, renders them liable to a number of serious diseases. The knee is the joint most often diseased, and after it, in order, the hip, ankle, and elbow. Although minor injuries may be followed by serious diseases, it is an important fact that very severe injuries, in which the skin remains unbroken, such as dislocations of, and fractures into, the joints rarely occasion any serious disease beyond stiffness and other direct results of the injury. On the other hand, penetrating wounds of joints are among the most serious of injuries, and require immediate and expert treatment. The following are some of the conditions from which joints suffer.

SYNOVITIS is the name given to any inflammation of the membrane lining the joint cavity. It may be acute, subacute or chronic.

Causes – The joints being much exposed to blows, wounds and strains, some injury often precedes the onset of inflammation. In many cases, the condition is due to some rheumatic condition such as rheumatoid arthritis osteoarthrosis (see RHEUMATISM), gout (qv) or tuberculosis.

Symptoms – In acute synovitis, following usually upon some injury, the synovial membrane becomes inflamed, thickened, and secretes an excessive amount of fluid into the joint. As a result, the joint becomes painful, red, swollen and hot to touch. It is usually kept more or less bent, and is painful to straighten and to handle. If the synovitis remains of a simple nature, these symptoms last some days and then gradually subside. Or the condition may persist for a long time, getting better for a little and then relapsing; or it may become chronic, and, whilst the heat and redness disappear, the joint remains stiff and distended with fluid. This condition most frequently affects the knee, and is then popularly known as water on the knee. On the other hand, in occasional cases which have begun in the simple form, and in cases due to a penetrating wound of the joint to which bacteria have gained entrance, a very serious inflammation occurs. Suppuration then takes place in the joint, an abscess forms with fever, great pain and other aggravated symptoms of abscess. A joint cavity is very difficult to render free from suppuration, and may even necessitate amputation of the limb in order to save life.

Treatment – In the early stages, complete rest of the joint, the limb being placed on a splint, together with the application of cold or of warm fomentations to soothe the pain, is alone necessary. Later, massage and compression of the joint by a bandage aid the absorption of the fluid and dispel the stiffness. When the condition becomes chronic, counter-irritation by iodine, blisters, etc., is necessary, and the joint is often punctured to draw off the fluid. Suppuration is, as already stated, a very serious matter, and is treated like an abscess elsewhere by opening, irrigation with antiseptics, drainage and the administration of antibiotics.

EPIPHYSITIS is the name given to an inflammation situated at the end of a long bone just outside the joint. An important point regarding this type of inflammation in children is that if the inflammation be severe it may permanently damage the plate of cartilage, situated close to the end of the bone, from which increase in length takes place, so that the child's limb may be seriously impaired in growth.

TUBERCULOUS DISEASE of a joint begins in the synovial membrane or in the end of the bone, and is popularly known as white swelling, on account of the characteristic appearance of the affected joint, particularly when the knee is involved. In many cases there are other manifestations of the disease, the lungs, for example, being affected, or the glands of the neck enlarged. Tuberculosis of the joints is commoner in children than in older persons. A proportion of cases, especially in children, are due to the drinking of tuberculous milk.

Symptoms – The condition is usually chronic, begins insidiously, sometimes being dated from a slight accident, and progresses slowly. Slight stiffness, wasting of the muscles in the affected limb, and pain and tiredness brought on by slight exertion, are the earliest symptoms. The joint later on assumes its characteristic appearance, becoming enlarged, losing the natural hollows about it, and appearing white and glistening, with large veins showing through the skin. The wasting of muscle above and below the joint causes it to look still more enlarged than it really is. Gradually the use of the limb is lost, and the general health deteriorates. Later in the disease, when the joint is becoming thoroughly disorganized, starting-pains at night, which waken the sufferer as he is dropping off to sleep, become troublesome. If the condition remains untreated after this stage is reached, an abscess forms in the joint and bursts through the skin, and hectic fever develops.

Treatment – In all cases of tuberculous disease rest of the joint is essential, the joint being fixed by a splint or other apparatus so that it cannot move to any great extent. As in all other tuberculous conditions, exercise and fresh air are of great importance, and therefore, when the disease affects a joint in the lower limb, some apparatus is devised whereby the patient can move about while the joint is still rigid. For the hip and knee this is secured by Thomas's splints, and for other joints by various pieces of apparatus. Fixation is sometimes effected by plaster bandages, though these have the great disadvantage of leaving the joint stiff and the limb weak. When a joint is thus fixed for a space of weeks or months, stiffness is apt to ensue, but the freedom of the joint must

often be sacrificed with the object of checking the disease. Care is taken that the position in which the joint is fixed shall be the most useful one, the knee being kept straight, the ankle at a right angle, the elbow a little more bent than a right angle, as the case may be. Sometimes in the case of the hip, especially if the pain be severe, the child is put in bed, and extension by means of a weight applied to the limb: by this means the deformity is corrected, the joint kept at rest, and the pressure of the diseased surfaces in the joint upon one another relieved. Massage, which is admirably adapted for the treatment of many joint conditions, is not suited for tuberculous disease while it is still active. Constitutional treatment must be energetically carried out, as in the case of tuberculosis elsewhere in the body.

Operative treatment is advisable for some tuberculous joints. The aim of surgical treatment is to secure fixation of the affected joint by bony ankylosis: ie. bringing together the ends of the damaged limb.

As in all other forms of tuberculosis the outlook has been revolutionized by the excellent results which have been obtained from the use of chemotherapy, giving combined therapy with streptomycin, PAS, and isoniazid for at least six months. The use of chemotherapy has not only reduced the time of treatment by one-half, but has resulted in a much larger number of patients being left with almost full range of movement of the diseased joints.

STIFFNESS OF JOINTS may be due to various causes. It may result from spasm of the muscles around the joint in cases of early tuberculous disease and of hysterical joints, or it may be due to permanent shortening in these muscles or contraction of the skin, due, for example, to a burn. Often a severe injury to the joint itself, such as a fracture of one of the bones that form it, or a dislocation, is followed by some stiffness. A large number of slight injuries, which set up a mild degree of inflammation, are followed by some adhesions in the joint, often of a painful nature. These limit the use of the joint considerably, but, when they are broken by forcible movements of the limb, recovery and relief are immediate.

LOOSE BODIES IN JOINTS result from inflammation of various types, the bodies being developed as projections on the synovial membrane or on the cartilages of the joint, and later pulled off by its movements. They bring on repeated attacks of synovitis, and often cause sudden locking of the joint, so that for a time it is immovable. They are removed by operation.

GOUT, RHEUMATISM AND RHEUMATOID ARTHRITIS are diseases of a constitutional nature which affect joints. (See under these headings.)

HYSTERICAL AFFECTIONS OF JOINTS are not uncommon, particularly in young women, although they are occasionally found in the opposite sex. The knee and hip are most often affected, but the ankle, wrist and elbow are also vulnerable. The affection takes many forms: stiffness, pain on movement, swelling, weakness, wasting of the limb may be complained of, and the appearances of tuberculous disease may be closely mimicked. As a rule there are no signs of general constitutional weakness; on the other hand, various other hysterical manifestations present themselves. (See HYSTERIA.)

SPRAIN is a vague popular term indicating the result of any slight wrench to a joint. A sprain consists generally of a mild attack of synovitis, or of tearing of ligaments with effusion of fluid into or round the joint. At the ankle, a twist of the foot inwards is followed by some tearing of the outer lateral ligament of the joint constituting a severe sprain, but a more serious accident, consisting of fracture at the lower end of the fibula, is apt to follow a wrench or twist of the foot outwards. (See FRACTURES.) In the knee, a sudden twist is occasionally responsible for loosening and rumpling up the inner of the two fibro-cartilages found in that joint. This accident has the awkward consequence of producing at subsequent times attacks of synovitis, or of sudden locking of the knee-joint. Behind the wrist and at the ankle, a sprain results sometimes in the displacement of some of the tendons which should be bound firmly to the bone, leading to occasional pain and a sense of weakness till the tendon happens to get replaced by another twist.

Treatment – When a sprain is of inflammatory character, the treatment is of the nature described under synovitis, and in the case of a bad sprain rest for a week or two may be essential. A sprain consisting in tearing of the ligaments round a joint, accompanied by effusion of blood beneath the skin, may be treated at the very beginning by applying wet compresses, or by holding the joint in a stream of cold water, which materially checks the effusion. After some time has elapsed, this form of treatment is of little use, and compression by a moderately tight, or by an elastic, bandage over the injured joint, together with elevation of the limb, forms a better line of treatment. When the pain is severe, fomentations of lead and opium lotion give relief. (See GOULARD'S WATER.) Massage is of great assistance in cases of sprain to prevent stiffness of the affected joint and to aid repair of injured tissues.

DISLOCATION (see DISLOCATIONS).

BURSITIS often occurs over the region of a joint. The prominences of several joints are protected by large bursae, and inflammation of these structures is sometimes mistaken for inflammation of the joint. (See BURSITIS.)

JOULE is the unit of energy in the International System of Units. The official abbreviation is J. 4186·8 J = 1 Calorie (or kilocalorie). (See also CALORIE; and WEIGHTS AND MEASURES.)

JUGULAR is a general name for any structure in the neck, but is especially applied to three large veins, the anterior, external and internal jugular veins, which convey blood from the head and neck regions to the interior of the chest.

JUNKET is the name of a food consisting of milk which has been acted upon by rennet. This forms a soft curd of the casein which is more easily digested than the curd which would naturally form in the stomach. Junket therefore forms a more easily digestible food than natural milk. If the curd is strained through muslin, whey is obtained which contains simply the water, sugar and albuminous materials of the milk and is very easily digestible. It is therefore used in the treatment of gastric ulcer and similar conditions. Half a pint (280 ml) of whey has an energy value of about 60 Calories.

K

KAHN REACTION is a substitute for the *Wassermann reaction* in the diagnosis of syphilis.

KALA-AZAR is another name for visceral leishmaniasis. (See LEISHMANIASIS.)

KANAMYCIN is an antibiotic derived from *Streptomyces kanamyceticus*. It is active against a wide range of organisms, including *Staphylococcus aureus* and *Mycobacterium tuberculosis*.

KAOLIN, or CHINESE CLAY, is a smooth white powder consisting of natural white aluminium silicate resulting from the decomposition of minerals containing felspar. It is used as a dusting powder for eczema and other forms of irritation in the skin. It is also used internally in cases of diarrhoea. The dose is 10 ml of Kaolin Mixture, B P C, best taken in water or milk before meals. Talc, French chalk and Fuller's earth are similar silicates.

Kaolin poultice contains kaolin, boric acid, glycerin and various aromatic substances.

KAOLINOSIS is a form of pneumoconiosis (qv) caused by the inhaling of clay dust.

KATA-THERMOMETER – A thermometer, invented by Sir Leonard Hill, which shows the rate of loss of heat, or cooling power, of the air. It is a spirit thermometer with a large bulb and marks on the stem at 95° F and 100° F. The thermometer, having been warmed up to above 100° F, is suspended in the air and the time taken in cooling from 100° F to 95° F is observed. Each instrument has marked on the stem a factor proportional to the total heat lost per square centimetre of the bulb in cooling from 100° F to 95° F. Dividing this factor by the number of seconds taken to cool gives a figure called the 'cooling power'.

KELOID is an overgrowth of fibrous tissue, usually on the site or scar of a previous injury. It gets its name from its claw-like off-shoots which pucker up the surrounding skin. It is sometimes painful, sometimes painless. It is much commoner in coloured than in white races. The most effective form of treatment is by injection of corticosteroids (qv) directly into the abnormal tissue. If this fails, then surgical excision is performed.

KERATIN is the substance of which horn and the surface layer of the skin are composed.

KERATITIS means inflammation of the cornea in front of the eye. (See EYE DISEASES AND INJURIES.)

KERATOMALACIA means softening of the cornea, as a result of a severe lack of vitamin A in the diet.

KERATOPLASTY is another term for a plastic operation in the eye. To a certain extent it is equivalent to corneal grafting (qv).

KERATOSIS is a disease of the skin characterized by overgrowth of the horny layer of the skin (qv). It is induced by exposure to sunshine and in temperate climates usually develops in older people. In sunnier realms it may develop much earlier particularly in sun-bathing enthusiasts who repeatedly over-expose their skin to the sin. It takes the form of firm, dry adherent scales with redness of the surrounding skin and patchy pigmentation of the skin exposed to sunlight. Treatment, and prevention, consist of avoiding overexposure to the sun.

KERION is the term applied to a suppurating form of ringworm (qv).

KERNICTERUS is the staining with bile of the basal nuclei of the brain, with toxic degeneration of the nerve cells, which sometimes occurs in HAEMOLYTIC DISEASE OF THE NEWBORN (qv).

KERNIG'S SIGN is a sign found in cases of meningitis, consisting in the fact that, whereas a healthy person's thigh can be bent to a right angle with the body when the knee is straight, in cases of meningitis the knee cannot be straightened when the thigh is thus bent, or intense pain is caused to the patient by doing so.

KETOGENIC DIET is one containing such an excess of fats that acetone and other ketone bodies appear in the urine. It is sometimes used in the treatment of epilepsy and chronic infections of the urinary tract by *Escherichia coli*. In this diet, butter, cream, eggs and fat meat are allowed, whilst sugar, bread and other carbohydrates are cut out as far as possible.

KETONE is another name for acetone or dimethyl ketone. The term, ketone bodies, is applied to a group of substances closely allied to acetone, especially β-hydroxybutyric acid and acetoacetic acid. These are produced in the body from imperfect oxidation of fats and protein foods, and are found in specially large amount in severe cases of diabetes mellitus, KETONURIA is the term applied to the presence of these bodies in the urine.

KHELLIN is a crystalline principle which has been isolated from the fruit of *Ammi visnaga*, an umbelliferous plant indigenous to the Mediterranean area, which has for long had a local reputation for the relief of renal colic. Khellin has been introduced to western medicine for the treatment of angina pectoris.

The principle of the artificial kidney is that the patient's blood circulates through it and there comes in contact with a dialysing membrane, on the other side of which is a specially prepared dialysing fluid. In this way the biochemical balance of the blood is restored to normal, just as it would have been had the kidneys been functioning normally. (See DIALYSIS; and HAEMODIALYSIS.)

KIDNEYS are a pair of glands situated close to the spine in the upper part of the abdomen. They are on a level with the last dorsal and upper two lumbar vertebrae, and each is, to a great extent, covered behind by the twelfth rib of its own side. They are kept in this position by a quantity of fat and loose connective tissue, in which they are embedded, by the large vessels which supply them with blood, and by the peritoneal membrane stretched over their front surface.

273 – A diagram showing the design of an artificial kidney. *The Practitioner.*

KIDNEY, ARTIFICIAL, is the term applied to an instrument (illustration 273) which has been introduced in recent years to take over temporarily the functions of the kidneys in cases of acute renal (kidney) failure. Such sudden failure of the kidneys may occur in a number of circumstances, including severe accidents such as the crush syndrome (qv), incompatible blood transfusions, mercury poisoning and severe haemorrhage in the later stages of pregnancy. It is also being used now in the treatment of chronic renal failure. In such patients the immediate results may be dramatic, but treatment has to be maintained more or less permanently.

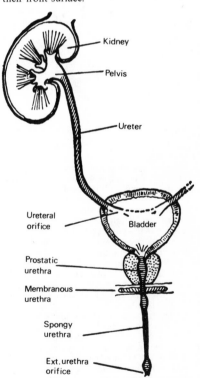

274 – Diagram of the male urinary system. From Boileau Grant, *An Atlas of Anatomy.* E. & S. Livingstone.

Structure – In size each is about 4 inches (10 cm) long, $2\frac{1}{2}$ inches wide (6·5 cm), $1\frac{1}{2}$ inches (5 cm) thick and weighs around 5 ounces (140 grams). The size, however, varies a good deal with the development, and probably with the habits of the individual. Kidney mass maintains a remarkably constant ratio to body weight. The left kidney is slightly longer and narrower, and lies a trifle higher in the abdomen than the right.

The kidney in adult human beings presents a smooth exterior, although in early life, as in many animals, it is divided up into distinct lobes, corresponding to the pyramids found in the interior. Enveloping it is a tough fibrous coat, which, in the healthy state, is bound to the kidney only

275 – Vertical section through the kidney. From Boileau Grant, *An Atlas of Anatomy*. E. & S. Livingstone.

by loose fibrous tissues and by a few blood-vessels that pass between it and the kidney. This capsule, which does not permit of much enlargement of the kidney, is an important factor with which to reckon when the kidney becomes congested in Bright's disease. The outer margin of the kidney is convex, the inner is concave, presenting a deep depression, known as the hilum, where the vessels enter its substance. At the hilum the renal vein lies in front of the renal artery, the former joining the inferior vena cava, and the latter springing from the aorta almost at a right angle. Here, too, is attached the ureter (illustration 274), which conveys urine down to the bladder. The ureter is spread out into an expanded, funnel-like end, known as the pelvis, to which the capsule of the kidney is firmly attached, and which further divides into little funnels known as the calyces. On splitting open a kidney, one finds it to consist of two distinct parts (illustration 275): a layer on the surface, about $\frac{1}{6}$ inch (4 mm) thick, known

as the cortex, and a part towards the hilum known as the medulla. The latter consists of pyramids, arranged side by side, with their base on the cortex and their apex projecting into the calyces of the ureter. The apex of each pyramid, of which there are about twelve in all, is studded with minute holes, which are the openings of the microscopic uriniferous tubes.

Each pyramid is, in effect, taken together with the portion of cortex lying along its base, an independent little kidney. About a score of small tubes open on the surface of each pyramid, and these, if traced up into its substance, divide again and again so as to form bundles of convoluted tubules (illustration 276), known as

276 – Diagram of renal tubules and blood supply of the kidney. P.C.T., proximal convoluted tubule; D.C.T., distal convoluted tubule. From Best and Taylor, *The Physiological Basis of Medical Practice*. The Williams & Wilkins Co.

medullary rays, passing up towards the cortex. If one of these be traced still farther back, it is found, after a very tortuous course, to end in a small rounded body: the Malpighian corpuscle or glomerulus (illustration 277). Each glomerulus and its convoluted tubule is known as a nephron (illustration 278), which constitutes the functional unit of the kidney. Each kidney contains around one million nephrons.

If the blood-vessels be now traced through the kidney their course is found to be as follows (illustration 276). The

Afferent vessel

Efferent vessel

Glomerular capsule

Capillary tuft

Capsule

Tubule

277 – Diagram of glomerulus. From Best and Taylor, *The Physiological Basis of Medical Practice*. The Williams & Wilkins Co.

renal artery splits up into branches, which form arches at the line of junction of cortex and medulla, and from these again spring vessels that run up through the cortex, giving off small branches in every direction. Each of these last ends in a little tuft of capillaries enclosed in a capsule (Bowman's capsule), that forms the end of the uriniferous tubule just described, and capillaries with capsule are known as a glomerulus (illustration 277). After circulating in the glomerulus, the blood emerges by a small vein, which again splits up into capillaries on the walls of the uriniferous tubules. From these it is collected finally into the renal veins and by them leaves the kidney. By means of the double circulation, first through the glomerulus and then around the tubule, it comes to pass that a large amount of fluid is removed from the blood in the glomerulus, and then the concentrated blood passes on to the uriniferous tubule for removal of parts of its solid contents. Other straight arteries come off from the arches mentioned above and supply the medulla direct, the blood from these passing through another set of capillaries and also finally into the renal veins. Although the circulation just described is confined entirely to the kidney, it has certain small connections both by arteries and veins which pass through the capsule and, joining the lumbar vessels, communicate direct with the aorta.

Function – The chief function of the kidneys is to separate fluid and certain solids from the blood. Briefly, the glomeruli filter from the blood the non-protein portion of the plasma. As this filtrate passes through the convoluted tubules, varying parts of it are reabsorbed. It is estimated that in 24 hours the total human glomeruli will filter between 150 and 200 litres, 99 per cent of which is reabsorbed by the tubules. The constituents of the filtrate may be grouped according to the extent to which they are reabsorbed by the tubules: (1) substances actively reabsorbed, such as amino-acids, glucose, sodium, potassium, calcium, magnesium and chlorine; (2) substances passing through the tubular epithelium by a simple process of diffusion when their concentration in the filtrate exceeds that in the plasma, such as urea, uric acid, phosphates; (3) substances not returned to the blood from the tubular fluid: eg. creatine.

When the kidneys are diseased and the number of glomeruli and tubules decreased in consequence, this alternating action is not so readily carried out, and therefore the work of the diseased kidney becomes increasingly embarrassed. When the blood-vessels of the kidney are partially closed by disease (arteriosclerosis), the general blood-pressure rises with the object of forcing more blood through the kidneys; in consequence, marked changes are produced upon the heart in this type of renal disease.

When the kidneys fail to act, these solid

DIAGRAM OF A NEPHRON

GLOMERULUS

PROXIMAL TUBULE

DISTAL TUBULE

278 – Diagram of a nephron. From Hanington, *Migraine*, 1974. Priory Press.

waste substances accumulate in the blood. The general 'poisoning' resulting from failure of renal function produces the clinical condition known as uraemia (qv).

KIDNEYS, DISEASES OF – The kidneys, being deeply buried in the abdomen, give little direct sign even when seriously diseased, although many of the effects upon the general constitution are sufficiently marked and serious.

General symptoms – The following are some of the general symptoms common to various types of kidney disease.

PAIN, of an aching nature, situated high up in the loins, is occasionally a symptom of inflammation of the kidneys, but pain in the lower part of the back is found in so many other diseases, and is so generally absent in serious kidney affections, that it is of little importance as a symptom. When a stone lodges in the ureter, however, there is a very definite type of pain known as renal colic. This pain is of an agonizing nature, shoots down from the kidney region to the groin, and usually appears with great suddenness. Also, when a kidney becomes movable and approaches the front of the abdomen, direct pressure upon it causes a sickening sensation of a type quite different from ordinary tenderness.

The URINE almost invariably shows changes in kidney diseases. In acute conditions it is diminished, generally contains albumin, and may be bloody. When unusual material is present in the kidney, careful examination of the urine generally reveals evidence of it: for example, pus in the urine points to a suppurative condition situated somewhere in the urinary tract; and when a stone is present in the kidney, its nature may often be conjectured by an examination of the crystalline deposit in the urine. In chronic Bright's disease the urine is generally increased in amount, pale and, as a rule, contains greater or less amounts of albumin. (See ALBUMINURIA.)

DROPSY, though due to many other conditions than Bright's disease, is a most important symptom of this and other kidney troubles. When dependent upon some defect in the kidneys, it appears generally in the morning after sleep, and affects the loose tissues of the body, such as the skin beneath the eyes and that on the back of the hands, which become swollen and puffy.

CHANGES IN THE CIRCULATION take place in chronic kidney disease. The signs of thickening in the arteries and in the heart-wall afford to the physician one of the most important signs both of the presence and of the severity of Bright's disease. These changes may produce pain in the chest, loss of mental power, bloodlessness, impairment of vision and may lead to apoplexy.

URAEMIA is a condition which is present in all cases in which the function of the kidneys is seriously impaired. It is a general poisoning of the system by waste products which the kidneys have failed to excrete, and may be acute or chronic in type. (See URAEMIA.)

The most important class of diseases affecting the kidneys is that comprising the changes grouped together as Bright's disease, in which albumin is excreted in the urine and dropsy is often present. (See BRIGHT'S DISEASE.) The following are some of the other important affections of the kidney. (See also PYELITIS.)

GRAVEL and *STONE* are produced by the deposit in the urinary passages of solid substances which are naturally present in the urine, and whose deposition depends upon their presence in excessive amount, or upon the failure of some condition which in general keeps them in solution. The most common constituents of such stones are ammonium phosphate, calcium phosphate and calcium carbonate, calcium oxalate, and uric acid and urates.

Among many factors responsible for the formation of stones in the kidneys is alteration in the reaction of the urine. Thus an excessive acid reaction may be accompanied by the formation of uric acid stones, whilst phosphate stones form in alkaline urine. Other factors which are associated with the formation of stones in the kidneys are prolonged recumbency, eg. following a fracture of the femur; infection of the kidney; lack of vitamin A in the diet; over-action of the parathyroid glands (qv) a high level of calcium in the urine; excessive sweating, as in hot climes, leading to a persistently concentrated urine; gout; and leukaemia. The most common cause in Britain is an abnormally high level of calcium in the urine: the condition known as hypercalciuria. They are more common in men than in women, and may occur at any age and particularly among sedentary workers. In cases in which the presence of a stone is suspected, X-ray examination is an important procedure in diagnosis.

Treatment – This depends upon the size of the stone. If it is large, then it has usually to be removed by operation. If it is small, it may be passed out in the urine following medical treatment. This consists of ensuring a large volume of urine by drinking large amounts of bland fluids. It is also helpful to alter the reaction of the urine. Thus, in the case of a uric-acid stone, the excessively acid urine is made alkaline by giving large doses of alkali: eg. 2 grams of sodium bicarbonate four times daily. In the case of stones associated with a high level of calcium in the urine, promising results are being obtained from the administration of either bendrofluazide, one of the benzothiazines (qv), or cellulose phosphate (qv), or a combination of the two. In the case of phosphate stones the excessively alkaline urine is made acid by the taking of 1 gram of ammonium chloride four times daily. Irrigation of the kidney with 'solution, G', which contains citric acid, magnesium oxide and sodium carbonate, is sometimes of value as it appears to dissolve small stones. If there is any infection of the kidney, this must be fully treated. The latest development is the use of ultrasonics to smash the stone into minute pieces which can then be passed in the urine. The efficacy and safety of this technique are under investigation.

RENAL CARBUNCLE is an abscess within the kidney. At one time the commonest cause was *Staphylococcus aureus* which reached the kidney via the bloodstream from staphylococcal infection elsewhere in the body. It is now more commonly due to infection spreading from the ureter or bladder. Patients debilitated by drug addiction and diabetes are especially at risk. The condition is characterized by pain in the loin and fever. The onset may be sudden with all the manifestations of septicaemia, or more gradual. Treatment consists of withdrawal of the pus and injection of the appropriate antibiotic into the abscess cavity.

TUBERCULOSIS of the kidneys is more common in adults than in children, and more common in men than in women. For a long time it may give rise to no symptoms or signs. It must therefore always be considered a possible diagnosis in cases in which urinary symptoms arise for which no cause can be found. Diagnosis partly depends upon the finding of *Mycobacterium tuberculosis* in the urine. As in other forms of tuberculosis, treatment has been revolutionized by the introduction of the anti-tuberculosis drugs: streptomycin, para-aminosalacylic acid and isoniazid. It is only in a minority of cases that surgical removal of the kidney is required.

MOVABLE KIDNEY is commoner in women than in men. The undue mobility of the kidney is part of a general visceroptosis (qv), and treatment should be directed to this. One risk of an abnormally mobile kidney is hydronephrosis (qv) from kinking of the ureter. Occasional kinking of the ureter may cause what are known as Dietl's crises: sudden attacks of intense abdominal pain radiating down the ureter, shivering, nausea, vomiting, fever, collapse. They are not common. If hydronephrosis develops, operation may be necessary.

INJURIES OF THE KIDNEY are very serious, although one of these organs may be completely shattered without a necessarily fatal result if the other kidney be healthy and uninjured. The kidney may be ruptured by a blow in the small of the back or when a person is run over, and death may result from the consequent loss of blood, which may appear in the urine.

TUMOURS of the kidney are not common, and, as a rule, they give little or no trouble till they have reached a large size. In the case of tumours growing in the pelvis of the kidney, large quantities of blood may be passed now and then in the urine with, however, no pain or other symptom referable to the kidney. *Congenital cystic kidney* is a form of tumour in the kidney which may last for many years with little trouble to the person in whom it occurs. *Hypernephroma* is a form of destructive tumour that occasionally develops in the kidney, being composed of cells resembling the suprarenal gland in appearance. *Nephroblastoma* (or *Wilms' tumour*) is the commonest kidney tumour in infancy. It is a malignant tumour, which occurs in around 1 per 10,000 live births. The survival rate with modern treatment (removal of the kidney followed by radiotherapy and chemotherapy) is now around 80 per cent.

HORSESHOE KIDNEY – Around 10 per cent of all live-born infants are born with malformations of the kidneys. Horseshoe kidney, so called because of its resemblance to a horseshoe, is among the commonest of these. It results from a partial fusion of the two kidneys, and is more common in males than females. In quite a number of cases, ranging from one-quarter to one-half according to different reports, the kidneys function normally. In the others the complications that are liable to occur are hydronephrosis (qv), pyelonephritis (see PYELITIS) and stones. Such kidneys are also more liable to develop cancer than normal kidneys. (See also TRANSPLANTATION.)

KILOGRAM is the basic unit of weight in the modern version of the metric system known as the International System of Units (SI). (See WEIGHTS AND MEASURES.) It is equivalent to 2·2 pounds.

KINAESTHETIC SENSATIONS is the descriptive term for those sensations which underlie muscle tension and position of joint and muscle. These sensations send impulses along nerves to the brain, and thus inform it of the position of the limb in space and of the relative position to each other of individual muscles and muscle-groups and of joints.

KING'S EVIL is an old name for scrofula, which was in olden times supposed to be curable by the touch of the royal hand. (See TUBERCULOSIS; and SCROFULA.)

KININS are substances present in the body which are powerful vasodilators (qv). They also induce pain and are probably involved in the production of the headache of migraine. In addition, they play a part in the production of allergy (qv) and anaphylaxis (qv).

KINO is the dried juice of *Pterocarpus marsupium*, an Indian tree. It contains an astringent principle, and its powder is useful in the treatment of diarrhoea, the tincture being also used as a gargle for relaxed throat.

KLEPTOMANIA is a psychological disorder in which the person afflicted has an irresistible compulsion to steal things, without necessarily having any need for the object stolen.

KNEE is the joint formed by the femur, tibia and patella (knee-cap). It belongs to the class of hinge-joints, although movements are much more complex than the simple motion of a hinge, the condyles of the femur partly rolling, partly sliding over the flat surfaces on the upper end of the tibia, and the acts of straightening and of bending the limb being finished and begun, respectively, by a certain amount of rotation. The cavity of the joint is very intricate: it consists really of three joints fused into one, but separated in part by ligaments and folds of the synovial membrane. The ligaments which bind the bones together are extremely strong, and include the popliteal and the collateral lig-

aments, a very strong patellar ligament uniting the patella to the front of the tibia, two cruciate ligaments in the interior of the joint, and two fibro-cartilages which are interposed between the surfaces of tibia and femur at their edge.

All these structures give to the knee-joint a great degree of strength, so that it is seldom dislocated. Its exposed position and the intricacy and consequent difficulty in cleansing its cavity, render this joint liable to be wounded, and make wounds of it very serious. The knee may also be affected by tuberculous disease.

A troublesome condition often found in the knee consists of the loosening of one of the fibro-cartilages lying at the head of the tibia, especially of that on the inner side of the joint. The cartilage may either be loosened from its attachment and tend to slip beyond the edges of the bones, or it may become folded on itself. In either case, it tends to cause locking of the joint when sudden movements are made. This causes temporary inability to use the joint until the cartilage is replaced by forcible straightening, and the accident is apt to be followed by an attack of synovitis, which may last some weeks, causing a certain amount of lameness with pain and tenderness especially felt at a point on the inner side of the knee. This condition can be relieved by wearing for a prolonged period of some months a bandage with pad or knee-truss which presses upon the inner side of the joint, or it may be more quickly remedied by an operation to remove the loose portion of the cartilage. (See also JOINTS, DISEASES OF.)

KNEE JERK (see REFLEX ACTION).

KNOCK-KNEE, or GENU VALGUM, is a deformity of the lower limbs in such a direction that when the limbs are straightened the legs diverge from one another. As a result, in walking the knees knock against each other. The amount of knock-knee is measured by the distance between the medial malleoli of the ankles, with the inner surfaces of the knee touching and the knee-caps facing forwards.

Causes – The condition is so common in children between the ages of 2 to 6 years that it may almost be regarded as a normal phase in childhood. When marked, or persisting into later childhood, it is usually due to faulty muscular tone. The condition is aggravated in children who are overweight or debilitated. At one time rickets was a common cause, but this is seldom the cause today in Great Britain.

Treatment – If rickets be the cause this must be treated. If, as is usually the case, there is no obvious cause, no treatment is required for knock-knee up to 3 inches (75 mm) in a child under 7 years of age. In the vast majority of cases it will have righted itself by this age. If the degree of knock-knee is more severe than this splints may be necessary, or even operation. When there is established bony deformity with over 4 inches (100 mm) of separation at the age of 4 years, or when there is still a considerable degree of knock-knee at the age of 9 years, operation should be performed. This may consist of cutting away the prominent part of the inner side of the lower end of the femora.

KÖHLER'S DISEASE is a not uncommon condition of the foot in younger schoolchildren, characterized by osteochondritis (qv) of the navicular bone. (See FOOT.)

KOILONYCHIA is the term applied to nails that are hollow and depressed like a spoon, a condition sometimes associated with chronic anaemia.

KOLA is the nut of *Kola acuminata*, a tree growing in various parts of Africa. It contains caffeine, upon which its action mainly depends, and also an astringent principle. Its action is a stimulating one, almost identical with that of tea or coffee. (See COFFEE.)

KOPLIK SPOTS are bluish-white spots appearing on the mucous membrane of the mouth in cases of measles about the third day, and forming the first part of the rash in this disease.

KORSAKOW'S SYNDROME is a term applied to a form of mental disturbance occurring in chronic alcoholism and other toxic states, such as uraemia, lead poisoning, cerebral syphilis. Its special features are talkativeness with delusions in regard to time and place, the patient, although clear in other matters, imagining that he has recently made journeys or been in distant places.

KOUMISS, or KEFIR, is a beverage made originally among the Kalmucks by fermenting mare's milk. It may be prepared from other kinds of milk also, and forms a stimulating and refreshing food which is sometimes better borne in weak states of the stomach than any other food. A home-made form of koumiss may be prepared as follows: mix 2 pints (1 litre) of buttermilk thoroughly with 3 pints (1·5 litres) of sweet milk, and add five lumps of white sugar. Place the milk in a bowl, cover with a towel, and let it stand in some warm corner of the kitchen for twenty-four hours: Then pour it into small bottles, cork them, and tie down the corks. Leave the bottles in the kitchen for three days, shaking occasionally. After this the koumiss is ready for use and should be kept in a cool place.

KÜMMELL'S DISEASE is a condition resulting from undiagnosed crush fracture of a vertebra, due to injury. The patient complains of backache, persistent rigidity of the spine and deformity.

KUPFFER CELLS are the star-shaped cells present in the blood-sinuses of the liver. They form part of the reticuloendothelial system (qv) and are to a large extent responsible for the breakdown of haemoglobin into the bile pigments.

KURU is a slowly progressive fatal disease due to degeneration in the central nervous system, particularly the cerebellum (qv). It is confined to the Fore people in the Eastern Highlands of New Guinea. It is believed to be due to a slow virus infection acquired from the cannibalistic rite of eating the organs, particularly the brains, of deceased relatives (out of respect). This origin of the disease was suggested by the fact that originally it was a disease of women and children, and it was they who practised this rite. Since the rite was given up, the disease has largely disappeared from children, but still occurs in women as it has an incubation period of up to 20 years.

KWASHIORKOR is one of the most important causes of ill health and death among children in the tropics. It is predominantly a deficiency disease due to a diet deficient in protein. There is also some evidence that there may also be a lack of the so-called essential fatty acids. It affects typically the small child weaned from the breast and not yet able to cope with an adult diet, or for whom an adequate amount of first-class protein is not available, and it is mainly found in the less well-developed countries.

The onset of the disease is characterized by loss of appetite, often with diarrhoea and loss of weight. The child is flabby, the skin is dry, and the hair is depigmented, dry, sparse and brittle. At a later stage oedema develops and the liver is often enlarged. In the early stages the condition responds rapidly to a diet containing adequate first-class protein, but in the later stages this must be supplemented by careful nursing, especially as the child is very liable to infections.

KYPHOSIS is the term applied to curvature of the spine in which the concavity of the curve is directed forwards. (See SPINE, DISEASES OF.)

L

LABETALOL is an alpha- and beta-adrenoceptor blocker (see ADRENOCEPTOR BLOCK) which is proving of value in the treatment of high blood pressure.

LABIUM is the Latin word for a lip or lip-shaped organ.

LABOUR, or PARTURITION, often popularly spoken of as the confinement, is the act of bringing forth young, and forms the end of the period of gestation or pregnancy during which the new individual is nourished from the maternal body. Parturition is a comparatively easy matter in lower animals and among primitive races. In the former the ease is dependent mainly upon the size and shape of the pelvic bones. In the latter this element is of course not present but, apart from purely anatomical differences, there is evidence that the higher we pass in the scale of civilization, the more difficult does the act of parturition become.

It is difficult to define an absolutely *normal labour* because individual labours differ so much in small details. Generally speaking, however, a normal labour is one in which the vertex of the child's head is born first, and the whole process ends favourably to mother and child within twenty-four hours, and without any operative interference. In the case of a first baby the confinement usually lasts from eight to sixteen hours, whilst the births of second and subsequent children tend to become progressively shorter processes. There are, of course, considerable variations in individual cases from these general statements. The majority of confinements end between midnight and 6 am. In 96 per cent of all cases the vertex of the child's head presents (that is, leaves the womb and descends through the vagina to the exterior first). In some cases, owing to a faulty position of the head or to the presentation of the child's face, the labour is considerably delayed, while for various reasons operative assistance may be necessary, in which case the labour is known as an instrumental one. The child may present quite another part than the head, the second most common presentation being the breech or buttocks. A rarer and more serious presentation is a transverse presentation or cross-birth, where the child lies obliquely across the womb. In these cases skilled assistance is specially necessary for the sake of both mother and child, and in the case of a cross-birth, assistance is imperative if the mother's life is to be saved. Finally, various complications, such as deformities of the mother and child, an excessive amount of bleeding, the birth of twins, and various general conditions of the mother, such as heart or kidney disease or convulsions, may influence the progress of the labour to an extreme degree.

Stages of labour – The process of labour is naturally divided into three stages. The *first stage* is that of dilatation of the neck of the womb to permit of the subsequent descent of the child. This is ushered in by the onset of the pains caused by the powerful intermittent contractions of the muscular wall of the womb. At first the pains come at considerable intervals – ten to twenty minutes – but as time passes the intervals become shorter and the pains become stronger. This stage is much the longest, particularly in the case of a first baby, when it may last for seven to fourteen hours. It is sometimes accompanied by sickness and vomiting. The full dilatation of the mouth of the womb is usually accompanied by the rupture of the amnion, the membrane containing the fluid in which the foetus moves, and the sudden escape of the amniotic fluid or 'waters'. The two events, however, do not necessarily take place at the same time, and sometimes the amnion ruptures at a much earlier, and sometimes at a later, period.

The *second stage* is the stage of expulsion of the child, during which the child's head, followed by the body and limbs, descends through the bony girdle of the pelvis and passes down through the vagina to the exterior. This process usually occupies two hours in a first labour, but, in the case of a woman who has had several children before, it may occupy a much shorter time. During this passage through the pelvis, the child's head goes through certain movements by which it adapts itself to the alterations in the shape of the pelvic canal as it passes down. The size of the head of an average child is such that there is just room for it to pass through the pelvis and no more. Accordingly the head is liable to be considerably pressed upon during this stage of labour, and this pressure manifests itself in the moulding of the child's skull. This moulding, which is rendered possible by the softness of the bones and by the presence of spaces between the bones, is a valuable provision of nature, and enables the head to pass down with the minimum of damage to the child and to the mother. In most cases the moulding disappears in the first day or two after birth. The second stage is one of strenuous muscular exertion, as not only the muscular wall of the womb, but the abdominal muscles and the diaphragm are all involuntarily called into play to aid the expulsion of the child. Pains are more severe, but at the same time the patient has a consciousness that she is making progress and this sometimes makes them more easily tolerated than the pains of the first stage. It is towards the end of the second stage that an anaesthetic is usually administered, the actual birth of the head being the time of greatest pain. Immediately thereafter there is a pause for a moment or two, and then the child's body is born, thus completing the second stage of labour. As soon as he is born the child usually cries loudly and in doing so establishes the function of respiration. The tying and cutting of the umbilical cord (see AFTERBIRTH) finally sever the child's vital connection with mother.

The *third stage* is the stage of delivery of the afterbirth. It begins immediately the child is born and rarely lasts more than half an hour. It is associated with the loss of a certain amount of blood: on average about 10 fluid ounces (280 ml). The great danger is from excessive haemorrhage associated with the separation of the afterbirth from the wall of the womb, and although the stage is much the shortest, yet this danger makes it imperative that it should be conducted with the greatest care.

Management of labour – In the absence of skilled assistance a normal labour will in all probability conduct itself to a successful issue, but it is always desirable that trained assistance should be obtained, both for the comfort as well as for the safety of the mother and the child. Obstetrical complications have a habit of arising suddenly and sometimes unexpectedly.

Where trained assistance is not at once available, the untrained person can still do much to help the prospective mother. As soon as the labour begins the mother should, if possible, have the lower bowel washed out with a soap-and-water enema, and if there is time it is advisable for mother to have a warm bath, or at least to have the genital regions thoroughly washed with soap and water. The bed upon which she is to be delivered should be prepared with a mackintosh sheet if possible, or failing that, one or two sheets

of glazed brown paper, placed across the middle of the bed and drawn well over the right-hand edge of it. A draw-sheet should be placed over this which can be changed afterwards. The clothing for the infant should be hung before the fire to be aired and warmed, and provision should be made for an ample supply of hot water and clean basins for the doctor or nurse, who should have been sent for. Ligatures should be prepared for tying the umbilical cord and these are best made of 3-ply linen thread twisted together and knotted at the ends so as to form a ligature of about 10 inches (25 cm) in length. Two of these are required, and should be sterilized by being boiled. The mother may, with advantage, remain up, either sitting or moving about her room as may be most comfortable for her, during the first stage; but when she feels fatigued and desires to lie down, and in any case when the membranes rupture and the 'waters' escape, she should lie down on the bed on her back.

During the second stage the mother will tend involuntarily to hold her breath and press down during the pains, and this down-bearing, as it is called, is helpful and should be encouraged, as it will expedite delivery. It is a mistake to urge a woman to bear down during the first stage, as it does no good and merely exhausts her strength. It helps the mother to be given something to hold on to during the down-bearing pains of the second stage, and it is a customary thing to tie a roller towel to the head of the bed and give her that to pull upon. This enables her to fix her abdominal muscles and to use her strength to the greatest advantage.

As soon as the child's head is born the eyes should be gently wiped clean with a pledget of cotton-wool or a clean soft linen handkerchief moistened in clean boiled water. After the child is born the cord should not be ligatured for two or three minutes until the pulsation in it is beginning to cease. One of the linen ligatures should then be tied tightly round the umbilical cord at a distance of about 2 inches (5 cm) from the child's navel. The other should be applied a few inches nearer the mother. With a clean pair of scissors which has been boiled, the cord should then be divided between the two ligatures. It is essential to make sure that there is no bleeding from the child's end of the cut umbilical cord. The infant should then be wrapped in a soft flannel or shawl and laid aside in some warm place until arrangements can be made for bathing. After the delivery of the child there will be an interval of some minutes before the uterine contractions start once more, and as a rule only a few contractions are needed to bring about the expulsion of the after-birth or placenta. This should be placed in a basin with some clean water and kept for inspection by the doctor or nurse.

All that now remains to be done is to clean the mother by gently swabbing her with pledgets of cotton-wool wrung out of clean boiled water, the hands of anybody who comes in contact with the patient having been previously most carefully and scrupulously scrubbed. The swabbing must be done from above downwards. A clean pad of cotton-wool, preferably scorched in front of a hot fire to sterilize it, should then be placed over the genitals and a firm binder drawn round the hips and over the lower part of the abdomen. A clean bolster slip serves this purpose admirably. After the confinement is over, the mother should be encouraged to sleep, or at least to rest quietly, and anything in the nature of excitement is to be avoided. For this reason friends and neighbours should as far as possible be excluded until the patient has had a good sleep.

Abnormalities and dangers of labour – These may rise in connection with the presentation or position of the child, with the uterus or maternal pelvis, or from the mother's health.

ABNORMAL PRESENTATIONS are relatively uncommon. The most frequent is a *breech presentation* (3 per cent of all labours). Here the labour is apt to be slow, but while there should be no increased risk to the mother (unless the labour happens to be a first labour), there is considerably greater danger to the child. Skilled assistance should always be obtained, but in the absence thereof the labour should be allowed to conduct itself without interference, until the lower limbs are born. These should then be wrapped in a warm flannel and gently supported, while steady pressure is applied to the top of the womb through the mother's abdominal wall. The after-coming head is thus gently pressed down into and through the pelvis. The main risk to the child is pressure on the umbilical cord during this stage, as it lies between the head of the child and the hard, bony pelvis. If this pressure is sufficient to impede the child's circulation for more than 8 or 10 minutes, the probability is that the child will be suffocated before he is born. (It must be understood that, until the head is born, the child obtains

the necessary oxygen by interchanges taking place between his blood and the blood of the mother in the placenta or after-birth, and that pressure on the cord prevents the passage of the foetal blood between the body of the foetus and the placenta.)

Face presentations occur but seldom (0·4 per cent of all labours). Usually the mother is able to deliver herself after a prolonged and tedious labour. The outlook is tolerably good for the child and should be satisfactory for the mother. There are, however, possibilities of serious danger, and medical help should always be sought.

The most dangerous mal-presentation is a *cross-birth*, where the child lies across the womb and the pelvis. None but an extremely premature child can be born in this position. If the condition is not corrected, the womb goes on trying to expel the child until it either becomes utterly exhausted and ceases to contract, or else it ruptures. In the former event, sufficient time may be gained – before the womb starts to contract again – in which to obtain skilled assistance to change the position of the child. In this way the mother's life may be saved, although the child will almost certainly have succumbed. In the second event, the shock and internal bleeding from the ruptured womb involve very grave risk to the mother's life, and delivery is impossible except by skilled assistance.

DEFORMITIES AND CONTRACTIONS of the mother's pelvis create great difficulty and may make natural labour impossible. The pelvis of every woman pregnant for the first time should be measured by a medical practitioner prior to labour with a view to the exclusion of any such possibility. Sometimes labour has to be induced early in these cases; in others, operative delivery at full time has to be arranged. (See CAESAREAN SECTION.)

HAEMORRHAGE during the last three months of pregnancy, or during labour, is always fraught with serious possibilities. It is due to the premature detachment of some portion of the placenta, which in many cases is situated too low down in the womb (*placenta praevia*). In the absence of skilled assistance, all that can be done is to keep the patient quite quiet in bed with the head low. No alcoholic stimulants should be given.

Bleeding during the third stage of labour or immediately after (*post-partum haemorrhage*) can be alarming and even fatal. In the absence of skilled assistance an attempt should be made to compress the womb forcibly by grasping it through the abdominal muscles. The foot of the bed may, with advantage, be raised and the patient provided with ample fresh air. No alcoholic stimulants should be given, as these only serve to increase the bleeding. Very hot applications to the vulva may help, and the doctor or nurse may administer a hot vaginal douche. (See DOUCHE.)

CONVULSIONS in association with pregnancy or labour, or occurring immediately after labour (*eclampsia*), constitute one of the most grave complications. Medical advice should be obtained without fail, and in the absence of such the patient should be kept absolutely quiet in a darkened room. No food, either solid or liquid, should be given. The actual convulsion should be treated on the ordinary lines, and if labour ensues, it also should be treated on the ordinary lines. (See ECLAMPSIA.)

PUERPERAL INFECTION is one of the most serious complications of labour. This is, in essence, the same as the infection of a wound, there being always a large raw surface in the interior of the uterus (the placental site), and in most cases innumerable small lacerations of the birth canal. All or any of these may be invaded by bacteria which subsequently tend to invade the blood-stream of the mother and give rise to acute septicaemia. About half the puerperal infections are due to the haemolytic streptococcus and about half to other organisms. The haemolytic streptococcus reaches the genital tract from the doctor, nurse, or midwife, from one of the patient's own household, or from the patient's own nasopharynx. The swabbing of throats, the exclusion from the patient's presence of streptococcal carriers and of anyone with a cold or sore throat, strict aseptic precautions during labour, will all help to diminish the incidence of haemolytic streptococcal puerperal infections. If infection occurs in spite of all precautions, then the sulphonamide drugs and penicillin are at hand as sovereign remedies. (See PUERPERAL FEVER.)

MATERNAL DEATHS – The number of mothers who die during pregnancy or childbirth, or the maternal mortality rate, is falling steadily in Britain. Thus, in the three-year period 1967–69, out of a total of 2,457,000 deliveries only 455 mothers died. This gives a rate of 18·5 deaths per 100,000 maternities, compared with a rate of 22·3 for the three years, 1964–66, and 53·3 for the three years, 1952–54. In England in 1977, the maternal mortality rate was 12 per 100,000 total births, there being 66 deaths, 10 due to abortion.

LACHESINE is a mydriatic: ie. it dilates the pupil of the eye. It is sometimes used for this purpose instead of atropine, as its action is of shorter duration.

LACRIMAL apparatus is the arrangement attached to the eye for moistening and cleansing the front of this organ. (See EYE.)

LACTATION is the period during which an infant is suckled on the mother's breast. (See BREASTS, DISEASES OF; INFANT FEEDING.)

LACTEAL is a lymphatic vessel that transmits chyle (qv) from the intestine. (See LYMPH.)

LACTIC ACID is a colourless, syrupy, sour liquid, which is produced by the action of a bacterium upon sugar of milk. The growth of this organism and consequent formation of lactic acid causes the souring of milk, and the same change takes place to a limited extent when food is long retained in the stomach.

Lactic acid ($CH_3 . CHOH . COOH$) is produced in the body during muscular activity, the lactic acid being derived from the breakdown of glycogen. Muscle fatigue is associated with an accumulation of lactic acid in the muscle. Recovery follows when enough oxygen gets to the muscle, part of the lactic acid being oxidized and most of it then being built up once more into glycogen.

LACTIC ACID BACILLI were introduced by Metchnikoff to prepare milk as a special article of diet, similar to koumiss (qv). The bacilli, which are issued in various forms, are added to fresh milk, allowed to act on it in a warm place for several hours (according to the degree of sourness desired), and the milk is then consumed with the active bacilli. These, after a course of such treatment, come to replace the bacteria naturally found in the intestines, and are supposed to be less injurious to the system. Sour milk forms a healthy article of diet; and the bacilli, which are harmless, have, in some cases of intestinal disease or of rheumatism, a beneficial action. Buttermilk has a similar effect. (See YOGHURT.)

LACTOMETER is the name of an instrument for ascertaining the specific gravity of milk.

LACTOSE is the official name for sugar of milk. (See SUGAR.)

LACUNA means a small pit or depression. Lacunar tonsillitis is a form of inflammation of the tonsils. (See TONSILLITIS.)

LAEVULOSE is the name of a sugar which forms one of the constituents of invert sugar. (See SUGAR.)

LAGOPHTHALMOS is the term describing the condition in which the eye cannot be completely closed.

LAMBLIA (see GIARDIASIS).

LAMELLA is a small disc of glycerin jelly, $\frac{1}{8}$ inch (3 mm) in diameter, containing an active drug for application to the eye. It is applied by inserting behind the lower lid.

LAMENESS (see GAIT; and JOINTS, DISEASES OF).

LAMINECTOMY is the term applied to an operation in which the arches of one or more vertebrae are removed so as to expose a portion of the spinal cord for removal of a tumour, relief of pressure due to a fracture, or similar reason.

LANOLIN is a fat derived from the wool of the common sheep. It is much used for ointments because it does not become rancid, and because it is supposed to have a special power of penetrating the skin. It is very sticky, and for use is mixed generally with an equal quantity of petroleum jelly to make it softer. Lanolin also possesses the valuable property of being able to mix with and absorb water to a considerable extent.

LAPAROTOMY is a general term applied to any operation in which the abdominal cavity is opened.

LARYNGECTOMY is the operation for removal of the larynx.

LARYNGISMUS STRIDULUS, or SPASMODIC CROUP, is a spasmodic condition in children, in which great difficulty of breathing, accompanied by a crowing noise, comes on as the result of partial clo-sure of the larynx. The children affected by it are generally suffering from rickets. It is rare over the age of 2 or 3 years. Attacks may be precipitated by fright, irritation or a cold draught. The attack may come on at any time during the day, or even during sleep; the spasm may amount only to difficulty of breathing or the stoppage may be almost complete.

Treatment is similar to that for croup. (See CROUP.)

LARYNGITIS, or inflammation of the mucous membrane of the larynx, may be either acute or chronic. (See also SINGER'S NODULE.)

ACUTE LARYNGITIS: **Causes** – This complaint is usually produced by exposure to infection: directly or through a catarrh extending from the nose above or from the bronchial tubes beneath to the mucous membrane of the larynx. It accompanies some of the infectious diseases in which the throat is liable to suffer, such as measles, scarlet fever, diphtheria, smallpox, and erysipelas. Excessive use of the voice, as in loud and prolonged speaking or singing, sometimes produces laryngitis. It therefore tends to be common among members of the acting and singing professions, as well as clergymen and other public speakers. Further, the inhalation of irritating particles and vapours, and the swallowing of very hot fluids are well recognized causes.

Symptoms – The chief changes in the larynx are great redness and swelling, which affect the whole interior of the cavity, but are specially marked where the tissues are loose, such as the neighbourhood of the epiglottis and of the vocal cords. The effect is to produce narrowing of the channel for the entrance of air, and to this the chief dangers are due. The symptoms vary with the intensity of the attack, but, along with more or less feverishness and constitutional disturbance, there is usually a sense of heat, dryness, and pain in the throat, attended by some difficulty in the act of swallowing. Cough is a constant symptom, and is either loud, barking, or clanging, or else husky and toneless. It is at first dry, but afterwards is accompanied with expectoration. The voice, like the cough, is rough, husky, or may for a few days disappear almost entirely. The breathing shows evidence of laryngeal obstruction, both inspiration and expiration being prolonged and difficult, with a somewhat hissing sound, and with almost no interval between the two acts. In severe cases, the face may become livid, and suffocation threatens, particularly during the paroxysms of coughing. In favourable cases, which form the majority, the attack tends to abate in a few days, but on the other hand, death may occur suddenly in a suffocative paroxysm, particularly in the case of children. Many cases of acute laryngitis are so comparatively slight as to make themselves known only by hoarseness and the character of the cough; nevertheless, in every instance, and particularly in children, the attack demands serious attention.

Treatment – The treatment consists in keeping the patient in bed in an atmosphere of 65° to 70° F (18·3° to 21° C), made moist by steam (see BRONCHITIS). The voice must be rested, and smoking is forbidden. The use of warm gargles, and the frequent inhalation of the vapour of hot water, containing such soothing substances as benzoin or menthol, and the application of hot fomentations to the front of the neck, will be found of much value. Spraying the larynx with a warm mixture of glycerin and water (1 part of glycerin to 2 parts of water) is also of value, particularly in children. Internally, diaphoretics, such as small doses of Dover's powder, are also to be recommended. In most severe cases the use of penicillin or the sulphonamides must be considered. Their efficacy is dependent upon the laryngitis being due to a penicillin- or sulphonamide-sensitive organism. Such remedies usually suffice to relieve the attack, but in very severe cases more active interference may be necessary. When there is much swelling of the mucous membrane in the upper portion of the larynx, as shown by great obstruction of the breathing, tracheostomy (qv) may have to be performed when death appears to be imminent from suffocation. Attacks of laryngitis may be largely prevented in those liable to them by a regimen calculated to invigorate the system, such as the cold baths, and regular open-air exercise.

CHRONIC LARYNGITIS: **Causes** – This may occur as a result of repeated attacks of the acute form, or may arise independently owing to such causes as habitual exposure (especially when along with this there is over-indulgence in alcohol) and the habitual over-use of the vocal organs. Any interference with the entrance of air through the nose, leading to the bad habit of mouth-breathing, has an influence in ·setting up chronic laryngitis. The changes taking place in the parts are more permanent than in the acute form, consist-

ing mainly in thickening of the mucous membrane and the vocal cords. Some cases are due to tuberculosis, syphilis, and other chronic inflammatory diseases, and these are apt to produce ulceration of the vocal cords and other parts of the larynx and ultimately destruction of its cartilages.

Symptoms – The symptoms vary according to the extent and amount, as well as the duration, of the inflammation. Thus there may simply be a certain huskiness or hoarseness on attempts at the use of the voice, this condition being well exemplified in the so-called clergyman's sore throat or *dysphonia clericorum* (see CLERGYMAN'S SORE THROAT); on the other hand, there may be not only complete loss of voice, but severe pain in the act of swallowing, and great difficulty in breathing, accompanied sometimes with expectoration of large quantities of matter in the cases in which ulceration is present. Under this variety of the disease may be included the ulceration due to syphilis and that occurring in the course of pulmonary tuberculosis. The diagnosis and the treatment of all such cases are greatly aided by the use of the laryngoscope (qv), by which a view of the affected parts can be obtained, and the proper remedies more readily applied.

Treatment – In the treatment of the chronic forms of laryngitis, rest to the parts is essential, any attempts at continuing the use of the voice only aggravating the condition. Antibiotics or sulphonamides may be called for if the condition is due to some antibiotic- or sulphonamide-sensitive micro-organism. Applications to the affected parts in the forms of solutions of lactic acid, nitrate of silver, alum, or tannin, either by means of a brush or syringe introduced into the cavity or by the simpler method of spraying, are often beneficial. Inhalations, as of eucalyptus or oil of pine, are also helpful. The diet must be made as simple as possible, and all irritating condiments such as mustard, pickles, and spices should be avoided. Alcohol is also highly prejudicial, especially in the form of strong spirits, and should be avoided. The habit of smoking must be abandoned. The improper use of the voice has been dealt with under the simple but very troublesome form of laryngitis known as CLERGYMAN'S SORE THROAT, which is prone to affect those who use the voice a great deal.

TUBERCULOUS LARYNGITIS practically always occurs as a result of infection spreading from the lungs. Until recently one of the most serious complications of pulmonary tuberculosis, the outlook has been completely changed by the introduction of streptomycin, as this has proved to be one of the forms of tuberculosis which responds best to streptomycin.

TUMOURS and various *inflammatory growths* are often met with in the larynx and may give rise to symptoms of chronic laryngitis. Such growths may be of simple character, in the form of isolated fibrous formations attached by a peduncle to some portion of the laryngeal mucous membrane, or as warty excrescences occurring upon or in the neighbourhood of the vocal cords. They are detected by means of the laryngoscope, and can often be dealt with effectually by a very slight operation, though one requiring great skill. Cancer of the larynx may often be removed successfully by means of the operation known as laryngectomy if the disease is detected in its early stages. *Hoarseness may then be the only symptom.* Hence arises the great importance of a careful examination of the larynx by an expert in every case of hoarseness which has lasted for some weeks or more.

Even in the more advanced cases satisfactory results can often be obtained either by supervoltage radiation therapy or by laryngectomy but, of course, the earlier the diagnosis and therefore the treatment, the better the results. Laryngectomee clubs are now being established throughout the country to advise and help patients who have had a laryngectomy. Details of these can be obtained from The National Association of Laryngectomee Clubs, Room 26, 38/39 Eccleston Square, London, S.W.1.

NERVOUS AFFECTIONS of the larynx occur independently of any local disease. One of the most important of these is *laryngismus stridulus*, otherwise called *child-crowing* or *spasmodic croup*. (See LARYNGISMUS STRIDULUS.)

Symptoms not unlike those of laryngismus sometimes occur in adults as the result of irritation of the recurrent laryngeal nerve, by the pressure upon it of an aneurysm or tumour situated in the chest. Such pressure, if long continued, results in paralysis of the nerve, with loss of voice. (See RECURRENT LARYNGEAL NERVE.)

In the condition known as *nervous aphonia*, which occurs mostly in women of hysterical temperament or in circumstances of enfeebled health, the voice becomes reduced to a whisper, but there is seldom any affection of the breathing, or cough, and the laryngoscope reveals a perfectly healthy state of the parts. In such cases the remedies must be directed to the improvement of the general health and reassurance of the patient that there is no disease underlying the loss of voice. The use of electricity (faradism) applied to the neck is often attended with marked benefit. Like other hysterical conditions, this condition may be present for years, causing even complete loss of voice, and

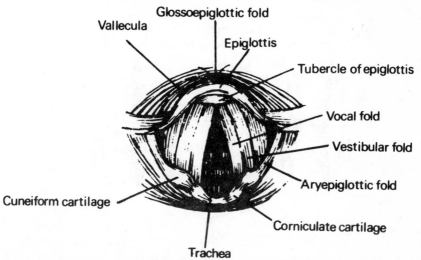

279 – A laryngoscopic view of the interior of the larynx. From *Gray's Anatomy*. Longman.

then may suddenly disappear as the result of a powerful mental impression.

LARYNGOLOGY is that branch of medical science which is concerned with disorders and diseases of the larynx and those parts of the respiratory tract immediately above and below it.

LARYNGOSCOPE is an instrument introduced by Signor Manuel Garcia, a London teacher of singing, about the middle of the nineteenth century, and first used for medical purposes by Türck and Czermak about 1858. The essential parts of the laryngoscope are a small mirror set upon a long stem at an angle of about 120°, for introduction into the back of the patient's throat, and a source of bright light placed close to the observer's eye. The light may be from a lamp placed by the side of the patient's head: the beam from this lamp is reflected by a mirror attached to a forehead-band or spectacle frame worn by the observer; more conveniently, the light may proceed from a small electric lamp directly attached to the observer's forehead. For the uses of the instrument, and the appearances observed by its help, see illustration 279 and LARYNX.

LARYNGO-TRACHEO-BRONCHITIS is an acute infection of the respiratory tract in infants and young children. It is usually a virus infection or caused by *Haemophilus influenzae*. In the old days it was often referred to as 'croup'. The onset is sudden, usually in a child who has had a cold to which little significance has been attached. Quite often the first sign is when the child wakens up with a loud inspiratory stridor and a harsh barking cough. Distress and restlessness ensue rapidly, and in some cases tracheostomy may be required as a life-saving measure. Because of the seriousness of the condition, these children should always be treated in hospital if at all possible, where the essentials of treatment are oxygen and humidification of the atmosphere, usually combined in an oxygen tent.

LARYNX is the organ of voice, and also forms one of the higher parts of the air passages. It is placed high up in the front of the neck, and there forms a considerable prominence on the surface. It is covered in front by the skin, a layer of fibrous tissue, and a thin layer of muscle, whilst its sides are protected by the lateral lobes of the thyroid gland, and by the large sternomastoid muscles.

The larynx (illustration 280) is almost 2 inches (5 cm) in height, and forms a sort of box, well protected in front by cartilages, rather more open behind, and communicating above with the throat at the root of the tongue, below with the windpipe. The larynx is enclosed by five large cartilages: the thyroid cartilage, whose prominent pointed front forms the Adam's apple; the

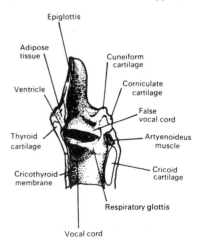

(A)   (B)

280 – (A) Vertical section of larynx seen from behind. (B) Vertical section of larynx seen from left side. From Stewart, *Logan Turner's Diseases of the Nose, Throat and Ear*. John Wright.

cricoid cartilage, a ring placed below it; the epiglottis, a leaf-like cartilage standing on the upper edge of the thyroid cartilage, and projecting up into the interior of the throat at the root of the tongue; and a pair of arytenoid cartilages jointed to the top edge of the cricoid cartilage behind, where the thyroid cartilage is deficient. There are

281 – Diagram of the opening of the larynx to show the action of the muscles. A horizontal section has been made at the level of the true vocal cords. *TT*, thyroid cartilage; *AA*, arytenoid cartilages with *aa*, vocal processes, and *ee*, muscular processes; *C*, upper border of cricoid cartilage; *v*, the vocal, and *r*, the respiratory part of the opening. The two cords are widely separated by the action of *pca*, the posterior crico-arytenoid muscles.

282 – Diagram of the opening of the larynx to show the action of the muscles. The letters indicate the same structures as in illustration 281, but the cords are now almost close together, by the action of *ta*, the thyroarytenoid, *lca*, the lateral arytenoid, and *ar*, the arytenoid muscles.

also four small nodules of cartilage above the arytenoids. The edges of the laryngeal cartilages do not fit closely together, and the spaces between are filled up by membranes. Certain of the ligaments which bind the cartilages together are of great importance. These pass along each side of the larynx, from the arytenoid cartilage behind to the thyroid cartilage in front, two bands of elastic fibres covered by the mucous membrane which lines the whole

larynx. One pair of these bands lies directly above the other, the upper pair being known as the false vocal cords; the lower pair are the true vocal cords (illustrations 281, 282). The latter are capable of various degrees of tenseness and slackness, and of approximation and separation, these results being achieved by several small muscles, which are attached to the arytenoid cartilages, and governed in their movements through branches of the vagus nerves. Between the true and false cord is a deep depression on each side, the ventricle or sinus of the larynx, from which a pouch, half an inch (12 mm) long, leads upwards exterior to the false cord. The larynx is lined throughout by mucous membrane, which generally is covered by ciliated cells (see EPITHELIUM); but over the true cords, which are subject to much friction in the production of the voice, the surface consists of flattened cells similar to those of the skin.

The vocal cords vibrating in different notes, according to their tenseness and the like, produce the sounds of voice and speech. (See VOICE AND SPEECH.)

LARYNX, DISEASES OF (see LARYNGISMUS; LARYNGITIS).

LASER stands for Light Amplification by the Stimulated Emission of Radiation. It is a potent form of energy which is proving of value in the treatment of detachment of the retina. (See RETINA, DISEASES OF.) Its three great advantages are its potency, the speed with which it acts and the facility with which it can be focused on a small area – even an area as small as 1 micrometre.

LASSA FEVER, which derives its name from the fact that it was first reported in Lassa in Nigeria, is a disease due to an arenavirus (qv). This may be transmitted by rodents or direct from an infected person to those around him. The incubation period is three to twenty-one days. It is characterized by headache, lethargy and severe muscular pains, and there is often a rash due to bleeding into the skin and mucous membranes. Sore throat is often present. It may carry a high mortality rate, particularly in pregnant women. As it is a virus infection, there is no specific treatment, and all that can be done is careful nursing, with rest in bed.

LASSAR'S PASTE, officially known as Zinc and Salicylic Acid Paste, B P, is the name given to a preparation used as a

517

remedy for eczema. It has a combined softening, antiseptic, astringent, and soothing action. It is made up of zinc oxide 24 grams; salicylic acid 2 grams; starch 24 grams; white soft paraffin 100 grams.

LATHYRISM is the term applied to a disease in which stiffness, pains in, and trembling and paralysis of, the legs are caused by varieties of lathyrus pea (chick-pea).

LAUDANUM is the popular name for tincture of opium. (See OPIUM.)

LAUGHING-GAS is a popular name for nitrous oxide (qv), which is used as an anaesthetic for short operations.

LAUREL is the name applied to two plants; one of these, *Laurus nobilis* or bay tree, affords leaves and berries from which an oil is extracted which is used for application in rheumatic and similar pains; the other, *Prunus laurocerasus* or cherry laurel, affords cherry laurel water, containing a small quantity of hydrocyanic acid, and is used for making up soothing solutions.

LAVAGE is the name applied to the washing out of the stomach.

LAXATIVES (see PURGATIVES).

LEAD has no action itself upon the system, but its salts, when absorbed in any quantity, or for any length of time, have very important effects. When a lead salt comes in contact with a wound or with any mucous surface, it combines with the albuminous material of the discharge or secretion to form a whitish glaze, which affords a degree of protection to the surface. Further, the lead salt has an astringent action upon the blood-vessels, and therefore helps to stop bleeding or relieve the congestion of inflammation. If one of the soluble lead salts be taken internally, in large amount, it has an irritant action, and the acetate (sugar of lead), subacetate, and nitrate of lead are irritant poisons when taken into the stomach, although their action is comparatively feeble.

Uses – Externally, subacetate of lead is used in the form of Goulard's water, for application to painful areas, such as inflamed joints, bruises, sprains. (See GOULARD'S WATER.) In eczema this solution, sponged upon the affected area, often

gives relief from itching. Lead lotion and lead and glycerin lotion are similarly used. Litharge, or lead monoxide, is used as a basis for many adhesive plasters, which are known as diachylon plasters. Lead with opium suppositories are used for the treatment of bleeding piles.

LEAD POISONING – Acute poisoning by lead acetate (sugar of lead) is an accident which sometimes, though rarely, happens to a child, and is treated, like cases of irritant poisoning generally, by administering diluents such as milk together with Epsom salts, which form an antidote, followed by emetics.

Chronic poisoning is apt to affect those who come in contact with lead or its salts, either in the production of these or in the course of their use in various arts and manufactures. Thus lead-smelters, plumbers, typefounders, compositors, filemakers, pottery workers who use lead in glaze, painters, dyers, above all, those who make white-lead, and also persons following various other callings, are liable to suffer. Another industrial lead health hazard is tetra-ethyl lead which is added to petrol as an 'anti-knocking' agent. The risk here is to workmen cleaning petrol storage tanks. Whether it has any effect on the general populace in this automobile-ridden age is still a moot point. Lead-containing paint is a common cuase of lead poisoning in children in the form of pica (qv) which manifests itself by the chewing of painted wood-work. Lead may also be introduced into the system through food and water, in those who have nothing to do with the metal in their work. For example, drinking-water is sometimes contaminated by lead which it has dissolved off the pipes through which it passes, or tinned fruits may dissolve lead out of the solder with which the tins are sealed. The solder used to weld the seam in such tins may contain up to 98 per cent lead. Cider, made in leaden presses, may so readily take up lead that 'Devonshire colic' was once a name given to lead-poisoning occurring in this part of the country, where cider forms a favourite beverage.

Control over lead in food in England and Wales is exercised by the Lead in Food Regulations 1961. These Regulations lay down a limit of 2 parts per million (p.p.m.) for most foods, with different levels for certain specified foods including canned meat and meat pastes, fish and fish pastes, for which a maximum of 5 p.p.m. is permitted. There are similar regulations for Scotland and Northern Ireland. Subsequent Regulations created a new category for foods specially prepared for infants and young children, and set a limit of 0·5 p.p.m. for this category. The upper allowable limit for lead in potable water is 0·1 mg per litre. Under an EEC directive the permitted quantity is 0·05 mg per litre. As regards drinking-water there is, in general, no danger, because the minerals in the water form, with the lead, insoluble compounds which are deposited in a thin coat upon the inside of the pipes. Pipes of bright untarnished lead, as in newly built houses, or an absolutely pure water which does not contain any mineral ingredients, may introduce an element of danger. But a greater danger exists in peaty or soft water, or in water contaminated by organic impurities, both of which give the water a high power of dissolving lead. Not only may the lead be introduced into the system through the skin of those who constantly handle lead-containing materials, and by way of the stomach, but in some of the most rapidly produced and serious cases – for example, among white-lead workers, and glazers of pottery – the lead is inhaled as dry dust. Lead is often similarly inhaled by men engaged in cutting up iron plates which have been fitted by the aid of red lead; this, being driven off by the heat of the blow-pipe employed, is apt to be inhaled.

Symptoms – Among the early symptoms of a chronic and insidious case are constipation, muscular weakness, and pallor of the skin. A blue line on the margin of the gums, due to deposit of lead sulphide in this locality, is also an important sign of the condition. Colic of a very painful nature, affecting the centre of the abdomen and lasting often for several days at a time, appears and forms one of the most prominent symptoms in almost every case. Lead has a specially injurious action upon the nervous system, causing an inflammatory process in the nerves, which results in tremors and paralysis, usually affecting the muscles on the back of the wrist first of all, and later those on the front and outer side of the leg, and causing wrist-drop and foot-drop. Convulsions, which may develop rapidly and may end in death, are also produced by poisoning of the nervous system, leading to a brain disorder known as lead encephalopathy. Occasionally, though fortunately rarely, affection of the optic nerve leads to blindness, which is either temporary or permanent. Owing to interference with the kidney functions, the urine becomes scanty, while a destructive action on the blood leads to anaemia.

Treatment – With regard to workers in lead and its salts, government regulations have been introduced which very effectively protect them. In 1970, 79 cases of lead poisoning were notified in Britain, and none of these was fatal. Among these preventive measures are included: personal cleanliness in washing the hands and changing the clothes before partaking of meals, the use of respirators by those who come in contact with white-lead dust, the provision of exhaust flues and electric fans beneath the tables at which pottery glazers work, and the drinking of at least a glass of milk daily. These and other measures confer a great degree of protection upon those engaging in these otherwise dangerous trades. Workers who begin to show symptoms of lead poisoning should at once undergo treatment. A frequent recurrence of symptoms shows a special liability to this form of poisoning, and indicates that the worker should seek some totally different employment. In the case of drinking-water the source of contamination must, of course, be removed. The drug which is of special use in treatment of lead-poisoning is calcium disodium versenate, by which lead salts deposited in the tissues are dissolved, to be afterwards excreted from the body. Colic is treated by hot fomentations, magnesium sulphate, and belladonna, and a high calcium diet.

In acute cases of lead colic the intravenous administration of calcium gluconate or calcium chloride gives immediate relief.

LEADERS is a popular name for the tendons or sinews at the wrist, ankle, etc. (See TENDON.)

LEBER'S DISEASE, or HEREDITARY OPTIC ATROPHY, is a hereditary disease in which blindness comes on at about the age of twenty.

LECITHIN is a very complex fat found in various tissues of the body, but particularly in the brain and nerves, of which it forms a large part. It is also found in large quantities in the yolk of an egg.

LEECHES are animals belonging to the class Vermes, provided with suckers and living a semi-parasitic life, their food being mainly derived from the blood of other animals. They abstract blood by means of a sucker surrounding the mouth, which is provided with several large sharp teeth. The medicinal leech, *Hirudo medicinalis*,

Skull

Cervical vertebrae

First and second
thoracic vertebrae

Clavicle

Scapula

Sternum

Humerus

Eleventh and twelfth
thoracic vertebrae

Lumbar vertebrae

Hip bone

Sacrum

Coccyx

Radius

Ulna

Carpus

Metacarpals

Phalanges

Femur

Patella

Tibia

Fibula

Tarsus

Metatarsals

Phalanges

s.w.w

Sesamoid

283 – The human skeleton, showing the bones of the leg. *Grays Anatomy*. Longman.

was formerly employed for the abstraction of small quantities of blood in inflammatory and other conditions.

LEG – This term is generally applied to the whole lower extremity but, properly speaking, includes that part between the knee and ankle joints. The lower limb is attached to the pelvic bones by strong muscles, especially the gluteal and hamstring muscles behind and the abductor

the tibia on the inner side and the fibula on the outer side. Seven tarsal bones comprise the hinder part of the foot, of which the talus takes the weight of the body from the tibia and fibula. There are five metatarsal bones in the front portion of the foot and each toe has three phalangeal bones, excepting the great toe, which has two. The powerful quadriceps extensor muscle in front of the thigh is attached to the

284 – Arteries of the lower limb. Anterior view (left) and posterior view (right).

muscles on the inner side of the thigh. The head of the femur, or thigh bone, lies in a deep cup-shaped hollow, the acetabulum, on the outer side of the pelvis (illustration 283). The femur, which is the longest and strongest bone in the body, forms at its lower end the joint of the knee with the tibia. The knee-joint is protected in front by the patella or knee-cap. Along the outer side of the tibia lies the smaller fibula, which does not extend up to the knee but which, along with the tibia, forms the ankle joint. The two prominences on the ankle (*malleoli*) are formed by

knee-cap, which in turn is attached to the front of the tibia by the patellar ligament. This muscle straightens the knee and keeps the body in an erect posture. Below the knee the muscles of the calf, attached to the heel through the tendo calcaneus, or tendon of Achilles, raise the heel off the ground in walking. In front of and to the outside of the leg lie the tibial and peroneal muscles, which bend the ankle upwards and raise the toes. In the sole of the foot are a number of small muscles which bend the toes downwards. The arch of the foot is a very important structure. (See FOOT.)

LEGIONNAIRE'S DISEASE

Most of the blood supply to the lower limb (illustration 284) is carried by the femoral artery, which issues from the abdomen in the middle of the groin where its pulse can be felt. This passes down the inner side of the thigh to reach the middle of the back of the knee, where it is known as the popliteal artery. Below the knee it divides into anterior and posterior tibial vessels. The former of these runs down the front of the leg and upper surface of the foot, and the latter, which is the larger, passes behind the inner ankle where its pulse can be felt about a finger's-breadth behind the bony prominence. The chief nerve in the lower limb is the sciatic nerve which runs down the middle of the back of the thigh deeply embedded in muscles. Above the knee it divides into two parts: the tibial and common peroneal nerves. The former of these runs down the back of the leg, deeply embedded in muscles, to the foot, and the latter passes round the upper end of the fibula on the outer side of the leg, where it can be felt and is liable to be damaged. The blood returns from the leg partly by deep veins lying alongside the arteries, but to a large extent by the great saphenous vein, which can be seen or felt under the skin for most of the distance from the inner ankle up the inside of the leg and thigh to the inner side of the groin, where it joins the femoral vein.

The arch of the foot is liable to give way, especially in debilitated or overworked persons, thus producing flat foot. The ankle joint is liable to sprains which consist of tearing of the ligaments, especially on the inner side. The fibula is liable to be fractured near its lower end, either by twists of the foot or by a blow on the outer side of the leg. Fracture of the tibia is also a common accident and, as the tibia lies immediately beneath the skin, this fracture is in danger of becoming compound. The knee-joint, by reason of its great strength, is seldom dislocated, but the partial displacement of a cartilage in the knee is a common occurrence. Fracture of the femur is a serious accident, requiring a period of several months for complete union of the bone. The long and poorly supported vein on the inner side of the leg and thigh is very apt to become distended along with its branches, producing the condition known as varicose veins with resultant eczema and ulcer. The bursa in front of the knee-cap, in persons who kneel much, readily becomes inflamed and thickened in the condition known as 'housemaid's knee'. (See also FOOT; FRAC-TURES; JOINTS; KNEE; LIMBS; VEINS, DISEASES OF.)

LEGIONNAIRE'S DISEASE is a form of pneumonia due to an unnamed bacillus. It has an incubation period of two to ten days. It starts with aches and pains followed rapidly by a rise in temperature, shivering attacks, cough and shortness of breath. X-rays show patchy areas of consolidation in the lungs. In those who recover the temperature usually begins to settle gradually after two or three days. The infection responds to treatment with erythromycin.

LEGUME is the pod or seed of a leguminous plant such as the pea or bean. As foods, legumes are of importance because of the relatively large amount of protein they contain. Peas in the fresh state may contain from 3 to 6 per cent of protein, which is from one-sixth to one-third the amount of protein contained in fish, beef, and similar animal foods. Beans contain rather more, and string or French beans somewhat less protein. They differ from meat foods in two important respects, however, one being that they contain from 5 to 15 per cent of carbohydrate, and the second difference being that vegetable protein does not contain all the amino-acids (qv) which are essential to health. They can never therefore completely replace animal protein. Legumes are not rich in vitamins, but they contain a varying amount of thiamine and riboflavine. They are fairly rich in iron, but contain little calcium. It is thus evident that legumes are a useful constituent of the normal diet. (See also DIET; and SOYA BEAN.)

LEIOMYOMA is the term applied to a tumour made up of unstriped or involuntary muscle fibres.

LEISHMANIASIS is a group of diseases due to infection with a number of parasites, of the genus known as Leishmania. The parasite is transmitted to man by the bite of certain sandflies.

VISCERAL LEISHMANIASIS, or KALA-AZAR, also known as DUM-DUM FEVER, occurs widely in tropical and sub-tropical Africa and Asia, the Mediterranean area and in tropical South America. It is caused by a parasite known as Leishmania donovani (illustration 285). The source of the infection, the type of sandfly that transmits it to man, and the common age of infection vary from one area to

285 – Leishmania. Mass of parasites inside a macrophage. From Blacklock & Southwell, *A Guide to Human Parasitology*. H. K. Lewis & Co. Ltd.

another. Thus, in the Mediterranean region it is predominantly a disease of infants, whereas in Africa it tends more to occur in adolescents and young adults. The onset may be sudden or gradual. In the well-established case there is enlargement of the spleen and of the liver, accompanied by fever and generalized glandular enlargement. The diagnosis is established by removing a piece of bone marrow, spleen or liver, and examining it for the presence of the causative parasite. Untreated the disease is usually fatal either in the acute stage or after two years or so.

Treatment – Sodium stibogluconate, a pentavalent antimonial compound, is the drug of choice. The response to treatment varies with the area in which the infection occurs. Thus, in India, the disease usually responds to one ten-day course of injections, whereas in the Mediterranean region two or three such courses may be needed. A high proportion of cases are cured in this way.

CUTANEOUS and MUCO-CUTANEOUS LEISHANIASIS is the form of the disease in which the parasite involves predominantly the skin and mucous membranes, and sometimes also cartilage. It is caused by a variety of species of Leishmania, and is known by different names in different geographical areas. Thus, in South America it is known as espundia, whereas in Asia it is known variously as oriental sore, Delhi boil, Aleppo boil, Baghdad boil, Biskra boil (or button). In the Old World it tends to be restricted to the skin, producing a chronic ulcer, whereas in the New World it tends to be more diffuse, involving the nose and throat, and leading to widespread erosion of the nasal cartilage; it may well terminate in a fatal broncho-pneumonia.

Treatment is by sodium stibogluconate, but most of the cases in the Old World heal spontaneously, and the affected area merely needs to be protected and kept clean.

LEMON is used in the form of the fresh peel, tincture, syrup, and oil. Its main value, however, is as a source of vitamin C (or ascorbic acid), the average content of ascorbic acid in the juice being 45 mg per 100 grams. (See also CITRIC ACID; and VITAMINS.)

LENS OF THE EYE is one of the refractive media through which light passes before reaching the retina. The lens is important, because its bulging and flattening, brought about by the ciliary muscle, automatically adjust the eye for focusing correctly on the retina rays of light from objects at varying distances. The lens begins to lose this power at the age of forty, hence the need of spectacles for near work as age advances. (See ACCOMMODATION.) The lens is the seat of the opacity which constitutes a cataract. (See CATARACT; EYE; and EYE, DISEASES OF.)

LENTIGO is another name for freckles (qv).

LENTILS are the seeds of *Lens esculenta* which originated around the Mediterranean. Esau sold his birthright to his brother Jacob 'for bread and pottage of lentiles'. It is used as soup or a flour. The latter makes an excellent nutritious lentil cake. (See PULSES.)

LEPROSY is a chronic disease which affects particularly the skin, mucous membranes, and nerves.

History – It has been said that 'leprosy is a disease as old as the world itself' (Cochrane). Some authorities say that it originated in the upper reaches of the Nile. Others claim that it originated in the region of the Indus. Wherever it originated, its subsequent history is difficult to trace because of the confusion as to what the older writers meant by the term 'leprosy'. The term is used in the Authorized Version of The Bible, but experts differ as to whether this is the correct translation of the Hebrew word, *Tsaraath*. As Sir William MacArthur, the medical historian, has pointed out, 'in the past "leprosy" and its equivalents had a multitude of meanings. It was used for the true disease and for every disorder that was formerly supposed to be leprosy'. In Europe it reached its highest incidence between 1000 AD and 1400 AD, thereafter slowly declining. The last indigenous case in Great Britain died in 1798 – in the Shetland Islands. So far as the American continent is concerned, the available evidence suggests that it was introduced there originally by Columbus's soldiers, and much later by the slave trade from West Africa.

Causes – The causative organism of leprosy is the *Mycobacterium leprae* which was discovered by Hansen in 1872. It is a straight or slightly curved rod which closely resembles the *Mycobacterium tuberculosis* in its size and acid-fast staining reaction.

The total number of cases in the world has been conservatively estimated at between 10 and 11 million: 6·5 million in Asia (mainly in the Indian Subcontinent and the Far East); 3·5 million in Africa; and 350,000 in the Americas (mainly Central and South America). In Europe it is largely confined to Portugal, Spain, the Balkan States, European Russia and European Turkey. It is estimated that there are 3000 cases in Portugal and probably as many in Spain. It has reappeared in Britain as a result of the recent influx of immigrants from countries in which leprosy is endemic. In 1977, in England there were 360 registered cases of leprosy, 258 of which were known to be quiescent; 21 cases were notified during the year. Since the disease became notifiable in Britain in 1951 no case has been reported of the disease being acquired in this country. All have been cases in which the infection was acquired overseas. The incubation period, or latent period between the infection being acquired and the disease manifesting itself is considered to be between 3 and 5 years or even longer. Males are more commonly infected than females. The variation of incidence among different races is due to contact rather than racial susceptibility, but the type of the disease varies in different races. Thus, the European and Mongol races appear to be more likely to acquire the serious lepromatous type of leprosy than the Indian and African races. There is no evidence that leprosy is in any way due to dietetic deficiencies. The disease is transmitted by contact with open cases of leprosy, but the precise method whereby this is achieved is still not quite clear. What is known is that only a few of the people exposed to infection develop the disease, and that those in contact with tuberculoid cases are much less likely to develop the disease than those in contact with lepromatous cases.

Symptoms – There are two distinct types of leprosy: tuberculoid and lepromatous. The differentiation is important because the former runs a relatively benign course and is often self-healing, whereas the latter is a steadily progressive form of the disease. The differentiation, however, is not always clear cut, and there is a group of 'indeterminate' or 'dimorphous' cases in which lesions similar to tuberculoid and lepromatous leprosy are seen in the same patient. The diffferentiation of those three types is a matter for the expert, and no attempt will be made here to go into the details of the different types.

Whatever form of leprosy may be present, the symptoms and signs can be divided into two main groups: those involving the skin and those arising from involvement of the nerves. The skin manifestations range from areas of whitening of the skin to massive nodules such as are so often shown in photographs of advanced cases of leprosy. The nerve manifestations range from localized swellings of the nerve to extensive areas of anaesthesia in the skin. The ultimate destruction of the nerves leads to the deformities which used to be such a marked feature of leprosy in the old days before adequate means of treatment became available. These included foot-drop, wrist-drop, claw-foot, extensive ulceration of the extremities leading to loss of the fingers and toes, and absorption of bone. The eyes may also be infected, leading to blindness, and ulcers may occur in the mouth and in the larynx. In the larynx they may cause hoarseness or even go on to the stage of producing complete blockage of it. These tragic cases of gross deformity, which in the past have made leprosy such a terrifying disease, should no longer occur. As Cochrane has pointed out: 'With the introduction of modern therapy the vast majority of cases, if treated adequately before extensive deformity has set in, should recover without any disability. Nevertheless, until adequate treatment and properly administered therapy are within the reach of all, the shadow of tragic deformity will remain, particularly where there is a failure to understand the importance of physiotherapy in preventing this'.

Treatment – For centuries chaulmoogra (hydnocarpus) oil was the great stand-by in the treatment of leprosy. There is an ancient Burmese folk-story that a Burmese prince, who discovered that he had leprosy, was directed by the gods to retire to the forest and there eat the seeds of the fruit of a certain tree. This he did and his leprosy was cured. Such is said to have been the introduction of chaulmoogra oil in the treatment of leprosy.

In 1941, the outlook was entirely changed by the discovery that a sulphone derivative was effective in the treatment. The sulphones can keep the disease under control and their widespread use has gone far to bringing leprosy under control. The most widely used sulphone is dapsone, which is given by mouth. Given over long periods of time, most cases of leprosy respond satisfactorily. Various other drugs have been introduced during recent years for the treatment of leprosy. The most promising are rifampicin, clofazimine, and thiacetazone. Unfortunately the *Mycobacterium leprae* is developing resistance to dapsone when this is given alone. To reduce this risk to a minimum, it is necessary to give it along with some other anti-leprosy such as thiacetazone. Preliminary results from Uganda suggest that BCG vaccine (qv) may be of value in the prevention of leprosy, but in the case of a disease like leprosy it is too early yet to assess the real significance of this observation. Hopes are also arising that it may be possible to produce an effective vaccine against the disease.

Chemotherapy, however, has not diminished the importance of physiotherapy in the treatment and prevention of deformity in leprosy. Equally important is the role of plastic and orthopaedic surgery in treating these deformities when they have reached a stage in which physiotherapy is of little use. Many patients with advanced leprosy, hitherto condemned to a life of chronic invalidism as a result of their deformities, are now being returned to the community as useful members who are able to use their hands and feet sufficiently to be able to earn a living and lead a reasonably active life.

The salient points about leprosy are summed up as follows in a *Memorandum on Leprosy* published by the Department of Health and Social Security.

(1) Leprosy is normally a curable disease.

(2) It is only slightly contagious and most people are, to some extent, naturally immune to the disease.

(3) If it is treated early enough, it can be arrested without deformity.

(4) Only a few people need to continue treatment for life.

(5) Leprosy is slow to develop and takes considerable time to treat.

(6) Patients with leprosy who are undergoing treatment for the disease can live at home, and continue normal family life and work.

LEPTAZOL is a synthetic organic drug introduced as a respiratory stimulant.

LEPTOMENINGITIS means inflammation of the inner and more delicate membranes of the brain or spinal cord.

LEPTOSPIRA is a group, or genus, of spiral micro-organisms, normally found in rodents and other small mammals in which they cause no harm. When transmitted to man by other animals, however, they give rise to various forms of illness.

LEPTOSPIROSIS is the disease caused by infection with Leptospira. It is an occupational hazard of farmers, sewage and abattoir workers, fish cutters and veterinary surgeons, but the infection can also be acquired from bathing in contaminated water. The disease varies in intensity from a mild influenza-like illness to a fatal form of jaundice due to severe liver disease. The kidneys are often involved and there may be meningitis. Penicillin is the great stand-by in treatment. (See also SPIROCHAETOSIS ICTEROHAEMORRHAGICA.)

LESION meant originally an injury, but is now applied generally to all disease changes in organs and tissues.

LETHARGY is a term applied to various disorders in which the affected person remains constantly asleep, though capable of being roused for short periods. It is a symptom of concussion of the brain and various mental diseases. (See BRAIN; HYPNOTISM; CATALEPSY.) Its most remarkable form is that observed in negro-lethargy or sleeping sickness. (See SLEEPING SICKNESS.)

LETTUCE is a green vegetable consisting of leaves of *Lactuca sativa*. It is a relatively rich source of vitamin A. The content of vitamin C is variable, ranging from 1 to 17 mg per 100 grams.

LEUCINE is one of the essential, or indispensable, amino-acids (qv). They are so called because they cannot be synthesized, or manufactured, in the body, and are therefore essential constituents of the diet.

LEUCOCYTE is the term applied to the white blood cells. Leucocytes differ from erythrocytes in that they contain no haemoglobin and are therefore colourless, and contain a well-formed nucleus. Most of them are larger than erythrocytes, being

LEUCOCYTOSIS

8 to 15 micrometres in diameter, and there are many fewer in the blood – usually about 8000 per cubic millimetre of blood. There are three main classes of white cells: granulocytes, lymphocytes, and monocytes. *Granulocytes*, or polymorphonuclear leucocytes as they are sometimes termed, which normally constitute 70 per cent of the white blood cells, have a lobed nucleus and a granular cytoplasm. They are divided into three groups according to the staining reactions of these granules: neutrophils, which stain with neutral dyes and constitute 65 to 70 per cent of all the white blood cells; eosinophils, which stain with acid dyes (eg. eosin) and constitute 3 to 4 per cent of the total white blood cells; and basophils, which stain with basic dyes (eg. methylene blue) and constitute about 0·5 per cent of the total white blood cells. *Lymphocytes*, which constitute 25 to 30 per cent of the white blood cells, have a clear non-granular cytoplasm and a relatively large nucleus which is only slightly indented. They are divided into two groups: small lymphocytes which are slightly larger than erythrocytes (about 8 micrometres in diameter); large lymphocytes, which are about 12 micrometres in diameter. *Monocytes*, which constitute about 5 per cent of the white blood cells, are 10 to 15 micrometres in diameter and differ from lymphocytes in having a rather smaller nucleus which tends to be more indented and to be placed more eccentrically. The cytoplasm is non-granular.

Site of origin – The granulocytes are formed in the red bone marrow. The lymphocytes are formed predominantly in lymphoid tissue. There is some controversy as to the site of origin of monocytes: some say they arise from lymphocytes, whilst others contend that they are derived from histiocytes: ie. the reticulo-endothelial system (qv).

Function – The leucocytes constitute one of the most important of the defence mechanisms against infection. This applies particularly to the neutrophil leucocytes. (See LEUCOCYTOSIS.)

(See also ABSCESS; BLOOD; INFLAMMATION; PHAGOCYTOSIS; WOUNDS.)

LEUCOCYTOSIS means a temporary condition in which the polymorphonuclear leucocytes in the blood are increased in number. It occurs in many different circumstances, and forms a valuable means of diagnosis in certain diseases. It may occur, however, as a normal reaction in certain conditions: eg. pregnancy, menstruation, and during muscular exercise. Apart from these conditions, leucocytosis is usually due to the presence of inflammatory processes. It is part of the body's defence mechanism against infection with micro-organisms, the purpose of the increase in the number of leucocytes being to help to destroy the invading bacteria. Thus, during many acute infective diseases, such, for example, as pneumonia, the number is greatly increased. Indeed, if it be found upon examination of the blood during a case of pneumonia that the number of white blood corpuscles is not increased, the sign is an ominous one, pointing to weakness in the body's power of resistance to the disease, and indicating a probably fatal result. In all suppurative conditions there is also a leucocytosis, and if it seems that an abscess is forming deep in the abdomen, or in some other site where it cannot be readily examined, as, for example, an abscess resulting from appendicitis, the examination of a drop of blood gives a valuable aid in the diagnosis, and may be sufficient, in the absence of other signs, to point out the urgent need of an operation. Typhoid fever constitutes the major exception to the statement that acute infective diseases show this increase of white corpuscles in the blood, and, accordingly, in the case of this disease, the presence of an increase is a specially reliable sign of abscess formation, or other severe complication.

Other infective conditions in which a leucocytosis does not occur include measles and influenza.

LEUCODERMA, or LEUCODERMIA, means a condition of the skin in which areas of it become white, as the result of various skin diseases.

LEUCOPENIA is a condition in which the white corpuscles of the blood are greatly reduced in numbers.

LEUCOPLAKIA means a chronic condition of the tongue in which, as the result of various forms of irritation, hard, smooth, whitish patches develop on its surface.

LEUCORRHOEA (see WHITES).

LEUCOTOMY is the operation of cutting the white nerve fibres in the frontal lobes of the brain. This operation severs the connections of the frontal cortex with other parts of the nervous system, especially the thalamus and the hypothalamus. The operation is done in psychotic patients who suffer from severe depression or tense obsessional states. It appears to relieve the symptoms, the patient becoming 'friendly, cheerful, agreeable, relaxed, and interested in what goes on about him'.

LEUKAEMIA, or LEUCOCYTHAEMIA, is a disease in which the number of white corpuscles in the blood is permanently increased. The disease is also characterized by great enlargement of the spleen, changes in the marrow of the bones, and by enlargement of the lymph glands all over the body. The condition may be either acute or chronic. According to the type of corpuscles chiefly present the acute form is called acute lymphoblastic leukaemia, or acute myeloblastic leukaemia. The names for the corresponding chronic forms of the disease are chronic lymphatic leukaemia, and chronic myeloid leukaemia. Acute lymphoblastic leukaemia is most common in the first five years of life, and rare after the age of 25. Acute myeloblastic leukaemia is most common in children and young adults, but may occur at any age. Chronic lymphatic leukaemia occurs at any age between 35 and 80, most commonly in the 60's, and is twice as common in men as in women. Chronic myeloid leukaemia is rare before the age of 25, and most common between 30 and 65. Men and women are equally affected.

Cause – The cause of the disease is unknown. In many ways it resembles a form of malignant disease characterized by uncontrolled over-production of the white blood corpuscles.

Symptoms – In the acute cases the patient shows pallor, occasional purpuric rash, and enlargement of the lymphatic glands and spleen. The temperature is raised, and the condition may be mistaken for general tuberculosis. Such cases usually run a rapid course, lasting a few weeks or months. In the chronic type of the disease the onset is gradual, and the first symptoms which occasion discomfort are either swelling of the abdomen and shortness of breath, due to painless enlargement of the spleen, or the enlargement of glands in the neck, armpits and elsewhere, or the pallor, palpitation, and other symptoms of anaemia which often accompany the malady. Occasional haemorrhages from the nose, stomach, gums, or bowels may occur, and may be severe. Dropsy of the feet and legs is not uncommon, from obstruction of the lymphatic vessels by the enlarged glands and spleen. Diarrhoea also may become very troublesome. Generally, there is a slight degree of fever. When the blood is examined microscopically, not only is there an enormous increase of the white corpuscles, which may be multiplied thirty- or sixty-fold, but various immature forms of corpuscles are found. In the lymphatic form of the disease the white corpuscles consist chiefly of corpuscles resembling in some measure the lymphocytes, which, in healthy blood, are present only in small numbers. In the myeloid form, myelocytes, or large immature corpuscles out of the bone-marrow, which are never present in healthy blood, appear in large numbers, and there may also be large numbers of immature, nucleated, red blood corpuscles.

Although there is still no cure, the outlook in both acute and chronic leukaemia has changed considerably for the better; particularly is this the case in the acute form of the disease. Thus, in the case of acute lymphoblastic leukaemia, which accounts for around 85 per cent of all childhood leukaemia, only 30 per cent of the cases seen at The Hospital for Sick Children, Great Ormond Street, London, in 1958–59 were alive after twelve months, and less than 10 per cent after two years. In 1966–67, however, 81 per cent survived for twelve months and 28 per cent were still alive three years later. In Britain as a whole the position today is that the chance of inducing a remission in children with acute lymphoblastic leukaemia is much better than 90 per cent, and they have a 50 per cent chance of a cure. The results in acute myeloblastic leukaemia are not nearly so satisfactory. In the case of chronic lymphatic leukaemia the average period from the time of diagnosis to death is around six years, although quite a number of cases, particularly the elderly, survive for ten years or more. In chronic myeloid leukaemia the average survival time is around three to four years, with 20 per cent surviving for more than five years.

Treatment – Unfortunately, there is no known cure for either the acute or the chronic forms of leukaemia but, as has been noted, promising results are being obtained in the control of the disease, especially by means of chemotherapy. In the case of acute leukaemia the drugs now being used include mercaptopurine, methotrexate, cyclophosphamide, and vincristine. But cortisone and its derivatives sometimes produce dramatic temporary improvement. Blood transfusion plays an important part in controlling the condition during the period before the response to chemotherapy or hormone therapy can be expected. Chemotherapy has almost completely replaced radiotherapy in the treatment of chronic leukaemia. For the myeloid form busulphan is the most widely used drug, replaced by hydroxyurea, mercaptopurine, or one of the nitrogen mustard derivatives (qv) in the later stages of the disease. For the lymphatic form the drugs used are chlorambucil, cyclophosphamide, and the nitrogen mustard derivatives.

LEVAMISOLE is a drug that is proving of value in the treatment of ascariasis. (See ASCARIASIS.) Its main advantage seems to be in mass treatment as one dose may prove effective. It is also being used in the treatment of a group of diseases of obscure origin including Crohn's disease (qv) and rheumatoid arthritis.

LEVODOPA is a drug that is being used in the treatment of Parkinsonism (qv).

LEVORPHANOL is a synthetic derivative of morphine. It is an effective analgesic but, like morphine, is a drug of addiction.

LICE (see INSECTS IN RELATION TO DISEASE).

LICHEN is a term applied to a group of chronic skin diseases characterized by thickening and hardening of the skin, with the formation of papules (qv). *Lichen simplex* develops as a result of persistent scratching. The cause of the itching is often obscure. The disease is more common in women than in men. In women it occurs most commonly in the nape of the neck. It also occurs on the back of the forearm, the inner part of the thigh, the back of the knee and around the ankle. The skin becomes thickened, and has been compared in appearance to that of morocco leather, but there are no papules. Treatment consists of that of the underlying condition if this can be recognized, and the application of corticosteroid cream. *Lichen planus* begins on the wrists and then spreads to the body and legs. The eruption is characteristic, consisting of purplish, shiny papules with thickening of the surrounding skin. The papules are often found as well in the mouth. The cause is obscure. In some it is apparently nervous or emotional in origin. In some it is due to drugs, including the organic arsenical drugs, gold, mepacrine,

chloroquine, and para-aminosalicylic acid (PAS). It usually persists for some three months, but occasionally it may last for years. Treatment consists of the corticosteroids (qv) given by mouth and applied locally.

LIENTERIC DIARRHOEA is a mild form of diarrhoea in which the bowels move soon after every meal.

LIGAMENTS are strong bands of fibrous tissue which serve to bind together the bones entering into a joint. They are, in some cases, cord-like, in others flattened bands, whilst most joints are surrounded by a fibrous capsule or capsular ligament. (See JOINTS.)

LIGATURE means a cord or thread used to tie round arteries in order to stop the circulation through them, or to prevent escape of blood from their cut ends. Ligatures are generally made of catgut or silk, and are tied with a reef-knot (illustration 286).

286 – A reef-knot or surgeon's knot half tied. This is the knot with which all ligatures are tied.

LIGHT DERMATITIS (see DERMATITIS).

LIGHT TREATMENT – The visible spectrum of white light, extending from red to violet, gives waves of different character, and beyond these, in the infra-red and ultra-violet regions, are numerous varieties of waves (illustration 287). Thus in the infra-red region we have radiant heat and electric waves, which are used for practical purposes in high-frequency apparatus and radio and television; in the ultra-violet region are the chemically active rays used in heliotherapy, and then, much higher in the series, X-rays and gamma rays emitted by radioactive substances.

From the point of view of treatment, radiant energy is utilized in the following ways:

(1) *Sunlight treatment* or heliotherapy.
(2) *Radiant heat*, obtained by artificial means from incandescent or arc lamps, or by diathermy.

287 – Spectrum of electromagnetic radiations.

(3) *Ultra-violet radiation.*
(4) *X-rays; radium; radiotherapy;* and *isotopes.*
The first three are treated here. For the fourth see X-RAYS AND RADIUM.

SUNLIGHT TREATMENT, or HELIO-THERAPY – Sunlight is essential to the well-being of all living things, both vegetable and animal. In the towns of Britain too much of the therapeutic efficiency of the solar rays is still filtered out by moisture, dust, and smoke. This has a specially harmful effect upon child life, and various disabling diseases, such as

529

tuberculosis and rickets, are traceable in part to lack of sunlight. On the other hand, in the clear air of high mountains, especially over snow, which acts as a reflector, the ultra-violet rays are at a maximum.

This is why it is essential that everyone, and especially children, should get as much sunshine as possible – by abolishing atmospheric pollution and by going to the country or seaside for an annual holiday. Much of the benefit of sunshine is derived from its ultra-violet rays, but natural sun-

therapeutic medicine, is obtained by ultra-violet irradiation of ergosterol.

Professor Finsen's discovery in 1893 that the rays in this part of the spectrum were bactericidal in their action induced him to try their local effect on lupus (tuberculosis of the skin), in which disease he recorded very happy results. In addition to the original Finsen lamps, the mercury vapour lamp and especially the Tungsten arc-lamp, which gives a very high proportion of ultra-violet rays, are favourite forms. In the use of these lamps, the

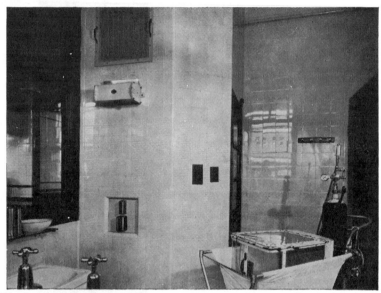

288 – A premature babies' ward showing a mercury vapour ray lamp controlling the air intake. *The Practitioner.*

light is preferable to ultra-violet rays produced by an ultra-violet lamp as it contains the complete spectrum of rays as well as those of light and heat. In Britain, however, sunshine is such a variable quantity that we are often dependent upon lamp-produced ultra-violet rays as a substitute for natural sunshine.

ULTRA-VIOLET RADIATIONS assist the natural defensive powers of the body and enable them to combat disease. They produce an erythema of the skin and, acting upon 7-dehydrocholesterol in the skin convert it into vitamin D_3, the natural vitamin D present in skin, milk, and fish-liver oils. Calciferol, or vitamin D_2, generally used in preventive and

patient's eyes are protected by wearing coloured glass goggles. A few minutes' exposure at a time is usually sufficient.

Excellent results were obtained by ultra-violet radiation in the treatment of lupus and some other forms of tuberculosis before the introduction of the anti-tuberculosis drugs. It is of use in hastening the cure of septic skin diseases, such as ulcers. Exposure to ultra-violet light is one way of treating rickets, as it converts the 7-dehydrocholesterol of the skin into vitamin D_3. Ultra-violet light is bactericidal, and ultra-violet-light 'barriers' have been used in children's wards (illustration 288) to prevent the spread of infection. Irradiation of the upper part of the atmosphere of schools have been used in an attempt to control the spread of common infections among school children.

INFRA-RED RADIATIONS employed in treatment are those with wavelengths immediately below those of luminous rays. Infra-red rays are emitted by all warm bodies, but the useful rays are given out only by bodies at a dull red or glowing temperature. The best source of these is sunshine, and they are also derived from incandescent light bulbs with tungsten filament, carbon arc lamps, and ordinary electric radiators at a red heat. These infra-red rays penetrate through the skin to a depth of $\frac{1}{4}$ to 1 inch (6 to 25 mm), and their action in moderate dosage is to dilate blood vessels and so produce an increased blood supply to the exposed part, and to exert a soothing action on its sensory nerves. They are useful therefore in rheumatic conditions, injury near the surface, to promote absorption and relieve pain, and in certain septic skin conditions such as boils and carbuncles. Apparatus is obtainable which supplies infra-red rays without luminous rays, but this has no advantage over sunshine or electric bulbs, which supply both infra-red and luminous rays, except in cases in which strong light is objectionable, as for example in treatment of conditions near the eyes. When deep penetration of heat is required, diathermy apparatus is used. (See DIATHERMY.)

LIGHTING – Daylight from a clear sky is the best illuminant, and in schools, offices and the like, the position of those working at desks should be arranged so that the light falls from behind, or from behind and to the left, and is not reflected straight up into the worker's eyes. Abundance of light, properly placed, is important, in order to avoid habitual strain of the eyes. The Illuminating Engineering Society Code (1973) recommends illuminance of 150 lux for casual reading, 300 lux for such activities as sewing and prolonged reading, and an increase of 50 to 100 per cent above these levels in old people's homes.

Electricity is the best form of artificial lighting. It is clean, free from any polluting action in the air, and easily adaptable. Fluorescent tubular lighting has been widely adopted as it so closely simulates natural lighting, reduces shadow formation and uses less electricity. If properly installed there is no evidence of any harm to the eyes.

LIGHTNING INJURIES are not uncommon – it is estimated that lightning strikes somewhere on the earth an average of 100 times a second, but the majority of those struck by lightning recover. A direct hit, however, means instantaneous death, with the clothes torn off, and the victim may be hurled quite a long distance. Even the individual who recovers falls unconscious the moment he is struck. Those who are a little farther away experience tingling of the skin and their hair may stand on end.

Preventive measures indoors during a lightning storm consist of keeping away from the fireplace, the main electrical switch, the bathroom, the kitchen sink and the television aerial. It is perfectly safe to use the telephone. There is no point in drawing the curtains, pulling down the blinds, covering mirrors or taking off metal-frame spectacles. Out of doors, solitary trees, walls, wire fences and other metallic structures such as sheds, park seats and tent-poles, ponds and river banks should be avoided. So also should flat open spaces, such as golf courses, where an individual may form the highest point. To use a metal-tipped umbrella or a golf club is asking for trouble. There is no risk inside a motor car, but it is wise to avoid moors or hills and make for the nearest low ground. If the storm is really severe, the safest thing is to lie down in a ditch. In Britain, there are around 10 deaths a year from being struck by lightning.

Treatment of an individual struck by lightning consists of artificial respiration, which may need to be prolonged for several hours.

LIGNOCAINE is a local anaesthetic. It is also used in the treatment of certain disorders of cardiac rhythm known as ventricular arrhythmias which may be particularly dangerous following a coronary thrombosis (qv).

LIMBS are outgrowths from the sides of the body, which, in man as in all the higher animals, number four. The limbs of all the higher animals, though differing much in outward appearance, are constructed on a similar plan, modified to suit the requirements of the owner, the forelimb, for example, developing in birds into a wing, in seals into a flipper. In all, however, the various muscles, bones, and blood-vessels, though differing in size and shape, correspond in arrangement. Also, between the upper and lower limb, a strict comparison is possible, and the bones, muscles, and main arteries of the arm, forearm, and hand have all representatives in the thigh, leg, and foot. (See ARM; and LEG.)

The union of the lower limb with the body is, however, more intimate than that of the upper limb. For, whilst the shoulder-blade and collar-bone of the upper limb are separated from the organs of the chest by the ribs and their muscles, the haunch-bone is applied on each side directly to the spine and forms the side of the pelvis.

In structure, each limb consists of four segments, the shoulder, arm, forearm, and hand in the case of the upper limb, corresponding to the haunch, thigh, leg, and foot in the lower limb. Upon the surface, the limb is enveloped by skin which, over the hand, is specially rich in its supply of sensory nerves. Beneath the skin is a layer of loose cellular tissue containing an amount of fat which varies with the corpulence of the individual. Next comes a strong layer of fibrous tissue, known as fascia, which provides a complete investment for the limb, and supplies a separate sheath for each muscle. The chief bulk of the limb is made up by the muscles or flesh. Finally, in the centre of the limb lie the bones which give it rigidity; and in general the large arteries and nerves are embedded among the muscles close to the bones.

The diseases affecting the limbs are those of the skin, muscles, bones, etc., forming them. (For injuries of the limbs see FRACTURES; HAEMORRHAGE; JOINTS, DISEASES AND INJURIES OF; and WOUNDS.)

LIME, CALX, QUICK LIME, or OXIDE OF CALCIUM, is a caustic, highly infusible solid which is prepared by calcining white marble, Iceland-spar, lime-stone shells or other forms of calcium carbonate ($CaCO_3$). Heating calcium carbonate drives off carbon dioxide, leaving lime or CaO. If water be sprinkled on it, the lime swells up, becomes hot, and breaks down into a white powder, known as calcium hydroxide or hydrated lime or slaked lime, the chemical formula of which is $Ca(OH)_2$. If a large quantity of water be added to this, a thick white liquid is formed, known as milk of lime, which is much used for whitewashing walls and the like. If the milk of lime be filtered, a clear liquid, having an alkaline reaction, and known as lime-water, is obtained. This lime-water contains a small amount of slaked lime in solution: about 1 part in 700 of water. Chlorinated lime is prepared by passing chlorine gas over slaked lime,

and is much used for bleaching and for disinfection. (See CHLORINATED LIME.)

When slaked lime is exposed to the air for some time it gradually hardens, as in mortar and plaster, changing into carbonate of lime. Carbonate of lime exists extensively also in a state of nature, being used in medicine in the form of chalk.

Action – Quick-lime has a caustic action upon parts of the body with which it is brought in contact. It is a fairly common accident for quick-lime or slaked lime to get into the eye, upon the delicate surface of which it exerts a destructive influence. (See EYE, DISEASES AND INJURIES OF.) Internally, lime-water and chalk exert a soothing and astringent action upon the bowels, although lime is absorbed only to a small extent into the blood.

Uses – Lime-water mixed with milk is administered to invalids and children in order to make the curd less hard and so render this food more easily digested, and also in order to exert a soothing action upon the stomach when there is a tendency to vomit. For this purpose two or three tablespoonfuls are generally added to a tumblerful of milk. (See INFANT FEEDING.) As an astringent in diarrhoea, Aromatic Chalk with Opium Mixture, BPC, is used in doses of 10 to 20 millilitres for an adult, and 2 to 5 millilitres for a young child.

LIME-JUICE is a yellow liquid obtained by squeezing lime-fruit, *Citrus limetta*. In common with lemon-juice, it is a rich source of vitamin C (16·8 to 62·5 mg per 100 ml) and contains a large quantity of citric acid. It is used as a refreshing drink and as a preventive of, and remedy for, scurvy. (See SCURVY.) Lime-juice which has been boiled, or preserved for a prolonged period, loses its anti-scorbutic properties.

LINCOMYCIN is an antibiotic derived from *Streptomyces lincolnensis*. It is active against a relatively limited number of bacteria, including staphylococci, streptococci, pneumococci and *B. anthracis*.

LINCTUS is a term applied to any thick syrupy medicine. Most of these are remedies for excessive coughing, of which the best is Gee's linctus, consisting of equal parts of paregoric, oxymel of squills, and syrup of tolu.

LINEA ALBA is the name given to the line of fibrous tissue stretching down the mid-line of the belly from the lower end of the sternum to the pubic bone. The linea alba gives attachment to the muscles of the belly wall.

LINEA NIGRA – During pregnancy the linea alba (qv) becomes pigmented and appears as a dark line down the middle of the belly, and is called the *linea nigra*.

LINEAR ACCELERATOR (see RADIO-THERAPY).

LINIMENTS, or EMBROCATIONS, are preparations intended for external application, generally with rubbing. Almost all are of an oily nature, and are highly poisonous, being dispensed therefore in green or blue bottles. Liniments should never be kept alongside medicines intended for internal use, because many fatalities occur through carelessness of administration, a dose being poured out of the wrong bottle. Among the chief liniments are aconite, belladonna, and camphor liniments, often mixed together in equal parts to form ABC liniment, which is extensively used for neuralgia, rheumatism, and other painful conditions; iodine liniment, used to paint over enlarged glands, and swollen joints; methyl salicylate liniment, used to apply in various painful rheumatic conditions; white liniment, which contains turpentine, used especially for sprains, bruises, and rheumatic conditions; liniment of ammonia, popularly known as 'hartshorn and oil', used for the same purpose; and soap liniment, known also as 'opodeldoc', of like application.

LINSEED is used either as the seeds or in the form of linseed meal obtained by grinding the seeds of *Linum usitatissimum*, the common flax.
Uses – Externally, linseed meal is used in poultices (qv); for internal use, linseed tea is an old domestic remedy for the treatment of cough.

LINT was originally made of teased-out linen; now it consists of a loose cotton fabric, one side of which is fluffy, the other being smooth and applied next the skin when the surface is broken. Marine lint consists of tow impregnated with tar, and is used where large quantities of some absorbent and deodorizing dressing are required. Cotton lint is impregnated with various substances, the most common being boracic lint. Lint containing perchloride of iron (15 per cent) is valuable as a styptic.

LIPAEMIA means the presence of an excessive amount of fat in the blood.

LIPASE is an enzyme widely distributed in plants, and present also in the liver and gastric and pancreatic juices, which breaks down fats to the constituent fatty acids and glycerol.

LIPID is a term which is used rather loosely. Strictly speaking, it means a substance which is insoluble in water but soluble in fat solvents such as alcohol and ether. The important lipids, so far as medicine is concerned, are the fats (or triglycerides), and the phospholipids which play an important part in the functioning of the membranes of the cells of the body.

LIPOCAIC is a hormone in the pancreas which plays a part in the metabolism of fat. In the absence of this hormone fat accumulates in the liver and seriously interferes with its function.

LIPODYSTROPHY means any disturbance of the body's economy which results from faulty metabolism of fat.

LIPOMA is the name given to a tumour mainly composed of fat. Such tumours arise in almost any part of the body, developing in fibrous tissues, particularly in that beneath the skin. They are simple in nature, and seldom give any trouble beyond that connected with their size and position. (See TUMOURS.)

LIPOSOMES are essentially tiny oil droplets consisting of layers of fatty material known as phospholipid separated by aqueous compartments. (Illustration 289.) Drugs can be incorporated into the liposomes, which are then injected into the bloodstreams or into the muscles, or given by mouth. Using this method of giving drugs, it is possible to protect them from being broken down in the body before they reach the part of the body where their curative effect is required: for example, in the liver or in a tumour.

LIPPITUDO means a chronic condition of inflammation at the margins of the eyelids, which ultimately renders the person 'blear-eyed'.

LIPS form a pair of curtains before the mouth, each composed of a layer of skin and of mucous membrane, between which lies a considerable amount of fat and of muscle fibres.

289 – Electron micrograph of a multilamellar liposome showing the bilipid layers separated by electron-opaque aqueous layers (sodium silicotungstate stain). (Medical Research Council)

The diseases to which the lips are liable are not numerous. *Fissures*, coming on in cold weather, form a troublesome condition often difficult to get rid of. *Herpes* often develops on the lip as a result of a cold or other feverish condition, but quickly passes off. (See HERPES.) *Ulcers* may form on the inner surface of the lip, usually in consequence of bad teeth or of dyspepsia, while in infants ulceration on the lips may be a sign of inherited syphilis. *Boils* sometimes form on the upper lip, and if large they produce a serious condition. (See BOILS.) *Cysts* of small size sometimes form on the inner surface of the lip, and are seen as little bluish swellings filled with mucus; they are of no importance. *Hare-lip* is a deformity sometimes present at birth. (See PALATE, MALFORMATIONS OF.) *Cancer* of the lip sometimes occurs, almost always in men, and usually on the lower lip. (See also MOUTH, DISEASES OF.)

LIQUOR, or SOLUTION as it is now known, is a solution of a drug in water. The majority of liquors are intended for internal use, but some of them are for external application only. (See also ALCOHOL.)

LIQUORICE is the root of *Glycyrrhiza glabra*, a plant of southern Europe and Asia. It is a mild expectorant, but is mainly used to cover the taste of disagreeable and more powerful drugs. Solid and liquid extracts are made from it, but the most commonly used preparation is compound liquorice powder, which contains also senna and sulphur. (See also GLYCYRRHETINIC ACID.)

LISTERIOSIS is an infectious, contagious disease of animals which is sometimes transmitted to man, in whom it usually affects the central nervous system, causing meningitis and encephalitis. It sometimes occurs in new-born babies as a result of infection through the placenta from the mother. The causative microorganism is *Listeria monocytogenes*. The infection responds well to penicillin and other antibiotics. There were 25 cases in the United Kingdom in 1973.

LITHAGOGUE is the term given to any agent which expels calculi from the body.

LITHIASIS is a general name applied to the formation of calculi and concretions in tissues or organs: eg. cholelithiasis means the formation of calculi in the gall-bladder.

LITHIUM CARBONATE is being used to an increasing extent in the treatment of mania and of recurrent depression.

LITHOLAPAXY is the term applied to the procedure of crushing a stone in the bladder and washing out the crushed fragments.

LITHOPAEDION is the term applied to a foetus which has died while in the mother's body and has become calcified.

LITHOTOMY is the term applied to the operation of cutting for stone in the bladder. The operation is of great historic interest, because more has probably been written about it in early times than about any other department of surgery, and because, for long, it formed almost the only operation in which the surgeon dared to attack diseases of the internal organs. It seems, from the fact that large numbers of people were cut for stone, and also from the fact that this operation remained, in France at least, in the hands of a special class of surgeons, referred to as lithotomists, that stone in the bladder must have been far commoner two or three centuries ago than it is today.

The bladder lies within the pelvis, protected in front by the pubic bones, but accessible above these through the lower part of the abdomen, or below them through the perineum. Operation by the former route is known as suprapubic lithotomy, and by the latter route as perineal lithotomy.

In the *suprapubic* operation a vertical opening is made through the lower part of the abdomen to reach the upper part of the bladder, and, with improved modern methods, it has practically displaced the perineal route for all bladder operations.

LITHOTRITY, or LITHOLAPAXY, is the term applied to the operation in which a stone in the bladder is crushed by an instrument introduced along the urethra, and the fragments washed out through a catheter. It has now, to a great extent, replaced lithotomy, except in cases where a stone is very hard and very large, and in boys whose urethra is too small to admit the passage of a lithotrite. The lithotrite, or stone-crusher, consists of two blades, one of which fits into a groove in the other, so that, when the inner blade is screwed home, the lithotrite is little larger than and similar in shape to a catheter, and can be easily passed along the urethra. The instrument is made of tough steel and provided with a powerful screw, so that when fragments of stone are caught between the blades they are easily crushed.

LITMUS, which is prepared from several lichens, is a vegetable dye-substance, which on contact with alkaline fluids becomes blue, and on contact with acid fluids, red. Slips of paper, impregnated with litmus, form a valuable test for the acidity of the secretions and discharges.

LITTLE'S DISEASE is a form of cerebral palsy. (See CEREBRAL PALSY.)

LIVE-FLESH is a popular term applied to fine muscular tremors or twitchings seen especially in the eyelids and muscles of the hands. It is usually due simply to tiredness caused by over-use of the twitching muscles, but when persistent it may be a sign of some serious nervous disorder, such as progressive muscular atrophy.

LIVER – The liver is a solid organ of dark-brown colour and the largest gland in the body. It discharges several functions, acting both as an excreting organ and as an elaborator and storehouse of nourishment.

Form – The shape of the liver is generally described as that of a right-angled triangular prism, with the right angle rounded off. It has five surfaces, superior, anterior, right, posterior, and inferior, of which the anterior and posterior surfaces are triangular, with the base towards the right side and tapering off to the left. The surfaces are separated from one another by rounded margins, except in the case of the lower surface, which is divided from the right, front, and upper surfaces by a sharp edge. The organ is divided also into four lobes. The great bulk of it constitutes the right lobe; the left lobe is small and extends a little way into the left half of the abdomen, to end in a sharp left border, whilst the quadrate, and caudate lobes are two small divisions upon the back and under surface. About the middle of the under surface, towards the back, is placed the porta hepatis, a transverse fissure, by which the hepatic artery and portal vein carry blood into the liver, and by which the right and left hepatic ducts emerge, carrying off the bile formed in the liver. The gall-bladder is attached to the under surface of the right lobe and projects from beneath the lower margin, where, if distended, it may be felt during life as a rounded swelling immediately beneath the end of the ninth rib. The connection of the gall-bladder – in which bile is stored – with the liver is rather complicated (illustration 227). The hepatic ducts emerge at the porta hepatis, one coming from the right and one from the left lobe. They immediately join to form the common hepatic duct, which is about 3 cm long, and joins the cystic duct, coming from the gall-bladder, at an acute angle. The hepatic and cystic ducts by their union form the bile duct, which is about 3 inches (75 mm) in length, and opens into the small intestine. Bile, which passes down from the liver by the hepatic duct, may either pass directly into the bile duct and so into the intestine, or it may pass upwards through the cystic duct into the gall-bladder, to be stored there, and later retrace its way through the cystic duct to the bile duct, and so to the intestine. The cystic duct and gall-bladder therefore together form a cul-de-sac upon the bile passages.

Position – The liver occupies the right-hand upper portion of the abdominal cavity (illustrations 290, 291). Its upper surface is in contact with the diaphragm, which also separates its right surface from the right lower ribs. About four-fifths of the organ lies to the right of the middle line of the body. As it is of a rounded shape it fills up the dome of the diaphragm, the lower part of the right lung being hollowed out to receive the liver, from which it is separated only by the diaphragm and pleural membrane. The liver, in turn, rests upon various abdominal organs, the right kidney and suprarenal gland the large intestine, the duodenum, and the stomach all making impressions upon it. In addition, the liver is swung from the walls of the abdomen by five ligaments, four of which consist of thickened parts of the peritoneal membrane lining the whole abdominal cavity, and reflected from the upper part of the liver to its walls. These are the coronary ligament, right and left triangular ligaments, falciform ligament, and a dense fibrous cord, the round ligament, or ligamentum teres.

Dimensions – The vertical thickness of the liver amounts, towards the right side, to over 5 inches (12 cm), and its extent from side to side is considerably more. Its weight is over 50 ounces (1·5 kg), varying with the size of the person, but making up about $\frac{1}{40}$ or thereabout of the whole body-weight. In young children it is relatively larger, accounting, to a large extent, for their protuberant abdomen, and making up about $\frac{1}{18}$ of the weight of the whole body.

Vessels – The blood supply of the organ (illustration 292) differs from that of any other part of the body, in that the blood collected from the stomach and bowels into the portal vein does not pass directly to the heart, but is distributed to the liver, in the substance of which the portal vein breaks up into capillary vessels. The effect of this is that some harmful substances, absorbed from the stomach and bowels, are abstracted from the blood-stream and destroyed, while various constituents of the food are stored up in the liver for gradual use. In addition, the liver receives a large hepatic artery from the coeliac axis, which also distributes branches to the stomach and pancreas, this blood supply serving to nourish the organ. After the blood has circulated through capillaries, it is collected together from both sources and emptied into the hepatic veins, which pass directly from the back surface of the liver into the inferior vena cava.

Minute structure – The liver is enveloped in a capsule of fibrous tissue, Glisson's capsule, from which strands run along the vessels, and, penetrating to the farthest recesses of the organ, bind its structure together. The hepatic artery, portal vein, and bile-duct divide and subdivide (illustration 293), the branches of each lying alongside corresponding divisions of the other two, till the finest divi-

290 – Chest with the skin and muscles removed from the front, showing the position of the heart, lungs and liver. *H*, Heart; *LL*, left lung; *RL*, right lung; *W*, windpipe; *L*, liver; *S*, stomach.

291 – A drawing of the abdominal contents, the anterior abdominal and thoracic walls having been removed. From J. Boileau Grant, *An Atlas of Anatomy*. E. & S. Livingstone.

sions of artery, vein, and bile-duct, known as interlobular vessels, lie between the lobules, of which the whole gland is built up. These lobules, each about the size of a pin's head, form each in itself a complete secreting unit, and the liver is built up of many hundred thousands of such exactly similar lobules.

A lobule has the following structure

292 – Diagram of the hepatic circulation. From Best and Taylor, *The Physiological Basis of Medical Practice*. The Williams & Wilkins Co.

(illustration 294). From the small vessels lying round its margin capillaries, or sinusoids, lined with stellate Kupffer cells (qv), are given off which run in towards the centre of the lobule, where they empty into a small central vein. These central veins from neighbouring lobules collect together, and ultimately the blood passes into the hepatic veins, and so leaves the liver. Between the capillaries, which radiate from the central vein to the edge of the lobule, lie rows of large liver cells, these forming the distinctive tissue of the organ, upon which its activity depends. Between the rows of cells also lie fine bile capillaries, which collect the bile produced by the cells and discharge it into the bile-ducts lying along the margins of the lobules. The liver cells are among the largest cells in the body, and each contains one or two large, round nuclei. In the cells can often be seen droplets of fat or granules of glycogen, ie. animal starch.

Functions – The liver is a vast chemical factory. The heat produced by the chemical changes taking place in it forms an important contribution to the general warming of the body. The liver secretes bile, the chief constituents of which are the bile salts (sodium glycocholate and taur-

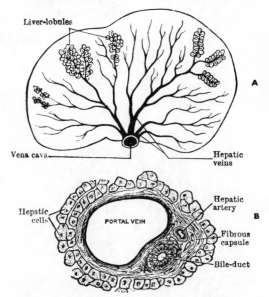

293 – Diagrammatic representation of liver structure. A, arrangement of liver lobules around the sublobular branches of the hepatic vein; B, section of a portal canal, showing branches of the portal vein, hepatic artery, and bile-duct surrounded by a prolongation of Glissons's fibrous capsule. From Cunningham, *Anatomy*, Oxford University Press.

537

ocholate), the bile pigments (bilirubin and biliverdin), cholesterol, and lecithin. The bile acids from which the salts are obtained are formed in the liver by the union of glycine and taurine with cholic acid. The bile salts are absorbed from the intestine and so find their way back to the liver again. The bile pigments are the iron-free and globin-free remnant of haemoglobin, being formed in the Kupffer cells of the liver. Bile pigments can, however, be formed in many other parts of the body: in the spleen, the lymph glands, bone-marrow, connective tissues (giving the colour to a bruise). Bile, then, serves to excrete pigment, the result of breakdown of old red blood corpuscles, and to aid the digestion of fat. Bile salts aid digestion of fat by emulsifying the fat, by activating

pancreatic lipase, and by promoting fat absorption. Bile is necessary for the absorption of vitamins D and E.

In addition to forming bile the liver has a number of important functions. These are enumerated briefly: (1) In the embryo it forms red blood corpuscles, and in the adult stores vitamin B_{12}, a substance necessary for the proper functioning of the bone-marrow in the manufacture of red corpuscles. (2) It manufactures the fibrinogen of the blood, and also the albumin and the globulin. (3) It stores iron and copper necessary for the manufacture of red corpuscles. (4) It produces heparin and, with the aid of vitamin K, prothrombin. (5) Its Kupffer cells in the liver blood-sinusoids are an important element in the reticulo-endothelial system, which breaks

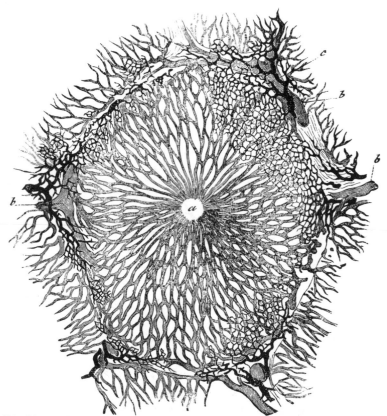

294 – Diagram of liver lobule. *a*, Central vein connected by network of sinusoids with *b*, *b*, peripheral or interlobular veins; *c*, interlobular bile-duct commencing in network of intercellular bile-canaliculi within the lobule. From Schafer, *Essentials of Histology*. Longman.

down red corpuscles, and probably manufactures antibodies. (6) It detoxicates noxious products made in the intestine and absorbed into the blood. (7) It stores carbohydrate in the form of glycogen, and maintains the two-way process: glucose ⇌ glycogen. (8) It forms vitamin A from carotene and stores the B vitamins. (9) It splits up amino-acids and manufactures urea and uric acid. (10) It plays an essential part in the storage and metabolism of fat.

LIVER DISEASES – The liver may be extensively diseased without any very urgent symptoms, unless the circulation through it be impeded, the outflow of bile checked, or neighbouring organs implicated. Jaundice, which is a symptom of several liver disorders, is dealt with elsewhere. Dropsy, which may be caused by interference with the circulation through the portal vein of the liver, as well as by other causes, is also considered separately. The presence of gall-stones is a complication of some diseases connected with the liver, and is treated under GALL-BLADDER, DISEASES OF. For hydatid cyst of the liver see TAENIASIS.

INFLAMMATION OF THE LIVER, or HEPATITIS, may occur as part of a generalized infection or may be a localized condition. Infectious hepatitis, which is the result of infection with a virus, is one of the most common forms of hepatitis. (See HEPATITIS, ACUTE INFECTIOUS.) In tropical countries amoebic hepatitis, which often goes on to abscess formation, is an important complication of amoebic dysentery. (See ABCESS, CHRONIC; DYSENTERY; ABSCESS OF THE LIVER.) Other tropical conditions in which the liver is always involved include malaria and yellow fever. Hepatitis may also occur if there is obstruction of the bile duct, as by a gallstone.

CIRRHOSIS OF THE LIVER – The cause of cirrhosis of the liver is still obscure. Experimentally it has been shown that the condition can be produced by a deficiency of certain of the amino-acids found in protein, but this only explains a small proportion of the cases found in man. It is probable that in most cases three factors are involved in varying degrees: a nutritional deficiency, a toxic factor, and an infective factor. The classical rôle of alcohol in its causation is probably an indirect one, accentuating a nutritional deficiency through its deleterious action on the digestive tract.
Symptoms – In one form of cirrhosis the liver is much contracted (atrophic or coarse cirrhosis), its blood-vessels are pressed upon, and dropsy results. In another form there is great enlargement of the organ (hypertrophic or biliary cirrhosis) and jaundice appears.

Treatment – Nothing can be done to repair a cirrhosed organ, but the cause, if known, must be removed and further advance of the process thus prevented. In the case of the liver a high-protein, high-carbohydrate, low-fat diet is given, supplemented by liver extract and vitamins B and K. The consumption of alcoholic liquors should be banned. In cirrhosis of the kidney, treatment is purely palliative, taking as much strain as possible off the kidneys.

ABSCESS OF THE LIVER – When an abscess develops in the liver, it is usually a manifestation of amoebic dysentery, appearing sometimes late in the disease, even after the diarrhoea is cured. It may also follow upon inflammation of the liver due to other causes; and abscesses may form in this organ as in other sites in cases of blood-poisoning. The symptoms of abscess are much the same as in other types of inflammation, only they are more pronounced, and accompanied often by rigors, severe pain over the liver which may also be referred to the right shoulder, and by great enlargement of the liver. In the case of an amoebic abscess treatment consists of aspiration of the contents of the abscess and the administration of either emetine or chloroquine.

CONGESTION OF THE LIVER is a term sometimes applied to the slighter forms of inflammation, in which the liver is said to be actively congested. But the term is generally reserved for a state of passive congestion, quite distinct from any inflammatory process, which often affects the liver to a marked extent in persons who are the subject of heart disease and some forms of lung disease. It arises in consequence of the close connection of the liver with the right side of the heart, through the inferior vena cava and the wide hepatic veins, which open into this vessel just before its entrance to the heart. When the right side of the heart is dilated, or there is some obstruction to the circulation through the lungs, or some valvular disease of the heart, the circulation of the blood is retarded and thus congestion of the liver results.

Symptoms – The liver becomes enlarged and causes a sense not so much of pain as of fullness and discomfort in the abdomen, which may be tender to the touch. The complexion is yellowish, the tongue furred, the appetite lost, and there are often both vomiting of bile and looseness of the bowels. There may also be headache, languor, and depression of spirits. At the same time the lung or heart condition which is responsible for the liver congestion gives rise to symptoms of its own. **Treatment** – The condition is usually a chronic one, with exacerbations from time to time. The treatment is that of the underlying cause, and as this is usually heart failure, the treatment consists principally of rest in bed, digitalis, and diuretics. (See HEART, DISEASES OF.)

FATTY DISEASE OF THE LIVER may consist of an infiltration of the cells of the liver with fat in those who eat to excess, particularly of rich, fat, or oily foods; or in wasting diseases there may be a degeneration in the liver-cells of this character. The liver is enlarged, and, though usually painless, it gives rise to discomfort and to embarrassment of breathing, particularly after meals. When due to over-eating, other organs, such as the heart, and the body generally, are also loaded with fat. A certain amount of indigestion and constipation is often present, and a person affected in this way can offer but feeble resisting power to any disease by which he may be attacked. (For treatment, see under CORPULENCE.)

ACUTE YELLOW ATROPHY, or ACUTE HEPATIC NECROSIS as it is now known, is a destructive and fatal disease of the liver which is very rare. It may be due to chemical poisons, such as carbon tetrachloride, chloroform, phosphorus and industrial solvents derived from benzene. It may also be the cause of death in cases of poisoning with fungi. Very occasionally it may be a complication of acute infectious hepatitis. It is also a rare complication of pregnancy. It sets in with a slight degree of jaundice, which cannot be distinguished from simple jaundice, and lasts several days. Then the jaundice suddenly deepens, there is pain in the region of the liver, convulsions and delirium appear, the heart grows very weak, and death ensues in a day or two. Crystals of leucine and tyrosine are found in the urine. The destruction of the liver as a secreting organ may be complete, but occasionally areas here and there only are affected, and recovery may then take place with restoration of the damaged areas after a prolonged illness.

CANCER OF THE LIVER is not uncommon, although it is rare for the disease to begin in the liver, the involvement of this organ being usually secondary to disease situated somewhere in the stomach or bowels. Cancer originating in the liver is more common in Asia and Africa. It usually arises in a fibrotic (or cirrhotic) liver. There is great emaciation, which increases as the disease progresses. The liver is much enlarged, and its margin and surface are rough, being studded with hard cancer masses of varying size, which can often be readily felt through the abdominal wall. Pain may be present. Jaundice and dropsy often make their appearance. (See also TRANSPLANTATION.)

LIVER-FLUKE is the popular name of *Fasciola hepatica*, a parasite which infests sheep, and which is occasionally found in the bile-passages and liver of man. (See FASCIOLIASIS.)

LIVER PILLS (see CHOLAGOGUES).

LIVER SPOT is a popular term applied to brownish marks which appear on the skin, especially of the face. This is sometimes caused by the growth of a parasite (*Tinea versicolor*) in the surface layers of the cuticle. It also frequently accompanies pregnancy or the presence of abdominal tumours. It may also be due simply to some long-continued form of local irritation.

LOBE is the term applied to the larger divisions of various organs, such as to the four lobes of the liver, the three lobes of the right and the two lobes of the left lung, which are separated by fissures from one another, and to the lobes or superficial areas into which the brain is divided. The term lobar is applied to structures which are connected with lobes of organs, or to diseases which have a tendency to be limited by the boundaries of lobes, such as lobar pneumonia.

LOBECTOMY is the operation of cutting out a lobe of the lung in such diseases as abscess of the lung and bronchiectasis.

LOBELIA is the name of a remedy used for asthma. It consists of the leaves and tops of *Lobelia inflata*, a common weed in the United States. In very large doses, it causes vomiting and paralyses the heart's action, being a dangerous poison, but in moderate doses it relieves the spasm to which asthma is due. It is a constituent of many burning powders made for smoking by asthmatics, but it is more commonly used in the form of tincture of lobelia combined with other drugs.

LOBELINE HYDROCHLORIDE is a derivative of α-lobeline, an alkaloid derived from lobelia. It is given by injection for the treatment of respiratory depression and for the resuscitation of the newborn.

LOBOTOMY is the cutting of a lobe. (See LEUCOTOMY.)

LOBSTER CLAW (see CLEFT FOOT).

the first four days it consists chiefly of blood; after the fifth day the colour should become paler, and after the first week the quantity should diminish and the appearance be creamy. There should at no time be any putrid odour, the presence of this being an indication of dangerous septic infection. The presence of blood after the second week indicates that the patient has been too active or that the natural absorptive changes are not duly taking place. (See PUERPERIUM.)

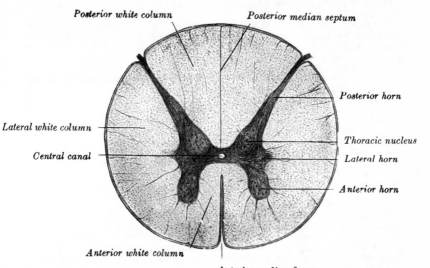

295 – Transverse section through the spinal cord in the thoracic region. Magnified eight times. From *Gray's Anatomy.* Longman.

LOBSTER FOOT (see CLEFT FOOT).

LOBSTER HAND (see CLEFT HAND).

LOBULE is the term applied to a division of an organ smaller than a lobe: for example, the lobules of the lung are of the size of millet seeds, those of the liver slightly larger. Lobules form the smallest subdivisions or units of an organ, each lobule being similar to the others, of which there may be perhaps several hundred thousand in the organ. The term lobular is applied to structures such as small blood-vessels belonging to individual lobules, or to disease which occurs in a scattered manner in organs, affecting lobules here and there.

LOCHIA is a term applied to the discharge which takes place during the first week or two after child-birth. During

LOCKJAW is a prominent symptom of tetanus and is the popular name for this condition.

LOCOMOTOR ATAXIA, also called TABES DORSALIS; POSTERIOR SPINAL SCLEROSIS, is a disease of the nervous system, manifesting itself principally by disordered movements of the limbs in walking. This is dependent on the loss of the power of coordinating the muscles into harmonious action, which is essential to the proper performance of the voluntary movements of the body, and the maintenance of its equilibrium.

Causes – The pathological condition giving rise to locomotor ataxia is disease of the posterior columns (illustration 295) of the spinal cord and the posterior nerve roots. These undergo chronic inflammatory changes, which result in their ulti-

541

mately becoming atrophied and indurated. When affecting, as this lesion most commonly does, the lower dorsal and lumbar regions of the cord, the ataxic symptoms are chiefly confined to the legs; but when it affects the cervical portion, the arms are involved. Occasionally the whole posterior columns of the cord are found diseased. It is a late result of syphilis.

Locomotor ataxia is much more common among men than among women, over 90 per cent of cases being males. It is a disease of middle life, most often occurring between the ages of 30 and 50.

Symptoms – Locomotor ataxia usually begins insidiously, and advances slowly. Among the earlier symptoms observed are a tendency to stagger in walking or standing, especially when the eyes are closed; disorders of vision, with occasionally temporary or permanent paralysis of some of the cranial nerves; violent shooting pains down the limbs, decreased or perverted sensibility in various parts of the body, and disturbance of the genito-urinary functions. Among the early signs of the disease discovered by the physician, two of the most important are: loss or diminution of the knee-jerks obtained on tapping the patellar tendon; and a sluggish condition of the iris of the eye, which, though altering the size of the pupil as the eye accommodates itself for vision of near objects, fails to contract normally when a bright light falls upon the eye. In the course of time, other symptoms are superadded. The sufferer feels as if some soft substance were interposed between his feet and the ground. His gait assumes a characteristic appearance. He begins the act of walking with evident difficulty, and his steps are short and hurried. Each foot is lifted well from the ground; but as he moves forward it is thrown out from him, and his heel descends forcibly, and is followed at a longer than the normal interval by the sole: the so-called stamping gait. In walking, he requires the aid of his vision to preserve his balance, and he therefore looks at his feet, or rather at the ground a little in front of them, as he advances. If asked to stand erect with his feet together, and then directed to close his eyes or to look upwards, he immediately begins to sway and totter, and would fall if not supported – a symptom known as Rombergism. Along with this there usually exists markedly diminished sensibility to touch and to painful impressions, such as a pin-prick. Sometimes the disorder implicates the upper extremities, and then the hands and fingers cease to per-

form their functions with precision, so that the patient is unable to pick up any small object from the ground, to button or un-button his clothing, and even sometimes to feed himself.

The patient's efforts to walk become more and more difficult, and ultimately he is compelled to lie in bed. In the later stages the patient has attacks of violent vomiting (gastric crises), of laryngeal spasm and difficulty in breathing (laryngeal crises), of inability to retain the urine (bladder crises). The shooting pains and violent jerkings of the limbs increase, motor power becomes impaired, and the patient sinks under the prolonged and exhausting course of discomfort, or dies from some intercurrent disease.

Treatment – The treatment has been revolutionized by the introduction of penicillin, which, when given in large doses for an adequate period of time, produces marked improvement in all but the late stages of the disease. In cases in which the gait is affected, much improvement in walking results from Frenkel's exercises (qv), a series of co-ordinated movements, such as walking carefully along a board on the floor.

LOGWOOD (see HAEMATOXYLON).

LOIASIS is the disease caused by the filarial worm *Loa loa*, a thread-like worm which differs from *W. bancrofti* in that it is shorter and thicker, and it is found in the blood-stream during the day, not at night. It is transmitted by the mango fly, *Chrysops dimidiata*, but other flies of this genus can also transmit it. It is confined to West and Central Africa. The characteristic feature of the disease is the appearance of fugitive swellings which may arise anywhere in the body in the course of the worm's migration through the body. These are known as Calabar swellings. The worm is often found in the eye, hence the old name of the worm in Africa – the eye worm. Satisfactory results are being reported from the use of diethylcarbamazine in the treatment of this form of filariasis.

LOIN is the name applied to the part of the back between the lower ribs and the pelvis. (For pain in the loins see BACKACHE; and LUMBAGO.)

LONG-SIGHT (see SPECTACLES).

LOPERAMIDE is a drug that is proving of value in the treatment of diarrhoea.

LORAZEPAM is a tranquillizer that is proving of value as a sedative for administration before operation. Its great advantage, compared with other similar drugs, is that it stimulates, rather than depresses, breathing.

LORDOSIS means an unnatural curvature of the spine forwards. It occurs chiefly in the lumbar region, where the natural curve is forwards, as the result of muscular weakness, spinal disease, etc. (See SPINAL COLUMN.)

LOSS OF BLOOD (see HAEMORRHAGE).

LOTION means a fluid preparation intended for bringing in contact with, or for washing, the external surface of the body. Lotions are generally of a watery or alcoholic composition, and many of them are known as 'liquors'. Those external applications which are of an oily nature, and intended to be rubbed into the surface, are known as liniments.

LOUSE (see INSECTS IN RELATION TO DISEASE).

LOZENGES also known as TROCHES, or TROCHISCI, consist of small tablets containing drugs mixed with sugar, gum, glycerin-jelly, or fruit-paste. They are used in various affections of the mouth and throat, being sucked and slowly dissolved by the saliva, which brings the drugs they contain in contact with the affected surface. Some of the substances used in lozenges are benzalkonium, benzocaine, betamethasone, bismuth, formaldehyde, hydrocortisone, liquorice, penicillin.

LUES is the Latin word for a serious infectious disease, the term being especially applied to syphilis.

LUGOL'S SOLUTION is a compound solution of iodine and potassium iodide.

LUMBAGO is a term applied to a painful ailment affecting the muscles of the lower part of the back, generally regarded as of rheumatic origin. In 1971–72, in England and Wales practically 7 million days were lost as a result of lumbago, prolapsed intervertebral disc and pain in the back, and it is considered that these figures almost certainly understate the problem. The cost of this incapacity is reckoned at around £75 million, to which has to be added direct costs to the National Health Service of some £25 million. (See also BACKACHE; PROLAPSED INTERVERTEBRAL DISC; and RHEUMATISM.)

Cause – Lumbago seems to be brought on by exposure to cold and damp, and by other exciting causes of rheumatism. Sometimes it follows a strain of the muscles of the loins. The pain accompanying rheumatic manifestations in this region is believed to be due to an inflammatory condition in the connective tissues of the muscles, causing congestion of the blood-vessels and consequent pressure upon the endings of the sensory nerves. To this condition the term, fibrositis, is applied. Lumbago is specially apt to occur in the back muscles after they have been the seat of a strain or other injury leading probably to a tear in the muscle fibres, and the pain in such a case is largely produced by violent spasm of the surrounding muscle. A not uncommon cause is a prolapsed intervertebral disc (qv). In other cases lumbago occurs in gouty subjects and the attacks take the place of an ordinary attack of gout.

Symptoms – An attack of lumbago may occur alone, or be associated with rheumatism in other parts of the body at the time. It usually comes on as a seizure, often sudden, of pain in one or both sides of the small of the back, of a severe cutting or stabbing character, greatly aggravated on movement of the body, especially in attempting to rise from the recumbent posture, and also in the acts of drawing a deep breath, coughing, or sneezing. So intense may it be that it is apt to suggest the existence of inflammation in some of the neighbouring internal organs, such as the kidneys or bowels. The attack is in general of short duration, but occasionally it continues for a long time, not in such an acute form as at first, but rather as a feeling of soreness and stiffness on movement.

Treatment – The treatment includes that for rheumatic affections in general (see RHEUMATISM), and the application of local remedies of counter-irritant nature, such as hot fomentations with turpentine or laudanum applied by means of flannel to the part; or the rubbing in, if this can be borne, of liniments. The old and homely plan of counter-irritation by applying a heated iron to the part with a sheet of brown paper or blanket interposed is often beneficial in chronic cases, as is also, on similar principles, Corrigan's button cautery. The hot-air bath, and various electrical applications, including faradization, static breeze, diathermy, and high-frequency currents, are also of value.

Should there be localized areas of tenderness, the injection into these of procaine may give relief. During the acute stages, relief is obtained from the taking of analgesics such as aspirin. (See BATHS; ELECTRICITY IN MEDICINE.)

LUMBAR is a term used to denote structures in, or diseases affecting, the region of the loins, as, for example, the lumbar vertebrae, lumbar abscess.

LUMBAR PUNCTURE is a procedure for removing cerebrospinal fluid from the spinal canal in the lumbar region in order: (1) to diagnose disease of the nervous system: (2) to relieve pressure when too much cerebrospinal fluid is being formed, as in meningitis; and (3) to introduce medicaments: spinal anaesthetics, or drugs, or serum.

LUMBRICUS is a name sometimes applied to the roundworm or *Ascaris lumbricoides*. (See ASCARIASIS.)

LUNAR CAUSTIC is another name for nitrate of silver.

LUNATIC is a general term applied to persons of disordered mind, because lunacy was supposed at one time to be largely influenced by the moon. (See MENTAL ILLNESS.)

LUNGS – The lungs form a pair of organs situated in the chest, and discharge perhaps the most important function of vital activity: respiration. (See RESPIRATION.) Whilst this is their primary function, they also act as a filter for the blood. The air, which enters through the nose and passes down the throat, larynx, and windpipe in succession (see AIR PASSAGES), reaches the lungs by the right and left bronchial tubes, into which the windpipe divides within the chest, at the level of the second rib. The texture of the lungs is very highly elastic, so that when the chest is opened each lung collapses to about one-third of its natural bulk.

Form and position – Each lung is roughly conical in shape, with an apex projecting into the neck, and a base resting upon the diaphragm (illustration 296). The rounded outer surface of each is in contact with the ribs of its own side, while the heart, lying between the lungs, hollows out the inner surface of each to some extent. There is an anterior border, along which the outer and inner surfaces meet, and the borders of the two lungs

touch one another for a short distance behind the middle of the breast-bone. The apex, which is blunt, extends $1\frac{1}{2}$ inches (35 mm) or more into the neck above the line of the collar-bone, being covered here by the muscles of the neck. The base is deeply hollowed, in correspondence with the domed shape of the diaphragm, which is pushed up by the liver on the right side, and by the stomach and spleen on the left. The right lung is split by two deep fissures into three lobes; the left has two lobes divided by a single fissure. The weight of the two lungs together is about 40 ounces (1·1 kg), the right being rather heavier than the left. The lungs of men are heavier than those of women. There is a tendency for lung mass to increase throughout life. Each lung is enveloped in a membrane, the pleura or pleural membrane, in such a way that one layer of the membrane is closely adherent to the lung, from which indeed it cannot be separated, while the other layer lines the inner surface of one half of the chest. These two layers form a closed cavity, the pleural cavity, which everywhere surrounds the lung except at the point where the bronchi and vessels enter it. This cavity is, in the natural state, a

296 – Chest with the skin and muscles removed from the front, showing the position of heart and lungs. *H*, Heart; *LL*, left lung; *RL*, right lung; *W*, windpipe; *L*, liver; *S*, stomach.

merely potential space, the two layers of pleural membrane being separated only by a thin layer of fluid, which enables them to glide with very little friction over one another as the lung expands and retracts in breathing; but, in certain states, fluid collects in the pleural cavity, so that several pints of fluid may be effused there, compressing the lung. In some circumstances air escapes into the pleural cavity, and the lung then collapses temporarily upon its root, but air in the pleural cavity is quickly absorbed, and the lung speedily comes to occupy its original volume.

Colour – In children, the colour of the lungs is rose-pink but, as life advances, they become more and more of a slaty hue, mottled with streaks and patches of dark grey and black, which are due to deposits in the lymph spaces of dust inhaled on the breath. Eskimos and others who live in an atmosphere free from dust retain the colour of childhood; on the other hand, the lungs of coal-miners become often of an almost uniform jet-black shade.

Changes at birth – Before birth, and in stillborn children, the lungs are of a yellowish colour, of solid gland-like appearance, and packed away in the back of the chest. Further, such lungs do not float in water, and their weight amounts to about $\frac{1}{70}$ of the whole body-weight. Immediately upon birth a remarkable change takes place: the tissue of the lungs expands, like the petals of an opening flower; the colour changes to rose-red, and the weight is suddenly doubled in consequence of the inrush of blood: the consistence becomes spongy, as air is drawn into the lungs, and if the child should die after drawing a few breaths, any portion of the lung which may be cut off floats in water. These changes are of importance, from the medico-legal point of view, in determining whether a dead infant was born alive or not.

Connections with heart – Not only does the heart lie in contact with the two lungs, so that changes in the volume of the lungs cannot fail to have an effect upon the heart's action, but the heart is also connected by vessels with both lungs. The pulmonary artery passes from the right ventricle and divides into two branches, one of which runs straight outwards to each lung, entering its substance along with the bronchial tube at the hilum or root of the lung. From this point also emerge the pulmonary veins, which carry the blood purified in the lungs back to the left atrium.

Minute structure – Each main bronchial tube, entering the lung at the root, divides into branches (illustrations 297 and 298), which subdivide again and again, to be distributed all through the substance of the lung, till the finest tubes, known as respiratory bronchioles, have a width of only $\frac{1}{100}$ inch (0·25 mm). In structure, all these tubes consist of a mucous membrane surrounded by a fibrous sheath. The windpipe as well as the larger and medium bronchi have in the fibrous layer large pieces of cartilage, which in the windpipe and largest bronchial tubes form regular hoops, and in the medium-sized tubes are disposed as irregular plates. These pieces of cartilage have the function of preventing the tubes from closing or being compressed, and so obstructing the passage of air. The larger and medium bronchi are richly supplied with glands secreting mucus, which is poured out upon the surface of the membrane. This surface is composed of columnar epithelial cells, which are provided with cilia. These have a co-ordinated beating action which sweeps expectoration upwards towards the throat. The wall of the bronchial tubes is rich in fibres of elastic tissue, and immediately beneath the mucous membrane is a layer of circularly placed unstriped muscle fibres, which is specially well developed in the smaller bronchi. This muscular layer plays an important role in the removal of expectoration by coughing; it is also of great importance in connection with the causation of asthma. (See ASTHMA.)

The smallest divisions of the bronchial tubes, or bronchioles, divide into a number of tortuous tubes known as alveolar ducts and these branch into expanded passages known as atria, each of which leads into a terminal air saccule (illustration 299). The walls of the alveolar ducts, atria and air saccules are covered with minute sacs, known as alveoli, of which there are around 300 million. Each alveolus consists of a delicate membrane composed of flattened, plate-like cells, strengthened by a wide network of elastic fibres, to which the great elasticity of the lung is due; and in these thin-walled air-cells the important function of the lungs is carried on.

The branches of the pulmonary artery accompany the bronchial tubes to the farthest recesses of the lung, dividing like the latter into finer and finer branches, and ending in a dense network of capillaries, which lies everywhere between the air-vesicles, the capillaries being so closely

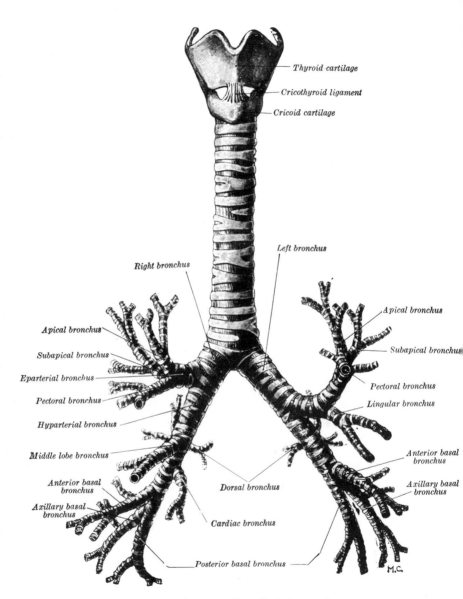

Thyroid cartilage

Cricothyroid ligament

Cricoid cartilage

Left bronchus

Right bronchus

Apical bronchus

Apical bronchus

Subapical bronchus

Subapical bronchus

Eparterial bronchus

Pectoral bronchus

Pectoral bronchus

Lingular bronchus

Hyparterial bronchus

Middle lobe bronchus

Anterior basal bronchus

Anterior basal bronchus

Axillary basal bronchus

Dorsal bronchus

Axillary basal bronchus

Cardiac bronchus

Posterior basal bronchus

M.C.

297 – The lower air passages. From *Gray's Anatomy*. Longman.

298 – The larynx, windpipe, bronchial tubes and lungs. *L*, larynx; *T*, thyroid cartilage; *C*, cricoid cartilage; *Tr*, trachea splitting at *B* into the two bronchi; *a*, apex; *b*, base of each lung.

placed that they occupy a much greater area than the spaces between them. The air in the air-vesicles is separated therefore from the blood only by two delicate membranes: the wall of the air-vesicle and the capillary wall, through which an exchange of gases readily takes place. The blood from the capillaries is collected by the pulmonary veins, which also accompany the bronchi to the root of the lung.

Another and much smaller set of bronchial blood-vessels runs actually upon the walls of the bronchial tubes, and these serve the purpose of nourishing the lung tissue.

299 – Diagram illustrating terminal divisions of the air tubes. *A*, respiratory bronchiole; *B*, alveolar duct; *C*, atrium; *D*, air saccule; *E*, alveolus. From *Hewer's Textbook of Histology*. William Heinemann, Ltd.

There is in the lung also an important system of lymph vessels, which start in spaces situated between the air-vesicles, under the pleural membrane and in the walls of the bronchial tubes. These vessels leave the lung along with the blood-vessels, and are connected with a chain of bronchial glands lying near the end of the windpipe.

LUNG DISEASES – The general symptoms and signs produced by disease of the lungs are mentioned under CHEST, DISEASES OF, and the chief affections to which these organs are liable are also treated under special headings. (See BRONCHIECTASIS; BRONCHITIS; CHEST, DEFORMITIES OF; CHILLS AND COLDS; EMPHYSEMA; EXPECTORATION; HAEMOPTYSIS; HAEMORRHAGE; PLEURISY; PNEUMONIA; OCCUPATIONAL DISEASES; PULMONARY EMBOLISM; TUBERCULOSIS.)

INFLAMMATION OF THE LUNGS is generally known as pneumonia, but may be of several different types. (See PNEUMONIA.)

ABSCESS OF THE LUNG is a comparatively rare condition, and consists, like abscesses elsewhere, of a collection of pus in one or more areas of the lung. It may result from an acute pneumonia which does not clear up properly, or it may be due to a wound of the lung from without, or to the presence of foreign bodies, such as buttons, pins, or fragments of food, which have been sucked down the air passages. An abscess may also occur in the lung, as in other organs, during the course of blood poisoning (pyaemia), or may be produced by the bursting of an abscess into the lung after its formation in some neighbouring organ. The condition may be difficult to differentiate from cavity formation due to tuberculosis; although the failure to find tubercle bacilli in the expectoration, after repeated examination, is an important point against the latter condition.

An abscess in the lung may burst into one of the bronchial tubes, and, after the pus is spat up, healing and recovery may take place. Most cases respond to appropriate antibiotics and postural drainage (qv) but occasionally it may be necessary to resort to surgery and drain the abscess through the chest wall.

GANGRENE OF THE LUNG is another result which may follow pneumonia in persons of poor constitution or debilitated by serious illness. Just as in the case of gangrene of the limbs, a portion of lung dies and putrefies, giving rise to a

547

most offensive smell, as the dead and broken-down lung tissue is spat up. The prospect of recovery is small, even when the portion of lung involved is very limited.

CONGESTION OF THE LUNGS is a term which is used in two quite different senses. In popular parlance, the term is used for acute inflammation of the lung in its early stages. When the patient recovers after a few days, the illness is often described as an attack of acute congestion.

In a strict medical sense, the term is used to mean quite a different condition of a more chronic nature: passive or mechanical congestion of the blood-vessels in the lungs due to some defect in the pumping action of the heart. Passive congestion arises under two sets of conditions. A very serious form, known as hypostatic congestion, arises when the heart is failing, towards the end of severe and long-continued fevers, such as typhoid fever; after severe surgical operations; and in old people who, for any reasons, such as the occurrence of a broken leg, are confined for some weeks to bed. It occurs in the back parts of the lungs, in consequence of the feeble heart being unable to drive out of them the blood which gravitates into these dependent parts. Inflammation is very apt to arise in these congested parts, and hypostatic pneumonia often ends the life of old or feeble persons confined to bed. The other form of passive congestion is due, not so much to weakness in the pumping action of the heart, as to some obstruction which hinders the escape of blood from the lungs into the left atrium of the heart. Narrowing of the opening which leads from the left atrium to the left ventricle (mitral stenosis) is the chief cause of this, and, although the condition is by no means so serious as the hypostatic form of congestion, it predisposes the persons affected by this form of heart disease to sharp attacks of blood-spitting on exertion, to bronchitis, and to pneumonia. The treatment, in both cases, must be directed towards the heart.

OEDEMA OF THE LUNGS is a condition in which these organs become dropsical. It occurs both when congestion is present as the result of heart failure, and also during Bright's disease, following dropsy in other parts of the body. It gives symptoms of its onset in constant rattling noises proceeding from the lungs and air passages of the affected person, whose face becomes gradually more livid, and who experiences great difficulty in breathing. The oedema may be accompanied by the collection of fluid in the pleural cavities (hydrothorax), and, if the condition be not speedily relieved, the person dies, literally drowned in the fluids of his own body.

COLLAPSE OF THE LUNG occurs under several conditions. The lungs are so resilient in consequence of the elastic fibres with which they are everywhere interspersed that, if air be admitted to the pleural cavities, the lungs immediately collapse to a third of their natural bulk. Accordingly, if one side of the chest be wounded and air be admitted (pneumothorax), the lung collapses, although, after the wound is healed, the air is absorbed from the pleural cavity and the lung quickly regains its size. Also, when fluid is effused into the pleural cavity the lung is compressed and collapses, and if the fluid be not absorbed or drawn off within some weeks, the collapse is apt to be permanent through the formation of adhesions round the lung. Again, if anything blocks a bronchial tube, the part of the lung to which it leads collapses, since these tubes do not communicate with one another. Thus, in children suffering from bronchitis or pneumonia areas of the lung may collapse through a plug of mucus sticking in a bronchus which the child is not sufficiently strong to free by coughing. A similar result is brought about by foreign bodies drawn into the air passages. It also occurs when the chest is opened on one side to drain away a collection of pus. The second lung, being healthy, is sufficient to overtake the needs of respiration, expanding as a rule somewhat in the process. The lungs of an infant at birth are collapsed in the sense that they have never been expanded, and any signs of expansion in the lungs of a dead infant form a sure token that he has been born alive. (See LUNGS.)

TUMOURS OF THE LUNG – Since the beginning of the twentieth century cancer of the lung has become increasingly frequent, particularly so in the last decade (table 36), and in 1977 was responsible for 32,273 deaths in England, compared with 10,570 deaths from carcinoma of the stomach and 11,172 deaths from carcinoma of the breast. Tumours may arise in the

Year	Males	Females
1951–55	16,678	2656
1956–60	22,670	3101
1961–65	29,974	3193
1966–70	33,430	4916
1971–75	37,258	5895

Table 36 – Cancer of the lung. The crude death rate per million living for each sex in England and Wales over the period, 1951–75.

mediastinum or in connection with the pleura. Hydatid cysts are found from time to time in the lungs.

WOUNDS OF THE LUNG are serious both by reason of the damage they may do to this organ and by admitting air into the pleural cavity, so that the lung collapses. The lung may be wounded by the end of a fractured rib, or by some sharp body pushed between the ribs, and it may also be torn as the result of disease: for example, a tuberculous and excavated lung may be perforated during a fit of coughing. If by any cause a free opening is made between the pleural cavity and air passages, immediate difficulty of breathing, due to collapse of the lung, ensues. Generally, however, the person recovers from the immediate symptoms, and, if the perforation be caused by a wound from without, the wound may heal without leaving any permanent damage. Frequently, in such cases, blood is effused into the pleural cavity (haemothorax). This is gradually absorbed, leaving usually some thickening of the pleural membrane and adhesions between the lung and chest wall. Such a wound is liable, at the time of infliction, to become infected by organisms, and empyema (qv) may then result, with a tedious illness.

Wounds of the lung are chiefly dangerous on account of the risk of wounding large blood-vessels. Spitting of blood in any quantity after a wound of the chest has been received is a sign that the lung has been injured. A stab or bullet wound, which does not injure any large vessel, may traverse the lung without any serious consequences, but if one of the main veins or arteries be torn, death is likely to ensue.

LUPUS is a term used to designate a group of skin diseases of intractable character. There are two chief types of the disease: *Lupus vulgaris*, which is due to the *Mycobacterium tuberculosis*; and *Lupus erythematosus*, which is of unknown origin.

LUPUS VULGARIS begins most commonly before the age of 20, and, not infrequently, persists all through life, healing in one place to break out a short distance off. The nose, cheeks, brow, and sides of the neck are most commonly attacked, although the hands and the mucous membrane inside the nose and mouth are also common seats of the malady. The first sign of the disease is a small, soft nodule of yellowish transparent appearance, on this account often called an 'apple-jelly' nodule. No pain or itching accompanies the disease, but the skin gradually becomes thickened and discoloured, other nodules appear, and finally ulcers or small abscesses form. The disease progresses very slowly, but, after it has been in existence some years, the deformity produced may be very great. The nose may be partly or wholly eaten away; the lower eyelids, if attacked, become drawn down, showing the red inner surface. The condition is of little infective power.

Treatment – These horrors have now been removed by the excellent results obtained from the use of isoniazid with or without streptomycin. In certain cases it is still sometimes helpful to remove individual nodules by excision or by curettage, followed by the application of trichloracetic acid. The local application of intensive ultra-violet light is also sometimes of value.

LUPUS ERYTHEMATOSUS is a disease of unknown etiology. It occurs in two forms. The more common form, discoid lupus erythematosus, which is more common in women, involves only the skin and consists of rounded, red, and slightly raised patches, which are distributed most commonly on the nose and cheeks. These patches, by fusing together at their edges, sometimes give a characteristic butterfly-like appearance to the reddened nose and cheeks. There is no tendency to the formation of ulcers, as in lupus vulgaris, and deformity in consequence does not result, although the patches of red alternating with white and atrophied skin can render the complexion quite unsightly.

The second form, disseminated, or systemic, lupus erythematosus, occurs predominantly in women. It tends to run an acute course and involves the joints as well as many of the internal organs of the body, including the kidneys, spleen, and heart.

Treatment – The treatment for the cutaneous form is the local application of corticosteroid (qv) ointment. If this fails, chloroquine (qv) may be given by mouth. The involved area of skin should be protected from sunlight. The only form of treatment which gives any relief in the disseminated form of the disease is one or more of the corticosteroid drugs.

LUX is the unit of illumination. The abbreviation is lx.

LUXATION is another word for dislocation. (See DISLOCATIONS.)

LYCANTHROPY is the term applied to the delusion entertained by an insane person that he or she is a wolf.

LYCOPODIUM is a fine, yellow powder, which consists of the spores of the club-moss, *Lycopodium clavatum*. It is used as a powder in which to roll pills, and is also a good dusting-powder for moist skin surfaces, such as the skin of infants.

LYING-IN (see LABOUR).

LYMPH is the fluid which circulates in the lymphatic vessels of the body. It is a colourless fluid, like blood plasma in composition, only rather more watery. It contains salts similar to those of blood plasma, and the same proteins, though in smaller amount: fibrinogen, serum albumin, and serum globulin. It also contains colourless lymph corpuscles, or lymphocytes as they are known, derived from the glands. In certain of the lymphatic vessels, the lymph contains, after meals, a great amount of fat in the form of a fine milky emulsion. These are the vessels which absorb fat from the food passing down the intestine, and convey it to the thoracic duct; they are called lacteals on account of the milky appearance of their contents. (See CHYLE.)

The lymph is derived, in the first place, from the blood, the watery constituents of which exude through the walls of the capillaries into the tissues, conveying material for the nourishment of the tissues and absorbing waste products.

The various gaps and chinks in the tissues communicate with lymph capillaries, which have a structure similar to that of the capillaries of the blood-vessel system, being composed of delicate flat cells joined edge to edge. These unite to form fine vessels, resembling minute veins in structure, to which the name of lymphatics is applied (illustration 300). These ramify all through the body, passing here and there through lymphatic glands, and ultimately discharge their contents into the blood circulation once more, by opening into the jugular veins in the root of the neck. Other lymph vessels commence in great numbers as minute openings on the surface of the pleura and peritoneum, and act as drains for these otherwise closed cavities. When fluid is effused into these cavities, as in dropsy or pleurisy, for example, its absorption takes place through the lymphatic vessels. The course of these vessels is described under GLANDS.

The circulation of the lymph is effected in some of the lower animals by lymph-hearts, which pump the lymph, just as the heart belonging to the blood-vessels keeps the blood in circulation. In man and most of the higher animals there is no heart for the lymph, which circulates partly by reason of the pressure at which it is driven through the walls of the blood capillaries, but mainly in consequence of accidental forces. The lymph capillaries and vessels are copiously provided with valves, which prevent any back flow of lymph, and every time these vessels are squeezed, as by the contraction of a muscle, or movement of a limb, the lymph moves on a little, leaving room for the exudation of fresh lymph.

300 – Diagram of the relation of the blood and lymph streams among the tissues. *A*, Small artery; *bc*, blood capillaries; *lc*, lymph capillaries; *V*, vein; *L*, lymphatic vessel; the arrows show the direction of the streams.

From this fact one can perceive the immense importance of regular exercise in maintaining the free circulation of lymph.

Lymph, like blood, possesses, in virtue of the fibrinogen which it contains, the power of clotting, forming, when it does so, a faintly yellow or colourless coagulum. This can be seen in the case of small wounds, after the blood has ceased to flow.

The term lymph is also applied to the serous fluid contained in the vesicles which develop as the result of vaccination, and used for the purpose of vaccinating other individuals. (See VACCINATION.)

The term lymph is also loosely applied to the layers and flakes of fibrin which are derived from the lymph and are found on the pleura and other serous membranes as the result of inflammation.

LYMPHADENITIS means inflammation of lymphatic glands. (See GLANDS, DISEASES OF.)

LYMPHADENOMA is another name for Hodgkin's disease (qv).

LYMPHANGIECTASIS means an abnormal dilatation of the lymph vessels, as in filariasis.

LYMPHANGIOGRAPHY, or LYMPHOGRAPHY, is the procedure whereby the lymphatics (qv) and lymphatic glands can be rendered visible on X-ray films by means of the injection of radio-opaque substances.

LYMPHANGITIS means an inflammation situated in the lymphatic vessels.

LYMPHATICS is the term applied to the vessels which convey the lymph (qv). (For an account of their arrangement, see GLANDS.)

LYMPHATISM, or STATUS LYMPHATICUS, is a condition characterized by enlargement of the lymphatic tissue throughout the body. The thymus gland is also usually enlarged. The real nature of the condition, which is usually found in children, is not known. Its importance is that such children are liable to sudden death under an anaesthetic.

LYMPHOCYTE is a variety of white blood corpuscle produced in the lymphoid tissues and lymphatic glands of the body. It contains a simple rounded nucleus surrounded by protoplasm generally described as non-granular. Two varieties of lymphocyte are described, small lymphocytes and large lymphocytes, and together they form over 20 per cent of the white corpuscles of the blood. They play an important part in the production of antibodies (qv), and in the rejection of transplanted organs such as the heart. (See TRANSPLANTATION.) This they do in two different ways. What are known as B lymphocytes produce antibodies, while T lymphocytes attack and destroy antigens (qv) directly. They are known as T lymphocytes because they are produced by the thymus gland. Their numbers are increased in tuberculosis and certain other diseases. Such an increase is known as lymphocytosis.

LYMPHOEDEMA means dropsical swelling of a part or organ due to obstruction to the lymph-vessels draining it.

LYMPHOGRANULOMA INGUINALE, LYMPHOGRANULOMA VENEREUM; PORADENITIS VENEREA; LYMPHOPATHIA VENEREUM, is a venereal disease in which the chief characteristic is enlargement of glands in the groin, the infecting agent being a virus.

LYMPHOMA is a tumour of lymphoid tissue, most commonly found in children in Africa; sometimes called Burkitt's lymphona after the surgeon who first described it. Because of its geographical distribution it is thought to be due to a virus which is transmitted by mosquitoes, but no virus has yet been definitely isolated from the tumour.

LYMPHOSARCOMA is a malignant growth of the lymphoid elements of the body, and is characterized by generalized enlargement of the lymphatic glands, spleen, and liver. The majority of cases – about 55 per cent – occur in the 60 to 70 age-group, but it may occur at any age. The prognosis is poor, 80 per cent of cases dying within six years. Treatment is by means of irradiation or chemotherapy.

LYSERGIC ACID, or LYSERGIC ACID DIETHYLAMIDE, popularly known as LSD, belongs to the ergonovine group of alkaloids. In minute doses it induces psychic states in which the individual becomes aware of repressed memories. Under the influence of the drug he feels he is watching himself and relives feelings from his childhood and infancy. It is proving of value in the treatment of certain anxiety states, but is a drug that must only be used under skilled supervision. (See DRUG ADDICTION.)

LYSIS means the gradual ending of a fever, and is opposed to crisis, which signifies the sudden ending of a fever. (See CRISIS.)
It is also used to describe the process of dissolution of a blood-clot, or the loosening of adhesions.

LYSOFORM is a liquid soap containing formalin, by virtue of which it possesses a strong antiseptic power.

LYSOL, or CRESOL or Soap Solution to give it its official *British Pharmacopoeia* name, is a brown, clear, oily fluid with antiseptic properties, made from coal-tar and containing 50 per cent cresol. When mixed with water it forms a clear soapy fluid which, in 1 per cent strength, is most useful for the disinfection of rooms and surgical instruments. It is used to a great extent in the same way as carbolic acid; it does not exert upon the skin so irritating and roughening an effect as the latter.

LYSOL POISONING – When lysol is swallowed there is a sense of burning about the mouth and throat. There are signs of corrosion around and in the mouth, with brown discoloration, and the characteristic smell of lysol is very evident in the breath. If the lysol is not speedily removed, unconsciousness and stupor gradually come on and death may occur within 24 hours. Septic pneumonia is also liable to supervene, and may produce death at a later period.

Treatment – If the skin has been contaminated with the lysol, it must be washed with water, and any lysol-contaminated clothing must be taken off. Large quantities of tepid water and salt may be given at once to dilute the lysol if it has been swallowed, and produce vomiting. The stomach may also be washed out with a solution of potassium permanganate. Subsequently, olive oil, white of egg, or milk and cream may be given to soothe the irritation, and the patient, on account of difficulty in swallowing, must be fed on fluid food for several days.

LYSOZYME is the name given to a bactericidal substance present in tears.

LYSSA is another term for rabies or hydrophobia.

M

McBURNEY'S POINT is an area of small size on the front of the abdomen, at which the tenderness experienced in appendicitis is felt with special keenness. It is situated between the navel and the prominent anterior superior spine of the right iliac bone, about 2 inches (50 mm) distant from the latter.

MACARONI is made from a hard variety of wheat (*Triticum durum*) which grows well in the hot dry Italian climate. Its characteristic shape results from its high gluten content. It has a low vitamin B content.

MACERATION is a term applied to the softening of a solid by soaking in fluid.

MACROCYTE is the term applied to an unusually large red blood corpuscle especially characteristic of the blood in pernicious anaemia.

MACROGLOSSIA means an abnormally large tongue.

MACROPSIA is the condition in which objects appear larger than they really are. It is due to disease of the retina. (See EYE; and RETINA, DISEASES OF.)

MACULES are spots or stained areas of brown or purplish-brown colour in the skin. They may be due to old haemorrhages, sunburn, disease of internal organs, pregnancy, skin diseases such as eczema and psoriasis, syphilis, and burns.

MADURA FOOT is the name given to a disease found in the Tropics in which the foot becomes swollen and its bones and other tissues riddled by sinuses. It is caused by the presence of a fungus.

MAGNESIUM is a light white metal which burns readily in the air with a brilliant white flame, and the production of a fine white powder. It is used for photographic purposes in the form of ribbon or powder, but the metal itself is not used in medicine. The salts of magnesium used as drugs are the hydroxide of magnesium, the oxide of magnesium, generally known as 'magnesia', and the carbonate of magnesium, all of which have an antacid action; also the sulphate of magnesium generally known as 'Epsom salts', which acts as a purgative.

Uses – Light and heavy carbonates of magnesia, are used to correct hyperacidity of the stomach, as are the hydroxide and the light oxide. They are also used as feeble laxatives. Cream of magnesia, the official *British Pharmacopoeia* name of which is Magnesium Hydroxide Mixture, is a widely used, effective antacid. In large doses it is a useful safe laxative.

Magnesium sulphate is the most commonly used saline purge. (See EPSOM SALTS.)

MAGNETISM (see ELECTRICITY IN MEDICINE).

MAIDISM is another name for PELLAGRA (qv).

MALACIA is a term applied to softening of a part or tissue in disease: eg. osteomalacia or softening of the bones.

MALABSORPTION SYNDROME includes a multiplicity of diseases, all of which are characterized by faulty absorption from the intestine of essential foodstuffs, such as fat, vitamins and mineral salts. Among the conditions in this syndrome are coeliac disease (qv) and sprue (qv).

MALAISE means a vague feeling of feverishness, listlessness, and languor, which often precedes the onset of serious acute diseases, or accompanies passing derangements, such as dyspepsia, chills, and colds.

MALARIA, which derives its name from *mala aria* – the Italian for bad air, and also known as AGUE, PALUDISM, JUNGLE FEVER, MARSH FEVER, PERIODIC FEVER, is a disease caused by the presence of certain parasites in the blood. It consists at first of a series of febrile attacks, which may come on every day, every second day, or every third day; later it assumes a chronic form, in which a poor state of health known as chronic malaria or malarial cachexia is developed, and there is a tendency towards frequent relapses.

History – It has been known from the earliest times, and not only is it described by many of the medical writers of antiquity, but numerous references to it exist in general literature, such as the works of Horace. From these it appears that its connection with swampy ground was quite well recognized even in ancient times.

The first important advance was made

in 1640, when the Countess of Cinchon, wife of the Viceroy of Peru, brought home to Europe the bark by which the South American Indians had learned to treat the disease successfully. From this bark, named after her Cinchona bark, and also known as Jesuit's bark, since the secret had been learned by priests from the Indians, quinine is derived. By this drug a means of treating the paroxysms of fever, as well as an aid in warding off the disease, was obtained. From the fact that quinine is an antiseptic it was assumed that the disease must be due to some poison circulating in the blood which the quinine could destroy.

Not till 1880 was the next great step taken when Laveran, a French military surgeon, discovered the presence of minute parasites in the corpuscles of blood drawn from malarious persons and examined them under the microscope. He described more than one form of the parasites, and subsequent observers demonstrated that the parasites go through a process of development, leading up to the production of spores, which are formed all through the blood of the affected person at one time, and from which a new set of parasites develops. Other observers were successful in finding similar parasites in the blood of lower animals, particularly of birds.

It had long been noticed, even by West African natives, that mosquitoes seem to flourish together with malaria, and several scientists endeavoured to establish a connection between the two. This was successfully proved by Manson in 1894, through bringing from Italy live mosquitoes which had been allowed to suck blood from malarious persons in that country, and allowing the insects to bite healthy people in London, who had no other possible connection with the disease. The experiment was successful, and those persons who had offered themselves for the experiment proved conclusively that malaria is carried by mosquitoes. Other persons proved the converse of this proposition, and showed, by living for some months in a malarious district, such as the Campagna at Rome, that infection does not take place provided mosquitoes be kept off by gauze and other means.

From the examination of the blood in malarious persons, Manson reasoned that the parasites go through a stage of their development in the bodies of the mosquitoes, passing, in the tissues of those insects, through a sexual stage, in which male and female forms unite in the production of

masses of new parasites. The arduous work of demonstrating this was undertaken by Ross, then a military surgeon in India. The difficulty of this work is understood when one considers that the dissection of a great number of mosquitoes and their examination under the microscope were necessary before Ross was able in 1898 to confirm the truth of Manson's theory, by demonstrating the genus Anopheles as the insect in which the development of the malaria parasite takes place. Other observers confirmed his observations, and traced out in detail the changes which the parasites undergo while in the mosquito.

301 – *Anopheles gambiae.* The most dangerous malaria-carrier in Africa. From Manson's *Tropical Diseases.* Cassell & Co. Ltd.

Causes – As shown by these discoveries, the presence of persons infected by the malarial parasite and the access of the Anopheles mosquito (illustration 301) to these and to healthy persons form two of the conditions producing infection of fresh cases. But there are various factors which aid or retard the development of the parasite and of the mosquito. The disease is known all round the world, but is chiefly found in tropical climates, spreading here and there into temperate regions, where it occurs in summer and autumn, if the other conditions are suitable. The presence of swamps, pools of surface water, rank vegetation, and a poorly fed population are also important factors. Its chief seats are India, south-east Asia, South China, and Central America. It is estimated that there are 2000 million people living in potentially malarious areas and in

1976 there were 5·8 million cases in India alone. There is a growing incidence of it in the United Kingdom in people who have acquired the disease abroad. In 1977, 1471 cases were reported in England, a 25 per cent increase on 1976. Eleven of these cases proved fatal.

The parasites of malaria are three in number, corresponding to the tertian fever, the quartan fever, and the aestivo-autumnal fever or subtertian or malignant tertian malaria. The parasites are protozoa, belonging to the order *Sporozoa*, and to the genus *Plasmodium*. The specific names for benign tertian, quartan, and malignant malaria are, respectively, *Plasmodium vivax*, *P. malariae*, and *P. falciparum*. As has been stated, the malarial parasite passes one phase of its life-cycle in man and the other in the stomach and tissues of the mosquito (the sexual phase). After sexual union of male and female forms in the mosquito's stomach, the resulting offspring – the asexual sporozoites – eventually find their way into the mosquito's salivary gland.

When the infected female mosquito bites a human being, these filamentous sporozoites are injected into the blood. They then find their way into the liver where they develop into what are known as schizonts. After a period ranging from six to sixteen days (depending on the species of plasmodium) these schizonts have reached maturity, and in the course of maturation each one has produced up to 40,000 merozoites (illustration 302). These merozoites are then released into the blood stream where they penetrate the red blood cells and form trophozoites or rings (illustration 303). These in turn enlarge, each to the capacity of the red corpuscle. The large trophozoite thus formed finally splits into numerous small parasites now called merozoites. These burst out of the red blood corpuscle into the blood stream and then attack other red corpuscles, the whole asexual cycle repeating itself once more. The paroxysm of malarial fever coincides with the bursting of the red blood corpuscles and the setting free of the merozoites into the blood-stream. Sexual forms – male and female gametocytes – also develop in the blood, but they undergo no

302 – A merozoite of *Plasmodium knowlesi* invading a red blood cell magnified × 35 000. (McLaren, Bannister, Trigg, Butcher) (NIMR 1977, Medical Research Council)

further change until a mosquito bite sucks them into the mosquito's stomach.

Symptoms – For a day or two before the actual fever sets in, there may be headache, vague pains about the body and limbs, chilliness, and slight rises of temperature. When the parasites have multiplied up to the stage already mentioned, the attack suddenly comes on.

The acute malarial attack has, in general, three stages, although in occasional cases one of the stages may be excessively marked or may be wanting. These are the

throughout the body, and sometimes even delirium. This stage may last several hours.

The sweating stage comes on after the fever reaches its height, as the temperature begins to fall. Profuse perspiration breaks out, the person begins to feel decidedly better, and the headache and pains at the same time pass off. Finally, after two or three hours the patient feels quite well, though much weakened, and remains so till the next attack begins.

If the parasite present be that of *quartan*

303 – Blood film from patient with malaria, showing a typical ring form inside a red blood cell.
Royal Army Medical College.

cold stage, the hot stage, and the sweating stage.

The cold stage begins with a feeling of chilliness even in the hottest weather. This increases till the person has to betake himself to bed and heap himself with clothes, face and nails being blue with cold, and the whole body shaken with shivering (rigors). Nevertheless, if the temperature be taken with a thermometer, it is found to be considerably raised. This stage lasts an hour or less.

The hot stage comes on as the temperature of the body rises, beginning with hot flushes, which lengthen till the body feels burning hot, the temperature rising to 105° or 106° F (40·5° to 41·1° C). There are also headache, dizziness, sickness, pain

fever there is an intermission of two days before the next attack: that is to say, if the first attack be on the 1st day of the month the succeeding ones are on the 4th, 7th, and so on. If the parasite be that of *tertian fever*, the attacks are on the 1st, 3rd, 5th, and so on; whilst in the severe *aestivo-autumnal fever*, each attack may last considerably over a day, so that there may not be time for one to pass off completely before the next begins. The patient then is in a continued state of fever, known as *subtertian fever*. A person may get a double or treble infection of the malarial parasites, and then the fever may also occur every day, although from the fact that the temperature on one set of days rises higher than it does on the set of alternate days, or from the time of the attacks being different, the attack beginning, for example, on the 1st, 3rd, 5th, etc., at 1 pm., and on the 2nd, 4th, 6th, etc., at 5 pm., it is clear that the person is affected by two agues running side by side. When the fever occurs every day, whatever be the cause, it is sometimes called a *quotidian fever*.

As a rule people, after passing through an ague, feel completely recovered till the next attack is due, but now and then the attack may develop seriously. For example, hyperpyrexia may develop, the temperature continuing to rise till death occurs before the sweating stage sets in. Insensibility may set in and the person die owing to blockage of the small vessels in the brain by immense numbers of the parasites; this is known as cerebral malaria. Severe vomiting or diarrhoea may also endanger the patient's life, or he may become very much collapsed during the sweating stage. One of the most dread complications of malaria is blackwater fever (qv).

If treatment be adopted between two attacks, the succeeding attack or the next after that is generally checked. Even when no treatment takes place, after a few weeks of the attacks these gradually get less and less marked and finally disappear, a rally taking place. The parasites become so diminished that they are unable to cause fever, but they are not entirely destroyed in the blood, and so the affected person is subject after some weeks or months to a relapse, when the attacks of ague are repeated as in the first seizure. These rallies and relapses may go on for several years, especially if the person leads an exposed, laborious life, or is poorly nourished. Anything which depresses the vitality, such as a chill, is apt to lead to a fresh relapse. On the other hand, under efficient treatment complete recovery occurs.

If the disease becomes chronic, various symptoms set in. The person becomes very anaemic in consequence of the large number of blood corpuscles destroyed by the parasites in each paroxysm of fever. A feeble state of health, accompanied by bodily wasting and yellow discoloration of the skin, ensues, and the spleen and liver, particularly the former, become enlarged.

Treatment – This falls into two important sections, preventive and curative.

PREVENTIVE TREATMENT may be directed either against the parasites or against the mosquitoes which convey them. Mepacrine, proguanil, pyrimethamine, chloroquine, and amodiaquine are effective prophylactics, and one of these should be taken regularly by all white people living in, or visiting, malarious districts. Full details as to which drugs to take and when, are given in two leaflets – *Notice to Travellers* published by the Department of Health and Social Security, and *Advice to Travellers* published by the Health Education Council – which are available from travel agencies. There is still some difference of opinion as to their relative efficacy. So far as mepacrine and proguanil are concerned, there is evidence suggesting that their efficacy depends upon the strain of parasite, and that this varies in different areas.

It is still more important to attack the mosquitoes in their developing stage. The eggs are laid on or near pools of stagnant water in which the larvae and pupae swim just below the surface, breathing through a tube which projects above the surface of the water. These larvae may be destroyed by pouring on the surface of these pools some fluid through which the breathing-tube of the larva cannot be protruded. Crude petroleum and a special oil known as 'malariol' are used for this purpose, and when poured upon pools the oil spreads out instantly into a film which will remain intact for several days if not destroyed by rain or wind. Further, all small pools in gardens should be filled up, tubs, flower-pots, cisterns, and other collections of water emptied regularly at least once a week, and in public works, such as railways, it should be made illegal, as is the rule in Italy, to leave holes and ditches where water can collect. Anopheline breeding grounds can be sprayed with Paris green. Fish which feed on the larvae can be introduced into ponds and lakes.

Although these methods are still of value, they have largely been replaced or supplemented by the use of insecticides such as DDT, benzene hexachloride (BHC) and dieldrin which have proved most effective in destroying mosquitoes.

Wire-gauze screens to all the windows of a house, and muslin mosquito netting over the beds, form an efficient protection, and it should be remembered that not only should mosquitoes be kept away from healthy people by these means, but that it is even more important that the insects should not gain access to those suffering from the disease, by whose blood they become infected and made carriers of malaria to the healthy.

CURATIVE TREATMENT depends upon a wide range of drugs, including chloroquine, primaquine, pyrimethamine, and quinine. In cases in which the malaria organism has become resistant to these the World Health Organization recommends amodiaquine or sulfadoxine. (See also BLACKWATER FEVER.)

MALATHION is one of the less toxic organo-phosphorus insecticides (qv).

MALE FERN, or FILIX MAS, is a remedy once widely used for the expulsion of tapeworms. It has now been largely displaced by dichlorophen (qv), mepacrine (qv) and niclosamide (qv).

MALFORMATION (see DEFORMITIES).

MALIGNANT is a term applied in several ways to serious disorders. Tumours are called malignant when they grow rapidly, tend to infiltrate surrounding healthy tissues, and to spread to distant parts of the body, leading eventually to death. (See CANCER AND SARCOMA.) The term is also applied to types of disease which are much more serious than the usual form, such as malignant hypertension, malignant smallpox. Malignant pustule is another name for anthrax. (See ANTHRAX.)

MALIGNANT HYPERTENSION has nothing to do with cancer. It derives its name from the fact that, if untreated, it runs a rapidly fatal course. It is still undecided whether it is a disease entity in itself or is merely a terminal stage in certain cases of essential hypertension (qv). Its characteristic features are that it occurs in a younger age-group than essential hypertension, there is a very high diastolic blood-pressure, with papilloedema (qv) and kidney failure. This is the type of hypertension in which the antihypertensive drugs (see ESSENTIAL HYPERTENSION) have proved so successful. Indeed, the introduction of these drugs has revolutionized the outlook. At one time an invariably fatal disease within two years, many patients with this condition can now enjoy many years of comparatively good health.

MALINGERING is a term applied to the feigning of illness. In the great majority of cases a person who feigns illness has a certain amount of disability, but exaggerates his illness or discomfort for some ulterior motive.

MALLEOLUS is the term applied to either of the two bony prominences at the ankle. (See LEG.)

MALLET FINGER is due to sudden forced flexion of the terminal joint of a finger, resulting in rupture of the tendon. As a result the individual is unable to extend the terminal part of the finger which remains bent forward. The middle, ring and little fingers are most commonly involved. A common cause in men is catching a cricket ball; in women the common cause is tucking the bedclothes under the mattress when bedmaking. Treatment is by means of splinting the finger. The end result is satisfactory provided the victim has sufficient patience.

MALLET TOE is the condition in which it is not possible to extend the terminal part of the toe. It is usually due to muscular imbalance but may be due to congenital absence of the extensor muscle. A callosity (qv) often forms on it which may be painful. Should this be troublesome, treatment consists of removal of the terminal phalanx.

MALT is a substance derived from barley by allowing a certain amount of growth to take place in the moistened grain, which is then dried and crushed. It contains a ferment named diastase, together with a large amount of malt-sugar and dextrin, the latter constituents being still further developed from the starch of the barley by the action of the ferment, when the malt is allowed to digest in water at a temperature approaching 104° F (40° C). Similarly, the ferment will convert into sugar a large amount of the starch in flour mixed with malt, and so perform some of the functions of the saliva and pancreatic juice.

For these reasons malt is mixed with various proportions of flour to form some of the popular foods for children. It is also used in the form of malt extracts, 1 ounce (28.3 grams) of which is equivalent to 80 Calories.

MALTA FEVER, also known as MEDITERRANEAN FEVER; ROCK FEVER; NEAPOLITAN FEVER; LEVANT FEVER; UNDULANT FEVER; and BRUCELLOSIS, is a long-continued fever which principally occurs on the shores and islands of the Mediterranean, but is found also in many other countries. (See BRUCELLOSIS.)

MAMMARY GLAND (see BREAST).

MAMMILLA is the Latin term for the nipple.

MAMMOGRAPHY is the term used to describe the special technique whereby X-rays can be taken that reveal the structure of the breast.

MANDELIC ACID is a non-toxic keto-acid used in the treatment of infections of the urinary tract, especially those due to the *Escherichia coli* and the *Streptococcus faecalis* or *Enterococcus*. It is administered in doses of 45 grains (3 grams) several times daily. As it is only effective in an acid urine, ammonium chloride must also be taken at the same time.

MANDIBLE is the name applied to the bone of the lower jaw.

MANDL'S PAINT consists of iodine 1·25 grams, potassium iodide 2·5 grams, water 2·5 ml, oil of peppermint 0·4 ml, alcohol (90 per cent) 4 ml, glycerin to 100 ml. It is used as a throat paint in pharyngitis and tonsillitis. It should be well shaken before use.

MANGANESE is a metal, oxides of which are found abundantly in nature. Permanganate of potassium is a well-known disinfectant. (See PERMANGANATE OF POTASSIUM.)

MANIA is a form of mental disorder characterized by great excitement. (See MENTAL ILLNESS.)

MANIC-DEPRESSIVE INSANITY, or CYCLOTHYMIA, is a form of madness characterized by alternate attacks of mania and depression.

MANIPULATION is the term applied to the forceful passive movement of joints. In skilled hands it is a most effective means of treatment of stiff joints or of pain in the back due to a prolapsed intervertebral disc (qv).

MANOMETER is an instrument for measuring the pressure or tension of liquids or gases. (See BLOOD-PRESSURE.)

MANTOUX TEST, also known as MENDEL'S TEST, is a test for tuberculosis. It consists in injecting into the superficial layers of the skin (ie. intradermally) a very small quantity of old tuberculin. A positive reaction of the skin – swelling and redness – shows that the person so reacting has been infected with the *Mycobacterium tuberculosis*. But it does not mean that such a person is suffering from active tuberculosis. (See TUBERCULIN.)

MANUBRIUM is the uppermost part of the breast-bone.

MANZULLO'S TELLURITE TEST consists in applying to the throat of someone suspected of having diphtheria a 2 per cent potassium tellurite solution. If diphtheria bacilli are present the solution blackens. But some other germs also reduce the tellurite solution. As a negative test it has some use, because if no reduction occurs it is highly improbable that the patient has diphtheria.

MAPLE-SYRUP URINE DISEASE is a condition in which there is an association between mental defect and a disorder of amino-acid metabolism. It is so named because the urine has the odour of maple syrup.

MARASMUS means progressive wasting, especially in young children, when there is no ascertainable cause. It is generally associated with defective feeding. (See ATROPHY; and INFANT FEEDING.)

MARBURG DISEASE, also known as GREEN MONKEY DISEASE and VERVET MONKEY DISEASE because the first recorded cases acquired their infection from monkeys of this genus, is a viral infection with a high mortality rate. The incubation period is 4 to 9 days. The onset is sudden with marked nausea and severe headache. This is followed by rising temperature, diarrhoea, vomiting. Towards the end of the first week a rash appears which persists for a week and is accompanied by internal bleeding. In those who recover convalescence is slow and prolonged. The world distribution of the causative virus is unknown.

MARCH FRACTURE is a curious condition in which a fracture occurs of the second (rarely the third) metatarsal bone in the foot without any obvious cause. The usual story is that a pain suddenly developed in the foot while walking (hence the name) and that it has persisted ever since. The only treatment needed is immobilization of the foot and rest, and the fracture heals satisfactorily.

MARGARINE (see DIET).

MARIHUANA is another term for CANNABIS INDICA, or hemp, or hashish. (See DRUG ADDICTION.)

MARRIAGE GUIDANCE COUNCIL –The idea of a marriage guidance council came from a group of doctors, clergy and social workers who were concerned for the welfare of marriage. It is based upon two major concepts: that marriage provides the best possible way for a man and woman to live and love together and rear their children, and that the counsellors share a basic respect for the unique personality of the individual and his (or her) right to make his (or her) own decisions. The organization consists of between 120 and 130 Marriage Guidance Councils throughout the country, comprising about 1250 counsellors. These Councils are affiliated to the National Marriage Guidance Council, which is responsible for the selection, training and continued supervision of all counsellors. Anyone seeking help can telephone or write for an appointment. No fees are charged, but those receiving help are encouraged to donate what they can. The address of the National Marriage Guidance Council is Herbert Gray College, Little Church Street, Rugby, Warwickshire CV21 3AP.

MARROW means the softer substance enclosed in the interior of bones. It is of two kinds: *yellow marrow*, which occupies the large tubular space in the shaft of a long bone, such as a limb bone, and *red marrow*, which fills up the spaces in the interior of the ribs, sternum, and vertebral bodies, as well as the ends of the shafts of the long bones such as the femur and humerus. There is no essential difference between the two, although yellow marrow owes its colour to the large amount of fat contained in it, whilst red marrow is of a highly cellular structure. The marrow is the site of formation of red blood corpuscles, platelets, and granular white blood cells.

MARSH FEVER (see MALARIA).

MARSHMALLOW ROOT is the root of *Althaea officinalis*, which has long been credited as a domestic medicine, with a soothing influence upon mucous membranes, as well as exerting a diuretic action. It is used chiefly as an ingredient of lozenges for cases of sore throat.

MASSAGE, or RUBBING, is a method of treatment in which the operator uses his hands, or occasionally other appliances, to rub, knead, or press the skin and deeper tissues of the person under treatment. It is often combined with (*a*) passive movements, in which the masseur moves the limbs in various ways, the person treated

making no effort; or (*b*) active movements, which are performed with the combined assistance of masseur and patient. Massage is also often combined with baths and gymnastics in order to strengthen various muscles. The beneficial effects of massage are exerted in different ways. Applied gently, it has a soothing action upon the nerves of sensation; applied more vigorously, certain methods have the effect of quickening the circulation of lymph and blood, and so leading to the rapid absorption of waste products in the muscles, and of the results of disease in various organs. Other forms of massage cause muscular contractions and so provide exercise for the muscles in cases where movements of the whole body are not desired.

Varieties – STROKING, or *effleurage*, consists of gentle pressure with the hand moved in one direction. It soothes the nerves of the part treated and empties the main lymph-vessels and veins, thus increasing the circulation locally. It is carried out either with the flat of the hand or with the edges of thumb and first finger widely separated.

KNEADING, or *pétrissage*, is the most commonly employed form, and consists of squeezing, kneading, rolling, or rubbing movements coupled with a considerable amount of pressure, effected, it may be, with the fingers or knuckles, but generally with the pulp or the ball of the thumb. It has a still greater effect than stroking in moving on the lymph and blood circulation of deep-seated parts, and so leading to the absorption of inflammatory thickenings in and around joints, tendon-sheaths, and muscles. The masseur in this method, as it were, tries to dispel inflammatory deposits by his own endeavours, although he knows that it is rather by the vital activity, which he merely assists, that the effect is gradually produced. (See LYMPH.)

STABILE MOVEMENTS include such applications as the following. *Pressing* may be done with the finger-tips or with the knuckles; it is usually combined with rubbing. *Tapping* is done with the points of the fingers from the wrist, and, when applied gently, has a soothing effect. *Thrusting*, which consists in poking up the deeper parts with the points of the fingers, and *hacking*, in which the muscles are struck with the inner edge of the hand, the arms moving from the elbows, are employed to cause muscular contractions.

VIBRATORY MOVEMENTS are made either by tapping (as above) or by special pads, to which a very rapid oscillation is communicated from an electric motor. This form of massage has been used in order to exert a soothing influence, for example, in cases of headache.

PASSIVE MOVEMENTS are made chiefly for their effect upon the joints. The synovial fluid is increased if scanty, and tends to be absorbed if excessive, while adhesions, which limit the motions of the joint or render these painful, are broken down by passive movements of a more forcible type. This type of massage is the form chiefly employed in the treatment of stiff joints by bone-setters.

ACTIVE MOVEMENTS of a carefully regulated type, in which the person's will is concentrated upon the movement made, are specially useful for developing the muscles brought into play thereby. The amount of muscular force required is graduated and increased by the masseur resisting the movements with varying degrees of force.

Uses – Massage can only be employed to full advantage by fully trained masseurs (or masseuses). A complete list of members of the Chartered Society of Physiotherapy who are qualified to give massage can be obtained on application to the Secretary of the Society, 14 Bedford Row, London, W.C.1. The types of case in which massage is useful are extremely various. Neuralgia, sciatica, and muscular rheumatism are among the painful conditions in which some relief is generally obtained. In muscular wasting, and paralysis due to nerve conditions – such as lead-poisoning, peripheral neuritis, crutch palsy, Bell's paralysis, and poliomyelitis – the muscles affected may be kept in a state of good nutrition till the nerve weakness has disappeared, and so recovery may be materially hastened. In various other nervous conditions, such as hysteria, chorea, loss of sensation, and writer's cramp, massage often proves of great benefit. Several types of joint disease, such as chronic rheumatism and stiffness due to previous slight injuries, such as sprains, are specially amenable to treatment by passive movements combined with deep rubbing, but any such interference with joints which have been recently the seat of tuberculous disease is very dangerous, as by these means the disease may be more widely spread. In several general conditions such as corpulence and constipation associated with a flabby state of body, massage may be of use.

Massage may be combined with electrical applications. For example, high-frequency and static electricity may be used along with gentle massage to obtain a soothing effect. The interrupted galvanic, sinusoidal, and faradic currents are useful combined with more forcible massage to stimulate muscular contraction in various cases of paralysis. (See also CARDIAC MASSAGE.)

MASS MINIATURE RADIO-GRAPHY is a method of obtaining X-ray photographs of the chests of large numbers of people at about the rate of two persons per minute. It has been used on a large scale of recent years as a means of screening the population for pulmonary tuberculosis.

MASTALGIA is the term applied to pain in the breast.

MAST CELLS are round or oval cells found predominantly in the loose connective tissues. They contain histamine (qv) and heparin (qv). Although thought to play a part in inflammatory reactions, allergy, and hypersensitivity, their origin and maintenance, as well as their precise function in health and disease are still not quite clear.

MASTECTOMY is the operation for removal of a breast. It is an operation that can cause considerable psychological disturbance. Those who find it difficult to adjust to the situation after the operation will obtain helpful advice from the Mastectomy Association, 1 Colworth Road, Croydon CR0 7AD.

MASTICATION is the act whereby, as a result of movements of the lower jaw, lips, tongue, and cheek, food is reduced to a condition in which it is ready to be acted on by the gastric juices in the process of digestion. Adequate mastication is an essential part of the digestive process. (See DIGESTION.)

MASTITIS is the term applied to inflammation of the breast. (See BREAST, DISEASES OF.)

MASTOID PROCESS is the large process of the temporal bone of the skull which can be felt immediately behind the ear. It contains numerous cavities, one of which, the mastoid antrum, communicates with the middle ear, and is liable to suppurate when the middle ear is diseased. (See EAR, DISEASES OF.)

MASTURBATION is the production of an orgasm, or at least a modicum of sexual pleasure, by self-manipulation of the penis or clitoris. It is a normal transitional stage of sexual development. Only when it is practised excessively does it become a condition requiring treatment.

MATCH-WORKERS' DISEASE (see PHOSPHORUS POISONING).

MATERIA MEDICA is that branch of medical study which deals with the sources, preparations, and uses of drugs.

MATERNITY and CHILD WELFARE – The high rate of infantile mortality which used to prevail in the larger towns drew attention to the great loss of infant life which was produced partly by ignorance on the part of the mothers and partly by poverty. A movement was accordingly begun early in the present century in some of the larger cities to provide trained women as health visitors for giving advice to working-class women on the proper methods of rearing their children. This was at first a voluntary effort conducted by philanthropic agencies, but it was soon taken up by local authorities throughout the country. The necessary information as to the existence of newly born infants was provided by the Notification of Births which was demanded by Acts passed in 1907 and 1915. Women health visitors were appointed to visit the homes of such newly born infants, and shortly afterwards INFANT CONSULTATION CENTRES and Clinics were established by various local authorities and voluntary agencies.

At first the movement for child welfare was limited to infants from birth to 1 year of age, but shortly afterwards the necessity for supervising the health of children until they came under school discipline at 5 years was recognized. Still later it became evident that it was desirable to watch over the health of the expectant mother and to provide skilled attendance prior to and during confinement. This led, accordingly, to the establishment of MATERNITY AND CHILD WELFARE CENTRES and CLINICS by many local authorities. The schemes which have now been devised for combating infantile mortality are very wide. They include better housing, health visitors, consultation centres for mothers, infant milk depots, the provision of milk, vitamin preparations and iron tablets for expectant and nursing mothers, and hospital accommodation for expectant mothers before and during confinement. The provision of Child Welfare Centres to which

parents may bring their infants at stated times produces valuable results, both by advice to the mothers and by keeping records of increase in weight and other important facts regarding the infants, and also by interesting and stimulating the mothers to greater efforts. The Centre also provides opportunities for giving instruction in health, cookery, sewing, etc., to the mothers, and for distributing food and clothing as may be necessary. Antenatal Clinics, which provide education and assistance for the expectant mother, form an important section of this work.

HEALTH VISITORS have been described as 'truly medico-social workers – playing a full part in both preventive medicine and social action'. Their duties include maternity and child welfare, school nursing, health education, tuberculosis, venereal disease, infectious diseases, mental illness, welfare of the aged and the handicapped, family welfare services, and cooperation with general practitioners. Health visitors must pass the examination for the Health Visitor's Certificate. Candidates for this examination must be either: (a) Nurses who have undergone a three-years' course of training at a recognized general or children's hospital, who have obtained Part I of the Certificate of the Central Midwife's Board, and who have attended an approved whole-time course in public health work lasting for nine months, or (b) Women, not being trained nurses, who have undergone an approved course of training in public health work for two years together with six months' training in hospital, and who have obtained Part I of the Certificate of the Central Midwifes Board.

ANTENATAL CLINICS are considered to be of great value, because the fatality among the unborn from stillbirth, abortion, etc., is higher than the mortality of infants during the first year of life; it is generally believed, further, that by the medical attention provided at such clinics many of these antenatal deaths could be prevented, and the number of infants born prematurely and of feeble constitution could be much reduced. Thus, it has been shown that the perinatal death rate (qv) is nearly five times higher in the children of mothers who are late in attending antenatal clinics than in the children of those who start attending early. Health visitors follow up cases seen at antenatal clinics and ensure that the medical instructions given at the clinic are carried out, and proper steps taken to prepare for the confinement.

Under the National Insurance Acts in Great Britain, a woman receives a maternity grant in respect of each child, and also a home confinement grant if the confinement takes place at home. A woman who ordinarily follows a gainful occupation is also given a maternity allowance for 18 weeks beginning about 11 weeks before her confinement provided that she abstains from work.

INFANT CONSULTATION CLINICS are conducted usually by local authorities, and, in cases where it is desirable, mothers are urged to bring infants to these clinics regularly. Many of the disabling illnesses of early childhood are thus prevented, and the attendance should continue as required during the first five years of the child's life.

DAY NURSERIES, or crèches, are provided in many places in connection with these clinics, at which children can be left when the mothers are out at work.

Most local authorities have schemes for supplying special foods or nutritious diet to mothers of children who after medical examination at the Clinic are found to require such assistance. SPECIAL TREATMENT CLINICS are also provided in many places for the examination and care of teeth, eyes, ears, nose, throat, and skin of children. Also there is at present a movement for the treatment of cases in which children are crippled as the result of early disease. Further, in connection with the clinics many local authorities possess convalescent homes, or arrange with voluntary agencies for admission to their convalescent homes of children who are in need of special care and open-air regime. Indirectly connected with these clinics in many places there have also been established play centres and kindergartens for young children.

Under the National Health Service Act, 1946, all these services were unified under Local Health Authorities. A statutory duty was imposed upon Local Health Authorities to provide health centres, maternity and child welfare, domiciliary midwifery, health visiting, home nursing, vaccination and immunization, and ambulances. They were also empowered to provide home-help services, and care and after-care. Maternity and child welfare covers the care of expectant and nursing mothers and of children under 5 years of age who are not attending school. It includes antenatal clinics, postnatal clinics, child-welfare clinics, and a priority dental service for both expectant and nursing mothers and young children. A further reorganization of the National Health Service introduced in 1974 aimed at a closer coordination of these services with the hospital service and the family doctor service.

MATTER (see PUS).

MATTOID is a term applied to a person who, though passing as sane, is eccentric or mentally unbalanced in some particular direction.

MAW-WORMS is another name for round-worms.

MAXILLA is the name applied to the upper jaw-bones, which bear the teeth.

MEASLES, also known as MORBILLI or RUBEOLA, is an acute infectious disease occurring mostly in children. It appears to have been known from an early period in the history of medicine, mention being made of it in the writings of Rhazes and others of the Arabian physicians in the tenth century. For long, however, its specific nature was not recognized, and it was held to be a variety of smallpox. Measles and scarlet fever were long confounded with each other; and in the account given by Sydenham of epidemics of measles in London in 1670 and 1674, it is evident that even that accurate observer had not as yet clearly perceived their pathological distinction, although it would seem to have been made a century earlier by Ingrassia, a physician of Palermo. The disease known as German measles, or rubella, is a much milder disease than measles. Measles is compulsorily notifiable in Britain.

Causes – Measles is a disease of the earlier years of childhood. Like most other infectious maladies, it is rare in infants under 6 months old on account of the antibodies that they have acquired from their mothers before birth. It is comparatively seldom met in adults, largely due to the fact that most persons have undergone an attack in early life, or have been repeatedly exposed to the infection of measles and so have probably acquired a certain amount of immunity, for, among communities where measles is not prevalent, the old suffer equally with the young, when infection is once introduced. Some countries enjoy long immunity from outbreaks of measles, but in such cases the disease, when introduced, spreads with great rapidity and virulence. Two classical examples of the last century were: the epidemic in the Faroe Islands in 1846, where, within six months after the arrival of a single case of measles, more than three-fourths of the entire population were attacked and many perished; and the similarly produced and still more destructive outbreak in Fiji in 1875, in which it was estimated that about one-fourth of the inhabitants were cut off by the disease within three months. In such cases it is generally held that epidemics arising on what may be termed a virgin soil are apt to possess a special severity.

In many lands, such as the United Kingdom and the United States, measles is rarely absent, especially from large towns, where sporadic cases are found in greater or less number at all seasons. But every two years, especially from December to February, epidemics arise and spread among the children who are not protected by a recent attack. In 1970 there were 289,893 cases in England with 40 deaths. One attack of measles does not give complete immunity from future attacks, but second attacks are rare.

There are few diseases so infectious as measles, and its rapid spread in epidemics is no doubt due to the fact that infection is most potent in the earlier stages, even for several days, before its real nature has been shown by the appearance of the rash. Hence the difficulty of timely isolation and the readiness with which the disease is spread, which is mostly by infected droplets from the nose and throat coughed or sneezed into the air. (See INFECTION.) Another fact, which sometimes assists the spread of measles, is that the temperature often falls to normal on the second day and the child appears to be much better, so that he is again allowed to mix with his play-fellows, owing to the mistaken idea that he is suffering merely from a cold, till the rash appears on the fourth day and shows the real nature of the malady. The infecting agent is a virus.

Symptoms – After the infection has been received into the system, a period of incubation or latency precedes the development of the disease, during which scarcely any disturbance of the health is perceptible. This period appears to vary in duration, but it may be stated as generally lasting for from ten to fifteen days, when it is followed by the invasion of the symptoms specially characteristic of measles. These consist in the somewhat sudden onset of acute catarrh of the mucous membranes. Sneezing, accompanied with a watery discharge, sometimes bleeding from the nose, redness and watering of the eyes, cough of a short, frequent, and noisy char-

acter, with little or no expectoration, hoarseness of the voice, and occasionally sickness and diarrhoea, are the chief symptoms of this stage. There is well-marked febrile disturbance, the temperature being elevated to 100° to 102° F (37·7° to 39° C), and the pulse rapid, while headache, thirst, and restlessness are usually present to a greater or less degree. In some instances these initial symptoms are so slight that they almost escape notice, and the child is allowed to associate with others at a time when the contagion of the disease is most active. In rare cases, especially in young children, convulsions usher in, or occur in the course of, this stage of invasion which lasts as a rule for three or four days, the febrile symptoms, however, showing a characteristic tendency to pass away temporarily (remission) on the second and sometimes also on the third day. About the fourth day after the invasion, sometimes later, rarely earlier, the characteristic eruption appears on the skin, being first noticed on the brow, cheeks, chin, also behind the ears, and on the neck. It consists of small spots of a dusky red or crimson colour, slightly elevated above the surface, at first isolated, but tending to become grouped together into patches of irregular, occasionally crescentic, outline, with portions of skin free from the eruption intervening. The face acquires a swollen and bloated appearance, which, taken along with the catarrh of the nostrils and eyes, is almost characteristic, and renders the diagnosis at this stage a matter of no difficulty. Even before it appears on the skin, the rash is sometimes visible within the mouth, as bluish-white spots on the mucous membrane, known as Koplik spots. The eruption spreads downwards over the body and limbs, which are soon thickly studded with the red spots or patches. Sometimes these become confluent over a considerable surface, giving rise to a larger area of uniform redness.

The rash continues to come out for two or three days, and then begins to fade in the order in which it first showed itself: namely, from above downwards. By the end of about a week after its first appearance, scarcely any trace of the eruption remains beyond a faint staining of the skin. Occasionally during convalescence slight peeling of the epidermis takes place, but much less distinctly than is the case in scarlet fever. At the start of the eruptive stage, the fever, catarrh, and other constitutional disturbances, which were present from the beginning, become aggravated, the temperature often rising to 105° F (40·5° C) or more, and there are headache, thirst, furred tongue, and soreness of the throat, upon which red patches similar to those on the surface of the body may be observed. These symptoms usually decline as soon as the rash has attained its maximum, and often there occurs a sudden and extensive fall of temperature, indicating that the crisis of the disease has been reached. In favourable cases, convalescence proceeds rapidly, the patient feeling perfectly well even before the rash has faded from the skin.

Measles may, however, occur in a very severe or malignant form, in which the symptoms throughout are of urgent character, the rash but feebly developed and of dark-purple hue, while there is great prostration of strength, accompanied with intense catarrh of the respiratory or gastro-intestinal mucous membrane. Such cases, always of serious import, are happily rare, occurring mostly in circumstances of bad hygiene, both as regards the individual and his surroundings. On the other hand, cases of measles are often met of so mild a form throughout that the patient can scarcely be persuaded to submit to treatment.

Measles derives its chief importance from the risk of certain complications which are apt to arise during its course, more especially inflammatory affections of the respiratory organs. These are most liable to occur in very young and delicate children. It has been already stated that irritation of the respiratory passages is one of the symptoms characteristic of measles, but that this subsides with the decline of the eruption. Not infrequently, however, these symptoms, instead of abating, become aggravated, and bronchitis of the capillary form (see BRONCHITIS); or pneumonia, generally of the diffuse or lobular variety (see PNEUMONIA), imparts to the case a gravity which it did not originally possess. By far the greater proportion of the mortality in measles is due to its complications, of which those just mentioned are the most common, but which also include infection of the ear (otitis media), infection of the eyes, diarrhoea, and encephalitis. A rare complication, except in grossly debilitated children, is a form of gangrene affecting the tissues of the mouth or cheeks and other parts of the body (CANCRUM ORIS), leading to disfigurement and even endangering life. (See also SUBACUTE SCLEROSING PANENCEPHALITIS.)

Treatment – The patient should be isolated, but quarantine of contacts is used much less than it used to be, though it is probably a wise precaution to keep infants away from the infected child. During an epidemic children under the age of 5 years should not be admitted to a nursery school, nursery class or infant school unless they are known to have had the disease or have been immunized against it. Child contacts of measles should be allowed to go to school provided they are sent home on the first suggestion of fever or malaise. Measles can be prevented or attenuated with gamma-globulin, and its use should be considered in young family contacts or older children suffering from some other disease. A vaccine is now available which gives a high degree of protection against the disease. It is usually given during the second year of life.

As regards special treatment, in an ordinary case of measles little is required beyond what is necessary in febrile conditions generally. Routine administration of sulphonamides or penicillin is not indicated, but the latter is indicated in: (a) children under 2 years of age; (b) children with previous middle-ear disease; (c) children suffering from some other disease; (d) children who are very ill. Confinement to bed so long as the temperature is raised; light, nourishing diet (eg. soups, milk puddings, glucose), and mild diaphoretics, such as Mindererus spirit and ipecacuanha (see DIAPHORETICS), are all that is necessary. There is no need to darken the room as used to be the practice. If the patient resents the light, he can easily turn his face away from it.

The serious chest complications of measles are to be dealt with by those measures applicable for the relief of pneumonia or bronchitis. (See BRONCHITIS; and PNEUMONIA.) Inflammation of the eyes is best soothed by washing several times daily with weak boric acid lotion, and thereafter smearing a little boric ointment on the edge of each lower lid. Ear complications, if they come on, usually appear with a discharge as the child is getting better (see EAR, DISEASES OF). Diarrhoea is treated by the usual remedies, including carefully administered doses of Dover's powder and kaolin mixture. (See DIARRHOEA.)

Isolation can end seven days from the appearance of the rash if all discharges have dried up.

MEASURES (see WEIGHTS AND MEASURES).

MEAT (see PROTEIN).

MEATUS is a term applied to any passage or opening: eg. external auditory meatus, the passage from the surface to the drum of the ear.

MECAMYLAMINE is one of the drugs introduced for the treatment of hypertension. It belongs to the group of ganglion-blocking drugs: ie. it acts by producing a block in the ganglion of the autonomic nervous system (qv). (See also ESSENTIAL HYPERTENSION.)

MECHANOTHERAPY is the provision of active physical exercise by means of a mechanical contrivance which necessitates the expenditure of physical work before it can be moved or used. Examples of mechanotherapy are dumb-bells, Indian clubs and parallel bars. One of the advantages of mechanotherapy, as opposed to other forms of physical exercise, is that it allows the amount of exercise performed to be accurately measured.

MECKEL'S DIVERTICULUM is a hollow process sometimes found attached to the small intestine. It is placed on the small intestine about 3 or 4 feet (90 to 120 cm) away from its junction with the large intestine, is several inches long, and ends blindly.

MECONIUM means the brown, semi-fluid material which collects in the bowels of a child prior to birth, and which should be discharged either at the time of birth or shortly afterwards. It consists partly of bile secreted by the liver before birth, partly of debris from the mucous membrane of the intestines.

MEDAZEPAM is a derivative of chlordiazepoxide (qv) which is proving of value in the treatment of anxiety neurosis.

MEDIASTINUM is the name given to the space in the chest which lies between the two lungs. It contains the heart and great vessels, the gullet, the lower part of the windpipe, the thoracic duct, the phrenic nerves, as well as numerous structures of less importance.

MEDITERRANEAN FEVER (see MALTA FEVER).

MEDULLA is another word for marrow. The term is usually restricted to the marrow of bones, or to designate a part of the brain, though the spinal cord is also sometimes known as the spinal medulla.

MEDULLA OBLONGATA is the hindmost part of the brain and is continued into the spinal cord. In it are situated several of the nerve-centres which are most essential to life, such as those governing breathing, the action of the heart, swallowing. (See BRAIN.)

MEFENAMIC ACID is a drug with pain-relieving, anti-inflammatory and antipyretic actions that is proving of value in the treatment of osteoarthrosis and rheumatoid arthritis.

MEGA- and MEGALO- are prefixes denoting largeness.

MEGALOMANIA is the term applied to a delusion of grandeur or an insane belief in a person's own extreme greatness, goodness, or power.

MEGRIM is another name for migraine (qv).

MEIBOMIAN GLANDS are the minute glands situated in the eyelids, in connection with which styes and cysts often arise. (See EYE DISEASES AND INJURIES.)

MELAENA means a condition of the stools in which dark, tarry masses are passed from the bowel. It is due to bleeding from the stomach or from the higher part of the bowel, the blood undergoing chemical changes under the action of the secretions, and being finally converted in large part into sulphide of iron.

MELANCHOLIA is a form of mental illness characterized by great mental and physical depression. (See MENTAL ILLNESS; and MANIC-DEPRESSIVE INSANITY.)

MELANIN is the dark pigment found in the skin and hair, as well as the choroid coat of the eye. It is the amount of melanin which decides the colour of the skin and hair. In white skin it occurs as granules in cells known as melanocytes situated in the stratum basale of the skin (qv). On exposure to ultra-violet light these granules are released and pass into the superficial layers of the skin where they produce the brown colour known as sun-tan which protects the skin against the harmful effects of continued exposure to the ultra-violet rays of the sun. Genetic factors play an important role in determining the distribution of melanin in the skin and hence its colour. Thus in those with genetically brown or black skin, as well as sun-tanned white-skinned people, there is a widespread distribution of melanin in the more superficial layers of the skin. This is due more to increased activity of the melanocytes than to an actual increase in their number.

MELANOMA is a tumour arising from the cells that produce melanin (qv). A highly malignant form, known as malignant melanoma, arises from the pigmented cells of moles (qv) or naevi.

MELORHEOSTOSIS is an abnormal condition of bone in which pathological hardening and denseness extend in a linear direction through one of the long bones of a limb, causing deformity and limitation of movement of the limb.

MELPHALAN is one of the alkylating agents (qv) which is proving of value in the treatment of certain forms of malignant disease.

MEMBRANES (see BRAIN; CROUP; DIPHTHERIA; and LABOUR).

MEMORY (see FORGETFULNESS).

MENAPHTHONE is a synthetic vitamin K₁ preparation. (See VITAMINS.)

MENARCHE is the term applied to the beginning of the menstrual function. The average age at which it occurs in British girls is 12½ years. In London girls it is 13·1 years. There is considerable racial and geographical variation: for example, from 12·4 in Cuban negroes to 18.8 in the Bundi tribe of New Guinea.

MENDELISM is the term applied to a law enunciated by G. J. Mendel that the offspring is not intermediate in type between its parents, but that the type of one or other parent is predominant. Characteristics are classed as either dominant or recessive. The offspring of the first generation tend to inherit the dominant characteristics, whilst the recessive characteristics remain latent and appear in some of the offspring of the second generation. If individuals possessing recessive characters unite, recessive characters then become dominant characters in succeeding generations. The law may be expressed by the following formula:

$$n(DD + 2DR + RR),$$

in which DD represents dominant

offspring, RR recessive offspring, and DR offspring with mixed characters.

MENIÈRE'S DISEASE, so called after the Frenchman, Prosper Menière, who first described it in 1861, is a disease characterized by tinnitus (qv), deafness and intermittent attacks of giddiness. Among the famous victims it has claimed are Julius Caesar, Martin Luther and Dean Swift. It usually occurs in middle age, and is slightly more common in men than in women. The first manifestation is usually deafness on one side. Then, as a rule many months later, there is a sudden attack, without any warning, of intense giddiness (or vertigo, as it is technically known). This often occurs during sleep, waking the patient up. It is soon followed by vomiting and sweating. The acute giddiness usually lasts for two to three hours but, after the attack, some unsteadiness persists for a few days. The time interval between attacks varies from a week to a few months. When they do recur, they tend to occur in clusters. The tinnitus, which tends to be high-pitched, comes on about the same time as the deafness. It is often described as being like rushing water or escaping steam. The deafness becomes gradually worse until it is complete. The condition is due to excessive fluid in the labyrinth of the ears (see EAR). The cause of this accumulation is not known, though it has been suggested that it might be a form of allergy, or might be due to spasm of the small blood-vessels.

Treatment consists of restricting the daily intake of fluid to 2½ pints (1·5 litres), and controlling the daily consumption of salt by not adding it to food at the table. A multiplicity of drugs has been recommended, including diuretics such as frusemide (qv), drugs to prevent vomiting such as dimenhydrinate (qv) and prochlorperazine (qv), and vasodilating drugs such as nicotinic acid (qv). If these all fail and the condition persists, then destruction of the labyrinth is carried out by operation or by ultrasound. An alternative is to cut the vestibular nerve; this has the advantage of preserving hearing, which the other surgical procedures do not do.

MENINGES are the membranes surrounding the brain and spinal cord (illustration 304). (See BRAIN.) The membranes include the dura mater, a tough, fibrous membrane closely applied to the inside of the skull; the arachnoid, a more delicate membrane, enveloping the brain but separated from its irregular surface by

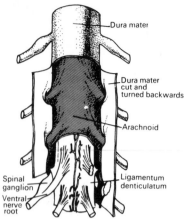

304 – The membranes of the spinal cord. From *Gray's Anatomy*, Longman.

spaces containing fluid; and the pia mater, a delicate network of fibres containing blood-vessels and uniting the arachnoid to the brain. The two latter are sometimes referred to as the pia-arachnoid. These membranes bear the blood-vessels which nourish the surface of the brain and the interior of the skull. Meningeal haemorrhage from these vessels forms one of the chief dangers arising from fracture of the skull.

MENINGISM is the name applied to a condition with symptoms closely resembling those of meningitis, but due simply to a feverish state.

MENINGITIS is a term applied to inflammation affecting the membranes of the brain (cerebral meningitis) or spinal cord (spinal meningitis), or both. Either the dura or the pia-arachnoid may be inflamed. In the former case the condition is known as pachymeningitis; in the latter, leptomeningitis. Pachymeningitis is the less common of the two, is often local and secondary to disease of the bone (eg. tuberculous or syphilitic), and may be cranial or spinal. Leptomeningitis is the more common, is usually extensive in distribution, greatly alters the composition of the cerebrospinal fluid, and may be primary or secondary to infection elsewhere in the body.

Meningitis may be classified according to the infecting organism as pneumococcal, pyogenic, tuberculous, syphilitic, meningococcal. The all-important evidence is gained by lumbar puncture and examination of the CEREBROSPINAL FLUID (qv). In meningitis the pressure of this fluid is increased, changes in its appearance and constituents occur, and the infecting agent can usually be isolated from it. In meningitis the protein and the number of cells increase and the glucose decreases. A decrease in the amount of chlorides of the cerebrospinal fluid is characteristic of tuberculous meningitis. Increase in the number of cells may make the normally clear cerebrospinal fluid opalescent, as in tuberculous meningitis, or turbid, as in pneumococcal and pyogenic meningitis. Clinically, the symptoms are due to irritation of the meninges and rise in the intracranial pressure: headache, vomiting, photophobia, rigidity of the neck, Kernig's sign (qv), convulsions, paralyses, coma.

In England, in 1974, there were 1985 cases of acute meningitis, 1105 of which were due to the meningococcus. (See MENINGOCOCCAL MENINGITIS.)

PNEUMOCOCCAL MENINGITIS is usually secondary to infection with the pneumococcus elsewhere: for example, empyema or otitis media. This formerly fatal condition is now in many cases successfully treated by the sulphonamide drugs or penicillin.

PYOGENIC MENINGITIS is due to secondary infection with staphylococci, streptococci, *H. influenzae*, gonococci, or anthrax bacilli – especially the first two. The introduction of the sulphonamides and of penicillin has altered the previously fatal prognosis of these cases. Satisfactory results are obtained from the use of chloramphenicol in the treatment of meningitis due to *H. influenzae*.

TUBERCULOUS MENINGITIS is an inflammation of the membranes caused by the *Mycobacterium tuberculosis*. The disease is most common in children under the age of 10 years, but is by no means confined to that period of life, and may affect adults. The determining factor in the disease is exposure to infection with the bovine or the human *Mycobacterium tuberculosis*. In numerous cases associated factors are bad hygienic conditions, with insufficient or improper feeding, or some disease of childhood, particularly measles or whooping-cough. When it occurs in adults it is usually secondary to some chronic manifestation of tuberculosis in another part of the body, especially in the lungs.

Symptoms – Tuberculous meningitis is usually described as passing through three stages; but its earlier manifestations are often vague.

The *premonitory symptoms* are mostly such as relate to the general nutrition. The patient, if a child, becomes listless and easily fatigued, loses appetite, and is restless at night. There is headache after exertion, and the temper often undergoes a marked change, the child becoming unusually peevish and irritable. These symptoms may persist during many weeks, or may be entirely wanting, the disease developing quite suddenly.

The onset of the *first stage*, or *stage of excitement*, is in most instances marked by the occurrence of vomiting, often severe, but sometimes only slight, and there is, in general, obstinate constipation. In some cases, the first symptoms are convulsions, which, however, may in this early stage subside, and remain absent, or reappear at a later period. Headache is one of the most constant of the earlier symptoms, and is generally intense and accompanied by sharper paroxysms, which cause the patient to scream with a peculiar and characteristic cry. There is great intolerance of light and sound and general nervous sensitiveness. The neck shows rigidity so that the head cannot be so readily bent forwards as usual, and similar rigidity in the lower limbs is almost invariably present. The latter symptom forms an important sign (Kernig's sign) of meningitis. If the knee is raised from the bed, stiffness and pain are experienced in the muscles behind the thigh when the attempt is made to straighten the leg at the knee-joint, whereas in the healthy child the whole lower limb can be readily flexed on the abdomen with the knee straight. Fever is present to a greater or less extent, the temperature ranging from 100° to 103° F (37·8° to 39·4° C); yet the pulse is not quickened in proportion, being on the contrary rather slow, but exhibiting a tendency to irregularity, and liable to become rapid on slight exertion. This slowness of the pulse is of great importance in distinguishing the disease from others which resemble it, and in which the heart beats more rapidly in proportion to the temperature. Symptoms of this character, constituting the stage of excitement, continue for a period varying from one to two weeks, when they are succeeded by the stage of depression.

In the *second stage*, or *stage of depression*, there is a marked change in the symptoms, which is apt to lead to the belief that a favourable turn has taken place. The patient becomes quieter and inclines to

sleep, but on careful watching it will be found that this quietness is but a condition of apathy or partial stupor into which the child has sunk. The vomiting has now ceased, and there is less fever; the pulse is slower, and shows a still greater tendency to irregularity than before, while the breathing is of markedly unequal character, being rapid and shallow at one time, and long drawn out and sinking away at another. There is manifestly little suffering, although the peculiar cry may still be uttered, and the patient lies prostrate, occasionally rolling the head uneasily upon the pillow, or picking at the bedclothes or at his face with his fingers. He does not ask for food, but readily swallows what is offered. The eyes present important alterations, the pupils being dilated or unequal, and scarcely responding to light. There may be double vision, or partial or complete blindness. Squinting is common in this stage, and there may also be drooping of an eyelid, due to paralysis of the part, and one or more limbs may be likewise paralysed.

To this succeeds the *third stage*, or *stage of paralysis*, in which certain of the former symptoms recur, while others become intensified. There is generally a return of the fever, the temperature rising sometimes to a very high degree. The pulse becomes feeble, rapid, and exceedingly irregular, as is also the case with the breathing. Coma is profound, but the patient may still be got to swallow nourishment, though not so readily as before. Convulsions are apt to occur, while paralysis, more or less extensive, affects portions of the body or groups of muscles. The pupils are now widely dilated, and there is often complete blindness or deafness. In this condition the sufferer's strength undergoes rapid decline and the body becomes markedly emaciated. Death takes place suddenly in a fit, or, more generally, from exhaustion. Shortly before the fatal event it is not uncommon for the patient, who, it may be for some days previously, lay in a state of profound stupor, to wake up, ask for food, and talk to those around. But the hopes which may be thus raised are quickly dispelled by the setting in of the symptoms of rapid decline.

The disease used to be invariably fatal, but the outlook has been entirely altered by the introduction of streptomycin. With modern treatment the mortality depends largely on the stage at which treatment is initiated. If this is in the early stages, 95 per cent recover, but if treatment is not started until later in the disease, only 60 per cent or fewer will recover.

Treatment – The only drugs of any value in the treatment of tuberculous meningitis are streptomycin and isoniazid. The administration of streptomycin and isoniazid in this condition requires skilled medical and nursing supervision such as is available only in hospital. Every child (or adult) with tuberculous meningitis, or suspected tuberculous meningitis, therefore should be examined as early as possible by an experienced children's (or tuberculosis) specialist, in order that an expert opinion may be obtained.

SYPHILITIC MENINGITIS is usually a chronic inflammation (but sometimes producing acute symptoms) occurring in most cases within the first four years of infection. It may spread from the pia-arachnoid into the brain – a meningo-encephalitis – or it may attack the dura mater and the overlying bone. The pressure of the cerebrospinal fluid is raised; the fluid itself is clear and contains an increased number of lymphocytes. Headache is a common symptom. Paralysis of cranial nerves (resulting, for example, in a squint) can occur as a result of strangulation of the nerve in inflamed meninges at the base of the brain. Hydrocephalus may arise suddenly, with headache, vomiting, sleepiness, mental changes, and congestion of the optic discs as symptoms and signs. Or syphilitic meningitis may come on acutely. The treatment is as for syphilis.

MENINGOCOCCAL MENINGITIS, also known as EPIDEMIC CEREBROSPINAL MENINGITIS, CEREBROSPINAL FEVER, SPOTTED FEVER, MALIGNANT PURPURIC FEVER, and POST-BASIC MENINGITIS, is a dangerous epidemic condition characterized by painful contractions of the muscles of the neck, retraction of the head, and mental symptoms. It was first distinctly recognized in the year 1837, when it prevailed as an epidemic, chiefly among troops in the south-west of France. In 1846 it appeared in Ireland, especially in the workhouses of Belfast and Dublin. Since that time it has appeared repeatedly both in Europe and America, notably in a severe epidemic in the large towns of Scotland in 1907–09, in a slighter form among the troops during the war of 1914–18, and a fair-sized epidemic in Great Britain in the winter of 1939–1940. In England there were 1105 cases in 1974. The disease is notifiable.

Causes – When an outbreak takes place, it usually occurs about the months of February, March, and April, and affects a closed community such as a school, garrison, camp, or prison. The direct cause is an organism, the *Neisseria meningitidis* or *meningococcus*, which is found in the exudation round the nervous system, in the blood, and often in the nasal discharge. The organism is of four different types. It is believed that the infection takes place through the nose and that a large number of persons who do not contract the disease harbour the meningococcus in the nasal discharge and form sources of infection to more susceptible people, especially children, by coughing and sneezing – they are known as carriers. Factors favouring infection are a high carrier-rate, the virulence of the organism, a closed community (eg. a camp), nasopharyngeal catarrh, bad ventilation, insufficient space between beds, introduction of susceptible persons into a closed community, season of the year (winter and spring). Young children are much more susceptible than adults. The incubation period is 2 to 10 days (commonly 2 to 5).

Symptoms – The onset is usually sudden, sometimes startlingly so. As a rule, vomiting, headache, and shivering first appear, followed in a few hours by stiffness of the neck. In children, convulsions are common. In a case of very sudden onset, the patient, while going about as usual, may fall down suddenly in a convulsion, or he may go to bed perfectly well and be found unconscious on the following morning. If the patient is not unconscious, headache and pain with stiffness in the back of the neck continue, squinting is often seen, the tongue is furred and dry, and there is a rise of temperature: 100° to 104° F (37·8° to 40° C). The patient is irritable, the body tender to the touch, and the limbs stiff so that bending up of the lower limbs on the abdomen with the knee straight becomes impossible (Kernig's sign). The patient is often sleepless or delirious, and there is a great tendency for the symptoms to go and come. The red spots, from which the disease takes its name of 'spotted fever', appear over the surface of the trunk during the first week of the disease in greater or less numbers in about one-quarter of the cases. Death occurs in a large number of the cases within a week of the onset, taking place very often suddenly from heart failure. After the first week, if life is prolonged, the disease usually abates gradually and in the course of some weeks the rigidity may have disappeared and the temperature may have become normal. On the other hand, the disease may pass into a chronic state with great wasting, and, if the patient be a young child, head retraction in these cases usually becomes very marked and the body is greatly bent backwards. The patient during the course of this chronic stage may become blind or deaf or may show marked mental deterioration. Very often the child falls a victim to some complication, such as bronchopneumonia.

In those patients who die, it is common to find the surface of the brain and the spinal cord covered with thick pus and the blood-vessels markedly congested. If death has occurred at a very early period, nothing more may be visible than very intense congestion of the membranes on the surface of the brain. The interior of the brain shows more than the usual amount of fluid.

The prognosis in this disease has been revolutionized by the introduction of the sulphonamides and penicillin. Formerly the mortality rate in epidemics was 70 to 80 per cent, whilst in fulminating cases it might even be 100 per cent. Today, with efficient treatment it has fallen to 7 to 10 per cent. The main factors governing the prognosis are: (1) The age of the patient: the disease is particularly dangerous in infants and old people. (2) The type of onset: a fulminating onset carries a bad prognosis. (3) The stage of the disease at which treatment is begun: the earlier the better.

Treatment – The patient must be isolated and, whenever possible, should be treated in hospital. Treatment consists essentially of the administration of full doses of sulphadiazine, sulphamerazine, or penicillin. The patient is confined to bed and given a light nutritious diet. For insomnia sedatives are usually required, whilst the pains in the joints and limbs are usually best relieved by warm baths. The headache usually responds to a combination of aspirin, paracetamol, and codeine but. if particularly severe, lumbar puncture may be necessary.

Quarantine of contacts is useless, but there is some evidence that, in the event of an outbreak in a semi-closed community (eg. a residential school or a military camp) the administration of sulphadiazine to all contacts may be of value.

MENINGOCELE is a protusion of the meninges of the brain through a defect in the skull. (See SPINA BIFIDA.)

MENINGOCOCCUS. (See NEISSERIA.)

MENINGOMYELOCELE is a protrusion of the meninges of the spinal cord

through a defect in the spine. (See SPINA BIFIDA.)

MENISCUS is the term applied to a crescentic fibro-cartilage in a joint, such as the cartilages in the knee-joint.

MENOPAUSE is the term applied to the cessation of menstruation at the end of reproductive life. Usually it occurs between the ages of 45 and 50, although in numerous women it occurs before 45 or after 50. It rarely occurs before 40 unless as the result of disease. It is a psychologically disturbing experience which is quite often accompanied by physical manifestations. These include hot flushes, tiredness, sleeplessness, irritability, lack of concentration, palpitations, aching joints and vaginal irritation. There may also be loss of libido, or sexual desire. Most women can, and do, live happy active lives through the menopause, the length of which varies considerably, without any support from drugs. What is too often forgotten is that it is a natural event, and it is those women who can accept it as such who are least likely to suffer from its manifestations. When drug treatment is required, it usually takes the form of short courses of an oestrogen (qv).

MENORRHAGIA means an over-abundance of the menstrual discharge.

MENSTRUATION is a periodic change occurring in human beings and the higher apes, and consists chiefly in a flow of blood from the cavity of the womb, and associated with various slight constitutional disturbances. It begins between the ages of 12 and 15, as a rule, although its onset may be delayed till as late as 20, or it may begin as early as 10 or 11. Along with its first appearance the body develops the secondary sex characteristics of the sex: eg. enlargement of the breasts, characteristic hair distribution. The duration of each menstrual period varies in different persons from two to eight days. It recurs in the great majority of cases with regularity, most commonly at intervals of twenty-eight days or thirty days, less often with intervals of twenty-one or twenty-seven days, ceasing only during pregnancy and lactation, till the age of 45 or 50 arrives, when it stops altogether, as a rule ceasing early if it has begun early, and vice versa. The final stoppage is known as the menopause or the climacteric (qv).

Menstruation depends upon a functioning ovary and this upon a healthy pituitary gland. The regular rhythm may depend upon a centre in the hypothalamus, which is in close connection with the pituitary. After menstruation the denuded uterine endometrium is regenerated under the influence of the follicular hormone, oestradiol. The epithelium of the endometrium proliferates, and about a fortnight after the beginning of menstruation great development of the endometrial glands takes place under the influence of progesterone, the hormone secreted by the corpus luteum. These changes are made for the reception of the fertilized ovum. In the absence of fertilization the uterine endometrium breaks down in the subsequent menstrual discharge.

Disorders of menstruation – In the majority of healthy women, menstruation proceeds regularly for thirty years or more, with the exceptions connected with childbirth. In many persons, as the result either of general or local conditions, the process may be absent or excessive, or may be attended with great discomfort or pain. The term *amenorrhoea* is applied to cases in which menstruation is absent, *menorrhagia* and *metrorrhagia* to cases in which it is excessive, the former if the excess occurs at the regular periods, the latter if it is irregular, whilst *dysmenorrhoea* is the name given to cases in which the process is attended by pain.

AMENORRHOEA may be due to general or to local causes. Among the former, anaemia, with the various conditions that lead to it, ranks perhaps first in importance in young women. Bad feeding, want of fresh air, and all causes which depress the system and cause loss of flesh tend to cause diminution and finally stoppage of the menses. In a similar manner, serious diseases, such as Bright's disease, tuberculosis, malaria, which weaken the constitution, lead to this result. Various influences which act through the nervous system, such as sudden fright, or great grief, may also cause stoppage for several months. Among the local causes of amenorrhoea, pregnancy, of course, stands first. Failure of menstruation to appear at all in a young woman may be due to slow or imperfect development of the ovaries or womb; and in occasional cases, although menstruation does take place regularly, the menstrual fluid does not escape but is retained and accumulates within the womb in consequence of some structural defect. (See HAEMATOCOLPOS.)

The treatment in all cases consists in removal of the cause and attention to the general health, remedies for the condition

of bloodlessness if present (see ANAEMIA), and, in the cause last mentioned, some operative interference.

MENORRHAGIA – Excessive menstruation may be due to the same general conditions which produce amenorrhoea, the same diseases, such as Bright's disease or tuberculosis, causing stoppage or excess in different persons. Thus, in some persons an excessive discharge is brought about by these conditions, and the bad effects of the general disease are much increased by the added drain upon the system, due to loss of blood. In heart disease, the womb may share in the general internal congestion, and the menses in consequence are increased. In some persons, menstruation at its first appearance is excessive; whilst this is so often the case as to be almost the general rule at the time when the menstrual periods are about to stop, ie. at the menopause, when they also tend to become irregular. But it is most often a local condition that produces menorrhagia: in this case, as a rule, not only is the periodic loss increased but there is bleeding at irregular times (metrorrhagia). Polypus, fibroid, and other tumours, displacements of the womb, and some inflammation consequent upon childbirth or miscarriage, are the most common causes of this type. In the treatment, rest and various internal remedies which check haemorrhage, together with careful attention to the general health between the periods, are essential. (See UTERUS, DISEASES OF.)

DYSMENORRHOEA may vary from mere discomfort to agonizing colic, accompanied by prostration and vomiting. Anaemia is sometimes a cause of painful menstruation as well as of stoppage of this function. Chills and exhaustion may produce pain for a single period in women whose periods are usually painless.

Inflammation of various internal organs, eg. of the womb itself, the ovaries, or the Fallopian tubes, is one of the commonest causes of dysmenorrhoea which comes on for the first time late in life, especially when the trouble follows the birth of a child. In this case the pain exists more or less at all times, but is aggravated at the periods. It is relieved by various local means directed towards checking the inflammation present.

Many cases of dysmenorrhoea appear with the beginning of menstrual life, and accompany every period. It has been estimated that 5 to 10 per cent of girls in their late teens or early twenties are severely incapacitated by dysmenorrhoea for several hours each month. Some of these are of an obstructive type, due to spasm of the neck of the womb, in consequence of which a severe uterine colic is set up. In many cases, the spasm appears to be one manifestation of a nervous temperament. In other cases the pain appears to be due to difficulty in the separation of the surface layer of mucous membrane, which comes away in healthy menstruation in fragments with the blood. In these cases, the lining of the uterus, after great difficulty, is finally expelled in the form of a complete membranous cast of the interior, and the pain then abates. In other cases, the spasm may be due in part to defective development of the womb, producing either narrowness of its mouth or causing it to be bent upon itself, and occasionally these cases are benefited, or cured by an operation designed to stretch the neck of the womb, or otherwise relieve the defect. Yet a further cause for this pain, it has been suggested, is an excessive production of prostaglandins (qv). In not a few – indeed some would say the majority – there is a large psychological factor. This may be the sole cause, or it may be an ancillary cause exacerbating the pain, or discomfort, induced by some physical cause. Whatever the psychological factor – whether due to inadequate sex instruction, fear, mental, domestic, or work disharmony – the sooner it is discovered and dealt with, the more likely is the dysmenorrhoea to come under control. For the temporary relief of dysemenorrhoea, rest in bed, or, at all events, in the recumbent position, a hot water bottle to the lower part of the abdomen, and aspirin internally, are the remedies which prove most useful.

MENTAL DEFECTIVENESS. (See MENTAL SUBNORMALITY.)

MENTAL ILLNESS arises from a multiplicity of causes, many unknown, and exists in an infinite variety of forms. So long as individual peculiarities occasioned by mental disorder do not result in conduct or behaviour which is markedly opposed to prevailing social custom, society does not interfere with the person. When the person's conduct becomes so far divergent from social usages that he becomes legally certifiable, he can be sent compulsorily to a mental hospital. It must be remembered, however, that there are all grades of mental disorder from slight peculiarities or temporary delirium, upwards. A great number of persons who do not reach a sufficiently abnormal grade of conduct to be regarded as certifiable are regarded by society as eccentric or peculiar, and a large number whose conduct shows them to be maladapted for social life, as the result of inferiority of mind, are classed, owing to circumstances, among criminals, paupers, vagrants, inebriates, and the like.

In primitive states of society mental disease is apt to pass unnoticed, and the more complex society becomes the more obvious is any maladaptation of an individual to his surroundings. By the old Greek physicians, in the time of Plato and Hippocrates, the brain was looked upon as the organ of intellect; sensation and the more purely animal functions being supposed to be situated in the thoracic region and in the lower part of the body, respectively. Mental disease was treated in a rational manner just as other bodily disorders. From the decline of the Roman Empire through the Middle Ages, various manifestations of insanity were regarded largely in the light of crimes or misdemeanours, and were treated with great harshness. In the course of the eighteenth century, opinion in regard to the treatment of mental disorders began to change, and the modern attitude, which regards mental disorder as a disorder or disease to be treated on the same lines as other diseases, is generally regarded as having begun with the publication of Pinel's *Traité medico-philosophique sur l'aliénation mentale ou la manie* in 1801. A great amount of attention was paid during the next fifty years to the study of mental diseases, and during this period a large number of asylums for the humane treatment of mentally disordered persons were founded.

The question of *responsibility in civil or criminal matters* is one of great importance in regard to mental disease. The question often arises in connection with the ability to make a valid will. The development of certifiable mental disease does not excuse the patient from the fulfilment of a contract, provided he was not certifiable at the time when the contract was entered into. When a crime is committed, the question of responsibility is often very difficult to decide. The general principle accepted is that, if the accused person suffers from a delusion, but is not insane in other matters, he is held responsible for his offence, unless he has acted in such a way as would have been permissible if the facts about which his delusion exists had been true. In other words, in order to establish a defence on the ground of insanity it must be proved that 'at the time of committing the act the party accused was labouring under such a defect of reason, from disease of the mind, as not to know the nature and quality of the act he was doing or, if he did know it, that he did not know he was doing it, or that he did not know he was doing what was wrong'. The principle is also recognized that, if the mind is so diseased or so defective that there is complete absence of the power of self-control, so that the person acts under an ungovernable impulse, then he is not held responsible. This inability to exercise self-control does not, however, exonerate a person in whom the loss of self-control is due to his own default, as, for example, when he is intoxicated.

Causes – The causes of mental disorder fall into two great groups. Certain persons go through life with a tendency to become disordered mentally when at any time certain causes arise, whilst other persons are subjected constantly to much greater strains of the same nature without developing any mental abnormality. It is necessary therefore to recognize (1) the nervous constitution or set of predisposing causes, and (2) the stresses which are particularly liable to unbalance the mind, or exciting causes.

(1) PREDISPOSING CAUSES – A nervous constitution may be inherited or acquired, and is the primary or essential reason of a mental breakdown. There may be some congenital nervous, mental or moral defect which is peculiar to the family of the person affected. This tendency may be broadly described as *heredity*. It may show itself in other members of the same family by various nervous diseases allied to mental instability, such as epilepsy or hysteria. The tendency may also show itself by such inability to regulate conduct as drunken habits or various moral delinquencies which have got other members of the patient's family into trouble. *Intermarriage* of near relations in a family in which neurotic tendencies are manifested often results in offspring showing characteristics which are natural enough in the parents, but are apt to be exaggerated to an unnatural degree in the children, so that they reach the stage of definite mental illness. A similar evolution of traits of character may be seen in the children of marriages between individuals of similar nervous temperament, though these be not related to one another.

How far 'nature' is to be blamed for insanity and how far 'nurture' is uncertain. At one time the hereditary factor is overstressed and at another the environmental factor. It is perhaps not far off the mark to state that in an unfavourable environment – using this word in a comprehensive sense to include the 'emotional' setting of family life as well as the physical environment – the person with an inherited unstable nervous system may break down with symptoms of mental illness. Bizarre, abnormal, or vicious behaviour is likely to be, not the cause, but a manifestation of innate mental instability.

The most important of the predisposing causes is the presence of an *abnormal disposition or temperament*, either inherited or acquired in the course of years. This is the most frequent sign of a nervous constitution. It may be acquired in childhood from habitual contact with abnormal older persons. It may also arise from a prolonged struggle between conflicting instincts. The instincts concerned are usually the two primitive instincts of the herd and self-preservation. The person is constantly attempting to conform to the rules and usages of society and, at the same time, striving for objects which conduce to personal well-being and satisfaction, and is constantly finding the two aims incompatible. Into this group fall the cases of anxiety and mental unrest derived from what, according to the Freudian conception, is a repressed and subconscious memory of sexual trauma. The resulting development of the abnormal temperament may show itself by some characteristic such as unusual irritability, jealousy, waywardness, unreasonableness, pessimism. All of these render the person more liable to mental breakdown when a sufficient exciting cause supervenes.

(2) EXCITING CAUSES – Among the most important of the stresses or exciting factors of mental disorder, in a person already predisposed, are other bodily diseases which produce defective nutrition, poisoning or exhaustion of the nervous system. These are sometimes grouped as toxic and exhausting causes.

Infectious diseases play an important part in this connection, especially when they are conjoined with some of the other stresses to be mentioned later. Puerperal sepsis occurring in connection with childbirth may act in this manner. A similar effect may be produced in occasional cases by attacks of influenza, pneumonia, erysipelas, typhoid fever, and tuberculosis. *Disorders of the endocrine glands*, which secrete substances that enter the circulation and produce important effects upon the nutrition of the body, have also a powerful effect on mental processes. The diseases arising from these defects, which are most often accompanied by mental disorder, are myxoedema and thyrotoxicosis. *Diseases of the blood and circulation* are liable, when they have been present for a considerable time, to produce mental changes: such diseases are anaemia, arteriosclerosis, and heart failure. The kidneys, in persons in whom they are diseased, may fail in their action of excreting waste products from the body, and these, circulating in the blood, produce deterioration in the action of the nervous system. External poisons may produce serious effects upon the nervous system as well as those developed within the body; such are especially the effects of *alcohol*, which is a common cause and which produces many different results on different brains, with different types of mental disorder. Other poisons which may produce similar effects in occasional cases are opium, cocaine and lead. The recognition of these toxic causes is of the greatest importance, because this opens up a wide field for treatment of the mental disorder, which is likely to improve when its cause is duly recognized and removed.

The most important type of stress productive of mental disorder is what may be called 'biological stresses', including those changes which occur in the body during the reproductive *epochs and crises of life* in both sexes, when changes also take place in the mental outlook. The most important of these epochs are: (1) *Adolescence*, the period when the body is attaining its maximum of activity and growth and when the function of reproduction is attaining full development. This adolescent change occurs in the female between the ages of 15 and 20, and in the male during a period about one or two years later. During this time emotional outbursts and other manifestations pointing to an unstable nervous system are particularly apt to show themselves. (2) *Childbirth* is an important crisis in the life of a woman, which may occur up to the age of 40 to 50. This process is accompanied by considerable stress during pregnancy, the puerperal state, and lactation; when to the biological stress is added a septic or exhaustive process, as sometimes occurs in the puerperal state, mental disorder may occur. This type of mental disorder is, however, one of the most curable forms. (3) The *climacteric period* is the time about the age of 50 when there is a distinct waning of the reproductive powers which have been fully developed during adolescence; it is earlier in the

female and associated with the cessation of menstruation; in the male it is more irregular and undefined. With its establishment the elasticity and enthusiasm of youth pass away; the strong passions of earlier life become feebler, and there are often marked nutritional changes in the body such as increase of corpulence with marked diminution of activity. Mental peculiarities are apt to set in at this time. (4) *Senility* may be regarded as starting in the 70's or 80's; it comes on prematurely with special readiness in persons whose arteries are diseased. It has been said that a 'man is as old as his arteries'; and if the arteries of the brain remain healthy, the mental faculties may remain healthy, the mental faculties may remain alert and the bodily functions active, long after the allotted span of threescore years and ten; if the arteries are diseased, the state of bodily and mental feebleness known as dementia is particularly apt to appear.

Hygienic stresses include privations or excesses in mode of life and exercise, productive of defective nutrition or exhaustion, thus leading to poisoning of the nervous system. These include want of food or of some essential element in the food such as vitamins; also excessive feeding and insufficient exercise, such as are apt to prevail in middle life. Physical or mental overwork – with want of sleep, rest, or recreation – and emotional stresses and strains may have a similar effect.

Energic stresses consist of external changes which produce shock to the nervous system such as head injuries, surgical operations, heatstroke, electric shock, and are occasionally productive of sudden mental disorder.

Psychic stresses may also produce mental disorder of sudden or gradual onset. These include shocks or exhaustion induced by such influences as fright, anxiety, grief, prolonged worry.

Organic disease of the nervous system, usually producing its effect by direct physical damage of the brain or by interference with its nutrition, forms another group of causes of mental disease which is then usually of a serious type as regards recovery. Such influences include syphilis, apoplexy, tumours of the brain, meningitis, cerebrospinal fever and encephalitis lethargica. Although the change that takes place in epilepsy is not definitely known, this disease as an associate of mental illness naturally falls into this group.

Symptoms of mental disorder – Before describing the chief varieties of mental illness with the main characteristics of each, we must refer to certain early symptoms, and also to some general symptoms which commonly accompany such disorders.

(a) EARLY SYMPTOMS – Mental illness rarely develops suddenly, and indications of an approaching mental breakdown may be gathered from some early premonitory symptoms, although these may be of so slight a character as to escape observation, or, if observed, to be considered as of no serious moment. Perhaps the most important is *alteration of disposition*: and this change may be either an exaggeration of the usual state of mind of the individual, or may be in a direction diametrically opposed to it. One man, for example, naturally of a suspicious nature, may begin to carry his suspicions so far as to imagine that people are talking evil about him, slandering him, and threatening him with violence; another, hitherto of a bright, cheerful disposition, becomes silent, moody, depressed, and self-depreciating to such an extent that he becomes quite unfitted for carrying on his ordinary work. In both these instances such symptoms may be the forerunners of mental illness, which may issue in homicide in the one case and suicide in the other. *Alterations of habit and conduct* also may be observed: a miser may become a spendthrift; a cool, calculating business man begins to indulge in foolish speculations; a hitherto temperate, upright man may give way to debauchery and depravity. In estimating these symptoms and attaching to them their proper significance, it is necessary always to bear in mind the social position and environment of the person, for it is obvious that a certain line of conduct would have a different meaning in an aristocrat from what it would have in a labourer. These early alterations of habit and conduct are often associated also with various *physical symptoms*, such as pains in the head, sleeplessness, disorders of digestion and loss of weight, these all pointing to disturbed and perverted physical health.

(b) GENERAL SYMPTOMS of mental illness fall under two divisions: (1) insane beliefs; (2) insane acts.

(1) *Insane beliefs* may be either of the nature of delusions or of hallucinations.

A *delusion* may be defined as 'a belief in a fact which, to a sane person of similar education, age, and race, appears certainly false, and of the falsity of which the person labouring under the insane delusions cannot be persuaded either by his own senses or by the arguments of others'. The presence of delusions is a strong proof of insanity, and in the investigation of any mental state special care must always be taken to find out their existence – a task which is often very difficult, as they may be carefully and skilfully concealed. They may be classified as follows. *Delusions of grandeur* accompany states of mental exaltation. A poor man thinks he is possessed of millions of money; another is the King of England; yet another is the King of the Universe, and can summon and hold converse at any time with the prophets of both the Old and the New Testaments. *Delusions of unseen agency* lead their victims to imagine that they are electrified by batteries; disturbed at nights by persons who attempt to mutilate or ravish them; or that, inside their body, they have a person or animal, and that all the food they take goes to nourish the intruder. *Delusions of suspicion and persecution* cause the persecutions to be attributed to actual known persons; the annoyance is not caused by something intangible and unknown, but certain persons, who can be named by the insane person, are supposed to have poisoned his food, called him bad names, or followed him about and annoyed him.

There are, in addition, numerous other delusions which cannot be classified under these heads, such as delusions of identity, the delusion of having no head, or no mouth, that speech is impossible. There is, indeed, no end to their variety.

Hallucinations are false perceptions of the senses, those of hearing and sight being the most commonly affected. *Hallucinations of hearing* are often found in chronic cases of mental illness and when the illness is insidious, free from acute symptoms, and slowly progressive, they often constitute very early symptoms. Patients complain that they hear voices speaking to them. These voices may be well known to them or unknown, may be in the same room in some corner or cupboard, or outside in the open air; they may rule their lives, compel them to eat or abstain from food, urge them to destroy themselves or to commit murder. These patients therefore are looked upon as dangerous both to themselves and to others. *Hallucinations of sight* are common in acute excitement, and always accompany, for example, acute alcoholism; the things that are seen may be animals, such as bats, mice, rats, or dogs; or there may be bright flashes of light, during which imaginary people are seen. *Hallucinations of smell* are important, and often indicate serious mental disease.

(2) *Insane acts* include suicide, homicide, and various other hurtful or bizarre forms of conduct.

Suicide may be the result of profound mental depression; it may be prompted by delusions of persecution, or by hallucinations of hearing, the sound of voices, for example, urging to self-destruction. It may accompany an acute illness, or may be the one outstanding feature of the illness, a true suicidal impulse. The idea is sometimes quite a sudden one, an attempt at self-destruction being made, and the patient being afterwards totally unable to account for it, or, on the other hand, the wish may have long been harboured and the details of the attempted suicide carefully planned.

Homicide, again, like suicide, may be the outcome of delusions, especially those of persecution and suspicion; or the act may be committed while the patient is under the influence of hallucinations. A genuine homicidal act is often committed by patients suffering from both delusions and hallucinations. A man believes, for example, that he is being persistently slandered and persecuted; he hears voices urging him to murder his persecutors, and he murders them, either suddenly under the influence of a genuine homicidal impulse, or deliberately after having carefully laid his plans.

Other insane acts may be mentioned briefly, such as constant tearing of clothes, fantastic and extravagant dressing, or, on the other hand, disregard of personal appearance, refusal of food, kleptomania, dipsomania, indecent exposure of the person, and the commission of revolting, unnatural sexual offences.

Varieties of mental disorder – NEUROSES and PSYCHONEUROSES form some of the milder types of mental disorder. The chief mental symptom is a general emotional tone of anxiety or apprehension; patients are afraid to open letters lest the contents convey bad news, and, for the same reason, they are terrified by telegrams; slight passing indispositions are feared to be symptomatic of some fatal disease; fleeting incidents are apt to be misinterpreted and worried over. Exophthalmic goitre, which is sometimes accompanied by mental symptoms, may in such cases be included in this group. Neurasthenia, hysteria, and various obsessions, including such symptoms as irrepressible thoughts, irrepressible fears, and irrepressible impulses, fall into the group of psychoneuroses.

PSYCHOSES include a group of the more serious and better-known types of mental disease, such as mania, melancholia or depression, paranoia, schizophrenia, and alcoholic psychosis.

MANIA – The term, mania, although applied commonly to various types of severe mental disorder, should, strictly, be reserved for the form characterized by mental exaltation. In *simple mania* the intellectual part of the cerebral function is in a state of over-activity, so that the patient is loquacious, garrulous, and often very clever in repartee; he flits, without apparent connection, from one subject to another; his mind never rests, and sleeplessness is a usual accompaniment. In the more pronounced form of *acute mania*, the motor functions of the brain are also affected; there is not only complete incoherence of speech, but there is intense restlessness and complete disappearance of will power; such a patient is popularly termed 'raving mad'. He seems to be insensible to fatigue, either of mind or body, and he gradually wears himself out. As a result, physical symptoms come on, especially loss of weight, and, if the condition be not relieved, a fatal result may ensue from exhaustion. The majority of cases, however, recover, sometimes quite abruptly, more often gradually after relapses. Some cases pass into *chronic mania*, in which the symptoms continue, but in a quieter form, with a tendency to occasional acute attacks. A few cases pass into dementia, in which the mental powers become completely enfeebled, and the patient is quiet.

MELANCHOLIA, or DEPRESSION, is characterized by a feeling of misery in excess of that which is justified by circumstances, and by physical weakness and loss of energy. In every person there is a tendency to fluctuate between times of mental elevation and times of mental lowness; an exaggeration and prolongation of this natural rhythm constitutes a mental disorder known as *manic-depressive psychosis*, in which the patient varies between mania and melancholia, at intervals of days, weeks, or months. In *simple melancholia* the depression is not very great, and the patient may be able to pull himself together in the presence of strangers, or at other times when it is necessary to do so, only his intimates knowing of his disinclination to work, lassitude, desire to be alone, and painful introspection. The reasoning power is still present, although it is perverted in the way of magnifying slight failings of character into vices and taking an unreasonably gloomy view of the future. At times the mental depression becomes more intense, and the danger, in such patients, is that it may culminate in suicide. In *acute melancholia* the willpower disappears, the mental anguish is greater, and there is no control over action. Sometimes, especially after the melancholy state has lasted for some time, such patients are completely apathetic, sit staring straight in front of them, and are persuaded with difficulty to take food; other patients show restlessness and agitation, wringing their hands, swaying the body, weeping, or showing inability for even the slightest concentration upon any one subject. Delusions may be present, and patients think they have wronged themselves and their family, that they are responsible for the illness or misfortune of other people, that they are going to be burned, tortured, or otherwise maltreated, and in such people the impulse to suicide may be very strong. Suicide more commonly takes place in people who say nothing about it than in those who threaten to take their own lives. Along with the mental symptoms, physical signs are always present, including especially greatly disordered digestion with constipation and muscular weakness. Recovery is usual in melancholia, but a person of melancholic temperament is liable to subsequent attacks of the disorder, which often become more prolonged as life advances. Some cases end in *chronic melancholia* with permanently fixed delusions of an unhappy nature, and a few pass into dementia.

PARANOIA is a condition in which there are delusions forming a system which gradually develops as a result of the disordered mind projecting its own ideas into the supposed motives and conduct of others. The patient takes a distorted view of his relationship to the world in which he lives. This form of psychosis is the outcome of a particular temperament, usually develops slowly, and is only noticed in middle life, the patient often having been previously regarded as merely eccentric or bad tempered. It is more common in men than in women, and among single persons and those who lead a solitary life. To begin with, such persons are often full of wild, altruistic, impersonal theories to which they give outlet in books, or by addressing crowds in open spaces. Many of the persons regarded as political cranks, who preach anarchy, revolution, and various anti-social projects, are subjects of this mental disease. Other paranoiacs

have delusions in which their own personality plays the most important rôle, and they usually believe themselves to be subjects of annoyance or persecution by other people. In this form of psychosis the patient is often very dangerous, because of the schemes he makes to revenge himself on his supposed persecutors or opponents.

SCHIZOPHRENIA (or DEMENTIA PRAECOX) is a mental disorder which appears in predisposed persons, most commonly during the twenties. Such persons usually come of a family with a history of mental disorder. The main characteristic of this disease is disorder of thinking and behaviour, with a progressive withdrawal from the real world into the unreal world of infantile fantasy. The patient may show numerous peculiar mannerisms, such as stilted methods of talking, negativism, (or a tendency to do precisely the opposite of what he is asked to do), an inclination to retain the limbs rigidly in any position in which they are placed, and to imitate any actions performed by other people in front of him. Meaningless repetition of actions, phrases, and words is also a characteristic. Some patients pass into a state of stupor (katatonia); others develop delusions, especially of persecution, or a double personality. Others experience hallucinations, most commonly in the form of threatening or unfriendly voices. The patient is convinced that his actions are controlled by some alien power, and that other people are putting thoughts into his mind and are able to read his thoughts. Many patients make a spontaneous recovery from the acute phase of the disease in three to nine months, and this recovery has been considerably facilitated by the introduction of the tranquillizer drugs. These drugs do not produce a radical cure of this little understood disease but do produce relief of the patient's delusions, hallucinations and alienation from reality.

ALCOHOLIC PSYCHOSIS – Alcoholism and drug habits are also of the nature of mental disorders, and alcohol in turn produces organic changes in the nervous system which lead to permanent mental disease. These are dealt with under ALCOHOLISM, CHRONIC; and DRUG HABITS.

CONFUSIONAL STATES – This type of mental disorder usually follows exhaustion due to over-exertion, or is due to poisoning, either by the toxins of fevers, or by poisons such as alcohol, introduced from outside. Such patients are anaemic, with pale, greasy complexion; the appetite is poor; the circulation feeble, and occasionally there is considerable weakness. There is great enfeeblement of intellectual power, so that the patient has difficulty in understanding simple questions. Hallucinations are common, and the patient may see faces in the air, insects crawling on the bedclothes, and mistake persons near him for old friends or enemies. It is common, too, that the patient has no idea where he is. Memory is much disordered, and if the patient is going about, he is liable, in some cases, to lose his identity, fail to recognize where he is, and may wander long distances from home, even to distant cities, and be quite unable to say who he is, or from where he comes. Usually there is a certain amount of depression and restlessness. This is one of the most curable forms of mental disorder, and the majority of cases make a complete recovery in six to twelve months, or sooner.

STATES OF MENTAL ENFEEBLEMENT – *Mental subnormality* (see MENTAL SUB-NORMALITY).

Dementia is a condition of great mental enfeeblement, usually the terminal stage of some more acute form of mental disorder. The patient in this condition shows great loss of perceptive and intellectual power as well as of bodily activity. It varies in degree, but when it is marked, the patient lives a vegetable existence, unable to converse or to work with any will-power, and he is usually of dirty habits. Recovery does not take place.

General paralysis of the insane, also known as paralytic dementia, is a mental and physical disease, due to syphilis of the nervous system. It is considered under the heading GENERAL PARALYSIS.

Treatment – (*a*) PREVENTION – The question of the prevention of mental illness entails two considerations: first, the counteraction of the various evil influences which impair the mental health of the social body generally; and secondly, the recognition of certain broad lines of living which should be followed by anyone who, on account of hereditary predisposition or abnormal temperament, is liable to become insane. In regard to persons predisposed to mental disorder, their adaptation to their surroundings is being increasingly effected by various agencies. These include the provision of institutions or homes for the mentally subnormal, and the setting up of departments of psychological medicine in general hospitals; and the general amelioration of social conditions and of uncertainty as regards wage-earning and maintenance. The provision of social workers in connection with out-patient mental clinics at hospitals, to investigate the social conditions operating upon the production of borderland cases of mental disorder, is also an important factor in preventing complete mental breakdown in many cases. Every effort should be made to encourage a healthy mode of living, to insist on the importance of good nourishing food, and to provide an education which shall be broad and liberal, and at the same time one that disciplines the mind in habits of self-control and self-denial. To those, however, in whom there is a strong hereditary tendency to mental disorder, life frequently resolves itself into a 'continual struggle to oppose the bent of their being'. Has such a person any power over himself to prevent his becoming mentally ill? That he is largely responsible for the preservation of his sanity there can be no doubt, and, in connection with this, the first truth for him to grasp is that his life must be lived under constant obedience to certain definite rules. Avoidance of psychic stresses, and especially those of an emotional character, is of particular importance.

(*b*) CURE – As the outcome of a more rational view of mental disease, the mentally ill are now regarded and treated as sick persons. The old methods of treatment by punishment, solitary confinement, manacles and strait-waistcoats have now disappeared. Many mentally ill patients can be treated at home, looked after and nursed by their friends, who must be warned, however, that they are responsible for their safety. Recently also there have been instituted, for the treatment of early mental cases, wards attached to the large general hospitals, and thereby the stigma of certification is avoided. More especially is this method of value in those illnesses which are likely to prove of short duration or of a mild character, and which are accompanied by bodily disease.

Home treatment is often, however, impossible, more especially if it becomes clear that the illness is going to be a protracted or violent one, if it is aggravated by home associations and surroundings, or if it is characterized by suicidal or homicidal tendencies. In this case the patient must be duly certified and admitted to a mental hospital. An increasing number of mentally affected persons are availing themselves of the possibility of entering a mental hospital voluntarily while they are still capable of understanding the advisability of doing so. This has the great advantage that patients secure admission at an early stage of their disorder, before they are certifiable, and the disease thus coming under treatment while it is still mild can be more easily and quickly cured.

The encouragement of this modern development of patients with mental illness seeking early admission to hospital is one of the keynotes of the 1959 Mental Health Act which came into force in 1960. The two principles upon which the Act is based are: (i) That as much treatment as possible, both in hospital and outside, should be given on a voluntary and informal basis. (ii) That the emphasis on mental cases should be shifted as far as possible from institutional care to care within the community. In other words, that a patient with mental illness should no more hesitate to go into hospital than a patient with appendicitis, but that so far as possible mentally ill patients should be looked after in the general community.

The actual treatment may be divided into (a) Moral; (b) Medical.

(a) By *moral treatment* is meant that personal influence which the mentally normal exercise over the mentally ill. In exercising this influence there must be constant kindness and perfect firmness. For this purpose it has been found that female nurses with thorough training in a general hospital are most satisfactory. The patient, whenever suitable, is given some liberty, he is allowed out on parole, he can visit places of amusement, he is encouraged to take exercise and recreation, and, above all, he is encouraged to work. In this respect, in mental hospitals, the inmates of which consist largely of those accustomed to manual labour, far more opportunities of bodily work are possible than in private hospitals. This *occupational therapy* is not only of benefit as exercise, but it provides the patient with an object upon which his mind can be concentrated, and so affords useful mental discipline. The work may include digging in the garden, and, in the case of a woman, employment in the kitchen or sewing-room. Useful work can often be produced by patients working at looms, making toys, baskets, and other simple articles. To enable this treatment to be properly carried out, the cooperation of good attendants and nurses is essential, and every effort is now made to have them in sufficient numbers and to encourage them in their work by good remuneration, lectures on the nursing and treatment of the mentally ill, and the granting of certificates of proficiency after examination.

(b) *Medical treatment* – The importance of absolute physical *rest* in the early and acute stages of the illness is now recognized; so is the importance of *fresh air and sunlight*. Good, plentiful food, of an easily assimilable kind, such as eggs and milk, is essential, and in those who refuse food, feeding through a tube passed through the nostril into the back of the throat is employed. The *control of excitement* and sleeplessness by various drugs, when simpler methods fail, is highly important. In patients who require soothing, especially in violent cases, it has been found that *prolonged baths*, at a temperature slightly below that of the body, have a beneficial effect. (See BATHS.)

Under such a regime there frequently come signs of improvement. Natural sleep gradually returns; the body weight increases; delusions become less prominent, are seldom spoken of, and finally disappear; a desire to get well returns; the manner becomes rational; conduct is no longer eccentric; the patient declares himself capable of earning his livelihood, and finally recovery becomes complete, and the patient is discharged.

Shock treatment consists in making the patient go through a number of violent convulsions. The convulsions are produced in various ways: by lowering the blood sugar by means of injections of insulin; by injections of convulsant drugs, such as leptazol; by passing an electric current through the brain. This last form of shock therapy is known as electro-convulsive therapy (ECT). Shock treatment is less useful in the treatment of schizophrenia than it was at first hoped to be. But it has proved valuable in the treatment of depressed or melancholic cases, especially in the form of ECT. A more drastic form of treatment is that known as *leucotomy* or prefrontal lobotomy. This is an operation in which the white nerve fibres in the frontal lobes of the brain are cut, the connections between these lobes and the thalamus and the hypothalamus being thus severed. Leucotomy (qv) has been found to relieve the symptoms of severely depressed or melancholic patients who did not respond to other treatment.

Tranquillizing drugs are being used to an increasing extent in the treatment of mental disease. These are not curative but they undoubtedly produce a marked improvement in a certain number of cases, and allow an increasing number of mentally ill patients to live happily in the community rather than in hospital.

The law and mental illness – Since 1948 the services provided by hospitals and local authorities for mental patients have been part of the National Health Service.

Considerable changes were introduced by the Mental Health Act, 1959. This repealed the Lunacy and Mental Treatment Acts and Mental Deficiency Acts which laid down special procedures for the admission of mental patients to hospital, for their detention in hospital, and for certain forms of control over those living in the community. So far as hospitals are concerned the main differences made by the new Act are freedom to provide psychiatric units in, or attached to, general hospitals for a wider range of mental patients, and the breaking down of the sharp distinction between mental illness and other forms of mental disorder. The main provisions of the Act are as follows. They are not applicable to Scotland and Northern Ireland.

The Board of Control has been dispensed with, and its functions divided between the Department of Health and Social Security, local authorities, and Mental Health Review Tribunals, of which there is one in each Regional Hospital Board Area. The single term, mental disorder, has been introduced to cover all forms of mental illness and disability, and mental disorder is divided into four categories: mental illness, severe subnormality, subnormality, and psychopathic disorder. It also allows for the informal admission of patients into any hospital or nursing home when powers of detention are not necessary. Further, it provides for the registration and inspection, under the Public Health Act, 1936, of all mental nursing homes other than hospitals or other premises managed by a Government department or provided by a local authority, and, under the National Assistance Acts, 1948, of all residential homes for the mentally disordered.

It provides for the compulsory admission of a patient to hospital for observation on the grounds: (a) that he is suffering from mental disorder of a nature or degree which warrants his detention under observation; and (b) that he ought to be so detained in the interests of his own health or safety or with a view to the protection of other persons. A patient admitted in this manner may not be detained for longer than 28 days unless he is in the meantime re-admitted as a result of an application for treatment. Compulsory admission to hospital for treatment is provided for on the grounds: (a) that he is suffering from mental disorder of a nature or degree which warrants his detention for treatment (i) in the case of a patient of any age, mental illness or severe subnormality;

(ii) in the case of a patient under 21 years, psychopathic disorder or subnormality; and (b) that it is necessary in the interests of his health or safety or for the protection of other persons that he should be so detained.

An application for admission of a patient for observation or for treatment may be made by the nearest relative of the patient or by a mental welfare officer (but, where treatment is applied for, the relative must normally concur) and must, except in emergency, be based on two medical recommendations. It must be addressed to the managers of the hospital to which admission is sought and the applicant must have seen the patient personally within the previous 14 days. In case of urgent necessity, application for admission for observation may be made on only one medical recommendation initially but will cease to have effect after 72 hours unless the remaining requirements are fulfilled.

A patient detained in hospital for treatment may apply to a Mental Health Review Tribunal within six months from the day of admission or the day on which he reaches the age of 16, whichever is the later. Authority to detain a patient admitted to hospital in pursuance of an application for treatment will lapse at the end of fixed periods, or at the age of 25 in respect of psychopathic or subnormal patients, unless reviewed. The first period will be one year, the second one year, and thereafter the periods will be of two years at a time. The discharge of a patient compulsorily detained for treatment may be ordered by the nearest relative, unless the medical officer at the hospital reports that the patient is dangerous; in this case the relative may appeal to the Mental Health Review Tribunal. The medical officer and the managers of the hospital have power to discharge the patient at any time.

For reception of a patient into guardianship of either a local health authority or any other person accepted by the local health authority and willing to act as guardian, the procedure is as follows. A guardianship application may be made on the ground of the patient's mental disorder, which may be: (i) in any case, mental illness or severe subnormality; (ii) in the case of a patient under the age of 21 years, psychopathic disorder or subnormality; and that it is necessary in the interests of the patient or for the protection of other persons that the patient should be received into guardianship. The provisions regarding application to a Mental

Health Review Tribunal and the periodic lapsing of authority to detain the patient are the same as in the case of patients detained for treatment, and the nearest relative has the same power of discharge.

Persons coming before the courts who are mentally disordered may be detained in hospital or received into guardianship if the court considers it a suitable course. In certain circumstances, higher courts may also make restriction orders, in which case the patient may not be discharged without the consent of the Home Secretary. Persons detained in prison or approved schools who are found to be mentally disordered may be transferred to hospital by the Home Secretary.

Provision is made for institutions, known as Special Hospitals, for mentally disordered persons who, in the opinion of the Minister, require treatment under conditions of special security on account of their dangerous, violent, or criminal propensities.

The Act continues the arrangements for the management of the property and effects of mentally disordered patients by nominated judges and the Court of Protection.

MENTAL SUBNORMALITY – This is the term introduced in the Mental Health Act, 1959, to replace the term mental defectiveness. In the Act, mental subnormality is subdivided into two categories:

Severe Subnormality – A state of arrested or incomplete development of mind so severe that a patient is incapable of living an independent life or of guarding himself against serious exploitation (or, in the case of a child, that he will be so incapable when adult).

Subnormality – A state of arrested or incomplete development of mind which includes subnormality of intelligence and requires special care or training, but does not amount to severe subnormality.

Causes – The term, mental subnormality, is largely a relative one, and the mentally subnormal individual must be compared with persons of his own race, age, and opportunities. Again, mental subnormality is not so evident in persons living in country districts, where suitable employment can be obtained, as it is among persons in towns, where the struggle for existence is more intense. Less importance than previously is now attached to heredity as a cause, although mentally subnormal children sometimes occur in a family of which other members

show evidence, for example, of insanity, epilepsy, alcoholism, especially when the parents are nearly related to one another. The descendants of mentally subnormal individuals have been traced and it has been found that among the descendants of a union between two mental defectives a high proportion of feeble-minded persons occurs.

Several varieties are recognized. The great majority of cases fall into the group of *simple primary amentia*, for which no further cause is evident than the hereditary consideration mentioned above. In these cases, the children show too little of the normal automatic movements of healthy infancy, and speech and walking fail to develop at the proper age, between 1 and 2 years. Many such children show peculiarity in gestures and behaviour even in early life, and are very late in gaining control over the bladder and bowels, if they do so at all. A proportion of such children also have epileptic attacks. Along with mental subnormality these children generally show much physical weakness, and they are more liable to die from slight disorders or injuries than are ordinary persons. Such children, even when the defect is not great, are difficult to teach, because they are unable to concentrate their attention on one subject for long. They are lacking in perseverance. Some are morbidly shy and self-conscious, or deficient in self-control so that they are constantly laughing, crying, and getting into unreasonable fits of passion. When these children go to school, the defect is soon noticed by comparison with other children of their own age, and in most large towns special schools are provided for mentally subnormal children, where they are taught by specially trained teachers and an attempt is made to fit them for taking up simple forms of employment. Whilst these children are generally benefited by contact with older persons who make allowances for them, their condition is usually made much worse by the teasing which they are apt to undergo at the hands of other children.

Other types of mental subnormality are those associated with *microcephaly*, in which the head is unusually small and the whole nervous system defective in development. Another type is that of *Mongolism*, in which there is some arrest or perversion of development prior to birth. These children often come at the end of large families. Still other cases are associated with gross disease of the nervous system in early life, such as *hydroce-*

phalus, haemorrhage on the surface of the brain at birth, *congenital syphilis* or disease of other organs, such as thyroid defect, which occurs in *cretins.* Children may also be mentally subnormal in cases where they have been deprived of some important sense, such as in blindness or deafness, but such mental subnormality is curable by special instruction.

Diagnosis – The symptoms by which the presence of mental subnormality is recognized in infants and young children are bodily as well as mental. At a later stage of life the degree of mental subnormality can be assessed by comparing the mental powers of the person in question with the capabilities of normal children of different ages.

Some children from birth present abnormalities of bodily structure which are commonly associated with mental defect. Thus, the conditions of microcephaly, mongolism, cretinism, chronic hydrocephalus, and various forms of paralysis can be recognized, and these are known to be commonly associated with mental defect. Other less marked bodily malformations may be found when careful search is made, such as unusual height of the palate, defects of the ear, defective formation of the head or spine, such as spina bifida, and congenital malformations of the heart. Any of these defects may be met in children of ordinary intelligence, but they are more common in the mentally subnormal, and, if noticed, should direct attention to the child's mental condition.

The occurrence in infants of convulsions may be associated with mental subnormality either as a cause of or produced by brain defect. Abnormal gestures and actions, such as constant crying, rolling of the eyes, or simply want of animation when the nurse or mother fondles a child, and, at a later stage, unmeaning laughter and grimaces, dirty habits, disgusting ways of eating, or dribbling of saliva from the mouth, are all signs of subnormal mentality.

Other significant signs are found in slowness of development as compared with other children. Thus the infant may be too long in learning to hold up the head, to use the hands for grasping objects, to stand, and to notice bright or attractive objects placed before him. Difficulty in learning to suck, backwardness in speaking, and delay in learning cleanly habits are all significant.

At a later age, in order to find out the degree of mental subnormality in a child or adult, a simple form of examination is set, questions being asked which have been found capable of being answered by a normal child at a given age. Various scales are employed, the best known being the Stanford revision of the Binet-Simon tests. Examples of these are given below. If the mentally subnormal person can only pass the test which a child of three would answer, his 'mental age' is said to be that of three years. If he can pass the test of a normal child of six, nine, etc., his 'mental age' is said to be six years, nine years, etc. The following are three examples:

Year 3 – A normal child of three should be able to do the following: (1) To point correctly to his nose, eyes, mouth, hair, etc., when asked to do so. (2) To name familiar objects like key, penny, knife, watch, pencil, etc., when shown to him. (3) To name three simple objects in a picture shown him. (4) To say whether he is boy or girl. (5) To tell his last name. (6) To repeat three numbers, eg. 6, 4, 1, when named to him.

Year 6 – A normal child of six should be able to do the following: (1) Point to right hand, left ear, etc., as named. (2) When shown a picture of a figure, from which parts have been left out, to name the missing parts. (3) To give an explicit reply to simple questions such as 'What should you do if you find that the house is on fire?' (4) To count objects up to 13. (5) To name correctly coins shown him. (6) To repeat correctly a simple sentence of 12 or 15 words. Incidentally it is of interest that an intelligent 6-year-old child knows the meaning of around 13,000 words. Two years later this figure has more than doubled.

Year 9 – A normal child of nine should be able to do the following: (1) To give the correct day, month, and year. (2) To arrange a series of weights in proper order. (3) To subtract two numbers from other two. (4) To repeat backwards four stated figures: eg. 6528. (5) To make a simple sentence containing three stated words. (6) To name the month coming before a stated month.

It must always be remembered that comparison with a normal child is only a rough index of the mental age of the subnormal person, who has reached a greater number of years and who has therefore had special experience along certain lines which the normal child has not yet had time to gain.

Treatment – In the great majority of cases, mental subnormality is incurable and children who are mentally weak will remain so throughout life. Nevertheless,

583

most mentally subnormal children, unless the defect is very great, are capable of improvement under suitable treatment, and may actually be able in later life to earn a satisfactory living at some simple automatic employment which a normally minded person would find depressing or even intolerable because of its monotony. Attention to the general health is of great importance, and when special conditions such as cretinism, syphilis, deafness, are found, these should receive appropriate treatment. Young children who are found to possess insufficient concentration for book work should be instructed in amusing kindergarten occupations, and bad and dirty habits should be gradually corrected. The child should be encouraged to do as much as he can for himself, and particular care should be exercised to promote self-control and to cultivate moral character.

If home conditions are satisfactory, the home is far the best place for a mentally subnormal child. At a later stage of childhood, however, he may become a drag upon normal children and be apt to be discouraged by ineffective competition with them, as well as by teasing to which they are very liable to subject him. He is then more happily placed with children about his own level of intelligence either in a special school or in an institution. Under the Mental Health Act, 1959, local health authorities have a duty to arrange for the care and training of these children. The Act gives them powers to require parents to ensure the attendance of children at Training Centres, unless the child is already receiving comparable training to that obtainable at the centre. At such a school or institution the attempt should be made to prepare him about the age of sixteen for taking up some simple form of productive work, if he is at all capable of such training. If he proves incapable of this, it is better for society – as well as for himself – that he should be maintained in some institution for the remainder of his life.

Parents or other relatives of mentally subnormal children can obtain helpful advice from the National Society for Mentally Handicapped Children, Pembridge Hall, 17 Pembridge Square, London W2 4EH, or the Scottish Society for the Mentally Handicapped, 69 West Regent Street, Glasgow G2 2AN.

MENTHOL is a white crystalline substance deposited from oil of peppermint when it is cooled. It comes principally from Japan, being derived from several species of *Mentha*. It dissolves freely in alcohol, ether, chloroform, and olive oil, and also to a slight extent in water, to which it gives a strong odour and taste of peppermint. Mixed with a little oil of peppermint, it can be moulded into cones, sticks, or pencils. When menthol is rubbed up with thymol, carbolic acid, chloral, or camphor, the two solids form a clear oily liquid which can be painted on the skin, exerting the effects of both drugs.

Action – Applied to the skin, menthol has weak antiseptic properties, and it acts upon the sensory nerves, causing first a hot, tingling sensation, followed quickly by a cool, numb feeling. When applied to inflamed mucous membranes, such as those of the nose and throat, menthol relieves irritability, diminishes congestion, and checks excessive secretion. Menthol has the merit of being non-poisonous.

Uses – In neuralgia, cones and sticks of menthol are used to rub over the affected part. In toothache, cotton-wool dipped in one of the oily fluids above named and placed in the cavity of the carious tooth quickly relieves the pain. In many itchy conditions of the skin a strong solution of menthol in olive oil (1 part in 10) relieves the sense of irritation at once. Menthol plaster is useful in gout, rheumatism, and neuralgia, and so are mixtures with chloral or camphor painted over the painful parts. For inflamed conditions of the nose and throat, the oily compounds of menthol are diluted with parolene and sprayed on the part affected, or in the case of the throat various lozenges and pastilles containing menthol are sucked. In bronchitis menthol crystals in hot water, from which the vapour is inhaled, give much relief.

MEPACRINE HYDROCHLORIDE is a synthetic acridine product used in the treatment of malaria. It came to the fore during the 1939–1945 War, when supplies of quinine were short, and proved of great value both as a prophylactic and in the treatment of malaria. It is also used in the treatment of infestation with tapeworms. (See TAENIASIS or TAPEWORMS.)

MEPROBAMATE is one of the tranquillizer drugs. It is mainly used for the relief of states of tension, mild anxiety states and persistent insomnia.

MEPYRAMINE MALEATE is one of the antihistamine drugs (qv).

MERALGIA PARAESTHETICA is a condition characterized by pain and paraesthesia (qv) on the front and outer aspect of the thigh. It is more common in men than in women, and the victims are usually middle-aged, overweight and out of condition. It is due to compression of the lateral cutaneous nerve of the thigh. It is exacerbated by an uncomfortable driving position when motoring long distances. Reduction in weight, improvement in general fitness and correction of faulty posture usually bring relief. If these fail, surgical decompression of the nerve may bring relief.

MERCAPTAMINE is a drug that is proving of value in the treatment of paracetamol poisoning.

MERCAPTOPURINE is one of a group of drugs known as antimetabolites which are proving of value in the treatment of certain forms of malignant disease, especially acute leukaemia. It is believed that they act by depriving rapidly dividing malignant cells of factors essential for their metabolism. Hence the generic name for the group of drugs – antimetabolites.

MERCUROCHROME is an organic salt of mercury with weak antiseptic action, which is sometimes used as an antiseptic to wash out the bladder when infected.

MERCURY, also known as QUICKSILVER or HYDRARGYRUM, is a heavy fluid metal which, with its salts, has been used in medicine for many centuries.

Action – The salts of mercury fall into two groups: the mercuric salts, which are very soluble and powerful in action; and the mercurous salts, which are less soluble and act more slowly and mildly. The mercuric salts are all highly poisonous both to man and to bacterial life, so that they are strongly antiseptic. In strong solutions, several act as caustics, and in weaker solutions they are irritants. Taken internally, the first effect of the mercuric, and to a less degree of the mercurous salts, is by their irritating action to set up copious purging. They are also credited with the power of increasing the flow of bile, and for this reason blue pill, which contains mercury, and mercurous chloride, ie. calomel, were at one time much used as purgatives.

Uses – Externally the mercuric salts are used as disinfectants and antiseptics. Ammoniated mercury ointment, or white precipitate ointment, is used in the treatment of impetigo. The yellow oxide of mercury ointment is used for an application to the eyelids when a mild antiseptic ointment is required. Internally, mercurial salts were widely used at one time as purges, particularly calomel, the dosage of which is ½ to 3 grains (30 to 200 mg) for an adult, and blue pill (4 to 8 grains) (250 to 500 mg). They are best taken at night, and followed by a saline draught in the morning. They are seldom used nowadays.

A complex organic salt of mercury (mersalyl) is used as a diuretic in the treatment of dropsy.

MERCURY POISONING is of two kinds: (1) acute mercury poisoning, due to swallowing one of the soluble mercury salts, such as perchloride of mercury or one of the organic mercury compounds used as fungicides; and (2) chronic mercury poisoning, produced either by continuing repeated medicinal doses of mercurials for too long a time, or by handling the metal or inhaling its fumes, as happens sometimes among mirror and barometer makers and dental technicians. The use of mercurial dusting powders in connection with the use of finger-prints in criminal investigations has also been reported as leading to mercury poisoning.

ACUTE POISONING. **Symptoms** – There is burning pain, first in the mouth, then in the stomach, followed by diarrhoea and vomiting. The lips and mouth are generally burned white, and a metallic taste is left in the mouth. Great collapse soon comes on, and the person may die in a few hours. If death does not take place at an early stage, the kidneys are liable to remain seriously damaged by the drug.

Treatment – The stomach should be washed out as quickly as possible with sodium bicarbonate. Some albuminous preparation, such as egg white or milk, should then be given, as, with corrosive sublimate, this forms an insoluble and harmless compound. Dimercaprol (BAL) (qv) should also be given. If signs of shock appear, the patient is treated accordingly. (See SHOCK.)

CHRONIC POISONING. **Symptoms** – When too much mercury is being taken into the system in small doses, the first signs are an excessive discharge of saliva into the mouth, and tenderness about the teeth when the mouth is tightly shut. Next, the odour of the breath becomes bad, the gums tender, spongy, and ready to bleed at the slightest touch, and the tongue swollen. Finally, the teeth become loose and drop out, the jaw-bone may become diseased, the person becomes generally weak and bloodless, and may indeed die. Persons who work with metallic mercury may develop these symptoms to some extent, and in addition they become affected by trembling and palsy in various parts of the body. Such trembling induced by mercury in the felthat industry was known as 'hatters' shakes', and was responsible for the phrase 'mad as a hatter'.

Treatment consists in stoppage of the mercury if it is being administered as medicine, and change of employment if the symptoms be due to work. Potassium iodide is often given, in addition to the good food and tonics which are necessary. If the condition is sufficiently severe, a course of injections of dimercaprol (qv) is given.

MERSALYL is a complex synthetic mercurial compound, used in the treatment of oedema (ie. dropsy) due to heart disease.

MERYCISM is another name for rumination, in which the contents of a meal are returned to the mouth some time after they have been swallowed and are once again chewed.

MESCALINE is derived from the Mexican peyote cactus, *Anhalonium lewinii*. It is probably the most powerful of all the hallucinogens and has been used from time immemorial almost by Indian tribes in Mexico as an intoxicant to produce ecstatic states for religious celebrations. (See DRUG ADDICTION.)

MESENCEPHALON is the term applied to the mid-brain connecting the cerebral hemispheres with the pons and cerebellum.

MESENTERY is the name given to the double layer of peritoneal membrane which supports the small intestine. It is of a fan shape, and its shorter edge is attached to the back wall of the abdomen for a distance of about 6 inches (15 cm), while the small intestine lies within its longer edge, for a length of over 20 feet (6 metres). The terms mesocolon, mesorectum, etc., are applied to similar folds of peritoneum that support parts of the colon, rectum, etc.

MESMERISM (see HYPNOTISM).

MESOCOLON is the name of the double fold of peritoneum by which the large intestine is suspended from the back wall of the abdomen.

MESTEROLONE is a synthetic androgen (qv) which is being used in the treatment of male infertility.

METABOLISM means tissue change and includes all the physical and chemical processes by which the living body is maintained, and also those by which the energy is made available for various forms of work. The constructive, chemical and physical, processes by which food materials are adapted for the use of the body are collectively known as anabolism. The destructive processes by which energy is produced with the breaking down of tissues into waste products is known as catabolism. *Basal metabolism* is the term applied to the energy changes necessary for essential processes such as the beating of the heart, respiration, and maintenance of body warmth. This can be estimated, when a person is placed in a state of complete rest, by measuring the amounts of oxygen and carbon dioxide exchanged during breathing under certain standard conditions. (See CALORIE.)

METACARPAL bones are the long bones, five in number, which occupy the hand between the carpal bones at the wrist and the phalanges of the fingers. The large rounded 'knuckles' at the root of the fingers are formed by the heads of these bones. (See HAND.)

METAPHYSIS is the extremity of a long bone where it joins the epiphysis (qv).

METAPLASIA is the term applied to a change of one kind of tissue into another.

METASTASIS and METASTATIC are terms applied to the process by which malignant disease spreads to distant parts of the body, and also to the secondary tumours resulting from this process. For example, a cancer of the breast may produce metastatic growths in the glands of the armpit, cancer of the stomach may be followed by metastases in the liver.

METATARSAL bones are the five bones in the foot which correspond to the metacarpal bones in the hand, lying between the tarsal bones, at the ankle, and the toes. (See FOOT.)

METATARSALGIA is the name applied to pain affecting the metatarsal region of the foot. It is common in adolescents associated with flat-foot (qv). In adults it may be a manifestation of rheumatoid arthritis. *Morton's metatarsalgia* is a form associated usually with the nerve to the second toe cleft often induced by the compression of tight shoes.

METATARSUS is the group name of the five metatarsal bones in the foot (qv). *Metatarsus varus* is the condition characterized by deviation of the forefoot towards the other foot. It is a common condition in new-born babes and almost always corrects itself spontaneously. Only in the rare cases in which it is due to some deformity of the bones or muscles of the foot is any treatment required.

METEORISM means the distension of the abdomen by gas produced in the intestines. (See FLATULENCE.)

METFORMIN is a biguanide (qv) which lowers the blood sugar. Its precise mode of action, however, is not known. It is active when taken by mouth and is proving of value in the treatment of certain cases of diabetes mellitus.

METHACHOLINE, is a derivative of acetylcholine (qv). It is more stable than acetylcholine. Its main use is in the treatment of paroxysmal atrial tachycardia.

METHADONE, or PHYSEPTONE, is an analgesic with morphine-like properties. It has much less hypnotic action than morphine, and is used as a linctus for the alleviation of troublesome cough. It has some of the addiction-forming properties of morphine.

METHAEMOGLOBIN is a modification of haemoglobin, the pigment of the blood. It is found in the blood and sometimes in the urine after taking large doses of certain drugs, such as acetanilide, and also in some diseases.

METHAQUALONE is a synthetic, non-barbiturate hypnotic.

METHICILLIN (see PENICILLIN).

METHISAZONE is a thiosemicarbazone derivative that is proving of value in the prevention of smallpox.

METHOHEXITONE is a recently introduced ultra-short-acting barbiturate which is proving of value as a short-acting anaesthetic – particularly in dentistry.

METHONIUM compounds are quaternary ammonium compounds which act by producing a block in the ganglia of the autonomic nervous system (qv) and can thereby produce a lowering of the blood-pressure and a lessening of the activity of the stomach. They therefore prove of value in the treatment of high blood-pressure. The preparations most widely used for this purpose are hexamethonium and pentolinium tartrate.

METHOTREXATE is an antimetabolite which is proving of value in the treatment of choriocarcinoma (qv).

METHOXYFLURANE is a general anaesthetic.

METHYL is the name of an organic radical whose chemical formula is CH_3, and which forms the centre of a wide group of substances known as the methyl group. For example, methyl alcohol is obtained as a by-product in the manufacture of beet-sugar, or by distillation of wood; methyl salicylate is the active constituent in oil of wintergreen: methyl hydride is better known as marsh gas.

Methyl alcohol, or wood spirit, is distilled from wood and is thus a cheap form of alcohol. It has actions similar to, but much more toxic than, those of ethyl alcohol. It has a specially pronounced action on the nervous system, and in large doses is apt to cause neuritis, especially of the optic nerves, leading to blindness, partial or complete.

METHYLDOPA is one of the drugs introduced for the treatment of high blood-pressure. Its mode of action is still obscure.

METHYLPHENOBARBITONE is a barbiturate used in the treatment of epilepsy.

METHYLPREDNISOLONE is a preparation with an action comparable to that of prednisolone, but effective at a somewhat lower dose.

METHYLTESTOSTERONE is a derivative of the testicular hormone, testosterone (qv), which is active when taken by mouth. About three to four times as big a dose is needed to produce the same effect as an injection of testosterone propionate.

METHYLTHIONIN CHLORIDE, or METHYLENE BLUE, is a dark powder forming a deep-blue solution, used for various tests.

METHYPRYLONE is a non-barbiturate sedative.

METHYSERGIDE is a drug that is being used in the prevention of attacks of migraine (qv). Its precise value is still not clear, and it has to be used with care because of the toxic effects it sometimes produces.

METOCLOPRAMIDE is a drug that is proving of value in the treatment of vomiting. It is said to restore normal co-ordination and tone to the upper digestive tract.

METOPROLOL is a drug that is proving of value in the treatment of angina pectoris (qv).

METRE is the basic unit of length in the modern version of the metric system, known as the International System of Units (SI). (See WEIGHTS AND MEASURES.) It is equivalent to 39·37 inches.

METRITIS means inflammation of the womb.

METRONIDAZOLE is a drug, administered by mouth, which is proving of value in the treatment of various diseases including balantidiasis (qv), giardiasis (qv), amoebic dysentery (see DYSENTERY) and trichomonal vaginitis. (See TRICHO-MONAS VAGINALIS.)

METROPATHIA HAEMORRHAG-ICA, or ESSENTIAL UTERINE HAEMORRHAGE, is the term given to a diseased state characterized by haemorrhage from the uterus, cysts in the ovaries, and thickening of the uterine mucosa.

METRORRHAGIA means bleeding from the womb otherwise than at the proper period. (See MENSTRUATION.)

METYRAPONE is a drug that is used in the treatment of Cushing's syndrome (qv).

MICONAZOLE is a drug that is proving of value in the treatment of the group of diseases known as the mycoses (qv).

MICROANGIOPATHY means disease of the capillaries (qv).

MICROBE (see BACTERIA).

MICROBIOLOGY is the branch of biology concerned with the study of micro-organisms. (See BACTERIOLOGY.)

MICROCEPHALY is a term applied to abnormal smallness of the head. (See MENTAL SUBNORMALITY.)

MICROCYTE means a small red blood corpuscle.

MICROGRAM is the $\frac{1}{1000}$th part of a milligram. The abbreviation for it is μg or mcg.

MICROMETRE, or MICRON, is the $\frac{1}{1000}$th part of a millimetre. The abbreviation for it is μm.

MICRO-ORGANISM (see BACTERIA).

MICROPSIA is the condition in which objects appear to be smaller than they really are. It is due to disease of the retina.

MICROSPORON is the genus of fungi which includes the fungi responsible for ringworm of the scalp. (See RINGWORM.)

MICTURITION means the act of passing water.

MIDGES (see BITES).

MIDWIFERY (see LABOUR).

MIGRAINE is a common condition characterized by recurring intense headaches, which has claimed many distinguished victims, including Prince Albert, the Prince Consort. It usually begins at puberty and often tends to stop in middle age: eg. in women attacks often cease after the change of life. It often disappears during pregnancy. In susceptible individuals attacks may be provoked by a wide variety of causes including:
Anxiety, worry, emotion, depression, shock, and excitement.
Overexertion.
Physical and mental fatigue.
Bending or stooping, as in gardening.
Lifting heavy weights, or straining of any sort.
Changes of routine: eg. holidays or change of job.
Late rising, especially at weekends or on holiday.
Travel.
Change of climate.
Changes in weather; eg. high winds.
Fluorescent lights, car headlights, direct

or interrupted bright sunlight and striped patterns.

Prolonged focusing on television or cinema screen.

Very hot baths.

Noise, especially loud and high-pitched sounds.

Penetrating smells.

Certain foods: eg. chocolate, cheese, citrus fruits, pastry.

Sleeping tablets.

Alcohol.

Prolonged lack of food.

Irregular meals.

Menstruation and the pre-menstrual period.

Menopause.

Continued use of oral contraceptives.

Toothache.

Indeed, it has been said that anything that can provoke a headache in the ordinary individual can precipitate an attack in a migrainous subject. It seems as if there is an inherited predisposition that triggers a mechanism whereby in the migrainous subject the headache, and the associated sickness persist for hours, a whole day or even longer.

The precise cause is not known, but the generally accepted view is that in susceptible individuals one or other of these causes produces spasm or constriction of the blood-vessels of the brain. This in turn is followed by dilatation of these blood-vessels which also become more permeable and so allow fluid to pass out into the surrounding tissues. This combination of dilatation and outpouring of fluid is held to be responsible for the headache. An alternative theory is that the fluid contains certain substances, such as prostaglandins (qv), which lower the threshold for pain and so increase the liability of the individual to feel pain. Recent work suggests that migraine may be due to a specific biochemical deficiency: namely, lack of a substance known as monoamine oxidase (see MONOAMINE OXIDASE INHIBITORS). This is an enzyme (qv) which destroys any excess which may accumulate in the body of what are known as vasoactive amines (see AMINES). These are substances responsible for controlling blood-vessels, causing them to dilate or constrict, and it is known that some of these vasoactive amines, including tyramine (which is found in cheese) and phenylethylamine (which is found in chocolate), can provoke attacks of migraine in susceptible people. The suggestion therefore is that these people are born with a lack of monoamine oxidase and are thus liable to develop an attack of migraine on eating cheese or chocolate. As there are other vasoactive amines that are concerned with attacks of migraine, this suggested that lack of monoamine oxidase may solve the age-old mystery of why some people develop migraine.

The typical attack is very characteristic. It consists of an intense headache, usually situated over one or other eye. The headache is usually preceded by a feeling of sickness and blurring of sight. In some cases this disturbance of sight takes the form of bright lights: the so-called aura of migraine. The majority of attacks are accompanied by vomiting. The duration of the headache varies, but in the more severe cases the victim is usually confined to bed for twenty-four hours.

Treatment consists, in the first place, of trying to avoid any precipitating factor. Patients must find out which drug, or drugs, give them most relief, and they must always carry them about with them wherever they go. This is because it is a not uncommon experience to be aware of an attack coming on and to find that there is a critical quarter of an hour or so during which their tablets are effective. If not taken within this period, they may be ineffective and the unfortunate victim finds himself prostrate with headache and vomiting. In addition he should immediately lie down, and at this stage a few hours' rest may prevent the development of a full attack. When an attack is fully developed, rest in bed in a quiet, darkened room is essential; any loud noise or bright light intensifies the headache or sickness. The less food that is taken during an attack the better, provided the individual drinks as much fluid as he wants. Group therapy, in which groups of around ten migrainous subjects learn how to relax, is often of help in more severe cases, whilst in others the injection of a local anaesthetic into tender spots in the scalp reduces the number of attacks. Drug treatment is not very satisfactory. Perhaps the most effective remedy for the condition is ergotamine tartrate which causes the dilated blood vessels to contract, but this must only be taken under medical supervision. In milder attacks, aspirin, with or without codeine and paracetamol, may be of value.

Migraine Clinics – There are five migraine clinics in London:

The Princess Margaret Migraine Clinic, 22 Charterhouse Square, E.C.1.

Charing Cross Hospital, Fulham Palace Road, W.6.

Elizabeth Garrett Anderson Hospital,

Euston Road, N.W.1. (Women only.)
King's College Hospital, Denmark Hill, S.E.5.
The National Hospital, Queen Square, W.C.1.

There are four in the provinces:

The Birmingham and Midland Eye Hospital, Church Street, Birmingham, B3 2NS.
Royal Surrey County Hospital, Farnham Road, Guildford, Surrey.
Hull Royal Infirmary, Anlaby Road, Hull.
Radcliffe Infirmary, Oxford.

There are two in Scotland:

Neurological Unit, Northern General Hospital, Ferry Road, Edinburgh, 5.
Southern General Hospital, Glasgow.

Patients must first obtain a covering letter from their general practitioner before requesting an appointment for consultation. All correspondence should be addressed to The Secretary, The Migraine Clinic.

People with migraine and their relatives can obtain help and guidance from the British Migraine Association, Evergreen, Ottermead Lane, Ottershaw, Chertsey, Surrey, KT16 0HJ.

MILIARIA is the name applied to the group of diseases of the skin caused by disturbances of perspiration. The best known is MILIARIA RUBRA, or PRICKLY HEAT (qv).

MILIARY is a term, expressive of size, applied to various disease products which are about the size of millet seeds: eg. miliary aneurysms, miliary tuberculosis.

MILIUM is the term applied to a small, whitish nodule in the skin, especially of the face. (See ACNE.)

MILK is the natural food of all animals belonging to the class of mammalia for a considerable period following their birth. It is practically the only form of animal food in which protein, fat, carbohydrate, and salt are all represented in sufficient amount, and it therefore contains all the constituents of a standard diet. Milk is important in human nutrition because it contains first-class animal protein of high biological value, because it is exceptionally rich in calcium, and because it is a good source of vitamin A, thiamine and riboflavine. It also contains a variable amount of ascorbic acid (vitamin C) and of vitamin D, the amount of the latter

being higher during the summer months than during the winter months (table 37). Raw milk yields 65 Calories per 100 millilitres, in which are present (in grams) 87·6 of water, 3·3 of protein, 3·6 of fat, 4·7 of carbohydrate, and 0·120 of calcium. Heat has no effect on the vitamin A or D content of milk, or on the riboflavine

	Human Milk	Cow's Milk
Vitamin A (summer)	450 μg	45 μg
Vitamin A (winter)		30 μg
Vitamin D (summer)	0·03 μg	0·04 μg
Vitamin D (winter)		0·01 μg
Thiamine	17 μg	40 μg
Riboflavine	30 μg	150 μg
Nicotinic acid	170 μg	80 μg
Vitamin C	3·5 mg	2 mg
Calcium	25 to 35 mg	120 mg

Table 37 – Vitamin and calcium content of human and cow's milk (per 100 millilitres).

content, but it causes a considerable reduction in the vitamin C and thiamine content.

The milk of different cows varies, especially in the amount of fat and of the fat-soluble vitamins A and D, but the mixed milk of a herd should reach a certain standard. It should contain over 12 per cent of solids, as shown in illustration 305. A pint (0·5 litre approximately) of milk provides about 400 Calories of energy value. The percentage of cream by volume should be not less than 10 per cent. The amount of cream contained in milk can readily be discovered by allowing the milk to stand overnight in a cylindrical graduated vessel, when the cream rises to the top, and its volume can be measured off.

The ready digestibility of milk, especially when mixed with lime water, or when 2 or 3 grains (125 to 200 mg) of citrate of soda have been added for each ounce (30 ml) of milk in order to soften the curd, makes it a specially suitable food for children, invalids, and persons suffering from fever; its blandness and the completeness with which it is absorbed and assimilated adapt it admirably for the general staple of nourishment in many diseases; and its high nutritive value compared with its cost renders it a valuable article of diet for the healthy. As a complete diet, for an adult doing hard work, about 9 pints (5 litres) of milk would be required daily; but for a person confined to bed and restricted in the matter of food, 3 pints (1·5 litres) daily afford sufficient nourishment for two or three weeks.

WATER   PROTEIN   FAT   CARBO-   ASH
                        HYDRATE

305 – Fresh milk
Fuel Value per pint
(560 ml) = 380 Calories.

	Per cent
Water	87·0
Protein	3·3
Fat	4·0
Carbohydrate	5·0
Ash	0·7

306 – Skim milk
Fuel Value per pint
(560 ml) = 210 Calories

	Per cent
Water	90·5
Protein	3·4
Fat	0·3
Carbohydrate	5·1
Ash	0·7

307 – Cream
Fuel Value per pint
(560 ml) = 1000 Calories

	Per cent
Water	74·0
Protein	2·5
Fat	18·5
Carbohydrate	4·5
Ash	0·5

Preparation of milk – Milk may be prepared for food in various ways. *Boiling* destroys the bacteria, especially any *Mycobacteria tuberculosis* which the milk may contain. It also partly destroys vitamin C and thiamine, as does *pasteurization*. *Curdling* of milk is effected by adding rennet, which carries out the initial stage of digestion and thus renders milk more suitable for persons who could not otherwise tolerate it. *Souring* of milk is practised in many countries before milk is considered suitable for food; it is carried out by adding certain organisms such as the lactic acid bacillus, the Bulgarian bacillus, and setting the milk in a warm place for several hours. (See LACTIC ACID BACILLI.) *Sterilization*, which prevents fermentation

and decomposition, is usually carried out by raising the milk to boiling temperature (100° C) for fifteen minutes and then hermetically sealing. *Condensed, unsweetened milk* – usually known as *evaporated milk* – is concentrated *in vacuo* at low temperature; the milk is then placed in tins, which are sealed, and is sterilized by heat at a temperature of 240° F (105° C). This destroys 60 per cent of the vitamin C and 30 to 50 per cent of the thiamine. *Sweetened condensed milk* is not exposed to such a high temperature. The sugar, which prevents the growth of micro-organisms, is added before the condensing, and finally reaches a concentration of about 40 per cent. In a good, well-prepared, sweetened condensed milk, only 15 per cent of vitamin C and 5 to 10 per cent of thiamine may be lost. The sweetened form is apt to lead in children to flatulence and diarrhoea. *Dried milk* is prepared by evaporating all the fluid so that the milk is reduced to the form of powder. In *spray-drying* a very fine spray of milk is forced into a heated chamber, where drying is almost instantaneous. Milk powder thus prepared is nearly completely soluble in water. During the drying process about 20 per cent of the vitamin C and 10 per cent of the thiamine are lost. There is about a 5 per cent decrease in the biological value of the milk proteins (casein, lactalbumin, lactoglobulin). The calcium is unaffected. *Roller-dried milk* is prepared by spreading a thin film of milk over steam-heated revolving metal cylinders; the powder is removed by a stationary scraper. Roller-dried milk is less soluble in water than spray-dried milk; in its preparation the loss of vitamin C and thiamine is higher and there is slightly greater deterioration of protein. *Peptonized milk* is prepared by treating fresh milk with peptonizing powder, and although the milk is rendered less palatable by this means, it is easily digested and is readily tolerated in weak conditions of the stomach and intestines. (See PEPTONIZED FOODS.) *Humanized milk* is cow's milk treated in such a way as to render it closely similar to human milk.

Grades of milk – In England and Wales the grades of milk that are now officially recognized are:

1. *Untreated milk.*

2. *Heat-treated milk*, which is divided into three categories: pasteurized, sterilized, and ultra heat-treated.

Pasteurized milk is milk that has been treated in one of two ways. One is the 'Holder Process', in which the milk is retained at a temperature of not less than

145° F (63° C) and not more than 150° F (65·5 C) for at least half an hour and then immediately cooled to a temperature of not more than 50° F (10° C). The other is the 'High Temperature Short Time Process', in which the milk is retained at a temperature of not less than 161° F (71·7° C) for at least fifteen seconds and then immediately cooled to a temperature of not more than 50° F (10° C). Pasteurization will not make satisfactory milk that was unsatisfactory in the first instance but, provided satisfactory milk is used in the first instance, it does provide a safe milk of good keeping qualities without affecting its nutritive value to any appreciable extent. *Sterilized milk* is milk that has been filtered or clarified, homogenized and then heated to, and maintained at, a temperature of at least 212° F (100° C) for such a period as to ensure that it complies with the turbidity test as described in the appropriate regulations. It is heat treated in bottles and after treatment the bottles are sealed with an airtight seal and labelled 'Sterilized Milk'. It is a perfectly safe milk though there is some decrease in the nutritive value. *Ultra heat-treated milk* is milk which has been retained at a temperature of at least 270° F (132° C) for not less than one second. It is required to satisfy the colony count test as laid down in the appropriate regulations. It keeps much better than pasteurized milk: packed in sterile cartons it will keep for several weeks without refrigeration.

In Scotland the grades of milk are:
1. *Untreated milk*, which is known as *Premium* or *Standard Milk*.
2. *Heat-treated milk*, which, as in England and Wales, is available as *Pasteurized*, *Sterilized*, or *Ultra heat-treated milk*.

MILK, DISEASES DUE TO – Milk has a remarkable power of absorbing gases and vapours to which it is exposed, so that it becomes readily tainted. Milk is also liable to be infected by dirt, or from water, or from the hands of milkers suffering from disease, and in these circumstances epidemics of enteric fever, scarlet fever, and diphtheria are traceable to the milk supply. It may also transmit *Brucella abortus*, the causative organism of undulant fever. Efficient protection against these diseases is obtained by boiling or pasteurizing the household supply of milk. Diarrhoea in children is often due to milk containing large quantities of bacteria. Tuberculosis may be communicated by the milk from disease affecting the cow itself. This risk is avoided by using milk from tuberculin-tested cows or by boiling or pasteurization.

MILK TEETH are the temporary teeth of children. (For the time of their appearance, see TEETH.)

MILLILITRE is the 1000th part of 1 litre. It is practically the equivalent of a cubic centimetre (1 c.c. = 0·999973 ml). Ml is the usual abbreviation for millilitre.

MIND DISORDERS (see MENTAL ILLNESS.)

MINDERERUS SPIRIT is an old name for *liquor ammonii acetatis*, a solution of ammonium acetate, which is much used in domestic medicine. It is a harmless substance, and acts as an antacid and diuretic, and helps to reduce feverishness. The usual dose is a dessert-spoonful or more, for colds and slight feverish conditions.

MINOCYCLINE is a long-acting tetracycline (qv) which is proving of value in the treatment of carriers of meningococci, or *Neisseria meningitidis* (see MENINGITIS), and in some cases of chronic bronchitis.

MIOSIS means a narrowing of the pupil. Some persons, largely on account of having a small amount of pigment in the eye, possess naturally small pupils but, apart from this, the condition is due usually to paralysis of the sympathetic nerve-fibres supplying the pupil, or to drugs such as opium and physostigmine.

MIOTIC means (*a*) causing the pupil of the eye to contract; (*b*) any agent which causes the pupil to contract such as physostigmine; (*c*) the pupil in the state of being contracted.

MISCARRIAGE (see ABORTION).

MITHRIDATISM is a term applied to immunity against the effects of poisons produced by administration of gradually increasing doses of the poison itself. The process is named after Mithridates, King of Pontus, who rendered himself immune against poisoning by this means.

MITOCHONDRIA are the rod-like bodies in the cells of the body (illustration 308) which contain the enzymes (qv) necessary for the activity of the cell. They have been described as the 'power plant of the cell'. (See CELLS.)

Mitochondria
Nucleus
Inclusion bodies
Golgi apparatus
Centrosphere
Nucleolus
Vacuole
Caryosome

308 – A semi-diagrammatic representation of a cell.

MITRAL STENOSIS is the term applied to the narrowing of the opening between the left atrium and left ventricle of the heart as a result of rigidity of, and adhesion between, the cusps of the mitral valve, due, almost invariably, to the infection of rheumatic fever.

MITRAL VALVE, so called from its resemblance to a bishop's mitre, is the valve which guards the opening between the atrium and ventricle on the left side of the heart. (See HEART.)

MOGIGRAPHIA is a term sometimes applied to writer's cramp. (See CRAMP.)

MOLAR TEETH are the last three teeth on each side of the jaw. (See TEETH.)

MOLE is a term used in two quite different senses. In the first place, a mole on the skin is a darkly pigmented spot, usually raised above the surrounding surface, rough, and covered with hair. These moles are of developmental origin, and malignant growths may spring from some of them late in life. Secondly the term hydatidiform mole is applied to cases in which, following upon conception, a degenerative mass forms in the womb, the embryo dying in the process; whilst the term, carneous mole, is applied to an ovum that has died in the early months of pregnancy.

MOLLITIES OSSIUM is another name for osteomalacia (qv).

MOLLUSCUM CONTAGIOSUM is the name given to a disease in which small tumours, seldom larger than peas, develop on the surface of the skin. It is due to a virus and is highly contagious, being most commonly conveyed from individual to individual in swimming baths and Turkish baths. Treatment is by freezing the nodules with liquid nitrogen. Alternatively, each nodule may be spiked with a sharpened orange stick which has been dipped in pure phenol.

MOLYBDENUM is a metallic element that occurs in all animal tissue. There is some evidence that deficiency of it plays a part in the causation of dental caries, and that a high intake of it, like fluorine, may protect against caries. There is also some evidence linking deficiency of molybdenum with cancer of the oesophagus (gullet).

MÖNCKEBERG'S SCLEROSIS (see ARTERIES, DISEASES OF).

MONGOLISM, or DOWN'S SYNDROME, is a variety of mental subnormality, in which the patient has Mongolian-like eyes, a snub nose, high cheek-bones, a large tongue, a small round skull, and short, thick hands and feet. Another characteristic feature is the palm print, which reveals distinctive markings: the most distinctive of these is the so-called four-finger line. The condition is often referred to as Down's syndrome (or disease) after Dr. J. L. H. Down, the London doctor who first described it in 1866.

The incidence is approximately 1 per 600 births, but the incidence in the community is lower than this, as many mongols die in infancy. This high death-rate is due partly to the fact that mongol children have a much higher incidence of other congenital deformities, such as malformations of the heart, than other children, and partly to their lower resistance to infection.

It is much commoner in children born to older women. Thus, the risk of having a mongol child in women over 45 is more than 1 in 60, compared with less than 1 in 1000 in women under 30. Fourteen per cent of children with mongolism are born to mothers over 40, 30 per cent to those aged 35 to 40. For mothers who give birth to a mongol child when they are younger the chances of a subsequent child being a mongol is relatively high. Precise figures in this respect can be misleading, and the best advice for a young mother who has had a mongol child, and who wishes to know the risk of her having another, is to go and discuss the matter with her family doctor.

In 95 per cent of cases the cause of mongolism is the presence of an extra chromosome (qv) in the ovum. The cause of this extra chromosome is not known. In the remaining cases the cause is a fault in the division of the germ cells known as translocation.

The degree of mental backwardness varies considerably. Up to a third of all severely mentally handicapped children of school age have mongolism. It has been estimated that 6 per cent of mongols are probably capable of profiting from attendance at schools for the educationally subnormal. Most mongols eventually acquire some degree of speech, and about 5 per cent learn to read. They practically never learn to write. Most learn to wash, dress and feed themselves, and many are able to run simple errands.

There is no known cure for the condition, but much can be done for them, especially if they can be kept at home rather than sent to an institution. Parents of mongol children seeking advice and help are recommended to get in touch with the Down's Children's Association, Quinborne Community Centre, Ridgacre Road, Quinton, Birmingham B32 2TW.

MONILIASIS is the infection caused by monilia, the genus of fungi now known as *Candida albicans*. The infection may occur in the mouth, where it is known as thrush [qv], lungs, intestine, vagina, skin, or nails.

MONKEYPOX is a smallpox-like disease, due to a virus which occurs in monkeys kept in captivity. Although a few cases have been reported in human beings in West and Central Africa, it is not at the moment considered to be a great risk to human beings.

MONKSHOOD (see ACONITE).

MONOAMINE OXIDASE INHIBITORS are drugs that destroy, or prevent the action of, monoamine oxidase (MAO). Monoamines, which include noradrenaline (qv) and tyramine, play an im-

portant part in the metabolism of the brain, and there is some evidence that excitement is due to an accumulation of monoamines in the brain. MAO is a naturally occurring enzyme (qv) which is concerned in the breakdown of monoamines.

An excessive accumulation of monoamines can induce a dangerous reaction characterized by high blood-pressure, palpitations, sweating and a feeling of suffocation. Hence the care with which MAO inhibitor drugs are administered. What is equally important, however, is that in no circumstances should a patient receiving any MAO inhibitor drug eat cheese, yeast preparations such as Marmite, tinned fish, or high game. The reason for this ban is that all these foodstuffs contain large amounts of tyramine which increases the amount of certain monoamines such as noradrenaline in the body. As can well be imagined such an increase in monoamines in a patient who is taking a full dose of a MAO inhibitor drug could be thoroughly unpleasant – if not disastrous.

There are also certain drugs, such as amphetamine and pethidine which must not be taken by a patient who is receiving an MAO inhibitor drug.

MONOMANIA means a kind of partial insanity, in which the affected person has a delusion upon one subject, though he can converse rationally and is a responsible individual upon other matters.

MONOPLEGIA means paralysis of a single limb or part. (See PARALYSIS.)

MONOSACCHARIDE is the term applied to a sugar having six carbon atoms in the molecule, such as glucose, galactose, and laevulose.

MONOSULFIRAM is a drug that is used in the treatment of scabies.

MOOREN'S ULCER is a degenerative ulcer of the eye.

MORBID means diseased.

MORBIFIC means disease-producing. For example, the *Vibrio cholerae* may be called the morbific agent in cholera.

MORBILLI is another name for measles.

MORBUS, the Latin word for disease, is used in such terms as morbus cordis (heart disease), morbus coxae (hip-joint disease).

MORON is the term applied to a feeble-minded person whose defect is relatively slight and whose mental age is somewhere between 8 and 12 years.

MORPHOEA is a form of circumscribed scleroderma. (See SCLERODERMA.)

MORPHINE, or MORPHIA, is the name of the chief alkaloid upon which the action of opium depends. (See OPIUM; and DRUG ADDICTION.)

MORTALITY (see DEATH, CAUSES OF; DEATH RATE; and INFANT MORTALITY).

MORTIFICATION is another name for gangrene. (See GANGRENE.)

MOSQUITOES. (See ANOPHELES; and BITES.)

MOTILIN is a hormone (qv) formed in the duodenum (qv) and the jejunum (qv) which plays a part in controlling the movements of the stomach and the gut.

MOTOR is a term applied to those nerves and tracts of fibres in the brain and spinal cord by which impulses are sent to the muscles, thus causing movements. (See SPINAL CORD.)

MOUNTAIN-SICKNESS is the name given to the group of symptoms which appear when people reach great heights, either in climbing mountains or in aeroplanes. Some persons suffer at lower altidues than others, but prolonged residence at a high level does not seem to prevent mountain-sickness when the person climbs higher. Persons who live habitually at a high altitude develop an increased proportion of red corpuscles in the blood and thus obtain a greater amount of oxygen from the rarefied air, and lose the tendency to mountain-sickness. Exhaustion, want of food, exposure to cold and a too rapid ascent bring it on sooner, but every one seems to begin to suffer when a height over 16,000 feet (4875 metres) is reached. Want of oxygen, in consequence of the rarefied atmosphere, is the cause. Weakness, difficulty of breathing, palpitation of the heart, giddiness, sickness, vomiting and finally unconsciousness, are the main symptoms, but these rapidly pass off, causing no per-

manent damage, when the person again reaches a lower level.

MOUTH is the cavity into which the food is first received, and where it is prepared by chewing and admixture with saliva for the early stages of digestion in the stomach. The mouth opens through the fauces, a narrow passage between the tonsils, into the pharynx or throat. The chief contents of the mouth are the edges of the jaw-bones bearing the teeth, and the tongue. The cavity is bounded above by the hard and soft palates, while beneath the tongue a layer of muscles, salivary glands, and other soft structures form the floor of the mouth. (See also TEETH; and TONGUE.)

MOUTH, DISEASES OF – The state of the mucous membrane lining the mouth as regards pallor, pigmentation, and other conditions gives a general idea of the extent to which other mucous membranes in the interior of the body are affected in, for example, anaemia, Addison's disease, jaundice. As the tongue consists essentially of a pointed mass of muscle wrapped round with mucous membrane, its condition as to shape and size gives valuable information regarding the general muscular state in debility, nervous diseases, and the like; while the mucous membrane covering it shows many marked changes in various diseases of the alimentary system and general maladies. (See also BURNING MOUTH.)

Conditions of the tongue – The *muscular condition* of the tongue is naturally such that the organ when at rest touches the lower set of teeth all round, and is slightly arched upwards. It should present a smooth surface, with a groove up the middle, and a sharp, even edge. Further, it is completely under control of the will, and can be moved in any direction. Now and then the tongue is too large for the mouth, rendering speech indistinct and even interfering with swallowing, or being so bulky that it is constantly protruded from the mouth. Such a condition, known as macroglossia, is either congenital or may result from inflammation. Tongue-tie is a congenital condition in which the band beneath the middle of the tongue uniting it to the floor of the mouth is either so short, or attached so far forwards, that the tongue cannot be fully protruded from the mouth, and cannot move with the freedom required for speech. This condition may be responsible for childish defects of speech but is much rarer than is popularly supposed. A flabby condition of the tongue, in which the organ is large, pale, and distinctly indented by the teeth along its edge, affords a sign of general debility. Tremulousness of the tongue when it is protruded is a sign of various nervous diseases, but by far its commonest cause is excessive indulgence in alcohol, of which it may form the only sign that cannot be concealed. After an apoplectic attack which has involved the nerve centre controlling one side of the tongue, this organ is protruded in a one-sided manner, pointing towards that side of the body which is paralysed, and the rapidity with which the person recovers the power to put the tongue out straight is a useful criterion of his progress towards recovery. Another important localizing sign in certain diseases of the brain and of the facial nerve is loss of the sense of taste on one side of the tongue.

A still more easily noticed sign is the presence or absence of *fur* on the tongue. This consists of a thickening of the superficial layers of the mucous membrane, due partly to increased growth, the result of fever and other conditions; partly to diminished use of the tongue, whose surface should constantly be rubbed down against the teeth and food. The fur is sometimes white, sometimes brown, or even black, from drying and the accumulation on it of materials derived from the food. It should be remembered that milk whitens the tongue and makes it look as if furred. Fevers of all sorts are associated with a furred tongue, and in typhoid fever perhaps, most of all, the fur accumulates till the tongue is covered with a thick mass, brown in the centre and yellow towards the edges, where the red mucous membrane is exposed. In scarlet fever there is often seen what is called a 'strawberry tongue', the general surface being covered with a white fur, through which project the red and inflamed points of the larger papillae with which the tongue is studded. Constipation and obstruction of the bowels are associated, as a rule, with a thick white or brownish fissured fur upon the tongue. Gastritis, particularly when due to excess in alcohol, is prone to cause a thin white fur; and the tremulous tongue coated in the mornings with fur, which wears off as the day advances, is one of the surest signs of habitual drinking. It is a noteworthy fact, however, that two of the most serious diseases of the stomach, cancer and gastric ulcer, are often associated with a remarkably clean tongue. All inflammatory affections of the throat, such

as tonsillitis, are apt to be accompanied by a thick, moist fur upon the tongue, very much resembling a layer of thick cream. In rheumatic fever a uniform yellowish fur often gives an appearance known as 'blanket tongue'. One half of the tongue may show a fur, while the rest of the surface is clean, and this is generally caused by neuralgia or by the presence of a bad tooth upon the furred side.

In some conditions the tongue may present a dry, red, *raw appearance*. An inflamed tongue ('beef tongue') is one of the characteristics of pellagra, a disease due to deficiency of nicotinic acid in the diet. A magenta-coloured tongue is said to be caused by deficiency of riboflavine in the diet.

Feeble children and persons brought very low by illness often develop small raised *white patches*, called thrush, upon the mucous membrane of the mouth and tongue. These are caused by the growth in its surface layer of a parasitic mould known as *Candida albicans*. Thrush is not of itself a serious condition, being easily removed by frequent application of borax-honey, or of glycerin of boric acid, to the affected spots. Nevertheless, the presence of this affection may indicate grave constitutional weakness.

A chronic condition, in which the tongue becomes studded with thickened, smooth, white patches, often separated by *deep fissures*, is known as leucoplakia. It develops gradually as the result of some long-standing irritation or inflammation of the tongue.

A slighter condition, in which the tongue shows white patches interspersed with sharply marked red, bare areas, is known as 'geographical tongue' or eczema of the tongue. It is a mild and usually transitory form of inflammation in which the surface layer of the mucous membrane on the tongue peels off, and it is usually associated with digestive disorders and a certain amount of general debility.

Ulcers on the tongue are common, but they generally remain of small size, and they do not differ from ulcers on other parts of the mouth, either in their cause or in their course. (See page 597.)

INFLAMMATION OF THE MOUTH, or STOMATITIS, arises from the same causes as inflammation elsewhere, but among the special causes may be noted a jagged or painful tooth, an ill-fitting plate, the cutting of teeth in children, alcohol, tobacco-smoking, digestive disturbance, and, in the special form of inflammation known as thrush (above mentioned), a parasitic mould. General ill-health plays an important part in the case both of children and of adults. Whatever be the cause, the mucous membrane becomes red, swollen, and tender, while small ulcers may in some cases develop here and there. Generally, the avoidance of highly spiced food, of alcohol, and of tobacco is sufficient to cure the condition, which may be soothed, while it lasts, by smearing on borax glycerin, or honey of borax.

The chronic inflammation of the gums (gingivitis) which arises in connection with unclean teeth, concealed inflammation within the sockets of the teeth, and pyorrhoea alveolaris, are forms of inflammation in the mouth which are treated under TEETH, DISEASES OF.

ULCERS OF THE MOUTH are usually of small size, and arise from a variety of causes. It is not at all uncommon in feeble, badly fed children for one or two ulcers to develop on the inside of the cheeks, on the gums, or on the tongue, causing pain in eating, profuse discharge of saliva, and great foetor of the breath. These ulcers generally heal when the child is well fed and a mouth-wash of chlorate of potash is often used, but they may pass on to the serious condition of cancrum oris. (See CANCRUM ORIS.) Single small ulcers arise in otherwise healthy people from the irritation of a jagged tooth, a small wound, or even apparently as the result of dyspepsia. These may be very troublesome, and, being generally situated in the groove between lip and gum, or on the tip and edge of the tongue, they are prevented from healing by the movement of the parts, and may remain very troublesome for weeks or even months. A small ulcer often develops beneath the tongue during the course of whooping-cough, as the result of friction against the lower teeth in coughing, and is prevented from healing by the same cause. The digestion must receive careful attention, the mouth must be kept clean by antiseptic washes and regular brushing of the teeth, and the ulcer may be touched with a strong astringent such as tincture of iodine or nitrate of silver every few days, and, in the interval, protected by occasional application of honey of borax or borax glycerin. Large ulcers may be of tuberculous, syphilitic or cancerous origin.

BAD TEETH form one of the commonest sources of complaint regarding the mouth. (See TEETH, DISEASES OF.)

GUMBOIL is a common minor disease. (See GUMBOIL.)

SALIVARY CALCULUS is a condition which sometimes occurs and may give rise to a good deal of trouble. (See CONCRETIONS.) The stone, if it lodges in one of the salivary ducts, may ulcerate out on the face, and then cause a fistula, from which saliva constantly trickles over the cheek. A fistula may be produced also by wounds of the cheek, involving the duct of the parotid gland. These fistulae are cured by an operation, which reopens a passage to the mouth and closes that upon the cheek.

RANULA is a clear, cyst-like swelling, appearing beneath the tongue in connection with the salivary glands in this region. It is a cyst full of saliva, and is treated by several minor surgical procedures, its obliteration being a simple matter.

MUMPS is an acute infective inflammation of the salivary glands. (See MUMPS.)

TUMOURS occur on the lips, on the alveolus bearing the teeth, arising either from the gums or bone, and most commonly on the tongue. Those which develop in the gum or bone beneath it go by the general name of epulis, whatever be their nature. Occasionally these are malignant; more often they are simple fibroid tumours, produced often by the irritation of decaying teeth. On extraction of the associated tooth or teeth and removal of the epulis it seldom gives more trouble. Growths upon the lips and tongue may be simple warts, or cysts may occasionally be found, but the commonest tumour of these parts is cancer. It seldom appears before the age of 40, and is much more common in men than in women. It is often associated with some form of *chronic* irritation such as a jagged tooth or smoking of a clay pipe. In other cases it follows prolonged chronic inflammation, such as syphilitic leukoplakia (qv). The glands on the front and sides of the neck in such cases soon become the seat of secondary malignant growths; and as the foul state of the interior of the mouth, after such a tumour ulcerates, causes much interference with the general health, the duration of life is not long, being little over a year after the tumour first appears if adequate treatment is not carried out. By modern surgical treatment, which aims at very free removal of the diseased part of the tongue and glands, life is prolonged, particularly in cases subjected to early operation, considerably beyond this period. The result of removal causes little or no disfigurement, and even when the whole tongue is removed the power of speech is often but little impaired. In cases which are detected early, satisfactory results are obtained from the use of radiotherapy.

MOVABLE KIDNEY (see KIDNEY, DISEASES OF).

MUCILAGE is prepared from acacia or tragacanth gum, and is used as an ingredient of mixtures containing solid particles in order to keep the latter from settling, and also as a demulcent. (See DEMULCENTS.)

MUCOCELE is an abnormally dilated cavity in the body due to the accumulation of mucus; such a 'cyst' may therefore form wherever there is mucous membrane.

MUCOCUTANEOUS LYMPH NODE SYNDROME is a disease that has been reported from Japan, Korea, Hawaii, Greece and the U.S.A., but not yet from Britain. The cause is not known. It occurs in young children, usually under the age of 5 years. It is characterized by fever, a generalized rash which becomes bright red on the hands and feet, and enlargement of the glands in the neck. Recovery usually occurs in two to four weeks. Complications sometimes occur in the form of meningitis, arthritis, jaundice, or myocarditis. The mortality rate is 1 to 2 per cent. There is no specific treatment.

MUCOLYTIC is the term used to describe the property of destroying, or lessening the tenacity of, mucus. It is most commonly used to describe drugs which have this property and are therefore used in the treatment of bronchitis (qv). The inhalation of steam, for example, has a mucolytic action.

MUCOMEMBRANOUS COLIC is the term applied to a disorder in which constipation, abdominal pain, and the passage of mucus or casts of mucus in the stools occurs in highly strung or neurotic people, especially women. The spasm of the colon causing these symptoms may be allergic in origin.

MUCOUS MEMBRANE is the general name given to the membrane which lines many of the hollow organs of the body. These membranes vary widely in structure in different sites, but all have the common character of being lubricated by mucus, derived in some cases from isolated cells on the surface of the membrane, but more generally from definite glands placed beneath the membrane,

and opening here and there through it by ducts (illustration 309). The air passages, the alimentary canal and the ducts of glands which open into it, and also the urinary passages, are all lined by mucous membrane.

309 – Section through the mucous membrane of the throat, showing two of the mucus-secreting glands. *e*, Epithelium of the surface; *ct*, connective tissue beneath it; *g*, gland; *d*, its duct opening on the surface; *a*, artery ending in a capillary network round the gland. Magnified 40 times.

In structure a mucous membrane consists of a basis of fibrous tissue resembling the true skin, though looser and lighter in texture, in which the blood-vessels, nerves, and mucous glands lie. This is covered on its surface by a layer of epithelium resembling the cuticle covering the skin, although the cells are in all cases of a more soft and succulent nature than those on the outer surface of the body.

It is in the character and properties of these cells that the various mucous membranes chiefly differ. In the air passages they are – almost everywhere except over the vocal cords – of a pillar-like shape and provided with thread-like processes, being known as ciliated cells (illustration 310). On the vocal cords the cells, which are exposed to constant friction, resemble those of the skin. In the alimentary system generally they are of a simple pillar-like

310 – Ciliated epithelial cells from the air passages.

311 – Columnar epithelium. *A*, side view of a group of cells; *B*, surface view of the ends of a group of cells; *C*, a columnar cell from the mucous membrane of the small intestine.

or columnar type (illustration 311), placed side by side, though in the mouth and gullet, where the food causes much friction, the surface, like that of the vocal cords, closely resembles the epidermis of the skin. In the urinary passages again the cells are ciliated, except in the bladder, where they approach in type to that of the skin epithelium.

Lying close beneath the epithelium there is, in most mucous membranes, a thin layer of involuntary muscle fibres, and to this, coupled with the extremely loose attachment of mucous membranes to the organs which they line, is due the great pliability and elasticity of these membranes.

MUCOUS PATCH is the name given to the syphilitic eruption as it affects mucous membranes. These patches are seen especially about the lips, mouth, and throat, and consist of slightly raised areas, reddish at the edge, and covered by a velvety whitish layer. They are very infectious. (See SYPHILIS.)

MUCOVISCIDOSIS (see FIBROCYSTIC DISEASE OF THE PANCREAS).

MUCUS is the general name for the slimy secretion derived from mucous membranes. It is mainly composed of a substance called mucin, which varies according to the particular mucous membrane from which it is derived, and it contains other substances, such as cells cast off from the surface of the membrane, ferments, and dust particles. From whatever source derived, mucin has the following characters: it is viscid, clear, and tenacious; when dissolved in water it can be precipitated by addition of acetic acid; and when not in solution already, it is dissolved by weak alkalis, such as lime-water.

Under normal conditions the surface of a mucous membrane is lubricated by only a small quantity of mucus; the appearance of large quantities is a sign of inflammation.

MULL is the name of a thin, soft muslin used in surgery. Plaster mull is the name given to a sheet of mull coated with gutta-percha and usually containing some drug or antiseptic for the treatment of skin disease.

MULTIGRAVIDA is a pregnant woman who has had more than one pregnancy.

MULTIPARA is a woman who has borne several children.

MULTIPLE BIRTHS – Twins occur about once in eighty pregnancies, triplets once in 6000, quadruplets about once in 500,000. Quintuplets are exceedingly rare. Such is the natural state of affairs. In recent years, however, the position has been altered by the introduction of the so-called fertility drugs, such as clomiphene (qv), which, through the medium of the pituitary gland, stimulate the production of ova. Their wide use in the treatment of infertility has resulted in an increase in the number of multiple births, a recognized hazard of giving too large a dose. So far as fraternal twins are concerned, multiple pregnancy may be an inherited tendency; it certainly occurs more often in certain families, but this may be partly due to chance. A woman who has already given birth to twins is ten times more likely to have another multiple pregnancy than one who has not previously had twins. In 1974, a Swedish mother, who had not had any fertility drugs, gave birth to her third lot of twin girls. Both she and her husband were twins themselves. The statistical chance of a third pair of twins was said to be 1 in 512,000. Identical twins do not run in families.

Twins may be binovular or uniovular. *Binovular*, or *fraternal*, *twins* are the result of the mother releasing two ova within a few days of each other and both being fertilized by separate spermatozoa. They both develop separately in the mother's womb and are no more alike than is usual with members of the same family. They are three times as common as *uniovular*, *or identical*, *twins*, who are developed from a single ovum fertilized by a single spermatozoon, but which has split early in development. This is why they are usually so remarkably alike in looks and mental characteristics. Unlike binovular twins, who may be of the same or different sex, they are always of the same sex.

The relative proportion of twins of each type varies in different races. Identical twins have much the same frequency all over the world: around 3 per 1000 maternities. Fraternal twins are rare in Mongolian races: less than 3 per 1000 maternities. In whites they occur two or three times as often as identical twins: between 7 (Spain and Portugal) and 10 (Czechoslovakia and Greece) per 1000 maternities. They are more common in Negroes, reaching 30 per 1000 maternities in certain West African populations. (See also SIAMESE TWINS.)

MULTIPLE SCLEROSIS is a disease of the brain and spinal cord, which, though slow in its onset, in time may produce marked symptoms, such as paralysis and tremors, and may ultimately render persons suffering from it confirmed invalids. It consists of hardened patches, from the size of a pin-head to that of a pea or larger, scattered here and there irregularly through the brain and cord, each patch being made up of a mass of the connective tissue (neuroglia), which should be present only in sufficient amount to bind the nerve-cells and fibres together. In the earliest stage, the insulating sheaths of the nerve-fibres in the hardened patches break up, are absorbed, and leave the nerve-fibres bare, the connective tissue being later formed between these.

Cause – Although this is one of the most common diseases of the central nervous system in Europe – there are around 50,000 affected individuals in Britain alone – the cause is still not known. The disease comes on in young people (onset being rare after the age of 40), apparently without previous illness. There may be a hereditary factor, but this is by no means proven. If such exists it is of an obscure nature and linked more to a defect in the individual's reaction to infection than to any precise defect in the nervous system. The actual changes in the nervous system appear to be due to the action of some substance which dissolves or breaks up the fatty matter of the nerve-sheaths.

Symptoms – These depend greatly upon the part of the brain and cord affected by the sclerotic patches. Temporary paralysis of a limb, or of an eye muscle, causing double vision, and tremors upon exertion, first in the affected parts, and later in all parts of the body, are early symptoms. Stiffness of the lower limbs causing the toes to catch on small irregularities in the ground and trip the person in walking, is often an annoying symptom and one of the first to be noticed. Great activity is shown in the reflex movements obtained by striking the tendons and by stroking the soles of the feet. The latter reflex shows a characteristic sign (Babinski sign) in

which the great toe bends upwards and the other toes spread apart as the sole is stroked, instead of the toes collectively bending downwards as in the normal person. Tremor of the eye movements (nystagmus) is usually found. Trembling handwriting, interference with the functions of the bladder, giddiness, and a peculiar 'staccato' or 'scanning' speech are common symptoms at a later stage. Numbness and tingling in the extremities occur commonly, particularly in the early stages of the disease. As the disease progresses, the paralyses, which were before transitory, now become confirmed, often with great rigidity in the limbs. Many cases progress very slowly and show little or no tendency to shortening of the duration of life.

People with multiple sclerosis, and their relatives, can obtain help and guidance from the Multiple Sclerosis Society. 4 Tachbrook Street, London SW1 1SJ. Another helpful organization is Action for Research into Multiple Sclerosis (71 Grays Inn Road, London WC1X 8TR) which provides a London-based telephone counselling service for those with the disease and their families. Those with sexual or marital problems arising out of the illness can obtain help from the Committee on Sexual Problems of the Disabled, 40 Victoria Street, London, SW1.

Treatment is unsatisfactory, because the most that can be done is, to lead a life as free from strain as possible, to check the progress of the disease. It is important to keep the nerves and muscles functioning, and therefore the patient should remain at his work as long as he is capable of doing it, and in any case should regularly exercise the lower limbs by walking and the upper limbs by carrying out movements requiring coordination, such as knitting or embroidery. In some cases protein shock by injections of peptone or anti-typhoid vaccine in doses sufficient to produce a moderate rise of temperature may help. (See PROTEIN SHOCK.) Arsenic, usually as Fowler's solution, is sometimes of temporary value. Injections of liver extract and vitamin B_1 have also been recommended, as have a host of different diets, but none of these has stood up to the test of time. Corticosteroids seem to be as effective a means as any of slowing up the progress of the disease, but they can only be used under skilled medical supervision.

MUMPS, also known as EPIDEMIC PAROTITIS, CYNANCHE PAROTIDEA, and popularly known as 'THE BRANKS', is an infectious disease characterized by inflammatory swelling of the parotid and other salivary glands, often occurring as an epidemic, and affecting mostly young persons.

Causes – Mumps is due to infection with a virus and is highly infectious from person to person. It is predominantly a disease of childhood and early adult life, but it can occur at any age. Epidemics usually occur in the winter and spring. It is infectious for two or three days before the swelling of the glands appears.

Symptoms – There is a long incubation period of two to three weeks after infection before the glands begin to swell. The first signs are fatigue, slight feverishness, and sore throat, which may precede the swelling by a day or two. The gland first affected is generally the parotid, situated in front of and below the ear. Along with the swelling there is often some face-ache and considerable rise of temperature to 101° or even 104° F (38·3° or 40° C). The swelling usually spreads to the submaxillary and sublingual glands lying beneath the jaw, and to the glands on the side opposite that first affected. There is hardly ever any redness or tendency to suppuration in the swollen parts, although interference with the acts of chewing and swallowing may occasion a good deal of trouble, and the swelling is tender to touch. After continuing four or five days, the swelling abates, the temperature having generally already fallen. In 15 to 30 per cent of males, inflammation of the testicles (orchitis) develops. This usually occurs during the second week of the illness, but may not occur until two or three weeks later. It may result in partial atrophy of the testicles, but practically never in infertility. In a much smaller proportion of females with mumps, inflammation of the ovaries or breasts may occur. Inflammation of the pancreas, accompanied by tenderness in the upper part of the abdomen and digestive disturbances, sometimes occurs. Meningitis is also an occasional complication. The various complications are found much more often when the disease affects adults than when it occurs in childhood.

Treatment – The patient must be confined to bed for at least a week or ten days, and kept in isolation for 14 days from the onset of the disease or 7 days from the subsidence of all swelling. Soft food, and the protection of the inflamed parts by a strip of flannel or by cotton-wool and a handkerchief are all the treatment usually required. If there be much face-ache, it is relieved by warm fomentations or aspirin.

MURIATIC ACID is an old name for hydrochloric acid.

MURMUR is the name given to an uneven, rustling sound heard by auscultation over the heart and various blood-vessels in abnormal conditions. For example, murmurs heard when the stethoscope is applied over the heart are highly characteristic of valvular disease of this organ.

MUSCAE VOLITANTES is a term signifying the floating specks which become visible when the eye looks steadily at a white ground in bright light. These specks are present in most eyes and can be seen at any time, but they become especially noticeable when the general health is depressed, and sometimes cause great annoyance through the fear that they may be the sign of some eye disease. They are due to the presence of filaments and cells in the vitreous humour of the eye, which, though transparent, are rather denser than the rest of the humour, and sufficiently opaque to cast a shadow upon the retina. These shadows are referred outwards as floating objects in the field of vision.

MUSCARINE is the poisonous principle found in some toadstools. (See FUNGUS-POISONING.)

MUSCLE, popularly known as FLESH, is the tissue by which, in virtue of its power of contraction, movements are made in the higher animals. Muscular tissue is divided, according to its function, into two great groups, *voluntary muscle* and *involuntary muscle*, of which the former is under control of the will, whilst the latter discharges its functions independently. The term *striped muscle* is often given to voluntary muscle, because under the microscope all the voluntary muscles show a striped appearance, whilst involuntary muscle is, in the main, unstriped or plain. There are exceptions to the latter statement, for the heart muscle, which is involuntary, is partially striped, while certain muscles of the throat, and two small muscles inside the ear, not controllable by will-power, are also striped.

Structure of muscle – VOLUNTARY MUSCLE is disposed in a regular method over the body, being mainly attached to the skeleton, and hence often called skeletal muscle. There are certain definite

312 – A muscle fibre splitting up into fibrils.

muscles, and these vary as to shape only slightly in different persons, although in one person particular muscles may be developed to a much greater bulk than in others. Each muscle is enclosed in a sheath of fibrous tissue, known as fascia or epimysium, and, from this, partitions of fibrous tissue, known as perimysium, run into the substance of the muscle, dividing it up into small bundles. Each of these bundles, if carefully examined, will be found to consist in turn of a collection of fibres, which form the units of the muscle. Each fibre is about 50 micrometres in thickness and ranges in length from a few millimetres to 300 millimetres. If the fibre be cut across and examined under a high-powered microscope, it is seen to be further divided into fibrils (illustration 312). Each fibre is enclosed in an elastic sheath of its own, which allows of its lengthening and shortening, and is known as the sarcolemma. Within the sarcolemma lie numerous nuclei belonging to the muscle fibre, which was originally developed from a simple cell. To the sarcolemma, at either end, is attached a minute bundle of connective-tissue fibres which unites the muscle fibre to its neighbours, or to one of the connective tissue partitions in the muscle, and by means of these connections the fibre produces its effect upon contracting. The sarcolemma is pierced by a nerve fibre, which breaks up upon the surface of the muscle fibre into a complicated end-plate, and by this means each muscle fibre is brought under the guidance of the central nervous system, and the discharge of energy which produces muscular contraction is controlled. When the muscle fibre within the sarcolemma is examined by a high magnifying power, it is found to show alternate light and dark transverse stripes, with a fine dotted line, called Dobie's line (illustration 313) or Krause's membrane, across the middle of each light stripe.

These appearances are due to the fact that the fibre is composed of segments made up partly of fibrous connective material, partly of semi-fluid contractile tissue, in which visible changes take place as the fibre contracts.

Between the muscle fibres, which have, on account of their relative length and width, a pillar-like shape, run many capillary blood-vessels. They are so placed that the contractions of the muscle fibres empty them at once of blood, and thus the active muscle is ensured a specially good blood supply. None of these vessels, however, pierces the sarcolemma surrounding the fibres, so that the blood does not come into direct contact with the muscular tissue, whose nourishment is carried on by the lymph that exudes from the blood-vessels. The lymph circulation is also automatically varied, as required, by the muscular contractions. Between the muscle fibres, and enveloped in a sheath of connective tissue, lie here and there special structures known as muscle-spindles. Each of these contains thin muscle fibres, numerous nuclei, and the endings of sensory nerves. They appear to be the sensory organs of the muscles. (See TOUCH.)

INVOLUNTARY MUSCLE includes, as already stated, the heart muscle and unstriped muscle. The heart muscle stands in structure between striped and unstriped muscle (illustration 314). Each fibre is short, has a nucleus in its centre, communicates with its neighbours by short branches, shows a faintly striped appearance near its exterior, and is devoid of sarcolemma.

Plain or unstriped muscle is found in the following positions: the inner and middle coats of the stomach and intestines; the ureters and urinary bladder; the windpipe and bronchial tubes; the ducts of glands; the gall-bladder; the uterus and Fallopian tubes; the middle

313 – Portion of a muscle fibre showing the alternate dark and light stripes, with Dobie's line in the clear stripe. Magnified about 500 times.

314 – Longitudinal section of human heart-muscle fibres. From *Hewer's Textbook of Histology*. William Heinemann, Ltd.

coat of the blood- and lymph-vessels; the iris and ciliary muscle of the eye; the dartos tunic of the scrotum; and in association with the various glands and hairs in the skin. The fibres are very much smaller than those of striped muscle, although they vary greatly in size. Each is pointed at the ends, has one or more oval nuclei in the centre, and a delicate sheath of sarcolemma enveloping it. The fibres are grouped in bundles, much as are the striped fibres, but they adhere to one another by cement material, not by the tendon bundles found in voluntary muscle.

Development of muscle – All the muscles of the developing individual arise from the central layer (mesoderm) of the embryo, each fibre taking origin from a single cell. Later on in life, muscles have the power both of increasing in size, as the result of use, for example, in athletes, and also of healing, after parts of them have been destroyed by injury. This takes place partly by the growth and splitting of the original fibres to form new fibres, and partly from reserve cells, known as sarcoplasts, which lie in every muscle between the muscle fibres. An example of the great extent to which unstriped muscle can develop, to meet the demands made upon its power, is given by the womb, whose muscular wall develops so much during pregnancy that the organ increases from the weight of 1 to 1½ ounces (30 to 40 grams) to a weight of around 2 pounds (1 kilogram), decreasing again to

its former small size in the course of a month after child-birth.

Physiology of contraction – A muscle is an elaborate chemico-physical system for producing heat and mechanical work. The total energy liberated by a contracting muscle can be exactly measured. From 25 to 30 per cent of the total energy expended is used in mechanical work. A steam engine puts out between 7 to 20 per cent of its energy in work. Muscle is therefore mechanically much more efficient. The heat of contracting muscle makes an important contribution to the maintenance of the heat of the body. (See also MYOGLOBIN.)

The energy of muscular contraction is derived from a complicated series of chemical reactions. Complex substances are broken down and built up again, supplying each other with energy for this purpose. The first reaction is the break-down of adenyl-pyrophosphate into phosphoric acid and adenylic acid (derived from nucleic acid); this supplies the immediate energy for contraction. Next phosphocreatine breaks down into creatine and phosphoric acid, giving energy for the resynthesis of adenyl-pyrophosphate. Creatine is a normal nitrogenous constituent of muscle. Then glycogen through the intermediary stage of sugar bound to phosphate breaks down into lactic acid to supply energy for the resynthesis of phosphocreatine. Finally part of the lactic acid is oxidized to supply energy for building up the rest of the lactic acid into glycogen again. If there is not enough oxygen, lactic acid accumulates and fatigue results.

There are some points to be noticed in this modern version of muscular activity. First, muscle contraction and relaxation take place in the absence of oxygen – the anaerobic phase. Secondly, oxygen comes into the picture in the phase of recovery, and by oxidizing some of the lactic acid winds up the contractile mechanism once more. Thirdly, the energy of contraction does not come directly from the break-down of glycogen.

The whole of the chemical changes are mediated by the action of several enzymes.

Involuntary muscle has several peculiarities of contraction. In the heart *rhythmicality* is an important feature, one beat appearing to be, in a sense, the cause of the next beat. *Tonus* is a character of all muscle, but particularly of unstriped muscle in some localities, as in the walls of arteries. Muscles are not held either slack or taut, but in a slightly stretched condi-

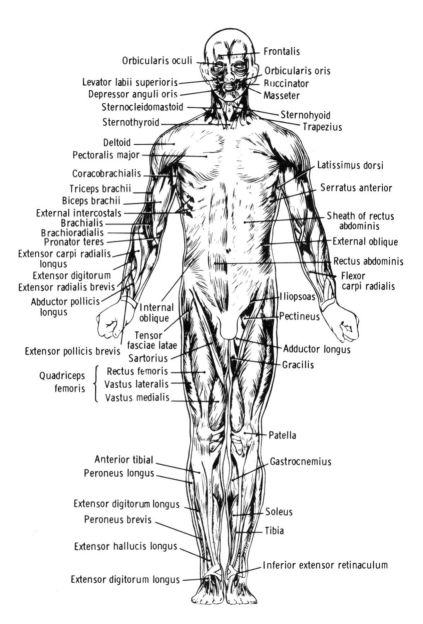

Orbicularis oculi

Levator labii superioris
Depressor anguli oris
Sternocleidomastoid
Sternothyroid

Deltoid
Pectoralis major
Coracobrachialis
Triceps brachii
Biceps brachii
External intercostals
Brachialis
Brachioradialis
Pronator teres
Extensor carpi radialis
longus
Extensor digitorum
Extensor radialis brevis
Abductor pollicis
longus

Internal
oblique

Tensor
fasciae latae
Extensor pollicis brevis
Sartorius

Quadriceps
femoris
Rectus femoris
Vastus lateralis
Vastus medialis

Anterior tibial
Peroneus longus

Extensor digitorum longus
Peroneus brevis

Extensor hallucis longus

Extensor digitorum longus

Frontalis
Orbicularis oris
Buccinator
Masseter
Sternohyoid
Trapezius

Latissimus dorsi
Serratus anterior

Sheath of rectus
abdominis
External oblique

Rectus abdominis
Flexor
carpi radialis

Iliopsoas
Pectineus

Adductor longus
Gracilis

Patella

Gastrocnemius

Soleus
Tibia

Inferior extensor retinaculum

315 – Muscles on the front of the body.

Sternocleidomastoid
Splenius capitis

Trapezius

Rhomboid major

Teres minor
Teres major

Latissimus dorsi

External abdominal
oblique

Gluteus medius

Gluteus maximus

Gracilis

Adductor magnus
Semitendinosus
Biceps femoris (long head)

Semimembranosus

Plantaris

Gastrocnemius

Soleus

Peroneus longus
Flexor digitorum longus
Peroneus brevis
Calcaneus tendon (Achilles)

Deltoid

Triceps brachii (long head)

Triceps brachii (lateral head)

Brachioradialis

Extensor carpi radialis
longus
Anconeus

Flexor carpi ulnaris
Extensor carpi ulnaris
Extensor digitorum

Extensor carpi radialis
brevis
Abductor pollicis longus

Extensor pollicis brevis

Iliotibial band

Biceps femoris (short head)

316 – Muscles on the back of the body.

605

tion, so that when occasion arises they are ready for instant action, while the arteries owe their elasticity and strength mainly to this fact. The involuntary muscle, forming the middle coat of the bowels, gland-ducts, and other tubes, contracts in the so-called *vermicular movement*, or peristalsis, which means that a ring of contraction passes slowly along the tube, at a rate of about 1 inch (25 mm) per second, the muscle relaxing as the ring of contraction passes on.

Fatigue of muscle comes on when a muscle is made to act for some time. It is due, not to wearing out of the muscle's power, but to the accumulation of waste products, especially sarcolactic acid, produced by the muscle's activity. These substances affect the end plates of the nerve controlling the muscle, and so prevent destructive over-action of the muscle. As they are rapidly swept away by the blood, the muscle, after a rest, particularly if the rest be accompanied by massage or by gentle contractions to quicken the circulation, recovers rapidly from the fatigue. After great muscular activity over the whole body, a more lasting fatigue is produced by the accumulation of these products, and by their action upon the central nervous system, this being recovered from after a prolonged rest, during which the waste substances are excreted by the lungs, kidneys, and other excretory organs.

Rigor mortis is a condition which comes on in the muscles after death, and to which the general stiffening of the body is due. It consists in a state of permanent, wasteful contraction, beginning in the muscles of the neck and lower jaw at a period which varies from ten minutes to seven hours after death, and spreading gradually over the whole body. It comes on quickest after death from exhaustion, or from some weakening disease; and, occasionally, after violent injuries causing death, it comes on instantaneously, so that the posture of the body is fixed in the attitude in which death occurs. The rigidity lasts usually from sixteen to twenty-four hours, but its duration is extremely variable, being longer, as a rule, when its onset has been slow. (See DEATH, SIGNS OF.)

Muscular system, popularly known as 'the flesh', comprises all the voluntary muscles (illustrations 315, 316), and amounts in an average man of 154 pounds (70 kg) to about 77 pounds (35 kg), or half of the whole body weight. The total number of the voluntary muscles, each of which is named, amounts to about 620, including the muscles of both sides.

Each muscle constitutes a separate organ, controlled by a special nerve or nerves, which connect it with the spinal cord and brain, where, however, actions and combined movements are represented rather than individual muscles. (See BRAIN.) The fleshy part of the muscle is known as its belly, and there is usually at either end a tendon, by which the muscle is inserted into bone or other structure, upon which it acts. One end is more fixed than the other, as a rule, the rigid end being known as the origin of the muscle, the more mobile end as its insertion.

UPPER LIMB – *Between the trunk and limb* run the following muscles: the trapezius, latissimus dorsi, large and small rhomboids, and levator of the angle of the scapula, behind; and the large and small pectoral, the subclavius, and serratus anterior muscles in front. *In the shoulder region* lie the deltoid, supraspinatus, infraspinatus, large and small teres, and the subscapular muscles. *In the upper arm* the coracobrachialis, biceps, and brachialis occupy the front, while the triceps fills up the back of the arm. *In the forearm* the muscles in front that bend the wrist and fingers, or turn the hand palm downwards, are the pronator teres, the radial flexor of the wrist, the long palmar, the ulnar flexor of the wrist, the superficial and deep flexors of the fingers, the long flexor of the thumb, and the pronator quadratus; while the muscles on the back of the forearm that extend the fingers and bend the wrist backwards, or turn the hand palm upwards, are the supinator, longer and shorter radial extensors of the wrist, extensor of the fingers, extensor of the little finger, ulnar extensor of the wrist, the extensors of the metacarpal bone, of the first joint, and of the second joint of the thumb, and the extensor of the forefinger. *In the palm of the hand* there are four lumbrical muscles, the short palmar muscle, three muscles each for the thumb and little finger, which respectively abduct, oppose, and flex these digits, an adductor of the thumb, and, in the spaces between the metacarpal bones, seven interosseous muscles.

LOWER LIMB – *Muscles of the hip* are the iliacus in front, and, behind, the three gluteus muscles forming the prominence of the buttock, with the pyriform, external and internal obturator, two gemelli, and quadratus femoris muscles under cover of the largest gluteal muscle, while to the outer side lies the tensor of the sheath of the thigh. *On the back of the thigh* lie the biceps, semitendinosus, and semimembranosus muscles, whose tendons, standing out prominently behind the knee, are known collectively as the ham-strings. *In front of the thigh* are placed the sartorius, which is the longest, and the quadriceps extensor of the leg, which is the largest muscle of the body. *On the inner side of the thigh* lie the gracilis and pectineus muscles, with the long, the short, and the large adductors. *On the front of the leg* are placed the tibialis anterior, the long extensor of the great toe, the long extensor of the toes, and the peroneus tertius muscles. *On the outer side of the leg* are two muscles, the long and short peroneal muscles, whose tendons pass down behind the outer ankle to the foot. *On the back of the leg* are two groups of muscles. The superficial group of three muscles, consisting of the gastrocnemius, a double-bellied muscle, and the soleus, which is flat and projects slightly beneath the gastrocnemius, together with the small plantaris muscle, forms the calf of the leg, and ends in the tendo Achillis behind the heel. The deep group lies close upon the bones, and consists of the popliteus, long flexor of the toes, long flexor of the great toe, and tibialis posterior muscles, the tendons of the last three passing down behind the inner ankle. *In the foot* there is one muscle, the short extensor of the toes, upon the 'dorsum' or upper surface; while in the sole of the foot are four layers of small muscles, comprising the short flexor of the toes, and abductors of the great and little toes; the accessory flexor of the toes, and four lumbrical muscles; the short flexor of the great toe, oblique and transverse adductors of the great toe, and short flexor of the little toe; and in the fourth layer seven interosseous muscles, as in the hand.

FACE AND HEAD – Attached to the auricle of the ear are three muscles of feeble power, which raise, draw back, and flatten the auricle. The eyelids, nose, and lips are provided with numerous flattened muscles, which dilate and draw together these openings, and which form the means by which varying facial expression is brought about.

The movements of the eye-ball are effected by six small muscles. (See EYE.) The movements of the lower jaw in chewing are controlled by four muscles on each side: the masseter muscle, which can be felt on the hinder part of the cheek as the jaws are closed; the temporal muscle, felt in the region of the temple; and the outer and inner pterygoid muscles, attached to the deep surface of the jaw-bone. Within the mouth the tongue consists of certain

intrinsic muscle bundles, together with four muscles on each side, which connect it with the lower jaw, hyoid bone, and base of the skull. The floor of the mouth is formed by four muscles, which pass from the hyoid bone in front of the neck up to the lower jaw and base of the skull. The throat or pharynx, which is open in front to the nose, the mouth, and the larynx, one beneath the other, is closed behind by three broad, flat muscles, the superior, middle, and inferior constrictors of the pharynx, and is swung from the base of the skull by the stylopharyngeus muscle on either side. The soft palate, which separates the hinder part of the cavities of nose and mouth from one another, consists of five muscles on each side covered by mucous membrane. The larynx is controlled by eleven small muscles, which open or close its opening, and render the vocal cords more or less tense in the production of the voice.

FRONT OF NECK – The most prominent feature of the neck is the thick sternocleidomastoid muscle, which on each side runs from behind the ear downwards and forwards to the breast-bone and collarbone. Partly under cover of these and protecting the front of the larynx are four small muscles on each side: the sternohyoid, sternothyroid, thyrohyoid, and omohyoid muscles. Deep in the neck, behind, and to either side of the windpipe, gullet, and large blood-vessels, lie the anterior, middle, and posterior scalene muscles, which pass from the spinal column to the upper two ribs. Lying close upon the spine are three rectus muscles on each side, which bend the head upon the spine, and the long muscle of the neck, which bends the spine in this region.

BACK OF THE NECK AND TRUNK – The muscles in this region form a very complicated system, most arising from the spines or transverse processes of several vertebrae or from a number of ribs, and running upwards to be attached to another series of vertebrae or ribs some distance above, whilst the upper muscles of the set are attached to the hinder portion of the skull. These muscles form a couple of strong columns running the whole length of the back from the loins to the head, with a groove between in which the line of vertebral spines can be felt. The upper and lower serrated muscles of the back are muscles of respiration passing from ribs to spine, and, together with the splenius muscle in the neck, form a superficial layer. Beneath them the erector spinae, the great muscle which supports the back, runs the whole distance from the sacrum to the skull, obtaining at numerous points attachments to the spines and transverse processes of the vertebrae and to the neighbouring portions of the ribs. This muscle, along with those about to be mentioned, is of great power, having, even in moderately strong persons, a lifting power of 200 to 400 pounds (90 to 180 kg). Covered by the erector is the transversospinalis group of muscles, in which all the muscles ascend with an inward inclination; a series of short muscles connecting succeeding vertebrae with one another; and four small muscles passing from the uppermost two vertebrae to the skull. These last-named muscles incline and rotate the trunk and head from side to side.

CHEST – The diaphragm is the chief muscle of this part of the body. (See DIAPHRAGM.) Next in importance come the outer and inner intercostal muscles, which form a double layer of oblique fibres filling up the gaps between the ribs, the fibres of the two muscles running in different directions. There are also levators of the ribs, which pass each from a vertebra to the rib beneath it, and subcostal muscles which are of feeble development. All these muscles share in the act of inspiration.

ABDOMEN – The sides and front of the abdomen, unprotected by any bone beneath the level of the ribs, are enclosed by thick muscular layers strengthened by sheets of fibrous tissue. On the sides of the abdomen are three muscles: the external oblique, consisting of fibres which run downwards and forwards from the lower eight ribs; the internal oblique, under cover of the first, consisting of fibres which run upwards and forwards from the haunch-bone, and fibrous layers in its neighbourhood; and thirdly, the transversalis muscle, the fibres of which run horizontally forward from the lower six ribs, the lumbar vertebrae, and the haunch-bone. The fibres of all three muscles end along a curved line, the semilunar line, which is plainly visible upon the surface of the abdomen, running with a curve from its upper to its lower end, and distant, at the level of the navel, some 4 or 5 inches (10 or 12·5 cm) from the middle line. From the curved line a sheet of dense fibrous tissue runs inwards, those of the two sides meeting down the middle line of the body. Embedded in this fibrous sheet is a strong muscle upon each side, the rectus abdominis, which is 3 or 4 inches (7·5 or 10 cm) broad, almost an inch (25 mm) thick in muscular persons, and runs vertically

from the front of the pelvis up to the lower part of the chest. It is a muscle of great strength, and is divided into four or five sections, by tendinous intervals, which run across the muscle, and which, in well-developed persons, form distinct transverse depressions on the front of the abdomen. The quadratus lumborum is still another muscle situated, behind, in the gap between the last rib and the haunch-bone. Other small muscles close the lower opening of the pelvis, and are associated with the functions of the bowel and genital organs.

MUSCLES, DISEASES OF – The muscles are singularly free from liability to diseases which commonly affect other tissues, this being the result, probably, of their activity, good blood supply, and the changes constantly taking place in them. Wasting of muscles sometimes occurs as a symptom of disease in other organs: for example, damage to the nervous system, as in poliomyelitis or in the disease known as progressive muscular atrophy. (See PARALYSIS.)

INFLAMMATION (myositis) of various types may occur. As the result of injury, an abscess may develop (see ABSCESS), although wounds affecting muscle generally heal well. Tuberculous inflammation in muscles is almost unknown. A growth due to syphilis, known as a gumma, sometimes forms a hard, almost painless swelling in a muscle. Rheumatism is a type of chronic inflammation (see RHEUMATISM) to which muscles are very liable. Fibroid and even bony degeneration may occur in muscles which are the seat of long-continued irritation, or which receive a poor blood supply, the former, for example, taking place under certain conditions in the heart, the latter affecting the thigh muscles of those who ride much.

RUPTURE of a muscle may occur, without any external wound, as the result of a spasmodic effort. It may tear the muscle right across, as sometimes happens to the feeble plantaris muscle in running and leaping, or part of the muscle may be driven through its fibrous envelope, forming a hernia of the muscle. The severe pain experienced in many cases of lumbago is due to tearing of one of the muscles in the back. These conditions give rise to considerable pain, but are relieved by rest and massage.

MYASTHENIA (see MYASTHENIA GRAVIS).

PAIN, quite apart from any inflammation or injury, may be experienced on exertion. This type of pain, known as myalgia, occurs especially in weakly persons, and is then relieved by rest and physiotherapy. It is also one of the common forms of rheumatism. In young children, pains of an aching character are often experienced in the muscles, especially of the legs and back, and are known as growing pains (qv). These come on especially after exertion and are relieved by resting.

CRAMP is a well-known condition due to spasm. (See CRAMP.)

MUSTARD is a yellowish powder, consisting of the dried, ripe seeds of *Brassica nigra* and *Brassica alba* mixed together. The former contains an active principle called sinigrin, the latter contains one named sinalbin, while both contain a quantity of a ferment named myrosin, which in the presence of water converts the two active principles into the volatile oil to which the action of mustard is due. This oil is extremely irritating to skin and mucous surfaces with which it is brought in contact.

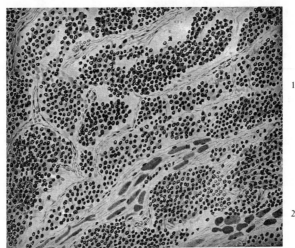

317 – Small round-celled sarcoma of muscle. (1) Sarcoma cells, (2) muscle fibres. Kettle's *Pathology of Tumours*. H. K. Lewis & Co. Ltd.

PARASITES sometimes lodge in the muscles, the most common being *Trichinella spiralis*, producing the disease known as trichinosis. (qv)

TUMOURS are occasionally met with, the most common being fibroid, fatty, and sarcomatous growths (illustration 317).

MYOPATHY is a term applied to a developmental defect in certain muscles. (See MYOPATHY.)

MUSCULAR DYSTROPHY (see MYOPATHY).

MUSHROOM POISONING (see FUNGUS-POISONING).

MUSHROOM-WORKER'S LUNG is a form of lung disease that occurs in mushroom workers as a result of their being hypersensitive to mushrooms. (See ALVEOLITIS.)

Uses – Externally mustard is used made into a paste with water and spread upon brown or cartridge paper, or made up with linseed into a poultice, for its irritant action upon the skin, in cases of rheumatism, inflamed joints, neuralgia, and for application to the chest and abdomen when organs in these cavities are inflamed. These applications should not, as a rule, last longer than twenty minutes. Liniment of mustard is used for similar purposes. In a hot or cold bath one or two tablespoonfuls of mustard have an invigorating effect. (For Mustard Pack, see WET PACK.) The effect of mustard, if too pronounced, may be relieved by applying olive oil.

Internally, mustard is used in small quantities as a stimulant to digestion, and in large quantities as an emetic, a tablespoonful of mustard powder being stirred up in a tumblerful of cold water for the latter purpose.

MUSTINE is the *British Pharmaco-poeia* name for the *bis* form of nitrogen mustard. The nitrogen mustards have an action comparable to that of ionizing radiation and inhibit cell division. Mustine is used in the treatment of chronic leukaemia and Hodgkin's disease.

MYALGIA means pain in a muscle. (See LUMBAGO; RHEUMATISM; BORNHOLM DISEASE.)

MYASTHENIA GRAVIS is the name given to a serious disorder, in which the chief symptoms are muscular weakness and a special tendency for fatigue to come on rapidly when efforts are made. The incidence is around 1 in 30,000.

The cause of the disease is not accurately known, but the symptoms are due to deficiency in the muscles of acetylcholine which is necessary for muscular contraction. It affects, as a rule, persons in early adult life. Not only the voluntary muscles, but those connected with the acts of swallowing, breathing, and the like, become infiltrated with small round cells and progressively weaker, though there is no very marked wasting. Rest and avoidance of undue exertion, so as carefully to husband the strength, are necessary, and regular doses of neostigmine bromide, or pyridostigmine at intervals enable the muscles to be used and in some cases have a curative effect. Good results are obtained in certain cases by surgical removal of the thymus.

MYCOPLASMA is a genus of micro-organisms which differ from bacteria in that they lack a rigid cell wall. They are responsible for widespread epidemics in cattle and poultry. The only member of the genus known to cause disease in man is *Mycoplasma pneumoniae* which is responsible for the form of pneumonia known as primary atypical pneumonia. (See PNEUMONIA.)

MYCOSIS is the general term applied to diseases due to the growth of fungi in the body. Among some of the simplest and commonest mycoses are ringworm, favus, and thrush. The Madura foot of India, actinomycosis, and occasional cases of pneumonia and suppurative ear disease are also due to the growth of moulds in the bodily tissues.

MYCOSIS FUNGOIDES is a rare neoplastic condition of the reticulo-endothelial system, characterized in its later stages by multiple tumours of the skin. The course is prolonged and almost invariably ends fatally.

MYDRIASIS means a state of unusual dilatation of the pupil. Drugs which cause dilatation of the pupil, such as belladonna and cocaine, are known as mydriatics.

MYELIN is the name given to the white fat-like substance forming a sheath round medullated or myelinated nerve-fibres in the nerves and in the central nervous system.

MYELITIS is inflammation of the spinal cord.

MYELOCYTE is the name given to one of the cells of bone-marrow from which the granular white corpuscles of the blood are produced. They are found in the blood in certain forms of leukaemia.

MYELOGRAPHY means the injection of a radio-opaque substance into the central canal of the spinal cord in order to assist in the diagnosis of diseases of the spinal cord or spine.

MYELOMA is the name of a tumour made up of bone-marrow cells and generally occurring in the marrow of more than one bone at the same time.

MYELOMALACIA is the term applied to morbid softening of the spinal cord as a result of injury, pressure, inflammation, or arterial disease.

MYELOMATOSIS is a malignant process involving the bone marrow. It runs an invariably fatal course.

MYIASIS is a term applied to any disease caused by maggots or flies.

MYOCARDIAL INFARCTION (see CORONARY THROMBOSIS).

MYOCARDITIS means inflammation of the muscular wall of the heart.

MYOCARDIUM is the name applied to the muscular substance of the heart.

MYOGLOBIN is the protein which gives muscle (qv) its red colour. It has the property of combining loosely and reversibly with oxygen. This means that it is the vehicle whereby muscle extracts oxygen from the haemoglobin in the blood circulating through it, and then releases the oxygen for use by the muscle.

MYOMA is the term applied to a tumour, almost invariably of a simple nature, which consists mainly of muscle fibres. These muscle tumours often occur in the uterus.

MYOPATHY also known as MUSCU-LAR DYSTROPHY or IDIOPATHIC MUSCULAR ATROPHY, is the term applied to a condition in which wasting takes place in certain muscles, with or without previous increase in bulk of these muscles, and apparently without any affection of the nervous system. The cause of the condition is still obscure, although the disease appears to run in families, being transmitted, like some other hereditary diseases, by the mother. Generally the disease appears in early childhood. The changes which are found after death show that a simple wasting away of the muscle fibres takes place, and that these are in some cases to a great extent replaced by fatty and fibrous tissue.
Symptoms – There are three chief types of myopathy. The commonest, known as pseudo-hypertrophic muscular dystrophy, affects particularly the upper part of the lower limbs of children. The muscles of the buttocks, thighs and calves seem excessively well developed, but nevertheless the child is clumsy, weak on his legs, and has difficulty in picking himself up when he falls. In another form of the disease, which begins a little later, as a rule about the age of 14, the muscles of the upper arm are first affected, and those of the spine and lower limbs become weak later on. In a third type, which begins about this age, the muscles of the face, along with certain of the shoulder and upper arm muscles, show the first signs of wasting. All the forms have this in common: that the affected muscles grow weaker till their power to contract is quite lost. In the first form, the patients seldom reach the age of 20, falling victims to some disease which, to ordinary persons, would not be serious. In the other forms the wasting, after progressing to a certain extent, often remains stationary for the rest of life.
Treatment – The general health must be well maintained. Massage, electricity and exercise short of fatigue are of the utmost importance, and above all, care must be taken that these invalids are not exposed unduly, as they succumb easily to chest affections.
The education and management of these unfortunate children raise many

difficulties. Much help in dealing with these problems can be obtained from the Muscular Dystrophy Group of Great Britain, 26 Borough High Street, London, SE1.

MYOPIA, or SHORT-SIGHT, is a condition in which, owing to the lens of the eye being too highly convex or the ball of the eye too long, rays of light are brought to a focus before they reach the retina, and so form circles of diffused light upon it. It is the opposite of hypermetropia or longsight. It is an important and common cause of visual impairment. It rarely occurs before the age of 6 years. A recent British survey has shown that it is more common in children from non-manual families than in those from manual families. At 11 years of age myopic children showed striking advantages in educational performance, over their normal-sighted peers, as judged by tests of reading, arithmetic and general ability. Children with myopia read more often in their leisure time than normally sighted children, but no evidence was found to support the old theory that children who are academically inclined and who are avid readers are more likely to develop myopia. Neither was any evidence found to support the old belief that short-sighted children tended to be more academic because defective distant visual activity prevented them from pursuing active physical lives, with the result that they spent more time reading. Indeed, it was found that, despite their visual impairment, they participated in outdoor sports as often as other children. (See SPECTACLES; VISION, DISORDERS OF.)

MYOSITIS means inflammation of a muscle. (See MUSCLES, DISEASES OF.)

MYOTONIA is a condition in which the muscles, though possessed of normal power, contract only very slowly. The stiffness disappears as the muscles are used.

MYRINGOTOMY is the operation of cutting the drum of the ear in cases of acute inflammation of the middle ear.

MYRRH is a gum-resin obtained from *Commiphora molmol*, an Arabian myrtle tree. It stimulates the function of mucous membranes with which it is brought in contact or by which it is excreted. Tincture of myrrh is used for a gargle in sore throat, as a tooth-wash when the gums are inflamed, and as an ingredient of cough mixtures.

MYXOEDEMA is a disease characterized by a swollen and degenerative condition of the subcutaneous and connective tissues throughout the body, due to a defect in the thyroid gland.

Causes – Beyond the fact that it is about seven times more common in women than in men, and that the great majority of cases arise in middle life, between the ages of 30 and 50, little is known as to the cause of the thyroid deficiency. In a small minority of cases it follows partial removal of the thyroid gland, a common form of treatment of thyrotoxicosis (qv).

The important part of the thyroid gland secretion is an iodine-holding body (thyroxine) which is concerned in the processes of nutrition. Deprivation of the secretion causes a deposition of fat, a varying degree of dropsy, and above all an excessive formation of loose connective tissue, from which there is often obtainable after death a considerable amount of mucoid material, a fact to which the disease owes its name. This connective tissue presses upon and destroys the proper tissues of the organs.

Symptoms – A person suffering from myxoedema to a marked degree presents a most characteristic appearance. The face is swollen, the features coarse, and the expression dull and unrelieved by any passing emotions or interests. The skin generally is dry and yellow, but the cheeks are usually bright red in contrast. The hair is thin, harsh and brittle, and the person may even be completely bald. The intellectual functions also are slow, the speech is deliberate, the formation of ideas, as for example in answer to questions, and indeed all the ordinary affairs of life, take far longer than in the case of healthy persons; but there is, nevertheless, in the early stages, no impairment in the quality of mental processes. Later, memory becomes bad, and the person grows deaf and very drowsy. Although at first the temper is placid and lethargic, in the later stages irritability and delusions appear, and the person, if untreated, may ultimately become mentally deranged.

Along with these more obvious changes there is general swelling all over the body. The hands assume the so-called spade-like appearance, and the person, partly in consequence of the slowness of his movements, partly as the result of weakness, becomes very ungainly. The cold is often complained of by the invalid, who has difficulty in keeping herself warm, and, if the temperature be taken, it is usually found to be subnormal: 96° to 98° F (25·5° to 36·7° C). A characteristic finding is a marked lowering of the basal metabolic rate.

Cases last for many years even when untreated, and the disease is seldom directly fatal. As a rule myxoedematous patients grow better and worse from time to time, although the trend is for the disease to get more marked. When the case is treated, improvement almost always takes place with great rapidity, and treatment is effective even after the person has been ill for many years.

Treatment – This consists of the administration of thyroxine sodium. The dosage depends upon the severity of the condition, but it is always advisable to start with a dose of 0·05 mg and increase this gradually. Some patients are sensitive to quite small doses, and if too big a dose is given initially there may be toxic effects. Most patients require to take a maintenance dose for the rest of their lives.

MYXOMA is the name applied to a tumour consisting of very imperfect connective tissue, and containing a peculiar mucus-like juice.

MYXOVIRUSES include the influenza viruses A, B and C; the para-influenza viruses, types 1 to 3; and respiratory syncytial virus which is an important cause of respiratory disease in the early years of life.

N

NAEVUS is the term applied to birthmarks, consisting of a mass of dilated blood-vessels. These structures may take the form of the large port-wine stain often seen upon the face, for which little can be done, or they may occur as swellings of a more restricted nature, usually of a red or bluish colour. Many naevi tend to decrease in size as the child advances in years; or if not, the blemish can often be removed by excision of the piece of skin that is involved, or by electrolysis.

NAIL-BITING is a common practice in schoolchildren, most of whom gradually give it up as they approach adolescence. Too much significance should therefore not be attached to it. In itself it does no harm, and punishment or restraining devices do nothing but harm. It is a manifestation of tension or insecurity, the cause of which should be removed. Otherwise a commonsense approach to discourage the habit, if excessive, can be made on the grounds of pride in the older child.

NAILS (see SKIN).

NAILS, DISEASES OF – The nails are subject to relatively few diseases. On the other hand, any interference with the natural appearance of the finger-nails is very unsightly, whilst the sensitive matrix of both finger- and toe-nails is extremely tender when diseased.

INFLAMMATION of the nails and of the bed in which they rest occurs in various skin diseases: eg. psoriasis, eczema, fungus infections (see RINGWORM). The nails then become rough, thickened, irregular, discoloured, and split readily into layers. Most acute febrile diseases are accompanied by irregularities in growth of the nails, producing a transverse furrow in the nail, as it grows onwards, and these furrows on the nails serve to date a severe illness fairly accurately, the furrow gradually approaching the free margin of the nail and disappearing in about six months' time. These transverse furrows must not be confused with furrows running lengthwise, which are said to indicate a gouty constitution.

Spoon-shaped or concave nails (KOIL-ONYCHIA) are often associated with anaemia, especially in middle-aged women, and become normal when this is treated.

ABSCESS may occur at the root of the nail (see WHITLOW) or underneath it near its edge. As a rule, these abscesses are caused by a minute poisoned wound, such as that due to a splinter of wood. The condition is generally very painful, but is relieved by opening, so as to allow free exit for the pus, the nail being snipped up with a pair of scissors if necessary. The nail in these cases is often cast off.

INJURY to the nail by a blow is often followed by an extravasation of blood beneath it, the nail first turning black, and then often being shed. In all these cases in which the nail is shed, a new nail generally appears quickly, and replaces the old one in six months, unless the matrix has been very seriously diseased or injured. While the new nail is growing, the point of the finger merely requires the protection of a finger-stall.

INGROWING NAIL is a troublesome condition affecting only the nails of the toes. It is due to a variety of causes, chief among which are the pressure of badly fitting shoes, cutting away of the corners in paring the nails, and want of attention to the nails, whereby scarf-skin and dirt collect beneath the nail, and by inflammatory changes causing ulceration of the skin at the sides. The condition commonly occurs in old, bedridden people, mainly for the last-named reason. The treatment is simple, though sometimes tedious. It consists in the wearing of well-made boots, cutting of the nails square across without paring away the corners (illustrations 318, 319) and the packing two or three times daily of a shred of boric lint between the corner of the nail and the skin which it is chafing. These measures are

318 – Finger-nail, showing method of cutting nail.

319 – Toe-nail, showing correct method of cutting nail straight across.

613

generally sufficient after a little time, but sometimes the nail is so much thickened that the edges cannot be raised up to admit the threads of lint. In this case the centre of the nail may be softened by dabbing on caustic potash, and then the nail is easily thinned down by scraping with a sharp knife till it becomes pliable. When the skin at the side of the nail bleeds very readily, this is remedied by touching with bluestone or with nitrate of silver. In severe cases a minor surgical operation may be required. Anyone having trouble with ingrowing toe-nails, especially elderly people, would be well advised to consult a chiropodist.

NALIDIXIC ACID is a recently introduced drug, active against Gramnegative organisms, which is proving useful in the treatment of infections of the urinary tract.

NALORPHINE HYDROBROMIDE reduces or abolishes most of the actions of morphine and similarly acting narcotics, such as pethidine. It is used as an antidote in the treatment of over-dosage with these drugs. It has no effect as an antidote to overdosage with barbiturates.

NALOXONE is a drug that has a similar action to that of nalorphine (qv). It is used as an antidote to morphine and similarly acting narcotics.

NANISM is another name for dwarfism (see DWARF).

NAPKIN RASH is the term applied to the eruption which tends to occur on the buttocks of infants, due to too infrequent changing of soiled napkins or inadequate laundering of napkins.
Prevention consists of four main measures. (i) When the baby is bathed, particular attention must be paid to the creases and folds of the skin which must be carefully washed, then equally carefully dried and sprinkled with a bland baby powder. (ii) Napkins must not be washed in strong soaps or detergent solutions. After washing they must be carefully rinsed out in several changes of clean water. (iii) Soiled napkins must be changed frequently. (iv) Waterproof drawers should be reserved for special social occasions, and not used all and every day.
Should the skin become inflamed, washing it with a 1 per cent solution of sodium sulphate, followed by careful drying and the application of calamine lotion, is often useful. An alternative application which has stood the test of time is zinc and castor oil ointment.

NAPRAPATHY is a system of healing which attributes disease to disorder in the ligaments and connective tissues.

NARCISSISM is an abnormal mental state characterized by excessive admiration of self.

NARCOLEPSY is a condition in which uncontrollable episodes of sleep occur two or three times a day. It starts at any age and persists for life. The attacks, which usually last for 10 to 15 minutes, come on at times normally conducive to sleep, such as during the sermon at church, after a meal, or sitting in a bus, but they may occur when walking in the street. In due course, usually after some years, they are associated with cataplectic attacks when for a few seconds there is sudden muscular weakness affecting the whole body. These attacks are commonly brought on by amusement with laughter. In others they may be induced by anger or by a sense of triumph. In the first of these groups the affected individual soon learns to sit down when jokes are going around. As one distinguished neurologist has put it, 'directly the subject's fancy is tickled, he weakens, sags at the knees and cannot hold the arms elevated or extended if they chance to be in either of these positions'. The attacks of narcolepsy seem to be reduced in number if the individual takes a 15-minute nap after meals. Affected people should carry 5 mg tablets of dexamphetamine about with them and take one or two to tide them over special occasions when an attack could be embarrassing. Some doctors recommend the regular taking of dexamphetamine, but this is deprecated by others in view of the possible adverse effect of such continued treatment on the mental state. The cataplectic attacks are controlled by imipramine or clomipramine.

NARCOSIS is a condition of profound insensibility, resembling sleep so far that the unconscious person can still be roused slightly by great efforts, or at all events is not entirely indifferent to sensory stimuli. It is most commonly produced by drugs, such as opium, but may also be due to poisons formed within the body, as in the uraemia of Bright's disease.

NARCOTICS (See HYPNOTICS).

NARES is the Latin word for the nostrils.

NASAL DISORDERS (see NOSE, DISEASES OF).

NASOPHARYNX is the upper part of the throat, lying behind the nasal cavity. (See NOSE.)

NATAMYCIN is an antibiotic isolated from *Streptomyces natalensis* which is proving of value in the treatment of moniliasis (qv).

NATIONAL LISTENING LIBRARY is a charity which produces recorded books for handicapped people who cannot read, with the exception of the blind who have their own separate organization, the Royal National Institute for the Blind. Otherwise it caters for all those who are deprived of the ability to read through any form of disability, including arthritis. Its catalogue includes over 700 titles, ranging from thrillers, to theology, as well as children's books. Its address, from which full details can be obtained, is: 49 Great Cumberland Place, London W1H 7LH. (See also CALIBRE.)

NAUSEA means a feeling that vomiting is about to take place. (See VOMITING.)

NAVEL, or UMBILICUS, is the scar on the abdomen marking the point where the umbilical cord joined the body in embryonic life. (See AFTER-BIRTH.)

NEAR-SIGHT (see MYOPIA).

NEBULA is the term applied to a slight opacity on the cornea producing a haze in the field of vision, and also to any oily preparation to be sprayed from a nebulizer, an apparatus for splitting up a fluid into fine droplets.

NECATOR AMERICANUS is the name of a hookworm, closely resembling but smaller than the *Ancylostoma duodenale*. (See ANCYLOSTOMIASIS.)

NECK is that portion of the body which extends from the upper limit of the chest to the base of the skull. Its main function is to support the head. Through its front part run the passages for the air and the food. The great bulk of the neck is composed of seven cervical vertebrae with the muscles attached thereto, in front and behind. (See MUSCLES.) Within the canal

formed by the rings of these vertebrae lies the cervical part of the spinal cord, from which proceed the nerves that control the movements of the neck and arms.

In front of the spinal column lies the pharynx, or throat-cavity, extending from the base of the skull above down to the lower edge of the sixth vertebra, where the gullet continues it directly downwards, while the larynx opens out of it in front (illustration 320). The larynx is close to the surface of the front of the neck, and the thyroid cartilage can be readily seen and felt beneath the skin. (See LARYNX.)

320 – Vertical section through the middle of the head and neck. The passages for air *a*, are indicated by a heavy dotted line, those for the food *f*, by a fainter line; *et*, Eustachian tube; *l*, larynx; *w*, windpipe; *t*, tonsil; *to*, tongue; *g*, gullet; *v*, vertebral column; *sp.c*, spinal cord. For other letters, see illustration 86.

The larynx is continued downwards by the windpipe, and just beneath the larynx the isthmus of the thyroid gland can be felt crossing the windpipe and connecting the two lobes of the gland which lie one on either side of the larynx. The strong sternocleidomastoid muscle is prominent on each side of the neck, running from the mastoid process of the skull down to the breast-bone and inner end of the clavicle; under cover of it lies a fibrous sheath containing the carotid artery, internal jugular vein and vagus nerve. The sternocleidomastoid muscle divides each side of the neck into two triangular areas, in which lie important nerves and branches

615

of these blood-vessels, as well as chains of lymphatic glands. Several large superficial veins run down the neck, and are of importance, because in wounds of the neck they may give rise to much bleeding. The chief of these are the external jugular vein, running straight downwards from the angle of the jaw, and the anterior jugular vein, running downwards from beneath the chin, not far from the middle line. At the root of the neck the apex of each lung projects a short distance from the chest into the neck.

NECROPSY is a post-mortem examination. It is carried out in such a way as to produce almost no disfigurement. The brain is examined by an opening across the scalp, afterwards hidden by the hair, and the contents of chest and abdomen are inspected through an opening down the middle line in front. If necessary minute pieces of organs are removed for microscopic examination. It is a social duty of the deceased person's relatives to permit or request a post-mortem examination in cases in which the disease was a matter of uncertainty. Nothing causes so much doubt in diagnosis, and therefore in treatment, as the inability of a medical man to confirm his opinions, owing to sentiment on the part of a deceased person's relatives.

NECROSIS means death of a limited portion of tissue, the term being most commonly applied to bones when, as the result of disease or injury, a fragment dies and separates. (See BONE, DISEASES OF.)

NEEDLING is the name for an operation performed by means of a needle, especially in the discission or tearing of a cataract so as to allow the fluid in the anterior chamber of the eye to dissolve it.

NEGATIVISM means a morbid tendency in a person to do the opposite of what he is desired or directed to do. It is specially characteristic of schizophrenia, but is not uncommon in non-psychotic persons.

NEGRO-LETHARGY is another name for sleeping sickness.

NEISSERIA is a group, or genus, of rounded bacteria that occur in pairs and are therefore known as diplococci (see BACTERIOLOGY). They are named after Albert Neisser, the German physician who discovered the gonococcus, the causative organism of gonorrhoea (qv), which is now known as *Neisseria gonorrhoea*. The group also includes the causative organism of cerebrospinal meningitis (see MENINGITIS): *Neisseria meningitidis*.

NEMATODE is a roundworm.

NEOMYCIN is an antibiotic derived from *Streptomyces fradiae*. It has a wide antibacterial spectrum, being effective against the majority of Gram-negative bacilli. Its use is limited by the fact that it is liable to cause deafness and kidney damage. For this reason it is never given by injections. Its main use is for application to the skin, either in solution or as an ointment, for the treatment of infection of the skin. It is also given by mouth for the treatment of certain forms of enteritis due to *E. coli*.

NEONATAL means pertaining to the first month of life.

NEONATAL MORTALITY is the mortality of infants under one month of age. In England and Wales this has fallen markedly during the last decade: from 28·28 per 1000 related live births in 1939 to 7·58 in 1977. This improvement can be attributed to various factors: better antenatal supervision of expectant mothers; care to ensure that expectant mothers receive adequate nourishing food; improvements in the management of the complications of pregnancy and of labour. Nearly three-quarters of neonatal deaths occur during the first week of life, and the chief causes of deaths in this period are immaturity of the infant, birth injuries, congenital abnormalities and asphyxia. After the first week the commonest cause is infection.

NEOPLASM, which means literally a 'new formation', is another word for tumour.

NEPENTHE is a solution of opium in alcohol and water given in the same dose as laudanum.

NEPHRECTOMY means the operation for removal of the kidney. (See KIDNEY, DISEASES OF.)

NEPHRITIS means inflammation of the kidneys. (See BRIGHT'S DISEASE.)

NEPHROLITHIASIS is the term applied to a condition in which calculi are present in the kidney.

NEPHROPEXY means the fixation of a floating kidney in its original position.

NEPHROPTOSIS means the condition in which a kidney is movable or 'floating'. (See KIDNEY, DISEASES OF.)

NEPHRORRHAPHY means the operation by which a movable kidney is fastened by stitches in its proper place.

NEPHROSIS is the term applied to a form of degeneration of the kidneys characterized by anaemia, widespread dropsy, and a high degree of albuminuria. (See also BRIGHT'S DISEASE.)

NEPHROSTOMY means the operation of making an opening into the kidney for the purpose of draining it.

NEPHROTOMY means the operation of cutting into the kidney, in search of calculi or for other reasons.

NERVES – The nervous system consists in part of cells and in part of fibres, each of which is a long process extending from a nerve-cell. The brain and spinal cord are often spoken of together as the central nervous system; the nerves which proceed from them, forty-three in number on each side, are named the cerebrospinal, or peripheral nerves; whilst the third great division, situated in the neck, thorax and abdomen, and intimately connected with the cerebrospinal nerves (though in its action largely independent of the brain and cord) is known as the autonomic nervous system. The last-named consists of ganglia containing nerve-cells, which are profusely connected by plexuses of nerve-fibres.

The nerve-cells originate, or receive, impulses and impressions of various sorts, which are conveyed from them to muscles, blood-vessels, and elsewhere, by efferent nerves, or received by them through afferent nerves coming from the skin, organs of sense, joints, etc. (illustration 321). The autonomic system is concerned mainly with the movements and other functions of the internal organs, secreting glands and blood-vessels, the activities of which proceed independently of the will.

Structure – (1) NERVE-FIBRES – The nerves vary much in size. The sciatic nerve, deeply buried in the muscles on the back of the thigh, is the largest nerve in the body, being of the thickness of a lead pencil or more; other nerves reach about the size of goose-quills, and from these there are all gradations, down to the minute single fibres distributed to muscle-fibres or to skin. A nerve, such as the sciatic, possesses a strong, outer fibrous sheath, called the epineurium, within which lie bundles of nerve-fibres, divided from one another by partitions of fibrous tissue, in which run blood-vessels that nourish the nerve. Each of these bundles is surrounded by its own sheath, known as the perineurium, and within the bundle fine partitions of fibrous tissue, known as endoneurium, divide up the bundle into groups of fibres. The blood-vessels and lymphatics of the nerves divide into fine branches, which run in these sheaths and partitions of fibrous tissue. The finest subdivisions of the nerves are the fibres, and these are of two kinds: medullated and non-medullated fibres.

321 – Diagram showing nervous connections between the central nervous system and muscle and skin. From Best and Taylor, *The Physiological Basis of Medical Practice*. The Williams & Wilkins Co.

The *medullated fibres* vary in thickness from $\frac{1}{12000}$ to $\frac{1}{1500}$ inch (2 to 15 micrometres), some nerves containing a greater proportion of the small fibres than others. Under the microscope, all have the appearance of tubes, this being due to the fact that each has an outer membranous sheath, the neurilemma, within which is a clear white material, the medullary (or myelin) sheath, in the centre of which runs the axis-cylinder or nerve-fibre proper (illustration 322). The neurilemma is a strong but thin sheath with nuclei at regular intervals on its inner surface. The medullary sheath is composed of fatty material containing lecithin and cholesterin, and to it the white colour of the nerves is mainly due. It is divided at regular intervals by short gaps, situated about $\frac{1}{20}$ inch (1 mm) apart, known as the nodes of Ranvier, but across these gaps the neurilemma and axis-cylinder are continuous. This medullary, or myelin, sheath is regarded as fulfilling a purpose similar to the insulating material upon electric wires

DENDRITES

CELL BODY

AXON

MYELIN SHEATH

NEURILEMMA

NODE OF RANVIER

BARE AXONS

322 – Diagrammatic representation of a nerve. From Best and Taylor. *The Physiological Basis of Medical Practice.* The Williams & Wilkins Co.

and preventing nerve impulses from passing beyond the nerve-fibre by which they are conveyed. The axis-cylinder, or axon, is the conducting part of the nerve, for whilst the neurilemma is absent from the fibre in its course through the brain and spinal cord, and the medullary sheath is absent from non-medullated nerves, the axis-cylinder never fails. It has a striped appearance, seeming to consist of a number of fibrils which, however, cannot be separated from one another. The *non-medullated fibres* are very much thinner than the average of medullated fibres, from which they differ only in the fact of not possessing a medullary sheath, and of being therefore greyish in colour.

(2) NERVE-CELLS, from one of which springs each nerve-fibre, are found in the grey matter of the brain and spinal cord. In the brain alone it is calculated there are some 600,000,000 of these cells. They also exist in the ganglia of the sympathetic system, in connection with some of the nerves of special sense, and on the posterior roots of the spinal nerves. The shape of these nerve-cells varies. The most common appearance is that of a large clear cell, containing an oval nucleus, and running out at various points into long processes, which, as a rule, branch again and again, after the manner of a tree, these dendritic processes, as they are called, meeting with similar processes from neighbouring cells (illustration 323). The ends of the branching processes from one cell meet the ends of similar processes from another cell, the points of apposition being known as *synapses.* The state of closure or openness of these synapses is believed to be of great importance in quickening or blocking nerve impulses. The body of the cell has a mottled appearance, owing to its containing many bodies, known as Nissl's granules (illustration 324), which appear to be of the nature of food material, destined to be used up when the cell is stimulated to work till reduced to a state of fatigue.

In the cerebrum, the cells are distinctly pyramidal in shape, and one of the processes of each cell is much longer than the rest, forming indeed a nerve-fibre, which may run a long distance down the spinal cord. Other cells are bipolar, ie. they possess but two processes, and others are unipolar, ie. they possess only one process, which, a short distance from the cell, divides in a T-shaped manner, as, for example, the cells in the ganglia upon the posterior roots of the spinal nerves. Other cells are found in the grey matter of the brain, which are known as neuroglia cells. These are provided with innumerable processes that form a supporting felt-work for the nerve-cells and nerve-fibres, and act merely as connective tissue cells.

(3) NERVE-ENDINGS – Each nerve-fibre proceeds from a nerve-cell to end in a definite organ, to or from which it carries a special form of nerve impulse. The manner in which the fibre ends in the organ to which it proceeds varies in different cases. The simplest mode of ending is that of the non-medullated fibres which proceed to the involuntary muscle-fibres, as, for example, those of the intestine. These fibres form a complex network between the layers of muscle, from which fine fibres pass between the muscle-fibres. In the heart the nerves end in a similar manner. In voluntary muscles the arrangement is more complicated. Each nerve-fibre splits up into numerous branches, which go to neighbouring muscle-fibres. Each branch pierces the membrane surrounding its muscle-fibre, and ends by spreading out into a plate composed of granular material and numerous nuclei. The endings of sensory nerves in the skin have a special arrangement (illustration 325). Most of these end, not in the cuticle, which is devoid

Axon

Axon

323 – Three nerve cells from the anterior column of the spinal cord. From Cunningham's *Anatomy*. Oxford University Press.

AXON

324 – A nerve-cell, showing Nissl's granules. From Best and Taylor, *The Physiological Basis of Medical Practice*. The Williams & Wilkins Co.

of sensation, but in the projections of the true skin beneath it, where each nerve-fibre enters a small rounded bulb. Some of these bulbs found beneath the skin of the fingers are known as Pacinian corpuscles: about $\frac{1}{10}$ inch (2·5 mm) long and half that in width. These consist of a large number of thin

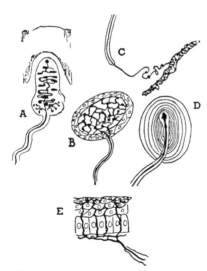

325 – some nerve endings. A. Meissner's corpuscle (touch); B. Krause's end bulb (cold); C. Ruffini's end organs (warmth); D. Pacinian corpuscle (deep pressure); E, bare nerve endings in cornea (pain). From Best and Taylor, *The Physiological Basis of Medical Practice*. The Williams & Wilkins Co.

coats enclosing the swollen end of a nerve-fibre. Other much smaller bodies, about $\frac{1}{300}$ inch (0·8 mm) long, known as touch-corpuscles, are found close beneath the cuticle all over the skin, and consist of a framework of connective tissue in which the nerve-fibre winds round and round. Similar bodies are found on the front of the eye (illustration 325 E). In other cases the nerves appear to end abruptly in cells situated in the deepest layer of the cuticle.

Development and repair – The whole nervous system is developed from the ectoderm or outer layer of the embryo, the brain and spinal cord arising from an infolding of the surface along the back to form a tube, and all the nerves being formed directly or indirectly as outgrowths from this tube, which increase in length till they reach the muscle, skin or other structure for which they are destined. Each nerve-fibre, as already stated, is the process of a nerve-cell, and if a nerve be cut, that portion of its fibres which is separated from the cells immediately starts to degenerate, the medullary sheath and axis-cylinder, as a rule, breaking up (illustrations 326, 327, 328). Within a few days or weeks, however, a bundle of small new fibres grows out from the cut end of each fibre in that portion which has not been cut off from connection with the nerve-cells, and these grow through the scar and down the sheath of the degenerated portion till they reach the organs to which the nerve originally proceeded. Thus the nerve is restored. This process is quickened when the cut ends have been carefully brought together, and indeed there are reasons for believing that, sometimes when this is done, no degeneration takes place, but the nerve heals and again transmits impulses at once.

Functions of nerves – The greater part of the bodily activity originates in the nerve-cells, food material being used up in the process. As a result of this activity, impulses are sent down the nerves, which act simply as transmitters. The impulse which passes from a nerve-cell along a nerve-fibre to a muscle may be compared to the electric spark which explodes a mine, since the nerve impulse causes sudden chemical changes in the muscles as the latter contract. (See MUSCLES.) Similarly, the impulse which passes from a sensory ending in the skin along a nerve-fibre to affect nerve-cells in the spinal cord and brain, where it is perceived as a sensation, may be compared to the electric current which passes along a telephone wire to affect the receiver. Nevertheless, it must be understood that the impulse passing along a nerve is a form of motion quite different from electricity: travelling at the slow rate of about 100 feet (30 metres) per second, and probably more nearly resembling the motion of air-particles which produces sound. (See NERVOUS IMPULSE.)

The important fact that the anterior root of each spinal nerve is motor in function was discovered in 1811 by Sir Charles Bell. This was confirmed by Magendie in 1822, and the discovery also made that the posterior roots are sensory in function. They therefore concluded that the anterior roots consist of motor fibres to muscles,

into sensations which furnish a sense of movement and locality, a sense of pain, and a sense of heat and cold. (See TOUCH.)

The connection between the sensory and motor systems of nerves is important. The simplest form of nerve action is that known as *automatic action*. In this a part of the nervous system, controlling, for example, the lungs, goes on rhythmically, making discharges from its motor cells sufficient to keep the muscles of respiration in regular action, influenced only by occasional sensory impressions and chemical changes from various sources, which increase or diminish its activity according to the needs of the body.

326 – A diagrammatic representation of a healthy nerve (for comparison with illustrations 314 and 315).

327 – Diagram of degenerating nerve cell after two days.

328 – Diagram of degenerating nerve cell after a week.

From Bradbury, *Hewer's Textbook of Histology for Medical Students.* Heinemann.

the posterior roots of sensory fibres from the skin. The terms, efferent and afferent, are applied to these roots more correctly, because, in addition to motor fibres, fibres through which blood-vessels are contracted and relaxed, and fibres which control secreting glands leave the cord in the anterior roots, while, in addition to sensory fibres, fibres which bring in impulses from muscles, joints and other organs, and inform the sense of locality as well as the sense of feeling, also enter the cord by the posterior roots.

Sensation is popularly supposed to be derived through five senses: smell, sight, hearing, taste and touch. In addition to these, impulses are brought by special nerve-fibres and converted in the brain

In *reflex action* (illustration 329), the parts engaged are a sensory ending, say in the skin; a sensory nerve leading from it to the spinal cord, where it ends by splitting up into processes near the nerve-cells; a nerve-cell which is stimulated by the sensory impulse, and which immediately sends a motor impulse down its nerve; and a muscle which contracts as the result. A simple example of reflex action is given by the drawing away of the hand when it is pricked with a pin, before and independently of the conscious perception of pain.

Voluntary acts are more complicated than reflex ones. The same mechanism is involved, but, in addition, the controlling power of its brain is brought into play. This exerts first of all an inhibitory or blocking effect, which prevents immediate reflex action, and then the impulse, passing up to the cerebral hemispheres, sets up activity in a series of cells there, the complexity of these processes depending upon the intellectual processes involved. Finally, the inhibition is removed and an impulse passes down to motor cells in the spinal cord, and a muscle or set of muscles is brought into play through the motor nerves.

The *trophic function* of nerves is another most important part of their activity, for it appears as if the constant passage of nerve impulses down the nerves of any part were important for its nutrition. Thus, if sensory nerves be diseased or injured, ulceration of the skin, bed sores and other changes are liable to occur, while muscles waste and disappear if their motor nerves be permanently destroyed.

upper four cervical nerves unite to produce the *cervical plexus*. From this the muscles and skin of the neck are mainly supplied, and the phrenic nerve, which runs down through the lower part of the neck and the chest to innervate the diaphragm, is given off. The *brachial plexus* is formed by the union of the lower four cervical and first dorsal nerves, and, in addition to nerves which proceed to some of the muscles in the shoulder region, and others to the skin about the shoulder and inner side of the arm, it gives off the following large nerves that proceed down the arm: the musculocutaneous nerve, the median nerve, the ulnar nerve, and the radial nerve, each of which is about the size of a goose-quill. The musculocutaneous nerve supplies the large muscles in front of the upper arm, as well as the skin on the radial side of the fore-

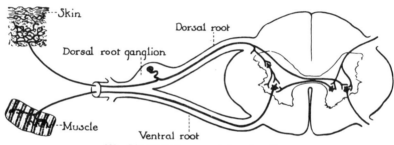

329 – Diagrammatic representation of a reflex arc.

Nervous system – The brain and its twelve pairs of cranial nerves are treated under BRAIN; the spinal cord and the origin of its thirty-one pairs of nerves are treated under SPINAL CORD.

Each of these spinal nerves arises by two roots (illustration 329), the posterior being larger than the anterior, and being furnished with a ganglion. Just before they emerge from the side of the spinal canal, the two roots unite to form a single nerve, their fibres mix, and then the nerve separates into two divisions.

One division immediately turns backwards to supply the skin and muscles of the back (posterior division), the other runs forwards (anterior division).

These anterior divisions supply the skin on the front and sides of the body and on the limbs, as well as all the muscles of the trunk and limbs, excepting those on the back. They do not run straight to these parts, but form a series of plexuses in which the nerve-fibres from different levels of the cord to the limbs are given off. The

arm as far as the wrist. The radial nerve winds round the back of the upper arm, where it supplies the triceps muscle, and then gives branches which innervate the skin on the outer side of the arm and forearm, the muscles behind the forearm, and finally the skin on the outer part of the back of the hand and fingers. The median nerve and the ulnar nerve run through the upper arm without giving off branches, and it is possible to feel the ulnar nerve as a cord running between the two marked bony prominences behind the elbow. The median nerve supplies most of the muscles in front of the forearm, a few of the small muscles in the hand and the skin of the palm and front of the thumb, index finger, middle finger and half of the ring finger. The ulnar nerve supplies two muscles in the forearm, most of the small muscles in the hand and the skin down the inner side of the forearm and palm and the skin in front of the little finger and half the ring finger.

The *thoracic* or *dorsal nerves*, with the

exception of the first, do not form a plexus, but each runs round the chest along the lower margin of the rib to which it corresponds, whilst the lower six extend on to the abdomen. In this course they supply both the skin and muscle of the trunk.

The *lumbar plexus* is formed by the upper four lumbar nerves, and its branches are distributed to the lower part of the abdomen, and front and inner side of the thigh.

The *sacral plexus* is formed by parts of the fourth and fifth lumbar nerves, and the upper three and part of the fourth sacral nerves. It gives branches directly to the muscles and skin about the hip and fork, and supplies the skin down the back of the thigh, but the main bulk of the plexus is collected into the sciatic nerve. This, the largest nerve in the body, is buried in the muscles on the back of the thigh, which it supplies. It continues down to the back of the knee, and there divides into two branches, the internal popliteal (tibial) nerve and the external (common) popliteal nerve, which between them supply all the muscles below the knee and the greater part of the skin covering the leg and the foot.

The *sympathetic system* is joined by a pair of small branches given off from each spinal nerve, close to the spine. This system consists of two great parts. There is, first, a pair of cords running down on the side and front of the back-bone, and containing on each side three ganglia in the neck, and beneath this a ganglion opposite each vertebra. From these two ganglionated cords numerous branches are given off, and these unite in the second place to form plexuses connected with various internal organs, and provided with numerous large and irregularly placed ganglia. The chief of these plexuses are the cardiac plexus, the solar or epigastric plexus, the diaphragmatic, suprarenal, renal, spermatic, or ovarian, aortic, hypogastric and pelvic plexuses, the name in each case indicating the organ upon which, or the part of the abdomen within which, the plexus is placed.

NERVE INJURIES are produced by several causes. Continued or repeated severe pressure may be enough to damage a nerve seriously, as in the case of a badly made crutch pressing into the armpit and causing drop-wrist. Bruising due to a blow which drives a superficially placed nerve against a bone may inflict severe damage upon a nerve such as the radial nerve behind the upper arm. A wound may sever nerves, along with other structures; this accident is specially liable to occur to the ulnar nerve in front of the wrist, owing to falls upon broken glass, and to various nerves in the armpit when the humerus is fractured near its upper end. Exposure to cold may also damage a nerve severely, as in the case of the facial nerve, when Bell's paralysis results. Or a nerve may be injured at its origin before it leaves the brain or cord, by haemorrhage in the substance of these organs.

Symptoms – When a sensory nerve is injured, sensation is immediately more or less impaired in the part supplied by the nerve. When the nerve in question is a motor one the muscles governed through it are instantly paralysed. In the latter case, the portion of nerve beyond the injury degenerates and the muscles gradually waste, and lose their power of contraction in response to electrical applications. Finally, deformities result and the joints become fixed. This is particularly noticeable when the ulnar nerve is injured, the hand and fingers taking up a claw-like position. The skin may also become cold, glossy and even ulcerate, owing to the loss of its nerve supply.

Treatment – The nerve, if wounded, should be carefully stitched with the ends touching one another, and, if injured by other causes, should be carefully protected from a repetition of the injury. In some cases recovery takes place within a few days, but usually, if the nerve be completely severed or seriously injured, the muscles supplied by it do not regain their power for several weeks at least. The reason of this is that the part cut off from connection with the brain and cord degenerates rapidly, and the new nerve has to grow all the way down the sheath of the old one. (See NERVES.) An operation designed to unite a damaged nerve and relieve paralysis may sometimes be successfully performed even some weeks or months after the wound has closed. When the ends of the damaged nerve are so shortened that they cannot be got to meet, a portion of a sensory nerve or of a nerve from an animal is sometimes inserted and carefully stitched between the divided ends. Nerve anastomosis is also sometimes practised by bringing the ends of the divided nerve up to a neighbouring nerve and carefully stitching them within its sheath. For example, the facial nerve when injured at the side of the face is sometimes anastomosed with the healthy hypoglossal nerve, and the facial paralysis which has resulted is thus relieved. Massage and galvanism of the muscles will keep them from wasting till the nerve is ready to take up its functions again. The power of the muscles to react again to faradic electricity is a most important sign, as showing that repair of the nerve is taking place.

NERVOUS DEBILITY (see NEURASTHENIA).

NERVOUS DISEASES – This class of disease is one of the most difficult to diagnose. The brain and spinal cord being enclosed in the skull and spine, beyond the reach of direct examination, and the nerves being almost everywhere deeply buried in the tissues, the nature of nervous diseases must be made out from the disturbances of organs governed by the affected nerves.

The following conditions are discussed under their individual headings: APHASIA; APOPLEXY; BRAIN DISEASES; CATALEPSY; CHOREA; CRAMP; EPILEPSY; FORGETFULNESS; HYSTERIA; LOCOMOTOR ATAXIA; MENTAL SUBNORMALITY; MENTAL ILLNESS; MULTIPLE SCLEROSIS; NERVE INJURIES; NEURALGIA; NEURITIS; PARALYSIS; SPINAL CORD, DISEASES OF.

Causes – Many factors contribute to the production of nervous diseases. That certain diseases are induced by a particular temperament, or by peculiar habits of life, is proved by the fact that some of the diseases are commoner among one race, others in another people. Heredity is, in several ways, an important matter. Some persons, particularly those of great intellectual power and of artistic temperament, seem born with a nervous constitution (see CONSTITUTION) which renders them more than ordinarily liable to the slighter nervous affections, such as headaches, neuralgia, hysterical manifestations and bizarre forms of mental activity. Those also who come of a degenerate stock seem to suffer very readily from nervous diseases of a severe type, probably not because these diseases are inherited, but because the nervous system is specially exposed to strain by the conditions of modern life, and, in such persons, gives way early. The great pressure at which modern commercial and intellectual life is carried on tends, undoubtedly, to exhaust the nervous system and bring on many diseases, such as neuralgia, anxiety states, digestive disturbances and various forms of mental disturbance. To counteract this a periodic rest and change of scene are of special importance, especially to those of

nervous temperament and those subjected to much strain in life.

Shocks both to mind and body, such as the loss of a relative, money reverses, an unfortunate love affair, an accident, may be the starting-point of many chronic nervous complaints. The nervous system seems to be specially prone to such injury about the critical periods of life (see CLIMACTERIC), while in young children the nervous system is always of a less stable character than in later life.

Many poisons, both of those produced within the body by disease and of those taken in from outside, have a specially harmful action upon the nervous system. Among these is syphilis, which plays an important part in the production of locomotor ataxia, general paralysis, and certain tumours (gummas) of the brain and spinal cord, while in advanced life it leads to degenerative changes that bring about premature loss of mental power. Chronic alcoholism may cause severe mental derangement and multiple neuritis. Lead-poisoning and diabetes are often accompanied also by multiple neuritis. Several of the acute infectious diseases such as diphtheria, are apt to be followed by loss of power in parts, due to affection of the nervous system, although such results are in general only temporary. The form of paralysis known as poliomyelitis (see POLIOMYELITIS) is also due to an infective process.

As to the changes in the nervous system which are caused by disease, and to which the symptoms are due, these are various in nature. There is a broad division of nervous diseases into organic, in which some change, visible either to the naked eye or on microscopic examination, is discoverable in the nervous system after death, and functional, in which no such change can be found. Into the latter class there fall, for example, hysteria, anxiety states and many cases of neuralgia. Among the organic changes is sclerosis, consisting of an overgrowth of the connective tissue framework of the brain, cord or nerves, accompanied by a disappearance of the nerve structures proper. Tumours, cysts, rupture or blocking of blood-vessels (with consequent loss of nutrition in a part of the nervous system), and local inflammatory processes may all be found constituting an organic change. In all cases the symptoms are dependent, not so much upon the nature of the disease as upon the part of the nervous system which it happens to affect.

Symptoms – Many slight affections of the nervous system are attributed to defects in the organs controlled by the affected nerves: for example, dyspepsia or palpitation may in some cases be due to weakness of the nervous system, and is then little or not at all benefited by remedies directed towards the stomach, heart or other organ in which the symptoms are manifested. It is specially important therefore that cases in which the nervous system is at fault should be early recognized.

There are two great symptoms of nervous disease: (1) disturbances of sensation in the direction either of loss of feeling, or of great pain, or of perverted sensation, such as tingling, hot flushes; and (2) the occurrence of more or less complete paralysis of groups of muscles, or of whole limbs. One or other of these types of symptoms predominates, according as sensory or motor nerves are chiefly affected. In addition to these, there is, in different diseases, more or less interference with the organs of special sense, the reflex actions, the nutrition of outlying parts of the body and the functions of internal organs.

With regard to *sensory symptoms*, loss of the sense of touch is found in locomotor ataxia, and, generally speaking, all maladies in which the posterior part of the cord or sensory nerves are affected. Syringomyelia is a disease affecting the central portion of the spinal cord, and characterized by loss of the power to feel pain and to recognize heat and cold in parts of the limbs. Painful sensations are present in many diseases, as, for example, shooting pains and the feelings of a tight band round the waist in locomotor ataxia.

As to *motor symptoms*, wasting of muscles and loss of power in parts of the body point usually to some affection of the motor nerves. Spasm as well as loss of power accompanies affections situated in the higher motor tracts of the brain and spinal cord, whilst flaccid palsy characterizes diseases and injuries in the grey matter of the cord or in the motor nerves. Conditions in which the nervous system is merely temporarily weakened are manifested by loss of tone in the muscular system, and speedy exhaustion on exertion. Twitchings in the muscular fibres, as in the condition popularly known as live flesh in the eyelids, are also found in this passing condition, as well as in more serious conditions, such as at the onset of progressive muscular atrophy. The impairment of the power of combination among muscles, known as incoordination, which produces trembling on exertion, staggering gait, difficulty in buttoning the clothes or in taking food, is found in multiple sclerosis, chorea, and paralysis agitans. Interference with the power of regulating the movements of the lower limbs is a common symptom of locomotor ataxia.

The *reflex functions*, tested by stroking the skin of various parts and observing the resulting muscular contraction beneath (superficial reflexes), and by tapping the tendons of muscles and watching the twitch that the latter give (deep reflexes), are, generally speaking, diminished when the sensory nerves, sensory paths in the spinal cord, or motor cells in the cord and their fibres are affected. They are increased when the higher motor paths in the cord are affected, as in multiple sclerosis.

Nutritional functions are impaired in all serious nerve diseases and injuries. As a result, localized sweatings, a glassy condition of the skin, bed sores, ulcers and even gangrene of the limbs are liable to appear in the final stages of nervous maladies.

The *functions of the internal organs*, being, as a rule, governed by the sympathetic system, are not in general affected unless this system be diseased. The movement of the bowel and bladder is, however, governed by spinal nerves, and thus these natural functions are impaired in all serious diseases of the spinal cord, so that difficulty of voiding or of retaining the stools and urine appears in such cases.

When the *cranial nerves* proceeding from the brain are involved, definite symptoms arise. Thus affection of the 1st nerve gives rise to loss of smell; of the 2nd nerve to impairment of vision; of the 3rd, 4th and 6th nerves to squints; of the 5th nerve to neuralgia; of the 7th nerve to Bell's paralysis; of the 8th nerve to deafness or giddiness; of the 9th nerve to loss of taste; of the 10th nerve to affections of the larynx, the heart and the stomach; of the 11th nerve to disordered action of the sternocleidomastoid muscle, causing wry-neck; and of the 12th nerve to interference with the movements of the tongue, and consequent difficulty in pronunciation. Many of these symptoms are discussed elsewhere.

Lumbar puncture and the examination of fluid withdrawn from the spinal canal are of great importance in the diagnosis of many serious nervous diseases. (See LUMBAR PUNCTURE.)

Treatment – Rest, which gives an opportunity for repair to the worn-out tissues, is the great remedy in all types of disease due to overstrain of body or mind, shock or inflammatory processes. Rest in its widest sense includes not merely cessation of activity, but suitable food, change of employment, and, it may be, active exercise in persons who have usually much mental work.

Where changes in the nervous system are the result of poisons, such as lead, appropriate drugs hasten their expulsion from the body, and thus check the progress of the disease. Similarly, if the changes be due to infection such as syphilis or tuberculosis, the appropriate antibiotics should be taken. Generally speaking, alcohol has a prejudicial effect in all forms of nervous disease, and particularly is this true in those diseases like polyneuritis, which are caused by it, and in which its use must be absolutely stopped.

There is no department of medicine in which the subconscious moral influence of a self-reliant and expert physician is more marked than in the treatment of functional nervous disorders, and the confidence reposed in the medical adviser and in the treatment employed is often sufficient, in these cases, to start the patient upon the road to improvement, which requires only time, rest and the constant exercise of a certain amount of will-power to complete.

NERVOUS IMPULSE – The effects of nervous activity are now believed in all cases to be transmitted chemically, by the formation at nerve-endings of chemical substances. When, for example, a nerve to a muscle is stimulated, there appears at the junction of nerve-ending and muscle the chemical substance, acetylcholine. Acetylcholine also appears at endings of the parasympathetic nerves and transmits the effect of the parasympathetic impulse. When an impulse passes down a sympathetic nerve, the effect of it is transmitted at the nerve-ending by the chemical liberated there: adrenaline or an adrenaline-like substance.

NETTLE-RASH, or URTICARIA, is a disorder of the skin characterized by an eruption resembling the effect produced by the sting of a nettle, namely, raised red or red-and-white patches, occurring in parts or over the whole of the surface of the body, and attended with great itching and irritation. It may be acute or chronic.

Causes – In some cases the attack appears to be connected with digestive derangements, or the taking of certain articles of diet particularly of a protein

nature, such as various kinds of meat, fish, shell-fish, also occasionally from the use of certain drugs, such as penicillin. In some it is due to the injection of sera, whilst in others it may follow the bite of an insect. In others it is due to exposure to cold: so-called cold urticaria, and occasionally may be the result of effort. There remains a considerable number of cases in which it is difficult to incriminate any one specific causal factor. The general consensus of opinion is that urticaria is an allergic reaction on the part of the affected individual to some substance to which he or she is hypersensitive. In other words, it comes into the same category as asthma and hay fever. In all three conditions the individual is allergic to some factor or factors, but the allergic response varies: in asthma it is the bronchioles of the lungs that are involved; in hay fever it is the mucous membrane of the nasopharynx, sinuses and eyes; whilst in urticaria it is the skin that gives the allergic response.

Symptoms – In severe cases there is at first considerable feverishness and constitutional disturbance, together with sickness and faintness, which either precede or accompany the appearance of the rash. The eruption may appear on any part of the body, but is most common on the face and trunk. In the former position it causes swelling and disfigurement while it lasts, and is apt to excite alarm in persons unacquainted with its nature. The attack may pass off in a few hours, or may last for several days, the eruption continuing to come out in successive patches. The lesions are accompanied by severe itching. Occasionally a similar process takes place in the throat, and there is then considerable danger from blockage of the larynx. (See also ALLERGY.)

Treatment – The treatment of urticaria has been revolutionized by the introduction of the antihistamine drugs. There is now a large number of these, and it is necessary to find which particular preparation suits a particular individual. In addition, it is necessary to discover, if possible, the causative factor and to remove it. For instance, if an attack always follows the taking of a certain article of diet, this should be carefully noted and avoided in future. The patient's general health should also be attended to, if this is not satisfactory. The local irritation is allayed by sponging with calamine lotion, a warm alkaline solution (a teaspoonful of soda or ammonia to a tumblerful of warm water), with Goulard's water, or by rubbing with menthol.

NEURALGIA, literally *nerve pain*, is a term which is often employed both technically and popularly in a somewhat loose manner, to describe pains the origin of which is not clearly traceable. In its strict sense it means the existence of pain in some portion of, or throughout the whole of, the distribution of a sensory nerve, without any distinctly recognizable structural change in the nerve or nerve-centres. This strict definition, if adhered to, however, would not be applicable to a large number of cases of nerve pain; for in many instances the pain is connected with pressure on, or inflammation of, the nerve. Hence the word is generally used to indicate pain affecting a particular nerve or its branches, whatever be the cause.

Causes – It may be generally stated that neuralgia rarely occurs in the midst of good health. Constitutional causes, hereditary or acquired, are among predisposing influences in its production. Thus it is often found to affect the rheumatic or gouty. In weakened conditions of the system from unsuitable or insufficient food, or as the result of any drain upon the body, or in anaemia from any cause, or when certain disease poisons are present, such as syphilis or malaria, it is common for neuralgia to come on. Further, any strain upon the nervous system, such as mental overwork or anxiety, is a powerful predisposing cause. Among the exciting causes of an attack of neuralgia, by far the most common is exposure to cold and damp, which seems to excite irritation in a nerve already disposed to suffer. But irritation may be produced by numerous other causes, such as bruising of a nerve by a blow, a decayed tooth, diseased bone, local inflammations in which nerves are implicated, or some source of pressure upon a nerve-trunk, such as swelling of the sheath in its passage through a bony canal. Also a foreign body, or even the scar of an old wound, has been found to be sufficient cause of irritation when situated close to a nerve. Further, there are causes of a reflex character which are capable of setting up neuralgia at a distance, such as intestinal or uterine derangements. Those cases in which, after removal of a piece of nerve, inflammatory changes and thickening of the nerve-sheath are found, receive the name of neuritis, but, as regards the question of pain, there is no difference between neuritis and neuralgia due to other causes, except that pain caused by neuritis tends to be continuous and is very difficult to treat.

The practical importance of ascertaining the probable nature of the cause is obvious.

Symptoms – Although the pain is generally localized, it may spread beyond the area where it first occurs. It is usually of paroxysmal character, and often periodic: that is to say, it occurs at a certain time of the day or night. It varies in intensity, being often of the most agonizing character, and again less severe and more of a tingling kind. Various forms of perverted nerve function may be found along with or following neuralgia. Thus there may be over-sensitiveness of the skin, loss of feeling, paralysis or alterations of nutrition, such as wasting of muscles, whitening of the hair. Attacks of neuralgia are apt to recur, particularly when the general health is low, and some persons unhappily continue to suffer from occasional attacks during the greater part of their lifetime.

Varieties – The nature of the disease is best described under the names of the forms in which it most commonly occurs. These are trigeminal neuralgia (qv) or tic douloureux; intercostal neuralgia; and sciatica (qv). Other forms, affecting other nerves, are of much less frequent occurrence.

INTERCOSTAL NEURALGIA is pain affecting the nerves which emerge from the spinal cord and run along the spaces between the ribs to the front of the body. This form of neuralgia affects the left side more than the right, is more common in women than in men, and occurs generally in enfeebled states of health. It might be mistaken for pleurisy or some inflammatory affection of the lungs; but the absence of any chest symptoms, its occurrence independently of the acts of respiration, and other considerations establish the distinction. The specially painful points are chiefly where the nerve issues from the spinal canal, and at the extremities towards the front of the body, where it breaks up into filaments which ramify in the skin. This form of neuralgia is occasionally the precursor of an attack of shingles (*herpes zoster*) as well as a result of it. (See HERPES.)

Treatment – With all forms of neuralgia it is of the first importance to ascertain, if possible, whether any constitutional condition is associated with the malady, and, if evidence of the presence of for example rheumatism, gout, or anaemia, be discovered, to administer along with the local remedies for neuralgia, the remedies required for the constitutional condition. Naturally also one looks for, and as speedily as possible removes, any source of local irritation, such as a decayed tooth, and also any such reflex source as uterine or intestinal disorder.

During the time an acute attack lasts, various local applications give relief, the most useful being, perhaps, hot fomentations applied over the painful part. Bathing with water as hot as can be borne is also beneficial in many cases. Rubbing or painting with anodyne liniment, such as a mixture of the liniments of aconite, belladonna and chloroform (ABC Liniment); or a mixture, in equal parts, of chloral, camphor and menthol, rubbed up together and painted over the part, is soothing, especially perhaps for those cases in which the pain begins as soon as the sufferer gets warm in bed at night. Ointment of aconitine is also recommended by some to be rubbed on the painful spot. Hypodermic injections of morphine, although they give temporary relief, are not to be recommended because of the great danger that their use will become a habit. In the case of purely sensory nerves, like the fifth nerve, injection of pure alcohol into the nerve has a deadening effect and often gives relief for a long time.

Internally, during an acute attack, many remedies are given. Those which are most generally useful, and which may be safely used without any tendency to bring about habitual use, are aspirin, paracetamol and codeine.

Local measures in the chronic state include the application of blisters or counter-irritation by touching the skin with the button-cautery. The blister is made of an oblong shape, with its length corresponding to the line of the nerve, and the spots at which the cautery is applied generally also follow the affected nerve. The use of galvanic electricity is often beneficial in both the acute and the chronic stage. (See ELECTRICITY IN MEDICINE.) Diathermy is also employed with soothing effect. (See DIATHERMY.) Baths of various sorts, particularly alternate hot and cold baths, or douches, and the hot-air bath, are sometimes of use. (See BATHS, DOUCHES.) Massage, though it increases the pain in the acute state, may be of great benefit in chronic cases due to some inflammatory process in the nerve.

Some cases resist all forms of medicinal treatment, and for these surgical procedures are sometimes tried, such as division and removal of a portion of the nerve, or injection of absolute alcohol into the nerve.

NEURASTHENIA means a condition of nervous exhaustion in which, although the patient suffers from no definite disease, he becomes incapable of sustained exertion. It was never a very well-defined entity, and the term has now been largely given up. The condition which it represented is now recognized to be a form of neurosis (qv) or psychoneurosis (qv).

NEURECTOMY is the term applied to an operation in which part of a nerve is excised: for example, for the relief of neuralgia.

NEURILEMMA is the name of the thin membranous covering which surrounds every nerve-fibre. (See NERVES.)

NEURITIS means inflammation affecting a nerve or nerves which may be localized to one part of the body, as, for instance, in sciatica, or which may be general, being then known as multiple neuritis, or polyneuritis. Owing to the fact that the most peripheral parts of the nerves are usually at fault in the latter condition, ie. the fine subdivisions in the substance of the muscles, it is also known as peripheral neuritis.

Causes – In cases of LOCALIZED NEURITIS the fibrous sheath of the nerve is usually at fault, the actual nerve-fibres being only secondarily affected. This condition may be due to inflammation spreading into the nerve from surrounding tissues, to cold or to long-continued irritation by pressure on the nerve, and the symptoms produced vary according to the function of the nerve, in the case of sensory nerves being usually neuralgic pain (see NEURALGIA), in the case of motor nerves more or less paralysis in the muscles to which the nerves pass. A typical example of this kind of neuritis is found in neuritis of the facial nerve. (See PARALYSIS.)

In POLYNEURITIS, which is always due to some general or constitutional cause, the nerve-fibres themselves in the small nerves degenerate and break down. Hence the very protracted nature of this malady, since, if recovery takes place, it must be brought about by the growth of new nerve-fibres from the healthy part of the nerve, down the sheath of the nerve, to the muscle. The cause of this degeneration may be said, in general terms, to be some poison either taken into or produced in the body, and circulating in the blood. By far the commonest of these poisons is alcohol, and the disease especially affects women who are quiet, steady tipplers. The condition also arises in men, though more rarely, the abuse of alcohol in this sex tending more to produce delirium tremens, from which women are almost exempt. Next in importance comes lead, wrist-drop and other features of neuritis being among the most prominent symptoms of lead-poisoning. (See LEAD-POISONING.) Arsenic is occasionally responsible for neuritis, particularly when the effect of arsenic is combined with over-indulgence in alcohol, as in an epidemic of neuritis, due to beer contaminated with arsenic, in the Midlands of England about the year 1900. Bisulphide of carbon, naphtha and other solvents of india-rubber are apt to produce the disease when inhaled in large quantity by the workmen engaged in india-rubber factories. Those who suffer from diabetes are prone to neuritis, the condition sometimes being the result of deficiency of thiamine in the diet. This deficiency probably also accounts for some cases of alcoholic neuritis. In both diabetes and chronic alcoholism the diet is far from normal. Gout, too, is occasionally accompanied by neuritis. Several of the acute infectious diseases, especially diphtheria and typhoid fever, are apt to be followed by neuritis. The disease known as beri-beri (see BERI-BERI) is a form of neuritis which persists in certain localities of the globe, in consequence of thiamine deficiency.

Symptoms – The chief symptom of a LOCALIZED NEURITIS, whether pain or paralysis, has been already stated to vary according to the functions of the nerve. In cases following diphtheria, or other infective disease, the neuritis of an outlying nerve often shows, as its most prominent and annoying feature, a paralysis of a group of muscles in the arm or leg, leading to weakness of the part concerned. This may cause inability for some months to grasp objects with the hand, to lift the foot in walking and similar troublesome symptoms. These, however, usually pass off completely in course of time. The area of skin associated with the affected nerve is, in addition, often much changed, becoming glossy, or developing an ulcer or, especially about the face and trunk, breaking out in shingles. (See HERPES.) A case of neuritis of this type may come on very quickly, developing fully in a few days.

POLYNEURITIS, as a rule, takes longer to show itself, even in the case of diphtheria, seldom developing till two or three weeks after the onset of the trouble in the throat. In most cases it begins with vague pains and tingling in the limbs; weakness and wasting of the muscles in the feet and legs, in the hand and arms, or in other parts, following later. Wrist-drop, the peculiar steppage gait in which the person lifts his feet as if he were constantly stepping over small obstacles, squinting, loss of voice, difficulty of breathing, enfeeblement of the heart's action appear according to the muscles whose nerves are affected. There is usually some loss of sensation in scattered areas over the skin, but a very characteristic sign, in the alcoholic form of neuritis at least, is that the muscles are extremely tender when squeezed. There is almost always some swelling of the feet, and in the neuritis of beri-beri dropsy is often a marked symptom. The knee-jerks and other deep reflexes are generally lost in all forms of neuritis, if severe in character. A peculiar feature of alcoholic neuritis is the wandering delirium from which the patient often suffers, her imagination conjuring up the most vivid delusions as to journeys she is making, and the mind being quite confused in matters regarding time and place especially.

The course of the disease is, usually very slow, and particularly is this the case when a poison, as in the case of alcohol or lead, has been taken into the system over a long period. Months, or even a year or two, may elapse before health is restored. The ultimate hope of recovery is, however, good. Except in the case of beri-beri, which is fatal unless treated, and in those cases of poisoning by alcohol, or of diphtheria, in which the mechanism of the heart or that of respiration becomes affected, the mortality is low.

Treatment – For the treatment of LOCALIZED NEURITIS see under NEURALGIA.

The first essential in the treatment of POLYNEURITIS is to discover and remove the cause by which the nerves are being poisoned. Particularly does this apply to alcoholism, lead-poisoning and neuritis due to manufacture of india-rubber. In the case of alcoholism there is always the moral difficulty of preventing the patient from obtaining fresh supplies of stimulants, so that treatment must be carried out in a hospital or nursing-home. Rest in bed is the next essential to prevent over-fatigue of the weakened nerves and muscles. In the early stages the muscles are too tender to permit of much handling, but, later on, massage helps to prevent wasting of muscles, and the deformities which arise through fixation of the joints in one position. These deformities must be prevented as far as possible during the earlier stages by frequently changing the position of the patient's limbs as he lies in bed. Electrical treatment may also help as recovery advances. Much benefit is sometimes gained from injections of thiamine or administration of foods containing it, such as Bemax or Marmite.

NEURODERMATOSES, sometimes grouped under the name of NEURODERMATITIS, and also known as ATOPIC DERMATITIS, are disorders of the skin in which stress is one of the important factors, if not the most important cause. In some conditions, such as pruritus (see ITCHING) and rosacea (qv) this is the principal cause. In others, such as atopic eczema (see ECZEMA) and lichen simplex (see LICHEN), it is a secondary, but nonetheless often important, factor, any mental or emotional stress or strain bringing on an exacerbation, or flaring up, of the skin condition. In others again, such as *dermatitis artefacta* the emotional, or mental, instability may be the sole cause, the individual deliberately damaging his or her skin, without divulging the cause. The extreme form of this manifestation of mental illness is parasitophobia, in which the individual has a morbid terror of parasites and is quite convinced that he or she is infested with some parasite which is causing the itching which in turn has been scratched until the skin has broken down.

NEUROGLIA is the name applied to a fine web of tissue and branching cells which supports the nerve fibres and cells of the nervous system. (See NERVES.)

NEUROLEPTIC is an anti-psychotic drug: ie., a drug used in the treatment of a psychosis (qv).

NEUROLOGY is the branch of medical practice and science which deals with the nervous system and its diseases.

NEUROMA means a tumour connected with a nerve, such tumours being generally composed of fibrous tissue, and of a painful nature.

NEUROMYASTHENIA is a disease, which often occurs in epidemics, and which is characterized by headache, stiffness of the neck and back, muscular weakness and pain, fever and often diarrhoea. When it occurs in epidemics it is known as epidemic neuromyasthenia, Icelandic disease or Royal Free disease. This last name results from an outbreak among the nurses at the Royal Free Hospital, London. The epidemic form is most common among women. The cause is not known but has been attributed to a virus or to hysteria.

NEURONE is the name given to a single unit of the nervous system consisting of a nerve cell with its various processes and the nerve fibre or fibres to which it gives origin. As applied to the motor part of the nervous system, two neurones are specially recognized: the *upper neurone*, which includes a cell on the surface of the brain and a fibre extending down into the spinal cord; the *lower neurone*, which consists of a cell in the grey matter of the cord with a nerve fibre extending outwards to end in a fibre of the muscle with which it is connected. The former has a controlling influence over the latter, whilst the latter is more directly concerned with the changes that result in the contraction of the muscle fibre and with nutritional influences over it. (See NERVES.)

NEUROSIS is a general term applied to mental or emotional disturbance in which, as opposed to psychosis, there is no serious disturbance of the personality. At one time the condition was differentiated from psychoneurosis, but it is now accepted that these two terms are synonymous, or at least merge into one another. As has been pointed out, 'there are few clearly defined boundaries in nature, and there is many a case of mental illness which it is difficult to assign definitely to the neurotic or psychotic group'. Speaking generally, however, a psychosis involves a change in the whole personality of the individual, whereas in a neurosis it is only part of the personality that is involved. Alternatively, it might be said that in a psychosis reality is changed and the individual acts accordingly. In a neurosis, on the other hand, reality is unchanged and the neurotic individual always acts as if reality had the same meaning for him as for the community at large.

Neuroses are usually classified into anxiety neuroses, hysteria (qv) and obsessional neuroses.

Anxiety neurosis constitutes the commonest form of neurosis. Fortunately, it is also almost the most responsive to treatment. It occurs in people of anxious personality – the timid worriers of this world who are always meeting trouble halfway. Once the neurosis develops, they are in a state of persistent anxiety and worry, 'tensed up', always feeling fatigued and unable to sleep at night. In addition, there are often complaints suggesting some physical disorder: eg. palpitation, flatulence or headache.

Obsessional neuroses are much less common, and constitute only about 5 per cent of all neuroses. Like other neuroses, they usually develop in early adult life. They are characterized by the individual developing a phobia or obsession about something, and this may be so persistent that life becomes almost unbearable. Again, as in almost the entire field of mental illness, the borderline between an anxiety neurosis and an obsessional neurosis may be far from clear, but in the latter the obsession interferes much more with the ordinary life of the patient.

NEUROSURGERY is surgery performed on some part of the nervous system, whether brain, spinal cord or nerves.

NEUROTIC is a general term of indefinite meaning applied to a person of nervous temperament, whose actions are largely determined by emotions or instincts rather than by reason.

NEUROTRANSMITTER is a substance which transmits the action of a nerve to a cell. It is now recognized that this is how nerves work. If there should be a lack or deficiency of the appropriate neurotransmitter, then the nerve cannot carry out its action. A classical example of this is dopamine (qv), lack of which is responsible for the condition, known as Parkinsonism (qv). Other neurotransmitters include acetylcholine (qv) which is the neurotransmitter for the parasympathetic system (qv) and noradrenaline which is the neurotransmitter for the sympathetic nervous system.

NEUTRON is one of the particles that enter into the structure of the atomic nucleus. (See RADIOTHERAPY.)

NEUTROPENIA denotes a reduction in the number of neutrophil leucocytes per cubic millimetre of circulating blood to a figure below that found in health. There is still some disagreement over the precise limits of normality, but a count of less than 2500 per c.mm would be generally accepted as constituting neutropenia. Several infective diseases are characterized by neutropenia, including typhoid fever, influenza and measles. It may also be induced by certain drugs, including chlor-

amphenicol, phenylbutazone, the sulphonamides and chlorpromazine.

NICLOSAMIDE is the drug of choice in the treatment of tapeworm infestation. It is also known as YOMESAN.

NICOTINAMIDE, the amide of nicotinic acid, is sometimes used instead of nicotinic acid.

NICOTINE is the active principle upon which the action of tobacco depends. (See TOBACCO.)

NICOTINIC ACID, or NIACIN, is a member of the vitamin B complex. It is essential for human nutrition, the normal daily requirement for an adult being about 15 to 20 mg. A deficiency of nicotinic acid is one of the factors in the etiology of pellagra (qv), and either nicotine acid or nicotinamide is used in the treatment of this condition.

NIGHT BLINDNESS, or NYCTALOPIA, is a condition in which a person becomes blind in dim lights, although able to see quite well in the full glare of sunlight or artificial light, in some cases inherited and in others the result of an insufficiency of vitamin A in the diet, this vitamin being essential for the formation of visual purple.

NIGHTMARE (see SLEEP).

NIGHT SWEATS consist in copious perspiration occurring in bed at night and found in conditions of general weakness, especially in tuberculosis.

NIGHT TERRORS form a kind of nightmare in children of nervous temperament. (See SLEEP.)

NIKETHAMIDE is a drug which stimulates the respiratory centre.

NIPPLES, DISEASES OF (see BREAST, DISEASES OF).

NIRIDAZOLE is a recently introduced drug which is proving of value in the treatment of schistosomiasis (qv) and guineaworm infections.

NITRATE OF POTASSIUM is the technical name for nitre. (See NITRE.)

NITRATE OF SILVER, also known as

NITRAZEPAM

LUNAR CAUSTIC, is a heavy crystalline salt of silver, very soluble in water and generally prepared in sticks. In weak solution it has a strong astringent action, and in the pure form it acts as a powerful caustic. It is very slowly discharged from the system, and, if used for any great length of time, it is apt to produce a brown discoloration of the skin all over the body, known as argyria.

Uses – Locally it is used as a caustic, acting painlessly on warts, and the like. As an astringent it is used in inflammatory conditions of mucous membranes, in the form of gargles, sprays and douches, usually in the strength of about $\frac{1}{2}$ to 2 grains (30 to 125 mg) to the ounce (28·5 ml) of distilled water, but often stronger. Its local action can be checked, and any pain it may cause can be stopped by simply moistening the part and placing common salt upon it. It is used to drop into the eye in cases of conjunctivitis, the usual strength for this purpose being from $\frac{1}{2}$ to 1 per cent.

NITRAZEPAM is a tranquillizer introduced as a hypnotic with a wide margin of safety.

NITRE, also known as SALTPETRE, NITRATE OF POTASSIUM and, in the form of sticks, as SAL PRUNELLE, is a crystalline substance of a sharp saline taste, found in India, Persia and other places. It is very irritating to the stomach and is not now used internally, but is of use for inhalation in the treatment of asthma, since the nitrate in burning gives off nitrites. Two and a half ounces (70 grams) of the saltpetre are dissolved in a tumblerful of water, and squares of thin white blotting-paper about 6 inches (15 cm) square are dipped in this brine and then allowed to dry. When used they are folded like a tent, set on a plate, and lighted at the edges. Several of these, burned in the room of a person suffering from asthma, often give relief.

NITRIC ACID is one of the strongest of the mineral acids, and is a clear, heavy liquid, becoming brownish with age. It is kept in dark, stoppered bottles, and immediately the stopper is removed from the bottle, irritating white fumes are given off.

Action – In its pure state, nitric acid acts as a powerful caustic upon the tissues of the body, which it turns a bright yellow colour. In weaker solution it is, like all acids, an antiseptic, but is very irritating. Internally, in small doses it has a stimulating action upon the gastric mucous membrane.

Uses – Nitric acid is one of the most effective caustics for warts, and is also used as a powerful antiseptic and caustic for destroying foul ulcers which threaten to spread, leaving clean ulcers in their place. It is applied to warts drop by drop with a glass rod, and its action can be checked by applying similarly a few drops of solution of common salt.

NITRITES are salts which have a powerful effect in paralysing the action of involuntary muscle, and they therefore dilate the blood-vessels, and check spasm of all sorts. The most commonly used nitrites are nitrite of amyl, of ethyl, and of sodium. Erythrol tetranitrate and nitroglycerin have a similar action. (See GLYCERYL TRINITRATE.)

NITROFURANTOIN is a synthetic nitrofuran derivative which has a wide range of antibacterial activity and is effective against many Gram-positive and Gram-negative organisms. It is used mainly in the treatment of infections of the urinary tract.

NITROGEN MUSTARDS are nitrogen analogues of mustard gas. They are among the most important alkylating agents (qv) used in the treatment of various forms of malignant disease. They include mustine, trimustine, uramustine, busulphan, chlorambucil and melphalan.

NITROHYDROCHLORIC ACID, or AQUA REGIA, so called because of its power to dissolve gold, is a yellow liquid prepared by adding 1 part of nitric acid to 4 parts of hydrochloric acid. It is a caustic in its pure state, but is only used for internal administration in a diluted form. It is used in the treatment of dyspepsia associated with a low gastric acidity.

NITROUS OXIDE GAS, also known as LAUGHING GAS, is, at ordinary pressures, a gas devoid of odour but of a slightly sweetish taste. It is kept under pressure in steel cylinders, from which it can be allowed to escape at any desired rate by turning a stop-cock. Its use in medicine is to produce insensibility to pain, which it does very quickly, and with a great degree of safety, though the effect is of very short duration, not extending beyond two or three minutes. Its use is therefore applicable only for short operations, such as extraction of a tooth, unless it be repeatedly administered in association with oxygen. (See ANAESTHETICS.)

NOCTAMBULATION is another name for sleep-walking. (See SLEEP.)

NOCTURIA, or NYCTURIA, is the term used to denote excess passing of urine during the night. Among its many causes are Bright's disease (qv) and enlargement of the prostate. (See also URINE, EXCESS OF.)

NOCTURNAL ENURESIS is the involuntary passing of urine during sleep. It is a condition predominantly of childhood. In a small minority of cases it is due to some organic cause such as infection of the genito-urinary tract, but in the vast majority of cases it is due to inadequate or improper training of the child or psychological ill health. Traditionally it is said to be associated with threadworms, but there is little, if any, evidence to support this tradition.

Before deciding that a child is suffering from nocturnal enuresis, it is necessary to remember that the age at which a child achieves full control of bladder function varies considerably. Such control is usually achieved in the second year, but more commonly in the third year of life, and there are some children who do not normally achieve such control until the fourth, or even fifth, year.

NODE – The term node is widely used in medicine. For instance, the smaller lymphatic glands (qv) are often termed lymph nodes. It is also applied to a collection of nerve cells forming a subsidiary nerve centre found in various places in the sympathetic nervous system, such as the sinu-atrial node and the atrio-ventricular node which control the beating of the heart.

NOISE (see DEAFNESS).

NOMA is another name for cancrum oris. (See CANCRUM.)

NON-SPECIFIC URETHRITIS is an inflammatory condition of the urethra (qv) due to infection with certain types of the micro-organism known as *Chlamydia trachomatis*. In England and Wales it is the commonest sexually transmitted disease: 74,000 cases were reported in 1976. Most cases respond well to tetracycline (qv). Children born to infected mothers may have their eyes infected during birth, producing the condition known as ophthalmia neonatorum (qv). This is treated by the application to the eye of chlortetracycline eye ointment. The lungs of such a child may also be infected, resulting in pneumonia. The eye may also be infected in adults with the disease or those who are in contact with infected sexual partners.

NORADRENALINE is a precursor of adrenaline (qv) in the medulla of the suprarenal glands. It is also present in the brain. Its main function is to mediate the transmission of impulses in the sympathetic nervous system (qv). It also has a transmitter function in the brain.

NORETHISTERONE is a synthetic preparation that has the action of progesterone (qv), but is active when given by mouth.

NORETHYNODREL is another synthetic substance which has a progesterone-like action. (See PROGESTERONE.) Originally – and still – used for the treatment of various menstrual disorders, at the moment the main interest of these progestogens, as they are known, is their property of inhibiting ovulation. It is this property that led to their use as oral contraceptives. (See CONTRACEPTION.)

NORMAL is a term used in several different senses. Generally speaking, it is applied to anything which agrees with the regular and established type. In chemistry the term is applied to solutions of acids or bases of such strength that each litre contains the number of grams corresponding to the molecular weight of the substance in question. In physiology the term normal is applied to solutions of such strength that, when mixed with a body fluid, they are isotonic and cause no disturbance: eg. normal saline solution. (See ISOTONIC.)

NORMOBLAST is the term applied to a red blood corpuscle which still contains the remnant of a nucleus.

NORTRIPTYLINE is an antidepressant drug which is also a sedative.

NORWEGIAN SCABIES is the name given in Scotland to the severe form of scabies (qv) in which the skin becomes greatly thickened and fissures develop.

NOSE – The nose has three main functions. It is the natural pathway whereby air enters the body in the course of respiration (qv). In the nose the incoming air is warmed, moistened and filtered before passing on into the lungs. It has also a protective function. Irritation of it by dust or the like induces sneezing (qv) which expels the irritant from the nose and so prevents it getting into the lungs. It is also the organ of smell (qv).

The *external nose* is formed partly of bone and partly of cartilage, covered by skin (illustration 330). In its upper part, the two nasal bones, one on each side, project downwards from the frontal bone for about an inch (25 mm), and, supported by a process of the upper jaw-bone, form

divided into two narrow cavities, one on each side, by a septum or partition running from front to back. This septum is a thin plate composed partly of bone, partly of cartilage, consisting in about its hinder two-thirds of the central plate of the ethmoid bone and of the vomer bone, and in about its anterior third of a four-sided plate of cartilage, which along one edge touches the nasal bones, the lateral cartilages, and the cartilages of the aperture. On both surfaces this septum is covered by the general mucous membrane that lines the nose.

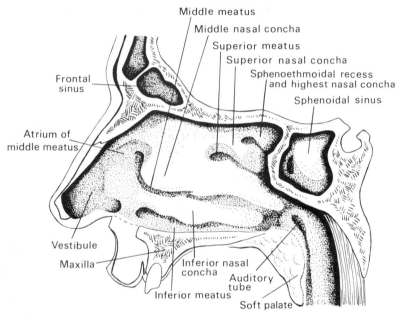

330 – The lateral wall of the right half of the nasal cavity. From *Gray's Anatomy*. Longman.

the hard bridge of the nose between the eyes. The ending of the bony part can be seen or felt on most noses, and, beneath this, two cartilages on each side, the lateral cartilages and the cartilages of the aperture give shape, firmness, and pliability to the lower two-thirds of the nose. The gap between the cartilages of the aperture can be distinctly felt on the point of the nose. The spaces between the cartilages are filled up and the cartilages firmly bound to the bones and to one another by fibrous tissue. When the nose is injured, some of the cartilages are apt to be dislocated, thus altering the shape of this organ.

In its *interior*, the nose is completely

The cavities on either side of the septum, known as the *nasal fossae*, are extremely narrow, being at their widest point less than $\frac{1}{4}$ inch (6 mm) in breadth, though in height they correspond to the length of the nose, and run directly backwards about 2 inches (5 cm). At its upper end each cavity is separated from the interior of the skull by a thin plate of bone containing many minute apertures for the passage of the filaments of the olfactory nerve. The front part of each cavity consists of the space enclosed by the cartilages of the nose, is lined by skin, which is furnished with stiff hairs that grow downwards and protect the entrance, and is known as the vestibule. Farther back the outer surface of each cavity is rendered very complicated, and the space in the cavity greatly filled up, by three projections known as the nasal conchae. These bones form ridges which run from before backwards with an inclination downwards, and, in section, each ridge is curled over so that its edge looks downwards. There are therefore three passages (meatus) running from before backwards, each under cover of a corresponding nasal

331 – Vertical section through the middle of the head and neck, showing the outer wall of the nose with the three nasal conchae. The passages for air, *a*, are indicated by a heavy dotted line; those for the food, *f*, by a fainter line; *et*, Eustachian tube; *l*, larynx; *w*, windpipe; *t*, tonsil; *to*, tongue; *g*, gullet. The sphenoidal and frontal sinuses are shown. Note the very thin plate of bone above the superior nasal concha which separates the cavity of the nose from the interior of the skull. (For other letters, *see* illustration 89.)

concha. As each of these bones, in common with the whole of the cavity, is covered with very vascular and thick mucous membrane, the air in its passage through the nose is by this arrangement brought into contact with a large surface of mucous membrane, and thus is considerably warmed before it enters the broncial tubes and lungs. In addition, this mucous membrane, which is covered with cilia (qv) secretes more than 500 millilitres of sticky mucus every 24 hours. This traps dust particles and the like, which are then moved on by the cilia and usually swallowed unnoticed. It is the excessive pro-

duction of this mucus, in response to irritations or infection, that is known as nasal catarrh (qv). The front portion of the inferior and of the middle nasal concha can be seen as two red projections by looking up the nostril with a bright light, when the nostril is slightly opened by a speculum. The superior meatus beneath the superior nasal concha is a narrow passage, and, upon this bone and passage as well as upon the corresponding part of the septum, the nerves of smell end in the mucous membrane. The wider and longer middle meatus and inferior meatus are the passages through which the air mainly passes out and in during respiration (illustration 331).

Certain *sinuses* lie concealed in the bones of the skull, into which air enters freely by apertures connecting them with the nose. These cavities occupy spaces in the frontal bone over the eyebrow (frontal sinus), in the upper jaw-bone, filling in the angle between the eye and the nose (maxillary sinus or antrum of Highmore), in the sphenoid bone (sphenoidal sinus), and in the lateral part of the ethmoid bone (ethmoidal sinus). These give both lightness to the skull and serve to diminish the violence of blows upon the face. The most capacious is the maxillary sinus, which is a cubical cavity, often over half an inch (12 mm) in measurement each way. The frontal sinus, maxillary sinus, and ethmoidal sinus open by small apertures about the centre of the middle meatus, the sphenoidal sinus above this. Into the front part of the inferior meatus opens the nasal duct, which carries the tears off from the eye. (See EYE.) The latter fact explains the frequent blowing of the nose which becomes necessary when a person is weeping. On a level with the inferior meatus, but situated in the part of the throat into which the nose opens, is placed the orifice of the Eustachian, or auditory, tube leading to the middle ear. (See EAR.)

NOSE, DISEASES OF – The nose, so far as the skin-covering is concerned, is subject to the same diseases as the skin of other parts. Redness of the skin of this part may, on account of its disfiguring character, be very annoying. It may be due to poor circulation in cold weather, partaking of the nature of a chilblain (see CHILBLAINS); occasionally it is due to constant indulgence in alcohol (see ROSACEA); habitual indigestion also tends to bring on a condition of redness, whilst any chronic state of inflammation or source of irritation in the interior of the nose may man-

635

ifest itself by redness on the surface. Among the skin diseases, acne (qv), lupus (qv), and erysipelas (qv) are specially prone to affect this site.

ACUTE INFLAMMATION of the nose (ACUTE RHINITIS) is generally a catarrhal condition affecting the mucous membrane, and is commonly known as a cold in the head. (See CHILLS AND COLDS.) It may be due, though less commonly, to the inhalation of irritating gases. Injuries to the nose are specially liable to be followed by erysipelas in some persons. (See ERYSIPELAS.) Boils occasionally develop just within the entrance to the nose, in connection with the hairs there, and in this locality give rise to great pain and considerable danger. (See BOILS.) Diphtheria is a form of acute inflammation which may spread to the nose. (See DIPHTHERIA.) Hay fever is a distressing form of acute rhinitis. (See HAY FEVER.)

CHRONIC INFLAMMATION of the nose (CHRONIC RHINITIS) is a common condition, and in a mild form may exist for years without attracting much attention.

Causes – Generally it follows upon repeated colds in the head, which do not pass off completely. It may also be due to the constant inhalation of dust or irritating vapours at work. There seems to be a hereditary tendency also for this type of inflammation to run in familes, probably in consequence of some peculiarity in the structure of the nose. The mucous membrane covering the nasal conchae swells up in consequence of the inflammation, and, by blocking the passage of the air to some extent, as well as by producing irritating discharges, forms a source of constant irritation which perpetuates the condition. Any malformation, such as great bulging of the septum to one side, or the presence on it of a spur, has a similar effect, and such malformations have often the effect of rendering persons who have a slight tendency to hay fever additionally liable to this malady, in consequence of the degree of chronic inflammation the malformations produce.

Symptoms – The most marked symptom is increased secretion from the swollen mucous membrane, causing constant running at the nose, together with a feeling of stuffiness. It is necessary to blow the nose very frequently, or the person is continually hawking mucus in the back of his throat. In some persons, however, instead of constant running of the nose, the inflammation is of a dry type, and the swollen mucous membrane becomes covered by crusts which are difficult to dislodge.

Sneezing is also a common symptom, resulting from the constant irritation in the nose, and a feeling of obstruction in the nose is usually experienced when the person lays his head down at night. The external nose, too, is liable to become large and red. When the condition becomes a little worse than usual, as the result, for instance, of a fresh cold, the person must breathe through his mouth, his voice takes on a nasal twang, and there is temporary loss of the senses of smell and taste. Occasionally the hearing is much impaired, and there may be neuralgia, aching over the bridge of the nose, and redness of the eyes.

Occasionally, in young persons of poor constitution, especially girls, the nose after suffering from this state for a short time takes on an atrophic process, and both the mucous membrane and the bones waste, so that the former loses its secretion and becomes covered by evil-smelling crusts, which make the breath very offensive, while the changes in the bones produce a small, tip-tilted nose. Happily, this condition, known as ozaena, is becoming less common.

Treatment – Care must be taken by those with a tendency to chronic inflammation of the nose to avoid catching colds. The condition of the mucous membrane can be greatly improved and the inflammation soothed by the use every night and morning of one of the following lotions, applied to the nose either by means of a hand-spray or from a nasal syringe or douche. (1) Sodium bicarbonate 30 grains (2 G), sodium chloride 30 grains (2 G), borax 30 grains (30 G), white sugar 60 grains (4 G), rose water 8 ounces (230 ml): a small quantity of this is mixed with an equal quantity of hot water before use. (2) A teaspoonful of sodium bicarbonate and common salt mixed in equal parts, added to a tumblerful of warm water. When the mucous membrane is much swollen and the nasal passage in consequence much blocked, it becomes necessary to reduce this swelling in order to relieve the inflammation. This is done most effectively by the galvano-cautery. Relief is often obtained from the inhalation of menthol. When the inflammation is perpetuated by the presence of malformations in the nose, such as spurs on the septum, polypi or suppuration in the sphenoidal or other sinuses, these conditions may be removed by operation.

In cases in which the inflammation is due to penicillin-sensitive organisms, a course of penicillin may be of value.

When dry crusts tend to form and block up the nose they may be removed by the same alkaline douches, and also by the simple expedient of plugging up the nostrils with pieces of cotton-wool for a quarter of an hour, just sufficiently tightly to prevent air from passing out and in. If the latter plan be adopted the crusts are softened, a watery secretion is produced, and the crusts can be got rid of by gently blowing the nose, after the cotton-wool has been removed.

MALFORMATIONS OF THE NOSE are of various kinds. The external nose varies much in shape in different races, even in different families, and persons who desire for aesthetic reasons to alter the character of this feature can mould the cartilages to a certain extent by constant manipulation or by wearing various appliances. Noses, which have become tiptilted through sinking in of the bridge, may, after the disease which has caused the sinking has subsided, be improved by the injection of paraffin under the skin. (See ARTIFICIAL LIMBS AND OTHER PARTS.) As to the interior of the nose, the two cavities are practically never of equal size, the septum always bulging to one or other side, so that the passage of air is freer on one side than on the other. When this bulging is so marked that the septum touches the nasal conchae on one side, or when, owing to injury or other cause, spurs and crests have developed on the septum, considerable irritation may arise, and this may form the starting-point for chronic inflammation of the nose, hay fever or asthma. These imperfections, though they often exist without the least ill-effect, and are only discovered accidentally, are readily removed by the specialist if necessary, such operations being attended by but little pain. A more common abnormality is that in which the nose becomes pinched and narrow as the result of blockage by polypi, adenoids and similar causes, and in consequence the person breathes through the mouth.

ADENOIDS, or ADENOID VEGETATIONS, means an overgrowth of the glandular tissue which is naturally found in small amount on the back of the upper part of the throat, into which the nose opens.

Causes – This glandular tissue is similar in structure to the tonsils and lymphatic glands, and in children between the ages of 5 and 12, particularly after some inflammatory condition of the respiratory passages or after one of the acute infections diseases, such as measles, it may develop to such an extent as to fill up this portion of the throat and obstruct the passage of air through the nose and into the Eustachian tubes.

Symptoms – Generally this overgrowth subsides as the child passes through his teens, but its continuance for even a few years may produce serious effects upon the child's physique and mental powers. The appearance of a child suffering from adenoids is highly characteristic. The mouth is kept constantly open, since breathing proceeds through it, and, as a result, the child is very liable to bronchitis, and he snores at night. The point of the nose is pinched and the nostrils narrow, since very little air passes through them, and the bridge of the nose is often flattened. The palate is highly arched and the front teeth often prominent. If the child be weak or rickety, the obstruction to the entrance of air into the chest is apt to produce a pigeon-breast. Deafness, as the result of inflammation spreading up the Eustachian tubes from the throat to the ear, is common, and may be permanent. There is also some interference with the senses of smell and taste, though this is not so serious as deafness. A typical mental condition is common among children thus affected, the child being generally listless and lacking in the power of concentration; a fact that is made more noticeable by the heavy, stupid look which the open mouth and the deafness give to the face. The irritability of the nervous system, occasioned by the difficulty of breathing during sleep, renders these children, much more than others, prone to suffer from nightmares and from the habit of wetting the bed at night.

Treatment – As already stated, it is not the occurrence but the overgrowth of adenoids that gives rise to trouble in children, and, even if large, they tend to subside as the child advances in years. It is often difficult to decide therefore whether an operation for their removal should be performed or not. Apart from any serious symptoms that may be occasioned, such as deafness or choking, which certainly call for operation, the usual test employed is the question as to whether the child can go about quietly without becoming short of breath, and can sleep with his mouth shut. The operation – which is simple, consisting in scraping the adenoids away with the curette or other instrument and in cutting out the tonsils, which, as a rule, are enlarged, along with the adenoids – is performed under an anaesthetic.

POLYPI are growths of a soft, jelly-like character, with more or less of a stalk, arising usually from the middle nasal concha. They are the result of chronic inflammation in the hinder part of the nasal cavity, produced by frequent colds, following on some of the acute infectious diseases, or due to suppuration in one of the air cavities adjoining the nose.

Symptoms – There is usually a sense of stuffiness, and obstruction to breathing through the nose; occasionally the patient may be conscious of movement of the polypus as he breathes or talks. Many of the symptoms mentioned under chronic inflammation are present, as this condition is found in a greater or less degree along with polypi and is the cause of their development. When the nose is examined with a bright light and mirror, part of the polypus is often seen, and being of a glistening, greyish colour, contrasts strongly with the red mucous membrane of the nose.

Treatment – These polypi occasion no danger to life. Malignant tumours are occasionally found growing in the nose, but are very rare, and when they do occur are hard in texture, unlike these soft mucous polypi. The polypi are, however, seldom or never single, and after a large one has been removed the smaller ones around grow into its place and must in turn be removed. The removal is generally effected, quite painlessly, by passing a wire snare along the corresponding nostril, catching the polypus, and tightening the wire around its stalk till it can be pulled off, and when periodically done, may at last result in a complete cure. Recurrence is also prevented in many cases by scraping the inflamed mucous membrane from which the polypi are growing, or, in cases due to suppuration in the ethmoidal air-cells, by a severer operation designed to remove completely the lateral part of the ethmoid bone.

BLEEDING FROM THE NOSE, or *EPISTAXIS* (See HAEMORRHAGE).

FOREIGN BODIES, such as buttons, slate-pencils, peas and small stones, are often pushed into the nose by children. In recent years the most commonly encountered ones have been the small cubes of plastic sponge used to stuff children's soft toys. As the floor of the nose slopes slightly backwards and downwards, they readily pass in beyond reach. Concretions form in the nose, as in other hollow organs: round small blood-clots, hairs, and the like and these may grow to a considerable size.

Symptoms – At first the foreign body, if smooth, may set up no symptoms, but soon swelling of the nose, discharge from one nostril, headache and various pains appear, especially if the body be one which swells, like a pea. These symptoms may to a certain extent pass off, and if the body be wedged in tightly beneath the inferior nasal concha, it may remain there for years, causing little discomfort, till a severe attack of inflammation comes on. When there is a constant discharge of matter from one nostril without any known cause, it is probably due to some foreign body which has previously been introduced into the nose.

Treatment – Tickling the nostril with a feather, or giving a large pinch of snuff, to provoke a vigorous sneeze, while the opposite nostril is closed by pressure with the finger, should be tried first of all. Very often this will drive out the stone or pea. If not, removal by a medical man, aided by a speculum and a bright light, is comparatively easy, much more so than in the case of bodies pushed into the ear. In the case of children, an anaesthetic is generally necessary, as the child will not remain still.

LOSS OF SENSE OF SMELL, or *ANOSMIA*, may be caused by conditions which block the lower part of the nose and produce a sodden condition of the mucous membrane in which the olfactory nerves end. Such conditions are polypi and chronic inflammation. Certain drugs, such as carbolic acid, are very destructive of this sense, and douching the nose with carbolic lotion has been known to produce loss of smelling power. A severe cold in the head causes temporary loss. It may also follow injuries to the brain and fractures of the skull involving the olfactory nerves. A powerful odour, when allowed to act upon the nose for long, may paralyse the sense of smell for that particular odour, although the sense may remain quite acute for all other smells. For this reason the nose is an uncertain guide to the presence of poisonous gases in the air, for the smelling power may quickly become numbed by such a gas as coal gas or prussic acid.

SUPPURATION IN THE SINUSES, or *SINUSITIS*, is of fairly frequent occurrence. Suppuration in the *frontal* sinus is rare, because of the very efficient drainage from this cavity straight downwards into the nose, whilst suppuration in the *cells of the sphenoid and ethmoid* bones, unless it causes polypi, is apt to escape notice, but the *maxillary sinus* lying in the maxillary bone close to the roots of the upper row of teeth, from which it is separated only by mucous membrane and thin bone, and opening only by its upper part into the nose, is liable to become inflamed and to have pus collect in it.

Symptoms – When suppuration occurs in the *frontal sinuses*, severe headache is apt to result as well as discharge from the nose. When suppuration takes place in the *sphenoidal sinuses*, there is constant purulent discharge either from the nose or into the throat, and there may be a state of general debility, or inflammatory changes may be set up in the eye or its optic nerve, which lie in close relation to these sinuses. The effects of a collection of pus in the *maxillary sinus*, or antrum, may be very slight; intermittent pain of a neuralgic character often felt above one eye, toothache and slight swelling of one cheek may be the only signs for a long time. Generally, however, attention is called to the nose by a slight intermittent discharge of matter from one nostril, especially when the head is laid upon the opposite side. The small operation of pushing a hollow needle through the plate of bone separating the nose from the sinus, which is no thicker than a playing-card, is bloodless and almost painless. If pus runs from the needle the diagnosis is confirmed.

Treatment – In the case of the maxillary sinus, the infection may respond to inhalations. In more severe cases it may be necessary to drain the sinus through an opening made between the sinus and the nose, as described in the preceding paragraph. Many different antiseptic solutions are used for washing out the sinus, including penicillin. It is sometimes advisable to give a course of penicillin by intramuscular injection, or a course of one of the sulphonamides, in addition to local treatment. Should the infection of the sinus be due to dental trouble, then this must be dealt with.

A more serious operation is necessary in order to explore and drain the frontal sinuses, the incision being made usually along the line of the eyebrow. In the case of the sphenoidal sinuses, these are explored and scraped out through the nose under a general anaesthetic. (See also HAY FEVER.)

NOSOLOGY is the term applied to scientific classification of diseases.

NOSOPHOBE is a person who has a morbid fear of contracting a certain disease.

NOSTALGIA means a form of melancholy or aggravated home-sickness occurring in persons who have left their home.

NOTIFIABLE DISEASES are diseases, usually of an infectious nature, which are required by law to be made known to a health officer or local authority. (See INFECTION.)

NOVOBIOCIN is an antibiotic derived from cultures of *Streptomyces spheroides* or *Streptomyces niveus*. It is particularly active against staphylococci, and has proved especially useful in the treatment of staphylococcal infections which have not responded to treatment with other antibiotics, or in which the causative organism is resistant to such antibiotics.

NUCHA is the Latin name for the back of the neck.

NUCLEAR MEDICINE is that branch of medicine that is concerned with the use of radioactive material in the diagnosis, investigation and treatment of disease.

NUCLEUS means the central body in a cell, which controls the activities of the latter. (See CELL.)

NUCLEUS PULPOSUS is the inner core of an intervertebral disc. (See SPINAL COLUMN.)

NULLIPARA is the term applied to a woman who has never borne a child.

NUMBNESS (see TOUCH).

NUMMULAR SPUTUM is expectoration which when spat into water flattens out into a shape like coins. (See EXPECTORATION.)

NURSING as a profession requires an elaborate training, although persons are often called upon to nurse relatives and friends without any previous experience of the subject. It is with reference to the latter contingency that the following remarks apply, as it would be quite impossible even to state briefly the many duties which hospital training teaches.

Professional nursing falls into four divisions: (*a*) *Hospital nursing*, which forms a training for all the other kinds of nursing. (*b*) *Private nursing*, ie. nursing of a single patient, to whom the nurse's undivided attention is given, at home. (*c*) *District nursing*, which is the most arduous, and requires the greatest skill in the nurse. In this type of nursing, patients are visited at home, and not only a long and varied training, but great self-reliance is required. (*d*) *Midwifery nursing*, which includes the care of mother and child for about a month after the latter is born. Full details about openings in nursing, details of training and of training schools can be obtained from the Royal College of Nursing, 1a Henrietta Place, London, W1.

Information on various special subjects arising in the course of a nurse's duties will be found under ANTISEPTICS; ASEPSIS; BATHS; BED; BED CHANGING; BED SORES; BLISTERS AND COUNTER-IRRITANTS; BLOOD-LETTING; CATHETERS; CHILDREN, PECULIAR-ITIES OF; CUPPING; DIET; DISINFECTION; DOUCHE; ELECTRICITY IN MEDICINE; ENEMA; FEEDING; FOMENTATIONS; GARGLES; HAEM-ORRHAGE; INFANT FEEDING; INFECTION; LIGHT; MASSAGE; PEPTONIZED FOODS; POUL-TICES; TEMPERATURE; VENTILATION; WET PACK; WOUNDS. The following remarks upon home nursing are made under the two headings of: (1) *the sick-room*; (2) *the patient*.

(1) **The sick-room** – The *situation* of the room is a matter of some importance. It must be bright and sunny, and should therefore, if possible, look to the south or south-west. It should be as much cut off from the general household as possible. Good drainage is of the utmost importance if there is a fixed basin in the room, particularly in the case of surgical or lying-in patients. The room should, in every case, be as large and airy as possible, for coldness is a minor danger and of far less importance than defective ventilation. The great test of *ventilation* is the presence or absence of the faintest 'stuffy' smell in the room. If the patient complains of any draught, the window should not be shut, but the stream of air is kept off the bed by a screen or a sheet supported on a clothes-screen. A thermometer should always hang on the wall, so that the *temperature* of the room can be kept fairly uniform, and a good average temperature is about 60° to 65° F (15·5° to 19·3° C), although in bronchitis and other chest complaints it may be advisable to keep the air warmer. Artificial lighting should be adequate, including a bedside lamp, but so arranged that it will not inconvenience the patient. There should be as little *furniture* as possible in a sick-room. A bed, a bed-side table or locker, a comfortable chair for the patient if out of bed, two plain chairs, and a table are all that are absolutely necessary, and there need be no carpet save a small piece of drugget at the bed-side. Fur-

niture should not be dusted, nor must the floor be swept during an illness, but the furniture may be wiped daily with a damp cloth, and the floor may be washed when required, or, preferably, gently swept with an oily mop. As to the disinfection of a room after the nursing of an infectious case, see DISINFECTION. When preparations are being made for a *surgical operation* at home a large but narrow strong deal table should be placed immediately before the window, and on it should be laid a couple of blankets, a large sheet of mackintosh, and a clean pillow. Several basins and a large supply of clean linen towels should be at hand, as well as a plentiful supply of boiling water, and a ewer full of water which has been boiled and set aside to cool, covered by a towel.

(2) **The patient** – In putting an injured person to bed, it is important to remove the *garments* first of all from the sound arm or leg, and lastly from the injured limb, which is then moved as little as possible. On the other hand, and for the same reason, in putting on garments the injured limb should be the first to have the garment drawn over it. While a patient, and especially one greatly prostrated, lies in bed, one of the chief duties of the nurse is the care of his *skin*. The patient should be washed daily all over with warm water. The ordinary bed-clothes are removed before commencing the washing; during the process of wash-ing the patient is covered by another blanket. During the washing it is quite un-necessary that the skin should be exposed, the blanket being raised over one part, which is washed and dried before the washing of another part is begun, so that there ought to be no risk of chill. Further, the back and all bony prominences must be examined at the same time for any trace of redness, which is the first sign of a bed sore, and treated promptly if any sign of a bed sore appears. (See BED SORES.) When the chest is affected, jackets made of two flaps of gamgee tissue, secured by tapes at the shoulders and beneath the arms, keep the chest warm, and are easily removed when necessary.

Hot water bottles are often put in bed for warmth; these should *never* be put in bed unprotected by a woollen covering. They may be placed in flannel bags, in stockings, or wrapped in shawls, and this precaution is specially necessary in the case of patients unconscious after a severe operation, or paralysed, and so to some extent insensible of heat. Otherwise very serious burns may result.

In cases of heart disease there should be a number of pillows, if not a *bed-rest*, breathing being easier when the patient reclines in a half-sitting posture. When the patient has to sit up for long periods, an *air-cushion* makes this position easier, or a high table placed across the bed and provided with a pillow upon which he can lean his arms. Care should always be taken to keep the shoulders warmly wrapped up. When the legs are swollen or inflamed, they should be raised on a pillow, or the foot of the bed may be tilted up on wooden blocks. Paralysed or helpless cases should be placed upon a *water-bed* from the first. A water-bed is most easily managed if it be in two sections, each covering half the bed. The water-bed is filled with water before the patient is laid upon it, and should not be quite tightly filled. It is separated from the patient by a blanket and sheet. The more modern *air-bed* is in many respects preferable to a water-bed (see BED). If, in paralysed or other cases, the weight of the bed-clothes be found irksome, they should be raised from the patient by an *iron-wire cage*, and it is then necessary to add an extra blanket to the coverings. Finally, it is well in nursing cases of long duration to have *two beds*, in one of which the patient spends the day and in the other of which he sleeps at night. Still better, if the circumstances of the house and the nature of the case permit, is the plan of having a day bedroom and a night bedroom.

Any *medicines* which the patient may have to take should be kept in a different part of the room from bottles containing lotions and other fluids intended for external application, and the nurse should never pour out a dose without previously reading the label on the bottle. All medicines, whether for internal or external use, should be poured out of the bottle with the label uppermost, so that the label is not rendered illegible by the medicine draining down over it.

In *dressing* surgical cases, the nurse should boil any instruments she uses every day, and should wash her hands thoroughly with an antiseptic such as hexachlorophane soap, and then steep them in an antiseptic lotion such as corrosive sublimate (1 in 4000) or lysol (1 in 100), or an alcoholic solution such as 75 per cent isopropyl alcohol before touching the injured part. She should also remember that abrasions or pustules upon her hands form a source of danger both to herself and still more to the patient, and these should be carefully covered with collodion.

The nurse attending an *infectious case* should wear a special gown which is taken off at the door before leaving the room, and hung up inside the room. The hands are washed every time the patient is handled and on leaving the sick-room. (See BARRIER NURSING.)

In order to discharge her duties well, in all cases the nurse must have good food, sleep eight hours in every twenty-four, quite free from any chance of being roused to attend the patient, and have two hours daily for exercise and relaxation. She must also remember, in the words of the authorized nursing manual of the St John Ambulance, St Andrew's Ambulance Association, and the British Red Cross Society that 'nothing is more nauseating than the smell of stale perspiration or smoke or both, and no patient should be subjected to this from the nurse who is attending him (or her)'.

NURSING-BOTTLE MOUTH is the state of rampant caries of the teeth induced in children who are allowed to suck a bottle when put to bed at night or in their prams during the day. While the caries is more likely to occur if the 'comforter bottle', as it is popularly known, contains a sweetened drink, as it all too often does, it may also occur if the contents are milk. The reason for this is that with the child lying down the drink, whatever it is, is not swallowed promptly but tends to remain in the mouth and thus damage the teeth. This bottle-induced caries is most likely to occur in children who are allowed to engage in this pernicious habit after they have been weaned on to an ordinary diet. In no circumstances should a 'comforter bottle' be used. The same applies to the so-called comforter or dummy, even though this 'accursed instrument', as it has been named, dates back to the days of the Romans. By itself it is not as dangerous as the comforter bottle but, if sweetened, it is truly 'accursed' and should never be used by any parent who has any respect for her (or his) children. (See also TEETH, DISEASES OF.)

NUTMEG is the kernel of the seed of *Myristica fragrans*, an East and West Indian plant, mace being its outside covering. It is seldom used now in medicine.

NUTS, which consist to the extent of one-half or more of vegetable fat, form a highly concentrated form of nourishment, and if suitably prepared, for example, by roasting to render them more digestible, become of higher nourishing value than cheese, and may to a considerable extent act as substitutes for meat.

NUX VOMICA is the seed of *Strychnos nux-vomica*, an East Indian tree. It has an intensely bitter taste. The medicinal properties of the plant are almost entirely due to two alkaloids, strychnine and brucine, which it contains. (See STRYCHNINE.)

NYCTALOPIA is another name for night blindness (qv).

NYSTAGMUS means a condition in which the eyeballs show constant, fine, jerky movements of an involuntary char-

acter. The movement may be from side to side, from above down, or rotary; and it may be present only when the person looks in a certain direction. It appears in children who have some defect in vision, such as that due to an opacity on the cornea, and it is caused by some occupations, such as that of miners, due principally to inadequate lighting. It also occurs in certain nervous diseases: eg. multiple sclerosis.

NYSTATIN is an antibiotic isolated from *Streptomyces noursei*. It was the first antibiotic to be isolated which was active against fungus diseases, and is proving particularly useful in the treatment of moniliasis (qv).

O

OATMEAL is a meal made from oats. Two-thirds of its weight consists of carbohydrate in the dry state, but when cooked in the form of porridge it contains in addition about seven times its weight of water. Dry oatmeal contains approximately 12 per cent of protein, 5 per cent of fat, and 70 per cent of carbohydrate; and 1 ounce (28·5 grams) has an energy-producing equivalent of over 100 Calories.

OBESITY (see CORPULENCE.)

OBSESSION in medicine means the sudden domination of the mind by an idea or emotion, leading to impulsive acts which are beyond the control of the will, the power of judgment being for a time lost.

OBSTETRICS means the art of midwifery. (See LABOUR.)

OBSTRUCTION OF THE BOWELS (see INTESTINE, DISEASES OF).

OCCIPUT is the name given to the lower and hinder part of the head where it merges into the neck.

OCCUPATIONAL DISEASES – The increasing complexity of industrial and manufacturing processes, and the large proportion of the population of the country who are employed in industry, render occupational or industrial diseases, of increasing importance. Whenever a new process is introduced into industry every care is taken to ensure that it will involve no hazards to those employed in it. Even so, it is not always possible to foresee all possible risks, and therefore the management and the industrial medical officer must always be on the look-out so as to be able to detect any such hazard at the earliest possible stage before irreparable harm is done to the health of men or women handling the process. In many cases freedom from the hazards to health inherent in industrial or manufacturing processes is, in part at least, dependent upon the active cooperation of workmen and involves such simple procedures as the wearing of respirators, careful washing of the hands before eating, the application of barrier creams to the hands and arms, and the like. The obtaining of such cooperation is one of the main aims of efficient industrial management at the present day.

The magnitude of the problem involved can be gathered from the fact that it is estimated that there are about 2000 diseases which can be attributed to an individual's occupation. It says much therefore for the efficiency of the precautionary measures, and the care and skill with which they are employed, that there are so relatively few industrial diseases in any given year in such a highly industrialized country as Great Britain. This satisfactory state of affairs is the result of close and cordial cooperation between employers, industrial medical officers, and the Chief Inspector of Factories and his staff.

Although many industrial diseases entitle the victims to compensation, only a few are compulsorily notifiable. The following are the diseases which, if contracted in a factory, must be notified by the medical practitioner to the Chief Inspector of Factories: poisoning by lead, phosphorus, manganese, arsenic, mercury, carbon bisulphide, and aniline; chronic benzene poisoning, toxic jaundice, anthrax, epitheliomatous ulceration, chrome ulceration, compressed air illness, byssinosis, asbestosis, nasal adenocarcinoma, and toxic anaemia.

Lead is used widely throughout industry, and the following are some of the occupations in which it constitutes a hazard to health unless adequate precautions are taken: smelting, plumbing and soldering, shipbreaking, printing, pottery industry, electric accumulator works, painting. In the case of pottery and printing the risk has been almost entirely eliminated by the use of modern methods. The lead salts used in industry which are most dangerous to health are the oxide, the carbonate, and the chromate. The lead usually enters the body by the inhalation of dust or fumes. One of the practical difficulties in detecting and preventing lead-poisoning is that it is often insidious in onset. (See LEAD POISONING.)

Phosphorus has practically been eliminated as a cause of industrial poisoning in Great Britain. The first cases to be reported in this country since 1919 occurred during the 1939–45 War – one in 1941 and 1944. Yellow and white phosphorus are the dangerous forms. The red phosphorus used in the making of safety matches is relatively harmless. The match industry, in the days when white phosphorus was used for this purpose, was the classical source of phosphorus poisoning. The phosphorus gained admission through abrasions in the gums and caused destruction of the jaw, the condition known as phossy jaw. Luminous paints are another potential source of danger, principally when used to paint luminous watch dials. (See PHOSPHORUS POISONING.)

Manganese is not a common cause of industrial disease, but it is important because the results are so serious. It affects the brain and causes a condition very like post-encephalitic Parkinsonism (qv) and leaves the victim a permanent invalid. The dioxide is the dangerous salt, and the risk occurs in the handling of manganese ore, or in the handling of manganese dioxide itself, from exposure to the dust.

Arsenic is encountered in industry in the smelting and refining of ores, the subliming of white arsenic, and the manufacture of sheep dip, Scheele's green, and Paris green. White arsenic is used as a preservative of furs, hides, and skins, whilst Paris green is used as an insecticide for fruit trees. The replacement of Scheele's green by aniline colours has abolished the historical rôle of the manufacture of green wallpapers and artificial flowers as a cause of arsenical poisoning. Poisoning from arsenic in industry usually results from inhalation of, or contact with, the dust of arsenic compounds, and results in eczema and neuritis. Occasionally it takes a more serious and acute form, when it results from the inhalation of arseniuretted hydrogen. (See ARSENIC; NEURITIS.)

Mercury constitutes an industrial hazard in three forms: (i) exposure to the dust or vapour of metallic mercury; (ii) contact with mercury fulminate; (iii) exposure to organic mercury compounds. The industries or processes in which exposure to mercury may occur include: mercury mining and the separation of the metal from the ore; the manufacture of barometers, thermometers, and certain types of electric bulbs; water gilding; the felt-hat industry; dental technicians. Mercury fulminate is used in the making of explosives, and is particularly liable to attack the skin. Organic mercury compounds are mainly used in the manufacture of seed dressings and fungicides, and in the pharmaceutical industry. (See MERCURY POISONING.)

Carbon bisulphide, for long used in the cold curing of rubber and as a solvent for rubber, oil, and fats, has in more recent years been used in large amounts in the manufacture of certain forms of artificial silk. One of its dangers is that it vaporizes at ordinary temperatures, and the breathing of 1150 parts per million parts of air for 30 to 60 minutes is dangerous. Its main effect is upon the nervous system: neuritis, anxiety, depression, and impairment of memory.

Aniline is used in a wide variety of industrial processes: dyeing, painting, varnishing, rubber processing, and the manufacture of dyes, explosives, pharmaceutical products, and photographic chemicals. Absorption takes place mainly through the skin but may also occur through the lungs. The chief early manifestation of poisoning is a greyish-blue colour of the skin followed by shortness of breath. In chronic cases anaemia develops.

Benzene, a coal-tar derivative, is used on a large scale: the distillation of coal tar, the blending of motor fuels, and in the chemical industry. It is also used as a solvent in the rubber, aeroplane, linoleum, and celluloid industries and in the manufacture of paints, varnishes, glue, and artificial manure. The main manifestation of chronic benzene poisoning is anaemia due to a toxic effect of the benzene upon the bone marrow. Benzene is absorbed by inhalation.

Cadmium may cause disease in two different ways. Its fumes, encountered in melting cadmium or cadmium alloy, or from the use of cadmium electrodes, and the manufacture of ceramics, may cause an influenza-like illness, with shortness of breath, cough, irritation of the throat and sickness. Cadmium oxide dust produces diarrhoea, pneumonitis (qv) and proteinuria (qv). There may be a long period between exposure to cadmium and the first signs of poisoning by it.

Nitrobenzene is used in the manufacture of aniline dyes and explosives, and is a constituent of shoe and floor polish. It is also used as a perfume in cheap soaps. The main route of absorption is through the skin. It acts upon the nervous system, causing headache, giddiness, and numbness in the limbs, and upon the blood, causing anaemia and cyanosis.

Dinitrobenzene, which is used in the manufacture of dyes and explosives, is absorbed through the skin. Its principal toxic effect is upon the blood, resulting in cyanosis, which manifests itself by a blue discoloration of the skin. It also causes anaemia.

Trinitrotoluene, better known as TNT, is used in the making of explosives. It is mainly absorbed through the skin, and causes dermatitis, jaundice, and anaemia.

Chrome, used in chromium plating, attacks the skin, causing dermatitis. It also attacks the septum of the nose, leading to chrome ulceration and perforation of the septum. It is the cartilaginous part of the septum and not the bone which is attacked.

Toxic jaundice may be caused by trinitrotoluene, tetrachloroethane, arseniuretted hydrogen, carbon tetrachloride, and certain benzene derivatives.

Epitheliomatous ulceration, a form of cancer, may arise among workers with tar, pitch, bitumen, or mineral oil. The best known form is mule-spinner's cancer.

Anthrax may occur among workers in wool, hides, and hair infected with the anthrax bacillus. The infection may be acquired through the skin, where it causes the so-called malignant pustule, or through the lungs by breathing in the bacillus, when pulmonary anthrax results. Its incidence among people handling infected wool gave rise to the name woolsorters' disease. (See ANTHRAX.)

Brucellosis is the disease caused by *Brucella abortus*, the micro-organism responsible for contagious abortion in cattle. It is a disease therefore to which farm workers, veterinary surgeons and abattoir workers are particularly susceptible. (See BRUCELLOSIS.)

Viral hepatitis is an inflammatory disease of the liver caused by a virus. Industrial injuries benefits are now payable to employees whose work brings them into close and frequent contact with human blood, human blood products or patients with viral hepatitis. The majority of people affected will be employed in the health sector, particularly doctors, nurses, laboratory technicians and similar groups of workers. (See HEPATITIS, ACUTE INFECTIOUS.)

Polymer fume fever is an influenza-like illness that occurs in people who work with polytetrafluoroethylene (Teflon). (See POLYMER FUME FEVER.)

Pneumoconioses – This is a group of diseases of the lungs due to the inhalation of dust (table 38). The most important dust in this connection is silica. The resulting disease is known as silicosis (qv). Other diseases in this category are asbestosis (qv), bagassosis (qv), berylliosis (qv), byssinosis (qv), siderosis (qv), stannosis (qv), and farmer's lung (qv).

Asbestosis is a form of pneumoconiosis, but its main hazard is the risk of cancer of the lung or pleura, or sometimes of the ovary. It is caused by the inhalation from asbestos dust, either in the mining or quarrying of it, or in one of the many industries in which it is used: eg. as an insulating material, in the making of paper, cardboard and brake linings. (See ASBESTOSIS.)

Byssinosis is another form of pneumoconiosis, caused by the inhalation of dust in textile factories. (See BYSSINOSIS.)

Kaolinosis is a form of pnuemoconiosis caused by the inhalation of clay dust.

Nasal adenocarcinorna is a form of cancer of the nose, and sometimes of the associated air sinuses, that sometimes develops in workers engaged in the manufacture of wooden furniture.

Vinyl chloride, which is used to make polyvinylchloride, one of the most widely used plastics today, is now known to cause cancer of the liver, and it may possibly cause cancer elsewhere in the body. There

Cause	Occupation	Disease
Coal dust	Coal mining	Coal-workers' pneumoconiosis
Silica	Gold mining	Silicosis
	Iron and steel industries (metal casting)	
	Metal grinding	
	Stone dressing	
	Pottery	
Asbestos	Asbestos mining	Asbestosis
	Manufacture of fireproof and insulating materials	
Iron oxide	Arc welding	Siderosis
Tin dioxide	Tin ore mining	Stannosis
Beryllium	Aircraft and atomic energy industries	Berylliosis
Cotton, flax or hemp dust	Textile industries	Byssinosis
Fungal spores from mouldy hay, straw or grain, bagasse, mushroom compost	Agriculture and related industries	Farmer's lung
		Metalworker's lung
		Bagassosis
		Mushroom worker's lung

Table 38 – Some occupational lung diseases. Davidson and Macleod.

is a long period between first exposure to vinyl chloride and the diagnosis of cancer: 12 to 29 years in one series of cases.

Tungsten carbide, which is used in metal machining and metal working, may cause a disease characterised by cough, shortness of breath and tightness of the chest. (See HARD METAL DISEASE.)

Dermatitis is now one of the most important industrial diseases. It may be caused by a wide variety of agents, including alkalis, oil, petrol, paraffin, French polish, various chemicals. Its importance lies in the fact that, with reasonable care, it can often be avoided, or, if it be detected early, it responds well to treatment. On the other hand, if allowed to persist for any length of time, it may become resistant to all but one form of treatment: ie. change of occupation to one in which the individual will not come into contact with the offending substance. Preventive measures ensure adequate washing facilities and their full use by all workpeople exposed to risk; maximum cleanliness at work, which reduces the risk of the individual coming into contact with the offending substance; the wearing of protective clothing; the use of barrier creams where this is possible. (See DERMATITIS.)

Cramps and paralyses – Cramps may occur in individuals whose work involves repeated use of the same groups of muscles. Perhaps the best known examples of this are *telegraphist's cramp* and *writer's cramp.* Another example is *twister's cramp* which occurs in the cotton and woollen industries among those whose job is the twisting of cotton or woollen yarns. Although in a somewhat different category, reference may also be made here to the painful condition which develops in the arms of those handling *powerful pneumatic tools.* This condition is liable to be accompanied by insomnia and tremors. No effective treatment is known.

Miner's nystagmus is a distressing condition, characterized by persistent uncontrollable movements of the eye, which occurs in coal-miners. It is now generally accepted that the main cause is inadequate illumination, and the introduction of adequate lighting into mines has gone far towards reducing its incidence. (See NYSTAGMUS.)

Compressed air illness, formerly known as caisson disease, occurs in divers and in those who work in caissons. It is due to the affected individuals being decompressed, or returned to atmospheric pressure, too quickly. Divers and caisson

workers work under high pressures, and if this pressure is reduced too quickly, bubbles of nitrogen are released in the body which cause pain in various areas – usually muscles or joints. These painful areas are known as bends. Adherence to official decompression tables should prevent such accidents, but when they do occur, the treatment consists of recompression until the pain goes, followed by slow decompression.

OCHRONOSIS is the term given to a very rare condition in which the ligaments and cartilages of the body, and sometimes the conjunctiva, become stained by dark brown or black pigment. This may occur in chronic carbolic poisoning, or in a congenital disorder of metabolism in which the individual is unable to break down completely the tyrosine of the protein molecule, the intermediate product, homogentisic acid, appearing in the urine – this being known as alkaptonuria.

OCULENTUM is an ointment for application to the eye.

ODONTALGIA is another name for toothache.

OEDEMA means dropsical swelling due to the passage of fluid through the walls of blood- or lymph-vessels into the spaces of cellular tissue beneath the skin, or beneath a mucous membrane, or into internal organs. (See DROPSY.)

OESOPHAGOSCOPE is an instrument constructed on the principle of the telescope, which on introduction into the mouth is passed down the oesophagus and enables the observer to see the state of the oesophagus.

OESOPHAGUS, or GULLET, is the tube which conveys the food and drink from the throat down to the stomach. It begins above at the level of the sixth cervical vertebra, and, lying close against the left side and front of the spinal column, passes downward through the neck and chest to pierce the diaphragm, and then opens into the stomach. It consists of three coats: a strong outer coat of muscle fibres in two layers, the outer running lengthwise, the inner being circular; inside this a loose connective tissue coat containing blood-vessels, glands, and nerves; and finally a strong mucous membrane lined by epithelium, which closely resembles that of the mouth and skin.

OESOPHAGUS, DISEASES OF – The oesophagus, or gullet, may be the seat of catarrhal or inflammatory conditions causing discomfort in swallowing, but the more important ailments are those which arise from local injuries, such as the swallowing of scalding or corrosive substances. This may cause ulceration followed by the formation of a scar which narrows the passage and produces the symptoms of *stricture* of the oesophagus: namely, pain and difficulty in swallowing, with regurgitation of the food. It is to be observed in all cases of organic stricture that the food does not necessarily return at once, but seems as if it has passed into the stomach. In reality, however, it has passed into the dilated or pouched portion of the gullet, which is almost always present immediately above the seat of stricture, where it remains until, from its amount, it regurgitates back into the mouth, when it can be seen, by the absence of any evidence of digestion, that it has never been in the stomach. The severity of the case will necessarily depend upon the amount of narrowing and consequent mechanical obstruction, but in some instances this has occurred to such an extent as practically to close the canal. Cases of oesophageal stricture of this kind may sometimes be dilated by the use of suitable instruments.

A still more serious and frequent cause of oesophageal stricture is that due to *cancer*, which may occur at any part, but is most common at the lower end, in the vicinity of the entrance into the stomach. The chief symptoms of this condition are increasing difficulty in the passage downwards of the food, steady decline in strength, together with enlargement of the glands in the neck, whilst the diagnosis is rendered the more certain by the absence of any cause, such as local injury, for the formation of a stricture, and by the age (as a rule at or beyond middle life) and the sex (usually men). In many cases treatment can only be palliative, but recent advances in surgery are producing promising results. In some cases treatment with irradiation produces relief, if not cure. In those in whom neither operation nor radiation can be performed life may be prolonged and freedom from pain obtained by fluid food which is either swallowed or passed down a tube. The operation of gastrostomy, by which an opening is made through the front of the abdomen, allows food to be directly introduced into the stomach.

Strictures of the oesophagus may also be produced by the pressure of tumours or aneurysms within the cavity of the chest but external to the canal.

An important cause of difficulty in swallowing is the condition known as *cardiospasm* or *achalasia of the cardia*. The latter is the more accurate description as the condition is due to failure of the cardiac sphincter (the sphincter at the lower end of the oesophagus) to relax when food is swallowed. The cause is not known. The condition occurs usually in young adults, who complain of food sticking behind the chest-bone. This results in vomiting and, of course, loss of weight. Treatment consists of passing special bougies down the oesophagus to dilate the sphincter. As this may need to be done before every meal for several months, the patient learns to pass the bougie himself. Such treatment, though prolonged, is usually successful.

Finally, difficulty in swallowing sometimes occurs in certain serious nervous diseases from paralysis affecting the nerves supplying the muscular coats of the pharynx, which thus loses its propulsive power (*bulbar paralysis*). When such complications occur, they usually denote an advanced stage of the brain disease with which they are connected, and a speedily fatal termination.

Foreign bodies which lodge in the respiratory part of the throat, ie. at the entrance to, or in the cavity of, the larynx, set up immediate symptoms of choking. (See CHOKING.) Those which lodge in the gullet, on the contrary, do not usually set up any immediately serious symptoms, although their presence causes considerable discomfort. Such bodies are divided, for practical purposes, into two classes. One class includes smooth bodies like coins or fruit stones, which may be pushed down into the stomach or pulled up into the mouth by means of a bougie or a special instrument known as a coin-catcher, or, better still, by forceps passed down under the direct guidance of the oesophagoscope. The other, and more dangerous, class comprises bodies which are too large to be pushed down into the stomach and safely passed by the bowels, or too rough to be pulled back into the mouth, such as large pieces of bone, or large plates of artificial teeth. In cases where it is impossible to dislodge a foreign body up or down, it becomes necessary to perform an operation in order to remove the body from the gullet directly through the side of the neck.

OESTRADIOL is the name given to

the oestrogenic hormone secreted by the ovarian follicle. Oestradiol is responsible for the development of the female sexual characteristics, of the breasts, and of part of the changes that take place in the uterus before menstruation.

OESTROGEN is the term applied to any substance that will induce oestrus or 'heat'. In human medicine it is applied to the substances, natural or synthetic, that induce the changes in the uterus that precede ovulation. They are also responsible for the development of what are known as the secondary sex characteristics in women: that is the physical changes that take place in a girl at puberty, such as enlargement of the breasts, appearance of pubic and axillary hair and the deposition of fat on the thighs and hips. They are used in the management of disturbances of the menopause, and also in the treatment of cancer of the prostate and certain cases of cancer of the breast. (See also DIENOESTROL; ETHINYLOESTRADIOL; OESTRADIOL; QUINESTROL; STILBOESTROL; MENSTRUATION.)

OFFICIAL is a term applied to drugs and preparations which are authorized by pharmacopoeias and other recognized lists.

OFFICINAL is a term applied to drugs and preparations which are regularly kept in stock for sale in the shops of druggists.

OILS are divided into *fixed oils* and *volatile* or *essential oils*. FIXED OILS are of the nature of liquid fats composed of a fatty acid and glycerin: for example olive oil, which consists of a mixture of glycerin compounds of oleic acid and palmitic acid. Other examples of fixed oils are almond oil, linseed oil, and cod-liver oil. Fixed oils are used as foods, and in large quantities as mild aperients. Some fixed oils have important special properties by virtue of active principles that they contain: for example castor oil, which acts as a purgative. Fixed oils are obtained from the fruits or seeds of plants or from animal tissues by pressure, or by boiling with water and skimming off the melted oil. Fats are fixed oils which are solid at ordinary temperatures and are extracted by combination of heat and pressure. An example of an animal fat is lard, and of a vegetable fat, cocoa butter. Fixed oils can be dissolved in ether and chloroform.

VOLATILE or ESSENTIAL OILS resemble fixed oils in being soluble in ether or chloroform and in being lighter than water. Examples of these are the oils of dill, anise, cajuput, caraway, cloves, cinnamon, eucalyptus, juniper, lavender, lemon, peppermint, rosemary, rue, mustard, and turpentine. The volatile oils have some actions in common by being in small doses antispasmodics and analgesics, and by possessing a mild antiseptic and disinfectant action. Most of them are prepared by distillation. Their composition varies considerably, some being of the nature of alcohols, others ketones, others allied to carbolic acid. Volatile oils can be dissolved to a small extent in water, to which they communicate their scent and other properties, and these aquae or waters are used in treating colic and other spasmodic conditions, usually in doses of one or two tablespoonfuls. Volatile oils are also readily soluble in spirit containing 90 per cent of alcohol, and these spirits usually contain about 10 per cent of the volatile oil and are given in doses of from 5 to 30 drops.

For oils of the petroleum series, see PARAFFIN.

OINTMENTS are semi-solid mixtures of medicinal substances with lard, benzoated lard, paraffin or yellow soft paraffin, and wool-fat (lanolin), intended for external application. They are used for three main purposes: (1) as emollients, that is to soften the skin; (ii) as a protective preparation to be applied to the skin; (iii) as a means for the local application of medicaments to be absorbed through the skin.

Other substances occasionally used to form the body of an ointment are almond oil, beeswax, camphor, glycerin, oleic acid, spermaceti, and prepared suet.

Among the most useful ointments are the following: *Simple ointment* B P, which contains 5 per cent each of wool fat, hard paraffin, and cetostearyl acid in white or yellow soft paraffin, and is used for application to chafed surfaces. *Cold cream*, made of beeswax, spermaceti, almond oil, rose water, and attar of rose, is used for a similar purpose. *Zinc and Castor Oil Ointment* B P, which contains 7·5 per cent zinc oxide and 50 per cent w/w castor oil has a well-earned reputation for the prevention and treatment of napkin rash. *Mercuric oxide eye ointment* B P C, or yellow oxide of mercury eye ointment as it is sometimes known, is used for treating inflammation about the eye.

OLD AGE (see AGE, NATURAL CHANGES IN)

OLEANDOMYCIN is an antibiotic derived from *Streptomyces antibioticus*. It is active against many Gram-positive organisms and some Gram-negative organisms.

OLEIC ACID is the commonest of naturally occurring fatty acids, being present in most fats and oils in the form of triglyceride. It is used in the preparation of ointments, but not eye ointments.

OLFACTORY NERVE, the nerve of smell, is the first cranial nerve.

OLIGAEMIA means a diminution of the quantity of blood in the circulation.

OLIGOMENORRHOEA is infrequent menstruation.

OLIGURIA means an abnormally low excretion of urine, such as occurs in acute nephritis.

OLIVE OIL is the oil obtained by pressure from the fruit of *Olea europaea*. It is practically a pure fat, and one ounce (28·5 grams) has an energy equivalent of about 270 Calories.

OMENTUM is a long fold of peritoneal membrane, generally loaded with more or less fat, which hangs down within the abdominal cavity in front of the bowels. It is formed by the layers of peritoneum that cover the front and back surfaces of the stomach in their passage from the lower margin of this organ to cover the back and front surfaces of the large intestine. Instead of passing straight from one organ to the other, these layers dip down and form a sort of fourfold apron. It is to the increasing deposit of fat in this structure that the prominence of the abdomen is largely due in persons of middle age who are large eaters. This omentum is often known as the great omentum, to distinguish it from two smaller peritoneal folds that pass from the stomach, the one to the liver (gastro-hepatic omentum), the other to the spleen (gastro-splenic omentum).

OMPHALOCELE is another name for exomphalos – a hernia of abdominal organs through the umbilicus.

OMPHALUS is another name for the navel or umbilicus.

ONCHOCERCIASIS is infestation with the filarial worm, *Onchocerca volvulus*. It is found in many parts of Africa, in Central and South America, and in the Yemen. It is estimated that there are more than 20 million victims of it. It is transmitted by gnats of the genus *Simulium*. Like loiasis, onchocerciasis is characterized by the appearance of nodules in various parts of the body. There may also be involvement of the eyes and the worm may invade the optic nerve and so cause blindness; hence the name of African river blindness. Treatment consists of removal of the tumours or nodules as they appear. Drugs of value are diethylcarbamazine and suramin, either alone or combined.

ONCOLOGY is that part of medical science which is concerned with the problems of tumours of the body.

ONYCHIA means an inflammation affecting the nails. (See NAILS, DISEASES OF.)

ONYCHOGRYPHOSIS is the term applied to a distortion of the nail in which it is much thickened, overgrown and twisted on itself. This usually affects a toenail and is the result of chronic irritation and inflammation.

ONYCHOLYSIS means separation of the nail from the nail-bed.

OÖPHORECTOMY is a term applied to removal, by operation, of an ovary. When the ovary is removed for the presence of a cyst, the term ovariotomy is usually employed.

OÖPHORITIS is another name for ovaritis or inflammation of an ovary.

OÖPHORON is another name for the ovary.

OPEN-AIR TREATMENT (see TUBERCULOSIS).

OPERATION – The general principles upon which an operation is conducted are mentioned under ANTISEPTICS and ASEPSIS. The preparations for an operation in a private house are mentioned in the article on NURSING. The method of healing after an operation is mentioned under WOUNDS.

OPHTHALMIA means inflammation of the eye, the term being used sometimes instead of conjunctivitis. (See CONJUNCTIVITIS under EYE DISEASES AND INJURIES.)

649

OPHTHALMOPLEGIA

OPHTHALMOPLEGIA means a paralysis affecting the muscles of one or both eyes. When the condition affects the muscles that move the eyeballs from outside, the term external ophthalmoplegia is applied to it; when the intrinsic muscles of the eye are affected, causing interference with the size of the pupil and with the accommodation of the eye for near and distant vision, internal ophthalmoplegia is the name given.

OPHTHALMOSCOPE is an instrument used for the examination of the back of the eye, and for the detection of defects in its transparent contents. Owing to the fact that the interior of the eye, like the inside of a camera, is black, and that the light enters only by a small opening in front, one cannot look into the eye under ordinary circumstances without, in the act of so doing, obstructing the entrance of direct light sufficient to light it up. It is to overcome this difficulty that an ophthalmoscope is used. Nowadays an electric ophthalmoscope, in which light is produced from a dry cell in the handle of the instrument, is used (illustration 332).

The ophthalmoscope is of immense value, not only to the ophthalmic surgeon, but also to the physician in the diagnosis of general diseases. The eye is the only position in the living body where the end of a nerve (optic nerve), together with an artery and vein (retinal artery and vein), is exposed to view (illustration 333); so that

332 – Ophthalmoscope. Keeler Instruments Limited.

the physician, by examining them, gains important information as to the general condition of the nervous and circulatory systems.

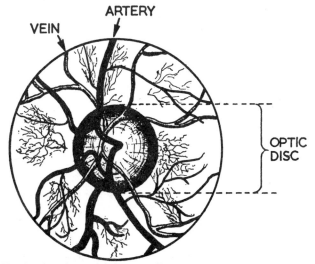

333 – The view through an ophthalmoscope. From Hanington, *Migraine*, 1974. Priory Press.

650

OPIPRAMOL is a drug with anti-depressant properties.

OPISTHOTONOS is the name given to a position assumed by the body during one of the convulsive seizures of tetanus. The muscles of the back, by their spasmodic contraction, arch the body in such a way that the person for a time may rest upon the bed only by his heels and head.

OPIUM, which is one of the most valuable remedies in the whole range of medicine, is the dried juice of the unripe seed-capsules of the white Indian poppy, *Papaver somniferum*. It is cultivated mainly in India, but it is also produced in Iran, China, and the Asiatic provinces of Turkey. Opium possesses its medicinal properties only when produced under favourable conditions of soil and climate, and the juice of other species of poppies grown in temperate climates is almost useless. The juice is obtained by scarifying the seed capsules of the poppies before they are ripe, and next day collecting the gummy sap which has exuded from the cuts. This is dried with great care, kneaded, and carefully tested. Good opium should contain about 10 per cent of morphine, to which its action is chiefly due. It is a brown, resinous-looking substance, or brown powder, with characteristic smell and bitter taste. The opium used in China is mixed with linseed oil, which renders it more suited for smoking. The action of opium depends upon the twenty to twenty-five alkaloids it contains. Of these, the chief is morphine, the amount of which varies from around 9 to 17 per cent. Other alkaloids include codeine, narcotine, thebaine, papaverine, and naceine, and as the action of these differs considerably, the effect of the opium naturally varies according to the proportion of each that it contains. Turkish opium, which is purest in morphine, is generally regarded as the best, the use of Indian opium, which contains a large proportion of narcotine, being more apt to cause sickness. Opium, which is exported from the country of its production in balls or cakes, is often adulterated with sugar, vegetable extracts, gum, molasses, and even stones concealed in the middle of the cakes, and it is therefore very carefully tested before sale.

The importation into Britain of opium is very carefully regulated under the *Dangerous Drugs Act*. Similar regulations govern the sale and distribution of any preparation of morphine or diamorphine (heroin) stronger than 1 part in 500.

The preparations of opium are numerous. Powdered opium (containing 10 per cent of morphine) is used in doses ranging from $\frac{1}{2}$ to 3 grains (30 to 200 mg). Among the other solid preparations are ipecacuanha and opium powder, better known as Dover's powder (containing 10 per cent of opium), in doses of 5 to 10 grains (300 to 600 mg); aromatic chalk with opium powder (containing 0·25 per cent of morphine), used for the treatment of diarrhoea, in doses of 8 to 75 grains (500 mg to 5 grams). Of the liquid preparations, the tincture of opium, better known as laudanum (containing 1 per cent of morphine), is the most used, in doses of 5 to 30 minims (0·3 to 2 ml); the camphorated tincture of opium, also known as paregoric (containing 0·05 per cent of morphine), is given in doses of 30 to 150 minims (2 to 10 ml). (See PAREGORIC.) A preparation of opium, known as nepenthe, is particularly useful in children, the dosage being 1 minim for each year of age.

The alkaloids, morphine and codeine, are administered in various forms. Morphine hydrochloride and morphine sulphate are given in doses from $\frac{1}{8}$ to $\frac{1}{3}$ grain (7·5 to 20 mg); codeine phosphate in doses from $\frac{1}{6}$ to 1 grain (10 to 60 mg). Morphine hydrochloride solution (containing 1 per cent of morphine) is used like laudanum, in doses from 5 to 30 minims (0·5 to 2 ml). A suppository of morphine (containing $\frac{1}{4}$ grain (15 mg) of morphine), is used for painful conditions of the lower bowel.

Action – The action of opium varies considerably, according to the source of the drug and the preparation used; it varies even more according to the age, race, and temperament of the individual. The unstable nervous system of children is profoundly affected by even the smallest doses, and the death of an infant has been caused by a few drops of laudanum, so that the drug is unsuited for use, except with great care, during childhood.

In small doses, opium produces a state of gentle excitement, the person finding his imagination more vivid, his thoughts more brilliant, and his power of expression greater than usual. This stage lasts for some hours, and is succeeded by languor. In larger, ie. medicinal, doses this stage of excitement is short and is followed by deep sleep, from which the person can still be aroused as from natural sleep. When very large, ie. poisonous, doses are taken, sleep comes on quickly, and passes into coma and death. The habitual use of opium obtains for it a great degree of tolerance, so that opium-eaters require to take large quantities, even many ounces, of laudanum daily, before experiencing its pleasurable effects. The need for opium also confers tolerance, so that persons suffering great pain may take, with apparently little effect beyond dulling the pain, quantities which at another time would be dangerous.

It checks all secretions, except the sweat, and slows the processes of tissue change, this action being sometimes useful, sometimes a hindrance to its employment.

Uses – Externally, opium was at one time widely used as an application to areas which are painful and inflamed, as in lumbago, inflammation of joints, pleurisy, peritonitis and shingles. There is, however, no evidence that it is of any value when used in this way.

Internally, its great use is to quiet severe pain, such as that of renal colic or cancer; for this purpose morphine is often given with atropine, which aids the effect in diminishing any spasm present, and at the same time is an antidote to the poisonous qualities of morphine. In conditions in which there is constant, irritating, useless cough, some preparation of opium or morphine may be used as an ingredient in cough mixtures to relieve this. In cases of pelvic pain, whether arising in the bowel, bladder, womb, or ovaries, morphine may be used in the form of suppositories to afford relief. All preparations of opium must be prescribed with the utmost discrimination, in view of the marked tendency to habit-formation. (See DRUG ADDICTION.)

OPIUM POISONING – Perhaps there is no drug in which the amount that can produce serious consequences varies so much as in the case of opium. Two drops of laudanum have been recorded as fatal to an infant, whereas addicts of the drug have been known to drink it like wine, with only a stimulating effect.

Symptoms – When a poisonous dose of any of the preparations of the drug has been taken, sleep rapidly comes on, becomes deeper and deeper, and passes gradually into a state of complete insensibility, usually within half an hour, although the effect may be postponed for several hours, particularly when the drug is taken along with spirituous liquors. Convulsions sometimes occur, especially in children, and vomiting may take place before sleep becomes deep, or as the person is recovering. The breathing is slow, quiet, and shallow; and these charac-

ters become more and more marked as death draws nigh, the person dying, indeed, as the result of paralysis of the respiratory centre in the brain. The lips and face become livid and covered with cold sweat, and the pupils are much contracted. As a rule, death occurs in from seven to eighteen hours after the dose has been taken.

It is important to distinguish opium poisoning from the effect of alcohol and from apoplexy in the case of persons found unconscious. If the person can be roused, the case is probably not one of apoplexy. Further, when apoplexy is the cause there is usually paralysis in one arm or leg, which lies perfectly helpless, or paralysis all down one side. In distinguishing the effect of alcohol from that of opium, the smell of the breath may give assistance, but the state of the pupils, which are contracted in opium poisoning and dilated in alcoholism, is more important. Help may also be gained from the facts that in opium poisoning the perspiration is greater and the person is at first more easily roused. In no case should the person be handled roughly, and if there be any doubt he should be treated as for opium poisoning.

Treatment – An emetic should be given as soon as possible (see EMETICS), and after this has acted, a cup of strong coffee should be swallowed. Even after an emetic has acted, and certainly if it fails to act, the stomach should be washed out with water containing potassium permanganate, which destroys the alkaloids of the opium. As an antidote, full doses of naloxone levallorphan or nalorphine should be given. Should none of these be immediately available, injections of caffeine sodium benzoate, amphetamine, or nikethamide may be given.

It is important to keep the patient awake; and for this purpose he must be walked up and down the room if possible, or one may tap him on the forehead with the finger-nails, flick him with wet towels, or apply other painful stimuli. From time to time strong coffee, and other stimulants may be given internally. If, in spite of all these measures, he becomes unconscious and the breathing begins to fail, artificial respiration must be performed. Generally speaking, by twelve hours after taking the poison the patient is either dead or is showing signs of recovery.

OPODELDOC is an old name for soap liniment.

OPSONINS are substances present in the serum of the blood which act upon bacteria, so as to prepare them for destruction by the white corpuscles of the blood.

OPTIC NERVE is the second cranial nerve, and connects the eye with the brain, conveying from the retina the impressions produced by light. (See EYE; and VISION.)

ORANGE is an excellent source of vitamin C: 100 millilitres of orange juice contain 50 mg of ascorbic acid (ie. vitamin C). It is also used as a flavouring agent in the form of infusion, tincture and syrup of the peel. Fresh orange is also employed, often mixed with glucose, in feverish conditions for the action of the citric acid it contains. (See CITRIC ACID.)

ORBIT is the pyramidal hollow in the skull, situated on each side of the nose, in which the eye is placed. In addition to the eye, each orbit contains the lacrimal gland, a quantity of soft fat upon which the eye rests, and various blood-vessels, nerves, and muscles.

ORCHIDECTOMY is the term applied to the operation for the removal of the testicles (one or both).

ORCHITIS means inflammation of the testicle. (See TESTICLE, DISEASES OF.)

ORCIPRENALINE is an adrenaline-like drug that is proving of value in the relief of the bronchial spasm in asthma. It is given either by mouth or by inhalation. One of its advantages is that it has relatively little action on the heart.

ORF is a widespread viral infection of sheep and goats which is sometimes transmitted to man, in whom it manifests itself as a skin eruption, usually on the hands, fingers, forearms and face.

ORGANIC DISEASE is a term used in contradistinction to the word functional, to indicate that some structural change is responsible for the faulty action of an organ or other part of the body.

ORGANIC SUBSTANCES are those which are obtained from animal or vegetable bodies, or which resemble in chemical composition those derived from this source. Organic chemistry has come to mean the chemistry of the carbon compounds.

ORGANISMS (see BACTERIOLOGY).

ORGANO-PHOSPHORUS INSECTICIDES are a group of insecticides which act by inhibiting the action of cholinesterase. (See ACETYLCHOLINE.) For this reason they are also toxic to man and must therefore be handled with great care. The most widely used are parathion (qv) and malathion (qv).
Some of them are of value in agriculture because, when applied to plants, they are absorbed, and distributed to all parts of the plant, where they may kill sucking insects such as aphids.

ORIENTAL SORE, also known as DELHI BOIL and as ALEPPO EVIL, is a disease of tropical climates in which an ulcer begins in a small pimple, spreads, and then heals very slowly, leaving an unsightly scar. (See LEISHMANIASIS.)

ORNITHOSIS is an infection of birds with the micro-organism known as *Chlamydia psittaci*, which is transmissible to man.

ORPHENADRINE is a drug used in the treatment of Parkinsonism (qv).

ORTHODONTICS is the branch of dentistry concerned with the prevention and treatment of dental irregularities and malocclusion.

ORTHOPAEDICS – Originally the general measures, surgical and mechanical, which can be used for the correction or prevention of deformities in children. Now, that branch of medical science dealing with skeletal deformity, congenital or acquired.

ORTHOPNOEA is a form of difficulty in breathing so severe that the patient cannot bear to lie down, but must sit or stand up. As a rule, it occurs only in serious affections of the heart or lungs.

ORTHOPTIC TREATMENT is the term applied to the treatment of squint by giving special exercises for the muscles of the eye. (See SQUINTING.)

OSMOSIS means the passage of fluids through a membrane, which separates them, so as to become mixed with one another. Osmotic pressure is a term applied to the strength of the tendency which a fluid shows to do this, and depends largely upon the amount of solid which it holds in solution.

OSSIFICATION means the formation of bone. In early life, centres appear in the bones previously represented by cartilage or fibrous tissue, and from these the formation of true bone and deposit of lime salts proceed. When a fracture occurs, the bone mends by ossification of the clot which forms between the fragments. (See FRACTURES.) In old age an unnatural process of ossification often takes place in parts which should remain cartilaginous, eg. in the cartilages of the larynx and of the ribs, making these parts unusually brittle.

OSTEITIS means inflammation in the substance of a bone.

OSTEITIS DEFORMANS (see PAGET'S DISEASE OF BONE)

OSTEITIS FIBROSA CYSTICA GENERALISATA is a disease characterized by the presence of cysts in bones, which thereby become weakened and may break. The cysts form because calcium salts are drained from the bone into the blood stream, the result of the action of a tumour of the parathyroid glands. (See PARATHYROIDS.)

OSTEOARTHROSIS, or OSTEOARTHRITIS, is a term applied to a chronic inflammation of the bones composing a joint, and leading to deformity. (See RHEUMATISM.)

OSTEOCHONDRITIS means inflammation of both bone and cartilage.

OSTEOGENESIS IMPERFECTA is a hereditary disease characterized by extreme fragility of the skeleton, resulting in fractures and deformities. It may be accompanied by blue sclera (the outermost, normally white coat of the eyeball), transparent teeth, hypermobility (excessive range of movement) of the joints, deafness, and dwarfism (shortness of stature). The cause is not known, though there is some evidence that it may be associated with collagen formation (see COLLAGEN). Parents of affected children can obtain help and advice from the Brittle Bone Society, 63 Byron Crescent, Dundee DD3 6SS.

OSTEOMALACIA is a disease, in which the bones become slowly softened as the result of the absorption of the lime salts they contain. The cause of the disease is a deficiency of vitamin D in the food, combined with lack of sunshine. It affects especially mothers who have borne many children in rapid succession. For long considered rare in Britain, it has recently come to be recognized as not uncommon among old people, in whom it is presumably due to a faulty diet containing inadequate vitamin D, and lack of sunshine.

The most serious feature of the disease is the deformity which occurs in the softened bones owing to the weight of the body and the action of the muscles. This deformity, when it affects the bones of the pelvis and spine, may cause difficulty in childbirth, and is a source of great danger to mother and child.

Treatment consists basically of giving large doses of vitamin D, and then ensuring that the individual has a balanced diet containing a full complement of all the vitamins, including vitamin D.

OSTEOMYELITIS means inflammation in the marrow of a bone. (See BONE, DISEASES OF.)

OSTEOPATHY is the name applied to a system of healing in which diseases are treated by manipulating bones and other parts with the idea of thereby restoring functions in the bodily mechanism that have become deranged.

OSTEOPHYTES are bony spurs or projections. They occur most commonly at the margins of points involved in osteoarthrosis (qv).

OSTEOPOROSIS means increased porousness of bone due to lack of calcium salts. It is one of the manifestations of the ageing process. In old people it is liable to be induced by prolonged periods of immobilization in bed. This is one reason why elderly people should never be kept in bed a moment longer than necessary. Another preventive measure is to ensure that the elderly consume an adequate amount of calcium. This is most simply done by their taking a pint (0·5 litre) of milk a day.

OSTEOSARCOMA is the most common, and most malignant, tumour of bone. It occurs predominantly in older children and young adults. The commonest site for it is at the ends of the long bones of the body: ie. the femur, tibia and humerus.

Treatment is by amputation of the limb followed by radiotherapy and chemotherapy. The 5-year survival rate is only 20 per cent.

OSTEOTOMY is the operation of cutting of a bone.

OTITIS means inflammation of the ear. (See EAR, DISEASES OF.)

OTOLOGY is that branch of medical science which is concerned with disorders and diseases of the organ of hearing, one practising this branch being called an OTOLOGIST.

OTOMYCOSIS (see EAR, DISEASES OF).

OTORRHOEA means discharge from the ear. (See EAR, DISEASES OF.)

OTOSCLEROSIS is the term applied to the condition in which spongy bone forms in the capsule of the labyrinth of the ear and progressive deafness develops. It is the commonest cause of deafness in active adult life, and is twice as common in women as in men. During the last twenty years surgical methods of treatment have been introduced, which restore hearing in 80 per cent of cases. Three forms of surgical treatment are now available, known, respectively, as fenestration, stapes mobilization, and stapedectomy. For those in whom operation is unsuccessful, hearing aids will enable them to hear again.

OUABAIN, or Strophanthin-G, is a glucoside first obtained from the African tree, *Acokanthera ouabaio*: it was used as an arrow poison in West Africa. It is now obtained from the African tree *Strophanthus gratus*. It is a cardiac stimulant, having a similar action to that of digitalis.

OVARIES – The ovaries are the glands in which are produced, in the female sex, the ova, capable, if fertilized, of developing into new individuals. They are situated, one on each side, in the cavity of the pelvis, corresponding on the surface of the body approximately to the centre of the groin. Each is shaped something like an almond, is about 1½ inches (37 mm) long, ½ inch (13 mm) wide, and ¾ inch (19 mm) in thickness, and is whitish in colour. It is attached to the broad ligament running from the womb to the side of the pelvis, by one edge along which blood-vessels and nerves enter. One end is connected to the expanded end of the

Fallopian tube, as well as by a ligament to the side of the pelvis, and the other end to a ligament to the side of the womb. The ovary therefore lies to a considerable extent free in the pelvis.

The chief bulk of the ovary is made up of connective tissue, which differs from ordinary fibrous tissue in being composed of spindle-shaped cells. On the surface is a layer of columnar cells, and beneath this a dense connective tissue layer, the tunica albuginea. Beneath the tunica albuginea the structure appears to the naked eye to be of a granular character, this appearance being due to the presence of a layer of follicles, estimated at around 800,000 in number in each ovary at birth. Each follicle contains one (seldom more) ovum, each of these ova being capable of developing into a new individual. Every follicle consists essentially of a hollow ball of cells, embedded in which is a single large cell, the ovum, and each ovary contains follicles in all stages of maturity, from the rudimentary ones described above to several which are greatly increased in size to 10 mm in diameter through multiplication of the cells surrounding the ovum and the formation among them of a cavity distended with fluid. One at least of these follicles comes to maturity, when it is known as a Graafian follicle, about half-way between two menstrual periods, distends till it reaches the surface of the ovary, and finally bursts allowing the escape of the contained ovum, measuring 110 mm in diameter, which finds its way down the corresponding Fallopian tube into the womb. This process is known as ovulation. (See MENSTRUATION.)

For ovarian secretions, see Ovaries under ENDOCRINE GLANDS, and also OESTRADIOL; OESTROGEN and PROGESTERONE.

OVARIES, DISEASES OF – Although many of the aches and pains to which women are heir are unjustifiably attributed to disease of the ovaries, there is no doubt that, when diseased, the ovaries can be responsible for much ill-health.

INFLAMMATION OF THE OVARY (OVARITIS) seldom, if ever, occurs alone and is usually associated with inflammation of the Fallopian tubes (ie. salpingitis) and of the pelvic peritoneum. It may be acute or chronic. The acute form is due to gonorrhoea, infection during the puerperium or following abortion, or infection from the alimentary tract: eg. the appendix. If the acute form is not successfully overcome, it is liable to become chronic with exacerbations. In the chronic stage adhesions form which bind down and displace the ovaries, the Fallopian tubes, and the uterus. Bladder function is also liable to be interfered with. In all cases of infection of the ovaries and Fallopian tubes the possibility of this being due to tuberculosis must be considered, particularly in young patients.

Symptoms – In the acute form these may be mild or severe, consisting of pain in the lower part of the abdomen, usually during or just after menstruation, prolongation of menstruation, and fever. There may also be pain on passing water, sickness and vomiting. In severe cases with high temperature there may be rigors. In chronic cases there may be backache, usually worse after a day's work, fatigue, excessive or painful menstruation, pain on passing water, sterility and debility. In more severe cases there may be a discharge from the vagina (ie. leucorrhoea) and anaemia. Sometimes an abscess develops in the ovary or in the Fallopian tubes, and in these cases the general health is more likely to suffer because of toxic absorption.

Treatment – In the acute cases this consists of rest in bed and the administration of penicillin or sulphonamides. Hot fomentations are useful to relieve pain. Hot douches to the vagina are not used as much as they were at one time, as they are sometimes liable to increase the pain. The diet should be light and nourishing. Care is necessary to ensure regular emptying of the bowels, but violent purgatives must not be used for this purpose. The majority of cases respond to such treatment. Operation is only indicated when there are signs of general peritonitis, or when there is no evidence of the condition responding to medical treatment in two to three weeks. The treatment of chronic cases is similar, but here hot douches to the vagina twice daily are also of value. Operation is required for chronic cases if the general health is affected, if there are acute exacerbations, or if there is much persistent local pain and menorrhagia.

OVARIAN TUMOURS may be of several kinds. Solid tumours, either simple or malignant, are relatively rare, though cancer of the ovary causes the death of more than 3000 women in Britain every year. Far commoner are the cystic forms, which often reach a huge size. These cysts are of several types, sometimes consisting of a distended condition of the Graafian follicles, at other times being simple cysts filled with a complex papillary growth, again being dermoid tumours and containing fat, hair, teeth, and other structures associated with the skin, and yet again arising from the distension of some part of the parovarium, a rudimentary structure attached to the ovary.

The fluid in these cysts is sometimes of a greenish-grey or brown colour and viscid, ropy consistence, at other times clearer and thinner, and, in the case of dermoid tumours, usually of a greasy nature.

Symptoms – These tumours generally remain quite painless till the weight and distension caused by their increasing size give trouble. They arise often in young women without any apparent cause. If they are not removed, some, which stand on the verge of being malignant tumours, increase rapidly in size, and all lead to great discomfort and loss of health, and finally shorten life.

Treatment – The one method of treatment adopted now consists in *ovariotomy*: ie. removal of the affected ovary. This operation should be performed early in the course of the disease, because, as the tumour grows, it contracts adhesions to surrounding organs, and these are the source both of the most distressing symptoms and of the chief difficulty and danger in a later operation. Most cases operated upon at an early stage recover well, the operation being one of the safest major operations in surgery.

OVARIOTOMY is the operation of removal of an ovary or an ovarian tumour.

OVERLAYING OF INFANTS is the term applied to the process whereby an infant sleeping in the same bed as an adult is suffocated as a result of the adult lying on top of the infant. In most cases the adult is under the influence of alcohol.

OVI ALBUMEN is a Latin term for white of egg; OVI VITELLUM is that for yolk of egg.

OVUM is the single cell derived from the female, out of which a future individual arises, after its union with the spermatozoon derived from the male. (See FOETUS; OVARIES)

OXALIC ACID is not used in medicine, but it is of importance because it is an irritant poison, and has a domestic use for cleaning purposes: eg. removing ink stains and iron mould, and cleaning leather. Oxalic acid, or binoxalate of potassium (salt of sorrel), is occasionally taken by mistake for Epsom salts or for cream of tartar. This substance is also important, because oxalate of lime is found in urinary sediment, and sometimes composes urinary calculi. (See BLADDER, DISEASES OF.) Oxalate of lime in the urine is derived partly from articles of food, like rhubarb, that contain it, and is partly produced within the body as the result of tissue change.

When poisoning is the result of taking oxalic acid or binoxalate of potassium, chalk or whiting well diluted with water should be given, and, if vomiting be not already present, an emetic; afterwards the irritation resulting in the stomach and bowels is to be soothed by demulcents. The antidote to oxalic acid is Calcium Gluconate Injection BP.

OXYCEPHALY, or STEEPLE HEAD, is the term for describing a deformity of the skull in which the forehead is high and the top of the head pointed. There is also poor vision and the eyes bulge.

OXYGEN is a colourless gas, devoid of smell, slightly heavier than common air. It was discovered by Joseph Priestley in 1772. It forms rather more than one-fifth by volume of the atmosphere. It may be obtained by the fractional distillation of liquid air, or by the electrolysis of water. It is stored at high pressure (up to 120 atmospheres) in steel cylinders, from which it is obtained at any desired rate by turning a stop-cock.

Action – Oxygen is necessary to life, and the process of respiration (see RESPIRATION) has, as one of its main objects, the supply of oxygen to the blood (see also HAEMOGLOBIN). Applied to the unbroken skin, oxygen has little effect, but when brought in contact with a wound or ulcer, it increases the circulation and acts as a stimulant.

The condition of oxygen want, or anoxaemia, may be produced by various conditions, such as damage to the lung by tumours, or defects of the circulation, eg. valvular disease of the heart, in which the circulation is so slow that the tissues do not receive their proper amount of oxygen, and in cases of anaemia and poisoning where the blood is not capable of carrying its normal amount of oxygen. In these states, and above all in cases of anaemia and valvular disease, when the pulse is quick and feeble, when the patient's lips and ears are blue, and when the breathing is rapid and shallow, the administration of oxygen gives great relief.

Uses – Oxygen is stored in cylinders which usually contain 20 or 40 cubic feet (0·5 or 1 cubic metre) of the gas, but larger cylinders containing 100 cubic feet can be obtained. In severe cases of anoxaemia the rate at which oxygen may require to be delivered to the patient is between 4 and 6 litres per minute. A rubber tube is attached to the head of the cylinder, which passes through the glass tubes of a washbottle and is continued to either a mask, which fits over the patient's nose and mouth, or to a rubber catheter which is passed into one of the nostrils and fixed in position at the side of his face by a strip of sticking plaster. The use of the latter is unaccompanied by any sense of oppression to the patient.

Great advances have been made in recent years in the development of both oxygen masks and tents. The advantage of the latter is that the patient is breathing all the time in an atmosphere saturated with oxygen. An example of a modern oxygen mask is shown in illustration 334.

A recent development in oxygen therapy is what is known as *hyperbaric oxygen*. This is the use of oxygen at high pressures, such as 3 atmospheres. Originally introduced as an adjunct to radiotherapy in the treatment of cancer, it is now being used in the treatment of carbon monoxide poisoning, *Clostridium welchii* infections (qv) and coronary thrombosis. The most

334 – Edinburgh Oxygen Mask. British Oxygen Co. Ltd.

convenient method of administering hyperbaric oxygen is in a special pressure chamber.

Substances which contain oxygen and are capable of giving it off, such as permanganate of potassium, and peroxide of hydrogen, have a powerful effect as disinfectants either by destroying organisms or oxidizing noxious products of their growth. Such substances are therefore used in the treatment of ulcers and various skin diseases and as antiseptics.

OXYMEL is an old-fashioned remedy for colds and sore throats, composed of vinegar and honey. It is given in doses of one or two teaspoonfuls.

OXYPERTINE is a tranquillizer that is proving of value in the treatment of anxiety neurosis.

OXYPHENBUTAZONE is a derivative of phenylbutazone that is proving of value as an anti-inflammatory and pain-relieving drug in the treatment of various forms of rheumatism.

OXYPHENONIUM is an anticholinergic drug which relieves spasm and hypermotility.

OXYTETRACYCLINE is an antibiotic derived from a soil organism, *Streptomyces rimosus*. Its range of antibacterial activity is comparable to that of tetracycline (qv).

OXYTOCIC means hastening parturition or stimulating uterine contraction, or a drug or procedure that has this effect.

OXYTOCIN is the extract isolated from the pituitary posterior lobe which stimulates the uterine muscle to contract. It can also be synthesized. (See PITUITARY BODY.)

OXYURIASIS is the condition of being infested with thread- or pin-worms.

OXYURIS is another name for the threadworm.

OZAENA is a chronic disease of the nose of an inflammatory nature, combined with atrophy of the mucous membrane and the formation of extremely foul-smelling crusts in the interior of the nose. (See NOSE, DISEASES OF.)

OZONE is a specially active form of oxygen in which three volumes of the gas are condensed into the space ordinarily occupied by two. It has a characteristic smell, which may be noticed in the neighbourhood of dynamos, as ozone is produced by the passage through the air of electric sparks. It exists free in small quantities in the air of pine-clad mountains and of the seaside, where the invigorating properties of the fresh air may be partly due to its presence. It has also a powerful deodorant action.

P

PACEMAKER (see CARDIAC PACEMAKER).

PACHYDERMIA means hypertrophy or thickening of the skin. PACHYDERMIA LARYNGIS is a name applied to thickening of the vocal cords due to chronic inflammation or irritation.

PACHYMENINGITIS means inflammation of the dura mater of the brain and spinal cord. (See MENINGITIS.)

PACINIAN CORPUSCLES, or lamellated corpuscles, are minute bulbs at the ends of the nerves scattered through the skin and subcutaneous tissue, and forming one of the end-organs for sensation (illustration 335).

335 – Pacinian corpuscle. From Best and Taylor, *The Physiological Basis of Medical Practice.* The Williams & Wilkins Co.

PACKS (see WET PACK).

PAEDIATRICS means the branch of medicine dealing with diseases of children.

PAGET'S DISEASE OF BONE, or OSTEITIS DEFORMANS, is the term applied to a chronic disease in which the bones – especially those of the skull, limbs, and spine – gradually become thick and also soft, causing them to bend. It is said to be the commonest bone disease in the world, and it is estimated that some 600,000 people in England may suffer from it. It seldom occurs under the age of 40. Pain is its most unpleasant manifestation. Evidence is now forthcoming that it responds well to calcitonin (qv).

PAIN is a necessary part of conscious existence, all our sensations being accompanied by more or less feeling of pleasure or pain. In the former case we seek the repetition of the sensations; in the latter case we instinctively avoid them, unless, by an act of will, we avoid the sense of pleasure or bear that of pain for some ulterior motive. The ability to perceive pain constitutes a special sense which the body has evolved, or with which it has been furnished, in order that it may preserve itself, by avoiding conditions that produce damage.

Pain is of various types. The most important is that caused by injury of the skin, as by a prick, burn, or pinch. This sense is quite distinct from that of touch. There are special nerve-fibres for the conduction of painful impressions running up the spinal cord near its central canal, while the fibres conveying the impressions for touch run up in the posterior part of the cord. This is proved by the destruction of the sense of pain in the disease known as syringomyelia (which affects the central part of the cord), notwithstanding the fact that the slightest touch can still be felt in the parts of the body incapable of feeling pain. It is probable that these nerves of pain have special endings in the skin, since pain does not appear to be felt uniformly, but, like the other senses, at special spots thickly scattered over the surface. And it is also likely that there is a special centre in the brain for the reception of painful impressions.

Internal parts are much less sensitive than the skin, and diseases in them usually give rise to quite a different sensation. Indeed these parts, not being liable to damage by external objects, are not endowed with the power of feeling pain due to sudden injury, so that the bowel, when brought out through the skin, may be cut with scissors or knife, though the individual, unless he sees it, is quite unaware of what is taking place; tendon, muscle, and bone are also very insensitive, so that the two former may be cut or scraped without more than a slightly sickening sensation, or the ends of a broken bone rubbed together without causing severe pain.

Nevertheless inflammatory changes in these deep-seated structures, and disturbances in their functions, are capable of influencing the brain so as to produce the severest type of pain. This inflammation, particularly when seated in dense structures which cannot expand so as to prevent the congested blood-vessels of the part from pressing upon its nerves, is accompanied by throbbing pain, and, in bone particularly, this is apt to be of a boring, excruciating character. The gnawing pain of a tumour invading surrounding tissues is of a similar nature, and any source of irritation on the course of a

659

nerve is apt to produce the severe pain of neuralgia. Over-action of a weak part or muscle leads to continued pain of an aching character, due probably to an irritating deposit of the chemical products of muscular activity, or may produce spasm, as in the stitch of the side caused by unwontedly violent exercise. Of a similar nature is the colic or griping pain, caused by irritation of the bowels, bile-ducts, and ureters, which in its severest forms may properly be designated agony. (See COLIC.) The burning pain of certain forms of dyspepsia is due to the action of an excessively acid gastric juice, and, like burns of the skin, is apparently due to irritation of the sensitive nerve-endings at points where the surface of the mucous membrane has become eroded.

Ordinary sensations of all sorts become painful when they are excessive, and thus liable to damage the organ in question: eg. bright light, loud sound.

Painful sensations depend much also upon the state of the nervous system, varying according to the power of the nerves to conduct, and of the brain to receive, impressions. Some persons are notoriously better at bearing pain than others, and the healthy and strong are less affected by trivial injuries than those whose nervous system is in a state of ready irritability through chronic ill-health. Persons of strong will-power can undoubtedly inhibit painful impressions, like those from a surgical operation, just as they can control irregular movements. Thus by a mental effort not only do such persons bear pain better, but they actually feel less pain. Similarly the mind that is dominated by an idea unconsciously inhibits painful impressions, so that they gain no entrance for the time, as in the case of soldiers wounded in the heat of battle, orators or preachers who are the victims of neuralgia, or even, in olden times, martyrs at the stake.

On the other hand, pain may be of a purely functional character, and a person with a highly strung or disordered nervous system may suffer pain without any external cause, the mind misinterpreting or exaggerating sensations which by the healthy person would not be noticed. (See HYSTERIA.)

These facts are well known to those faith-healers and others who attempt to cure by a direct mental impression, and who by this means often succeed in alleviating pain, although only in special cases, such as the functional pains just mentioned, are they successful in curing the disease to which the pain is due, and of which it is the warning.

Pain in a certain part is not necessarily due to disease in the same part. In the case of injury to the skin covering the body, the mind, as the result of experience, very accurately refers the painful impressions down the nerves which bring them, to the parts from which they come. But when impressions come to the central nervous system from organs or parts of the body not usually liable to injury or disease, the mind is apt to refer the pain to some other part which is more commonly the seat of pain, and whose nerve-fibres enter the same part of the brain or spinal cord as do those coming from the part which is really affected. For example, in the early stages of hip-joint disease, the pain is more often felt down the inner side of the thigh and knee than in the deep-seated hip-joint, since branches from the same nerves (obturator and femoral) supply the hip-joint and the skin of this particular area. For the same reason, the pain of spinal disease, due to pressure upon the large nerve roots close to the point where they enter the cord, is often referred, not to this unfamiliar seat of pain, but to the sides and front of the body where these nerves end in the skin. In this connection it may be stated that pain felt equally on both sides of the body is almost always due to some affection of the central nervous system.

In the case of the internal organs whose nervous control is derived from the sympathetic nervous system (in the case of the heart, lungs, stomach, and bowels partly also from the tenth cranial, or vagus, nerve), through which they often obtain complicated and very distant connections with the brain and cord, pain is often referred, in what seems at first sight to be a bizarre manner, to distant points. *Referred pain* is often, in the case of the heart, stomach, liver, and bowels, felt on the surface situated over these organs, and the skin may be so tender that gentle pressure or even the slightest touch cannot be borne. Heart conditions are liable also to cause pain running down the inner side of the left, and in some cases of the right, arm to the elbow. In dyspepsia, due to irritation of the stomach, the pain is often referred to the pit of the stomach or middle of the back. In conditions affecting the liver there may be pain in the region of the right shoulder. Affections of the lower end of the bowel commonly cause pain down the back of the thighs, especially of the left thigh, to the knee. Pain due to disorders of the womb is felt internally much less often than in the lowest part of the back and the thighs; and, when the ovaries or Fallopian tubes also are affected, the pain may have a wide distribution, including the small of the back, the groin, and the front of the thigh, or it is occasionally referred to the hip or knee-joint, so that the case may for a time be mistaken for disease in one of these joints.

Treatment of pain – There are three general principles by which the relief of pain may be attempted. (1) The most natural way is to remove the cause of pain, such as a decayed tooth, ulcer, abscess, or inflammatory condition of some internal organ, or to soothe the nerves of the affected part by warmth or some other means. (2) The nerves which convey impressions from the affected region may be treated so that their conducting power is lessened or stopped, as, for example, by administration of sedatives, use of electricity, local anaesthetics, or by chordotomy (qv) (see NEURALGIA). (3) The part of the brain which receives the impressions of pain may be dulled by drugs, or the influence of these impressions may be inhibited by powerful mental impressions, as, for example in hypnotism, faith-healing. (See also ANAESTHETICS; ANALGESICS; ANODYNES; and under the headings of the various diseases that give rise to pain.)

PAINS (see LABOUR).

PAINTER'S COLIC (see COLIC; LEAD-POISONING).

PALATE is the partition between the cavity of the mouth, below, and that of the nose, above. It consists of the *hard palate* towards the front, which is composed of a bony plate covered below by the mucous membrane of the mouth, above by that of the nose; and of the *soft palate* farther back, in which a muscular layer, composed of nine small muscles, is similarly covered. The hard palate extends a little farther back than the wisdom teeth, and is formed by the maxillary and palate bones. The soft palate is concave towards the mouth and convex towards the nose, and it ends behind in a free border, at the centre of which is the prolongation known as the uvula. When food or air is passing through the mouth, as in the acts of swallowing, coughing, or vomiting, the soft palate is drawn upwards so as to touch the back wall of the throat and shut off the cavity of the nose. Movements of the soft palate, by changing the shape of

the mouth and nose cavities, are important in the production of speech.

PALATE, MALFORMATIONS OF – The palate is subject to certain alterations, as the result of defective development. The hard palate may be much more arched than usual; this is sometimes due to failure to breathe through the nose, caused by the presence of adenoid vegetations in the throat. (See NOSE, DISEASES OF.)

In early embryonic life (see FOETUS) there are certain clefts in the region of the throat and face, the nose being formed by the junction of one process which grows down from between the eyes (fronto-nasal process) and two which grow in, one from either side (maxillary processes). The fronto-nasal process produces the external nose, the septum of the nose, the central part of the upper lip, and that part of the upper jaw which carries the two front teeth. The maxillary processes form the remainder of the upper jaw and the palate on each side. These three should unite completely prior to birth, but if they fail to do so, a Y-shaped gap is left. This gap runs from the back of the palate forward to a point a little distance behind the front teeth, from which point a limb of the gap runs forwards to each nostril and through the upper lip. This complete state of cleft palate may occur; or there may be only a partial gap in the soft palate, the parts having closed in front (illustration 336a); or again, there may be closure behind and only a notch be left in the lip or a single cleft in the edge of the upper jaw. The notch of the lip is known as hare-lip, from a fanciful resemblance to the hare, which has a notch in the centre of its lip (illustration 336b).

The incidence of cleft lip (hare-lip) and cleft palate seems to be increasing and one child in approximately 700 normal births has some degree of cleft lip and palate. The increase is probably due to more of these babies surviving, as a result of improved surgical techniques, and getting married and having children. As a rough guide, it can be said that if a child is born with a cleft, and there is no family history as far back as the parents' grandparents, the chances of another malformed child is about the same as in the general population. When one parent is affected, the risk is around 1 in 80 but, when a mother with a cleft palate produces a daughter with a cleft palate, the risk to a second daughter is as high as 1 in 7.

Cleft-palate and hare-lip should, if possible, be rectified by operation, because

(a)

(b)

336 – Cleft palate (*a*) and hare-lip (*b*). From Peet and Patterson, *Essentials of Plastic Surgery.* Blackwell Scientific Publications.

both are a serious drawback to feeding in early life, while later, hare-lip is a great disfigurement, and cleft-palate gives to the voice a peculiar twang. When there is merely a slight degree of hare-lip, it is usual to operate a few weeks or even some days after birth, although, when the notch is very large, it may be necessary to wait till the child is several months old. The closure of a large cleft in the palate, which is a more formidable operation, is usually deferred till the child has gained some strength, and the most suitable time is generally held to be between eighteen months and two and a half years of age, because the fault must be remedied before the child has learned to speak. The operations performed vary greatly in details, but all consist in paring the edges of the gap and drawing the soft parts together across it.

Until a hare-lip has been remedied, it is often necessary to feed the child with a spoon, as he cannot suck. When a cleft palate is too wide for operation, its effects can be diminished in later life by wearing an artificial palate.

Parents of such children can obtain help and advice from the Cleft Lip and Palate Association, The Hospital for Sick Children, Great Ormond Street, London WC1N 3JH.

PALINDROMIC RHEUMATISM is a form of rheumatism in adults characterized by multiple, afebrile attacks of acute arthritis, and inflammation of the surrounding tissues, with pain, swelling, redness, and disability of one or more small or large joints, the attacks coming on suddenly, lasting a few hours to a few days then disappearing completely, to recur at irregular intervals.

PALLAESTHESIA means sensibility to the vibrations of a tuning-fork applied to the neighbourhood of a bone. Loss of this sense is an early feature of certain nervous diseases, such as locomotor ataxia.

PALLIATIVE is a term applied to the treatment of incurable diseases, in which the aim is to mitigate the sufferings of the patient, not to effect a cure.

PALPATION means the method of examining the surface of the body and the size, shape, and movements of the internal organs, by laying the flat of the hand upon the skin.

PALPITATION is a condition in which the heart beats forcibly or irregularly, and the person becomes conscious of its action.

Causes – As a rule we are quite unconscious of the beating of the heart, but when the nervous system is unduly excited its action may become unpleasantly palpable. It is liable to come on at the time of puberty or of the change of life, and also in the weak state of body that accompanies great anaemia, acute fevers, or neurasthenia. Sudden emotions, such as fright, and occasionally dyspepsia, may bring it on. A common cause consists in over-use of tobacco, tea, coffee, or alcohol. Sometimes it may appear in cases of organic heart disease.

Symptoms – There may simply be a fluttering of the heart and a feeling of weakness, which is often expressively described as 'gone-ness'; or the heart may be felt pounding and the arteries throbbing, causing great distress to the affected person. In some cases the subject of palpitation is conscious of the heart missing beats.

Treatment – Mental quietness is the great requisite to still the overaction, and all sources of excitement must be avoided. The person should understand that, however unpleasant the condition may be, there is no danger from it, and that serious disease is not usually the cause. Moderate exercise is a good thing. If the person be a heavy smoker, this is probably the cause, and tobacco should be given up. Similarly tea, coffee, and alcohol should be partaken of sparingly, and any food likely to cause flatulent dyspepsia should be avoided. In the cases due to organic disease, the condition causing palpitation must be treated.

PALSY is another name for paralysis. (See PARALYSIS.)

PALUDISM, or PALUDAL FEVER, is another name for malaria.

PALUDRINE (see PROGUANIL).

PAN- is a prefix meaning all or completely.

PANACEA is a term applied to a remedy for all diseases, or more usually to a remedy which benefits many different diseases.

PANARITIUM is a term applied to a whitlow which remains chronic and destroys part of the finger.

PANCARDITIS means inflammation of the pericardium, myocardium, and endocardium at the same time.

PANCREAS, or SWEETBREAD, is a long secreting gland situated in the back of the abdomen, at the level of the first and second lumbar vertebrae (see plate II). It lies behind the lower part of the stomach, an expanded portion, called the head of the pancreas, occupying the bend formed by the duodenum or first part of the small intestine, whilst a long portion known as the body extends to the left, ending in the tail, which rests against the spleen. A duct runs through the whole gland from left to right, joined by many small branches in its course, and, leaving the head of the gland, unites with the bile duct from the liver to open into the side of the small intestine about 3 or 4 inches (7·5 to 10 cm) below the outlet of the stomach.

Minute structure – The gland resembles one of the salivary glands, being composed of tubes of columnar cells bound together by loose connective tissue. These cells are arranged with one end abutting on a central lumen into which the secretion of the cells passes, and each group of tubes ends in a small duct, which

unites with other small ducts to join the main pancreatic duct running to the intestine. The cells present an outer, clear zone, and an inner zone filled with granules of the materials secreted by the activity of the cell. Blood-vessels and nerves in large numbers run in the connective tissue of the gland.

Scattered through the pancreas are collections of cells known as the islets of Langerhans, of which there are around a million in a normal individual. These do not communicate with the duct of the gland, and the internal secretion of the pancreas – insulin – is formed by these cells and absorbed directly into the blood.

Functions – The most obvious function of the pancreas is the formation of the pancreatic juice, which is poured into the small intestine after the partially digested food has left the stomach. This is the most important of the digestive juices, is alkaline in reaction, and contains, in addition to various salts, three enzymes. These enzymes are: trypsin, which digests proteid bodies; amylase, which converts starchy foods into the disaccharide maltose; lipase, which breaks up fats. For the action of these see DIGESTION.

Inadequate production of insulin by the islets of Langerhans leads to the condition known as diabetes mellitus (qv). In addition to insulin, another hormone believed to be produced by the pancreas has been called LIPOCAIC (qv); it is thought to play a part in fat metabolism.

PANCREAS, DISEASES OF – Abscesses, cysts, calculi, and tumours may occur in the pancreas as in other organs, but are not very common. The most important disease of the pancreas, though again, fortunately, not very common, is acute pancreatitis. This is sudden in onset, accompanied by acute pain, and causes severe shock and collapse. It carries a mortality rate of around 20 per cent, even when treated adequately and early. Chronic pancreatitis is a much more indeterminate disease, commonly associated with disease of the gall-bladder, particularly gall-stones, and chronic alcoholism. Pancreatitis may occur as a complication of mumps. Cancer of the pancreas is on the increase; from 3070 deaths in England and Wales in 1962 to 4414 cases in 1970. In 1977 it was responsible for 5313 deaths in England. There is an established association with heavy cigarette smoking, and it is twice as common in patients with diabetes mellitus as compared with the general population. Reference has already been made to the association between the islets of Langerhans and diabetes mellitus (qv).

PANCREATIN (see PEPTONIZED FOODS).

PANDEMIC is the term applied to an epidemic which affects a vast area, such as a country or a continent.

PANHYSTERECTOMY is the term applied to an operation by which the uterus is completely removed.

PANNICULITIS means inflammation of the subcutaneous fat, and may occur anywhere on the body surface.

PANNUS is the name applied to the growth across the cornea of an abnormal opaque membrane with minute blood-vessels, due to some serious form of irritation. It is found especially in cases of trachoma and tends gradually to cause blindness.

PANTOTHENIC ACID, which has now been prepared synthetically, is part of the vitamin B complex. It is known as the chick anti-dermatitis factor because if it is absent from the chick's diet the bird develops dermatitis, and degeneration of nerve-fibres in the spinal cord also occurs. In rats lack of pantothenic acid produces greying of the hair, but there is no evidence that in man greying is due to lack of this vitamin. Indeed, little is known about the significance of pantothenic acid in man, except that it is one of the essential constituents of the diet. The daily requirement is probably around 10 milligrams. It is widely distributed in foodstuffs, both animal and vegetable. Yeast, liver, and egg-yolk are particularly rich sources.

PAPAIN, PAPYAOTIN, and PAPOID are names given to a ferment, or mixture of ferments, obtained from the juice of the pawpaw, the unripe fruit of *Carica papaya*, which has an action similar to that of the ferments of the gastric and pancreatic juices. It is accordingly sometimes used to peptonize foods for invalids, as it does not give them the same bitter taste that pepsin gives. It is widely used as a meat tenderiser.

PAPILLA means a small projection, such as those with which the true skin is covered, and which project into the scarf-skin and make its union with the true skin

more intimate; or those covering the tongue and projecting from its surface.

PAPILLITIS is the term applied to inflammation of any papilla, but especially of the prominence formed by the end of the optic nerve in the retina, also known as optic neuritis.

PAPILLOEDEMA is the term applied to congestion and swelling of the optic disc, at the point of entry of the optic nerve into the interior of the eyeball. Such congestion is the result of increased pressure within the skull: eg. from a cerebral tumour. It also occurs in malignant hypertension (qv) and occasionally, in the late stages of chronic nephritis. (See BRIGHT'S DISEASE.)

PAPILLOMA means a tumour composed of papillae growing from the surface of skin or mucous membrane. These tumours may be either simple or malignant in nature. Such a tumour is found occasionally in the bladder, and the chief symptom of its presence is the painless presence of blood in the urine.

PAPOVA VIRUS is a group of viruses, one of which is responsible for warts (qv).

PAPULE means a pimple.

PARA- is a prefix meaning near, aside from, or beyond.

PARA-AMINOSALICYLIC ACID has a marked bacteriostatic action against the *Mycobacterium tuberculosis*, and is now one of the standard drugs used in the treatment of tuberculosis. Because of the tendency for the *Myco. tuberculosis* to develop resistance to it, PAS, as it is often referred to, is always given in conjunction with streptomycin and/or isoniazid.

PARACENTESIS is the puncture by hollow needle or trocar and cannula of any body cavity (eg. abdominal, pleural, pericardial), for tapping or aspirating fluid pathologically accumulated. (See ASPIRATION.)

PARACETAMOL has antipyretic and analgesic actions similar to those of aspirin. The dose is 500 to 1000 milligrams.

PARACETAMOL POISONING – Paracetamol is one of the safest of drugs when taken in correct dosage. When an overdose is taken, however, it is a very dangerous one because of the toxic effect on the liver. This is why cases of poisoning with it must be taken to hospital as quickly as possible. In the early stages there is only sickness and vomiting without any loss of consciousness. Once in hospital, treatment consists of washing out the stomach, and the administration of certain drugs, such as cysteamine and acetylcysteine, to protect the liver.

PARACUSIS means any perversion of the sense of hearing.

PARAESTHESIA is a term applied to unusual feelings, apart from mere increase, or loss, of sensation, experienced by a patient without any external cause: for example, hot flushes, numbness, tingling, itching. Various paraesthesiae form a common symptom in some nervous diseases.

PARAFFIN is the general name used to designate a series of saturated hydrocarbon bodies, discovered by Reichenbach in 1830 and first produced as a commercial product by Young in 1850. The higher members of the series, paraffin-waxes, are solid at ordinary temperatures, some being hard, others soft. Lower in the scale comes petroleum, which is liquid at ordinary temperatures. Naphtha, petroleum spirit, and hydramyl are lower members of the series which are very volatile, and lowest comes methane, better known as marsh-gas, which is a gaseous body.
Uses – In the form of the *British Pharmacopoeia* preparation, liquid paraffin, it is used in the treatment of habitual constipation.
Externally, the hard and soft paraffins are used in various consistencies, being very useful as ointments and lubricants by reason of their apparently harmless nature.

PARAFORMALDEHYDE is used as a source of formaldehyde. For disinfecting rooms it is prepared in the form of tablets which are vaporized on an electric hot-plate. It is also used as lozenges. To keep catheters and other surgical instruments aseptic, it is enclosed with them in airtight containers.

PARAGANGLIOMA is the term used to describe two types of tumour. One known as a CHROMAFFINOMA or PHAEOCHROMOCYTOMA, is a tumour containing chromaffin cells (qv), most often found in the medulla of the suprarenal gland, where

chromaffin cells are normal constituents. An important sign of these tumours is paroxysmal high blood-pressure. The other, also known as a CHEMODECTOMA, occurs in the carotid body (qv) and the comparable aortic body. It is usually quite small and is more common in women than men.

PARAGONIMIASIS is the condition caused by *paragonimus*, a genus of Trematode or fluke, the most common being *Paragonimus westermani*, which is most often found in the Far East, but is also found in India, South America and parts of Africa. The disease is also known as endemic haemoptysis, as the presenting feature is haemoptysis, or the coughing up of blood, due to the worm settling in the lungs. The infection is acquired by eating inadequately cooked crayfish or crab. Bithionol is the drug most commonly used in treatment. Chloroquine is also used.

PARAGRAPHIA is misplacement of words, or of letters in words, or wrong spelling, or use of wrong words in writing as a result of a lesion in the speech region of the brain.

PARALDEHYDE is a clear, colourless liquid with a penetrating ethereal odour, and a burning taste followed by a cool sensation in the mouth. Although in small quantities it may cause excitement, in larger doses it is a soporific, with little depressing effect, and productive of quiet, refreshing sleep.
Uses – It is given when a powerful hypnotic action is required, and is particularly useful in inducing sleep in mentally unstable patients. Its unpleasant taste restricts its use, but has the compensatory advantage that it usually prevents the patient receiving paraldehyde from becoming an addict. It is sometimes given per rectum as a general anaesthetic.

PARALYSIS, or PALSY, means loss of muscular power due to interference with the nervous system. When muscular power is weakened as the result of some affection of the nervous system, but not entirely lost in the parts concerned, the term *paresis* is often used instead of paralysis. Various terms are used to designate paralysis distributed in different ways. Thus *hemiplegia* is the term applied to paralysis affecting one side of the face, with the corresponding arm and leg, as the result of disease on one side of the brain; *diplegia* means a condition of more or less

665

337 – Diagram of the brain and spinal cord, showing the motor paths, and the positions of injuries causing different forms of paralysis. The front half of the brain is supposed to have been removed and the reader is looking at its interior. *CH*, cerebral hemisphere; *Cb, cerebellum; T, thalamus; LN*, lentiform nucleus; *M, medulla oblongata; P, pons; SC*, spinal cord; 1, position of a haemorrhage causing paralysis of left arm; 2, position of a haemorrhage causing complete paralysis of the left side; 3, position of a haemorrhage followed by paralysis of left arm and leg, with right side of face (crossed paralysis); 4, position of the disorder causing paralysis of both lower limbs (*paraplegia*); 5, position of the disease responsible for poliomyelitis in the left leg.

total paralysis, in which both sides are affected in this manner; *monoplegia* is the term applied to paralysis of a single limb; and *paraplegia* signifies paralysis of both sides of the body below a given level, usually from about the level of the waist; *quadriplegia* is paralysis of all four limbs.

Certain descriptive terms are used in popular language in connection with the word paralysis; thus *creeping paralysis* is a vague term applied most often to locomotor ataxia, *shaking paralysis* is the popular name for paralysis agitans or Parkinsonism, and *wasting paralysis* commonly means progressive muscular atrophy.

Paralysis should be regarded rather as a symptom than as a disease by itself, and it is generally connected with well-marked disorder of some portion of the nervous system. According to the locality and extent of the nervous system affected, so will be the form and completeness of the paralysis. It is usual to classify paralysis according to whether it depends upon disease of the brain, of the spinal cord, or of the nerves; and hence the terms: *cerebral, spinal,* and *peripheral paralysis.* The distribution of the paralytic condition may be very extensive, involving more or less all the functions of the body. as in *general paralysis of the insane* (see GENERAL PARALYSIS), or it may, as already stated, affect half the body, or only certain limbs, or it may even be restricted to single muscles or single groups of muscles supplied by a particular nerve (illustration 337).

Reference can here be made only to the more common types of paralysis, and that merely in general terms.

1. PARALYSIS DUE TO BRAIN DISEASE – Of this, by far the most common form is palsy affecting one side of the body, or **Hemiplegia.** It usually arises from disease of the hemisphere of the brain opposite to the side of the body affected, such disease being in the form of haemorrhage into the brain substance (*cerebral haemorrhage*), or the plugging up of blood-vessels by a locally formed clot (*cerebral thrombosis*) or by a clot dislodged from some other part of the body (*cerebral embolism*), and consequent arrest of blood supply to an area of the brain; or again, it may result from an injury, or be due to a tumour in the tissues of the brain. The character of the seizure and the amount of paralysis vary according to the situation of the disease or injury, its extent, and its sudden or gradual occurrence. The attack may come on as a stroke of apoplexy (see APOPLEXY), in which the patient becomes suddenly unconscious, and loses completely the power of motion of one side of the body, or a like result may arise more gradually and without loss of consciousness. In either type of complete hemiplegia, the paralysis affects on one side the muscles of the face, tongue,

1 *Conscious muscle sense; direct touch*

1 Posterior columns

2 Dorsal spinocere-
/ bellar tract

3 Lateral cortico-
spinal tract
(Pyramidal)

2 *e 6 Unconscious
muscle sense*

4 Rubrospi-
nal tract
(Extrapyramidal)

3 *e 8
Voluntary
control of
striated muscle*

4 *Involuntary
control of
striated
muscle*

5 Lateral
spinothalamic
tract

6 Ventral spino-
cerebellar tract

5 *Pain, heat,
and cold*

7 *Crossed touch*

8 Ventral
corticospinal
tract (Pyramidal)

7 Ventral spino-
thalamic tract

338 – Diagrammatic representation of cross section of spinal cord. The nerve tracts are shown on the right and their function on the left. From Choffre and Greisheim, *Basic Physiology and Anatomy.* Lippincott.

body, and limbs. Speech is indistinct and thick, and the tongue, when protruded, points towards the paralysed side owing to the unopposed action of its muscles on the unaffected side. The muscles of the face implicated are chiefly those about the mouth. The paralysed side hangs loose, and the corner of the mouth is depressed, but the muscles closing the eye are, as a rule, unimpaired, in consequence of the fact that movements like that of shutting the eyes, which are performed usually on both sides together, are controlled from either side of the brain. As a result the eye on the paralysed side can be shut, unlike what occurs in another form of facial paralysis (Bell's palsy), in which the fault lies in the nerve. The muscles of respiration on the affected side are seldom more than slightly weakened for deep breathing, but those of the arm and leg are completely powerless. Sensation may at first be impaired (anaesthesia), but as a rule returns soon, unless the portion of the brain involved be that which is connected with this function. Rigidity of the paralysed members is usually present as a later symptom. In many cases of even complete hemiplegia, improvement takes place after the lapse of weeks or months, and is in general indicated by a return of motor power, first in the face, next in the leg, while that of the arm follows after a longer

or shorter interval, and is rarely complete. Such recovery of movement is, however, only partial in a large proportion of cases and the side remains weakened. In such instances the gait of the patient is characteristic. In walking, he leans to the sound side and swings round the affected limb from the hip, the foot scraping the ground as it is raised and advanced. The paralysed parts retain their contractility when stimulated by electric currents, but they are apt to suffer in their nutrition from disuse and to assume an attitude of rigidity unless treatment is carefully carried out.

In many instances the hemiplegia is only partial, and instead of the symptoms of complete paralysis just described, there exist in varied combination only certain of them, their association depending on the extent and locality of the damage to the brain. Thus there may be impairment of speech and some amount of facial paralysis, while the arm and leg may be unaffected, or the paralysis may be present in one or both extremities of one side while the other symptoms are absent. Further, the paralysis may be incomplete throughout, and the whole of the side be weak, but not entirely deprived of motor power. To partial paralysis of this latter description the term PARESIS is applied.

Besides hemiplegia, various other forms

667

of paralysis may arise from cerebral disease. Thus occasionally there is CROSSED PARALYSIS, one side of the face and the opposite side of the body being affected simultaneously. Or again, as is often observed in the case of tumours of the brain, the paralysis may be limited to the distribution of one or more of the cranial nerves, and may produce a combination of symptoms (such as squinting, drooping of the eyelid, and impairment or loss of vision) which may enable the seat of the disease to be accurately localized. The condition of DIPLEGIA, in which both sides are affected, sometimes occurs in infants, and is due generally to some inflammation of the brain occurring soon after birth.

Trembling palsy, PARALYSIS AGITANS; PARKINSONISM or SHAKING PARALYSIS (see PARKINSONISM).

Cerebral palsy (see CEREBRAL PALSY).

Functional paralysis includes other forms of paralysis which, being of cerebral origin, should be mentioned here, although they are not connected with any discoverable disease of the brain. These forms of paralysis are amenable to psychological treatment, the cause of the paralysis often being traceable to some deep-seated mental conflict having its origin in childhood. (See HYSTERIA; CRAMP; NEURASTHENIA.)

2. PARALYSIS DUE TO DISEASE OF THE SPINAL CORD – Of paralysis from this cause, there are numerous varieties, depending on the nature, the site, and the extent of the disease. Frequently defects in muscular action, due to disease in the spinal cord, are not of a paralytic nature, and these must be carefully distinguished. For example, in disease of the posterior part of the cord, involving the sensory paths, the condition of *ataxia* is produced, and the patient, though sufficiently strong, cannot control his movements, as he is unconscious of the directions in which his limbs move till he sees the movements made. Or again, in disease of the lateral parts of the cord, involving the controlling motor paths from the brain, the condition of *spasticity* results, and when muscles contract they do so excessively, so that freedom of movement is impossible (illustration 338).

Paraplegia, paralysis of both lower extremities, including usually the lower portion of the trunk, and occasionally also the upper portion – indeed, all the parts below the seat of the disease in the spinal cord – is a form of paralysis which is a common result of injuries or disease of the vertebral column; also of inflammation affecting the spinal cord (myelitis), as well as of haemorrhage or tumours involving its substance. When it is due to disease, this is generally situated in the lower portion of the cord. The symptoms necessarily vary in relation to the locality and the extent of the disease in the cord. Thus, if in the affected area the posterior part of the cord, including the posterior nerve roots, suffer, the function of sensation in the parts below is impaired because the cord is unable to transmit the sensory impressions from the surface of the body to the brain, and the condition of ataxia affects the power of motion. If, on the other hand, the anterior portion of the cord and the anterior nerve roots be affected, the motor impulses from the brain cannot be conveyed to the muscles below the seat of the injury or disease, and consequently their power of movement is abolished. Whilst, if the lateral portions of the cord be affected, a condition of spastic paralysis is set up. In many forms of this complaint, particularly in the case of injuries, the whole thickness of the cord is involved (transverse myelitis), and both sensory and motor functions are lost below the level at which the cord is affected. Further, the functions of the bladder and bowels are apt to suffer, and either spasm, or more often paralysis, of these organs is the result. The nutrition of the paralysed parts tends to become affected, and bed sores and wasting of the muscles are common. Occasionally, more especially in cases of injury, recovery takes place, but in general this is incomplete, the power of walking being more or less impaired. When the paralysis is due to pressure caused by a diseased or injured spine, an operation designed to relieve this pressure is often completely successful, and entire power is restored, even after the paralysis has lasted for several months. On the other hand, the patient may linger on for years bedridden, and at last succumb to bed sores or to a septic affection of the paralysed bladder spreading up to the kidneys. Advances in recent years, however, have gone a long way towards ameliorating the lot of the paraplegic patient and allowing him or her to lead a reasonably active life at home and in the community.

Infantile paralysis (see POLIOMYELITIS).

Motor neurone disease is a disease usually occurring in middle life. Pathologically it is characterized by degeneration: (*a*) of the motor cells of Betz in the cerebral cortex, with corresponding degeneration of the pyramidal tracts; (*b*) of the anterior horn cells of the grey matter of the spinal cord, with corresponding degeneration of the peripheral motor nerves and wasting of the muscles innervated by them; (c) of the nerve cells in the bulb of the brain from which the motor cranial nerves arise: hypoglossal, facial, trigeminal, oculomotor, accessory, glossopharyngeal, vagus. There is diffuse atrophy of the white matter of the spinal cord, excepting the posterior, sensory columns. The cause of the degeneration is not known.

From this it can be seen that spastic paralysis and profound wasting of muscle may be combined, as in amyotrophic lateral sclerosis (qv); that a purely spastic paralysis may occur when the degenerative process affects principally the motor cells of the cerebral cortex; that a wasting of groups of muscles will occur when predominantly the anterior horn cells of the spine are involved as in progressive muscular atrophy; and that the clinical picture will be that of a bulbar paralysis when the motor nuclei of cranial nerves degenerate.

Progressive muscular atrophy is characterized by the gradual wasting of certain muscles or groups of muscles, loss of power in them, fibrillation (fine twitching of muscle fibres), alteration of tendon and skin reflexes. It is insidious in its onset, and usually first shows itself in the prominent muscular masses in the palm of the hand, especially the ball of the thumb, which becomes wasted and deficient in power. The other palmar muscles suffer in like manner, and as the disease advances the muscles of the arm, shoulders, and trunk become implicated if they have not themselves been the first to be attacked. The malady tends to spread symmetrically, involving the corresponding parts of both sides of the body in succession. It is slow in its progress, but, although it may occasionally undergo arrest, it tends to advance and involve more and more of the muscles of the body, until the sufferer is reduced to a condition of extreme helplessness. Should some other ailment not be the cause of death, the fatal result may be due to the disease extending so as to involve the muscles of respiration.

In bulbar paralysis, the muscles of facial expression, of mastication, of articulation, and of swallowing suffer progressive loss of power.

Progressive muscular dystrophy, MYOPATHY, or PSEUDOHYPERTROPHIC MUSCULAR DYSTROPHY, is another form of paralysis, in certain respects resembling progressive muscular atrophy, although in it the change occurs in the muscles themselves, not in the nervous system. (See MYOPATHY.)

3. *PERIPHERAL PARALYSIS*, or local paralysis of individual nerves, is of frequent occurrence. Only the most common and important examples of this condition can be briefly referred to.

Facial paralysis and BELL'S PALSY are the terms applied to paralysis involving the muscles of expression supplied by the seventh cranial nerve. It is unilateral. The cause is not known, but it sometimes follows exposure of one side of the head to a draught of cold air, which sets up inflammation of the nerve. It may also be due to injury or disease either affecting the nerve near the surface or deeper in the bony canals through which it passes, or in the brain itself, involving the nerve at its origin. The paralysis is manifested by a marked change in the expression of the face, the patient being unable to move the muscles of one side in such acts as laughing, and whistling, or to close the eye on that side. The mouth is drawn to the sound side, while, although the muscles of mastication are not involved, the food in eating tends to lodge between the jaw and cheek on the palsied side. Occasionally, when the nerve is injured as it passes through the skull, the sense of taste is impaired. In the ordinary cases of this disease, such as those due to exposure, recovery usually takes place in about six weeks, the improvement being first shown in the power of closing the eye, which is soon followed by the disappearance of the other signs. Recovery may be speeded up by the administration of prednisolone (qv), especially if this is given at an early stage of the disease. It is more effective in younger patients (under the age of 45) than older ones. When the paralysis proceeds from wounding of the nerve, disease of the temporal bone, or from tumours in the brain, it is more apt to be permanent, and is in many cases of serious import.

Lead palsy is a common form of local paralysis. It is due to the poisonous action of lead upon the system, and, like the other symptoms of lead poisoning, affects chiefly workers in that metal. (See LEAD-POISONING.)

A form of peripheral paralysis, resembling this often results from chronic alcoholism. Other poisons also act similarly, as, for example, arsenic. (See NEURITIS.) Injury to a nerve may cause paralysis in the muscles which it should supply, and this may follow on wounds, severe bruises, or even long-continued pressure, as in crutch-palsy. (See DROP-

WRIST; NERVE INJURIES.) The paralysis occurring after diphtheria, another example of the peripheral variety, has been already mentioned, and similar paralyses, for example of the foot, follow sometimes on other infectious diseases. (See DIPHTHERIA; DROP-FOOT.)

Treatment – It is impossible in a brief notice like the present to enter at any length into the treatment of the different varieties of paralysis. Generally speaking, the treatment consists of measures which aim at supporting the patient's strength and maintaining his health while the nervous system is slowly restoring itself so far as may be. The conditions of the disease in any particular case can only be understood and appreciated by the medical expert, under whose direction alone treatment can be advantageously carried out.

An important point in the treatment is that, since paralysed muscles tend to undergo degenerative changes, their action should be maintained as long as possible. With the view of improving the circulation in the muscles, and also in order to prevent stiffening of the joints, massage is very useful. In order to exercise the muscles, the faradic current or, failing it, the interrupted galvanic current, may be applied daily.

In the case of paraplegia there is a necessity for highly skilled nursing, since not only the patient's comfort but his life depends upon careful management, directed towards preventing bed sores (see BED SORES), and inflammation of the bladder (see CATHETERS) in cases where the act of urination is interfered with. A similar remark applies to bulbar palsy, in which special care is necessary in feeding the patient, owing to his difficulty in swallowing.

PARAMETRITIS means inflammation in the cellular tissue at the side of the womb.

PARAMNESIA is the term applied to a derangement of the memory in which words are used without a comprehension of their meaning; it is also applied to illusions of memory in which a person in good faith imagines and describes experiences which never occurred to him.

PARAMYOCLONUS is the name applied to an affection in which paroxysmal jerking contractions of the muscles of the limbs take place; it is sometimes due to organic disease of the nervous system, sometimes hysterical.

PARANOIA is the term applied to a form of fixed delusional insanity in which the delusions, usually of persecution, all centre round some perverted idea and have an important bearing upon the person's actions. Heredity plays an important part, recovery is unlikely, and in marked cases restraint is often necessary to prevent criminal acts. Many paranoic persons, however, are able to go about freely and transact business, with which their delusions do not interfere, and are regarded simply as eccentric persons. (See MENTAL ILLNESS.)

PARAPHASIA is misplacement of words, or use of wrong words, in speech as a result of a lesion in the speech region of the brain.

PARAPHRENIA is a form of paranoia (qv). (See also MENTAL ILLNESS.)

PARAPLEGIA means paralysis of the lower limbs, accompanied generally by paralysis of bladder and rectum. (See PARALYSIS.)

PARAQUAT is a contact herbicide widely used in agriculture and horticulture. A mouthful is enough to kill. The eyes and skin must also be carefully protected so as not to come into contact with it.

PARASITICIDE is a general term applied to agents or substances destructive to parasites.

PARASITOSIS means infestation with a parasite or parasites. It is a not uncommon delusion in mentally or emotionally unstable individuals.

PARASYMPATHETIC NERVOUS SYSTEM is that part of the autonomic nervous system which is connected with the brain and spinal cord through certain nerve centres in the mid-brain, medulla, and lower end of the cord. The nerves from these centres are carried in the 3rd, 7th, 9th, and 10th cranial nerves and the 2nd, 3rd, and 4th sacral nerves. The action of the parasympathetic system is usually antagonistic to that of the sympathetic system. Thus it inhibits the action of the heart and augments the action of the intestine, whereas the sympathetic augments the action of the heart and inhibits that of the intestine.

PARATHION is one of the organophosphorus insecticides (qv). It is highly toxic to man and must therefore be handled with the utmost care.

PARATHORMONE is the name of the hormone secreted by the parathyroid gland (qv).

PARATHYROID is the name applied to four small glands which lie to the side of and behind the thyroid gland. These glands regulate the metabolism of calcium and of phosphorus. If for any reason there is a deficiency of the secretion of the parathyroid glands, the amount of calcium in the blood falls too low and the amount of phosphorus increases. The result is the condition known as tetany (qv), in which there is great restlessness and spasm of muscles. The condition is checked by the injection of the parathyroid hormone – parathormone – which causes an increase in the amount of calcium in the blood. If there is over-activity of the parathyroids there will be an increase of calcium in the blood. This extra calcium is drawn from the bones, in which, as a consequence, thin cysts form and greatly weaken the bones, these breaking easily as a result. This cystic disease of bone has the elaborate title of GENERALIZED OSTEITIS FIBROSA CYSTICA. Tumours of the parathyroid glands result in this over-activity of the parathyroid hormone, and the resulting increase in the amount of calcium in the blood leads to the formation of stones in the kidneys. (See KIDNEYS, DISEASES OF.)

PARATYPHOID FEVER (see ENTERIC FEVERS).

PAREGORIC, or CAMPHORATED OPIUM TINCTURE, is a preparation of opium much used for cough mixtures. It contains 5 per cent of tincture of opium, together with oil of anise, benzoic acid and camphor. The dose is 2 to 10 ml. Scotch paregoric, or ammoniated opium tincture, contains 10 per cent of tincture of opium, together with dilute ammonia solution, oil of anise and benzoic acid. The dose is 2 to 4 ml.

PARENCHYMA is a term meaning originally all the soft tissues of internal organs except the muscular flesh, though now reserved for the secreting cells of the glandular organs.

PARENTERAL is the word applied to the administration of drugs by any route other than by the mouth or by the bowel. Parenteral methods of giving drugs include injection under the skin or into

muscle, inunction, and intrathecal injection.

PARESIS means a state of slight or temporary paralysis. (See PARALYSIS.)

PARIETAL is the term applied to anything pertaining to the wall of a cavity: eg. parietal pleura, the part of the pleural membrane which lines the wall of the chest.

PARKINSONISM, or PARKINSON'S DISEASE, so called after the London general practitioner who first described the condition in 1817, is also known as PARALYSIS AGITANS. It is a progressive disease of insidious onset which comes on in the second half of life, and is due to degenerative changes in the ganglia at the base of the cerebrum. This results in a deficiency of a neurotransmitter (qv) known as dopamine (qv), and it is this deficiency of dopamine which is responsible for most cases. In some, however, deficiency of neurotransmitters other than dopamine may be the cause. It is much commoner in men than in women. In some cases the disease is a sequel to encephalitis lethargica. The disease first manifests itself by increasing rigidity of the muscles. In the face this results in a loss of the natural play of expression and produces a mask-like expression. The voice is also affected by the rigidity of the muscles of the larynx, tongue and lips, loses its tone and inflexion and develops into a monotone. Later the limbs become rigid, and this is typified by the peculiar running gait. The patient always seems to be tottering and taking short steps as if running after himself. Later a coarse tremor develops in the muscles, best typified in the rolling movements of the fingers as if a cigarette was always being rolled. The tremor is exaggerated by excitement and self-consciousness and ceases during sleep. In the hands and arms it may interfere grossly with eating and dressing.

Treatment – There is now an increasing number of drugs that keep the condition under control. None of them is curative, and the effort to find the most suitable one for any given individual is usually a matter of trial and error, the successful outcome of which depends largely upon understanding cooperation between family doctor and patient. The most promising one at the moment is levodopa which is a precursor of dopamine. Its introduction has revolutionized the outlook in this disease and has almost done away with the need for stereotactic surgery. Unfortunately it is not curative and has considerable side-effects, which means that it must only be administered under skilled medical supervision. Current opinion is that it produces spectacular improvement in one-fifth of patients, moderate improvement in two-fifths, modest improvement in one-fifth, and no improvement in one-fifth. Patients with the disease and their relatives, seeking advice and help, are recommended to get in touch with the Parkinson's Disease Society, 81 Queens Road, London SW19 8NR.

PAROMOMYCIN is an antibiotic derived from a sub-species of *Streptomyces rimosus*, which is proving of value in the treatment of certain cases of both bacillary and amoebic dysentery.

PARONYCHIA is the term applied to inflammation near the nail. In the *acute* form it is usually due to infection with *Staphylococcus aureus*, and is most often seen in nurses and others handling septic material. It usually starts at one corner of the nail-fold and then spreads to the other side and deeply under the base of the nail. There is local pain and tenderness, with swelling of the nail-fold. Treatment in mild cases consists of applying an adhesive dressing and giving penicillin. In more severe cases the swelling has to be opened. A new nail grows in two or three months displacing the old one in front of it. *Chronic paronychia* occurs usually in women who have their hands much in water. In men it occurs in fishmongers and chefs. It may affect one or more fingers. Treatment consists of keeping the finger dry and giving a suitable antibiotic. (See WHITLOW.)

PAROSMIA means a perverted sense of smell; everything usually smells unpleasant to the affected individual. The most common cause is some septic condition of the nasal passages, but it may occasionally be due to a lesion in the brain involving the centre responsible for the sense of smell.

PAROTID GLAND is one of the salivary glands. It is situated just in front of the ear, and its duct runs forwards across the cheek to open into the interior of the mouth on a little projection opposite the second last tooth of the upper row. The parotid gland is generally the first of the salivary glands to become enlarged in mumps. (See MUMPS.)

PAROTITIS means inflammation of the parotid gland. Epidemic parotitis is another name for mumps (qv).

PAROVARIUM is the name of a rudimentary structure situated near the ovary, in which tumours sometimes arise.

PARSLEY is the leaves and fruit of *Apium petroselinum*. It has a stimulant and diuretic action. It should not be confused with *fool's parsley*, or lesser hemlock, *Aethusa cynapium*, which is highly poisonous.

PARTHENOGENESIS is non-sexual reproduction. In other words, development of the ovum into an individual without fertilization by a spermatozoon. It is a rare spontaneous event but has been produced in animals experimentally. There is, however, no certain record of the birth of a parthenogenetic animal. The most that has been achieved is that parthogenetic mice and rabbit embryos have developed normally to about halfway through pregnancy but have then died and been aborted.

PARTOGRAM is a method of recording the degree of dilatation, or opening, of the cervix (or neck) of the uterus in labour, which is of value in assessing how labour is progressing.

PARTURITION (see LABOUR).

PARULIS is another name for gumboil or abscess of the gum.

P.A.S. is a commonly used abbreviation for para-aminosalicylic acid (qv).

PASTEURELLA is a group of bacilli. They are essentially animal parasites that under certain conditions are transmitted to man. They include the micro-organism responsible for plague and tularaemia.

PASTEURIZATION is a method of sterilizing milk which is not open to some of the objections attending boiling. The boiling of milk gives it a taste and smell which are disagreeable to some persons. In many parts of the world pasteurization has done away with milk-borne infections, of which the most serious is bovine tuberculosis, affecting the glands, bones, and joints of children. Other infections conveyed by milk are scarlet fever, diphtheria, enteric fever (typhoid and paratyphoid), undulant fever (brucellosis), and food poisoning (eg. from the toxins of the staphylococcus). The case therefore is very clear for the compulsory pasteurization of all milk. Pasteurization destroys about 20 per cent of vitamin C, but it should be remembered that we do not rely upon milk to protect us from scurvy, but on fresh fruit and vegetables, such as oranges, lemons, currants, potatoes, and green vegetables.

HIGH-TEMPERATURE SHORT-TIME (HTST) PASTEURIZATION consists in heating the milk at a temperature not less than 161° F (71·7° C) for at least fifteen seconds, followed by immediate cooling to a temperature of not more than 50° F (10° C).

LOW-TEMPERATURE PASTEURIZATION, or 'HOLDER' PROCESS, consists in maintaining the milk for at least half an hour at a temperature between 145° F and 150° F (63° to 65° C), followed by immediate cooling to a temperature of not more than 50° F (10° C). This has the effect of considerably reducing the number of bacteria contained in the milk and of preventing the diseases conveyed by milk referred to above. This procedure is sufficient for the sale of milk as 'pasteurized milk' in England.

PATELLA, also known as the knee-pan or knee-cap, is a flat bone shaped somewhat like an oyster-shell, lying in the tendon of the extensor muscle of the thigh, and protecting the knee-joint in front. (See BONES; KNEE; FRACTURES.)

PATHOGENIC means disease-producing, and is a term, for example, applied to bacteria, capable of causing disease.

PATHOGNOMONIC is a term applied to signs or symptoms which are specially characteristic of certain diseases, and on the presence or absence of which the diagnosis depends. Thus the discovery of the *Mycobacterium tuberculosis* in the expectoration is said to be pathognomonic of pulmonary tuberculosis.

PATHOLOGY is the science which deals with the causes of, and changes produced in the body by, disease.

PAUL-BUNNELL TEST is a test for glandular fever (qv) which is based upon the fact that patients with glandular fever develop antibodies which agglutinate sheep red blood cells.

PEANUTS, also known as GROUND-NUTS and MONKEY NUTS, are the seeds of a leguminous plant, and therefore pulses (qv) and not nuts. They differ from other pulses in their high fat content – around 40 per cent. This is twice the amount in soya beans. They are cultivated mainly for their oil which is used as cooking oil and also making margarine and soap. The residual cake, as it is known, is an excellent cattle food. Hitherto its unpleasant taste has rendered it unfit for human use, but this difficulty is now being overcome and palatable foods are being produced, in which a significant proportion of the protein comes from groundnuts.

PEAS (see PULSES).

PECTIN is a polysaccharide substance allied to starch, contained in fruits and plants, and forming the basis of vegetable jelly. It has been used as a transfusion fluid in place of blood in cases of haemorrhage and shock.

PECTORAL means anything pertaining to the chest, or a remedy used in treating chest troubles.

PECTORILOQUY means the resonance of the voice, when spoken or whispered words can be clearly heard through the stethoscope. It is a sign of consolidation, or of a cavity, in the lung.

PEDICULOSIS is infestation with lice.
Pediculi, or lice, are of three species, which vary in shape and size as well as in the area of the body they infest.

PEDICULUS HUMANUS var. CAPITIS (*Pedicalus capitis*), or the head louse, is similar in practically all respects to the body louse, except that it occurs in the head and not on the trunk of the body. The eggs, commonly known as nits and visible as little white specks, are usually laid in the hairs of the back of the head; behind the ears is also a favourite site. On infested heads the hairs are often matted together by the exudate which results from irritation and scratching. The glands behind the ears and in the back of the neck are often enlarged.

PEDICULUS HUMANUS var. CORPORIS (*Pediculus vestimenti*), or the body louse (illustration 339), is found on the underclothing on the trunk and upper arms, rather than on the skin. The female louse, which has a life of almost a month, lays seven to ten eggs a day. The eggs hatch out in 7 to 10 days and become mature in another week. Without food the adult dies in nine days and the newly hatched louse in two days. The eggs are viable for much longer (up to a month) and are usually

339 (*left*) – The female *Pediculus humanus* var. *corporis.*

340 (*above*) – The female *Phthirus pubis*, or crab louse.

found in the more inaccessible parts of the clothing: eg. the seams.

PHTHIRUS PUBIS, popularly known as the crab louse (illustration 340), is broader and shorter than the pediculi. It is found predominantly on the short hairs of the pubic region, to which it adheres very tenaciously. It causes intense itching. So far as is known, it does not carry any disease. It is most commonly transmitted from one person to another by sexual contact. Live lice have been found on lavatory seats, and the eggs may be spread from a lousy person by attachment of their infected hairs to towels and clothing.

(For further details, see INSECTS IN RELATION TO DISEASE.)

PELLAGRA is a nutritional disorder, showing a number of nervous, digestive, and skin symptoms.

Causes – It occurs in those parts of the world where the inhabitants live on a diet of maize without adequate first class protein in the form of milk and meat. It is due to deficiency of the nicotinic acid component of the vitamin B complex, in association with deficiency of protein. For long the puzzling feature was that it occurred predominantly in maize-eating areas of the world, yet maize has as much nicotinic acid as wheat but the disease did not occur in wheat-eating areas. The explanation is that the nicotinic acid in maize is in a bound form that the consumer cannot utilize. Further, maize is deficient in the amino-acid, tryptophan, from which the human body can make nicotinic acid.

Symptoms – Pellagra is known as the disease of the three D's: dermatitis, diarrhoea and dementia. The course of pellagra lasts many years, with digestive disturbances including loss of appetite and diarrhoea or constipation, headache, and irritability of temper. The skin symptoms consist at first of redness resembling severe sunburn on the parts of the body exposed to the sun, such as the hands, forearms, chest, neck, and face. The irritation usually lasts about a fortnight, is followed by desquamation, and the skin remains rough, thickened, and permanently brownish in colour. This brownish and roughened appearance on the hands is the most prominent feature of the disease, and from this the disease takes its name. Tremors, sleepiness, and weakness of the legs also appear. For several years the disease may recur in this manner every spring, the attacks gradually becoming more severe, the patient slowly growing emaciated and in some cases completely paralytic or demented.

Treatment – The disease is prevented or cured by adding to the diet foods such as fresh meat, eggs, milk, liver, and yeast extracts, and nicotinic acid, as well as by improvement of the general conditions of life.

PELOTHERAPY is the therapeutic use of mud or peat. It is prescribed either as general or local baths or in the form of a pack.

PELVIS is that division of the skeleton which is made up of the haunch-bones, one on each side, and the sacrum and coccyx behind. It connects the lower limbs with the spine. Each haunch-bone is composed of three originally separate bones, in the adult pelvis firmly fused together: the ilium; the ischium, with a rounded part below, the tuberosity, upon which the body rests in sitting; and the pubis in front. The expanded parts of the iliac bones incompletely surround the lower part of the abdomen, known as the false pelvis, and are separated by a distinct line, known as the brim or inlet, from the true pelvis beneath. The true pelvis, as its name implies, is basin-shaped, and though in the dried state it has a wide outlet beneath, yet in the living body it is well closed and rounded off by ligaments and muscles so as to leave small openings only for the urinary and genital passages and for the rectum. This soft floor of the pelvis is composed mainly of two muscles, the levators of the anus, whilst the deep notch, between the haunch-bone and sacrum behind, is closed in by a pair of strong sacro-sciatic ligaments.

The pelvis varies considerably in the two sexes. In the female it is shallower and the ilia are more widely separated, giving great breadth to the hips of the woman; the inlet is more circular and the outlet larger; whilst the angle beneath the pubic bones (subpubic angle), which is an acute angle in the male, is obtuse in the female. All these points are of importance in connection with the subject of child-bearing.

The contents of the pelvis are the urinary bladder and rectum in both sexes, and in addition the male has the seminal vesicles and the prostate gland surrounding the neck of the bladder, whilst the female has the womb, ovaries, and their appendages.

In addition to these sex differences, there are differences in the pelvis of different races, those of certain races, such as the Negro race, being, generally speaking, longer from before back and from above down than those of Caucasians: the so-called anthropoid pelvis.

PELVIS OF THE KIDNEY, or RENAL PELVIS, is the cavity of the kidney, lined by mucous membrane, in which the ureter commences. (See KIDNEYS.)

PEMPHIGUS is a skin condition characterized by the appearance of large blebs. *Pemphigus neonatorum,* the form of the disease which appears in young infants, is really a form of impetigo (qv). It is liable to occur in nurseries and maternity hospitals, and is highly infectious. Strict isola-

tion of cases is essential, and the prognosis is satisfactory provided active treatment is started at an early stage. In addition to the local treatment recommended for impetigo in older children and adults, an antibiotic or sulphonamide should be given provided the staphylococcus responsible for the condition is sensitive to it. Unfortunately, *Staphylococcus aureus,* especially that which occurs in hospital, is so often resistant to penicillin, that this antibiotic is of no avail, and some other has to be used. *Pemphigus vulgaris,* which occurs in the middle-aged, particularly Jews, is a comparatively rare condition. The skin eruption is accompanied by marked constitutional disturbances, and until the introduction of the corticosteroids (qv) it was almost invariably fatal. With large doses of corticosteroids, however, the condition can usually be kept under control. The local application of zinc cream or calamine lotion is soothing. *Pemphigus foliaceus,* in which practically the whole of the skin may be involved, is not marked by such constitutional disturbances. Treatment is as for pemphigus vulgaris. *Pemphigoid* is the form of the disease as it occurs in old age. It responds well to corticosteroids.

PEMPIDINE is a drug for the treatment of hypertension. It closely resembles mecamylamine (qv) in its action. (See ESSENTIAL HYPERTENSION.)

PENICILLIN is the name given by Sir Alexander Fleming, in 1929, to an antibacterial substance produced by the mould *Penicillium notatum.* This mould was first described in 1911 in Scandinavia, where it was discovered in decaying hyssop. The story of penicillin is one of the most dramatic in the history of medicine, and its introduction into medicine initiated a new era in therapeutics comparable only to the introduction of anaesthesia by Morton and Simpson and of antiseptics by Pasteur and Lister. The two names that will always be primarily associated with penicillin are those of Sir Alexander Fleming, of St Mary's Hospital, London, who discovered its anti-bacterial action, and Lord Florey, of Oxford, who did so much to develop its practical use during the 1939–45 War. The two great advantages of penicillin are that it is active against a large range of bacteria and that, even in large doses, it is non-toxic. Among the organisms against which it is active are: staphylococcus, streptococcus, pneumococcus, meningococcus, gonococcus, and the organisms responsible for syphilis, and for gas gangrene.

Penicillin has been synthesized in the laboratory, but it is such a complex and unstable substance that there is no reason to believe that it will be possible to synthesize it on a commercial scale – at least not for a long time to come. This means that the main method of obtaining penicillin is by the laborious technique of cultivating the penicillin mould, *Penicillium chrysogenum*. Partial synthesis of penicillin, however, has been achieved by the isolation of the penicillin nucleus – 6-aminopenicillanic acid. This can still only be obtained by culture of the penicillin mould but, now that the nucleus can be isolated, it has proved possible to add side-chains to it and so produce a large number of different – semi-synthetic as they are known – penicillins.

Various forms of penicillin are now available. *Benzylpenicillin* is available as the sodium or potassium salt. It is given intramuscularly, and is the form that is used when a rapid action is required. It can also be given by mouth but, as the proportion absorbed varies greatly, it is unreliable in action when given in this way. *Procaine penicillin* is a relatively insoluble form of penicillin. A single daily intramuscular injection of 600,000 units will maintain a bacteriostatic level in the blood for twenty-four hours. *Benzathine penicillin* is a relatively insoluble derivative of penicillin which is often given by mouth. When given intramuscularly it gives low but very prolonged blood levels of penicillin. *Phenoxymethylpenicillin* is given by mouth and produces higher blood levels than benzathine penicillin.

Phenethicillin is the first of the new penicillins obtained by adding a side chain to the penicillin nucleus. It is effective when taken by mouth and produces a blood concentration of penicillin which is twice as great as that following a comparable dose of phenoxymethylpenicillin. *Ampicillin* is another of the new penicillins derived by semi-synthesis from the penicillin nucleus. It, too, is active when taken by mouth, but its special feature is that it is active against Gram-negative organs such as *E. coli* and the salmonellae. *Cloxacillin* is yet another of the semi-synthesized penicillins. It has a relatively weak antibacterial action, but has the advantage of being active against penicillin-resistant staphylococci. *Propicillin* is α-phenoxypropyl penicillin, which is active when taken by mouth, and against penicillin-resistant staphylococci. *Phenbenicillin* is

potassium phenoxybenzylpenicillin and is active when taken by mouth.

Methicillin is another of the new penicillins derived from the penicillin nucleus. It is active against penicillin-resistant staphylococci but has to be given by injection as it is destroyed by the acid secretion of the stomach. *Carbenicillin*, yet another of the new semi-synthetic penicillins, must be given by injection, which may be painful. Its main use is in dealing with infections due to *Pseudomonas pyocanea*. It is the only penicillin active against this micro-organism. *Carfecillin* is another semi-synthetic penicillin. It is given by mouth and in the body is converted into carbenicillin, to which it owes its antibiotic properties. It is proving of particular value in the treatment of infection of the urinary tract such as cystitis and pyelonephritis. *Flucloxacillin*, also a semi-synthetic penicillin, is active against penicillin-resistant staphylococci and has the practical advantage of being active when taken by mouth. *Amoxycillin* and *talampicillin* are orally administered semi-synthetic penicillins with the same range of action as ampicillin but less likely to cause side-effects. *Mezlocillin*, another semi-synthetic penicillin, is comparable to ampicillin in its range of action, but is particularly active against *H. influenzæ*, gonococci, and *Proteus* micro-organisms. *Mecillinam* is yet another in this series, though of slightly different chemical origin. It is proving of value in the treatment of infections with Salmonellae (see SALMONELLA INFECTIONS), including typhoid fever, and with *E. coli* (see ESCHERICHIA). It is given by injection. There is a derivative, *Pivmecillinam*, which can be taken by mouth.

PENIS is the organ down which, in the male, passes the urethra, the tube by which the contents of the urinary bladder and those of the seminal vesicles escape.

PENNYROYAL is a popular name for several plants such as *Mentha pulegium* (European pennyroyal) and *Hedeoma pulegioides* (American pennyroyal). These plants contain a volatile oil which is used for rubbing into the skin to prevent the bites of midges and mosquitoes and to allay the itching caused by them.

PENTAMIDINE is a drug that is used in the prevention and treatment of African trypansomiasis, and in the treatment of leishmaniasis.

PENTAZOCINE is a pain-relieving drug with similar actions and uses to those of morphine, but much less likely to lead to addiction. It is used, usually by injection, for the relief of moderate to severe pain, especially postoperative pain, and to relieve the pain of myocardial infarction, or coronary thrombosis.

PENTOLINIUM TARTRATE is a methonium compound which is used as a hypotensive agent in the treatment of high blood-pressure.

PEPPER is the unripe fruit of *Piper nigrum*, a vine of the East Indies, and possesses an active principle, piperine. It is used externally as a counter-irritant and internally as a stimulant to digestion.

PEPPERMINT is the leaves and tops of *Mentha piperita*. It has an aromatic odour, due to the presence of an oil from which is obtained menthol, a camphorlike substance. (See MENTHOL.) Peppermint water is a useful remedy for flatulence and colic in infants. Oil of peppermint is used like the other volatile oils.

PEPSIN is the name given to a ferment found in the gastric juice which digests proteins by converting them into albumose and finally into peptones. Pepsin is used in medicine in cases of weak digestion either to digest food before it is taken or more frequently to administer after meals. It is a light yellowish-brown or white powder prepared from the fresh mucous membrane of the stomach of pigs, sheep, or calves, and it can dissolve from 2500 to 5000 times its weight of hardboiled white of egg. (For the predigestion of food, see PEPTONIZED FOODS.)

PEPTIC ULCER is the term commonly applied to ulcers in the stomach and duodenum. (See DUODENAL ULCER.)

PEPTIDE is a term applied to a compound formed by the union of two or more amino-acids.

PEPTONE is a whitish soluble powder prepared from meat which has been peptonized either by the action of acids or by artificial digestion with pepsin or trypsin. It is used as a food, especially in the form of freshly peptonized milk or beef, and it is also injected subcutaneously in the treatment of disease. (See PROTEIN SHOCK.)

PEPTONIZED FOODS – Pepsin and pancreatin are extracts made from the stomach and pancreas, respectively, of newly killed animals, and at one time widely used by persons of weak digestion, or those recovering from a severe illness, or those devitalized by age, in order to assist in the digestion of the food by converting its insoluble proteins into peptones. They may be added to the food before it is taken into the stomach, being allowed to act upon it at a temperature a little above that of the body for a period of some minutes to several hours, or they may be given in solution, or as a powder in cachets along with the food.

PEPSIN is extracted with weak alcohol from the stomach of the pig, and is then dried to a light yellow powder. (For its use, see PEPSIN.)

PANCREATIN contains three ferments, trypsin, lipase, and amylase (see DIGESTION), and is made by macerating pancreas in alcohol. Pancreatin has the advantages over pepsin that it acts more quickly, digests all kinds of food, does not require an acid to assist it, and does not unpleasantly change the taste of food unless allowed to act upon it too long. Beef-jelly, chicken-jelly, wheat flour, and other foods are sold, predigested to some extent by pancreatic extract, for the use of invalids.

Peptonized milk is made by taking a quarter of a pint (140 ml) of cold water, mixing with it two Compound Pancreatin Tablets, B.P.C., adding this to a pint (570 ml) of fresh milk in a quart bottle, and finally placing the bottle in a pan of water just so hot that the hand can be immersed in it without pain. The bottle of milk is left in this bath according to the amount of digestion desired, but not longer than fifteen minutes. If the milk be not immediately used, it must be placed upon ice, having been brought quickly to the boil in order to stop the action of the peptonizing ferment. In any case it should be used within twenty-four hours of preparation. It is often sufficient to administer one or two teaspoonfuls of liquor pancreaticus along with the milk without any digestion outside the body.

Peptonized beef is prepared as follows: A quarter of a pound (115 grams) of finely minced lean beef is mixed with half a pint (280 ml) of cold water, and cooked gently over the fire till it has boiled a few minutes. The liquor is then poured off, and the meat rubbed or beaten to a paste. The liquor and meat are placed next in a clean jar, and half a pint (280 ml) of cold water

677

containing two crushed Compound Pancreatin Tablets, B.P.C. (or a teasponful of Pancreatin Solution, B.P.C.) and half a teaspoonful of bicarbonate of soda are added. The jar with its contents is covered and set aside in a warm place for three hours, and then boiled quickly to stop further peptonization. The resulting liquid is seasoned with salt, and, if necessary, strained before use.

Other foods are peptonized in a similar manner. These artificially digested foods should never be used for longer than necessary, except in the relatively rare cases of deficiency of the pancreatic secretions, when it may be necessary to continue their use for long periods as a form of substitution therapy. Except in such cases, peptonized foods are seldom used now.

PERCUSSION is an aid to diagnosis practised by striking the body with the fingers or with an instrument known as a plessor, in such a way as to make it give out a note. It was introduced in 1761 by Auenbrugger of Vienna. According to the degree of dullness or resonance of the note, an opinion can be formed as to the state of consolidation of air-containing organs, the presence of abnormal cavities in organs, and the dimensions of solid and air-containing organs, which happen to lie next one another. Still more valuable evidence is given by auscultation (qv).

PERCUTANEOUS is a term applied to any method of administering remedies by passing them through the skin, as by rubbing in an ointment or carrying in drugs on the galvanic current.

PERFORATION is one of the serious dangers attaching to any ulcerated condition of the stomach or bowels. When a perforation from one of these hollow organs takes place into the peritoneal cavity, many bacteria, together with putrescible material, are poured into this cavity and there set up peritonitis. (See PERITONITIS.) The immediate signs that a perforation has taken place are usually a state of collapse, and increase of pain over the abdomen, together with, in some cases, the evidence of free fluid and gas in the peritoneal cavity.

PERHEXILINE is a drug used in the treatment of severe cases of angina pectoris (qv).

PERI- is a prefix meaning around.

PERIARTERITIS NODOSA (see POLYARTERITIS NODOSA).

PERICARDITIS means inflammation of the pericardium. (See HEART DISEASES.)

PERICARDIUM is the smooth membrane that surrounds the heart. (See HEART.)

PERIHEPATITIS means inflammation of the peritoneal covering of the liver.

PERIMETRITIS means a localized inflammation of the peritoneum surrounding the womb.

PERINATAL MORTALITY consists of deaths of the foetus after the 28th week of pregnancy and deaths of the new-born child during the first week of life. Today, more individuals die within a few hours of birth than during the following forty years. It is therefore not surprising that the perinatal mortality rate, which is the number of such deaths per 1000 total births, has come to be looked upon as a valuable indicator of the quality of care provided for the mother and her new-born baby. In 1976, the perinatal mortality rate was 17·6 in England and 19·0 in Wales, compared with a combined rate for the two countries of 62·1 in 1931. This is still much higher than in several other countries. Thus, in 1976, the perinatal mortality rate was 10·7 in Sweden and 13·3 in Norway. In Northern Ireland it was 22·3. Overall, in 1975, the latest year for which comparable figures are available, the perinatal mortality rate for England was the 15th lowest (jointly with France and West Germany) of the 31 countries for which statistics were available.

The causes of perinatal mortality include intrapartum anoxia (that is, difficulty in the birth of the baby, resulting in lack of oxygen), congenital abnormalities of the baby, antepartum anoxia (that is, conditions in the terminal stages of pregnancy preventing the foetus getting sufficient oxygen), and injuries to the brain of the baby during birth.

In England and Wales, in 1967, the four chief causes of deaths during the first week of life were: asphyxia and atelectasis which were responsible for 2204 of the 8945 deaths during the first week of life, immaturity of the infant which was responsible for 2156 of the deaths, birth injuries which were responsible for 1438 of the deaths, and congenital malformations which were responsible for 1521 of the deaths. (See also INFANT MORTALITY.)

PERINEPHRITIS means inflammation in the cellular tissue round the kidney, often leading to formation of an abscess. (See ABSCESS, ACUTE.)

PERINEUM, or FORK, or CROTCH, is the region situated between the opening of the bowel behind and of the genital organs in front. In the female it is apt to be lacerated in the act of childbirth.

PERIOD (see MENSTRUATION).

PERIOSTEUM is the membrane surrounding a bone (illustration 341). The periosteum carries blood-vessels and nerves for the nutrition and development of the bone. When it is irritated, an increased deposit of bone takes place beneath it, and, if it is destroyed, the bone may cease to grow and a portion may die and separate as a sequestrum. (See BONE.)

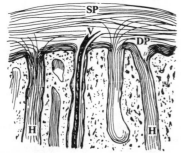

341 – Surface of a growing bone. *SP*, superficial fibrous layer of periosteum; *DP*, deep cellular layer next the bone; *V*, blood-vessel entering the bone; *HH*, Haversian canals. Magnified by about 200.

PERIOSTITIS means inflammation on the surface of a bone affecting the periosteum. (See BONE, DISEASES OF.)

PERIPHERAL NEURITIS means inflammation of the nerves in the outlying parts of the body. (See NEURITIS.)

PERISTALSIS is the term applied to the worm-like movement by which the stomach and bowels propel their contents. It consists of alternate waves of relaxation and contraction in successive parts of the tube. When any obstruction to the movement of the contents exists, these contractions become more forcible and are liable to be accompanied by the severe form of pain known as colic.

PERITONEOSCOPY is viewing of the peritoneal cavity through a tube fitted with mirrors and light. The instrument (resembling a CYSTOSCOPE, qv) is entered just below the umbilicus. The peritoneal cavity is then inflated with air. This simple operation may obviate a more drastic one: for example, if peritoneoscopy shows deposits of cancer in the peritoneum or the liver. Colour photographs of the liver have been taken through the peritoneoscope.

PERITONEUM is the membrane lining the abdominal cavity, and forming a covering for the organs contained in it. That part lining the walls of the abdomen is called the parietal peritoneum, and that part covering the viscera is known as the visceral peritoneum. The two are continuous with one another at the back of the abdomen, and form a closed sac. One may understand its relation to the organs by conceiving them to have been pressed against the outside of this sac from behind, and each to have become wrapped up in the hinder part of the sac without being forced through to its interior, while the front wall of the sac remains quite smooth. The folds of peritoneum passing from one organ to another are thus very complicated, and receive special names in various parts. (See MESENTERY; OMENTUM.)

It is stated that the peritoneum forms a closed sac, but to this there is an exception in the female, the Fallopian tube on each side having an opening into the cavity at its end large enough to admit a bristle. There is, however, no large outlet for drainage of fluid, so that a small amount is always present to lubricate the membrane, while a large amount collects in conditions that are associated with dropsy. From this arises one great reason for the danger of inflammation affecting this membrane, since there is no escape from it for the pus and other products of inflammation, which accumulate and increase the state of irritation.

In structure the peritoneum consists of a dense, though thin and elastic, fibrous membrane covered, on its inner side, by a smooth glistening layer of plate-like epithelial cells. Here and there between the cells are minute openings (stomas), each of which communicates with a lymphatic vessel, so that the fluid in the cavity is constantly draining off into the general lymphatic circulation.

PERITONITIS means inflammation of the peritoneum or membrane investing

679

the abdominal and pelvic cavities and their contained viscera. It may exist in an acute or a chronic form, and may be either localized in one part or generally diffused. Inflammation of this membrane varies much as regards its causes, severity, and danger, according as it is acute or chronic.

ACUTE PERITONITIS: **Causes** – As a rule it arises in consequence of the entrance of micro-organisms into the peritoneal cavity, which gain entrance through wounds from the exterior or pass out of some of the abdominal organs. The great danger which follows upon stabs and other penetrating wounds of the abdomen originates from the risk of peritonitis. On the other hand, the danger may come from within, and all conditions which lead to perforation of the stomach, bowels, bile-ducts, bladder, and other hollow organs may produce it. Thus gastric ulcer, typhoid fever, gall-stones, rupture of the bladder, strangulated hernia, and obstructions of the bowels may end in peritonitis. Again, abscesses and cysts developed in connection with various organs may burst and so produce it, appendicitis, abscesses of the ovary and Fallopian tubes being specially dangerous. Peritonitis may also arise within a few days after delivery.

The changes which take place in the peritoneum are similar to those undergone by other serous membranes when inflamed: (1) congestion; (2) exudation of fibrin in greater or less abundance, at first greyish in colour and soft, thereafter yellow and becoming tough in consistence, causing the folds of intestine to adhere together, and so tending to limit the spread of the inflammation; (3) effusion of fluid, either clear, turbid, bloody, or purulent; (4) absorption, more or less complete, of the fluid and fibrin, or, in cases which proceed to a serious issue, the formation of grey or greenish-grey pus. Occasionally shreds or bands of unabsorbed fibrin remain, and become converted into fibrous tissue, thus producing adhesions which constitute a subsequent danger of strangulation of the bowel, although this risk follows more often upon recovery from the chronic form.

In some cases the peritonitis becomes *localized* by adhesions between neighbouring organs due to the deposit of fibrin upon their surface. This process takes place with great rapidity, and it makes a good deal of difference to the result of the disease whether it be thus shut in to one part of the abdomen or whether it spreads so rapidly, or is of so virulent a type, as quickly to become *general*.

The bacteria causing peritonitis are numerous, but among the most common are the *Escherichia coli*, which is always a denizen of the intestine; streptococci, which produce the most virulent form of inflammation; and the gonococcus.

Symptoms – The symptoms usually begin by a rigor, together with vomiting and pain in the abdomen of a peculiarly severe and sickening character, accompanied with extreme tenderness, so that the slightest pressure causes intense aggravation of the pain. The patient lies on the back with the knees drawn up, and the hands often rest upon the head, and it will be noticed that the breathing is rapid and shallow and performed by movements of the chest only, the abdominal muscles remaining rigid, unlike what takes place in healthy respiration. The abdomen becomes swollen by flatulent distension of the intestines, which increases the patient's distress. There is usually constipation. The skin is hot, and the temperature rises to 104° or 105° F (40° to 40·5° C), although there may be no perspiration; the pulse is small, hard, and wiry; the urine is scanty and high coloured, and passed with pain. The patient's aspect is one of anxiety and suffering. These symptoms may subside in a day or two, but if they do not, the case is apt to go on rapidly to a fatal termination. In such an event, the pain and tenderness subside, the abdomen becomes more distended, hiccough and vomiting of brown or blood-coloured matter occurs, the temperature falls, the face becomes pinched, cold, and clammy, the pulse exceedingly rapid and feeble, and death takes place from collapse, the patient's mental faculties generally remaining clear till the close. When the peritonitis is due to perforation, as may happen in the case of a gastric ulcer, or the ulcers of typhoid fever, the above-mentioned symptoms and the fatal collapse may all take place in from twelve to twenty-four hours. But usually the disease lasts four or five days, and the patient sometimes survives as long as a week. The puerperal form of this disease, which comes on within a day or two after parturition, is always very serious.

Treatment – The patient should lie recumbent on the back, with a pillow beneath the knees, so as to bend up the thighs, and a cage over the abdomen to support the weight of the bed-clothes. Externally, either an ice-bag or hot laudanum fomentations give relief, though sooner or later morphine or pethidine is necessary to give relief from the pain. The patient must be given ample fluid, but this must not be given by mouth or in the form of enemas. It must be given parenterally – preferably intravenously but, if facilities for this are not available, it can be given subcutaneously. The fluid may be normal saline (see ISOTONIC) or one-fifth normal saline with 4·2 per cent dextrose. If it is to be given intravenously, plasma or blood is given. Once vomiting occurs, it is usual in hospital to pass a tube through the nose into the stomach (a naso-gastric tube) and keep the stomach clear by aspirating the stomach contents through this tube.

The introduction of the antibiotics and of the sulphonamides has resulted in a great improvement in the outlook for this serious condition.

The question of operation arises in every case of peritonitis. In cases due to perforation of the stomach or intestine which are discovered early, operation is always advisable, because there is a good prospect of freeing the abdomen from the septic material which has entered it, and, if no operation be performed, the patient will almost certainly die. In cases in which peritonitis has become localized the question of when to operate is often a difficult one and can only be answered by an experienced doctor or surgeon. The operation consists in making an opening into the abdomen, carefully cleansing the outer surface of the bowels, and attending to the original cause of the peritonitis, whether it be a perforation, obstruction, abscess, or appendicitis, after which it is usual to insert drainage tubes.

CHRONIC PERITONITIS: **Causes** – In the great majority of cases this is tuberculous in origin and secondary to tuberculous disease of bones, joints, glands, or bowels. There is also a localized form of chronic peritonitis, which is non-tuberculous. This latter form is due to long-continued inflammation in an abdominal organ or to ulceration which threatens to perforate. This type of peritonitis is advantageous, because it produces great thickening and adhesions over the part in question, thus lessening the risk of perforation or of infection of the general peritoneal cavity: eg. in appendicitis.

Symptoms – The chief symptoms of tuberculous peritonitis are abdominal pain and distension, along with disturbance of the functions of the bowels, there being either constipation or diarrhoea, or each alternately. Along with these local manifestations, there exist the usual phenomena of tuberculous disease: fever, with emaciation and loss of strength. The abdominal pain may, however, be so slight as

only to reach a feeling of uncomfortable weight and fullness.

The simple localized form is characterized mainly by recurring attacks of sharp pain, and sometimes the thickening of the peritoneum is so great as to resemble and be mistaken for a tumour.

Treatment – The same rules, as to diet and a healthy life, that pertain to the treatment of pulmonary tuberculosis, apply to tuberculous peritonitis (see TUBERCULOSIS). In addition, the patient is treated with a combination of streptomycin, para-aminosalicylic acid and isoniazid.

PERITONSILLAR ABSCESS is the term applied to an attack of tonsillitis which results in an abscess near the tonsil, forming the condition known as QUINSY. It usually points and bursts through the soft palate.

PERITYPHLITIS means inflammation round the region of the caecum, that part of the large intestine situated in the lower right-hand corner of the abdomen from which the appendix vermiformis springs. The name is now little used, having been introduced before people came to recognize the fact that inflammation in this region usually originates in the appendix. (See APPENDICITIS.)

PERLÈCHE (see CHEILOSIS).

PERMANGANATE OF POTASSIUM is a crystalline substance of brilliant purple hue. Permanganate of sodium is red in colour, and is the chief ingredient in Condy's disinfectant fluid, having an action similar to that of the potassium salt. Potassium permanganate dissolved in water is of a brilliant purple colour, and has a powerful oxidizing action, in exerting which it disintegrates alkaloidal poisons, foul and decomposing organic bodies, and kills low forms of life, such as bacteria. It is therefore a powerful antiseptic. It is non-volatile, and therefore has not the penetrating power of carbolic acid, and in exerting its oxidizing power it is itself reduced, so that it gradually loses strength. *Green Condy's fluid* contains sodium manganate, which has a similar action.

Uses – Permanganate of potassium is a cheap disinfectant, and is conveniently kept in a saturated solution (1 part of potassium permanganate to 20 parts of water). If this be diluted with water twenty-five times (1 in 500), that is, to a crimson tint, or in the proportion of about a tablespoonful of the strong solution to a tumblerful of water, it forms an excellent lotion for washing ulcers and suppurating wounds, and, diluted to a pale pink colour, makes a good gargle for an ulcerated throat. In the latter strength, it may be poured down drains, when it both purifies them and destroys the smell proceeding from them. If the hands become brown after its use, this discoloration may be removed by oxalic acid. As a hair-dye, potassium permanganate gives a rich chestnut-brown colour. As an antidote to poisoning by opium, strychnine, colchicum, oxalic acid, and toadstools (muscarine), potassium permanganate is most valuable if administered at once; 3 or 4 grains (200 or 250 mg) may be given well diluted in water. A pale pink solution of potassium permanganate is also a test for the purity of drinking-water; a drop or two allowed to fall into a glass of water should tinge the latter pink, but, if the pink colour disappear, it indicates the presence of organic impurities.

PERNICIOUS ANAEMIA is a severe form of anaemia also known as ADDISONIAN ANAEMIA. (See ANAEMIA.)

PERONEAL is the name given to structures, such as the muscles, and nerves, on the outer or fibular side of the leg.

PERPHENAZINE is one of the many tranquillizers now being used.

PERSEVERATION is the term for describing the senseless repetition of words or deeds by a person with a disordered mind.

PERSPIRATION, or SWEAT, is an excretion from the skin, produced by microscopic sweat-glands scattered over the surface. There are two different types of sweat-glands, known as eccrine and apocrine. Perspiration takes place constantly by evaporation from the openings of the sweat-glands, and this insensible perspiration amounts in twenty-four hours to considerably over a pint (570 ml). Under certain circumstances, as when the skin is heated or the person exerts himself, drops of sensible perspiration appear on the skin; to these the term sweat is generally confined, and the amount of sweat secreted may become very large: up to 3 litres an hour for short periods of time.

Sweat is a faintly acid, watery fluid containing less than 2 per cent of solids, made up mainly of salts and to a slight extent of fatty material, and including 0.3 per cent amount of urea (about the same concentration as in the blood), the substance which the kidneys excrete in large amount. When the action of the kidneys is defective, for example in Bright's disease, urea and other substances, which the kidneys normally excrete, pass out in increased amounts through the skin. This action of the skin is so marked that in a case of uraemia crystals of urea may be deposited on the surface as the sweat evaporates.

The eccrine sweat-glands in man (illustration 342) are situated in greatest numbers on the soles of the feet and palms of the hands, and with a magnifying glass their minute openings or pores can be seen in rows occupying the summit of each ridge in the skin. Perspiration is most abundant in these regions, though it also occurs all over the body. Different animals perspire in different regions; thus rabbits and rats do not sweat at all, oxen very little, pigs mostly on the snout, dogs and cats chiefly from the pads of the feet.

The chief object of perspiration is to regulate the amount of heat lost from the surface of the body and so maintain an even body temperature. Accordingly muscular activity, which sets free a great deal of heat, is the chief cause of sweating, and external heat is another. The process is regulated by nerves, some of which are the nerves controlling the size of the blood-vessels (vasomotor), and therefore the amount of blood in a part, whilst other nerves proceed to the sweat-glands (secretory) and directly influence secretion. These are presided over by centres in the spinal cord and medulla.

The apocrine sweat-glands are found in the armpits in association with the external genitalia and in the areola and nipple of the breast. (The glands that produce wax in the ear are modified apocrine glands.) They are developed in close association with hairs and their ducts often open into hair follicles. They do not start functioning until puberty. In animals they subserve a sexual function. It is the decomposition of apocrine sweat in the armpits by the bacteria of the skin that produces the characteristic smell of armpit sweat.

Abnormalities of perspiration – LESSENED sweating under certain conditions may occur, as in the early stages of fever, in diabetes, and in some forms of Bright's disease. Certain persons are peculiar in the fact of being unable to sweat copiously after muscular exertion, or when exposed to heat, and such persons are often seriously affected by exposure to a hot sun or

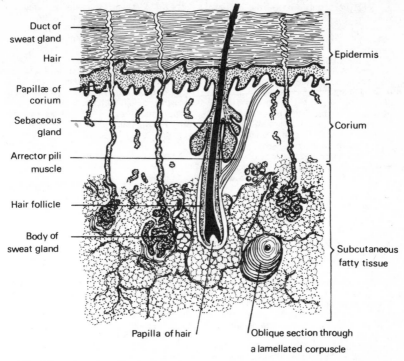

Duct of
sweat gland

Hair

Papillæ of
corium

Sebaceous
gland

Arrector pili
muscle

Hair follicle

Body of
sweat gland

Epidermis

Corium

Subcutaneous
fatty tissue

Papilla of hair

Oblique section through
a lamellated corpuscle

342 – Schematic vertical section of skin. From *Gray's Anatomy*, 35th edition, 1973. Longmans.

to the heat of an engine-room. (See HEAT-STROKE.)

EXCESSIVE sweating or HYPERIDROSIS, may take place in any feverish condition, tending to be particularly marked in rheumatic fever, and, above all, in advanced pulmonary tuberculosis, where the night-sweats are often copious enough to drench the patient's night-clothes and bedding. Such copious night-sweats also occur in certain cases of undulant fever. In a slighter degree, persons of feeble muscular power are apt to perspire very freely on exertion or when exposed to heat. It may also be due to hyperthyroidism, obesity, diabetes mellitus, or an anxiety state. Rickets is another disease in which children perspire copiously when asleep, and in this disease the sweating is mainly about the head. There is also a form of hyperidrosis, which may be localized or generalized, due to some disturbance of the nervous control of the sweat-glands. The troublesome form of excessive sweating in the armpits tends to run in families. Rare in children and the aged, it is usually induced or exacerbated by emotional stress.

OFFENSIVE perspiration, or BROMIDROSIS, is not uncommon. In rheumatic conditions the sweat has a peculiar, sour smell. Dyspeptics, too, are sometimes troubled by an unpleasant odour of the skin. But it is sweating of the feet or armpits that is most offensive of all, this condition being often due to decomposition of the skin secretions by bacteria.

COLOURED perspiration is a rare peculiarity, the sweat being tinged blue by indigo, or red by altered blood pigment.

Treatment – LESSENED perspiration is treated when necessary by various drugs known as diaphoretics (see DIAPHORETICS), and by hot-air baths (see BATHS; BRIGHT'S DISEASE).

EXCESSIVE sweating occurring in febrile diseases, eg. pulmonary tuberculosis, is diminished by treatment of the condition responsible for the fever. In conditions such as pulmonary tuberculosis, in which the sweating is liable to be prolonged and is

683

particularly irritating to the patient, sponging the skin with vinegar in water may be helpful. In other cases the administration of extract of belladonna by mouth may help.

Hyperidrosis, in which the perspiration is often offensive, is best treated by frequent baths. Regular shaving of the axillary, or armpit, hair is also helpful. If indigestion is present, this should also be treated. The feet, armpits, and other sources of perspiration should be washed daily with hexachlorophane, coal-tar, or other mildly antiseptic soap, carefully dried, and thereafter dusted with talcum powder or bathed with hydrogen peroxide. The stockings must be frequently changed. Shoes should be worn in preference to boots, so as to allow freer access of air to the feet, and for the same reason it is a good plan not to wear rubber soles. Sandals should be worn in hot weather. Sweating may also be considerably checked, if it is very copious, by rubbing the feet and armpits with liniment of belladonna or with spirit. Another useful plan in the case of excessive sweating of the feet is to soak the soles (not the entire foot) in 3 per cent formalin solution for five to ten minutes every night. There is also available a wide range of antiperspirant preparations, the active ingredient of which is often an aluminium salt. One of the most effective of these aluminium salts, is 25 per cent aluminium chloride hexahydrate in absolute alcohol, but this must only be used under medical supervision. In severe cases of localized excessive sweating, treatment by X-rays may be necessary and may give satisfactory results. Alternatively, in cases of excessive sweating in the armpits, which fails to respond to any other form of treatment, removal, by surgery or cryosurgery (qv) of a small area of skin (4 × 2·5 cm) at the dome of the armpit, where 70 to 80 per cent of the sweat-glands are present, may bring the condition under control.

PERTHES' DISEASE is an affection of the hip in children, due to fragmentation of the epiphysis (or spongy extremity) of the head of the femur. No active treatment is called for, as the condition settles spontaneously in a few years.

PERTUSSIS is another name for whooping-cough. (See WHOOPING-COUGH.)

PERUVIAN BARK is another name for cinchona bark, from which quinine is derived.

PES CAVUS is the technical name for claw-foot (qv).

PES PLANUS is the technical name for flat-foot (qv).

PESSARIES are either instruments designed to support a displaced womb, or solid bodies suitably shaped for insertion into the vagina, which are made of oil of theobromine or a glycerin basis and are used for applying local treatment to the vagina.

PEST is an old name for plague. (See PLAGUE.)

PETECHIAE are small spots on the skin, of red or purple colour, resembling flea-bites. They may be due to minute areas of inflammation, as in typhoid fever, or to small haemorrhages in the skin, as in purpura.

PETHIDINE HYDROCHLORIDE is a synthetic analgesic and antispasmodic drug, which is used in the treatment of painful and spasmodic conditions in place of morphine and atropine. It was at first thought that the drug would have an advantage over morphine in not encouraging addiction, but this has not proved to be the case.

PETIT MAL means the lesser type of epileptic seizure. (See EPILEPSY.)

PETRI DISHES are shallow, circular glass dishes, usually 4 inches (10 cm) in diameter, which are used in bacteriology laboratories for the growth of micro-organisms.

PETROLATUM is another name for soft paraffin. (See PARAFFIN.)

PEYER'S PATCHES are conglomerations of lymphoid nodules in the ileum, or lower part of the small intestine. They play an important part in the defence of the body against bacterial invasion, as in typhoid fever.

PHAGEDAENA means a process of ulceration of so severe a type that pieces of skin become gangrenous and slough off. It is due either to great weakness on the part of the person attacked, or to excessive virulence of the bacteria concerned.

PHAGOCYTOSIS is the name applied to a process by which the attacks of bacteria upon the living body are repelled and the bacteria destroyed through the activity of the white corpuscles of the blood.

The first observations upon this point were made by Metchnikoff in the case of the Daphnia or water-flea. This little animal, which exists in large numbers in pools of stagnant water, may often be observed to devour the large spores of a species of fungus. Metchnikoff observed that these spores, perforating the intestine of the Daphnia, found their way into its body cavity and there multiplied. They were, however, attacked at once by the white corpuscles circulating in the creature's vessels, which surrounded and took into their substance these spores, apparently in time digesting them, so that they broke down and disappeared. In some cases, however, he found that the spores developed quickly, the white corpuscles appeared to be sluggish in attacking them, and the creature died.

Similar observations have been made in the case of other bacteria in higher animals. The processes which precede phagocytosis – the slowing of the blood-stream in the part, collection of the white corpuscles on the walls of the vessels, their passage out of the vessels into the tissues (diapedesis), and their approach to the bacteria – are described under ABSCESS and INFLAMMATION. When bacteria are very virulent they seem to repel the white corpuscles instead of attracting them, and no phagocytosis takes place, but the bacteria develop unimpeded. (See OPSONINS.)

It should be stated that some hold that these white corpuscles do not devour and digest the living bacteria, but simply take up dead ones, just as they absorb particles of carbon, fragments of dead bone, and the like. These authorities suppose that the death of the bacteria is due to some chemical products formed by the body in response to the poisonous substances set free by the bacteria.

PHALANX is the name given to any one of the small bones of the fingers and toes. The phalanges are fourteen in number in each hand and foot, the thumb and great toe possessing only two each, whilst each of the other fingers and toes has three.

PHANTASY, or FANTASY, is the term applied to an imaginary appearance or day dream.

PHANTOM LIMB – Following the amputation of a limb it is usual for the patient to experience sensations as if the limb were still present. This condition is referred to as a phantom limb. In the vast majority of cases the sensation passes off in time.

PHARMACOLOGY is the part of medical science dealing with knowledge of the action of drugs.

PHARMACOPOEIA is an official publication dealing with the recognized drugs and giving their doses, preparations, sources, and tests. Most countries have a pharmacopoeia of their own. That for Great Britain and Ireland is prepared by the British Pharmacopoeia Commission under the direction of the Medicines Commission. Many hospitals and medical schools have a small pharmacopoeia of their own, giving the prescriptions most commonly dispensed in that particular hospital or school.

PHARMACY is the term applied to the art of preparing and compounding medicines, or to a place where this is carried out.

PHARYNGITIS is an inflammatory condition affecting the wall of the pharynx or throat proper. It may be due to infection, which may either be confined to the pharynx (the common 'sore throat') or may also involve the rest of the upper respiratory tract: ie. the nose and larynx. It may be associated with derangements of the digestive organs, or be caused by the irritation of highly spiced food or of constant spirit-drinking, or by excessive tobacco-smoking. On looking into the back of the throat, while the tongue is held down, one sees the mucous membrane unduly red and glazed, with enlarged lymph-follicles like sago-grains scattered over it. Small varicose veins are often seen here and there, and when these burst, the person may spit up blood, which he is apt to attribute wrongly to some disease in his lungs. It produces considerable irritation, cough, tickling in the throat, and discomfort, which may last long if not treated. Treatment consists in the use of gargles or sprays, whilst much relief may be obtained from the sucking of medicated pastilles or lozenges. In more acute cases a short course of penicillin or sulphonamides may be necessary. The diet should be bland, and the use of irritants such as smoking and highly spiced foods should be forbidden.

PHARYNX is another name for the throat. The term throat is popularly applied to the region about the front of the neck generally, but in its strict sense it means the irregular cavity into which the nose and mouth open above, from which the larynx and gullet open below, and in which the channel for the air and that for the food cross one another. It extends from the base of the skull down to the 6th cervical vertebra, separated from the upper six vertebrae only by some loose fibrous tissue, and is about 5 inches (12·5 cm) long (illustration 343).

343 – Vertical section through the middle of the head and neck. *a*, Is a heavy dotted line indicating the air passages; *f*, a lighter line shows the food passages. The two cross in the throat; *et*, Eustachian tube; *t*, tonsil; *to*, tongue; *g*, gullet; *l*, larynx; *w*, windpipe. For other letters, see illustration 89.

It is completely closed behind by a layer of muscles, and by mucous membrane, but in front it opens into the nose, mouth, and larynx in succession from above down. In its upper part, the Eustachian tubes open one on either side, and between them on the back wall grows a mass of glandular tissue known as the third tonsil, which, if enlarged, produces the condition known as adenoids. (See NOSE, DISEASES OF.) The muscles which close in the sides and back of the pharynx are three in number on each side, and spring, one from the jawbone, the second from the hyoid bone, the third from the side of the larynx, each of these constrictors spreading out like a fan

on the back of the pharynx. Two other small muscles run downwards on each side.

PHENACETIN is a white crystalline coal-tar product, at one time much used in fevers, influenza, headaches, and neuralgias of all kinds, on account of its power of reducing temperature and of deadening pain. As its regular use is not without danger, particularly to the kidneys, it is gradually being discarded, and in Britain is only now available on a doctor's prescription.

PHENAZOCINE is a powerful pain-reliever, or analgesic, which is said to be more potent, but less habit-forming, than morphine.

PHENAZONE, also known as ANTIPY-RIN, is an antipyretic and analgesic. Its indiscriminate use is not without danger.

PHENBENICILLIN (see PENICILLIN).

PHENELZINE is one of the widely used antidepressant drugs which are classified as monoamine oxidase inhibitors (qv).

PHENETHICILLIN (see PENICILLIN).

PHENETHYLDIGUANIDE is one of the oral hypoglycaemic agents. Unlike carbutamide (qv), chlorpropamide (qv) and tolbutamide (qv), it is not a sulphonamide derivative. Its action does not appear to depend upon the presence of insulin, as is the case with the sulphonamide derivatives. The reduction in blood sugar is effected by the process known as anaerobic glycolysis. (See also DIABETES MELLITUS.)

PHENINDIONE is a synthetic anti-coagulant (qv) which is effective by mouth, and is used for the same purpose as heparin. It is slower in action than heparin, the full anticoagulant effect not being obtained until 36 to 48 hours after the initial dose.

PHENMETRAZINE is a drug chemically related to ephedrine (qv) and amphetamine (qv), but has no effect on the heart and much less stimulant action on the central nervous system. For reasons that are not precisely known, it is a potent appetite-suppressant. Its use, however, is not without danger, and it is therefore only available now on a doctor's prescription, and is prescribed with increasing caution because of its addiction-forming propensities.

PHENOBARBITONE is the *British Pharmacopoeia* name for what is probably the most widely used of all the barbiturate group of drugs. It is given in doses of $\frac{1}{2}$ to 2 grains (30 to 125 mg). Phenobarbitone Sodium is a soluble preparation which can be given by injection.

PHENOL is another name for carbolic acid (qv).

PHENOLPHTHALEIN is a substance much used as an indicator of reaction in urine, and gastric juice, for example, being colourless in acid media, brilliant red with alkalis, and varying in tint according to the acid concentration. It is also given internally in 1 to 5 grain (60 to 300 mg) doses as an aperient.

Phenolsulphonephthalein is used to test the power of the kidneys, a measured quantity being injected intramuscularly or intravenously and the amount excreted in the urine during the next few hours carefully estimated by a colour scale. *Phenoltetrachlorphthalein* is a coal-tar derivative used as a diagnostic agent for the estimation of the functional power of the liver by intravenous injection.

PHENOXYMETHYLPENICILLIN (see PENICILLIN).

PHENSUXIMIDE is a succinamide derivative used in the treatment of *petit mal* and the psychomotor type of epilepsy.

PHENYLBUTAZONE has proved to be a useful drug for relieving the pain and discomfort in chronic rheumatic disorders such as rheumatoid arthritis, but it must only be used under medical supervision on account of the toxic effects which it sometimes produces.

PHENYLKETONURIA is one of the less common, but very severe, forms of mental deficiency. The incidence in populations of European origin is around 1 in 15,000 births. It is due to the inability of the baby to metabolize the amino-acid, phenylalamine. Its outstanding interest lies in the fact that, if it is diagnosed soon after birth – and this can be done by a simple urine test or by a test carried out on a drop of blood – and the infant is then given a diet low in phenylalamine, the chances are that the infant will grow up mentally normal. Parents of children with phenylketonuria can obtain help and information from the National Society for Phenylketonuria and Allied Diseases, 26 Towngate Grove, Mirfield, W. Yorks.

PHENYTOIN SODIUM is one of the most effective drugs for the treatment of epilepsy. One of its advantages is that it does not make the patient feel particularly sleepy. Its use is not without risk and it must therefore be used only under medical supervision.

PHEROMONES are chemicals produced and emitted by an individual which produce changes in the social or sexual behaviour when perceived by other individuals of the same species. The precise role of these odours, for it is by their smell that they are recognized, in man is still not clear, but there is growing evidence of the part they play in the animal kingdom. Thus if a strange male rat is put into a group of female rats, this may cause death of the foetus (qv), and this is attributed to the pheromones emitted by the male rat.

PHIMOSIS is the name applied to a condition of great narrowing at the edge of the foreskin, for which the operation of circumcision is necessary.

PHLEBITIS means inflammation of a vein. (See VEINS, DISEASES OF.)

PHLEBOGRAPHY is the study of the veins, particularly by means of X-rays after the veins have been injected with a radio-opaque substance.

PHLEBOLITH is the term applied to a small stone formed in a vein as a result of calcification of a thrombus.

PHLEBOTOMY is an old name for the operation of blood-letting by opening a vein. (See BLOOD-LETTING.)

PHLEGM is a popular name for mucus, particularly that secreted in the air passages. (See BRONCHITIS; EXPECTORANTS; MUCUS.)

PHLEGMASIA DOLENS is another name for white leg (qv).

PHLEGMON is an old term for inflammation.

PHLYCTENULE is a small inflammatory swelling situated on the conjunctiva or on the cornea in front of the eye. Phlyctenules are found especially in ill-nourished, weakly children, and cause a great deal of irritation, pain, running at the eyes, and inability to face the light. (See EYE, DISEASES OF.)

PHOLCODINE is the 3-(2-morpholinoethyl) ether of morphine. As it resembles codeine in suppressing cough, it is used for the relief of unproductive coughs.

PHONOCARDIOGRAPH is an instrument for the graphic recording of heart sounds and murmurs.

PHOSPHATES are salts of phosphoric acid, and, as this substance is contained in many articles of food as well as in bone, the nuclei of cells, and the nervous system, phosphates are constantly excreted in the urine. In certain diseased conditions, such as gout, the amount of phosphates excreted rises above the 2 to 3·5 grams daily excreted in health, but it is only in diseased conditions of the urinary passages that these give rise to trouble. The continued use of an excess of food containing alkalis, such as green vegetables, and still more the presence in the urine of bacteria which lead to its decomposition, produce the necessary change from the natural mild acidity to alkalinity, and lead to the deposit of phosphates and to their collection into stones.

PHOSPHATURIA means the presence in the urine of a large amount of phosphates.

PHOSPHORIC ACID, either as the dilute acid or in the form of phosphates, forms a constituent of many so-called 'tonics'. Phosphate of lime is used in cases of debility and especially of bone disease. Sodium phosphate and effervescent sodium phosphate are much used as mild aperients, and acid sodium phosphate is used in cases of cystitis.

PHOSPHORUS BURNS – If particles of phosphorus settle on or become embedded in the skin, the resulting burn should be treated with a 2 per cent sodium bicarbonate solution, followed by application of a 2 per cent solution of copper sulphate. Fats and oils should not be employed.

PHOSPHORUS POISONING is now rare, and is produced only by the yellow,

soluble form of phosphorus. Red phosphorus, from which safety matches are made, is harmless or nearly so. The main cause of acute phosphorus poisoning at the present moment is the swallowing of a rat poison containing phosphorus. When taken internally phosphorus acts first as an irritant poison, and, being thereafter absorbed, produces profound degenerative changes in the liver and other abdominal organs. There is also a chronic form of phosphorus poisoning, usually due to exposure to phosphorus fumes in chemical works. This consists of profound debility, and the occurrence of disease in the lower jaw-bone (phossy jaw), which necroses and comes away in large fragments, over a period of months or years. It is now believed by some authorities that this disease in the bone is due partly to infection occurring in the jaw as a result of toxic effects produced by the phosphorus.

Symptoms – When a child, for example, has taken a large dose he speedily suffers from pain, vomiting, colic, diarrhoea, and perhaps convulsions, and may die in a few hours. Or partial recovery may take place, and the sufferer survive for several days, later developing jaundice and blood-stained urine.

Treatment – As phosphorus is absorbed slowly, washing out the stomach may succeed in removing the poison up to two hours after it has been swallowed. Copper sulphate, $1\frac{1}{2}$ to 3 grains (100 to 200 mg) in water, may be given every ten minutes until vomiting occurs. Gastric lavage with a 1 in 5000 solution of potassium permanganate or with hydrogen peroxide solution may be tried instead. After emesis and gastric lavage two or four ounces (56 or 112 ml) of liquid paraffin and a big dose of a saline purge should be given. No oils, fats, or milk should be taken so long as any phosphorus remains in the gastrointestinal tract, for phosphorus is soluble in fats. If damage to the liver is threatened then treatment with sodium bicarbonate, glucose and insulin is indicated.

Chronic poisoning is prevented in chemical works dealing with phosphorus, by free ventilation, cleanliness, and periodic examination of the teeth of the match-workers.

PHOTOCOAGULATION is a method of producing controlled burns of the retina, usually using a zenon arc, but the laser ophthalmoscope can also be used for this purpose. It is proving of value in the treatment of the form of blindness, or impaired vision, known as diabetic retinopathy, as well as the treatment of retinal detachment. (See RETINA.)

PHOTODERMATOSIS, or PHOTO-DERMATITIS, is the term applied to an eruption on areas of the skin exposed to sunlight, caused by sensitivity to sunlight. In some cases the sensitivity is caused by certain drugs, cosmetics or chemicals.

PHOTOPHOBIA means a condition in which a person shrinks from letting bright light fall upon the eye. It is a symptom of inflammation of the eye, and occurs especially when the iris is inflamed.

PHOTOTHERAPY is treatment by means of light rays, the source of which is usually fluorescent light strips. Its main use is in the treatment of jaundice in the newborn infant.

PHRENIC NERVE is the nerve which chiefly supplies the diaphragm. It springs from the 3rd, 4th, and 5th cervical spinal nerves, and has a long course down the neck, and through the chest, where each nerve lies between the heart and corresponding lung, to the diaphragm. Phrenicectomy is an operation performed to divide this nerve in the neck. (For its object, see under TUBERCULOSIS.)

PHRENOLOGY is an old term applied to the study of the mind and character of individuals from the shape of the head. As the shape of the head has been shown to depend chiefly upon accidental characteristics, such as the size of the air spaces in the bones, and not upon development of special areas in the contained brain, this branch of science is now generally discredited.

PHTHALYLSULPHATHIAZOLE is a sulphonamide drug similar to succinyl-sulphathiazole (qv). Because of its slow absorption from the gut it is used as an intestinal antiseptic.

PHTHIRIASIS means the condition of eczema, matted hair, dirt, and enlarged glands caused by the crab louse (*Phthirus pubis*). (See PEDICULOSIS.)

PHTHISIS means wasting, and is the general term applied to that progressive enfeeblement and loss of weight that arise from tuberculous disease of all kinds, but especially from the disease as it affects the lungs. The term is also used, in a more limited sense, to designate that variety of tuberculous disease of the lungs in which rapid breaking down of the lung tissue takes place, with the formation of a cavity.

PHYLACOGEN (see VACCINES).

PHYSIOLOGY is the branch of medical science that deals with the healthy functions of different organs, and the changes that the whole body undergoes in the course of its activities.

PHYSIOTHERAPY is the form of treatment involving the use of physical measures, such as exercise, heat and massage in the treatment of disease. An alternative name is PHYSICAL MEDICINE.

PHYSOSTIGMINE, or ESERINE, is an alkaloid obtained from Calabar bean, the seed of *Physostigma venenosum*, a climbing plant of West Africa. Calabar bean is known also as the ordeal bean, because preparations derived from it were at one time used by the natives of West Africa to decide the guilt or innocence of accused persons, the guilty being supposed to succumb to its action, while the innocent escape. Its action depends on the presence of two alkaloids, the one known as physostigmine or eserine, the other as calabarine, the former of these being much the more important.

Action – Physostigmine produces the same effect as stimulation of the parasympathetic nervous system (qv): ie. it constricts the pupil, stimulates the gut, increases the secretion of saliva, stimulates the bladder, and increases the irritability of voluntary muscle. In poisonous doses it brings on a general paralysis.

Uses – It is used in medicine in the form of physostigmine salicylate. Its main use is to contract the pupil and thereby reduce the pressure inside the eyeball. For this purpose it is used as eye-drops or as lamellae. It is also given by subcutaneous injection to stimulate the gut when this is paralysed or atonic.

PHYTOMENADIONE is the *British Pharmacopoeia* name for vitamin K. (See VITAMIN.)

PIA MATER is the membrane closely investing the brain and spinal cord, in which run blood-vessels for the nourishment of these organs. (See BRAIN; SPINAL CORD.)

PICA is a term which means an abnormal craving for unusual foods. (See APPETITE.)

PICORNAVIRUSES derive their name from pico (small) and R N A (because they contain ribonuleic acid). They are a group of viruses which includes the enteroviruses (qv) and the rhinoviruses (qv).

PICRIC ACID, or TRINITROPHENOL, is used for preparing explosives, and so is employed in medicine only in solution. As it coagulates albumin, it produces a soothing pellicle over any raw surface with which it is brought into contact. It has antiseptic properties, but is rapidly going out of use because of its toxic effects.

PICROTOXIN is a bitter crystalline principle obtained from the fruit of *Anamirta cocculus*. By virtue of its stimulating action upon the respiratory centre, it is an antidote in poisoning from barbiturate drugs.

PIGEON BREAST (see CHEST DEFORMITIES).

PIGEON-BREEDER'S LUNG, or BIRD FANCIER'S LUNG as it is sometimes known, is a form of extrinsic allergic alveolitis resulting from sensitization to pigeons. In pigeon fanciers skin tests have revealed sensitization to pigeons' droppings, eggs, protein and serum, even though there has been no evidence of any illness. (See ALVEOLITIS.)

PIGMENT is the term applied to the colouring matter of various secretions, blood, etc.; also to any medicinal preparation of thick consistence intended for painting on the skin or mucous membranes.

PILES, or HAEMORRHOIDS, consist of a varicose and often inflamed condition of the veins about the lower end of the bowel, known as the haemorrhoidal veins.

Varieties – It is usual to divide haemorrhoids into external piles, internal piles, and mixed piles. To understand this division, it is important to remember that at the margin of the anus the skin joins the mucous membrane of the bowel in a sharp line, and that the bowel is kept closed by two circular muscles, the external sphincter and internal sphincter. The external sphincter is a weak muscle situated immediately beneath the skin, while the internal sphincter is a stronger circular band, extending up the bowel for an inch. External piles are found outside the bowel, and are covered by skin, being brown or dusky purple in colour; internal piles are within the opening, covered by mucous membrane, and are bright red or cherry-coloured. Mixed piles are those situated just on the margin, and covered half by skin, half by mucous membrane. Even internal piles do not extend more than an inch up the bowel, corresponding to the position of the internal sphincter muscle.

Causes – There is always a tendency for the veins in this situation to become distended, partly because they are unprovided with valves, partly because they form the lowest part of the portal system and are very apt to become overfilled when there is the least interference with the circulation through the portal vein, and partly because the muscular arrangements for keeping the rectum closed interfere with the circulation through the haemorrhoidal veins. Probably most people of middle life are troubled by this condition to some extent, especially men of sedentary habits who indulge in over-eating and are troubled by constipation, as well as women who have borne many children. Habitual constipation is perhaps the principal cause of the presence of piles, and sitting on a cold stone or damp seat, or even a general chill, may suffice from time to time to irritate them and bring on what is popularly known as an 'attack of piles'.

It must be remembered, however, that in a certain number of cases piles are merely a symptom of disease higher up on the portal system, causing interference with the circulation. They often come on during pregnancy, passing off when this condition has terminated. They are common in heart disease, liver complaints, such as cirrhosis or congestion, and any disease affecting the bowels.

Symptoms – EXTERNAL PILES may be present for years and give no trouble whatever, beyond occasioning pain of a cutting or burning character now and then when a very costive motion is passed. When, in consequence of a chill or other cause, they become inflamed, they are very painful and tender from chafing against the thighs and clothing in walking, and from pressure upon the chair on which the person sits. The pile, or piles, in these circumstances become enlarged and red, and give off a thin blood-stained discharge. They may become so badly inflamed as to suppurate, and this sometimes results in a natural cure, or they may cure by filling with blood-clot and shrivelling up into hard little knots. Such an 'attack of piles' lasts generally a week or two, and then subsides till another chill is caught.

INTERNAL PILES may be slight, and may give no sign of their presence beyond occasional bleeding, which may vary from a mere streak, when the bowels are opened, to a discharge of several ounces of dark blood. They are apt to produce a constant discharge of mucus tinged with blood which soils the linen, but unless very severe are not, as a rule, painful. These discharges of blood may, when copious and frequent, cause anaemia and become a serious menace to the health, though they are never fatal. On the other hand, in plethoric, overfed people, they may be a salutary thing, warding off apoplexy, or relieving the heart when it is failing. When internal piles are large they may come down with the movement of the bowels, and may then become inflamed and painful from time to time, just like external piles.

Treatment – Constipation must, in the first place, be guarded against. While the use of violent and irritating purgatives, like aloes, should be avoided, care must be taken, by regulation of the diet and other means, to secure soft motions. (See CONSTIPATION.) The diet should include plenty of fruit, vegetables, and butter, and should in all cases be of a simple nature. Alcoholic beverages tend to produce and perpetuate piles, and should therefore in bad cases be entirely abandoned. Regular exercise is necessary in order to carry off the blood to the limbs and so relieve the portal circulation.

Locally, great care must be taken not to irritate the piles, and when they are inflamed they should be washed with water and cotton-wool every time the bowels move. Bleeding and the tendency to inflammation may be controlled by applying a sponge full of very hot water, or by smearing on cocaine or adrenaline ointment after the motion. In the case of internal piles which come down at stool it is very important that they should be returned within the bowel each time by gentle steady pressure with the fingers. If they are down and inflamed, a hot bath followed by a cocaine and morphine suppository gives relief.

Often these means suffice to keep the piles from causing trouble or to cure them completely, but occasionally surgical means are had recourse to. The external piles are simply removed. Internal piles require, according to their size and position, to be ligatured, destroyed by clamp and cautery, or, when they extend all round the bowel, to be removed *en masse* along with the last inch of mucous membrane lining the bowel. In many cases, however, the most satisfactory treatment of internal piles consists of injecting them with a 5 per cent solution of phenol in arachis oil, to which 0·5 per cent of menthol has been added, or some other comparable solution. Alternative non-surgical methods of treatment that are now being advocated are ligation of the piles with rubber bands, cryosurgery (qv), and manual dilatation of the anus.

PILLS are small round masses containing active drugs held together by syrup, gum, glycerin, or adhesive vegetable extracts. They are sometimes without coating, being merely rolled in French chalk, but often they are covered with sugar, gelatin, or gilt. Some pills, designed to act upon the bowels only, are coated with keratin, salol or other substances which are insoluble in the gastric juice.

PILOCARPINE is an alkaloid derived from the leaves of *Pilocarpus microphyllus* (jaborandi). It produces the same effects as stimulation of the parasympathetic nervous system: ie. it has exactly the opposite effect to atropine (qv), but cannot be used in the treatment of atropine poisoning as it does not antagonize the action of poisonous doses of atropine on the brain. Its main use today is in the form of eye-drops to decrease the pressure inside the eyeball in glaucoma (qv).

PIMENTO, or ALLSPICE, is the dried fruit of *Pimenta officinalis*, a Central American shrub, from which oil of pimento, a volatile oil, is obtained. It is used in the form of aqua pimentae, or water of allspice, in doses of a tablespoonful or more in cases of colic, and to make up various medicines.

PIMPLES, technically known as papules, are small, raised, and inflamed areas on the skin. On the face the most common cause is acne (qv). Boils (qv) start as hard pimples. The eruption of smallpox and that of chickenpox begin also with pimples. (See also SKIN DISEASES.)

PINE OIL is a nearly colourless oil with aromatic odour, distilled from the fresh needles of *Pinus silvestris*, the Scotch fir. Its action is similar to that of turpentine, and it is mainly used as an inhalation, prepared by adding a few drops to hot water.

PINEAL BODY is a small reddish structure, 10 mm in length and shaped somewhat like a pine cone (hence its name), situated on the upper part of the mid-brain. Many theories have been expounded as to its function, but there is increasing evidence that, in some animals at least it is affected by light and plays a part in hibernation and in controlling sexual activity and the colour of the skin. This it seems to do by means of a substance it produces known as melantonin. A body resembling an imperfect third eye is found in its position in some of the lower vertebrate animals, as, for example, in the lizard, Hatteria.

PINK DISEASE (see ERYTHROEDEMA).

PINK-EYE is the name given to an acute muco-purulent conjunctivitis caused by various germs and highly contagious from such things as towels. (See EYE DISEASES.)

PINS AND NEEDLES is a form of paraesthesia (qv), or disturbed sensation, such as may occur, for example, in neuritis (qv) or polyneuritis (qv).

PINT is a measure of quantity containing 16 fluid ounces (wine measure) or 20 fluid ounces (Imperial measure). The metric equivalent is 568 millilitres. (See WEIGHTS AND MEASURES.)

PIPERAZINE is a substance which was credited with the power of dissolving uric acid. It was therefore widely used at one time for the treatment of gout and of uratic stones in the kidneys and bladder, but there is no evidence that it is capable of dissolving uric acid in the body. It has recently come back into use, however, for the treatment of threadworms and ascariasis. (See ENTEROBIASIS; ASCARIASIS.)

PIRQUET'S REACTION is a test for tuberculosis. A solution of old tuberculin is gently rubbed into a patch of scarified skin on the arm. The subsequent appearance of a raised reddened papule (positive test) shows that the person tested has been infected by the *Mycobacterium tuberculosis* but not necessarily that he has active tuberculosis. (See TUBERCULIN.)

PITHIATISM is a name applied to a group of disorders in which the patient is subject to cure by persuasion or suggestion, the term being used as an equivalent for hysteria. (See HYSTERIA.)

PITUITARY BODY, also known as the PITUITARY GLAND and the HYPOPHYSIS, is an ovoid structure, weighing around 0·5 gram in the adult, attached to the base of the brain, and lying in the depression in the base of the skull known as the sella turcica on account of its resemblance to a Turkish saddle. It consists of an anterior and a posterior section divided by a clear line of cleavage. For long these two parts were known, respectively, as the anterior and the posterior lobes of the pituitary body, and the part of the gland that connected it to the brain was known as the stalk or infundibulum. This, however, was too simple a classification to be accurate, as was realized once information concerning the multifarious functions of the gland began to accumulate. It was therefore decided to divide it up according to its origin. The reason for this is that the pituitary has a double origin. The anterior part is derived in the embryo from the ectoderm (see FOETUS) of the primitive mouth, and this part of the gland is now known as the adenohypophysis. The posterior part is derived from the brain and is now known as the neurohypophysis. The gland is connected to the hypothalamus (qv) of the brain by a stalk known as the hypophyseal or pituitary stalk. The confusing thing about this new 'classification' of the pituitary is that it involves a certain amount of overlapping with the old classification. Thus, the adenohypophysis is made up of the anterior lobe which, in turn, is subdivided into a pars distalis and a pars tuberalis, and the pars intermedia of the posterior lobe. The neurohypophysis is also made up of three parts: the infundibular process (or neural lobe) of the posterior lobe, the nervous part of the stalk known as the infundibular or neural stalk, and the median eminence of the tuber cinereum.

The pars distalis, which accounts for the greater part of the gland, is composed of masses of cells which fall into three main groups: (1) chromophobe cells which do not stain and constitute about 50 per cent of the total; (2) acidophil cells which stain with acid dyes and constitute about 35 per cent of the total; and (3) basophil cells which stain with basic stains and constitute about 15 per cent of the total. The pars intermedia consists only of a few cells, whilst the pars tuberalis contains nongranular cells. The neurohypophysis is composed of nerve fibres and brown granular cells known as pituicytes.

The pituitary gland is the most important ductless, or endocrine, gland in the body. (See ENDOCRINE GLANDS.) It has been described as the master gland of the endocrine system, or the conductor of the endocrine orchestra. This over-all control it exerts through the media of a series of hormones which it produces. The adenohypophysis is the major producer of these, and those it produces will be dealt with first. Those which function through the media of other endocrine glands are known as trophic hormones and have therefore been given names ending with 'trophic' or 'trophin'. The thyrotrophic hormone, or thyroid stimulating hormone (abbreviated to TSH) as it is also known, exerts a powerful influence over the activity of the thyroid gland. The adrenocorticotrophic hormone, also known as corticotrophin (ACTH), stimulates the cortex of the adrenal glands. The growth, or somatotrophic, hormone, also known as somatotrophin (SMH), controls the growth of the body. There are also two gonadotrophic hormones which play a vital part in the control of the gonads: these are the follicle stimulating hormone (FSH), and the luteinizing hormone (LH) which is also known as the interstitial cell stimulating hormone (ICSH). (See GONADOTROPHINS.) The lactogenic hormone, also known as prolactin, mammotrophin and luteotrophin, induces lactation. The neurohypophysis produces two hormones. One is oxytocin which is widely used because of its stimulating effect on contraction of the uterus. The other is vasopressin, or the antidiuretic hormone (ADH), which acts on the renal tubules and the collecting tubules (see KIDNEYS) to increase the amount of water that they normally absorb.

Gigantism is the result of the overactivity of, or tumour formation of, the acidophil cells in the adenohypophysis which produce the growth hormone. If this over-activity occurs after growth has ceased a condition known as acromegaly (qv) arises, in which there is gross overgrowth of the ears, nose, jaws, and hands and feet. Dwarfism may be due to lack of the growth hormone. Diabetes insipidus (qv), a condition characterized by the passing of a large volume of urine every day, is due to lack of the antidiuretic hormone. Various other disorders are the result of disturbed pituitary function, such as: premature senility, extreme wasting, development of painful growths of fat, and various disturbances of growth and sexual development.

PITYRIASIS ROSEA is a skin eruption of unknown origin that occurs in young people. It starts characteristically with an oval, slightly red and scaly area – known as the herald patch – between the shoulder blades or on the lower abdomen. Three or four days later the eruption spreads all over the trunk. It consists of pink papules (qv) and oval brownish macules (qv), which tend to itch considerably. It usually lasts about six weeks, and does not usually recur. No specific treatment is called for. Hot baths should be avoided as they tend to accentuate the itching. If this is unpleasant, it can be relieved with calamine lotion to which 1 per cent phenol has been added.

PIVMECILLINAM is a derivative of the antibiotic, mecillinam (qv). It differs from the latter in being active when taken by mouth. (See PENICILLIN.)

PIX is another name for tar.

PLACEBO is the term used to describe a medicine (or pill) given to a patient, not because it will have any definite action but because the patient will not be satisfied unless he (or she) receives some active treatment.

PLACENTA is the technical name for the afterbirth. (See AFTERBIRTH.)

PLACENTOGRAPHY is the procedure of rendering the placenta, or afterbirth (qv), visible by means of X-rays. This can be done either by using what is known as soft-tissue radiography, or by injecting a radio-opaque substance into the bloodstream or into the amniotic cavity. (See AMNION.) The procedure is not without danger to both mother and foetus, and must therefore only be carried out under expert supervision but it is sometimes of value in assessing the cause of antepartum haemorrhage.

PLAGUE, or BUBONIC PLAGUE, is the name of an infectious epidemic disease common to man and many of the lower animals. Its main characters are fever, swelling of the lymphatic glands, a rapid course, and a very high mortality, which has made it a much-dreaded scourge. In the Middle Ages it was known as the BLACK DEATH, which again and again ravaged Europe, though for the past century it has been almost confined to warm climates. The ancients referred to a disease which they called 'pestis', a term which possibly included several severe epidemic maladies; but, according to Hirsch, there is a recognizable description of an epidemic of what we know as plague infesting Libya, Egypt, and Syria between the second and third centuries BC. The first occurrence of the disease in Europe was the plague of Justinian, which swept through the Roman Empire in AD 542, devastating cities and country as it spread. Subsequently it periodically invaded Europe from the east, and spread westward, though with lessening severity in successive epidemics. The last occasion on which England was seriously invaded was at the time of the Great Plague in 1664–65, when 70,000 people died in London out of the total population of 460,000. In Glasgow a small outbreak occurred in 1900, which was quickly suppressed. The disease had not invaded America till 1899–1900, when it broke out in Brazil, the Argentine Republic, San Francisco, and Mexico. At the present day 1000 to 6000 cases occur annually, with 100 to 200 deaths.

Causes – The disease is probably always present (endemic) in certain localities. such as in the south-west of China, among the hill people of India, and in East Africa. From these areas it spreads outwards at intervals, sometimes creeping from village to village, at other times being disseminated widely along trade-routes. The bacillus (*Yersinia pestis*) which is the immediate cause was discovered independently by Kitasato and Yersin in 1894. (See BACTERIOLOGY.) It is found in the enlarged lymphatic glands, and the sputum in pneumonic cases, as well as in the blood of septicaemic cases.

Plague occurs first as an epizoötic (qv) in rats: especially in the black rat, *Rattus rattus*. The infection is then conveyed to man by the rat flea, especially *Xenopsylla cheopis*. The plague bacilli multiply in the gastro-intestinal tract of the flea, which may remain infectious for as long as six weeks. In pneumonic plague the bacillus may pass from man to man as a droplet infection.

The rat is not the only rodent which serves as a reservoir for *Yersinia pestis*. In the Caucasus, Siberia, and Manchuria the marmot is an important reservoir, whilst in Argentina it has been found in wild guinea-pigs. In the USA between the Rocky Mountains and the west coast plague is widespread among ground squirrels, wood rats, and prairie dogs. Between 1900 and 1951 rodent plague had spread through fifteen of the western states of the USA. This carries with it the risk of starting plague in any city with a large rat population. In South Africa, too, plague is prevalent in rodents, and human cases have cropped up from time to time. In England the last outbreak was in Suffolk in 1910.

Symptoms – A graphic description of the symptoms of the disease is given by Defoe in his *Story of the Great Plague*, through which he lived as a child in London in 1664–65.

After infection, an incubation period, varying from two to six days for bubonic plague, and three to four days for pneumonic plague, elapses, and then the disease sets in suddenly with fever, headache, great lassitude, and aching of the limbs. The temperature soon rises to 103° F (39·5° C) or more, the skin is hot and dry, the tongue furred, while thirst, prostration, and a feeling of utter weakness assail the sufferer. His features become drawn, his eyes sunken, and he sinks into a state of stupor or passes sometimes into wild delirium. There is often also sickness and vomiting.

In over two-thirds of all cases there are swollen glands, known as buboes, from which the malady has received the name of *bubonic plague*. These are situated most commonly in the groins, less often in the armpits, and give sometimes the first sign that the person has contracted the plague. There are also haemorrhages under the skin in many cases, which sometimes produce black gangrenous patches that lead to large ulcers, and hence the old name of black death. In favourable cases the fever abates at about the end of a week, the strength gradually returns, and the buboes soften, burst, and discharge foul-smelling pus.

There is a rapidly fatal form, associated with great weakness, in which the bacteria enter the blood, and the person dies on the second or third day, sometimes even in a few hours, before the buboes have time to form (*septicaemic plague*).

In other cases the lungs especially become affected, and pneumonia comes on, with death on the fourth or fifth day. This is said to be both the most infectious and the most fatal form of the disease (*pneumonic plague*).

In all epidemics, especially at the beginning and end of the epidemic, mild cases occur, in which the persons continue to go about, the buboes being almost the only sign of the malady. The matter from the buboes of such slight cases is, nevertheless, infectious, and these cases are therefore specially dangerous to other people.

The death-rate in untreated cases varies in different epidemics from 25 to 50 per cent. Untreated septicaemic plague and pneumonic plague is usually fatal, but modern treatment has reduced the fatality considerably, even in pneumonic plague.

Treatment – Preventive treatment is all-important in this disease. Plague is one of the six internationally quarantineable diseases, the others being cholera, louse-borne relapsing fever, smallpox, louse-borne typhus, and yellow fever. Contacts of plague are quarantined for six days. The strictest quarantine is apt to be ineffective, and measures directed against the spread of plague are essential. This includes the disinfestation of all contacts with insecticide powder. such as 5 to 10 per cent DDT powder. Clothes, skins, any soft merchandise which have been in contact with the plague-stricken preserve the bacilli, and consequently their infectiousness, for several months. Such articles must therefore be either destroyed or disinfected with DDT. Houses or huts in which plague has occurred should either be carefully disinfected with DDT or, if valueless, burned to the ground. The inhabitants of a plague-infected village or district are not allowed to migrate, carrying infection with them, to other localities, but all who have been in contact with a plague-stricken person should be isolated as contacts or suspects in special houses or camps and dusted with DDT.

In time of plague, or when plague is approaching, a war of extermination should be waged against rats and other rodents which are responsible for spreading the disease, and the bodies should also be carefully examined. Various devices are adopted against the rats on ships. Thus the ships are generally moored a little way distant from the quay, the hawsers are rendered 'rat-proof' by slipping hollow metal cones round them, and sulphurous acid gas or hydrocyanic acid is pumped into the holds under closed hatches to kill vermin which may be among the merchandise.

Personal protection is gained by good feeding, and by living in bright, well-ventilated rooms or out of doors. The wearing of high boots and special clothing impervious to fleas is important for those who go into the neighbourhood of plague cases. The use of antiseptics for the hands and of disinfectant mouth-washes is important for those nursing the plague-stricken, and special precautions must be taken to seal up any small wounds on the hands, and so guard against inoculation.

Vaccination affords partial protection for six months, and is used in the control of local outbreaks of plague. The administration of the sulphonamides, sulphadiazine, sulphamerizine, or sulphadiamine, is recommended for the protection of those who have been exposed, particularly to pneumonic plague.

In the treatment of the disease the best results are obtained from streptomycin or one of the broad-spectrum antibiotics.

PLASMA is the name applied to the fluid portion of the blood composed of serum and fibrinogen, the material which produces clotting. When the plasma is clotted, the thinner fluid separating from the clot is the serum.

PLASMA TRANSFUSION is sometimes used instead of blood transfusion. Plasma, the fluid part of blood from which the cells have been separated, may be dried and in powder form kept almost indefinitely; when wanted it is reconstituted by adding sterile distilled water. In powder form it can be transported easily and over long distances. Transfusion of plasma is especially useful in the treatment of shock. One advantage of plasma transfusion is that it is not necessary to carry out testing of blood groups before using it.

PLASMODIUM is the general term applied to minute protoplasmic cells, and particularly to those which cause malaria and allied diseases. (See MALARIA.)

PLASMON is a term applied to a flour-like food consisting of the protein materials of milk.

PLASTER OF PARIS is a form of calcium sulphate, which, after soaking in water, sets firmly. For this reason it is widely used as a form of splinting in the treatment of fractures. It is used for this purpose in the form of bandages which consist of bleached cotton cloth impregnated with the plaster and suitably adhesive. Its great advantage, compared with an ordinary splint, is that it can be moulded to the shape of the limb.

PLASTERS (see ADHESIVE PLASTERS).

PLASTIC SURGERY is that branch of surgery which is concerned with the reformation and restoration of parts of the body which are damaged, lost, or deformed.

PLASTRON is the term applied to the skeleton on the front of the chest consisting of the breast bone and attached rib cartilages.

PLATELETS – Blood platelets, or thrombocytes, are small spherical bodies in the blood, which play an important part in the process of blood coagulation. Normally, there are around 300,000 per cubic millimetre of blood.

PLATING is a term used in connection with bacteriological investigation to mean the cultivation of bacteria on flat plates containing nutrient material. The term is also applied in surgery to the method of securing union of fractured bones by screwing to the sides of the fragments narrow metal plates, which hold them firmly together while union is taking place.

PLEOPTICS, which literally means full sight, is a form of treatment of an eye which has become amblyopic (see AMBLYOPIA) due to a squint.

PLETHORA means a condition of fullness of the blood-vessels in a particular part or in the whole body. Persons who consume much more food and drink than that necessary for the work they do, and who tend to the development of gout, apoplexy, and other diseases of allied nature, are commonly classed as plethoric. The term is applied to a condition in which the volume of the blood is increased above normal; there may or may not be an increase in the total number of red blood corpuscles.

PLETHYSMOGRAPH is an apparatus for estimating changes in the size of any part placed in the apparatus; in this way changes in the volume of blood in a part can be measured.

PLEURA, or PLEURAL MEMBRANE, is the name of the membrane which, on either side of the chest, forms a covering for one lung. The two pleurae are distinct, though they touch one another for a short distance behind the breast-bone. (See LUNGS.)

PLEURISY, or PLEURITIS, means inflammation of the pleura or serous membrane investing the lung and lining the inner surface of the ribs. It is a common

condition, and may be either acute or chronic, the latter being usually tuberculous in origin.

The changes which take place are as follows. (1) Inflammatory congestion and infiltration of the pleura, which may spread to the tissues of the lung on the one hand, and to those of the chest wall on the other. (2) Exudation of fibrin on the pleural surfaces. This exudation is of variable consistence, sometimes composed of thin and easily separated pellicles, or showing itself in the form of a membrane. It is of greyish-yellow colour, and, microscopically, consists mainly of coagulated fibrin along with epithelial cells and red and white blood corpuscles. Its presence causes roughening of the two pleural surfaces by material which may later break up or may become organized by the development of new blood-vessels and formation of fibrous tissue. This, by forming permanent adhesions, may obliterate the pleural sac throughout a greater or less space, and interfere to some extent with the free play of the lungs. (3) Effusion of fluid into the pleural cavity. This fluid may vary in its characters. Most commonly it is clear or slightly turbid, of yellowish-green colour, sero-fibrinous, and containing flocculi of fibrin. In cases in which the pleurisy complicates some severe form of disease, eg. the acute infectious maladies, it is deeply coloured, bile-stained, sero-purulent, purulent, or bloody, occasionally containing bubbles of air from decomposition. The amount may vary from an almost inappreciable quantity to a gallon (4·5 litres) or more. When large in quantity, it may fill the pleural sac to distension, bulge out the thoracic wall externally, and compress more or less completely the lung, which may in such cases have all its air displaced and be reduced to a mere fraction of its natural bulk lying squeezed up upon its own root. Other organs, such as the heart and liver, may in consequence of the presence of the fluid be shifted away from their normal position. In favourable cases the fluid is absorbed more or less completely and the pleural surfaces may unite by adhesions; or, all traces of inflammatory products having disappeared, the pleura may be restored to its normal condition. When the fluid is not speedily absorbed, it may remain long in the cavity and compress the lung to such a degree as to render it incapable of re-expansion as the effusion passes slowly away. The consequence is that the chest wall falls in, the ribs become approximated, the shoulder is lowered, the spine becomes curved and internal organs permanently displaced, while the affected side scarcely moves in respiration. Sometimes the unabsorbed fluid becomes purulent, and an *empyema* is the result. In such a case the matter seeks outlet in some direction, and it may point as an abscess upon the chest or abdominal wall, or, on the other hand, burst into the lung and be discharged by the mouth, if it is not evacuated by surgical means.

Many cases of pleurisy are associated with only a little effusion, the inflammation consisting chiefly in exudation of fibrin. To this form the term *dry pleurisy* is applied. Further, pleurisy may be limited to a very small area, or, on the contrary, may affect, throughout a greater or less extent, the pleural surfaces of both lungs.

Causes – Pleurisy is often associated with other forms of inflammatory disease within the chest, more particularly pneumonia, bronchiectasis, and tuberculosis, and also occasionally accompanies pericarditis. It may also be due to carcinoma of the lung, or be secondary to abdominal infections such as subphrenic abscess. Further, wounds or injuries of the thoracic walls are apt to set up pleurisy. The connection of pleurisy with tuberculosis is important. Sometimes it happens that an attack of pleurisy, which apparently has passed off, returns and is eventually followed by tuberculosis, it may be after several years.

Symptoms – The symptoms of pleurisy vary, being generally well marked, but sometimes obscure.

DRY PLEURISY – In the case of dry pleurisy, which is, on the whole, the milder form, the chief symptom is a sharp pain in the side, felt especially on breathing. Fever may or may not be present. There is a slight, dry cough, which the individual does his best to suppress because of the pain which it causes. The breathing is quicker than normal and shallow. Should a deep breath be taken, it ends with a characteristic catch, due to the pain which it causes. If much pain is present, the body leans somewhat to the affected side, to relax the tension on the intercostal muscles and their covering, which are even tender to touch. On listening to the chest with the stethoscope the physician recognizes sooner or later friction, a superficial rough rubbing sound, occurring only with respiration and ceasing when the breath is held. It is due to the coming together during respiration of the two pleural surfaces which are roughened by the exuded fibrin. The patient may himself be aware

of this rubbing sensation, and its vibration or fremitus may be felt by the hand laid upon the thoracic wall during breathing. This form of pleurisy may be limited or may extend over the greater part of one or both sides. It is a frequent complication of pulmonary tuberculosis. In general it disappears in a short time, and complete recovery takes place; or, on the other hand, extensive adhesions may form between the surfaces of the pleura covering the ribs and the lung, preventing uniform expansion of the lung in respiration, and leading to emphysema. Although not of itself attended with danger, dry pleurisy must always be treated as a serious condition, as it may be accompanied by disease in the underlying lung.

PLEURISY WITH EFFUSION is usually more severe than dry pleurisy, and, although it may in some cases develop insidiously, it is in general ushered in sharply by shivering and fever, like other acute inflammatory diseases. Pain is felt in the side or breast, of a severe cutting or stabbing character, referred usually to the neighbourhood of the nipple, but it may be also at some distance from the affected part, such as through the middle of the body or in the abdominal or iliac regions. This transference of the pain occasionally leads to errors in diagnosis, the patient being supposed to be the subject of appendicitis, gastric ulcer, or some other serious abdominal condition. The pain is greatest at the outset, and tends to abate as the effusion takes place. A dry cough is almost always present, which is particularly distressing, owing to the increased pain the effort excites. The breathing is painful and difficult, tending to become shorter and shallower as the disease advances, and the lung on the affected side becomes compressed. The patient at first lies most easily on the sound side, but as the effusion increases he finds his most comfortable position on his back or on the affected side. When there is very copious effusion and, as is apt to happen, great congestion of the other lung, or disease affecting it, the patient's breathing may be so embarrassed that he cannot lie down.

In most instances the termination is favourable, the acute symptoms subsiding, and the fluid (if not drawn off) gradually or rapidly becoming absorbed, sometimes after re-accumulation. On the other hand, it may remain long without undergoing much change, and thus a condition of *chronic pleurisy* becomes established. Such cases are to be viewed with suspicion, particularly in those who are predisposed to tuberculosis, of which it is sometimes the precursor.

Pleurisy may exist in a *latent form*, the patient going about for weeks with a large accumulation of fluid in his thorax, the ordinary acute symptoms never having been present in any marked degree. In some cases the pleurisy is on the under surface of the lung. This condition, known as *diaphragmatic pleurisy*, gives few signs on examination and is liable, when the symptoms are severe, to be mistaken for some acute inflammation of the abdomen.

The chief dangers in pleurisy are the occurrence of a large and rapid effusion, particularly if both sides be affected, causing much embarrassment to the breathing, and tendency to collapse; the formation of an *empyema* (often marked by recurring rigors and hectic symptoms); severe collateral congestion of the other lung; imperfect recovery, and the supervention of tuberculosis.

Acute pleurisy is often merely an accompaniment of the severer condition of lobar pneumonia, the disease really being a *pleuro-pneumonia*.

Treatment – The treatment varies greatly with the form and severity of the attack. If it is tuberculous in origin, a full course of chemotherapy is given as for pulmonary tuberculosis. (See TUBERCULOSIS.) Should it be associated with an underlying infection of the lung, such as pneumonia, the appropriate antibiotics are given.

So far as the treatment of the pleurisy itself is concerned, in the early inflammatory stage, one of the chief symptoms calling for treatment is the pain, which may be soothed by opiates in the form of morphine or Dover's powder, along with the application to the chest of heat in the form of hot poultices, fomentations or a rubber hot water bottle. Instead of these, an ice-bag may be applied to the side, and this has the effect of almost immediately soothing the acute pain. Another plan consists in the fixing, as far as possible, of one side of the chest by means of overlapping cross strips of adhesive plaster. Cases of simple dry pleurisy usually soon yield to such treatment.

In the case of pleurisy with effusion, in addition to these measures, aspiration of the fluid may be required. (See ASPIRATION.) All the more necessary does the operation become if the accumulated fluid is interfering with the function of other organs, such as the heart, or is attended with marked embarrassment of the breathing. The chest is punctured in the lateral or posterior regions, and most

physicians prefer to draw off not more than 30 ounces (850 ml) or thereabout at one time and to repeat the operation if necessary. In general, the operation is unattended with danger, although not entirely exempt from such risks as sudden fainting. In many instances, not only is the removal of distressing symptoms speedy and complete, but the lung is relieved from pressure in time to enable it to resume its normal expansion. When there is any evidence that the fluid is purulent, the operation should be performed early. In such cases it is sometimes necessary to establish for a time a drainage of the pleural cavity by introducing a drainage tube through an opening in the lower part of the side, a portion of a rib being usually removed to admit the tube. The pleural cavity is then irrigated through the opening at regular intervals, and treated exactly as any other large abscess cavity. (See EMPYEMA.)

The convalescence from pleurisy requires care, and the expansion of the lung may be assisted by suitable breathing exercises (see CHEST DEVELOPMENT), or by connecting two wash-bottles in such a way that a quantity of fluid can be blown over from one to the other repeatedly. The latter exercise is graduated by blowing the fluid from one bottle to the other an increasing number of times on each successive day.

After an attack of pleurisy, and particularly after a second attack, the person should submit himself from time to time to medical examination, in order to make sure that tuberculosis does not develop in the lung. He will thus be enabled, if this serious disease should show itself, to start its treatment at an early stage, when a cure may be expected.

PLEURODYNIA means a painful condition of the chest-wall. It may be due to rheumatism of the intercostal muscles or to neuralgia of the intercostal nerves, or, when of the sharp nature popularly known as a 'stitch in the side', to cramp.

PLEURO-PNEUMONIA means a combination of pleurisy with pneumonia. Acute pneumonia is practically always accompanied by a certain amount of pleurisy, to which the pain experienced in pneumonia is mainly due. The epidemic disease known as pleuro-pneumonia, which is so fatal to horned cattle, does not affect man.

PLEXIMETER is the name applied to a small plate of ivory or similar material laid upon the skin to be struck in percussion. The small hammer used to strike it is called a plexor or plessor.

PLEXUS is the name applied to a network of nerves or vessels: eg. the brachial and sacral plexuses of nerves and the choroid plexus of veins within the brain.

PLICA is the term applied to various folded structures in the body.

PLICATION is the operation for taking tucks in the walls of a hollow organ.

PLOMBIERES DOUCHE is a term applied to lavage of the lower bowel by means of a soft rubber tube which is inserted into the rectum to a distance of 3 to 6 inches (7·5 to 15 cm). Several pints of fluid are slowly allowed to run in by gravity, the patient reclining on the left side with the hips raised, and later turning on the back so that the fluid may penetrate throughout the large intestine. The fluid is retained as long as possible and returned by the ordinary movement of the bowels. Various fluids, but especially normal saline solution, are used for this purpose.

PLUMBISM is another name for lead-poisoning. (See LEAD-POISONING.)

PLUMMER'S PILL is another name for compound calomel pill. It contains calomel, antimony, and guaiacum.

PLUMMER-VINSON SYNDROME is a syndrome associated with certain cases of hypochromic anaemia. It consists of hypochromic anaemia, difficulty in swallowing, and enlargement of the spleen. It is found practically only in women. (See ANAEMIA.)

PLURIGLANDULAR means derived from several glands.

PNEUMOCONIOSIS is the general name applied to a chronic form of inflammation of the lungs which is liable to affect workmen who constantly inhale irritating particles at work. It has been defined by the Industrial Injuries Advisory Council as: 'Permanent alteration of lung structure due to the inhalation of mineral dust and the tissue reactions of the lung to its presence but does not include bronchitis and emphysema'. It is liable in certain cases to develop into pulmonary tuberculosis. Some of the trades liable to suffer are those of stone-masons, potters, steel-grinders,

ganister workers, colour-grinders, coal-miners, millers, and workers in cotton, flax, or wool mills. In 1976, there were 935 cases of pneumoconiosis in Britain, 575 of these in coalworkers and 189 in asbestos workers. (See OCCUPATIONAL DISEASES; TUBERCULOSIS.)

PNEUMOGASTRIC, or VAGUS, nerve is the tenth cranial nerve. (See VAGUS NERVE.)

PNEUMONECTOMY is the operation of removing an entire lung in such diseases as bronchiectasis, tuberculosis, and cancer of the lung.

PNEUMONIA or inflammation of the substance of the lungs, manifests itself in several forms which differ from each other in their nature, causes, and results: (1) *Acute lobar*, or *pneumococcal, pneumonia*, the most common form of the disease, in which the inflammation affects a limited area, usually a lobe or lobes of the lung, and runs a rapid course. (2) *Broncho-pneumonia, catarrhal pneumonia*, or *lobular pneumonia*, which occurs as a result of bronchitis, and is more diffuse in its distribution and longer in duration than the former. (3) *Primary atypical pneumonia*.

In addition to these three principal types, pneumonia may arise as a part of other diseases of which it forms a serious complication: for example, it may occur in the course of typhoid fever, anthrax or plague, in each case being caused by the special bacteria associated with the disease in question. Pneumonia may also supervene in a person suffering from serious heart trouble or in old and devitalized persons, coming on gradually as the result of lying for a long time on the back with resultant congestion of the lower and back portions of the lungs. This type of pneumonia is known as *hypostatic pneumonia*, but is essentially of the same nature as broncho-pneumonia.

ACUTE LOBAR PNEUMONIA is the disease commonly known as inflammation of the lungs. The changes that take place in the lung are chiefly as follows. (1) *Congestion*, or engorgement, is the first stage, the blood-vessels being distended and the lung more voluminous, heavier than normal, and of dark-red colour. Its air-cells still contain air. The inflammation may pass off without proceeding further and the symptoms then abate after two or three days' duration. This is what tends to happen at the present day since the introduction of antibiotics (2) *Red hepatization* is so called from the resemblance that it gives the lung to liver tissue. (3) *Grey hepatization* is the next stage in which the lung retains its solid liver-like consistence, but the colour of a cut section is now grey. (4) *Resolution* is the final stage which occurs in all cases which run a satisfactory course. The exudation now undergoes a process of liquefaction, and the material is either completely reabsorbed into the blood-vessels or to a certain extent is expectorated. Air again enters them and they resume their normal function. This is the manner of termination in the great majority of cases of acute lobar pneumonia, but it sometimes happens that this favourable result is not attained, and that further changes take place in the inflamed lung in the form of suppuration ending in abscess or gangrene. In such cases there usually exists some serious constitutional cause which contributes to an unfavourable termination to the course of the disease, such, for example, as pre-existing diabetes or Bright's disease, or even the presence of old and partially healed tuberculosis in the lung. In occasional cases the pneumonia may become chronic, the lung never completely clearing up but continuing to discharge small quantities of pus which are brought up in expectoration, and to undergo a gradual fibrous change (*interstitial pneumonia*).

Acute lobar pneumonia is usually limited to a portion of one lung, the commonest part being the lower lobe on one or other side. Occasionally the pneumonia spreads throughout the whole of one lung, or it may affect both lungs, when it is called *double pneumonia* and is a serious and sometimes dangerous condition. The apex of the lung is sometimes the only part affected (*apical pneumonia*), and this type seems especially to affect alcoholics, in whom pneumonia is often a fatal malady. The right lung is more often affected by pneumonia than the left lung.

Causes – The *pneumococcus*, or *Diplococcus pneumoniae* as it is technically now known, is the specific infecting microorganism in about 95 per cent of all cases of lobar pneumonia. The death-rate from pneumonia is highest in the first five years of life and after the age of 60.

The disease may occur at any age, but is most common during the active years of life from 20 to 50. Among the aged the other type of pneumonia, *bronchopneumonia*, is much more common. During the prime of life the disease affects men much more commonly than women.

It appears to be a more serious disease among the darker races than in white men. There is a distinct tendency for pneumonia to be more prevalent during the late winter and early spring months, February, March, and April, but it is not specially associated with very low temperatures.

Symptoms – After an incubation period of two to six days, the attack usually begins with shivering (or in young children with a convulsion), and this is speedily followed by pain in the chest and sometimes by vomiting. The temperature almost at once rises to 101° or even 104° F (38·3° or 40° C), the pulse is quickened, and the breathing is rapid, shallow, and sometimes laboured. Occasionally the development is less abrupt, and the patient, although not feeling well, may remain at work for two or three days after the onset. The lips are dark and the face has a dusky flush. Cough is an early symptom, at first frequent, hacking, and accompanied by only a little clear, tough expectoration, but later bringing up a copious, rusty-brown material which is generally very tenacious, sticking to the sputum-dish even when the latter is turned upside down ('rusty sputum'). Occasionally the expectoration contains bright red blood, and this is by no means a bad sign. The temperature may abate a little after the initial rise, but usually continues between 103° and 105° F (39·5° and 40·5° C) for about a week, when it falls with considerable suddenness (crisis) to normal. The crisis generally takes place between the seventh and tenth day of the illness, most commonly about the eighth. At the crisis the pulse rate drops from about 120 to 80, and the respirations diminish from about 36 per minute to 24 or less. At the time of crisis the skin, which was previously dry and hot, perspires freely. Pain, which is an almost constant feature at the beginning of pneumonia, due to the accompanying pleurisy, tends to abate as the disease advances. It is specially felt on coughing or drawing deep breaths. Pain is usually felt in the side, but may be referred by the patient to the pit of the stomach or even to the lower part of the abdomen. In the latter case the symptom is apt to lead to a mistaken diagnosis of some acute abdominal disorder. Although the breathing is rapid, the patient is not usually breathless unless a large area of the lungs is affected, and he lies on the back or on the affected side. Sleeplessness is often a troublesome feature of the disease, and tends to exhaust the patient unless it is relieved by hypnotics or other means. Delirium is occasionally present, but, so long as it is mild, affords no cause for anxiety. An eruption of herpes is often noticed about the lips. Certain physical signs are usually present. Diminished movement of the affected side is noticeable, the healthy side of the chest performing most of the respiratory function. On percussion over the affected area a dull note is obtained, which becomes particularly marked if fluid has collected in the pleural cavity. On auscultation over the affected area, the breathing is usually harsh and high pitched (tubular breathing), but it sometimes shows no deviation from the normal, especially in cases in which the deeper parts of the lung only are affected. Accompanying the breathing in the early stages of the disease, crackling sounds known as crepitations are commonly heard. These disappear during the period in which the lung remains solid, but reappear (redux crepitations) when resolution begins to take place. All these physical signs disappear with remarkable rapidity in about two days after the crisis has taken place. A moderate increase in the number of the white blood corpuscles is a favourable sign. An increase to too large an extent in the later stages is a sign that suppuration is taking place.

In unfavourable cases, death may take place either from the extent of the inflammatory action, especially if the pneumonia is double, from exhaustion due to excessive fever, sleeplessness, and similar causes, or from failure of the heart's action in cases in which a great amount of general poisoning is present, or again from the disease assuming from the first a low adynamic form, with delirium and great prostration. Such cases are found in persons worn out in strength, in the aged, and in persons suffering from alcoholism or chronic conditions like Bright's disease and diabetes. Some of the unfavourable signs are extremely rapid and shallow breathing with accompanying lividity, delirium of wildly excited type in which the patient becomes excited by struggling, persisting sleeplessness, a rapid and feeble pulse indicating impending heart-failure, excessive sweating, and the occurrence of complications such as pericarditis. Death may also take place at a later stage from the development of empyema, abscess, or gangrene of the lung. In a small number of cases, recovery may be imperfect, the disease gradually passing into a chronic interstitial pneumonia.

Treatment – Good nursing is all-important. Pain and difficulty of breathing may be relieved by the application of rubber hot water bottles, or ice-bags to the affected side. Cough is relieved by expectorants (qv). Any tendency to excessive fever may often be held in check by sponging with tepid water. Cases in which the disease is extensive in the lungs or in which the heart is feeble and the blood in consequence not properly oxygenated, as shown by blueness of the face and lips, obtain great relief and benefit from the inhalation of oxygen. As regards feeding, the digestive powers being much reduced, the patient should be fed with milk, soups, and other light forms of nourishment frequently administered. Sleeplessness is sometimes relieved by sponging the body with tepid water or, if more troublesome, by a sedative or hypnotic, or, if delirium be also present, by morphine.

The prime agent in treatment is penicillin. Indeed, the introduction of penicillin has completely changed the outlook for the better in this disease. So much is this the case that very few doctors today have seen the disease run the course just described. If the condition is diagnosed on the first day or so, and penicillin given immediately, the whole disease is over in a few days. At one time one of the most common serious diseases encountered in temperate climates, it is now a relatively mild one.

After the acute symptoms disappear, the patient must remain in bed for some time. The occurrence of empyema (qv), which, when it takes place, is indicated by hectic rise of temperature every day, sometimes follows or prevents the crisis and requires aspiration or surgical drainage of the pleural cavity. After recovery is complete, a period of approximately a month's convalescence is advisable.

BRONCHO-PNEUMONIA, BRONCHIAL PNEUMONIA, CATARRHAL or LOBULAR PNEUMONIA, differs from acute lobar pneumonia in several important points. The inflammation is more diffuse, and tends to affect small patches or lobules of lung tissue here and there, rather than one or more lobes. If the condition becomes extreme, the affected parts may join so that the whole lung is affected, but there are still certain important differences.

In favourable cases, resolution takes place after a longer or shorter interval. At the same time, a large amount of the material filling the lungs is gradually expectorated by the patient. On the other hand, when the illness is prolonged, degenerative changes may take place in the lung tissue, small abscesses may form, and a condition of chronic interstitial pneumonia or bronchiectasis (qv) may develop. In the great majority of instances bronchopneumonia occurs as an accompaniment or sequel of bronchitis, either from the inflammation passing from the finer bronchi to the air-vesicles or from its affecting portions of the lung which have undergone collapse through obstruction of their bronchial tubes by secretion. It occurs commonly in children, often following upon some previous acute illness in which the bronchi are inflamed, such as measles or whooping-cough. It also tends particularly to affect old people in a more chronic form as the result of bronchitis, and it forms one of the chief causes of death among the aged. Hence its title of 'the old man's friend', as it so often brings old age to a peaceful end – or at least did before the introduction of the sulphonamides and antibiotics.

Symptoms – The symptoms of bronchopneumonia in its more acute form are the occurrence, during an attack of bronchitis, of a sudden and marked rise of temperature, together with quickened pulse and increased difficulty of breathing. The cough becomes short and painful unless the child or aged person is too feeble to bring up expectoration, when the cough becomes of a suffocative type, which forms a bad sign. Vomiting sometimes occurs in children and may be a salutary symptom because it aids in freeing the lungs from the accumulating secretion. In a severe case of broncho-pneumonia the dusky red colour of the lips, cheeks, and ears is also present as noticed in acute lobar pneumonia, due to defective oxygenation of the blood.

Physical signs of a somewhat vague character are found over the chest. The note obtained by percussion is duller at some points than at others; the breathing is harsh with the signs of bronchitis, which is also present, and here and there breathing may be tubular, with fine crackling sounds (crepitations).

The illness does not end by a crisis as in the case of lobar pneumonia, but the temperature tends for an indefinite period, it may be of several weeks, to remit and rise again with a gradual fall to normal.

Broncho-pneumonia must be regarded as a condition of serious import. It is apt to run rapidly to a fatal termination in weakly persons, the inflammation spreading and the lungs filling up with secretion.

After its occurrence there is a tendency in susceptible individuals to the development of tuberculosis. On the other hand, a favourable result is frequent if the condition is recognized in time to admit of efficient treatment.

Treatment – The treatment is essentially that for the more severe forms of bronchitis (see BRONCHITIS), where, in addition to expectorants intended to help the freeing of the chest from secretion, various stimulants and good nourishment are of great importance. Ample fresh air in broncho-pneumonia following whooping-cough, measles, and similar diseases is of great importance, the patient at the same time being protected by light warm applications, such as a gamgee-tissue jacket on the front and back of the chest. Administration of oxygen is of great value in cases showing duskiness of the lips and face. The antibiotics are important drugs in treatment, and must be given in full doses, the choice of antibiotic depending upon the infecting micro-organism. The posture of the patient in bed is a matter of importance; whilst in the case of lobar pneumonia the patient obtains most relief from lying on his back or on the affected side, in broncho-pneumonia with an excessive amount of secretion the patient is usually most comfortable and breathes most easily when kept constantly in a half-sitting posture with the shoulders raised high by pillows placed behind the back. Because of this excess secretion patients with broncho-pneumonia must never be given morphine for the relief of pain or as a sedative.

PRIMARY ATYPICAL PNEUMONIA, is due to *Mycoplasma pneumoniae*. A disease of winter, it occurs most commonly in children and young adults. Epidemics are liable to occur in barracks and institutions.

Symptoms – The incubation period is very variable: from 2 to 21 days, or even longer. The onset is usually insidious. Apart from general malaise, the presenting symptom is cough, accompanied by a varying amount of sputum. The temperature is usually in the region of 100° to 103° F (37·8° to 39·5° C). Features which may help to differentiate it from other forms of pneumonia include a normal white blood cell count, a relatively slow pulse in relation to the temperature, and a typical agglutination reaction in the blood in the second to fourth week of the illness. The prognosis is good, but the condition tends to drag on for several weeks.

Treatment – Promising results are now

being obtained from the use of the antibiotics, particularly oxytetracycline.

PNEUMONITIS means inflammation of the lungs that does not go on to pneumonia (qv).

PNEUMOPAROTITIS is the term applied to inflammation of the parotid glands (qv) caused by the presence of air in the glands. It has been reported in glassblowers and in players of wind instruments.

PNEUMOPERITONEUM means a collection of air in the peritoneal cavity. Air introduced into the peritoneal cavity collects under the diaphragm which is thus raised and collapses the lungs. This procedure is sometimes carried out in the treatment of pulmonary tuberculosis as an alternative to artificial pneumothorax.

PNEUMOTHORAX means a collection of air in the pleural cavity, into which it has gained entrance by a lesion in the lung or a wound in the chest wall. When air enters the chest the lung immediately collapses towards the centre of the chest, but, air being very quickly absorbed from the pleural cavity, the lung expands again in a short time. (See LUNGS, DISEASES AND INJURIES OF.)

Artificial pneumothorax is an operation by which in a case of pulmonary tuberculosis or of bronchiectasis air may be run into the pleural cavity so as to cause collapse of one lung, which rests it and allows cavities in it to heal.

PODAGRA is another name for gout affecting the foot. (See GOUT.)

PODOPHYLLIN is a resin derived from the root of *Podophyllum peltatum*, a plant of the United States and Canada, or from *Podophyllum emodi*, a plant which grows in the Himalayas. It has a purgative action but must be combined with hyoscyamus or belladonna, as by itself it causes severe griping and it is seldom used for this purpose now. It is also used as a local application in the treatment of venereal warts.

POIKILOCYTE is the name applied to a malformed red blood corpuscle found in the blood in various types of anaemia.

POISON IVY (*Rhus* (or *Toxicodendron*) *toxicodendron*), POISON OAK (*Rhus* (or *Toxicodendron*) *radicans*) and POISON SUMAC (*Rhus* (or *Toxicodendron*) *vernix*) are plants which grow widely in North America. In Britain, poison ivy and, less often, poison sumac, are grown in gardens for their attractive autumn tints. They contain a poisonous principle, urushiol, which induces a severe dermatitis in half the people who come in contact with the plant, and many severe effects, including kidney trouble, in 10 per cent. Treatment of the dermatitis consists of immediately washing the skin with soap and water to remove all the poison. This is followed by the application of wet dressings such as 1 per cent aluminium acetate, or 1 in 10,000 potassium permanganate.

POISONS – It is difficult to give a concise definition of the word, poison, because substances which are injurious by their mechanical action, such as steel filings or powdered glass, cannot be classed as such; nor is boiling water a poison; nor can a substance be regarded as a poison if it owes its effect to some bodily peculiarity: as, for example, a draught of cold water taken by an overheated person. The following definition is, however, given by Guy: 'A poison is any substance or matter (solid, liquid, or gaseous) which, when applied to the body outwardly, or in any way introduced into it, can destroy life by its own inherent qualities, without acting mechanically, and irrespective of temperature'. Even this definition is not quite satisfactory, because many substances are poisonous in large quantities, harmless in smaller amounts: eg. saltpetre, tartaric acid, Epsom salts. Further, a substance originally poisonous in a certain dosage may be tolerated in increasingly large doses as the individual continues to take it over a period of time, as in the case of arsenic and opium. (See OPIUM.) Again, different persons and animals vary widely in susceptibility to poisons, the old adage that 'one man's meat is another man's poison' being literally true. Many herbivorous animals, like the cow, feed upon the deadly nightshade with impunity, and pigeons are almost entirely unaffected by opium.

Varieties – Many substances which are poisonous are valuable remedies when used in small quantities or properly applied externally. Others are common household substances or garden plants, and many have important uses in the arts. Under the heading of poisons must be included bacteria and the harmful substances which their growth produces, such as the poisons found in decomposing meat. (See BACTERIOLOGY; FOOD POISON-ING, and other headings.) The injuries in-flicted by insects, snakes, and other animals which introduce some poison into the body are considered under BITES.

Leaving these out of account, we may classify poisons either according to their source or to their mode of action. Clas-sified according to their source they are: *animal*, like cantharides; *vegetable*, like deadly nightshade; *mineral*, like sulphuric acid or perchloride of mercury; and *aerial*, like carbon monoxide gas. By this classifi-cation, however, substances with the most diverse actions are included in each group. A more practical arrangement is made, according to the mode of action, into:

Corrosives, which burn and destroy the parts with which they come in contact.

Irritants, which have generally an irritant action upon the stomach and bowels.

Narcotics, which affect the brain and spinal cord, causing a stuporous state.

Narcotico-irritants, which produce first of all an irritative effect upon the stomach or upon the nervous system, and finally act as narcotics.

The two last-mentioned groups are by some authorities placed together as *narcotics*.

(1) CORROSIVES go so far as to corrode, ulcerate, or even perforate the organs with which they come in contact. The chief cor-rosives are the strong mineral acids, like sulphuric, nitric, hydrochloric; the alkalis, like caustic soda or potash, their carbon-ates, and ammonia; and certain strong salts, like corrosive sublimate.

(2) IRRITANTS include vegetable acids and some acid salts, such as tartaric acid, white arsenic (arsenious acid), yellow arsenic (orpiment), acetate of lead (sugar of lead), sulphate of copper (blue vitriol), subacetate of copper (verdigris), arsenite of copper (Scheele's green), tartarated antimony (tartar emetic), chloride of anti-mony (butter of antimony), chloride of zinc (Burnett's disinfectant), nitrate of silver (lunar caustic), bichromate of potas-sium, sulphate of iron (green vitriol or copperas); also the leaves, roots, berries, or resins of many plants taken in large amount, such as colocynth, savin, gamboge, aloes, croton oil, elaterium.

(3) NARCOTICS include a large range of substances ranging from the age-old opium to the modern synthetic drugs produced so freely by the modern phar-maceutical company. Few poisons have a purely narcotic action, most producing also sickness, delirium, or other signs of irritation. Among the narcotics are opium

and its preparations, prussic acid (hydro-cyanic acid), cyanide of potassium, alco-hol, ether, chloral, chloroform. Most poisonous gases also belong to this group, the chief among them being carbon dioxide, carbon monoxide, water gas, sulphuretted hydrogen, sulphide of ammonium, and other sewer gases. The amount of these which is necessary in the air in order to produce serious symptoms, or even to cause death if breathed for long, is very small. (See ASPHYXIA.)

(4) NARCOTICO-IRRITANTS form a large group in which the individual substances cause varied symptoms of irritation, such as delirium and excitement, convulsions, or sickness and vomiting. The group in-cludes carbolic acid, oxalic acid, binoxa-late of potash (salt of sorrel), nux vomica, strychnine, meadow saffron (*Colchicum autumnale*), white hellebore (*Veratrum album*), foxglove (*Digitalis purpurea*), monkshood (*Aconitum napellus*), henbane (*Hyoscyamus niger*), deadly nightshade (*Atropa belladonna*), black or garden nightshade (*Solanum nigrum*), woody nightshade or bittersweet (*Solanum dulca-mara*), potato tops and seeds (*Solanum tuberosum*), tobacco (*Nicotiana tabacum*), Indian tobacco (*Lobelia inflata*), thorn apple (*Datura stramonium*), spotted hem-lock (*Conium maculatum*), water hemlock or cowbane (*Cicuta virosa*), hemlock-water dropwort (*Oenanthe crocata*), five-leaved water hemlock (*Phellandrium aquaticum*), fool's parsley (*Aethusa cynapium*), yew leaves and berries (*Taxus baccata*), laburnum seeds and bark (*Cytisus laburnum*), and many species of poisonous fungi. (See FUNGUS POISONING.)

Symptoms – The symptoms of poison-ing, which come on soon after a meal, or at least after some substance has been swallowed, are of great importance, be-cause the treatment varies according to the type of poison taken, as shown by the symptoms.

CORROSIVE POISONS produce immediate pain and swelling of the lips, mouth, and throat, which also show signs of discolora-tion, depending on the poison taken. If the dose be large, there may be speedy col-lapse and death.

IRRITANT POISONS produce vomiting, purging, and abdominal pain. In the case of the milder irritants, the results may be deferred for a few hours, particularly when a full meal has been taken along with the poison. Later, in very serious cases, col-lapse and insensibility come on.

NARCOTICS produce giddiness, head-

Poison	Treatment	Poison	Treatment
Acids: Hydrochloric Nitric Sulphuric	Give lime-water, magnesia, chalk, whitening, or bicarbonate of soda in water, oil, or barley water; then albumin water.	**Digitalis** (Foxglove)	Give emetics; wash out stomach with permanganate of potassium.
Aconite	Lay patient down; give stimulants; wash out stomach with permanganate of potassium; give injection of atropine.	**Ether**	Wash out stomach; cold douches.
		Iodine	Give flour or other form of starch in water; wash out stomach.
Alcohol	Wash out stomach; give stimulants.	**Lead acetate** (sugar of lead)	Give magnesium sulphate or Glauber's salt; wash out stomach; then give albumin water or barley water.
Alkalis: Caustic soda Caustic potash Ammonia	Give vinegar in water, lemon juice, or dilute hydrochloric acid then linseed or olive oil.		
Arsenic	Wash out stomach; give Glauber's salt; then magnesia or hydrated oxide of iron, prepared by mixing solution of perchloride of iron with solution of ammonia in equal parts, straining through a handkerchief, and stirring up the precipitate in water; then albumin water or barley water; give dimercaprol; give laudanum if much colic.	**Laudanum:** Morphine Opium, etc.	Give emetic; wash out stomach with permanganate of potassium; give strong coffee; keep patient awake; artificial respiration.
		Lysol	(See CARBOLIC ACID above.)
		Mushrooms: Fungi	Give emetic; hypodermic injections of atropine and nikethamide.
Belladonna and atropine	Give emetic; wash out stomach with permanganate of potassium; neostigmine as antidote; artificial respiration.	**Oxalic acid** and binoxalate of potassium (salt of sorrel)	Give magnesia, chalk, or whitening (*not* bicarbonate or carbonate of soda); wash out stomach; give albumin water or milk.
Camphor	Give emetic, then a stimulant.	**Phosphorus** (matches, etc.)	Give sulphate of copper as emetic; wash out stomach with potassium permanganate; give albumin water; avoid oils.
Carbolic acid, Cresol, Lysol, etc.	Give magnesium sulphate or Glauber's salt, then albumin water or milk; wash out stomach.		
Chloral	Give emetic; wash out stomach with potassium permanganate; give stimulants; artificial respiration.	**Silver nitrate** (lunar caustic)	Give salt in water; wash out stomach; give albumin water or milk.
Cocaine	Give stimulants; wash out stomach; artificial respiration.	**Strychnine**	Wash out stomach with permanganate of potassium; give chloral.
Corrosive sublimate (mercuric chloride)	Give albumin water or milk; wash out stomach with sodium bicarbonate; give dimercaprol.	**Turpentine**	Give emetics, then magnesium sulphate and albumin water or milk.
		Zinc chloride	Wash out stomach; then give albumin water or milk.

Table 39 – Table of common poisons and their treatment.

ache, interference with sight, stupor, preceded occasionally by convulsions, followed by deepening insensibility ending in coma and death. No pain is produced by these. (For the means by which narcotic poisoning is distinguished from apoplexy, or alcoholic intoxication, see OPIUM.)

NARCOTICO-IRRITANTS produce at first the symptoms of the irritant poisons: vomiting, abdominal pain, and in many cases purging. Later, delirium or convulsions appear, ending in stupor and death.

Further details as to the symptoms and treatment connected with the more important poisons will be found under the headings of these poisons.

Treatment – The first essential in the first-aid treatment of a case of poisoning is to arrange for the casualty to be seen by a medical practitioner, or removed to hospital as quickly as possible. If he is conscious he should be asked what poison he has taken, as he may lose consciousness any moment. If he is unconscious, or even semi-conscious, no attempt should be made to give him anything by mouth, as this may cause choking or asphyxia. He should be placed in what is known as the recovery position (illustration 344), which ensures that an open airway is maintained. This is done as follows:

(1) Kneel beside him.

(2) Turn him gently on his side by grasping the clothing at the hip.

(3) Draw up the upper arm until it makes a right angle with the body and then bend the elbow.

(4) Draw up the upper leg till the tight makes a right angle with the body and then bend the knee.

(5) Draw out the under arm very gently backwards to extend behind his back.

(6) Bend the undermost knee slightly.

When a CORROSIVE POISON has been taken, one should first of all administer the chemical antidote to the poison, if there be one; and thereafter soothing substances should be given to allay the irritation in the mouth, throat, and stomach. The following corrosive poisons have such chemical antidotes. When acids have been taken, give a dilute alkali, such as lime-water,

344 – Recovery position.

magnesia, chalk, whitening, or even plaster scraped from the walls and mixed with water. When caustic alkalis have been taken, give weak acids, such as copious draughts of vinegar in water or lemon juice in water. When corrosive sublimate is the poison, white of egg in water or milk combines with it to form a harmless substance.

After the poison has been neutralized, milk, white of egg in water, or other bland fluid may be given to mitigate the irritation it has caused.

In the case of the IRRITANT POISONS, draughts of water or milk to dilute the poison, together with an emetic consisting of a tablespoonful of mustard in water, or of 20 grains (1·2 grams) of sulphate of zinc in water, should be given as soon as possible. Still better is it to wash out the stomach with the stomach tube at the earliest possible moment.

The following irritant poisons have chemical antidotes, which may be given before the stomach is emptied. When oxalic acid or salt of sorrel has been taken, give chalk or magnesia, which forms in the stomach the harmless oxalate of lime. If lunar caustic should have been swallowed, common salt in water neutralizes it by forming the inert chloride of silver. When sugar of lead has been swallowed, Epsom salts is an efficient antidote, producing the insoluble sulphate of lead in the stomach. Carbolic acid also has Epsom salts as an antidote. Arsenic is neutralized by a solution of hydrated peroxide of iron, when this is obtainable.

In the case of NARCOTIC AND NARCOTICO-IRRITANT poisons, an emetic administered at once is beneficial, and it is the usual practice for a medical man to wash out the stomach with a weak solution of permanganate of potassium, when he sees the case. Permanganate of potassium has the power of destroying many of these vegetable poisons which are of an alkaloidal nature. Many of these poisons, whose deadliness depends upon active principles, can be neutralized to some extent by other drugs.

WHEN THE POISON IS UNKNOWN, but the fact of poisoning suspected, the safest course is to administer tepid water containing common salt (sodium chloride) (see EMETICS), in order to expel the contents of the stomach, thereafter administering a drink of milk. The drink of salty water must not be repeated as too much salt may be harmful. Above all things is it necessary to keep all vomited matter and the remains of food that the poisoned person has been taking till the arrival of a medical man.

POLDINE, or POLDINE METHYLSULPHATE to give it its full name, is a synthetic drug, with an atropine-like action (see ATROPINE), which is used in the treatment of gastric and duodenal ulcers.

POLICLINIC is the name applied to a hospital or clinic belonging to a city. POLYCLINIC is the term applied to a clinic where diseases of all kinds are studied and treated.

POLIOMYELITIS, or INFANTILE PARALYSIS, is an infectious disease involving the spinal cord and the brain.

Cause – The first epidemic of poliomyelitis to be recorded occurred in Sweden in 1881. The disease then became of increasing importance, particularly in Scandinavia, USA and Australia, but with the successful introduction of poliomyelitis vaccination it rapidly became a relatively rare disease. In Great Britain the disease has been notifiable since 1912. Although sporadic cases may occur at any time, there is a definite seasonal incidence, epidemics tending to occur in the late summer and early autumn in the northern hemisphere and in March and April in the southern hemisphere. In the tropics infection continues throughout the year. In 1977, there were only 14 cases in England and Wales, compared with 3200 in 1956.

The infecting organism is a virus, of which there are three types. Infection occurs from ingestion of the virus by mouth. The virus then passes to the lower alimentary tract and is excreted in the stools. It has been shown that the viruses are excreted by 90 per cent of paralytic cases, particularly children, and they are also excreted in the stools by healthy contacts of cases. It is in this way that the disease is spread: through contaminations of the hands and then contamination of the mouth from such contaminated hands. Children are the most susceptible members of families, but during recent years there has been a definite tendency to severe paralytic cases occurring among young adults. One attack usually produces permanent immunity; second attacks are rare.

Pathology – The sites of selection for the virus are the motor cells in the anterior horn of the spinal cord, and there is a tendency for this to be more marked in the lumbar part of the cord. The cranial nerves and certain nuclei in the brain are also involved in some cases.

Symptoms – The incubation period is 3 to 21 days, commonly 7 to 12 days. The onset may be either sudden or gradual. In the case of the latter the child may merely be 'off colour' for a day or two and complain of aches or pains in the limbs; there may be only a slight rise in temperature. This may gradually pass into the stage of weakness, and then paralysis, of the limbs. In other cases, after a few days' vague illness, the paralysis of the limbs may come on quite suddenly, usually with a sharp rise in temperature. In cases of sudden onset, the victim complains of headache and aches and pains, and the temperature rises to 103° F (39·5° C) or higher. In other cases, particularly in children, the limbs may be found to be paralysed when the child wakens in the morning, although he was apparently quite well when he went to bed the previous evening.

The site and the distribution of the paralysis depend upon the extent to which the spinal cord and brain are involved. The most serious cases are those in which the diaphragm and the muscles of respiration (the intercostal muscles) are involved, as this prevents the patient breathing, and he may die in a very short space of time unless he is placed in a respirator. When the cranial nerves and brain are involved, there may be nystagmus (qv), hoarseness, and difficulty in swallowing. Convulsions may occur in young children. The cerebrospinal fluid contains an excess of cells in the first and second weeks and an increased amount of protein in the third week.

Prophylaxis – A high degree of protection is given by poliomyetis vaccine. This is now given by mouth, and its use has practically banished the disease. Of the 14 cases in England and Wales in 1977, 11 had not been immunized. The vaccine is given in childhood, but a booster dose should be given to adults, particularly young adults, when they are going to a country of high poliomyelitis incidence, which in practice means any country outside Europe and North America.

In the presence of an epidemic the following measures should be taken. Children should not be allowed to go into crowded buildings such as cinemas. Public swimming baths should be avoided. Children, especially younger ones, should not be allowed to get overtired, particularly in hot weather. Particular care should be taken to protect food from flies and to ensure that the highest standards of cleanliness are observed in the handling of food. No operations for the removal of tonsils or adenoids should be performed. Immunization against diphtheria and whooping-cough and smallpox vaccination should, if at all possible, be postponed until the epidemic is over.

Treatment – The patient must be put to bed on the first sign of the disease, and the affected limbs completely rested. This is the one definite practical fact that has resulted from all the careful investigation of the disease during recent years: that the earlier the disease is detected, and therefore the earlier the patient is put to bed and the affected parts rested, the better the ultimate result. Splints may be necessary at this stage to give adequate rest to the affected muscles. Later, careful physiotherapy is necessary. If the breathing is affected, it may be necessary to put the patient in a respirator or iron lung. To ensure the best possible results, after-treatment may need to be continued for two or three years. In cases in which severe paralysis and wasting of limbs persist, surgical treatment may be necessary to reduce the resulting disability to a minimum.

POLIOSIS means premature greying of the hair. It is also the term applied to whitening of the hair in segments, such as a forelock.

POLITZER'S BAG is an india-rubber bag with nozzle intended for inflation of the middle ears by blowing air up one nostril while the other is closed, and so clearing a blocked Eustachian tube. (See EAR, DISEASES OF.)

POLLEN consists of microspores formed in flowering plants and conifers. Between 4 and 7 million tons of it are said to be shed throughout the world. From ancient days it has had the reputation of being a specific against old age, and recent reports from Russia claim that bee-keepers live longer because they eat pollen. It contains protein, vitamins A, B, C, D and K, small amounts of minerals including calcium, copper, iron, magnesium, manganese, phosphorus, potassium, and sulphur, as well as several enzymes. It has a bitter taste, which is traditionally disguised by honey – the ambrosia of the Bible, the Koran and the Talmud. Sufferers from hay fever should not eat it during the hay-fever season as it may induce allergic reactions.

POLLEX is a Latin term for thumb.

POLYARTERITIS NODOSA, or PER-IARTERITIS NODOSA as it is sometimes known, is a disease of unknown origin, in which prolonged fever and obscure symp-toms referable to any system of the body are associated with local areas of inflammation along the arteries, giving rise to nodules in their walls. Recovery occurs in about 50 per cent of cases.

POLYCHROMASIA and POLY-CHROMATOPHILIA are terms applied to an abnormal reaction of the red blood corpuscles in severe anaemia, whereby they have a bluish tinge instead of the normal red colour in a blood film stained by the usual method. It is a sign that the cell is not fully developed.

POLYCYTHAEMIA is the name applied to excess in the number of red corpuscles in the blood.

POLYDACTYLY means the presence of extra, or supernumerary, fingers or toes.

POLYDIPSIA means excessive thirst, which is a symptom of diabetes and some other diseases.

POLYGRAPH is the term applied to an instrument for making simultaneous tracings of the pulse in two different parts of the circulation at one time.

POLYMER FUME FEVER occurs in people who work with polytetrafluoroethylene (PTFE, Teflon). The fever is caused by degradation products, including hydrofluoric acid, which are produced at temperatures of 170° C and upwards. The likeliest source of these injurious products is cigarette smoking. Even the tiniest particles of PTFE on a burning cigarette will yield sufficient of these degradation products to cause fume fever.

The illness consists of an influenza-like illness, which lasts for a few hours.

POLYMORPH is a name applied to certain white corpuscles of the blood which have a nucleus of irregular and varied shape. These form between 70 and 75 per cent of all the white corpuscles.

POLYMORPHIC LIGHT ERUPTION is a photodermatosis (qv) which occurs predominantly in females, appearing first as a rule in adolescence or early adult life. The eruption, which consists of a mixture of erythema (qv), papules (qv) and vesicles (qv), occurs on those parts of the body exposed to the sun, mainly the back of the hands, the forearms, the front of the neck, the cheeks and the nose. There are usually several attacks a year, depending on the amount of sunlight. The attacks start in the spring and continue until the winter. Apart from the fact that the rash is provoked by sunlight, the precise cause is not known. Treatment consists of avoiding sunlight, wearing protective clothing, and using sunscreening preparations. (See SUNBURN.)

POLYMYALGIA RHEUMATICA is a form of rheumatism characterized by gross early morning stiffness, which tends to ease off during the day, and pain in the shoulders and sometimes round the hips. It affects women more than men, and is rare under the age of 60. The cause is still obscure. It responds well to prednisolone (qv), but treatment may need to be long continued. On the other hand the condition is not progressive and does not lead to crippling.

POLYMYXIN is the name applied to the group of antibiotics derived from various species of *Bacillus polymyxa*. Polymyxin B is the one available commercially, and is the antibiotic of choice in the treatment of infections due to *Ps. pyocyanea*.

POLYNEURITIS means an inflammatory condition of nerves in various parts of the body. (See NEURITIS.)

POLYPHARMACY is a term applied to the administration of too many drugs in one prescription.

POLYPOSIS means the presence of a crop, or large number, of polypi. The most important form of polyposis is that known as *familial polyposis coli*. This is a hereditary disease characterized by the presence of large numbers of polypoid tumours in the large bowel. Every child born to an affected parent stands a fifty-fifty chance of developing the disease. Its importance is that sooner or later one or more of these tumours undergoes cancerous change. If the affected gut is removed surgically before this occurs, and preferably before the age of 20, the results are excellent.

POLYPUS is a general name applied to tumours which are attached by a stalk to the surface from which they spring. The term refers only to the shape of the growth and has nothing to do with its structure or nature. Most polypi are of a simple nature, though malignant polypi are also found. The usual structure of a polypus is that of a fine fibrous core covered with epithelium resembling that of the surrounding surface. The sites in which polypi are most usually found are the interior of the nose, the outer meatus of the ear, and the interior of the womb, bladder, or bowels (see POLYPOSIS).

Their removal is generally easy, as they are simply twisted off, or cut off, by some form of snare or ligature. Those which are situated in the interior of the bladder or bowels, and whose presence is usually recognized by the presence of blood in the urine or stools, may require a more serious operation to reach the organ into which they project.

POLYTHELIA is the term applied to the condition in which extra or supernumerary nipples appear along a line between the armpit and the groin.

POLYURIA means the passage of an amount of urine considerably in excess of the fifty ounces (1500 ml) or thereabout which is the usual daily quantity. It is a symptom of diabetes, certain forms of Bright's disease, and some nervous diseases.

POMPHOLYX is a form of eczema characterized by the appearance of deeply set vesicles (qv) on the palms and soles, fingers and toes. When it occurs on the fingers and hands it is known as CHEIRO-POMPHOLYX. On the toes and feet it is known as PODOPOMPHOLYX.

PONS VAROLII is the bridge of the brain, mainly composed of strands of white nerve-fibres which unite various parts of the brain. (See BRAIN.)

POPLITEAL SPACE, or HAM, is the name given to the region behind the knee. The muscles attached to the bones immediately above and below the knee bound a diamond-shaped space through which pass the main artery and vein of the limb (known in this part of their course as the popliteal artery and vein), the tibial and common peroneal nerves (which continue the sciatic nerve from the thigh down to the leg), the external saphenous vein, as well as several small nerves and lymphatic vessels. The muscles, which bound the upper angle of the space and which are attached to the leg bones by strong prominent tendons, are known as the hamstrings. The lower angle of the space lies between the two heads of the gastrocnemius muscle, which makes up the main bulk of the calf of the leg.

POPPY as used in medicine is of two species: *Papaver somniferum*, the white opium-poppy (see OPIUM), and *Papaver rhoeas*, the red corn-poppy. The corn-poppy is chiefly used as a colouring agent, the syrup made from it having a brilliant crimson colour.

PORENCEPHALY, or PORENCEPH-ALIA, is a term applied to the presence of cysts in the surface of the brain due to an arrest of development or to birth haemorrhage. The condition is generally associated with serious mental defect.

POROPLASTIC is the name of a thick kind of felt which is easily moulded into splints when softened by hot water and used for surgical purposes.

PORPHYRIA is a condition, or rather a series of conditions, characterized by an excessive production and excretion of porphyrins. Porphyrins are constituents of various blood and respiratory pigments found throughout the animal kingdom, including human beings. They are also found in plants and micro-organisms.

In porphyria there is some disturbance of their metabolism and this results in a variegated picture which includes discoloration of the urine due to excessive excretion of porphyrins, skin rashes due to sensitization of the skin to light, various forms of indigestion and mental disturbances.

PORRIGO is a general term applied to diseases of the skin covering the head, such as ringworm.

PORTAL VEIN is the vein which carries to the liver blood that has been circulating in many of the abdominal organs. It is peculiar among the veins of the body in that it ends by breaking up into a capillary network instead of carrying the blood directly to the heart, a peculiarity which it shares only with certain small vessels in the kidneys. The portal system begins below in the haemorrhoidal plexus of veins round the lower end of the rectum, and from this point, along the whole length of the intestines, the blood is collected into an inferior mesenteric vein upon the left, and a superior mesenteric vein upon the right side. The inferior mesenteric vein empties into the splenic vein, and the latter, uniting with the superior mesenteric vein immediately above the pancreas, forms the portal vein. The portal vein is joined by veins from the stomach and gall-bladder, and finally divides into two branches which sink into the right and left lobes of the liver. (For their further course, see LIVER.)

The organs from which the portal vein collects the blood are the large and small intestines, the stomach, spleen, pancreas, and gall-bladder.

POSOLOGY means the science or system of dosage in regard to medicines.

POSSETTING is the technical term used to describe the quite common habit of healthy babies to regurgitate, or bring up, small amounts of the meal they have just taken.

POST- is a prefix signifying after or behind.

POST-MORTEM EXAMINATION (see NECROPSY).

POST-PARTUM is the term applied to anything happening immediately after child-birth: for example, post-partum haemorrhage.

POSTURAL DRAINAGE is the process whereby the drainage of secretions from dilated bronchi of the lungs is facilitated. The patient lies on an inclined plane head downwards and is encouraged to cough up as much secretion from the lungs as possible. The precise position depends on which part of the lungs is affected. It may need to be carried out for up to three hours daily in divided periods. It is of particular value in bronchiectasis (qv) and lung abscess.

POTASH, or POTASSA, is the popular name for potassium carbonate. Hydrated oxide of potassium is usually known as caustic potash, and its solution as potash solution.

POTASSIUM is a metal which, on account of its great affinity for other substances, is not found in a pure state in nature. Its salts are used to a great extent in medicine but, as their action depends in general not on their metallic radicle but upon the acid with which it is combined, their uses vary greatly and are described elsewhere. (Thus for the uses of potassium bromide, see BROMIDES, for those of potassium iodide, see IODIDES, for those of potassium permanganate, see PERMANGANATE OF POTASSIUM, for those of the bicarbonate, citrate, and tartrate of potassium, see

CITRIC ACID, and for those of nitrate of potassium, see NITRE.)

All salts of potassium have a depressing effect on the heart's action by virtue of the potassium ion.

POTASSIUM CHLORATE, in addition to the general actions exerted by potassium salts, has a soothing action upon inflamed mucous membranes, and is used for a gargle in sore throat of every description.

POTASSIUM PERCHLORATE is an antithyroid drug used in the treatment of hyperthyroidism. It acts by inhibiting the mechanism in the thyroid gland for collecting inorganic iodine from the blood supply to the gland.

POTT'S DISEASE is a name often applied to the angular curvature of the spine which results from tuberculous disease. (See SPINAL DISEASES.) The disease is named after Percivall Pott, a famous English surgeon (1714–88), who first described the condition.

POTT'S FRACTURE is a term applied to a variety of fractures around the ankle, accompanied by a varying degree of dislocation of the ankle. In all cases the fibula is fractured. Named after Percivall Pott, who suffered from this fracture and was the first to describe it (see FRACTURES), it is often mistaken for a simple sprain of the ankle.

POULTICES (see also FOMENTATION) are soft moist applications to the surface of the body, generally used hot. They soften the parts with which they come in contact, soothe irritated nerve-endings, relax spasmodically contracted muscle-fibres, and, after being applied for some time, dilate the vessels of the part they cover and increase the circulation through it. These applications are consequently used in all stages of inflammation to soothe pain and promote resolution, or in the late stages, when pus is forming, to aid the rapid formation of an abscess. (See ABSCESS.)

Poultices should on no account be applied to open wounds, for their warmth and moisture favour the growth of bacteria.

Variety and uses – LINSEED POULTICE made from crushed linseed is one of the most commonly used, and is applied hot in cases of inflammation. OATMEAL POULTICE is used in precisely the same conditions. MUSTARD POULTICE is used where it

is desired to combine a counter-irritant action with the warmth of a poultice. BREAD POULTICE and STARCH POULTICE are used at the body temperature, generally in order to remove the crusts of skin eruptions or soften a hardened surface. CHARCOAL POULTICE was formerly much used to diminish the smell from foul ulcers. Hot fomentations for acute pain are now used in preference to the more cumbersome and less cleanly poultices.

Method of application – LINSEED POULTICE should be made of freshly crushed linseed as the meal soon grows rancid if kept. About half a pint (280 ml) of boiling water is poured into a small basin, already warmed, and the linseed is slowly added to it, stirring all the while. Enough meal, about 4 ounces (112 grams), is added to make a mass sufficiently thick to adhere together, but thin enough to spread. This may be judged by the mass being sufficiently coherent to allow a spoon or spatula to stand upright in it. A linen, or better a flannel, rag is laid by the basin and the hot linseed quickly spread on it with a spatula or tableknife. It may be covered with a piece of thin muslin, or the linseed may be applied directly to the skin. On the outer surface of the poultice a piece of macintosh or oil-silk should be placed, and outside of this a thick piece of cotton-wool to retain the warmth. The whole is fixed in place by a flannel bandage or binder. Such poultices become cold in two hours or so and should then be renewed, but the cold poultice should not be taken off till the new one is ready to lay on. In changing the poultice great care should be taken that the patient is not exposed to chill.

MUSTARD POULTICE is made by mixing 2½ ounces (70 grams) of linseed with half a pint (280 ml) of boiling water as above, adding to it 2½ ounces (70 grams) of mustard flour which has already been mixed with lukewarm water, and stirring the two together. This is spread and applied in the same way as the linseed poultice, but must not be left on longer than twenty minutes to half an hour. There must be a piece of muslin on the surface in order to keep the mustard from adhering to the skin. The patient's sensations form the best guide as to the length of time over which such a poultice should be left on. The place of this poultice is now to a great extent taken by mustard leaves, which simply require to be wetted and applied.

BREAD POULTICE is made by breaking up stale bread in a basin, pouring boiling water over the crumbs sufficient to soak them, allowing to cool, draining off superfluous moisture, spreading on a cloth, and covering with muslin.

STARCH POULTICE – Add a teaspoonful of powdered boric acid to four tablespoonfuls of cold-water starch, mix with a little cold water, then pour in a pint (570 ml) of boiling water, and stir till thickened; let stand till cold; spread the cold starch *thickly* on pieces of cotton, cover with muslin, and apply to the part, changing the poultices every few hours and wiping the skin gently each time the poultices are reapplied. Starch poultices are used for the removal of crusts or scales on the skin.

CHARCOAL POULTICE is made by preparing a bread poultice and sprinkling it with dry powdered charcoal.

KAOLIN POULTICE is a paste which is applied by heating the pot containing it in a pan of boiling water, and spreading thickly on lint.

POUPART'S LIGAMENT, also known as the inguinal ligament, is the strong ligament lying in the boundary between the anterior abdominal wall and the front of the thigh.

POWDERS form a method in which drugs are prescribed, powerful drugs being made up with inert substances like sugar, gum, or ginger in order to give them sufficient bulk. The best known powders are Dover's powder (ipecacuanha and opium powder), containing opium; Gregory's powder (compound rhubarb powder); and Seidlitz powder (compound effervescent powder). Powders have largely been replaced by tablets.

Method of use – If the powder be small and tasteless, a little water is poured out into a teaspoon, the powder shaken out on the surface of the water and swallowed. If it be large and nauseous, the best plan is to envelop it in a rice-paper. A little water is placed in the bottom of a saucer and the circular rice-paper laid upon it, when it quickly softens. The powder is shaken out upon the centre of the rice-paper, and the edges of the latter are quickly turned over it with a teaspoon. The soft mass is then pushed on to the spoon and is easily swallowed, being thus untasted.

PRE- is a prefix meaning before.

PRECORDIAL REGION is the area on the centre and towards the left side of the chest, lying in front of the heart.

PREDNISOLONE, is a derivative of cortisone, which is five or six times as active as cortisone and has less of the salt-and water-retaining properties of cortisone. It is given by mouth.

PREDNISONE is the official name for deltadehydrocortisone, and has the same action as prednisolone.

PRE-ECLAMPSIA is a complication of pregnancy characterized by oedema, high blood-pressure and the presence of albumin in the urine. It is so called because, unless adequately treated in time, it may be a prelude to the onset of eclampsia (qv).

PREFRONTAL LOBOTOMY (see LEUCOTOMY).

PREGNANCY – This state is a natural one, although it sets up great changes, not only in the womb, but throughout the whole body. Most of these changes subside quickly after delivery is accomplished, and though a few minor alterations persist throughout life, the mother returns to her normal state within about one month after the child is born.

Duration of pregnancy – It is generally accepted that pregnancy lasts about 280 days from the first day of the last menstrual period. In exceptional cases there may be considerable variation, but it is generally agreed that the shortest duration of a normal pregnancy is 240 days and the longest duration 313 days. The cause of these variations is not understood. The longest period of gestation that has ever been admitted in the Law Courts in Great Britain is 349 days, whilst the shortest that has been accepted is 174 days. For the purpose of calculating the probable date of confinement, it is usual to take the first day of the last period that occurred, to allow seven days for the duration of this and then to add 273 days for the duration of gestation, making in all 280 days from the beginning of the last menstruation. The actual date can be estimated roughly by adding seven days and then counting forwards nine calendar months; for example, supposing the last menstrual period began on 3rd October, adding seven days makes the 10th October, and nine months forwards from this gives the date of probable confinement as the 10th of July. It is usual to say that this day is the middle of the week in which the confinement may be expected.

Signs of pregnancy – (*a*) The stoppage of

the menstrual flow is the sign which first attracts attention. This symptom may, however, be due to many other causes (see MENSTRUATION), but if it occurs quite suddenly it may usually be counted upon as an important sign. It is a popular mistake to suppose that pregnancy cannot occur in a woman while she is suckling a previous child, for this does occur even while the menses are in abeyance. (b) Swelling of the breasts is another important sign, appearing even in the second or third month of pregnancy. A thin fluid, known as colostrum, can, even at this early stage, be pressed from the nipples. At the same time the veins on the breasts become enlarged and visible, and the pigmented ring round the nipple (areola) becomes much darker than before, as well as showing small nodules (Montgomery's tubercles) round its edge. (c) Sickness in the mornings immediately on rising is also a common sign, occurring in about two-thirds of all women, though it may be absent, and even if present may be due simply to dyspepsia When the sickness is marked, however, it is a valuable sign, because it appears early in the course of pregnancy, during the second month, and lasts usually about a couple of months. (d) Quickening, or the fluttering sensation felt by the mother in consequence of the child's rapid movements, is a very important sign, though it does not usually occur till some time during the fifth month of pregnancy or even later. It is the first sign of life felt by the mother, though it is a popular error to suppose that the child only then begins to live. (e) Enlargement of the abdomen is a pronounced sign, though for the first three months the enlargement is not apparent. It must not be forgotten, however, that enlargement may be due to other causes, such as tumours, dropsy, and even constipation or increasing development of fat. It is not an uncommon mistake for an elderly childless woman to delude herself with the hope that she is about to bear a child, when the abdomen is enlarging simply for the last-named reason. This condition is known as pseudocyesis or false pregnancy. (f) The only absolutely certain sign of pregnancy is obtained when the medical attendant hears the beating of the foetal heart by auscultation over the lower part of the abdomen. The heart-sounds are rapid, much resembling the ticking of a watch, and are heard, in general, from the middle of the fifth month onwards. (g) There are various minor signs which are sometimes present, sometimes absent, some of which are noticeable by the mother, others appreciable only by the medical attendant. Such are the occurrence of varicose veins, mucous discharge from the vagina, changes in the neck of the womb.

Hygiene of pregnancy – It is unnecessary for a healthy woman to make any great change in her ordinary mode of life during pregnancy. Her diet must be good, but should be simple and moderate. Alcoholic liquors and smoking should preferably be abandoned during pregnancy. Because of the possible risk to the unborn child, no drugs should be taken during pregnancy except on medical advice. A pregnant woman should drink at least one pint (0.5 litre) of milk a day, on account, amongst other things, of the calcium it contains. Cheese should also be taken for its calcium. (The foetus in the uterus needs calcium for its bones.) Iron-containing foods are also important for the development of the foetus's red blood corpuscles. Iron is present in such foods as eggs, green leafy vegetables, and in liver and meat. Vitamins are also of great importance to the pregnant woman, and these are present in such foods as eggs, milk, cheese, butter, wholemeal bread, brown bread, fresh vegetables, and fruit (especially oranges, lemons, currants, potatoes, and tomatoes), and fat fish, such as herring and salmon; in the winter months cod-liver oil or hali-but-liver oil may well be taken in addition. Constipation should be avoided by a suitable diet containing vegetables, fruit, and the like, or by mild aperients. The skin should be kept in good condition by regular bathing. Moderate exercise should be taken every day and late hours avoided. The dress should be loose and comfortable. During pregnancy a healthy woman gains an average of 12.5 kg (28 pounds), but this varies considerably.

Special ailments – The misfortune which specially attaches to the condition of pregnancy is miscarriage (see MISCARRIAGE), but this is not likely to occur in healthy persons. Digestive disturbances are common. Thus the natural morning sickness may become very troublesome, or even dangerous, and require special treatment. Constipation or diarrhoea may be troublesome, but either of them is treated much as under ordinary circumstances. Varicose veins in the legs, piles, swelling of the feet, and cramps in the legs are all liable to be caused in the later months by pressure of the increasing womb upon the large vessels and nerves within the pelvis. These, however, are not serious signs, and must simply be tolerated till after the child

713

is born, when they quickly improve. Varicose veins, if very severe, should be supported by elastic stockings or by bandaging the legs, and cramps may be relieved by the usual means. (See CRAMP.) Irritability of the bladder, showing itself by frequency of making water, is also a temporary inconvenience, similarly due to pressure.

More serious symptoms occasionally arise, such as those of kidney disease, various nervous disorders, and especially the condition known as eclampsia, in which convulsions occur. A sudden gain in weight in late pregnancy may indicate the onset of pre-eclampsia (qv). Displacements of the womb, which have existed prior to pregnancy, may also give trouble and it may be necessary for the subject of such displacements to wear a pessary during the earlier months. As a rule, however, the displacement rights itself as pregnancy proceeds.

It is because of the possibility of such ailments, whether mild or serious, occurring during pregnancy that every pregnant mother should be seen by her doctor, or attend an antenatal clinic, at regular intervals throughout pregnancy.

PREGNANCY TESTS – There are several tests for pregnancy in its early stages.

The Aschheim-Zondek test – This was the first to be introduced and depends upon the fact that in the first few months of pregnancy there is a greatly increased secretion of chorionic gonadotrophin (see GONADOTROPHINS), of which the excess is discharged in the urine. A small quantity of urine passed by the woman whom it is desired to test is sent to a laboratory, where a few drops are injected on several successive days into a young and immature female mouse or other small animal. The animal is killed five days later, and if the person whose urine is being tested is pregnant, it is found that the ovaries of the immature mouse have been stimulated into a state of full maturity; but if the urine has come from a non-pregnant person, the young mouse's ovaries remain unchanged. The test is highly accurate but slow and each test involves the use of five or six animals.

The Friedman test – The test animal is the rabbit. The isolated rabbit does not ovulate spontaneously, but ovulation can be induced within twenty-four hours by the intravenous injection of pregnancy urine. This test thus gives a result within twenty-four to forty-eight hours, and with

an accuracy similar to the Aschheim-Zondek test.

The rat hyperaemia test – The subcutaneous injection of pregnancy urine induces hyperaemia of the ovary in the immature rat. This test gives a result within ten hours, which is as accurate as the Aschheim-Zondek test.

The Hogben test – This test is based upon the observation that the injection of pregnancy urine promotes ovulation in the female South African clawed toad (*Xenopus laevis*). It gives a result within twenty-four hours and has an accuracy similar to that of the Aschheim-Zondek test.

The Kapeller-Adler test – This is a chemical test based upon the identification of histidine, which is a normal constituent of the urine throughout pregnancy. It is said to be 100 per cent accurate in normal pregnancy, but non-pregnancy urine sometimes gives a positive reaction.

The Haemagglutination Inhibition test – This, and the subsequent tests to be mentioned, are known as immunological tests, as opposed to those already mentioned which are known as biological tests. They are known as immunological tests because they are based upon the effect of the urine from a pregnant woman upon the interaction of red-blood cells, which have been sensitized to human gonadotrophin (qv), and anti-gonadotrophin serum. They have the great practical advantage of being performed in a test-tube or even on a slide, and therefore not requiring animals. Because of their ease and speed of performance (a result can be obtained in two hours), these tests are being used on an increased scale. Their degree of accuracy is not quite as high as the Hogben test, and the current recommendation is that while a negative result may be accepted, a positive result (ie. one indicating that the woman is pregnant) should be confirmed by a Hogben test. With this combination an accuracy of over 99 per cent has been reported.

The *Latex test* and the *Gravindex test* are modifications of the haemagglutination test.

PREGNANDIOL is the excretion product of the hormone, PROGESTERONE (qv), manufactured by the corpus luteum of the ovary. Pregnandiol is excreted in the urine during the second half of the menstrual period, and its excretion rises steadily throughout pregnancy.

PREMATURE BIRTH (see ABORTION; BIRTH; FOETUS) is one that takes place before the end of the normal period of gestation. In practice, however, it is defined as a birth that takes place when the baby weighs less than $5\frac{1}{2}$ pounds (2·5 kilograms).

PRENYLAMINE is a drug that is proving of value in the treatment of angina pectoris (qv).

PREPUCE is the free fold of skin that overlaps the glans penis.

PRESBYACUSIS is the deafness that comes on with increasing years. It is caused by increasing loss of elasticity in the hearing mechanism combined with the slowing down of the mental processes that accompanies old age. It is characterized by particular difficulty in hearing high notes such as the telephone and the voices of women and children. Hearing in a background of noise, such as a cocktail party, is also early affected. Modern, miniaturized, transistor hearing aids are of little help in this form of deafness. One of the older, more robust types is usually more successful. (See also DEAFNESS; and HEARING AIDS.)

PRESBYOPIA is the general term used to indicate the changes that take place naturally in the eye with the advance of age, and quite apart from any disease. The chief of these changes consists in decreasing elasticity of the lens, so that it becomes increasingly difficult to use the eyes for near work. At the age of 40 this change has proceeded so far that the lens can just manage to accommodate itself for vision of objects at around 10 inches (25 cm), the distance which is most convenient for reading or other close work. After the age of about 45, therefore, much work must be done at an uncomfortable distance, or glasses must be worn in order to aid the natural lens. Persons who, during youth, have a slight degree of short-sight, may in old age not require any glasses for near work.

PRESCRIPTION means the written direction given by the doctor to the chemist for the compounding of medicine suitable to a patient's case. It was long customary to write prescriptions in Latin, a usage which came down from mediaeval times, and which had a parallel in ancient Greece, where the practitioners at Athens are said to have written their prescriptions in the Doric dialect. The quaintest part of this traditionary usage lies in the R which heads every prescription, and which was

at first probably the eye of the god Horus, a charm used by the ancient Egyptians, and later the sign of the planet Jupiter. It now stands for the initial of the word *recipe* meaning 'take', and ‚introduces the directions to the dispenser.

At the present day the official recommendation is to prescribe in terms of milligrams and grams rather than grains and ounces, millilitres rather than minims, and in the *British Pharmacopoeia* dosages are given in terms of the metric system only. Further, in the *British Pharmacopoeia* names of drugs are given in English, and not in Latin. (See also DOSAGE; and DRUGS.)

PRESENTATION means the appearance in labour of some particular part of the child's body at the mouth of the womb. This is a head presentation in 96 per cent of cases, but in a certain number the breech (or buttocks) may present, or the face, or foot, or even a part of the trunk is cases of cross-birth.

PRESSOR is the term applied to anything that increases the activity of a function: for example, a pressor nerve or pressor drug.

PRESSURE SORES (see BED SORES).

PRICKLY HEAT, or MILIARA RUBRA, is a troublesome skin condition affecting Europeans in tropical climates. It consists in the appearance of numbers of minute vesicles, produced by blocking of the outlet of the sweat or sebaceous glands in the skin, and accompanied by intolerable itching.

Causes – Nearly every European suffers from prickly heat during the early years of residence in the tropics, when the hot season comes round. It is due probably to the cells on the surface of the skin becoming sodden by the constant perspiration, and so swelling and blocking the outlets of the minute gland-ducts. Anything that leads to perspiration, such as hot drinks, hot soup, close rooms, or warm clothing, aggravates the condition.

Symptoms – The surface is covered by minute vesicles which cause extreme itching and pricking. The scratching which this entails often leads to the formation of boils and pustules, but the condition is not in itself a dangerous one. The extreme discomfort, and the loss of sleep arising from it, may, however, be a serious matter for invalids.

Treatment – The most important point

is to avoid, so far as possible, all causes of excessive perspiration, such as warm drinks and rough underclothing. Curtailing the intake of salt and maintaining an adequate intake of fluid are also said to be helpful. Common soap should not be used in the bath, and each time after bathing, the skin should be dusted with an astringent and antiseptic dusting powder, such as one composed of boric acid, zinc oxide, and starch in equal parts. Equally effective is the use of an emollient cream or bath oil. If nothing else is immediately available, the application of olive oil is often helpful.

As a preventive, rubbing the body over after the bath with the juice of a lemon has been recommended. Calamine lotion (either alone or incorporating some menthol crystals) or carbolic acid lotion relieves the itching temporarily.

PRIMIDONE is a drug used for the treatment of epilepsy.

PRIMIPARA is the term applied to a woman who has given birth, or is giving birth, to her first child.

PRO- is a prefix meaning forwards.

PROBE is the name of a slender, flexible instrument usually made of metal designed for introduction into a wound or cavity either to explore its depth and direction, to discover the presence of foreign bodies, or to introduce medicinal substances.

PROBENECID is a benzoic acid derivative. It interferes with the excretion by the kidney of certain compounds, including penicillin and *para*-aminosalicylic acid, and was originally introduced into medicine for this reason, as a means of increasing and maintaining the concentration of penicillin in the body. It has also proved of value in the treatment of chronic gout.

PROCAINAMIDE is a derivative of procaine, which has been introduced for the treatment of certain cardiac arrhythmias.

PROCAINE, or PROCAINE HYDROCHLORIDE, is a synthetic substance having a similar action to the natural alkaloid, cocaine. It is a powerful local anaesthetic with transitory effect. Procaine possesses the anaesthetic properties of cocaine, but has an advantage over the latter in being very much less poisonous, so that it can be

administered in larger doses, and also in producing no tendency to contract a habit for its use.

PROCAINE PENICILLIN (see PENICILLIN).

PROCARBAZINE is a drug that is proving useful in the treatment of various forms of tumour, especially Hodgkin's disease (qv). It acts by interfering with the process of mitosis (qv), whereby the cells of the body, or tumours, reproduce themselves.

PROCHLORPERAZINE is a tranquillizer. It is also an effective drug for the prevention or treatment of vomiting, and has therefore been used in the treatment of Menière's disease (qv). It is available in two forms: as the maleate which is taken by mouth, and the mesylate which is given by intramuscular injection.

PROCIDENTIA is another term for prolapse (qv).

PROCTALGIA is neuralgic pain in the anus or rectum. The term is usually reserved for rectal pain without local disease in the rectum to account for it. *Proctalgia fugax* is a condition characterized by cramp-like pains in the rectum which may be excruciatingly painful. They are more common in men than women. They occur during the night, last up to fifteen minutes and may be accompanied by a feeling of faintness. The cause is not known. The taking of food or drink may bring relief, as may pressure on the perineum (eg. by sitting astride the edge of the bath). A finger in the rectum may also bring relief. The sucking of a 1 mg tablet of glyceryl trinitrate is said by some to bring prompt relief. The attacks are said to cease after the age of 50.

PROCTITIS means inflammation situated about the rectum or anus.

PRODROMATA is a term applied to the earliest symptoms of a disease, or those which give warning of its presence. For example, vomiting and headache may be prodromata of scarlet fever.

PROFLAVINE is a valuable antiseptic. It is an acridine derivative, its chemical description being 2:8-diaminoacridine sulphate. Like all the acridine derivatives it is effective against both Gram-positive and Gram-negative bacteria and is not inactivated by body fluids or pus. It is also non-toxic and non-irritating.

PROGERIA is a term for premature old age. When the physical appearances of old age occur in children the condition is believed to be due to disease of the pituitary gland (qv).

PROGESTOGEN is a preparation with an action like that of progesterone (qv).

PROGESTERONE is the hormone of the corpus luteum (qv). After the escape of the ovum from the ruptured follicle, the corpus luteum secretes progesterone, which stimulates the growth and secretion of the endometrial glands of the uterus during the fourteen days before menstruation. In the event of pregnancy, the secretion of progesterone continues until parturition. (See also ETHISTERONE; NORETHISTERONE; NORETHYNODREL; PREGNANDIOL; CONTRACEPTION; MENSTRUATION.)

PROGLOTTIS is a term applied to the segment of a tapeworm.

PROGNOSIS is the term applied to a forecast as to the probable result of an illness or disease, particularly with regard to the prospect of recovery, based upon the nature and symptoms of the case.

PROGRESSIVE MUSCULAR ATROPHY (see PARALYSIS).

PROGUANIL HYDROCHLORIDE is a synthetic antimalarial drug which has proved of value both in the treatment and the prevention of malaria, particularly the form known as malignant tertian malaria.

PROLACTIN is the name of the pituitary hormone which initiates lactation. The development of the breasts during pregnancy is ascribed to the action of oestrogens (qv). Prolactin starts them secreting. If lactation does not occur or fails, it may be started by injection of prolactin.

PROLAPSE means slipping down of some organ or structure. The term is applied chiefly to downward displacements of the rectum and womb. When the lower end of the bowel prolapses each time the bowels move – as may occur in children – it should be carefully sponged with cold water, replaced, and, if necessary, retained in place by a soft pad and bandage attached to a waist-belt, or by strapping the buttocks together with plaster. The condition tends to pass off as the child grows older. Prolapse which affects the womb may, in the earlier stages, cause protrusion of a fold of the bowel or bladder through the vagina, and in the later stages the womb itself may protrude to the exterior. The condition, which affects elderly women, is mainly due to injuries caused by childbirth. It may often be remedied by wearing a suitably shaped pessary, or by an operation designed to unite the torn parts.

PROLAPSED INTERVERTEBRAL DISC – The spinal column (qv) is built up of a series of bones, known as vertebrae, placed one upon the other. Between these vertebrae lies a series of thick discs of fibro-cartilage known as intervertebral discs. Each disc consists of an outer portion known as the annulus fibrosus, and an inner core known as the nucleus pulposus. The function of these discs is to give flexibility and resiliency to the spinal column and to act as buffers against undue jarring. In other words, they are most efficient shock absorbers. They may, however, prolapse (illustration 345), or protrude, between the two adjacent vertebrae. If this should happen they press on the neighbouring spinal nerve and cause pain. As the most common sites of protrusion, or prolapse, are between the last two lumbar vertebrae and between the last lumbar vertebra and the sacrum, this means that the pain occurs in the back, causing lumbago (qv) or down the course of the sciatic nerve causing sciatica (qv).

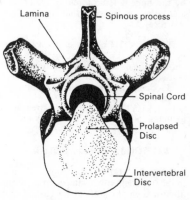

Lamina — Spinous process

Spinal Cord

Prolapsed Disc

Intervertebral Disc

345 – Diagrammatic representation of prolapsed intervertebral disc.

The prolapse is most likely to occur in middle age, which suggests that it may be associated with degeneration of the disc involved, but it can occur in early adult life as well. It usually occurs when the individual is performing some form of exercise which involves bending, as in gardening. The onset of pain may be acute and sudden, or gradual and more chronic in intensity.

Treatment varies, depending, amongst other things, on the severity of the condition. In the acute phase rest in bed is essential. Later, exercise and physiotherapy are helpful, and in some cases manipulation of the spine brings relief by allowing the herniated, or prolapsed disc to slip back into position. The injection of a local anaesthetic into the spine (epidural anaesthesia) is yet another measure that often helps the more chronic cases. The ultimate form of treatment is an operation to remove the prolapsed disc, but this is a procedure that is not now performed nearly as often as it once was. An alternative form of treatment is the injection into the disc of chymopapain, an enzyme (qv) obtained from the paw-paw, which dissolves the disc.

PROMETHAZINE HYDRO-CHLORIDE is a widely used antihistamine drug with a prolonged action and a pronounced sedative effect. (See ANTI-HISTAMINE DRUGS.)

PROMETHAZINE THEOCLATE, or AVOMINE, is a drug that is widely used in the alleviation or prevention of sea-sickness.

PRONATION is the movement whereby the bones of the forearm are crossed and the palm of the hand faces downwards.

PROPANTHELINE, or PROPANTHEL-INE BROMIDE, is a substance with an anticholinergic, or atropine-like action, which is used in the treatment of conditions such as duodenal ulcer and spastic colon.

PROPHYLAXIS means treatment or action adopted with the view of warding off disease.

PROPICILLIN (see PENICILLIN).

PROPRANOLOL is a drug that is used in the treatment of angina pectoris, certain abnormal rhythms of the heart, and high blood-pressure. It is also proving of value in preventing attacks of migraine, and in certain anxiety states, particularly those associated with unpleasant bodily sensations, such as palpitations.

PROPTOSIS means undue prominence of the eyeballs.

PROSTACYCLIN is a substance produced by the endothelial lining of the blood vessels. It inhibits the aggregation of platelets (qv), and thereby reduces the likelihood of the blood clotting. It is also a strong vasodilator.

PROSTAGLANDINS, so called because they were first discovered in the semen and thought to arise in the prostate gland, are a group of recently discovered substances with a wide range of activity. The richest known source is semen, but they are also present in many other parts of the body. Their precise mode of action is not yet clear, but they are potent stimulators of muscle contraction and they are also potent vasodilators (qv). They cause contraction of the womb and have been used to induce labour. They are also being used as a means of inducing therapeutic abortions. They play an important part in the production of pain, and it is now known that aspirin relieves pain by virtue of the fact that it prevents, or antagonizes, the formation of certain prostaglandins. In addition, they play some, though as yet incompletely defined, part in producing inflammatory changes. (See INFLAMMATION.) One of them is a powerful inhibitor of the secretion of gastric juice, which opens up the interesting possibility that it may be of value in the treatment of peptic ulcers. (See DUODENAL ULCER.)

PROSTATE GLAND is a structure which lies at the neck of the bladder in men and surrounds that part of the urethra lying within the pelvis. This gland is of importance, especially because in late life it is apt to increase in size and change in shape in such a way as to obstruct the exit of water from the bladder. Accordingly, great difficulty occurs in making water. In the large majority of cases, however, in which enlargement of the prostate produces such obstruction, removal by means of operation is now recommended. At the present day this operation, if performed by experienced surgeons, carries a relatively low mortality rate – 0·75 to 1 per cent, even though it is often carried out on old men who are far from fit. It has been estimated that one in every ten men will undergo this operation. The prostate is also one of the common sites of cancer in the male, and it is in the control, though unfortunately not the cure, of this form of cancer that such dramatic results have been obtained from the use of the synthetic oestrogens, such as stilboestrol (qv).

PROSTHESIS is an artificial replacement, such as an artificial limb or eye, or a denture.

PROTAMINES are a class of proteins found in combination with nuclei and in the heads of fish spermatozoa. They have two main uses in medicine. When combined with insulin they produce a compound which exerts a slower and more prolonged anti-diabetic action. (See INSULIN.) They also act as an antidote to heparin (qv).

PROTEIN is the term applied to members of a group of non-crystallizable nitrogenous substances widely distributed in the animal and vegetable kingdoms and forming the characteristic materials of their tissues and fluids. They are essentially combinations of amino-acids. They mostly dissolve in water and are coagulated by heat and various chemical substances. Typical examples of protein substances are white of egg and gelatin.

Proteins constitute an essential part of the diet as a source of energy and for the replacement of protein lost in the wear and tear of daily life. Their essential constituent from this point of view is the nitrogen they contain. To be absorbed, or digested, proteins have to be broken down into their constituent amino-acids. The adult human body can maintain nitrogenous equilibrium on a mixture of eight amino-acids, which are therefore known as the essential amino-acids. They are isoleucine, leucine, lysine, methionine, phenylalanine, threonine, tryptophan and valine. In addition, infants require histidine. It is because some of these essential amino-acids, particularly lysine are lacking in cereals and pulses that these cannot alone constitute an adequate diet. Generally speaking, the major source of protein is animal food, although some vegetables, notably the pulses, contain protein. The use of a certain amount of nitrogenous food is necessary to the system, as from this source alone can the body derive all the building material it requires to repair daily waste. (See DIET.) Even carbohydrate foods contain a certain amount of protein, but if all the necessary protein were to be obtained from these it would incur the waste of much starch, or its formation into fat in the bodily tissues. Hence the main value of a mixed diet. The nitrogenous foods may be grouped as follows:

Meat, including beef, mutton, pork and other forms of flesh, poultry, game and the internal organs.
Soups and beef-extracts.
Fish.
Milk and cheese.
Eggs.
Pulses and other nitrogenous vegetables.

Meat in structure consists of long cylinders of semi-fluid, protein material enclosed in thin, fibrous tubes, and known as muscle fibres. (See MUSCLE.) These are bound together by fibrous tissue, enclosing more or less fat in its meshes. The protein material consists mainly of myosin, which clots when the muscle dies, and contains also albumin and haemoglobin. In addition, there are several chemical substances which can be extracted by steeping the meat in hot water, and which are therefore known as extractives. To these the flavour of meat is due, and the varying taste of different meats is to be explained by slight chemical differences in the extractives present. The feeding and habits of animals have much to do with these differences, and explain the variety in taste between the flesh of wild and tame rabbits, and of grouse and poultry. The shape of the muscle fibres has much to do with the digestibility of meat, short or fine fibres, as in poultry, being the most quickly dissolved. The fatness of meat, or rather the extent to which the fat is interspersed between the meat fibres, is of more importance in connection with digestibility and explains why pork, duck, and goose have a reputation for being indigestible. Sweetbreads and tripe, being held together by loose connective tissue, are, on the other hand, quickly digested, and therefore suitable for invalids. Liver and kidney, which contain much nuclein, a substance closely allied to uric acid, are bad for gout.

Jellies contain little but gelatin, obtained from the fibrous tissue of meat and sinews, and when made with a large quantity of water, ie. weak in gelatin, they are easily digested. Gelatin is of little or no use as building material, and the main value of jellies is to add bulk and variety to the invalid diet.

Soup consists of a small quantity of gelatin, fat, salts and extractives in hot water.

To make soup or beef-tea from meat does not remove the nutritious materials, although it extracts all the flavour and hardens the meat. Clear soup contains practically no nourishment, although it is stimulating to the digestion by reason of the extractives it contains. Thick soup is nutritious only by reason of the vegetables and gelatin added to it. The same is true of the extract of meat introduced by Baron Liebig in 1865, and of its many more recent imitations. Each pint of beef-tea made from this extract represents the salts and extractives in about half a pound of lean meat, although it contains little or none of the nutritive materials. Its use is valuable, because it appears to play a part in helping on the processes of nutrition. It is useful therefore in fevers and in feeble conditions, when little food is needed, or when the digestive powers are weak. Beef-juice, obtained by chopping meat up finely, mixing with a little water and squeezing out cold, is quite another article, and contains a larger proportion of the nutritive materials as well as extractives.

Fish is an excellent source of protein, and, in the case of fatty fish, such as herring and mackerel, has the additional advantage of containing vitamins A and D. Haddock and whiting are among the most digestible fish, some of which, like cod, have a coarse fibre, and others, like salmon, are very fat. Herring is one of the cheapest as well as one of the most palatable forms of nitrogenous food, and two herrings contain as much animal protein as need enter into the daily dietary of an ordinary working man.

Milk is practically the only form of animal food in which protein, fat, carbohydrate and salt are all represented in sufficient amount. It contains 2 to 3 per cent of casein, from which cheese, an almost purely protein and fatty food, is made; a small quantity of milk-albumin; 4 per cent of fat in the form of a fine emulsion, which gradually rises to the surface as cream; and 4 to 5 per cent of milk-sugar, to the decomposition of which souring of milk is due. (See DIET; INFANT FEEDING; MILK.)

Eggs, each of which contains the material necessary to form a chicken, present the building material for the formation of bone and muscle in an easily convertible form, and are therefore an excellent food for convalescents, and for children. They do not contain any carbohydrate material, and therefore, to form a good article of general diet, should be mixed with rice, flour or other cereals, as is done in the shape of puddings. The digestibility is increased when an egg is beaten up with milk or water, and still more when the eggs are lightly boiled. One egg corresponds in nutritive value to about half a tumblerful of good milk, or to about 1 ounce (28·5 grams) of meat.

Pulses, of which the chief are peas, beans and lentils, have been called the 'poor man's beef'. This, however, is misleading, because, though they are cheap, they are not so digestible, contain little first-class protein, and are far from being so completely absorbed as meat unless carefully cooked, while in some persons the gases formed by their decomposition in the bowels give rise to great flatulence. They are also poor in fat, hence the habit of eating them combined with fat foods, as pork and beans, duckling and peas, and butter with beans. Nevertheless, the pulses form a valuable form of food.

The necessity for protein and the reason for its combination with other foods is described under the article on DIET.

PROTEIN SHOCK is a method of treatment by intramuscular or intravenous injection of protein material. Its object is to cause a reaction accompanied by moderate rise of temperature which produces stimulation of the general chemical processes of the body and of its absorptive and healing powers. Various protein substances are used for this purpose, including 5 per cent peptone solution, sterilized milk, and bacterial vaccines in large doses. Somewhat similar effects are produced by injection of certain metallic salts. This method is sometimes used in treatment of chronic diseases such as multiple sclerosis and rheumatoid arthritis though much less commonly than at one time.

PROTEINURIA is the condition in which proteins are found in the urine. It is usually referred to as ALBUMINURIA (qv), but this is not strictly correct, as both of the two blood proteins – albumin and globulin – may be found in the urine.

PROTO- is a prefix signifying first.

PROTOPLASM is the viscid, translucent, glue-like material containing fine granules and composed mainly of proteins, which makes up the essential material of plant and animal cells and has the properties of life.

PROTRIPTYLINE is an antidepressant drug.

PROUD FLESH is the popular name given to the unhealthy granulations which sometimes arise from an ulcer which is inflamed and is not healing properly, or from the margins of a sinus. It is checked by applying to it some astringent like nitrate of silver solution or copper sulphate.

PROXIMAL is a term of comparison applied to structures which are nearer the centre of the body or the median line as opposed to more distal, or distant, structures.

PRURIGO is the name of a chronic skin disease in which small papules (qv) develop in the skin, accompanied by intense itching. The condition may either be permanent or may come and go.

PRURITUS is another name for itching (qv).

PRUSSIC ACID POISONING – Prussic, or hydrocyanic, acid is a very deadly poison with a sweet smell and pleasant taste, paralysing every part of the nervous system with which it comes in contact. In its dilute state it was once widely used as a remedy for irritable conditions of internal mucous membranes, such as that of the stomach, and for irritable skin diseases, being used in small doses to check vomiting or cough, and applied in lotions to relieve itching. It exerts this curative action by numbing the sensory nerves with which it is brought in contact. At the present day it is seldom used for therapeutic purposes.

As a poison it acts with great rapidity, and, since potassium cyanide is much used in the processes of electroplating and photography, and is almost as deadly in its effects as the acid, persons using the cyanide should be acquainted with the treatment which may be of avail to save life in a case of poisoning.

Symptoms – After a large dose, the poison is very rapidly diffused through the body, and only a few minutes or seconds elapse before the symptoms appear. These are slowness of breathing, slowness and irregularity of the heart's action, and blueness of the face and lips. In a few minutes, insensibility with gradual stoppage of breathing and of the heart's action comes on, preceded in some cases by convulsions.

The suddenness and character of the symptoms and the sweet smell of prussic acid on the breath make the cause evident.

Treatment – This is based upon the administration of nitrites, which convert cyanide in the blood into the harmless cyanmethaemoglobin. Amyl nitrite is given by inhalation for 30 seconds every two minutes and also, if the victim can still swallow, 0·5 gram of sodium nitrite in 10 millilitres of water, by mouth. Artificial respiration (see DROWNING, RECOVERY FROM) is started immediately, preferably by the Holger-Nielsn method (*not* by the mouth-to-mouth method), and oxygen is administered. Injections of sodium nitrite and sodium thiosulphate are then given, as well as analeptics. An 'Ampin' Cyanide Emergency Kit is available which allows these injections to be given quickly. The victim must be watched carefully for forty-eight hours. Another antidote that is proving of value is cobalt edetate.

PSAMMOMA is the name given to a small hard tumour of the brain containing calcareous matter.

PSEUDOCYESIS means spurious or false pregnancy, a condition characterized by enlargement of the abdomen, and even enlargement of the breasts and early morning sickness, the unfortunate woman being quite convinced that she is pregnant.

PSEUDOHYPERTROPHIC MUSCULAR DYSTROPHY, or PSEUDO-HYPERTROPHIC PARALYSIS, is a condition in which certain muscles enlarge owing to a fatty and fibrous degeneration, giving a false appearance of increased strength. (See MUSCLES, DISEASES OF.)

PSILOSIS is another name for sprue (qv).

PSITTACOSIS is a contagious infection of parrots sometimes communicated to man and caused by a micro-organism known as *Chlamydia psittaci*.

PSOAS is the name of a powerful muscle which arises from the front of the vertebral column in the lumbar region, and passes down, round the pelvis and through the groin, to be attached to the inner side of the thigh-bone not far from its upper end. The act of sitting up from a recumbent posture, or that of bending the thigh on the abdomen, is mainly accomplished by the contraction of this muscle. Disease of the spine in the lumbar region is apt to produce an abscess which lies within the sheath of this muscle and makes its way down to the front of the thigh, where it threatens to burst. Such an abscess is known as a psoas abscess. (See ABSCESS, CHRONIC.)

PSORIASIS is a disease of the skin in which raised, rough, reddened areas appear, covered with fine silvery scales. This eruption consists of a chronic inflammatory process in the corium, the papillae of which become considerably lengthened and more vascular than usual, together with changes in the epidermis which cause a defect in the horny formation that naturally takes place on the surface and results in an increased production of epidermal cells. The nails are also involved in about 50 per cent of cases. (See SKIN.)

Causes – The condition generally appears for the first time around adolescence or early adult life and, it has been estimated, affects around 2 per cent of the population in Britain. It is often a family disease. A child with one affected parent has a 25 per cent chance of developing the disease. The risk rises to 60 per cent if both parents are affected. If parents without the disease have a child with psoriasis the risk for a subsequent child is 17 per cent. It may be associated with gout or rheumatism. In some persons, psoriasis appears repeatedly at a particular season of the year, especially in the spring and autumn, but it is not infectious. Depressing influences seem to have something to do with its appearance, and people who are liable to it are troubled by its reappearance at any time when the general health is below par.

Symptoms – The eruption almost always appears first round the back of the elbows and front of the knees. It begins as small pimples, each covered with a white cap of scales, which enlarge in breadth till they form patches 2 or 3 inches (5 or 7·5 cm) wide. At the same time, patches appear on other parts of the body, the scalp and face especially. The disease is divided into several varieties according to the size, shape, and distribution of these patches.

Treatment – It is essential first of all to attend to the general health. There is no cure for the condition and the best that can be hoped for is that it can be kept under control. Tar and dithranol are among the chief and most successful external applications. Satisfying results can also be obtained from the use of creams or ointments containing one or other of the corticosteroid preparations. Natural sunlight, or ultra-violet light, alone or in combination with tar preparations, produces a marked improvement in many cases. The latest form of treatment is that known as PUVA (qv). Patients with psoriasis can obtain help and advice from the Psoriasis Association, 7 Milton Street, Northampton NN2 7JH.

PSYCHASTHENIA is a condition in which the mind becomes temporarily weakened, the person a prey to anxieties and impulsive acts, the power of concentration poor, and the judgment capricious, without definite delusions or other signs of insanity. The condition is a form of neurosis. (See NEUROSIS.)

PSYCHEDELIC DRUGS are drugs, such as lysergic acid diethylamide (LSD), that expand consciousness and perception. (See DRUG ADDICTION.)

PSYCHIATRY is that branch of medical science which treats of mental disorder and disease.

PSYCHO-ANALYSIS is the term applied to the theories and practice of the Freudian school of psychology. It depends upon the theory that states of disordered mental health have been produced by a repression of painful memories or of conflicting instincts. By such repression these hurtful memories or instincts are kept constantly in a subconscious condition. As a result, the individual's mental power is needlessly occupied and diverted from the proper objects with which it should be concerned, and he finds difficulty in concentrating his attention upon and adapting himself to the practical realities of everyday life.

Psycho-analysis aims at discovering these repressed memories which are responsible for the perversion of mental power and of which the affected person usually is only dimly aware or quite unaware. The fundamental aim of psychoanalysis as a method of treatment is the free expression of thoughts, ideas, and fantasies on the part of the patient. To facilitate this, he lies on a couch to relax mind and body, and the analyst may sit so as to observe the patient but not to be observed by him. The analyst's task is to adopt a neutral attitude to the patient, to encourage the free association of ideas, and to explain where explanation is necessary for the continuance of free association. The analyst will become a part of the patient's fantasies and represent in them from time to time objects of love and hate – especially members of the patient's family. In the course of analysis the patient will, so to speak, sink back into childhood and re-enact his early emotional attitudes, the analyst representing in this phase father, mother, or brother or sister. In this re-enactment various infantile emotional tensions are released, and relief of painful mental symptoms secured.

There is much that is highly speculative in the theories of psycho-analysis, but at the same time its fundamental conceptions have been widely adopted by other schools of psychology to their enrichment, and the new approaches to the study of the mind in health and disease opened up by the concepts of Freud have changed the attitude of the lay and the medical public to the problems of the neurotic, the morbidly anxious, the fearful, and the mental and emotional development of the child.

PSYCHOLOGY is the branch of science that deals with the mind and its methods of working.

PSYCHONEUROSIS is a general term applied to various functional disorders of the nervous system. (See NEUROSIS.)

PSYCHOPATHIC – Psychopathic states are defined by the Mental Health Act 1959 as 'persistent disorders of mind (whether or not accompanied by subnormality of intelligence) which result in abnormally aggressive or seriously irresponsible conduct on the part of the patients, and require or are susceptible to medical treatment'. The cardinal features have been summarized by Blair as follows: (1) Lack of a normal conscience. (2) Absence of such normal feelings for other people as love, affection, sympathy and condolence. (3) A tendency to antisocial impulsive acts with no forethought of the consequences. (4) A failure to learn by experience and to be deterred from crime by punishment. (5) Freedom from any other form of mental disorder.

PSYCHOSIS is a term applied to serious disorder of the mind, amounting to insanity.

PSYCHOSOMATIC is a term applied to diseases in which the physical manifestations are in part, at least, due to emotional or mental factors. For instance, an attack of lumbago may be due not to any disease of the muscles of the back, but to emotional disturbances which literally prevent the individual from standing up to the stresses and strains of life.

PSYCHOTHERAPY is the term applied to any form of treatment in disease which operates through the mind. Almost every form of disease or injury has a certain mental aspect, even if this relates only to the pain or discomfort that it causes. In some diseases, and with some temperaments, the mental factor is much more pronounced than in others; and for such cases psychotherapy is particularly important. The chief methods employed are the following:

Suggestion is the most commonly employed method. Indeed, it is used in almost every department of medicine. It may consist, in its simplest form, of a mere reiteration of the statement that the health is better, either by the medical attendant or by the patient, so that this idea becomes fixed in the patient's mind. Or a suggestion of efficacy to cure may be conveyed by the taste or other physical properties of a medicine or by the imposing appearance of some apparatus used in treatment. Again, suggestion may be conveyed through an emotional channel, such as that of religious fervour. In occasional cases the result is secured when the suggestion is made to the patient in the hypnotic state.

Persuasion is a method of treatment in which appeal is made to a patient's reasoning faculties. It presupposes a higher type of mentality than that required for simple suggestion treatment.

Analysis consists in the elucidation of the half-conscious or subconscious repressed memories or instincts that are responsible for some cases of mental disorder. (See PSYCHO-ANALYSIS.)

Group therapy is a method of treatment being used to an increasing extent whereby, instead of receiving individual treatment, patients are treated in small groups, and encouraged to participate actively in the discussion and arguments which ensue among themselves and the participating doctors. A modification of group therapy which is proving of increasing value is *drama* therapy.

Education and employment are important factors in psychotherapy, and employment should be of a congenial character and one which the patient can carry out without great effort.

PTERYGIUM is the name applied to a patch of opaque tissue gradually extending over part of the clear cornea.

PTISAN is another name for barley water.

PTOSIS means drooping of the upper eyelids. It is a sign of paralysis of the third cranial nerve, which governs the muscle that elevates the upper lid.

PTYALIN is the name of the enzyme contained in the saliva, by which starchy materials are changed into sugar, and so prepared for absorption. It is identical with the amylase of pancreatic juice. (See DIGESTION; and PANCREAS.)

PTYALISM is a condition characterized by excessive production of saliva.

PUBERTY means the change that takes place when childhood passes into manhood or womanhood. This change is generally a very definite one, taking place at about the age of fourteen years, although it is modified by race, climate, luxurious habits, and bodily health, so that it may appear a year or two earlier or several years later. At this time the sexual functions attain their full development, the contour of the body changes from a childish to a more rounded womanly, or sturdy manly form, and great changes take place in the mode of thought and feeling. In girls it is marked by the onset of menstruation and development of the breasts. Development of the breasts is usually the first sign of puberty to appear, and may occur from $8\frac{1}{2}$ years onwards. Most girls show signs of breast development by the age of 13. The time from the beginning of breast development to the onset of menstruation is usually around two years but may range from six months to five years. The larynx enlarges in boys, so that the voice, after going through a period of 'breaking', finally assumes the deep manly pitch. Hair appears on the pubis and later in the armpits in both boys and girls, whilst in the former it also begins to grow on the upper lip, and skin eruptions are not uncommon on the face. (See ACNE.)

The period is one of transition from a physical, mental, and moral point of view, and the pressure of physical and intellectual work should not be made too hard, care being rather taken that good habits and modes of thought are formed at this impressionable time.

Puberty is not to be regarded as a physiological 'coming of age', for full development and vigour are not attained till between twenty and thirty years of age. (See also MENARCHE; MENSTRUATION.)

PUBIS is the bone that forms the front part of the pelvis. The pubic bones of opposite sides meet in the symphysis and protect the bladder from the front.

PUBLIC HEALTH (see SANITATION; also DISINFECTION; INFECTION; SEWAGE AND SEWAGE DISPOSAL; VENTILATION; WATER SUPPLY).

PUERPERAL FEVER, or CHILD-BED FEVER, was in former times the great dread of those whose duty it was to attend women in child-birth, both in private practice and to a much greater extent in public hospitals.

Causes – This fever is of various types and grades of severity. After the birth of a child, the mother is specially liable, for several reasons, to contract any infectious disease to which she may be exposed. In the first place, she is weakened by the strain through which she has passed, and often by the loss of a considerable quantity of blood. In the second place, the injuries incidental to child-birth produce raw surfaces in the genital tract, from which absorption occurs with great facility. The organism most commonly involved is the *Streptococcus haemolyticus* (qv). (For causation, see LABOUR.)

Symptoms – The symptoms vary according to the form that the infection takes, and most commonly appear on the second or third day after labour, the first three days being regarded as the critical period in recovery. Thus the organisms may, in the mildest form, develop on the raw or wounded surface, to which they gain access without entering the system. In such a case, there are general discomfort and feverishness, rise of temperature, and quickening of the pulse.

When the organisms gain access to the surrounding lymphatic vessels and veins, inflammation in the cellular tissue of the pelvis results, and may be followed by abscesses, peritonitis, either localized or general (see PERITONITIS), or, later on, by the condition known as white leg, caused by blocking of the veins in one lower limb. In these conditions, which are less common, the symptoms are more severe. There are considerable fever, shivering, prostration, and quickening of the pulse as early signs, together with pain in the lower part of the abdomen, followed later on by the symptoms belonging to peritonitis, white leg, or other condition set up by the inflammation. The condition may be recovered from in a week or two, or long-continued ill-health may result, or the patient may speedily succumb.

If the organisms gain access to the general circulation, the serious condition known as septicaemia results (see BLOOD-POISONING), and is accompanied by high fever, great prostration, delirium, and increasing feebleness of the heart's action.

Treatment – The prevention of the condition is of the greatest importance. For this reason, care in the choice of a lying-in room, great care to shield the patient from every risk of infection, and above all, scrupulous cleanliness on the part of all the attendants, are necessary. (See also LABOUR.)

Treatment resolves itself into careful nursing, blood transfusion if haemoglobin falls below 40 per cent, and administration of penicillin or the appropriate sulphonamide drug. The recognition of the bacteria responsible for puerperal infection and the introduction of the sulphonamide drugs and of penicillin in treatment have gone a long way to remove the terrors of this grim attendant upon child-birth.

PUERPERIUM is the period which elapses after the birth of a child until the mother is again restored to her ordinary health. It is generally regarded as lasting for a month. One of the main changes that occur is the enormous decrease in size that takes place in the muscular wall of the womb. (See MUSCLE.) There are very often afterpains during the first day in women who have borne several children, less often after a first child. (See AFTERPAINS.) The discharge is blood-stained for the first two or three days, then clearer till the end of the first week, after which it becomes thicker and less in quantity, finally disappearing altogether, if the case goes well, at the end of two or three weeks. The breasts, which have already enlarged before the birth of the child, secrete milk more copiously, and there should be a plentiful supply on the third day of the puerperium.

Management – It is now realized that prolonged rest in bed is not necessary for the mother after a normal birth. Indeed, it may be harmful. In the United States of America it is common practice to get the mother up on the first day, but in Britain it is most common to get her up on the second or third day. Soon thereafter she should start practising exercises to help to ensure that the stretched abdominal muscles regain their normal tone. There is no need for any restriction of diet, but care must be taken to ensure an adequate intake of fluid, including at least a pint

(580 ml) of milk a day. The bowels are generally sluggish and it is usual to take an aperient on the second or third day.

Milk, as already stated, appears copiously on the third day, but this is preceded by a secretion from the breast, known as colostrum, which is of value to the new-born child. The child should therefore be put to the breasts within six to eight hours of being born, in order to obtain the small amount of fluid they are secreting, and also because suckling stimulates both the breasts and the natural changes taking place during this period. Suckling is beneficial for both child and mother.

PULEX IRRITANS is the common human flea. It is between 2 and 4 mm in length. Of more importance is *Xenopsylla cheopis*, the rat-flea which transmits plague. Both are destroyed by DDT: 5 per cent solution in kerosene for buildings and furniture: 10 per cent powder for clothing. For pet animals DDT should be used as a powder and not as a solution. (See BITES AND STINGS.)

PULLED ELBOW (see ELBOW).

PULMONARY DISEASES (see LUNG DISEASES).

PULMONARY EMBOLISM is the condition in which an embolus (see EMBOLISM), or clot, is lodged in the lungs. The source of the clot is usually the veins of the lower abdomen or legs in which clot formation has occurred as a result of the occurrence of thrombophlebitis. (See VEINS, DISEASES OF.) Thrombophlebitis, with or without pulmonary embolism, is a not uncommon complication of surgical operations, especially in older patients. This is one reason why nowadays such patients are got up out of bed as quickly as possible, or, alternatively, are encouraged to move and exercise their legs regularly in bed. The severity of a pulmonary embolism, which is characterized by the sudden onset of pain in the chest, with or without the coughing up of blood, and a varying degree of shock, depends upon the size of the clot. If large enough it may prove immediately fatal. In other cases immediate operation may be needed to remove the clot, whilst in less severe cases anticoagulant treatment, in the form of heparin (qv), is given to prevent extension of the clot.

PULSATION, or throbbing, is an appearance seen or felt naturally below the fourth and fifth ribs on the left side, where the heart lies, and also at every point where an artery lies close beneath the surface. In other situations, it may be a sign of aneurysm. In nervous persons, particularly if thin, great pulsation can often be seen and felt in the upper part of the abdomen, due to the throbbing of the normal abdominal aorta.

PULSE – If the tip of one finger be laid gently on the front of the forearm, about one inch (25 mm) above the furrows that mark the wrist, and about half an inch (12 mm) from the outer edge, the pulsations of the radial artery can be felt. This is known as *the pulse*, but a pulse can be felt wherever an artery of large or medium

to 100, and is quicker in childhood and slower in old age than in middle life; it increases in all feverish states.

Further, the character of the vessel wall is of great importance. In childhood and youth the vessel wall is so thin that, when sufficient pressure is made to expel the blood from it, the artery can no longer be felt. In old age, however, and in some degenerative diseases, the vessel wall becomes so thick that it may be felt like a piece of whipcord rolling beneath the finger. The extent to which this change has taken place gives the physician valuable information as to the state of the arteries.

The size of the column felt also gives information. For example, after great muscular exertion, or when the heart is

346 – Pulse tracing, taken by the sphygmograph on smoked paper, from a case of atrial fibrillation in disease of the mitral valve. The pulse shows considerable irregularity.

347 – Pulse tracing from a case of incompetence of the aortic valve, showing the great extent to which the artery fills at each beat and empties between the beats.

size lies near the surface. (See HAEMORRHAGE.)

The cause of the pulsation lies in the fact that, at each heart-beat, 80 to 90 millilitres of blood are driven into the aorta, and a fluid wave, distending the vessels as it passes, is in consequence transmitted along the arteries all over the body. This pulsation gets less and less marked as the arteries grow smaller, and is finally lost in the minute capillaries, where a steady pressure is maintained. For this reason, the blood in the veins flows steadily on without any pulsation. Immediately after the wave has passed, the artery, by virtue of its great elasticity, regains its former size. In this wave the physician has a valuable means of studying both the state of the artery as regards elasticity and the heart's action.

The pulse rate is usually about 70 per minute, but it may vary in health from 50

beating strongly, the vessels of the limbs are full and the pulse is large.

Different types of heart disease have special features of the pulse associated with them. In atrial fibrillation the great character is irregularity (illustration 346). In cases in which the aortic valve is incompetent, the pulse has the peculiarity of rising very quickly and collapsing suddenly, suggesting the pulsation observed in the toy known as the water-hammer, after which this type is named (illustration 347). In persons of habitually relaxed physique, or suffering from some weakening fever, the pulse is apt to become dicrotic. (See DICROTIC.)

An instrument known as the sphygmograph has been devised, whereby the artery is made to register these waves. Another instrument known as the polygraph enables tracings to be taken from the pulse at the wrist and from the veins in the neck and simultaneous events in the two compared. The pressure of the blood in various arteries is estimated by an instrument known as the sphygmomanometer. (See BLOOD-PRESSURE.)

PULSES are the seeds of the *Leguminosa* family. They include peas, beans and lentils and constitute a valuable source of food. Most contain around 20 grams of protein per 100 grams of dry weight but the biological value of this protein requires supplementation to ensure an adequate intake of first class, or essential, amino-acids (qv). They have been described as 'the poor man's protein', and a combination of pulse and cereal proteins may have a nutritive value comparable to that of animal protein. (See also DIET.)

PUNCTATE BASOPHILIA (see BASOPHILIA.)

PUNCTUM is the term applied to a minute spot or puncture, especially to the lacrimal punctures near the inner end of the upper and lower eyelids. (See EYE.)

PUPIL is the opening in the centre of the iris through which rays of light pass into the eye. (See EYE.)

PURGATIVES are drugs or other measures which produce evacuation of the bowels.

Varieties and action – Purgatives are divided into several groups, according to the manner and degree of violence with which they act.

LAXATIVES are those which gently stimulate the bowels and render the motions slightly more frequent and softer without causing any griping. Most articles of food that leave a large indigestible residue upon which the intestine can contract, such as cabbage, brown bread, and oatmeal porridge, act in this way. Those fruits which contain rough seeds, sugar, and vegetable acids act similarly. Among the laxatives are honey, tamarinds, figs, raspberries, strawberries, prunes, stewed apples, senna and magnesia. Liquid paraffin also produces this effect.

SIMPLE PURGATIVES, or APERIENTS, produce one or more copious and slightly liquid movements, often accompanied or preceded by griping pains. Examples of this class are aloes, rhubarb, cascara sagrada, senna, castor oil.

DRASTIC PURGATIVES cause a violent action of the bowels, accompanied by considerable griping. In small doses many of them have a simple aperient action, while in excessive doses most are irritant poisons. Such are elaterium, colocynth, jalap, scammony, croton oil. Many of these produce very copious watery evacuations, and, since they remove a considerable quantity of water from the system, are known as *hydragogues*. These drastic purgatives are seldom used nowadays.

SALINE PURGATIVES are salts of the alkaline metals and alkaline earths. Such are sulphate of potassium, sulphate of sodium (Glauber's salt), sulphate of magnesium (Epsom salts), phosphate of sodium, bitartrate of potassium (cream of tartar), tartrate of potassium and sodium (Seidlitz powder), and citrate of magnesium. Taken in large doses, many of these salines also act as hydragogues.

Purgatives produce their effects either by stimulating the mucous membrane so that the amount of fluid in the intestine becomes larger, or by stimulating the muscular coat so that peristaltic contractions become more vigorous. Most purgatives have the double action, though one or other preponderates. Further, certain purgatives act all along the intestine, such as Epsom salts, whilst others, such as cascara, are almost devoid of action until they reach the large intestine. Castor oil, on the other hand, acts mainly on the small intestine.

Uses – The most common use of purgatives is to remove the contents of the bowels when their action is sluggish. (See CONSTIPATION.) In many cases of diarrhoea, due to the presence of irritating material in the intestine, a single dose of purgative medicine, such as castor oil, is given with the object of getting rid of the offending material, after which the diarrhoea ceases. In cases of inflammation affecting the bowels, saline purgatives are often given with the view of diminishing the congestion in the bowel-wall. In plethoric persons or persons for whom any strain may be harmful, such as in cases of threatened apoplexy, and, in persons suffering from hernia or aneurysm, laxatives are given to prevent straining at stool.

A protest must be entered against the common domestic practice of administering purgatives on every occasion of slight illness, especially in children, regardless of the complaint or symptoms. Undoubtedly some cases of malaise are due simply to constipation; but care must be taken that no serious trouble is present, for many persons have undoubtedly died through receiving only an aperient whom timely medical aid might have saved. (See

ABDOMEN, DISEASES OF.) Equally reprehensible is the still all too common practice, again especially in children, of giving a laxative simply because the child has missed emptying his or her bowels on one day. Nothing is more guaranteed to produce constipation, or irregular bowel action in later life, than this indiscriminate use of laxatives in childhood.

PURPURA is a disease characterized by the occurrence of purple-coloured spots upon the surface of the body, due to extravasations of blood in the skin, associated occasionally with haemorrhages from mucous membranes.

Causes – The condition is due either to an increased permeability of the smallest blood-vessels (ie. the capillaries) which allows blood to pass through their walls, or to a shortage of blood platelets which normally play an important part in sealing off any damage which may occur to the walls of the capillaries. The damage to the capillary wall may arise as a result of an infection, eg. scarlet fever; a toxic factor, eg. certain drugs; malnutrition or wasting, eg. in the terminal stages of cancer; or in scurvy. Such cases are described as *secondary purpuras*.

There are two other conditions in which purpura occurs and in which the cause can often not be found. One, sometimes known as *idiopathic thrombocytopenia*, or *primary thrombocytopenic purpura*, is definitely associated with a marked diminution in the number of blood platelets or thrombocytes (hence the name). The other, known as *anaphylactoid purpura*, is supposed to be an allergic condition, the increased permeability of the capillary wall being due to the individual coming in contact with, inhaling, or ingesting, some substance to which he is sensitized. Two special forms of anaphylactoid purpura are recognized. One is *Henoch's purpura*, in which the purpuric haemorrhages occur in the wall of the intestine, causing symptoms resembling an acute abdominal emergency. This form occurs in children and young adults. The other is *Schönlein's purpura*, in which the purpura occurs around the joints causing them to be painful and tender. This form principally affects young adults.

Symptoms – The complaint is usually ushered in by lassitude and feverishness. This is soon followed by the appearance on the surface of the body of the characteristic spots in the form of small red points scattered over the skin of the limbs and trunk. They are not raised above the surface, and they do not disappear on pressure. Their colour soon becomes deep purple or nearly black; but after a few days they undergo the changes which are observed in the case of an ordinary bruise, passing to a green and yellow hue and finally disappearing. When of minute size they are termed petechiae, when in patches of considerable size ecchymoses. They may come out in fresh crops over a lengthened period.

The form of the disease above described is that known as *purpura simplex*. A more serious form of the malady is that to which the term *purpura haemorrhagica* is applied. Here there is a tendency to the occurrence of haemorrhage from mucous surfaces, especially from the nose, but also from the mouth, lungs, stomach, bowels, kidneys, and womb, sometimes in large and dangerous amount. Great physical prostration is apt to attend this form of the disease, and a fatal result sometimes follows the successive haemorrhages, or is suddenly precipitated by the occurrence of an extravasation of blood into the brain.

Treatment – The treatment of *secondary purpura* consists of that of the underlying cause: eg. scurvy. The treatment of *primary thrombocytopenic purpura* consists of the administration of one of the cortisone-like drugs: eg. prednisolone. In cases which do not respond to such therapy, removal of the enlarged spleen is often helpful, especially in children. The treatment of *purpura haemorrhagica* is similar, except that surgical removal of the spleen is more likely to be called for. In severe cases, with heavy loss of blood, blood transfusion may be necessary. The treatment of *anaphylactoid purpura* consists of the administration of antihistamine drugs. If these fail, then it is worth trying the effect of prednisolone. If, as is often the case, there is any anaemia, this must be treated by the administration of full doses of iron: eg. ferrous sulphate.

PUS or MATTER, is a thick, white, yellow, or greenish fluid, which is found in abscesses, on ulcers, and on inflamed and discharging surfaces generally. Its colour and consistence are due to the presence, in great numbers, of pus corpuscles. These are derived mostly from the white corpuscles of the blood, and consist also of the superficial cells of granulation tissue or of a mucous membrane which die and are shed off in consequence of the inflammatory process. (See ABSCESS; PHAGOCYTOSIS.)

PUSTULE means a small collection of pus. (See ABSCESS.) Malignant pustule is one of the forms taken by woolsorters' disease. (See ANTHRAX.)

PUTREFACTION is the change that takes place in the bodies of plants and animals after death, whereby they are ultimately reduced to carbonic acid gas, ammonia, and other simple substances. The change is almost entirely due to the action of bacteria, and, in the course of the process, various offensive and poisonous intermediate substances are formed. In the case of the human body, putrescine,

When bodies decompose in water, particularly that drained from peaty soil, the skin becomes white and sodden and the changes take place more slowly. Sometimes, in these circumstances, instead of going through the usual changes, the body undergoes a process of saponification, and the tissues are converted into a mixture of soaps, fatty acids, and volatile substances known as *adipocere*. This does not readily undergo further changes, and so bodies lying in ponds or damp graves may become changed in the course of some months or years into this wax-like substance, after which they may be

348 – PUVA unit at the Institute of Dermatology, London. (Medical Research Council)

cadaverine, and other alkaloids are among these intermediate products.

The first sign of putrefaction is the appearance of a greenish tinge over the lower part of the abdomen, visible on the second or third day after death. This is not to be confused with the lividity seen on the back, due to the blood running down into the dependent parts, which is visible within eight or twelve hours. In from two to three weeks the body is greenish-brown throughout, the skin beginning to give way, and the features almost unrecognizable. By the end of one year, none of the organs is recognizable. After the lapse of four to seven years, bodies buried in gravel or sandy soil have lost all trace of the soft parts, the bones alone remaining.

preserved with the smallest details of feature for many years.

Mummification may prevent putrefaction in the dry air of deserts, and even in the case of a body lying in a strong draught of air these changes may be indefinitely postponed by gradual drying. A similar result has been known to occur in the bodies of persons who have taken antimony for a long period prior to death, the antimony deposited all through the body acting as an antiseptic.

PUTRID FEVER is an old name for typhus fever.

PUVA is a method of treating severe cases of psoriasis which do not respond to other forms of treatment. This consists of giving the patient a tablet of a psoralen preparation which sensitizes the skin cells to sunlight and then exposing him in a special cubicle (illustration 348) to high-intensity long-wave ultraviolet radiation (UVA). Hence the name PUVA: a combination of P for psoralen and UVA. Initially this treatment is given twice a week. Although not curative, it has proved highly effective, but can only be carried out in specially equipped hospital departments.

PYAEMIA means a form of blood-poisoning in which abscesses appear in various parts of the body. (See BLOOD-POISONING.)

PYELITIS means inflammation of that part of the kidney known as the pelvis, which is connected with the ureter. It is now realized, however, that the infection is seldom restricted to the pelvis, but involves the kidney tissue as well. In other words the correct diagnosis is pyelonephritis.

The inflammation may spread upwards from the bladder or may follow on febrile diseases in which bacteria leave the body by the urine. One of the commonest organisms productive of this condition is the *Escherichia coli*, which produces a highly acid state of the urine accompanied by the presence of pus. Pyelitis sometimes occurs as a complication of pregnancy. There are generally symptoms of feverishness, general malaise, loss of weight, discomfort in the region of the loins, and frequency in passing water. Examination reveals the presence of the infecting organism and of pus in the urine.

Treatment – In some cases the administration of alkalis and the drinking of ample bland fluids are all that is required. As a rule, however, more active treatment is necessary and this consists of the administration of mandelic acid, one of the sulphonamides, or an antibiotic. As pyelitis may be due to some other condition of the kidney, such as a stone, a full investigation is necessary, as such cases will not clear up unless the underlying cause is removed.

PYELOGRAPHY is the term applied to the process whereby the kidneys are rendered radio-opaque, and therefore visible on an X-ray film. It constitutes a most important part of the examination of a patient with kidney disease. (See SODIUM DIATRIZOATE.)

PYELONEPHRITIS (see PYELITIS).

PYKNOLEPSY is the term applied to a type of epilepsy in which the only manifestation is a sudden and temporary loss of consciousness. There are no convulsions and the attacks tend to disappear in time.

PYLEPHLEBITIS means inflammation of the portal vein. It usually results from disease in the intestine and is part of a general blood-poisoning.

PYLOROSPASM means spasm of the pyloric portion of the stomach. This interferes with the passage of food in a normal, gentle fashion into the intestine and causes the pain that comes on from half an hour to three hours after meals and is associated with severe disorders of digestion. It is often produced by an ulcer of the stomach or duodenum.

PYLORUS is the lower opening of the stomach, through which the softened and partially digested food passes into the small intestine.

PYO- is a prefix attached to the name of various diseases to indicate cases in which pus is formed, such as pyonephrosis.

PYOGENIC is a term applied to those bacteria which cause the formation of pus and so lead to the formation of abscesses. Although many bacteria have this property, the most common cause of abscess is one of the rounded forms of bacterium (eg. streptococcus).

PYORRHOEA is the name given to any copious discharge of pus. For *Pyorrhoea alveolaris* see under TEETH, DISEASES OF.

PYRETOTHERAPY is the term applied to the treatment of disease by raising the temperature of the body above normal.

PYREXIA means fever. (See FEVER.)

PYRIDINE is an alkaloidal substance derived from coal-tar and tobacco. It is added to methylated spirit in order to render this undrinkable.

PYRIDOXINE, or vitamin B_6, plays an important part in the metabolism of a number of amino-acids. Deficiency leads to atrophy of the epidermis, the hair follicles, and the sebaceous glands, and peripheral neuritis may also occur. Young infants are more susceptible to pyridoxine deficiency than adults: they begin to lose weight and develop a hypochromic anaemia; irritability and convulsions may also occur. Liver, yeast, and cereals are relatively rich sources of it. Fish is a moderately rich source, but vegetables and milk contain little. The minimal daily requirement in the diet is probably about 2 mg.

PYRIMETHAMINE is an antimalarial drug which is particularly valuable as a prophylactic.

PYRO- is a prefix meaning anything connected with fire or produced by heating.

PYROGALLIC ACID is a substance derived from gallic acid and used in the treatment of psoriasis. It has the disadvantage of staining the skin a deep brown colour.

PYROXYLIN is another name for gun-cotton, which is used for producing collodion. (See COLLODION.)

PYROSIS, or WATERBRASH, is a symptom of dyspepsia consisting of an irritable, burning pain in the throat, accompanied by the constant secretion of mouthfuls of saliva. (See DYSPEPSIA.)

PYURIA means the presence of pus in the urine, in consequence of inflammation situated in the kidney, bladder, or other part of the urinary tract. (See URINE.)

Q

Q FEVER is a disease of world-wide distribution, due to the *Coxiella burneti*. The disease is primarily one of animals, involving cattle, sheep and goats; half the cases reported in England have been due to drinking unpasteurized milk. In 1972, there were 59 cases in England, Wales and Northern Ireland. The disease occurs in small epidemics, and is characterized by fever, severe headache and some form of infection of the lungs, often pneumonia. The incubation period is two to three weeks, and the disease lasts for about a fortnight. It responds well to chloramphenicol, chlortetracycline, or oxytetracycline.

QUADRICEPS is the name of the large four-headed muscle occupying the front and sides of the thigh, which straightens the leg at the knee-joint and maintains the body in an upright position.

QUADRIPLEGIA means paralysis of the four limbs of the body.

QUADRUPLETS (see MULTIPLE BIRTHS).

QUARANTINE means that principle of preventing the spread of infectious disease by which persons, baggage, merchandise, and so forth likely to be infected or coming from an infected locality are isolated at frontiers or ports till their harmlessness has been proved to the satisfaction of the authorities. (See INFECTION.)

Originally quarantine, as its name implies, involved detention for forty days; but, as this proved intolerable for persons engaged in business, the time of detention is now calculated so as simply to cover the incubation period of the disease, the presence of which is suspected.

Numerous international conferences upon the subject have been held with the view of arriving at a uniform practice as regards quarantine in different countries. The diseases to which quarantine applies are cholera, yellow fever, plague, smallpox, typhus and relapsing fever.

The general practice with regard to quarantine is that when a serious disease breaks out in any country, the government of that country notifies surrounding governments as to the ports and other places that have become centres of infection. Any persons travelling from these centres and attempting to enter another country, are subject to measures prescribed in the appropriate Regulations. These measures vary with the disease involved; as often as not, today they merely involve keeping under the surveillance of the local medical officer through the incubation period of the disease in question.

QUARTAN AGUE is that form of malaria which returns after intermissions of two days: ie. every fourth day. (See MALARIA.)

QUASSIA is the wood of *Picrasna excelsa*, a large West Indian tree. Its virtues depend upon the presence of an active principle, quassin, which is excessively bitter and also irritating. The various preparations of the wood are mainly used as a bitter tonic. (See BITTERS.)

QUICKENING (see PREGNANCY).

QUILLAIA is the bark of *Quillaja saponaria*, or soapbark, a South American tree. Tincture of quillaia is used in cases of bronchitis, pleurisy, and for making emulsions, in doses of about 60 minims (4 ml).

QUINESTROL is a synthetic, long-acting oestrogen (qv).

QUINETHAZONE is a moderately powerful diuretic, active when given by mouth, with an action extending over eighteen hours.

QUINIDINE is an alkaloid obtained from cinchona bark and closely related in chemical composition and in action to quinine. It is commonly used in the form of quinidine sulphate in doses of 3 to 10 grains (200 to 600 mg). It is used in the treatment of the cardiac irregularity known as atrial fibrillation, being particularly useful in cases of recent onset.

QUININE is an alkaloid obtained from the bark of various species of cinchona trees. This bark is mainly derived from Peru and neighbouring parts of South America and the East Indies. For the story of its introduction see MALARIA. Other alkaloids and acid substances are also derived from cinchona bark, such as quinidine and cinchonine, but these closely resemble quinine in action.

Quinine is generally used in the form of one of its salts, such as the sulphate of quinine, or dihydrochloride of quinine. All are sparingly soluble in water, much more so when taken along with an acid.

Action – Quinine lessens the activity of lowly forms of life. It is therefore a powerful antiseptic. Its best-known action is in checking the recurrence of attacks of malaria, and this action it exerts by virtue of its destructive power against the malarial parasite in the blood. In fevers it acts as an antipyretic (qv).

In small doses it has a stimulating effect upon the stomach, although larger doses are capable of acting upon an irritable stomach to produce nausea and vomiting. Small doses have also a stimulating action upon the nervous system and a general tonic effect, whilst large doses cause decided depression of the respiration and the heart's action.

Among the other unpleasant effects, due to large doses, are ringing in the ears, temporary impairment of vision, and sometimes irritation of the kidneys: all these pass off when the drug is discontinued.

Uses – The most important use of quinine is its original one in malaria, attacks of which it quickly cuts short or prevents altogether, but it has largely been replaced by the more effective and less toxic antimalarial drugs now available. (See MALARIA.) For hypodermic injection, when this is necessary in cases of malaria, a soluble form of quinine, the dihydrochloride, is used in doses of 5 to 10 grains (300 to 600 mg). Blackwater fever has by some been attributed to the excessive use of quinine in severe cases of malaria. Ammoniated solution of quinine given in teaspoonful doses in water is a favourite household remedy in feverish colds and other mild febrile attacks. Quinine and urea hydrochloride is employed as a local anaesthetic with a prolonged effect. Quinine hydrochloride has been used with urethane as a sclerosing agent in the treatment of varicose veins (qv).

As a 'tonic', minute doses of quinine are used. For example, a single grain of quinine is often given after meals, or it is more commonly combined with other tonics, as in the citrate of iron and quinine, or in syrup of the phosphate of iron with quinine and strychnine.

QUINSY is a corruption of *cynanche*, and is an old name for a peritonsillar abscess (qv).

QUINTUPLETS (see MULTIPLE BIRTHS).

QUOTIDIAN AGUE means a type of malaria in which the attack recurs daily. (See MALARIA.)

R

RABIES is an acute and very fatal disease which affects the lower animals, particularly carnivora, and may be communicated from them to man. Infection from man to man is very rare, but those in attendance on a case should take precautions to avoid being bitten or allowing themselves to be contaminated by the patient's saliva as this contains the causative virus.

Cause – The disease is in existence constantly among dogs and wolves in some countries, and from these it spreads widely now and then in epidemics. It also occurs in foxes, coyotes and skunks, as well as vampire bats. Thanks to quarantine measures, it has been practically stamped out in Great Britain since 1897. The last case of human infection contracted in Britain was in 1911. Since 1946, thirteen cases have been diagnosed in Britain, in all of which the infection was acquired overseas. Recent cases of rabies in dogs in this country demonstrate that continuing. indeed increasing, vigilance is necessary if the United Kingdom is to be protected from the ravages of this dread disease. Particularly is such vigilance necessary in view of the way that the disease in animals is now spreading across Europe. Thus in France and West Germany 7,750 cases of rabies in animals were reported in 1975. In Europe, in 1974, there were 21 deaths from rabies, mainly in Poland, Turkey and Yugoslavia. In 1977, a man died of rabies in Switzerland after being bitten by a cat and a dog. In the whole of Western Europe, only Denmark and Britain are now free of rabies. Restrictions have accordingly been tightened up and under The Rabies Act 1974, which came into force in February 1975, all mammals, except farm livestock, brought into the country must come through designated ports (Dover [Eastern Docks], Harwich [Navy Yard Wharf], Hull, Liverpool, Southampton, and International Hoverport at Ramsgate) and airports (Birmingham, Edinburgh, Glasgow, Leeds, London [Gatwick and Heathrow], Manchester and Prestwick), have an import licence and undergo a compulsory six months' quarantine. Any animals brought in illegally may be destroyed on the spot, and the offender fined an unlimited amount, sentenced up to a year's imprisonment, or both. It also empowers the Government, in the event of the disease being confirmed in Britain again, to destroy foxes, control movement of domestic pets, ban hunts and dog and cat shows, and destroy stray animals.

It is highly infectious from the bite of an animal already affected, but the chance of infection from different animals varies. Thus only about one person in every four bitten by rabid dogs contracts rabies, whilst the bites of rabid wolves and cats almost invariably produce the disease. Bites on exposed parts, like the face, are more dangerous than those through the clothes. The disease is due to a virus which has a special affinity for attacking the nervous system. The test as to whether a dog, which has died, suffered from rabies, is to inject a preparation made from part of its brain into another animal, and to watch the latter for signs of the disease. In the brain of an affected animal, certain microscopic appearances known as *Negri bodies* can usually be found. The saliva of infected animals is highly poisonous.

Symptoms – In animals there are two types of the disease: mad rabies and dumb rabies. In the former, the dog runs about, snapping at objects and other animals, unable to rest; in the latter, which is also the final stage of the mad type, the limbs become paralysed, and the dog crawls about or lies still.

In man the incubation period is usually six to eight weeks, but may be as short as ten days or as long as two years. The disease begins by mental symptoms, the person becoming irritable, restless, and melancholy. At the same time, feverishness and difficulty of swallowing gradually come on. After a couple of days or so, the irritability passes into a state of wildness or terror, there is great difficulty in swallowing either food or drink. Even the mere sight of fluid may induce spasm of the muscles of the mouth and throat: hence the common name for the disease: hydrophobia (fear of water). Breathing, too, becomes difficult, because of spasm of the respiratory muscles. The flow of saliva is great, and therefore the patient is constantly spitting, and has a dry, short cough, which has given rise to the popular idea that he barks like a dog. A loud noise, a bright light, and particularly any attempt to drink are sufficient to throw the person into a convulsion. Convulsions and attacks of maniacal excitement become more frequent, and although between these the patient may be quite sensible and able to talk rationally, he becomes gradually weaker. Finally, about four days after the onset of the disease, the patient dies of exhaustion.

Treatment – The best treatment is, of course, preventive, and this may be attained by strict quarantine regulations and the slaughter of all animals bitten by, or coming into contact with, rabid dogs. The current regulations in the United Kingdom are a quarantine period of six months, and that the animal be given a dose of an inactivated rabies vaccine on entry into quarantine and another dose 28 days later. If a person has been bitten by a dog supposed to be rabid, the dog should not be killed at once, but should be carefully isolated for ten days; if, after this period it is still alive, it was non-infective at the time of biting.

Local treatment consists of immediate, thorough, and careful cleansing of the wound surfaces and surrounding skin with 20 per cent soap solution or any other detergent followed by flushing out with some antiseptic such as benzalkonium or cetrimide. Special attention should be paid to any deep fang punctures, which should be carefully probed with a swabstick dipped in strong nitric acid. Immediate suture of lacerations should not be carried out.

This is followed by a course of rabies vaccine therapy. Only persons bitten or in certain circumstances licked, either by a rabid animal or by one thought to be infected with rabies need treatment with rabies vaccine and antiserum and immunoglobulin (qv). The usual course is six injections given intramuscularly. A dose of rabies antiserum may be given with the first dose of vaccine, depending on the circumstances, such as the severity of the bites, whether located about the face and neck, whether the animal is known to have rabies and if it is a wild animal. The vaccine is also used to give protection to those liable to infection, such as kennel workers and veterinary surgeons: two intramuscularly injections four weeks apart, followed by a third a year later.

When the bitten person develops the disease, all that can be done is to quieten the convulsion by intravenous injections of a barbiturate, and to keep him as comfortable as possible by good nursing.

RACHIANAESTHESIA is the method of producing anaesthesia of a part of the body by the injection of anaesthetic drugs into the space round the spinal cord.

RADIATION SICKNESS is the term applied to the nausea, vomiting, and loss of appetite which may follow the use of radiotherapy in the treatment of cancer and other diseases. The antihistamine drugs, as well as one known as cysteamine, are proving of value in its prevention and treatment.

RADICULITIS is the condition in which the root or roots of a spinal nerve is or are inflamed.

RADIOACTIVE ISOTOPES (see ISOTOPES).

RADIOGRAPHY (see X-RAYS).

RADIONUCLIDE is another word for a radioactive isotope. (See ISOTOPES.)

RADIOTHERAPY is the term applied to treatment by radium or other radioactive matter, including X-rays. For long, radium and X-rays were the only sources available. Developments in our knowledge of atomic energy, however, have changed the picture entirely, and we have now at our disposal radioactive isotopes (see ISOTOPES) and X-ray machines which have largely replaced radium, except in the case of certain tumours.

Supervoltage X-ray machines are now available capable of producing X-rays generated at up to 22 million electron volts (22 MeV). These include linear accelerators (illustration 349) which produce X-rays at four or more million electron volts, and betatrons which produce X-rays at 22 million electron volts. The advantage of these supervoltage machines is that it is predominantly γ-rays they produce, which are penetrating rays and can therefore be used to treat deep-seated tumours.

Almost equally high concentrations of γ-rays can now be obtained from the use of certain radioactive isotopes, particularly cobalt and caesium. Thus a telecobalt machine (illustration 350) is now in use which contains 2000 curies or more of radioactive cobalt (Co^{60}), an amount equivalent to 3000 grams of radium (an unheard-of amount – the ordinary radium beam units contained only 10 grams of radium). Not only does this machine give a high concentration of γ-rays (equivalent to that from a 3 million-volt X-ray machine), it is absolutely safe for both patient and operators, and allows the beam to be directed accurately on the tumour.

Other forms of radiant energy are now coming into use in radiotherapy. One of

349 – The Dynaray 4 clinical linear accelerator. Radiation Dynamics Ltd.

these is electron-beam therapy. The usual source of electrons, one of the particles in the atomic nucleus, is the betatron, which can produce either electrons or X-rays at energies ranging from 18 to 42 MeV. Whilst the effect of electrons in the tissues of the body is the same as that of X-rays, their great practical advantage is that their effect can be concentrated on the part being treated, without any adverse effect on the surrounding normal tissue. The other form of radiant energy now being used is neutron therapy. Neutrons of 6 MeV energy are obtained from a cyclotron. One of the advantages of neutron therapy is that even if a cell is only partially damaged by neutrons it never recovers, but inevitably dies.

RADIUM – The radiations of radium consist of: (1) α-rays, which are positively charged helium nuclei; (2) β-rays, negatively charged electrons; (3) γ-rays, similar to X-rays but of shorter wave-length.

Treatment by radium – Radium salts are applied enclosed in various forms of applicator, most commonly a thin tube or plaque enclosed within a capsule of aluminium or platinum. External screens are made to enclose these fine tubes, serving the double purpose of filtration of the less penetrating rays and strengthening the applicators against damage when inserted into a tumour.

At the present day the use of radium is largely restricted to the treatment of carcinoma of the neck of the womb, the tongue, and the lips.

Neither X-rays nor radium supersede active surgical measures when these are available for the complete removal of a tumour.

RADIUS is the outer of the two bones in the forearm. (See BONE.)

RAG-SORTERS' DISEASE is another name for anthrax. (See ANTHRAX.)

RAILWAY SPINE is a form of compensation neurosis, in which the victim of a railway accident persists in complaining of pain in the back even though no cause for this can be found.

RANULA is the name given to a swelling which occasionally appears beneath the tongue, caused by a collection of saliva in the distended duct of a salivary gland. (See MOUTH, DISEASES OF.)

RAPHE means a ridge or furrow between the halves of an organ.

RAREFACTION is the term applied to the diminution in the density of a bone as a result of withdrawal of calcium salts from it.

RASH (see ERUPTION).

RAT-BITE FEVER is an infectious disease following the bite of a rat. There are two causative organisms – *Spirillum minus* and *Actinobacillus muris* – and the incubation period depends upon which is involved. In the case of the former it is 5 to 30 days; in the case of the latter it is 2 to 10 days. The disease is characterized by fever, a characteristic skin rash and often muscular or joint pains. It responds well to penicillin.

RAUWOLFIA is a drug used in the treatment of high blood-pressure, and as a tranquillizer. It is derived from the root of *Rauwolfia serpentina*, a plant which grows widely in India, Ceylon, Burma, and Malaya. The active medicinal properties, which reside mainly in the root of the plant, have been recognized for centuries in India, where extracts of the root were used for the treatment of fevers, insomnia, and nervousness.

It is mainly used in the form of reserpine, which is an alkaloid obtained from the root of the plant. (See ESSENTIAL HYPERTENSION; TRANQUILLIZERS.)

RAY-FUNGUS is the organism that causes woody tongue. (See ACTINOMYCOSIS.)

RAYNAUD'S DISEASE, so called after Maurice Raynaud (1834–81), the Paris physician who published a thesis on the subject in 1862, is a condition in which the circulation becomes suddenly obstructed in outlying parts of the body. It is supposed to be due to spasm of the smaller arteries in the part affected, as the result of nervous influences, and its effects are increased both by cold and by various diseases involving the blood-vessels. It is predominantly a disease of women, the majority of cases occurring before the age of 40.

Symptoms – The condition is most commonly confined to the occurrence of dead fingers, the fingers or the toes, ears, or nose becoming white, numb, and waxy-looking. The circulation is often so much reduced that the part does not bleed if pricked or cut. This condition may last for some minutes, or may not pass off for several hours, or even for a day or two. Persons affected in this way are often of a decidedly nervous temperament, and

350 – Mobaltron-80 rotational cobalt therapy unit, complete with counterweight and removable treatment table TEM Instruments Ltd.

737

suffer from 'bilious attacks' and other nervous disturbances.

In a more severe type, which depends apparently upon irregular contractions of the veins as well as of the arteries, periodic attacks come on in a similar manner, but the fingers and other parts affected, instead of being cold and white, are swollen, purple and tingling.

In a third form, which is fortunately rare, after repeated attacks of one of the other forms, the circulation becomes so much cut off that the part dies and a localized gangrene results.

Treatment – Persons who are subject to these attacks should be careful in winter to protect the feet and hands from cold, and should always use warm water when washing the hands. In addition, the whole body should be kept warm, as spasm of the arterioles in the feet and hands may be induced by chilling of the body. Victims of this disease should be advised to give up smoking. Iodides are also of value in early cases. In all cases which do not respond to such medical treatment, surgery should be considered in the form of sympathectomy: ie. cutting of the sympathetic nerves to the affected part. This results in dilatation of the arterioles and hence an improved blood supply. This operation is more successful in the case of the feet than in the case of the hands.

RAYON, OILED, consists of rayon fabric made waterproof with drying oils or oil-modified synthetic resins.

RECTUM is the last part of the large intestine. It pursues a more or less straight course downwards through the cavity of the pelvis, lying against the sacrum at the back of this cavity. This section of the intestine is about 9 inches (23 cm) long. Its first part is freely movable and corresponds to the upper three pieces of the sacrum, the second part corresponds to the lower two pieces of the sacrum and the coccyx, whilst the third part, known also as the anal canal, is about 1 inch (25 mm) long, runs downwards and backwards, and is kept tightly closed by the internal and external sphincter muscles which surround it. The opening to the exterior is known as the anus. The structure of the rectum is similar to that of the rest of the intestine. (See INTESTINE.)

RECTUM, DISEASES OF – Owing to the fact that this part of the intestine is more exposed to external influences than the rest of the bowels, and that it forms the place of lodgment of the stools prior to the evacuation of the bowels, and is therefore often subject to considerable irritation, the rectum is specially liable to various diseases.

Peculiarities of the motions are treated under STOOLS, while PILES and FISTULA are described under these headings. DIARRHOEA and CONSTIPATION are also treated separately.

IMPERFORATE ANUS, or absence of the anus, may occur in newly born children, and, unless the condition be relieved by operation within a few days, the child dies.

ITCHING at the anal opening, or PRURITUS ANI, is often very troublesome. It may be due to slight abrasions, piles, the presence of threadworms, and sometimes sexual irregularities. All stimulants, mustard and pepper must be avoided in the diet. After evacuation of the bowels, the part should be bathed with cotton-wool and warm or cold water; it is sometimes an advantage to add starch to the water. Toilet paper should not be used. In addition, the area should be bathed once or twice a day. Clothing should be loose and smooth – preferably cotton or linen next to the skin. Calamine lotion, containing 1 per cent phenol, or 0·1 to 0·5 per cent camphor, is soothing – applied as a compress on gauze at night and dabbed on during the day. The local application of hydrocortisone ointment is often effective.

PAIN of an acute cutting character, at stool, is often due to the presence of a small ulcer or 'fissure', which, owing to movements of the sphincter, will not heal; it is treated by rubbing the ulcer with a caustic point or injecting into it a local anaesthetic of prolonged action. The pain soon disappears. Pain of an aching nature is not uncommonly caused by the presence of piles. (See also PROCTALGIA.)

ULCERATION may occur here in the course of tuberculous disease of the bowels, in dysentery, or even as the result of the constant irritation due to long-continued constipation. Ulcers in this locality cause a discharge of matter and often streaks of blood mixed with the motions. If the ulcer lasts a long time it may lead to narrowing and obstruction of the bowel.

ABSCESS in the cellular tissue at the side of the rectum, known from its position as an ischio-rectal abscess, is fairly common. It often arises at a late stage in the course of pulmonary tuberculosis, and is a serious sign with regard to hope of ultimate cure of the disease. It may also arise, like an abscess elsewhere, as the result of injury, exposure to cold, and other debilitating influences. In any case it is likely to produce a fistula. (See FISTULA.)

PROLAPSE or protrusion of the rectum is sometimes found in children, usually between the ages of 6 months and 2 years. In slight cases, where a ring of bright red mucous membrane half an inch or an inch (12 or 25 mm) in width protrudes as the result of straining at stool, the condition is generally easily curable. Any irritable condition of the bowels due to diarrhoea, constipation or worms, must be removed and the evacuations regulated by diet and laxatives, so as to avoid all straining. Each time the bowels move, the protruded portion must be returned by steady pressure with a cloth or sponge wrung out of cold water. If the bowel comes down when the child runs about, the wearing of a suitable pad is necessary, or the buttocks are strapped together and the child must lie down for some time each day. The general health is attended to by suitable treatment. When the protruded part is very large and the condition does not yield to simple treatment it can be remedied by operation but this is not usually necessary, as the prolapse ceases to occur as the child grows older.

TUMOURS of small size situated on the skin near the opening of the bowel, and consisting of nodules, tags of skin, or cauliflower-like excrescences, are common, and may give rise to pain, itching, and watery discharges. These are easily removed if necessary. Polypi occasionally develop within the rectum, and may give rise to no pain, though they may cause frequent discharges of blood. Like polypi elsewhere, they may often be removed by a minor operation. (See POLYPOSIS.)

CANCER of the rectum is fairly common, this part of the bowel being one of the chief sites of this disease. In 1977, in England there were 5757 deaths from cancer of the rectum. It is a disease of later life, seldom affecting young people, and its appearance is generally insidious. The tumour begins commonly in the mucous membrane, its structure resembling that of the glands with which the membrane is furnished, and it quickly infiltrates the other coats of the intestine and then invades neighbouring organs. Secondary growths in most cases occur soon in the lymphatic glands within the abdomen and in the liver. The symptoms appear gradually and consist of diarrhoea, alternating with attacks of constipation, and, later on, discharges of blood or of thin blood-stained fluid from the bowels, together with increasing loss of weight and weakness, and pains about the lower part of the back and down the thighs. Upon examination, the tumour can be felt projecting from one side or in a ring-form into the interior of the bowel. These cases are usually far advanced before they give rise to much disturbance, but much can now be done to help them by surgical operation. In the majority of cases this consists of removal of the whole of the rectum and the distal two-thirds of the sigmoid colon, and the establishment of a colostomy (qv). Approximately 50 per cent of the patients who have this operation are alive and well after five years. In some cases in which the growth occurs in the upper part of the rectum it is now possible to remove the growth and preserve the anus so that the patient is saved the discomfort of having a colostomy.

RECURRENT LARYNGEAL NERVE is a branch of the vagus nerve which leaves the latter low down in its course, and, hooking round the right subclavian artery on the right side and round the arch of the aorta on the left, runs up again into the neck, where it enters the larynx and supplies branches to the muscles which control the vocal cords. The importance of this nerve consists in the fact that it is apt in this long course to be pressed upon, especially when aneurysm of the aorta or right subclavian artery is present, and thus defects of vocalization may point to disease situated within the chest.

RED GUM is the popular name for a red rash that often appears in children about teething-time, generally associated with diarrhoea. It is treated by care in dieting.

The term is also applied to the gum of the eucalyptus tree, which has astringent properties and is much used in throat pastilles.

RED LOTION is a lotion containing sulphate of zinc, compound tincture of lavender which gives it a red colour, and water. It is used as an astringent application to ulcers.

REDUPLICATION is a term applied to a peculiarity in the heart-sounds as heard by auscultation. Whilst it is found in certain diseases of the heart, such as obstruction at the mitral valve, it also occurs in normal hearts.

REDUX is a term applied to the reappearance of certain signs or symptoms which are absent at the height of a disease, and the reappearance of which indicates that the disease is passing off. Such are redux crepitations at the end of pneumonia.

REFLEX ACTION is one of the simplest forms of activity of the nervous system. (For the mechanism upon which it depends, see NERVES.) Reflex acts are divided usually into three classes. *Superficial reflexes* comprise the sudden movements which result when the skin is brushed or pricked, such as the movement of the toes that results from stroking the sole of the foot. *Deep reflexes* depend upon the state of mild contraction in which muscles are constantly maintained when at rest, and are obtained, as in the case of the knee-jerks, by sharply tapping the tendon of the muscle in question. *Visceral reflexes* are those connected with various organs, such as the narrowing of the pupil when a bright light is directed upon the eye, and the contraction of the bladder when distended by urine.

Faults in these reflexes, both in the direction of excess and of diminution, give valuable evidence as to the presence of nervous diseases and the part of the nervous system in which such disease is situated. Thus, absence of the knee-jerk, when the patellar tendon is tapped, means some interference with the sensory nerve, nerve-cells, or motor nerve upon which the act depends, as, for example, in poliomyelitis, or peripheral neuritis; whilst an excessive jerk implies that the controlling influence exerted by the brain upon this reflex mechanism has been cut off, as, for example, by a tumour high up in the spinal cord, or in the disease known as multiple sclerosis.

The condition of the plantar reflex (obtained by stroking the skin of the sole of the foot) is an important point in diagnosing organic disease of the nervous system. The normal reflex consists in bending downwards of the toes towards the sole. In organic disease of the higher parts of the nervous system the great toe tends to bend upwards with spreading out of the other toes (Babinski's sign).

The reflex of the pupil to light is also of great diagnostic importance. The pupil quickly contracts when light falls upon the eye or when the eyes are directed suddenly to a near object. In certain serious diseases of the nervous system, especially in general paralysis and locomotor ataxia, the contraction on looking at a near object remains, while the effect of light is lost (Argyll-Robertson pupil).

REFRACTION (see SPECTACLES).

REFRIGERANTS are substances which relieve thirst and give a feeling of coolness. The chief refrigerants are acidulous drinks such as lemon juice, weak mineral acids, and tartaric acid, in water. The parched condition of the mouth and throat that arises during hard work in a dry and dusty atmosphere is best relieved by water to which has been added some demulcent substance which forms a coating on the dried mucous membrane. Such liquids are obtained by mixing oatmeal or milk with water. (See also CITRIC ACID; and IMPERIAL DRINK.)

REFRIGERATION ANAESTHESIA (see CRYMOTHERAPY).

REGIONAL ILEITIS (see under ILEITIS).

REGURGITATION is a term used in various connections in medicine. For instance, in diseases of the heart it is used to indicate a condition in which, as the result of valvular disease, the blood does not entirely pass on from the atria of the heart to the ventricles, or from the ventricles into the arteries. The defective valve is said to be incompetent, and a certain amount of blood leaks past it, or regurgitates back, into the cavity from which it has been driven. (See HEART, DISEASES OF.) The term is also applied to the return to the mouth of food already swallowed and present in the gullet or stomach.

REHABILITATION is the restoration to health and working capacity of a person incapacitated by disease, mental or physical, or by injury. It is a word that came into prominent use during the 1939–45 War, reflecting the growing awareness of the medical profession that the treatment of a sick or injured person does not end at the moment of recovery from the immediate effects of illness or injury. For example, a man with a fractured limb or spine has to recover full use not only of the injured part but of his whole body; and he has to recover confidence in his ability to work and enjoy life. (See DISABLED PERSONS; REMPLOY.)

REITER'S DISEASE is a condition characterized by arthritis, urethritis, and conjunctivitis. The cause of the condition is not known.

RELAPSE means the return of a disease during the period of convalescence. Many relapses are due to some injudicious exposure or exertion on the patient's part, or to some error in diet, although certain diseases, such as typhoid fever, are particularly liable to relapses.

RELAPSING FEVER, so-called because of the characteristic temperature chart (illustration 351) showing recurring bouts of fever, is an infectious disease caused by spirochaetes. There are two main forms of the disease.

ture subsides after five or six days, to rise again in about a week (illustration 351). There may be up to four such relapses.

Treatment – Preventive measures are the same as those for typhus (qv). Rest in bed is essential, as are good nursing and a light, nourishing diet. There is usually a quick response to penicillin. The tetracyclines and chloramphenicol are also effective. Following such treatment the incidence of relapse is about 15 per cent. The mortality rate is low, except in a starved population.

TICK-BORNE RELAPSING FEVER is an endemic disease which occurs in most tropical and sub-tropical countries.

351 – Temperature chart in a case of louse-borne relapsing fever.

LOUSE-BORNE RELAPSING FEVER is an epidemic disease, usually associated with wars and famines, which has occurred in practically every country in the world. For long confused with typhus and typhoid, it was not until the 1870's that the causal organism was described by Obermeier. It is now known as the *Borrelia recurrentis*, a motile spiral organism 10 to 20 micrometres in length. The organism is transmitted from man to man by the louse. *Pediculus humanus.*

Symptoms – The incubation period is up to 12 days, usually 7 days. The onset is sudden, with high temperature, generalized aches and pains, and nose-bleeding. In about half the cases a rash appears at an early stage, beginning in the neck and spreading down over the trunk and arms. Jaundice may occur; and both the liver and the spleen are enlarged. The tempera-

The causative organism is *Borrelia duttoni,* which is transmitted by a tick, *Ornithodorus moubata.* David Livingstone suggested that it was a tick-borne disease, but it was not until 1905 that Dutton and Todd produced the definite evidence.

Symptoms – The main differences from the louse-borne disease are: (*a*) the incubation period is usually shorter, 3 to 6 days, but may be as short as 2 days or as long as 12; (*b*) the febrile period is usually shorter and the afebrile periods are more variable in duration, sometimes only lasting for a day or two; (*c*) relapses are much more numerous.

Treatment – Preventive measures are more difficult to carry out than in the case of the louse-born infection. Protective clothing should always be worn in 'tick country'. Old, heavily infected houses should be destroyed. Curative

741

treatment is the same as for the louse-borne infection.

RELAXED THROAT (see THROAT, DISEASES OF; and CLERGYMAN'S SORE THROAT).

REMITTENT FEVER is the term applied to the form of fever in which, during remissions, the temperature falls, but not to normal.

REMPLOY is a company set up under the provisions of the Disabled Persons (Employment) Act 1944 to provide employment for severely disabled persons. A person seeking employment with Remploy must be on the Disabled Persons Employment Register, which is maintained by the Manpower Services Commission through its Employment Services Agency. Those employed by Remploy are people who, because of the nature and degree of their disability, would find it difficult or impossible to obtain and retain work in open industry. In its 87 factories scattered throughout England, Scotland and Wales it provides work at as near normal industrial conditions as possible. Employees work a normal 40-hour week for an agreed basic wage. In 1966–67 over 153 different products and services were being made and provided in its factories by 8,200 disabled employees, with sales running around £24 million. Full details can be obtained from Remploy Ltd., 415 Edgware Road, Cricklewood, London NW2 6LR. (See also DISABLED PERSONS.)

RENAL DISEASES (see KIDNEYS, DISEASES OF).

RENIN is a protein-like substance extracted from the kidney which, when injected into animals, causes a rise of blood-pressure. This it does, apparently, by reacting with a substance normally present in the blood plasma to produce angiotonin. Angiotonin has been obtained in crystalline form, and it is angiotonin which causes the rise in blood-pressure. This work may have an important bearing on the problem of high blood-pressure in man.

RENNET is a substance prepared from the stomach of the calf, in order to curdle and partially digest milk. Its activity depends upon a ferment known as rennin. Rennet is used for the preparation of junkets and in the making of cheese.

REPAIR of tissues after injury is described generally under WOUNDS, and the repair of special tissues which present various peculiarities is described under BONE; MUSCLES; NERVES, etc.

RESECTION is the name given to an operation in which a part of some organ is removed, as, for example, the resection of a fragment of dead bone.

RESERPINE is an alkaloid obtained from the root of Rauwolfia (qv), and is used as an anti-hypertensive and a tranquillizing agent.

RESINS are solid or semi-solid exudations from plants, which are insoluble in water, mostly soluble in alcohol or ether, soften or melt at moderate temperatures, and burn with a smoky flame. They are transparent when pure, but opaque when they contain water. They are non-conductors of electricity. Some of them are acids and combine with alkalis to form soaps. A *natural resin* is one that occurs as an exudation, such as mastic. A *prepared resin* is made from a drug, such as podophyllin, or from a natural oleoresin such as rosin which is obtained from various species of *Pinus*. Oleoresins may be either natural oleoresins, which are mixtures of volatile oils and resins generally obtained by incising trunks of trees, such as turpentine and copaiba; or prepared oleoresins which are concentrated liquid preparations made from drugs containing both volatile oil and resin, such as capsicum. *Gum resins* are natural mixtures of gums and resins, usually obtained as exudations from plants, such as myrrh and asafoetida. (See also ION EXCHANGE RESINS.)

RESOLUTION is a term applied to infective processes, to indicate a natural subsidence of the inflammation without the formation of pus. Thus a pneumonic lung is said to resolve when the material exuded into it is absorbed into the blood and lymph, so that recovery takes place naturally; an inflamed area is said to resolve when the inflammation fades away and no abscess forms; a glandular enlargement is said to resolve when it decreases in size without suppuration. Resolvents was an old term applied to procedures capable of assisting this process. (See BLISTERS; and INFLAMMATION.)

RESONANCE means the lengthening and intensification of sound produced by striking the body over an air-containing structure. Decrease of resonance is called dullness and increase of resonance is called hyper-resonance. The process of striking the chest or other part of the body to discover its degree of resonance is called percussion, and according to the note obtained, an opinion can be formed as to the state of consolidation of air-containing organs, the presence of abnormal cavities, and the dimensions and relations of solid and air-containing organs lying together. (See also AUSCULTATION.)

RESORCIN, or RESORCINOL, is a white, crystalline, antiseptic substance soluble in water, alcohol, and oils. It is mainly used in skin diseases which require a stimulating and antiseptic application.

RESPIRATION is the process in which air passes into and out of the lungs with the object of allowing the blood to absorb oxygen and to give off carbon dioxide and water. This occurs 18 times a minute in a healthy adult at rest, this being known as the respiratory rate. In other words we inspire more than 25,000 times a day and during this time inhale around 35 pounds of air.
Mechanism of respiration – For the structure of the respiratory apparatus see AIR PASSAGES; CHEST; LUNGS. The air passes rhythmically into and out of the air passages, and mixes with the air already in the lungs, these two movements being known as inspiration and expiration.
INSPIRATION is due to a muscular effort which enlarges the chest in all three dimensions, so that the lungs have to expand in order to fill up the vacuum that would otherwise be left, and the air accordingly enters these organs by the air passages. It must be understood that there is no direct pull upon the lungs, each of which is simply suspended within the corresponding pleural cavity by its root, and made to fill this cavity in all conditions of the chest by the pressure of the outer air exerted through the nose, mouth, and air passages. The increase of the chest in size from above downwards is mainly due to the diaphragm, the muscular fibres of which, by their contraction, reduce its domed shape and cause it to descend, pushing down the abdominal organs beneath it. The increase from before back is mainly due to a tilting forwards of the lower end of the breast-bone, and of the lower rib cartilages. The increase from side to side can best be understood by examining a skeleton, noting the very oblique position of the lower ribs, and observing how greatly the capacity of the chest is increased when each is raised, in the manner of a bucket-handle, taking its fixed points at the spine and breast-bone. (See RIBS.)

The muscles which chiefly bring about these changes in ordinary quiet inspiration are the diaphragm, intercostal muscles, and levators of the ribs, whilst in forced or extraordinary inspiration, when a specially deep breath is taken, the sternocleidomastoid, serratus magnus, trapezius, and pectoral muscles are also brought powerfully into play. Many other muscles take part to a slight extent, steadying the spine and the upper and lower ribs, while even the muscles of the face and of the larynx are thrown rhythmically into activity, dilating the nostrils and the entrance to the larynx at each breath.
EXPIRATION is in ordinary circumstances simply an elastic recoil, the diaphragm rising and the ribs sinking into the position that they naturally occupy, when muscular contraction is finished. Expiration occupies a slightly longer period than inspiration. In forced expiration many powerful muscles of the abdomen and thorax are brought into play, and the act may be made a very forcible one, as, for example, in coughing.
Nervous control – Respiration is usually either an automatic or a reflex act, each expiration sending up afferent, sensory impulses to the central nervous system, from which efferent impulses are sent down various other nerves to the muscles that produce inspiration. It appears that there are several centres which govern the rate and force of the breathing, although all are presided over by a chief respiratory centre in the medulla oblongata, which is sometimes spoken of as the vital knot (*noeud vital*). Although this centre appears to be absolutely essential to life, it in turn is under the control of the higher centres in the cerebral hemispheres, through which the will acts, so that breathing can be voluntarily stopped, quickened, or otherwise changed at will. It would be impossible, however, to cause death by voluntarily holding the breath, because, as the blood becomes more venous, the vital centre in the medulla again assumes control and breathing starts again. Apart from changes due to will-power, the respirations follow one another rhythmically at the rate of about 18 per minute, being in general one for every four heart-beats.
Quantity of air – The lungs do not by any means completely empty themselves

at each expiration and refill at each inspiration. An amount equivalent, in quiet respiration, to less than one-tenth of the total air in the lungs passes out and is replaced by the same quantity of fresh air, which mixes with the stale air in the lungs. This renewal, which in quiet breathing amounts to about 500 millilitres, is known as the *tidal air*. By a special inspiratory effort, one can, however, draw in about 3000 millilitres, this amount being known as *complemental air*. By a special expiratory effort, too, after an ordinary breath one can expel much more than the tidal air from the lungs, this extra amount being known as the *supplemental* or *reserve air*, and amounting to about 1300 millilitres. If one takes as deep an inspiration as possible and then makes a forced expiration, one breathes out the sum of these three, which is known as the *vital capacity*, and amounts to about 4000 millilitres in a healthy adult male of average size. These figures all apply to a man of average height. Figures for women are about 25 per cent lower. The vital capacity varies with size, sex, age and ethnic origin. The following formulae, incorporating age, height and sex, give an approximate guide to the vital capacity:

Men:

vital capacity (in millilitres)
$$= [27.63 - (0.112 \times \text{age})] \times \text{height}$$
(in centimetres)

Women:

vital capacity (in millilitres)
$$= [21.78 - (0.101 \times \text{age})] \times \text{height}$$
(in centimetres)

Over and above the vital capacity, the lungs contain air which cannot be expelled by the strongest possible expiration. This *residual air*, as it is known, which remains in the lungs even after death, amounts to another 1500 millilitres.

Tests of respiratory efficiency are being increasingly used to assess lung function in health and disease. The most widely used one is based on an analysis of a single forced expiration after a maximal inspiration. The volume expelled in the first second of expiration (known as FEV_1) correlates well with the respiratory efficiency. Normal values for FEV_1 vary with age, sex and, to a lesser extent, with the size of the body but, by and large, healthy persons can breathe out 15 per cent or more of vital capacity within the first second.

Abnormal forms of respiration – Apart from mere changes in rate and force, respiration is modified in several important ways, either involuntarily or voluntarily. *Sighing* is a long-drawn inspiration following a pause when breathing has been checked by mental preoccupation. This form of breathing also characterizes some conditions of extreme weakness of the nervous system, such as shock and diabetic coma. *Sobbing* is a series of convulsive inspirations, at each of which the larynx is partially closed; it follows grief or great exertion. *Snoring*, or stertorous breathing, is due to a flaccid state of the soft palate causing it to vibrate as the air passes into the throat, or simply to sleeping with the mouth open, which has a similar effect. *Coughing* is a series of violent expirations, at each of which the larynx is suddenly opened after the pressure of air in the lungs has risen considerably; its object is to expel some irritating substance from the air passages. *Sneezing* is a single sudden expiration, which differs from coughing in that the sudden rush of air is directed by the soft palate up into the nose in order to expel some source of irritation from this narrow passage. *Cheyne-Stokes' breathing* (qv) is a type of breathing found in persons suffering from apoplexy, Bright's disease, heart disease, and some other conditions, in which death is impending; it consists in an alternate dying away and gradual strengthening of the inspirations. Other disorders of breathing are found in LARYNGISMUS STRIDULUS and in ASTHMA (qv).

RESPIRATORY DISTRESS SYNDROME (see HYALINE MEMBRANE DISEASE).

RESPIRATORY SYNCYTIAL VIRUS, or RS VIRUS as it is usually known, is one of the myxoviruses (qv). It is the major cause of bronchiolitis and pneumonia in infants under the age of 6 months.

RESUSCITATION (see DROWNING, RECOVERY FROM).

RETCHING is an ineffectual form of vomiting. (See VOMITING.)

RETE MUCOSUM is an old name for the true skin. (See SKIN.)

RETENTION OF URINE (see URINE, RETENTION OF).

RETICULOCYTES is the name given to newly formed red blood corpuscles, in which a fine network can be demonstrated by special staining methods.

RETICULO - ENDOTHELIAL SYSTEM consists of highly specialized cells scattered throughout the body, but found mainly in the spleen, bone marrow, liver, and lymph glands. Their main function is the ingestion of red blood cells and the conversion of haemoglobin to bilirubin. They are also able to ingest bacteria and foreign colloidal particles.

RETICULOSES is the term used to describe a group of conditions characterized by progressive widespread proliferation of the cells of the reticuloendothelial system. The two most important members of this group are Hodgkin's disease (qv) and lymphosarcoma (qv).

RETINA is the innermost and light-sensitive coat of the eyeball. (See EYE.)

RETINA, DISEASES OF – Diseases of the retina are often part and parcel of some general disease; particularly is this the case when the disease involves the blood-vessels, as, for instance, in high blood-pressure. This is why careful examination of the retina by means of the ophthalmoscope (qv) is an essential part of the medical examination of anyone who is found to have high blood-pressure, nephritis (Bright's disease), or diabetes mellitus, for instance. The changes induced by disease of the retinal blood-vessels used to be described as retinitis. This, however, is not an accurate description as it suggests some inflammatory process. The term more generally used now is retinopathy, which merely indicates some disturbance of the retina.

RETINOPATHY due to degenerative changes in the retinal blood-vessels occurs predominantly in three conditions: hypertension (or high blood-pressure), diabetes mellitus, and toxaemia of pregnancy. These changes result in the vessels becoming permeable so that exudates (qv) are formed in the retina. Because of their characteristic appearance they are known as cotton-wool patches. There may also be haemorrhages. These, along with the thickening of the walls of the blood-vessels, can be seen quite distinctly with the ophthalmoscope (qv). The changes produced by different diseases are often quite distinctive. The treatment is that of the underlying disease.

In some cases of arteriosclerosis, with or without high blood-pressure, there may be sudden blockage of one of the arteries of the retina. If the central artery of the retina is involved, the eye becomes suddenly blind. Whether or not sight returns to the affected eye depends largely upon how long the obstruction persists.

RETINITIS PIGMENTOSA, or PIGMENTARY RETINAL DYSTROPHY, is a hereditary, slow degenerative disease of the retina, beginning in childhood and often resulting in blindness in middle age. Methods are now available whereby carriers of the disease (that is, people who do not suffer from the disease but are capable of transmitting it to their children) can be diagnosed. The disease can be detected in children before any signs of it appear, by means of electro-oculography (qv) and electro-retinography (qv). Those suffering from the disease and their relatives can obtain information and advice from the Retinitis Pigmentosa Society, 12 Ridge Green, South Nutfield, Nr Redhill, Surrey RH1 5RN. The first evidence of it is usually night blindness. There is no effective treatment.

DETACHMENT OF THE RETINA takes two forms. *Simple Detachment* is due to the formation of a hole in the retina, which allows fluid from the vitreous to leak through and raise the retina from its base. The hole or tear is usually due to degenerative changes in the retina, which are most common in short-sighted people and in those who have had a cataract (qv) removed. It may also be due to localized disease of the retina. The actual detachment is usually produced by some special form of exertion such as heavy lifting. The condition manifests itself by transient flashes of light, or as if a cloud has come over the front of the eye. Treatment consists of fixing the retina. This is done by a variety of means, including diathermy, light coagulation, or laser (qv). The prognosis is good in healthy individuals who are operated on at an early stage: from 75 to 90 per cent of cases recover a satisfactory degree of vision. *Secondary Detachment* is due to the retina being pushed away from its bed by a tumour or a haemorrhage, or being pulled away by some form of disease of the retina. The outcome in these cases is steadily improving as a result of advances in treatment.

RETROLENTAL FIBROPLASIA is a disturbance of the retina which was responsible for a high proportion of blindness in children. It is almost entirely confined to premature infants, and is now known to be due to the administration of excessive amounts of oxygen to premature infants. Since oxygen concentrations have been restricted to below 35 per cent, the condition has practically disappeared.

RETRO- is a prefix signifying behind or turned backward.

RETROBULBAR NEURITIS is the term applied to inflammation of the optic nerve just behind the eyeball.

RETROFLEXION means bending of an organ so that its top is thrust backwards. Retroversion is a similar displacement in which the whole organ is turned backwards. These terms are particularly applied to the uterus.

RETROPHARYNGEAL ABSCESS is the name given to an abscess occurring in the cellular tissue behind the throat. It is the result in general of disease in the upper part of the spinal column.

RETROPULSION is the term applied to the involuntary act of running backwards which occurs in patients suffering from rigid paralysis: for example, paralysis agitans or Parkinsonism.

RHABDOVIRUSES is a group of viruses which includes the rabies virus.

RHATANY is the root of *Krameria triandra*, a South American plant, which contains an astringent principle. It is mainly used in diarrhoea in the form of a tincture or extract, and to make lozenges for use in cases of relaxed throat.

RHESUS FACTOR (see BLOOD GROUPS).

RHEUMATIC FEVER is another term for acute rheumatism. (See RHEUMATISM.)

RHEUMATISM is a general term applied to a group of diseases, which have for their chief manifestations inflammatory or degenerative affections of the fibrous textures of joints, muscles, and other parts. The term is a very old one based upon the idea that the disease was of a moist nature leading to watery deposits in the joints. The parts affected may be the joints alone, either in acute or chronic form; or various other tissues, especially the fibrous tissues and nerves, may be affected, either with or without disorder in the joints. No satisfactory classification of this heterogeneous collection of diseases has yet been evolved, but the following, recommended by the Royal College of Physicians of London, is probably the best: (1) acute rheumatism (or rheumatic fever) and subacute rheumatism; (2) non-articular rheumatism; (3) gout; (4) chronic arthritis, which includes rheumatoid arthritis and osteoarthrosis. Gout is described elsewhere (see GOUT), and the remaining conditions will be noticed here.

ACUTE RHEUMATISM, or RHEUMATIC FEVER, is a general disorder accompanied by much pain in the joints, feverishness, and copious perspiration, with a tendency to spread in an erratic manner, and to involve the smooth membranes lining various cavities of the body, particularly the heart.

Causes – The nature of this disease is still unknown, but there appears to be a definite association with streptococcal infections. There is, for example, the common association of recurrent attacks of streptococcal tonsillitis with subacute rheumatic fever and the streptococcal tonsillitis which so often precedes the attack of acute rheumatic fever. This, however, is not the whole story, and the reports on the effect of cortisone, a hormone produced by the cortex of the suprarenal glands, suggests that the underlying cause of rheumatic fever may be some biochemical or metabolic disturbance of the tissues due to lack of this hormone.

Certain predisposing causes are generally admitted. The disease is prevalent in the late autumn, October, and November in Britain, but in other countries reaches its chief frequency about March. It is rare before the age of 3 years, occurs most commonly in childhood and adolescence, and becomes increasingly less common after adult life is attained. If chorea be excluded, the disease is equally common in the two sexes. There is some evidence that the disease tends to occur in certain families and the suggestion has been put forward that there is a genetic constitution that favours the rheumatic response to infection with streptococci. The condition tends to occur more commonly in children with a high complexion and a reddish tint in their hair. The disease is more common among the poorer classes. Any depressing cause acting upon the general health, such as overwork or anxiety, may precipitate an attack in persons predisposed to them. Attacks of acute rheumatism may follow exposure to cold and damp and excessive fatigue. Persons who have once suffered from this disease are liable to a recurrence.

The relationship to diseases caused by the haemolytic streptococcus is particularly important. Thus, an attack of rheumatic fever is often preceded by a sore throat or tonsillitis due to this organism. This is especially apt to occur with recurrent attacks. Occasionally rheumatic fever follows an attack of scarlet fever, which is a disease due to the haemolytic streptococcus. Chorea (qv) is a manifestation of rheumatic fever; in 25 per cent of rheumatic children it is the first sign of the disease. In recent years there has been a marked decline in the incidence of the disease and in its severity in Britain and in other parts of the Western world.

Symptoms – An attack of acute rheumatism usually begins with chilliness or rigors, followed by feverishness and a feeling of stiffness or pain in one or more joints, generally those of larger size, such as the knee, ankle, wrist or shoulder. The pain soon becomes intense and is accompanied by severe constitutional disturbance. The patient lies helpless in bed, restless, but afraid to move or to be touched, and often unable to bear even the weight of the bed-clothes. The face is flushed, and the whole body bathed in perspiration, which has a sour, disagreeable odour and highly acid reaction. The temperature is elevated: usually about 103° F (39·5° C); the pulse is rapid, full, and soft; the tongue is coated, and there are thirst, loss of appetite and constipation. At first the pain is confined to only one or two joints, but soon others become affected, very commonly similar joints on the two sides of the body. Flitting joint pains, as they are known, are very characteristic of the disease. The affected joints are red, swollen, hot and excessively tender. In mild cases one or two joints only are affected, but in severe cases scarcely a joint, large or small, may escape, and the pain, restlessness, and fever then render the patient's condition extremely miserable.

An attack of acute rheumatism is of variable duration, sometimes passing away in the course of a few days. The usual period during which the temperature remains elevated is a week or less, and, if the temperature subsides to normal and again rises, or if it continues elevated beyond ten days, some complication, such as involvement of the heart, may be suspected. Such cases may last for many weeks with relapses, in which all the former symptoms return and prolong the illness.

If no complication has arisen, there may be complete recovery in the course of about three weeks. Sometimes, when all the acute symptoms have disappeared, the joints remain swollen, stiff, and painful on movement, but this condition may also gradually pass away, or, on the other hand, the rheumatism may become chronic. In any case there always remains a liability to subsequent attacks.

In certain cases small subcutaneous nodules develop on the extensor aspect of certain joints, especially the back of the wrist, the back of the elbow, and the knee. They may also occur on the back of the neck. The significance of these rheumatic nodules, which are about the size of a split pea, is that they tend to occur in the more severe cases.

Complications – This disease derives much of its serious import from certain complications which are apt to arise during an attack. Among these the most frequent and the most serious is heart disease. This occurs in about 45 to 55 per cent of children with first attacks of acute rheumatism. The incidence of rheumatic heart disease rises from around 20 per 100,000 population at the age of 6 to 150 at the age of 14 years, and around 8000 people, many young, die each year in Britain from rheumatic heart disease. If the heart is involved in a first attack of acute rheumatism, it is liable to become more seriously involved in subsequent attacks. Pericarditis (inflammation of the membrane covering the heart), endocarditis (inflammation of the lining membrane of the heart), and myocarditis (inflammation of the heart muscle) may all develop. (See HEART DISEASES.) The risk of cardiac complications seems to be greater the younger the patient, and, indeed, in children the joint pains are often so slight as to be overlooked, and the valvular disease may only be discovered accidentally at a later period of life. Pericarditis occurs less often, but is more serious as regards the patient's immediate prospect of recovery.

Amongst other serious complications is excessive fever (hyperpyrexia), which sometimes develops in a sudden and alarming manner, the temperature rising rapidly to 106° to 108° F (41° to 42° C), or even higher, and thus endangering life unless prompt treatment be resorted to. Complications connected with the lungs, such as pleurisy, pneumonia, and bronchitis, sometimes arise in the course of the disease. Certain skin conditions may also occur, including purpura, erythema nodosum, and erythema marginatum. Chorea (St. Vitus's dance) sometimes follows after the acute symptoms have subsided.

Treatment – Rest in bed is essential until all signs of activity of the disease have subsided. Movements of all kinds should be avoided so far as possible during the first few days. In view of the pain the child should be handled with particular care, and the weight of the bedclothes should be kept off him by means of a cradle. The skin requires special care, with frequent sponging, in view of the excessive sweating that tends to occur. The diet should consist entirely of milk, glucose, and fruit juices in the acute stage of the disease.

The affected joints should be wrapped in cotton-wool or gamgee tissue, kept in position by a light bandage or by tapes. If the pain is very great, relief is sometimes obtained by wrapping the painful parts in flannel cloths wrung out of a strong (5 per cent) solution of washing soda in water, to which some laudanum has been added. Methyl salicylate painted on the painful joints and covered with oil-silk and cotton-wool, and a mixture in equal parts of chloral, menthol and camphor, are similarly soothing applications. Relief from very acute pain is obtained in all cases by fixing the joint by means of splints.

Penicillin should be given for the first week, to kill off any haemolytic streptococci that may be present in the throat. Sodium salicylate forms the sheet anchor of drug treatment, the usual dose being equivalent to 120 mg per kg of body weight every day. Some authorities prefer aspirin (80 to 100 mg per kg of body weight). In severe cases one or other of the corticosteroid drugs may be given. In the dangerous complication of hyperpyrexia, the cold bath, in which the water is quickly cooled down from 94° to 68° F (34·5° to 20° C), or the cold pack, is often successful in lowering temperature and saving life. In order to reduce the risk of permanent damage to the heart, it is essential that every patient with rheumatic fever should be kept at complete rest in bed for ten days following the return of the temperature to normal. It should be another two or three weeks before the patient is allowed out of bed. For some time following recovery special care should be taken in avoiding exposure to cold and damp, crowds, and over-exertion.

SUBACUTE RHEUMATISM is a name sometimes applied to mild attacks of acute rheumatism, in which the temperature does not exceed 101° F (38·3° C), and which respond quickly to treatment by sodium salicylate. These cases are often of long duration and they may be accompanied by endocarditis, especially in the case of children. The significance of these attacks is that, no matter how mild they may appear to be, they may involve the heart. Treatment should be instituted immediately by putting the patient to bed, and full doses of aspirin or sodium salicylate should be given. Experience in this country and in the United States has shown that the incidence of such recurrent attacks is reduced by giving children who are susceptible to, or who have had an attack of, rheumatic fever regular small daily doses of a sulphonamide drug or of penicillin over a long period.

NON-ARTICULAR RHEUMATISM includes all those forms of rheumatism which do not involve the joints. Classification is difficult as the cause is not known. Many different names have been given to the various manifestations of this group: eg. fibrositis, bursitis, myalgia, muscular rheumatism, neuritis, lumbago, sciatica, pleurodynia, panniculitis. Although the cause is obscure, there is no doubt about the practical importance of this group of diseases. In the United States of America it accounts for about 30 per cent of all rheumatic diseases, and in Great Britain the incidence is even higher.

Causes – Only certain predisposing factors are known. The actual cause is still to be found. The onset may be acute, as in certain cases of lumbago, or gradual. It may be generalized, eg. involving the muscles of the back and shoulders, or it may be localized. Exposure to cold or damp is a common predisposing factor. Undue exertion may precipitate an attack. In other cases it appears to be associated with a focus of infection somewhere in the body, eg. septic teeth, but the importance of this factor has been grossly over-rated in the past. The condition is much more apt to occur in middle-age than in young adults. Certain individuals are much more likely to suffer from the condition than others, and it is in these susceptible individuals that the factors already mentioned are most likely to induce an attack.

Symptoms – These consist of pain and stiffness which range in intensity from the agonizing pain of acute lumbago, which literally immobilizes the victim for a time, to a vague sense of discomfort which the individual may have difficulty in localizing precisely. The pain and stiffness are usually worst after resting and tend to improve with exercise. Thus, they tend to be worst on awakening in the morning. Damp and cold weather make them worse, whilst they improve in dry warm weather. Tender spots can sometimes be felt in the affected muscles, and the detection of these is of importance from the point of view of treatment. There is seldom any wasting or atrophy of muscle and the joints are not involved. The general health is not affected.

Treatment – This depends upon the acuteness of the condition. If very acute, a period of rest in bed may be necessary, but as a rule this is not essential. Avoidance of strenuous physical exertion is advisable, but moderate exercise is advantageous as it prevents the affected muscles becoming stiff. For the relief of pain, heat in some form is used. This may consist of hot baths, hot packs, hot water bottles or diathermy. Warming the affected part gently in front of a gas-fire is as useful a way as any. In more severe cases some form of counter-irritation, eg. a mustard plaster, may be necessary. Electricity in the form of faradism, galvanism, or high-frequency currents is often useful. Massage is usually helpful. In severe cases analgesics are required, and the best of these is aspirin, with or without paracetamol. If localized tender spots are found, the injection into them of procaine often gives relief which is sometimes dramatic.

Individuals who are susceptible to non-articular rheumatism often benefit from a stay at a spa: eg. Bath. Advice which is becoming increasingly difficult to follow, is for such individuals to live, or holiday, in warm dry climes: eg. South Africa, Egypt, California. More practical advice is that in cold damp weather they should wear warm clothing and take particular care to avoid undue exposure to cold or damp: eg. they should be especially careful about changing their clothes if they get wet.

LUMBAGO – This is myalgia or fibrositis occurring in the strong and dense sinews of the erector spinae muscles of the back, and is considered separately because of its great frequency and importance in regard to occupation, and because it is readily distinguishable. (See LUMBAGO.)

SCIATICA AND BRACHIAL NEURITIS – The rheumatic processes may affect the fibrous tissues of various nerves, the nerves of the arm and the sciatic nerve running down the back of the thigh being especially liable to this affection. The causes described above under myalgia are also operative in producing neuritis, and, in the case of the nerves of the arm, overstrain at work, eg. in hammermen, plays an important part. The treatment of this condition is described under NEURALGIA. (See also SCIATICA.)

RHEUMATOID ARTHRITIS, also known as ATROPHIC ARTHRITIS, is one of the most crippling of all the rheumatic diseases.

Causes – For many years regarded as an infective condition, evidence is now accumulating that it is due to some fundamental biochemical or immunological disturbance associated with deficient production of certain hormones in the cortex of the suprarenal glands. The precise nature of this disturbance is not understood, and it must be admitted that the brilliant researches of Dr Hench and his colleagues at the Mayo Clinic, which have shown that a dramatic, but only temporary, improvement in patients with rheumatoid arthritis can be produced by the administration of cortisone, one of the hormones of the suprarenal cortex, have raised almost as many problems as they have solved. The majority current concept at the moment is that it is a manifestation of auto-immunity (qv). The disease is one of temperate climates and is more common in women than in men. The majority of cases occur between the ages of 35 and 40. It is uncommon under the age of 25, and first attacks seldom occur after the age of 50. A form of rheumatoid arthritis known as Still's disease (qv) occurs in children. Another form occurs in association with psoriasis (qv).

Pathology – The first change in the affected joints consists of thickening of the synovial lining of the joint. This is followed by involvement of the articular cartilage, which becomes ulcerated, covered with granulation tissue, and ultimately destroyed in severe cases. There is an overproduction of connective tissue and in due course the joint becomes ankylosed and fixed. There is also rarefaction of the bone adjoining the joint, and marked wasting of the adjoining muscles. This last change is due, in part at least, to disuse: because of the painful state of the joint the individual uses it as little as possible.

Symptoms – The disease has usually a gradual onset. There is pain, swelling, and redness of the affected joints. The condition usually begins in the small joints of the hand, especially in the fingers. Later, almost any joint in the body may be involved, but the condition tends to spread from the smaller joints to the larger joints. Thus, the shoulder and the hip joint are usually affected last. Even mild attacks are usually accompanied by fever, and in acute attacks the rise in temperature may be quite considerable and accompanied by the rise in pulse-rate and all the other accompaniments of fever: eg. prostration, loss of appetite, sweating, and the like. With recurrent attacks the affected joints tend to become chronically swollen and fixed. The position in which fixation of the joint occurs depends upon the relative strength of the muscles around the joint. In the case of the hand this results in the characteristic deformity – with the hand deviated towards the little finger side. In comparison with the swelling of the joints, the wasting of the surrounding muscles shows up particularly markedly, and gives a characteristic appearance, which in the case of the fingers justifies the description of spindle-shaped. X-ray examination reveals the presence of well-marked changes in the joints, including widening of the joint space and decreased density of the bones adjoining the joints. The sedimentation rate (qv) is raised, and, though this is of little help in diagnosis, the course of the sedimentation rate over a period of time is a useful guide as to how the disease is responding to treatment. With recurring attacks the patient's general health tends to become affected with anaemia, loss of weight, loss of appetite, and lassitude. The outlook, or prognosis, is satisfactory in so far as this is not a killing disease, but it is unsatisfactory in that, up to date, no effective treatment is available and the disease tends therefore to be chronic and recurrent. It has been estimated that a quarter of the patients show marked improvement approaching a cure, a half show slight or moderate improvement, and a quarter fail to improve, or become worse.

Treatment – It is now clear that cortisone is not a cure for the condition. Increasing experience has shown that its use is not without danger. Used with circumspection, under skilled supervision, it is undoubtedly a useful adjunct in the treatment of rheumatoid arthritis, but it by no means replaces the well-tried measures which are summarized in the remainder of this section.

These consist, in the first place, of rest, the degree of rest depending upon the severity of the condition. Rest, however, must never be absolute, even in the acute stages, as this may lead to unnecessary stiffness in the joints. It must be accompanied by exercises to keep the joints as mobile as possible. During the more acute phases, when it is necessary to keep the patient in bed, the affected joints should be splinted so as to prevent deformities developing. Heat, in the form of hot water bottles, wax baths, or diathermy, is useful in relieving pain and discomfort, and this may be supplemented by the administration of aspirin or sodium salicylate. Spa

treatment is also of value. Satisfactory results have been obtained from the use of certain salts of gold. Although gold does not produce a cure, it is the one agent which, apart from the cortisone group of drugs, has been shown to improve the condition. Its use, however, is not without risk, and it must therefore only be used under medical supervision. Surgery is only required to correct any deformity which is crippling the patient, provided this crippling is confined to one or two joints. The general health of the patient must also be attended to by ensuring that he or she has an adequate nutritious diet, containing plenty of milk, fruit, and vegetables. Dental care is necessary, but it is now recognized that there is no justification for the wholesale extraction of teeth which was fashionable at one time. Removal to a dry, warm climate is beneficial, but economically this is seldom advice that can be followed by the affected individual.

OSTEOARTHROSIS, or OSTEOARTHRITIS, is the most common disorder of joints and is estimated to be present in 80 to 90 per cent of people over the age of 60 years. It is characterized by gradual destruction of the central part of the cartilage lining the affected joint, whilst at the same time there is overgrowth of the outer part of the cartilage which ultimately results in the growth of bony spurs or osteophytes. The condition is probably a degenerative one, but it is accentuated or accelerated by trauma. Thus, it is liable to occur in a knee in which there has been cartilage trouble which has not been treated adequately. Obesity, accompanied as it so often is by faulty posture, results in abnormal stresses and strains being applied to the hip joints and knees, and this in due course results in osteoarthritic changes in these joints. There is some evidence that there may be a hereditary predisposition. The condition is more common in women than in men, and the joints mainly involved are the hip, the knee, and the shoulder joint. The terminal joints of the fingers are also quite a common site. Pain and stiffness in the affected joints are the usual manifestations of the disease. A creaking sensation (crepitus) is felt in moving the joint in the more advanced cases. In chronic cases the joint becomes enlarged. There is seldom any generalized disturbance such as fever or malaise. The diagnosis is confirmed by X-ray examination.

Treatment consists of rest and graduated exercises. A course of spa therapy is often helpful. When the joints are painful the local application of heat is beneficial: eg. hot towel packs or infra-red light. Aspirin or sodium salicylate also relieves the pain temporarily. If the individual is overweight, a reducing diet is necessary to bring the weight down. In the more advanced cases, surgery is often of value. The essence of treatment, however, has been aptly summarized as follows: 'The obvious thing to do is to "spare" the joints, just as one spares a horse that is "a bit gone in the forelegs" or a car with a worn transmission'.

GOUT (see GOUT).

RHEUMATOID ARTHRITIS (see RHEUMATISM).

RH FACTOR (see BLOOD GROUPS).

RHINITIS means inflammation of the mucous membrane of the nose. (See NOSE, DISEASES OF.)

RHINOPHYMA is the condition characterized by enlargement of the nose due to enormous enlargement of the sebaceous glands which may develop in the later stages of rosacea (qv).

RHINOPLASTY means the repair of the nose or the modification of its shape by operation. The operation is carried out by obtaining a flap of skin from the forehead or from the forearm. In milder cases of deformity the shape is often improved by injection of paraffin under the skin of the nose, or by insertion of a piece of cartilage taken from one of the ribs. (See ARTIFICIAL LIMBS AND OTHER PARTS.)

RHINOVIRUSES are a large group of viruses; to date around 80 distinct rhinoviruses have been identified. Their practical importance is that some of them are responsible for around one-quarter of the cases of the common cold.

RHIZOTOMY is the surgical operation of cutting a nerve root, as, for example, to relieve the pain of trigeminal neuralgia.

RHONCHI is the term used to denote the harsh cooing, hissing, or whistling sounds (wheezing) heard by auscultation over the bronchial tubes when they are the seat of infection. (See BRONCHITIS.)

RHUBARB is the root of *Rheum palmatum*, a plant originally derived from China and Tibet, and other species of Rheum. It has a gentle purgative action.

RHUS is the name for a genus of trees and shrubs, some of which are used as astringents, while others, particularly *Rhus toxicodendron*, or poison oak, and *Rhus radicans*, or poison ivy, are poisonous.

RIBOFLAVINE is the *British Pharmacopoeia* name for what used to be known as vitamin B_2. Riboflavine belongs to a group of animal and plant pigments which give a greenish fluorescence on exposure to ultra-violet rays. It is present especially in milk, and is not destroyed during pasteurization. Other rich sources are eggs, liver, yeast and the green leaves of broccoli and spinach. It is also present in beer. Deficiency of riboflavine in the diet is thought to cause inflammation of the substance of the cornea, sores on the lips, especially at the angles of the mouth (cheilosis (qv)), and dermatitis.

The minimal daily requirement for an adult is 1·5 to 3 mg, but is greater during pregnancy and lactation.

RIBS are the bones, twelve on each side, which enclose the cavity of the chest (illustration 352). The upper seven are joined to the breast-bone by their costal cartilages and are therefore known as true ribs. The lower five do not reach the breast-bone, and are therefore known as false ribs. Of the latter, the 8th, 9th and 10th are joined by their costal cartilages, each one to the

352 – The ribs. The shaded portions of the ribs are the costal cartilages. The central shaded structure is the sternum, or breast-bone. From *Gray's Anatomy*. Longman.

rib immediately above it, while the 11th and 12th are free from any such connection, and are therefore known as floating ribs. Each rib is possessed of a head, by which it is jointed to the upper part of the body of the vertebra with which it corresponds, as well as to the vertebra immediately above. Next comes a narrow part known as the neck, and then a tubercle, by which the rib is joined to the transverse process of the corresponding vertebra. Finally, the greater part of the bone is made up of the shaft, which runs at first outwards and at the angle turns sharply forwards. On the lower margin of the shaft is a groove, which lodges the corresponding intercostal artery and nerve.

RICE DIET – A diet containing a minimum amount of sodium is a valuable adjunct in the treatment of heart failure. It is also used in the treatment of high blood-pressure. The rice diet was introduced for this purpose. It consists of rice cooked in unsalted water, fruit, fruit juice and sugar, and contains less than 0·5 gram of sodium per day. Its practical disadvantage is its unpalatability.

RICE-WATER forms a useful diluent drink for invalids, similar to barley-water. To prepare rice-water take 6 tablespoonfuls of rice, wash it in cold water, then place it in a saucepan with 1½ pints (850 ml) of water and allow to simmer for an hour or two, until the bulk of fluid is reduced to about a pint (570 ml). The rice-water is then cooled, strained, and, if desired, sweetened with sugar and flavoured with lemon.

RICKETS is a disease of childhood characterized chiefly by a softened condition of the bones, and by other evidence of perverted nutrition.
Causes – This disease is found chiefly among the ill-fed children of the poor, and is the result of deficiency of vitamin D in the diet, and also of deficiency of calcium. Healthy bones cannot be built up without calcium (or lime) salts, and the body cannot utilize these salts in the absence of vitamin D. Want of sunlight and fresh air in the dwellings where the children are reared is also of importance. Once a common condition in industrial areas, it had almost disappeared in Great Britain, but there has been a recurrence of it in recent years that is giving rise to concern.
The changes that take place in the bones are due to an irregular process of bone formation. The periosteum, the

membrane enveloping the bones, becomes inflamed, and in consequence the bone formed beneath it is defective in lime salts and very soft. At the growing ends of the bones there is an even more striking change. The epiphyseal plate of cartilage, from which growth takes place, is much thickened, the cellular elements in it much increased in number, and the bone which it produces markedly deficient in lime salts. The new bone shows a deficiency of lime amounting to 25 or 35 per cent, and this, too, notwithstanding the fact that there is abundance of lime in the body, as shown by its excessive excretion in the urine. The disease rarely occurs under the age of 6 months, from which it may be assumed that exposure to unsuitable conditions for several months is necessary before rickets ensues. It is most common between 1 and 2 years of age and is increasingly rare after the age of 3.
Symptoms – The symptoms of rickets most commonly attract attention about the end of the first year, and the disease rarely appears for the first time after the age of 5. The symptoms, which precede the outward manifestations of the disease, are marked disorders of the digestive and alimentary functions. The child's appetite is diminished; there is frequent vomiting and diarrhoea; or irregularity of the bowels appears, the evacuations being clay-coloured and unhealthy. Along with this the child ceases to gain in weight or actually falls away in flesh. One of the most noticeable symptoms is profuse sweating of the head and upper parts of the body, particularly during sleep, with a tendency in the child to kick off the bed-clothes and expose the limbs. Bronchitis is also a common early symptom and often the first to attract attention. In infants, convulsions are sometimes a symptom of rickets and disappear under the treatment appropriate to this disease. At the same time there is tenderness of the bones as shown by crying when the child is moved or handled. A little later it is noticed that there is delay in learning to sit up and walk, so that the child who has begun to walk loses this power.
Gradually changes in the shape of the bones become visible, first chiefly noticed at the ends of the long bones, as in those of the arm, causing enlargement at the wrists, or in the ribs, producing a row of knobs at the junction of their ends with the rib cartilages (rickety rosary). Because of their softened condition the bones also tend to become distorted and bent both by the action of the muscles and by the weight of

the body resting upon them. Those of the legs are bent outwards and forwards and the child becomes bow-legged or knock-kneed, often to an extreme degree. The trunk of the body likewise shows various alterations and deformities owing to curvatures of the spine, flattening of the lateral curves of the ribs, and the projection forward of the breast-bone. (See CHEST DEFORMITIES.) The cavity of the chest may thus be contracted and interference produced with the development of the thoracic organs, whose functions thus become embarrassed. The liver is pushed outwards and the abdomen becomes protuberant (pot belly). The pelvis undergoes distortion which may reduce its capacity to such a degree that in females serious difficulties may arise later in life in the course of labour. The head of the rickety child is square with high 'intellectual' forehead; the individual bones of the cranium remain long ununited, while the soft fontanelle remains unclosed long after the end of the second year, the time by which it should have disappeared; the face is small and ill-developed; and the teeth appear late and fall out or decay early.

The disease usually terminates in recovery with more or less of deformity and dwarfing, the bones, although altered in shape, becoming ultimately firmly ossified. On the other hand, during the progress of the disease, various intercurrent ailments are apt to arise which may cause death, such as bronchitis and other chest complaints, meningitis, convulsions, laryngismus. Another disease for which rickets is apt to be mistaken is infantile scurvy (qv).

Treatment – The treatment of rickets is more hygienic and dietetic than medicinal. The specific remedy is vitamin D, given in the form either of cod-liver oil, halibut-liver oil, or calciferol (vitamin D_2). A full diet is of course essential, with emphasis upon a sufficient supply of milk. Rickets practically does not occur in breast-fed children but it is a wise precaution to give breast-fed babies supplementary vitamin D. (See INFANT FEEDING.) After the child is weaned, the provision of suitable food is of the greatest importance, supplemented by the administration of cod-liver oil or some other source of vitamin D. (See INFANT FEEDING.)

General hygienic measures, including abundance of fresh air and sunshine, cleanliness, warm clothing, and attention to regularity in all the child's functions, are of the greatest importance.

While the disease is advancing, it is desirable to restrain the child from walking, and this must sometimes be achieved by the use of splints and other apparatus as supports of the limbs and body. This enables the child to move about without risk of bending and deformity of the bones, which would otherwise probably result. If deformities of the legs have occurred, operative treatment may be necessary at a later period of life in order to straighten the limbs.

RICKETTSIA is the general term given to a group of micro-organisms, which are intermediate between bacteria and viruses. They are the causal agents of typhus and a number of typhus-like diseases, such as Rocky Mountain spotted fever, Japanese River fever, and scrub typhus. These micro-organisms are usually conveyed to man by lice, fleas, ticks, and mites.

RIFAMPICIN is an antibiotic derived from *Streptomyces mediterranei*, which is proving of value in the treatment of tuberculosis and leprosy.

RIGG'S DISEASE is another name for pyorrhoea alveolaris. (See TEETH, DISEASES OF.)

RIGOR means shivering. If prolonged, it is generally accompanied by raised temperature, and may be a sign of the onset of some acute febrile disease, such as influenza, pneumonia, or some internal inflammation. *Rigor mortis* is the name given to the stiffness that ensues soon after death. (See DEATH, SIGNS OF.)

RIMA is a term, meaning a crack or fissure, applied to any narrow natural opening: eg. rima glottidis, the chink between the vocal cords.

RINGWORM, or TINEA, is the name given to inflammatory affections of the skin produced by moulds. The main forms of ringworm in man are: (i) *Tinea tonsurans*, or ringworm of the scalp; (ii) *Tinea barbae*, or ringworm of the beard; (iii) *Tinea cruris*, or ringworm of the groin, and also known as dhobie itch; (iv) *Tinea pedis*, or ringworm of the feet; (v) *Tinea circinata*, or ringworm of the body; (vi) ringworm of the nails; (vii) *Tinea favosa*, favus, or honeycomb ringworm; (viii) *Tinea versicolor.*

RINGWORM OF THE SCALP, a disease of childhood, is usually due to a human species of fungus, *Microsporon audouini*; some five per cent of cases are

753

due to infection by microspora acquired from cats and dogs. Boys are more infected than girls, and in both it disappears spontaneously at adolescence, being excessively rare in adults. It is most contagious. The incidence of the disease fell rapidly in the 1920–30's, and by 1939 was a rare condition in many parts of the country. During the 1939–45 War, however, its incidence increased, and epidemics in schools and institutions are still not uncommon. The typical appearance is that of circular patches of lustreless, greyish, broken hairs scattered over the scalp. The scalp itself is covered with fine greyish-white scabs. Under Wood's light (the rays of a mercury vapour lamp screened through a special glass) the infected hairs have a bright green colour, which is diagnostic.

Treatment – As in all other forms of ringworm, the outlook has been radically changed by the introduction of the antibiotic, griseofulvin (qv). When used under medical supervision, this is the most effective method of treatment yet discovered, curing the condition in a high proportion of cases. Treatment should be continued for four weeks or until there is complete cure. In order to prevent reinfection, the infected hairs should be removed either manually, or by clipping and shaving, after three weeks' treatment with griseofulvin. A daily application of an antifungal preparation is not essential but is of value in preventing the spread of infection to other parts of the scalp or to other children. The child should be excluded from school until cured.

RINGWORM OF THE BEARD is one of the forms of barber's rash. There is a form occurring in grooms and cattlemen, in which the infection is acquired from animals.

Treatment – This consists of the administration of griseofulvin (qv). If suppuration is also present, hot fomentations of 2 per cent sodium thiosulphate should be applied.

RINGWORM OF THE GROIN, or DHOBIE ITCH, is caused by a fungus of the same group as is responsible for ringworm of the foot: *Epidermophyton*. It occurs at any age, but is most common in young adult males. The eruption is a sharply defined, slightly raised reddish area, which begins in the inner aspect of the upper third of the thigh and tends to spread over the perineum (or crutch) and to involve the scrotum. It is accompanied by considerable irritation.

Treatment – This consists of the administration of griseofulvin (qv). In addition, the prevention of reinfection is essential by the individual always wearing cotton underpants night and day, and sterilizing them by boiling every evening. This means, of course, that at least two pairs of pants must be in use, so that one is always available to wear while the other is being sterilized.

RINGWORM OF THE FOOT, or athlete's foot as it is often known, is one of the most common forms of ringworm at the present day. It is due to an *Epidermophyton*. Most common among adolescent and young adult males, the infection is usually acquired by walking with bare feet on infected floors: eg. hotel and school bathrooms, public swimming baths, and pithead baths. The eruption begins between the toes as a rule, but may also be found on the soles of the feet. There are two main forms of eruption: (a) the *vesicular*, in which the affected area is covered with small blisters – this form begins on the sole; (b) the *intertriginous*, in which the skin between the toes becomes white and sodden, and peels off, leaving a raw red area. Before beginning to treat this type of ringworm it is particularly important to demonstrate the fungus in material removed from the affected area, as a superficially similar appearance may be produced by other infecting organisms or even by excessive sweating alone.

Treatment – Careful hygiene of the feet, particularly by those who tend to perspire freely in the feet, is essential: (a) to prevent infection; (b) to aid in curing the condition once acquired; (c) to prevent relapses. Such hygiene consists of washing the feet every night in warm water, drying them thoroughly but carefully, and then powdering them with a bland dusting powder. A fresh pair of socks should be worn at least every other day, and rubber footwear should not be used. Once the infection is acquired, the treatment depends upon the local condition. In mild and moderate cases in which the epidermophyton alone is responsible, an ointment or powder containing salts of undecylenic acid or propionic acid is probably best. Good results are sometimes obtained from the use of phenyl mercuric nitrate (or acetate) as an ointment or powder. Another useful preparation is tolnaftate applied as a powder.

Griseofulvin has not proved as effective in this form of ringworm as in other forms, but it is always worth trying if the methods described fail to clear the infection.

RINGWORM OF THE BODY, which may occur with ringworm of the scalp, may be due to either a microsporon or a tricophyton. The eruption consists of circular discs, usually red in colour at first, but later tending to become pale in the centre, and blisters may appear in the surrounding ring. There is considerable itching.

Treatment is as for other forms of ringworm of the skin.

RINGWORM OF THE NAILS is not common but is most resistant to treatment. Several nails are usually affected, and they turn a greenish-grey colour, and become brittle and separated from the nail-bed.

Treatment consists of the administration of griseofulvin, but treatment may need to be continued for long periods: for up to six months. Toe-nails are particularly resistant to griseofulvin. Expert opinion is still divided as to whether or not the infected nail should be removed.

FAVUS is due to a fungus of the genus, *Tricophyton*. It occurs on the scalp, skin, and nails, and consists of thick yellow cups of crust. It is rare in Great Britain. It responds to griseofulvin.

TINEA VERSICOLOR, due to *Malassezia furfur*, is characterized by thin, greenish-yellow patches on the chest and abdomen. Treatment consists of the local application of a saturated solution of sodium thiosulphate night and morning, or the daily application of a lotion of selenium sulphide (qv).

RISUS SARDONICUS is the term used for describing the facial appearance when the muscles of the forehead and the face go into spasm in tetanus, giving the effect of a sardonic grin.

ROCHELLE SALT, SEIGNETTE SALT, and TARTRATED SODA are names for sodium potassium tartrate, a saline purgative which forms the chief constituent of Seidlitz powder. The dose of Rochelle salt as an aperient is 120 to 240 grains (8 to 16 grams) or a heaped dessert-spoonful.

ROCKY MOUNTAIN SPOTTED FEVER is a fever of the typhus group. It received its name from the fact that it was first reported in the Rocky Mountain states of USA. These are still the most heavily infected states, but it is now found in all parts of the United States. The causative organism is *Rickettsia rickettsi*, which is transmitted to man by tics. (See also TYPHUS FEVER.)

RODENT ULCER is the name given to a chronic form of ulcer, which is found chiefly about the nose and face of elderly persons, and which gradually increases in size. It stands between a simple chronic ulcer and a cancer, being much slower in its growth than the latter. Treatment consists in cutting out the ulcer with the healthy skin for a little distance all round. It is also very amenable to treatment by X-rays, radium, and other forms of radiant energy.

ROENTGEN RAYS (see X-RAYS).

ROETHELN, is another name for GERMAN MEASLES (qv).

ROMBERGISM is a term applied to marked unsteadiness in standing with the eyes shut. It is found as a symptom in some nervous diseases, such as locomotor ataxia.

RORSCHACH TEST is a method of investigating the personality and disorders of personality. It was devised by a Swiss psychiatrist, Hermann Rorschach (1884–1922), who determined individuals' reactions to a series of symmetrical ink-blots, ten in number and standardized by him. The person investigated is shown the ink-blots in a defined order and is asked to describe what he sees. His descriptions and ideas about the blots are noted and an elaborate system of scoring is said to afford indications of the kind of personality and psychological make-up of the person investigated. Much work has been done on the test and it is thought highly of by experienced psychiatrists.

ROSACEA, or ACNE ROSACEA as it is sometimes known, is a condition in which there is chronic congestion of the flush areas of the face and forehead, leading to the formation of red papules. In the earlier stages the erythema, or redness of the skin, tends to wax and wane, being more marked after a meal or excessive drinking of alcohol. Ultimately, however, the erythema becomes permanent, and may be accompanied by gross enlargement of the sebaceous glands (see SKIN), leading to the gross enlargement of the nose known as rhinophyma (qv) or grog blossoms.

Causes – Although the condition is often associated with dyspepsia, the main cause is stress (see NEURODERMATOSES).

Symptoms – In the milder forms there is simple redness, burning, and tingling of the nose, the redness lasting at first only for a few hours every day, but later tend-

ROSE

ing to become permanent, and also to appear upon the cheeks. In the severer form the nose becomes very red and the skin thick and lumpy, while the openings of the sebaceous glands are seen as quite wide pits. In exceptional cases, more commonly in men than in women, there may be enormous enlargement of the sebaceous glands of the nose, the condition known as rhinophyma.

Treatment – The mild form is lessened by attending to the dyspepsia which is its cause; avoiding exposure to cold winds; and by painting with some sulphur preparation, such as 2 per cent Precipitated Sulphur B P in Hydrous Ointment B P, or calamine lotion. In the more severe forms the dilated veins may be destroyed by electrolysis. When there is much overgrowth of the skin, it may be necessary to remove some of the overgrown tissue.

ROSE, or ST. ANTHONY'S FIRE, is an old name for erysipelas. (See ERYSIPELAS.)

ROSEMARY is a plant affording a fragrant volatile oil which is used in the form of spirit of rosemary.

ROSEOLA is a term applied to any rose-coloured rash.

ROSEOLA INFANTUM is an acute infectious disease of infancy, with an incubation period of ten to fifteen days. It is probably due to a virus. The onset is sudden, with a fever of around 102°–105° F (39°–40·5° C), which drops as quickly as it rose after three days. As the temperature falls, a rose-coloured rash appears on the trunk, where it may stay, but it sometimes spreads to the face, neck and limbs. It fades and disappears in forty-eight hours. The glands in the neck may become enlarged, and there may be a sore throat. No special treatment is required. The child should be kept warm and quiet while the temperature is raised, and allowed to drink plenty of fluids, including warm milk, and fruit drinks containing glucose.

ROSE-RASH, or ROSEOLA, is an old name used to describe any eruption of a very faint red character. The term, erythema, is now generally used in its place. (See ERYTHEMA.)

ROSE-WAALER TEST is a blood test which is proving of value in the diagnosis of rheumatoid arthritis. It is positive in over 70 per cent of patients with this

756

disease, compared with only 4 per cent of people not suffering from rheumatoid arthritis.

ROSE-WATER is prepared by soaking rose-petals in water and distilling over part of the fluid. It is used as an ingredient of cold-cream, etc. Rose oil, or attar of rose, is prepared by distilling the fresh flowers of *Rosa damascena*, about 180 pounds (82 kg) of roses being required in order to yield an ounce (28·5 ml) of this oil. It is largely used in perfumery, and in lozenges, dentifrices and ointments.

ROSIN, or COLOPHONY, is the name of a resinous substance remaining after oil of turpentine has been distilled from the pitch of pine wood. It is used for making plasters.

ROTAVIRUSES are a new group of viruses which have been reported as being a common cause of gastroenteritis (qv) in infants. They are rarely found in children over 6 years of age. They are related to the viruses which cause diarrhoea in mice, and Nebraska calf scour.

ROTENONE is the name of a substance obtained from derris root (qv).

ROUGHAGE, or dietary fibre, has long been known to affect bowel function. The Romans, for instance, knew that wholemeal flour increased the output of faeces. How it does this is still not quite clear but the probability is that it achieves this through its capacity to hold water in a gel-like form. But fibre is not an inert substance as was long thought to be the case. It is digested and metabolized in the colon by the micro-organisms there. This digestive process alters the properties of dietary fibre, including an increase in the amount of bile acids in the stools. The full significance of these changes is not yet known. Many claims are being made for the value of dietary fibre in maintaining health and preventing disease. What does seem to be clear is that it plays a role in the prevention of constipation, diverticular disease (see DIVERTICULOSIS) and the irritable bowel syndrome (qv). There is also some evidence that it may reduce the incidence of cancer of the colon. Be all that as it may, though bran is not the panacea it is made out to be by some, there seems little doubt that modern western diets do not contain as much roughage, such as wholemeal flour, as they should.

ROULEAUX is the term applied to the heaps into which red blood corpuscles collect as seen under the microscope.

ROUNDWORMS (see ASCARIASIS).

ROUS SARCOMA is a malignant tumour of fowls which is caused by a virus. This tumour has been the subject of much experimental work bearing upon the nature of cancer.

RUBBING (see MASSAGE and LINIMENTS).

RUBEFACIENTS (see BLISTERS AND COUNTERIRRITANTS).

RUBELLA is another name for GERMAN MEASLES (qv).

RUBEOLA is another name for MEASLES (qv).

RUE is the name of a herb, *Ruta graveolens*, from which a volatile oil with irritating properties is produced.

RUPIA is the term applied to an eruption characterized by the accumulation of thick crusts. Apart from the original cause of the eruption, the accumulation of the crusts is due to want of cleanliness.

RUPTURE is a popular name for hernia. (See HERNIA.) The term is also applied to the tearing of a muscle or ligament, bursting of a blood-vessel, etc.

S

SACCHARIN is a soluble coal-tar product of white crystalline appearance. It has an extremely sweet taste, being prepared in various strengths so as to equal in sweetness from 300 to 500 times its own weight of cane-sugar. It escapes from the body unchanged, having practically no effect upon the tissues beyond its influence upon the sensation of taste. Accordingly it is used by diabetics, corpulent persons, and others to whom sugar is harmful. It tends to give a bitter flavour to drinks to which it is added.

SACCHAROMYCES is another name for yeast.

SACCHARUM is the Latin name for ordinary cane-sugar or beet-sugar. (See SUGAR.)

SACRUM is the name given to a portion of the spinal column near its lower end. The sacrum consists of five vertebrae fused together to form a broad triangular bone which lies between the two haunch-bones and forms the back wall of the pelvis.

SADISM (Marquis de Sade) is the term applied to a form of sexual perversion, in which satisfaction is derived from the infliction of cruelty upon another person.

SAFE PERIOD is that period during the menstrual cycle when fertilization of the ovum is unlikely to occur. Ovulation usually occurs about 15 days before the onset of the menstrual period. A woman is commonly believed to be fertile for about 11 days in each menstrual cycle: ie. on the day of ovulation and for 5 days before and 5 days after this. This would be the eighth to the eighteenth day of the usual 28-day menstrual cycle. Outside this fertile period is the SAFE PERIOD: the first week and the last ten days of the menstrual cycle. On the other hand, there is increasing evidence that the safest period is the last few days before menstruation. In the case of irregular menstruation it is not possible to calculate the safe period. In any event the safety is not absolute.

SAFFRON, or CROCUS, is a yellow powder derived from the dried stigmas and styles of the flower of *Crocus sativus*. It is used as a 'tonic' and colouring matter, and there is a popular superstition that its administration is useful in bringing out the rash of measles.

SAGITTAL is the term applied to a structure or section running from front to back in the body.

SAGO is the name of a starch derived from the pith of various species of palm. (See CEREALS.)

ST ANTHONY'S FIRE is an old name applied both to erysipelas and to ergot-poisoning.

ST JOHN LONG'S LINIMENT is an old name for acetic turpentine liniment, containing oil of turpentine, liniment of camphor, and glacial acetic acid. It is used as an application for chronic rheumatism.

ST VITUS'S DANCE is another name for CHOREA (qv).

SAL AMMONIAC is another name for chloride of ammonium, which is widely used in cough mixtures and lozenges as an expectorant.

SALBUTAMOL is a drug that is proving of value, and safe, for the relief of spasm of the bronchi in asthma.

SALEP is a mucilaginous substance derived from the dried tubers of various species of orchid. It is used to allay irritation of the stomach and bowels, and in India constitutes an article of diet.

SALERATUS is another name for bicarbonate of potassium.

SALICIN is an active principle derived from the bark of several species of poplar and willow trees. It is a crystalline powder of bitter taste and slight solubility. It has been used for the treatment of acute rheumatism, just as sodium salicylate is used.

SALICYLATE OF SODA is a white crystalline substance which is prepared from salicylic acid. It is very soluble in water, and has a sweet, mawkish taste, which to most people is very unpleasant.
Action – When taken internally in the course of acute fevers, and especially of acute rheumatism, it has the effect of reducing temperature, diminishing pain, and causing profuse sweating. Its action is sim-

ilar to that of aspirin. When taken for some time, it causes fullness in the head, deafness, buzzing in the ears, curious disturbances of sight (so that the person may fancy he sees people in the room who are not there), and, if excessive doses be taken, great depression of the heart's action and of respiration.

Uses – The main use is in acute rheumatism, doses of 10, 15, or more grains (600 mg, 1 G or more) being given several times daily, according to circumstances. It not only diminishes pain and reduces temperature, but may help to cut short an attack of acute rheumatism. In other rheumatic conditions its use is also followed by great benefit.

SALICYLIC ACID is a white substance in fine crystals, of sweetish taste, and sparingly soluble in water.

Action – Salicylic acid is an antiseptic. Externally it is used in ointments to check various skin affections due to bacteria, and, since it has in addition a softening action on the surface of the skin, salicylic acid plasters are used to remove corns and various other superficial overgrowths.

SALINES are purgatives belonging to the class of salts which produce watery evacuations. (See PURGATIVES.) For normal or isotonic saline solution see ISOTONIC.

SALIVA is the fluid which is always present to some extent in the mouth, and is secreted in specially copious amount during a meal, or when the salivary glands are stimulated, as for example by an acid substance placed in the mouth. Saliva contains much mucus, a ferment known as ptyalin, which changes starch into dextrin and maltose (see DIGESTION); also many cells of different types. About 750 millilitres are produced daily.

The principal function of saliva is to aid in the initial processes of digestion. When food is taken into the mouth, an increased output of saliva is evoked. This saliva is essential for the process of mastication (qv), whereby food is reduced to a homogeneous mass before being swallowed. In addition, the ptyalin in the saliva initiates the digestion of starch in the food.

An excessive flow of saliva known as *salivation* occurs as the result of taking certain drugs over a considerable period. Salivation also occurs as the result of irritation in the mouth, as for instance, in the teething child, and from dyspepsia. Dribbling of saliva is a common symptom of bulbar paralysis.

SALIVARY GLANDS are the glands situated near, and opening into, the cavity of the mouth, by which the saliva is manufactured. They include the *parotid gland*, placed in the deep space that lies between the ear and the angle of the jaw; the *submandibular gland*, lying beneath the horizontal part of the jaw-bone; and the *sublingual gland*, which lies beneath the tongue.

Each gland is made up of branching tubes closely packed together, and supported by strong connective tissue. These tubes are lined by large cells that secrete the saliva, and from their interior lead ducts that unite with one another to form ultimately the large main ducts that open into the mouth. The appearance and character of the secreting cells vary in different glands. In the parotid gland they secrete a clear fluid containing the ferment, ptyalin: in the sublingual gland they mainly produce mucus, whilst the submandibular gland contains cells of both types.

SALMON PATCHES are small pink patches found in a certain number of new-born infants – on the eyelids, on the forehead between the eyes, and on the nape of the neck. Those on the first two of these three sites have usually faded by the baby's first birthday, but those on the nape of the neck may be more persistent. (See also BIRTH-MARKS.)

SALMONELLA INFECTIONS, or SALMONELLOSIS (see FOOD POISONING).

SALOL is a white, crystalline, tasteless substance with faint aromatic odour. It was used as an intestinal antiseptic at one time, but its main use now is in sun-screen lotions.

SALPINGITIS is the name applied to inflammation situated in the Fallopian tubes.

SALPINGO- is a prefix indicating a connection with either the Fallopian (or uterine) tubes or the Eustachian (or auditory) tubes.

SALT is the substance produced by the replacement of the acidic hydrogen of an acid by a metal or basic radical. It is also a synonym for common salt or sodium chloride.

SALTPETRE (see NITRE).

SALUTARIUM is the name applied to a resort for the preservation of health.

SAL VOLATILE is another name for aromatic solution of ammonia, a liquid of burning taste and great stimulating powers. Its action depends upon various volatile oils, ammonia, and bicarbonate of ammonia which it contains. It is used as a stimulating expectorant in cough mixtures, and is valuable as a stimulant in faints. The dose is from half to one teaspoonful (1 to 5 millilitres) in a wineglassful of water. (See AMMONIA.)

SANATORIUM is the name applied to an establishment for the treatment of sick persons, especially convalescents or those who are not extremely ill. The term is applied particularly to institutions for the open-air treatment of tuberculosis. (See TUBERCULOSIS.)

SANDALWOOD OIL is a yellowish, fragrant-smelling oil with bitter taste obtained from the wood, *Santalum album*, by distillation. It has an antiseptic action and was at one time widely administered in doses of 0·3 to 1 ml for inflammation of mucous membranes, particularly those of the urinary organs. It is also used in perfumery.

SANDFLY FEVER, also known as PHLEBOTOMUS FEVER, THREE-DAY FEVER, and PAPATACI FEVER, is a short, sharp fever occurring in many parts of the tropics and subtropics, including most of the Mediterranean littoral, due to a virus conveyed by the bite of a small hairy midge or sandfly (*Phlebotomus papatasi*). The incubation period is three to seven days.
Symptoms – There are headache, feverishness, general sensations like those of influenza, flushed face and bloodshot eyes, but no signs of catarrh. The fever passes off in three days, but the patient may take some time to convalesce.
Treatment – As there is no specific remedy, prophylaxis is important. This consists of the spraying of rooms with DDT or Gammexane; the application of insect repellents such as dimethyl phthalate to the exposed parts of the body (eg. ankles, wrists and face), particularly at sunset; and the use of sandfly nets at night. Once the infection is acquired, treatment consists of rest in bed, light diet and aspirin and codeine.

SANGUINEOUS means containing blood.

SANIES means an evil-smelling, thin discharge from a wound or ulcer.

SANITATION, or the science which aims at the prevention of disease, although only fully developed during the last hundred years, was recognized in ancient times. So well were its fundamental principles understood, that even in the Mosaic days isolation of infectious cases, disinfection of infected materials by burning, and regulations for the abatement of nuisances, were in force. The importance of adequate water supplies was appreciated even before the days of the Roman Empire, and the sewers of Nineveh point to the beginnings of the drainage systems of cities.

At first, preventive medicine took cognizance only of the preventable or infectious diseases, but in its vast ramifications at the present day it aims also at the improvement of the general health of the populace, by the mitigation of all external conditions which tend to disease in individuals. It is not a science independent or standing alone. It is the handmaiden of various sciences. It embraces a knowledge of medicine, bacteriology, engineering, meteorology, architecture and geology. It aims at the reduction of infectious diseases, but these have been its greatest advisers and teachers. The recurrent epidemics of cholera which formerly invaded Britain forced the hands of the populace to remedy their water supplies and remodel their systems of drainage. Smallpox and its long roll of victims forced on the compulsory adoption of Jenner's discovery of the value of vaccination. These sowed the seed, and other infectious diseases have brought it nearer maturity. Improved sanitation in matters of ventilation, sewerage, water supply, hospital accommodation, the abatement of nuisances and the inspection of meat has naturally followed from the first step in advance. Its value has been shown in the improved hygiene of the factory, where sanitation has been called in to save the workers from the dangers of their occupation, in meeting the demands of modern civilization, and in the improved conditions of life in dwellings and in general surroundings. It aims at correcting the evils arising from the aggregation of people in cities and towns. It benefits the country dweller and the resident in town by improved methods of sewage and refuse disposal.
Sanitary law – Numerous laws dealing with sanitary matters have been put in force in recent years. The general public health administration of the country is based, in England on the Public Health Act of 1875, and in Scotland on that of

1897, but into many Acts not primarily dealing with sanitation, sanitary provisions have been introduced, as in the various Factory and Workshop Acts. Special local Acts have also been obtained by various authorities, and almost every year some Act is passed by Parliament giving greater sanitary control.

In the various Public Health Acts, which constitute the basis of sanitary administration, machinery is provided for dealing with:

1. General nuisances and offensive trades. Offensive trades include the trades of blood boiler, blood drier, bone boiler, fat extractor, fat melter, fellmonger, glue maker, gut scraper, rag and bone dealer, size maker, soap boiler, tallow melter or tripe boiler.
2. Scavenging and cleansing and the formation of scavenging districts.
3. The seizure of unsound food.
4. The general prevention and mitigation of infectious diseases, including the provision of isolation hospitals, ambulances, disinfecting stations and apparatus. The diseases defined by Act of Parliament in Britain as infectious are: smallpox, cholera, diphtheria, membranous croup, erysipelas, scarlet fever; and the fevers known by any of the following names – typhus, typhoid, enteric, relapsing, continued and also any infectious disease to which the Act has been applied by the local authority in manner provided by the Act. (See INFECTION.)
5. The regulation of common lodging-houses and houses let in lodgings.
6. The provision of water and sewers and the formation of special districts for water supply and drainage.
7. The regulation of buildings.
8. The constitution of port sanitary authorities.
9. Prevention of pollution of rivers by sewage.
10. Regulations as to sale and adulteration of foods.
11. Dairies, cowsheds and milkshops Orders.
12. Various Acts for housing of working classes, including Town Planning Acts.
13. Tuberculosis Orders, Factory and Workshop Acts.
14. Cleansing of persons.
15. Notification of births, Children's and Midwives' Acts.

Community Physician – Under the National Health Service Reorganization Act 1973, the post of Medical Officer of Health was abolished, and his duties were largely taken over by what are now known as Community Physicians. It is therefore now the Community Physician who is required to acquaint himself with the general sanitary condition of his district, to suggest the steps he considers might be taken for its improvement, and to advise the local authority in all sanitary matters. He is expected to investigate all outbreaks of infectious disease, report upon them, and recommend and see carried into force such preventive measures as he deems necessary. He must, if it is advisable, or if he is directed by the sanitary authority, himself inspect any article exposed for food, and deal with it, if it is unsound. He advises also as to nuisances injurious to health. He is also expected to inform the Department of any outbreak of dangerous infectious disease.

Environmental Health Officer – The Environmental Health Officer, formerly known as the Public Health Inspector, and before that as the Sanitary Inspector, attends to the general sanitation of the district, investigates all conditions of nuisances, sees that the regulations and by-laws relating to offensive trades are observed, and that all unsound meat is dealt with. He takes, if authorized by the sanitary authority to do so, samples under the Sale of Food and Drugs Acts, and if these be found adulterated, he takes action under the Act. He reports to the Community Physician any infectious disease, coming under his notice, occurring in the district. He is required to preserve records of his inspections and actions.

Nuisances – A large number of objectionable processes are declared by the Public Health Acts to be 'Nuisances or injurious or dangerous to health'. Houses badly constructed or overcrowded, streets, ditches, water supplies, stables and byres, if foul and unclean, accumulations of filth, factories overcrowded, ill ventilated and filthy, furnaces not consuming their smoke as far as possible, overcrowded cemeteries, all constitute nuisances.

Every sanitary authority is required to have its district inspected for the detection of nuisances. Any person, however, who suspects the presence of a nuisance may complain to the sanitary authority, who will at once have the matter investigated. If the authority is convinced of the existence of a nuisance, a notice will be served on the person responsible, or, if the author cannot be found, on the owner or occupier of the premises, requiring the removal of the nuisance within a specified time. If the sanitary authorities fail to discharge their duty with reference to nuisances, individuals can appeal to the Department of Health and Social Security, who may issue an order to be enforced in a High Court of Justice, or may direct any police officer of the district to institute the ordinary legal proceedings in case of nuisances. The most expeditious method, however, for individuals to gain redress in case of default by the sanitary authority, is to complain direct to a justice, and the court may make orders and exact penalties, just as if the complaint had been made by the sanitary authority.

If the nuisance is then not removed, or is likely to recur, the sanitary authority may apply to a justice, who will require the presence of the person responsible before a court of summary jurisdiction. If satisfied that the nuisance exists, or is likely to recur, the court may at once decern (or decree), or may remit to a special inspector to report. When the court is satisfied of the existence of the nuisance, an order will be granted for its removal, and for the performance of such works as will prevent its recurrence. The court has the further power, if convinced that the nuisance arises from wilful fault or negligence, to fine the author of the nuisance. Where the author is not known, the local authority may be directed to remove the nuisance themselves. Special by-laws are also made by local authorities with reference to their own towns.

Houses and sites for building – The health of the community depends in a large measure on the condition of its housing. Several factors contribute to the healthiness of a dwelling. The site must be suitable, the ventilation and water supply adequate, the construction must ensure the absence of dampness, and the sewage and refuse must be efficiently removed.

The site should be preferably on porous soil, such as gravel or sand, whence water can easily be carried away. In every case, whether on porous soil or on clay, the ground should be well drained. In towns, no choice can usually be made in the site, and houses are placed wherever convenient. Many are placed on 'made soils', but care ought to be taken that all organic matters have been completely decayed, a process which takes at least three years for completion, and not until that period has elapsed can a building be safely placed on a site of made soil. The site of the house should be covered by a layer of concrete to prevent the ground air and moisture gaining entrance into the house. The house should be so placed as to allow sufficient air to circulate around it, and to have abundance of light, and so elevated as to allow for proper drainage arrangements.

In the construction of houses, several points must be noted. The foundations must be strong enough to support the building upon them, while the walls should be built on a special basis of

concrete. To obviate dampness further, an impervious layer of slates bedded in cement, or of lead, or asphalt, known as the *damp-proof course*, should be inserted in the wall, at least 6 inches (15 cm) above the ground level. This may also consist of a layer of perforated stoneware tiles, embedded in cement, which not only act as a hindrance to damp, but ventilate the area between the ground and the floor (illustration 353).

353 – Foundation of a building in which the floor is above the level of the ground. The wall should rest on a concrete foundation.

The walls of the house may be built of stone, bricks, mortar or wood. Stones tend to absorb moisture, but not nearly so freely as bricks. Thus, a brick should not absorb more than 15 per cent of its own weight of water. The corresponding figures for limestones and sandstones are 10 and 8 per cent, respectively. Bricks also permit of the free percolation of air. Wood should be reserved for the inner fittings of houses. It is desirable that the height of each room should be at least 10 feet (3·5 metres). Each room should be supplied with adequate windows equal in area to at least one-tenth of the floor space, while no boxed-in, ill-ventilated, and sunless apartments should be permitted. Special ventilators should be fitted for each room, independent of the personal control of the occupants. (See VENTILATION.)

Dampness in houses may arise from moisture finding its way up the walls where damp-proof courses are not provided; and, where the house is in an exposed position, by rain being driven through the walls. This dampness arising from the driven rain can be prevented by covering the walls with some impervious material, as glazed tiles or Portland cement. Defective mortar, broken rain-pipes and gutters, choked gutters and drains, leaks in water and drainage pipes, and defects in the roof and the slating may all lead to dampness.

Streets and open spaces – Streets not only act as thoroughfares for traffic, but also provide for ventilation and admission of sunlight to buildings, in addition to constituting the course for the main sewers and water-supply pipes. The width of the street is important with reference to the height of the houses along it. Too narrow a street with high buildings implies dingy, dark, ill-ventilated dwellings. Considerable powers have therefore been given to sanitary authorities under the various Public Health Acts to regulate the width of the street, the height of the buildings, and as to repair. More important still is the regulation dealing with the air-space required in the rear of the new house.

Air and ventilation – Pure atmospheric air contains a little over 20 per cent by volume of oxygen, about 78 per cent of nitrogen, and about 0·04 per cent of carbon dioxide, together with traces of water vapour and some inert gases. The carbon dioxide present is generally accepted as the standard of impurity, but this is only a guide. There is no evidence that the discomfort experienced in badly ventilated rooms is due to lack of oxygen or excess of carbon dioxide. It is more closely associated with heat stagnation due to excess of moisture and lack of air movement. The air is naturally purified by winds driving the impurities away and allowing fresher air to take its place; by rain removing dissolved gases and washing away suspended impurities; and by vegetable life absorbing carbon dioxide in the day-time and giving off oxygen. Fogs tend naturally to pollute it. It is vitiated by respiration, combustion, putrefactive processes of animal and vegetable matters, and by the products of trades and industries, such as the mineral particles set free in grinding and the organic effluvia given off in soap-making, bone-boiling and tannery work.

Smoke from factories and open fires is a serious problem in diminishing the sunshine of large towns, but is being gradually lessened by the increasing use of gas and electricity and by the enactments of the Clean Air Acts, whereby air pollution, with all its accompaniments of fog, dirt and lack of sunshine is becoming a thing of the past, with a well-nigh revolutionary change in those towns and cities with enlightened local authorities who have applied the enactments of these Acts. Thus the pea-souper fogs which once were world famous as one of the banes of life in London are now a thing of the past, and the inhabitants of cities like Stoke and Sheffield can now bask in summer sunshine instead of a perpetual pall of smoke.

Water and water supplies – An adequate supply of water is necessary for every condition of life. Its importance has been recognized and appreciated from earliest times, and is closely bound up with the industrial activity and progress, as well as the health of communities. The increase in the purity of the supplies of this country has undoubtedly lessened the occurrence of water-borne epidemics of disease. Every township of any importance at the present time aims at possessing a pure and abundant supply. This supply is utilized for domestic, municipal and trade purposes. The domestic supply must be liberal for cleanliness, cooking, drinking and sanitary requirements. Municipal requirements for washing the streets, flushing the sewers, and extinguishing fires, absorb a considerable quantity. Trade processes vary in their demands, according to the nature of the industries.

The original source of all water supply is the rain and the dissolved snow. This may be gathered and used. Part, however, may sink through the soil, to reappear in the form of springs, or to be reached by means of wells. Part may flow on the surface as rivers and streams, or may be collected together in lakes. All these may form the source of supply. (For further details consult the article on WATER SUPPLY.)

Refuse and sewage disposal – The subject of refuse and sewage disposal is concerned with removal from towns and from buildings of waste matters. These waste matters consist chiefly of two distinct kinds: the excreta and waste waters, commonly dealt with as one in the sewage (qv); and, secondly, the dry refuse. The dry refuse includes the dust, ashes and debris of vegetable and animal food from households, the sweepings of streets and the dust and mineral particles of trade processes. The liquid and solid excreta and the waste water of houses have to be dealt with in sewage disposal. All the dry refuse is usually removed by dust carts and street sweepers.

Food and disease: BUTCHER MEAT – Butcher meat, if good, should be firm and elastic, marbled with fat, light red in colour, neither purulent, livid nor too moist. Various parasites may be present in meat which is diseased. The *Trichinella* *spiralis*, may be found in the muscles of the pig, and so infect man; while cysticerci in the ox and the pig produce tapeworms in man.

Meat which is infected or contaminated with bacteria, or their toxins, if eaten, may cause alarming symptoms of vomiting, diarrhoea and colic. (See FOOD POISONING.) Anthrax and tuberculosis may be spread to man from meat affected with these diseases.

Meat may be preserved by salting, pickling or canning.

MILK – Milk, being one of the chief articles of food, is often suspected of being the means of carrying disease. Milk may convey the infecting organisms of bovine tuberculosis, scarlet fever, enteric fever, diphtheria, undulant fever, septic sore throat, and of FOOD POISONING (qv). Being so largely used as a food, it may be adulterated, water being the commonest adulterant, whilst cream may be abstracted. Occasionally such articles as borax, salicylic acid and boric acid may be added in order to preserve the milk fresh and sweet. (See MILK.)

BUTTER – Butter may be adulterated with foreign fats and additional water. Margarine is occasionally substituted.

COFFEE – Coffee may contain excess of chicory.

WHEAT FLOUR – Wheat flour is sometimes adulterated with other grains.

Foods are now rigidly inspected. Samples are taken for analysis, and if these are found to be adulterated the vendors or suppliers are prosecuted, and may be heavily punished. At every slaughterhouse, inspection of meat is carried through as a matter of routine, and no meat declared unsound is allowed to be sold. (See also ADULTERATION OF FOOD.)

Infectious diseases are due to the entrance into the body of certain bacteria or their toxins, or of viruses which multiply in the system, and can be given off from the person affected, and thus may be received into the body of other individuals, in whom they may reproduce the disease. Hence the diseases are known as infectious diseases.

The infectious diseases may be spread from a person in various ways.

1. By the breath, as, for example, in scarlet fever, measles and whooping-cough. In many cases the expired air gathers its infection from the throat.

2. By particles of skin and the dried purulent crusts of smallpox.

3. By excretions and secretions. The discharges from the throat and nose are highly infectious in scarlet fever, diphtheria and measles. The faecal excretions in enteric fever and cholera contain the infection. The purulent discharges of abscesses and pustules in certain diseases carry infection. The sputum of tuberculous patients contains the tubercle bacillus, or *Mycobacterium tuberculosis* as it is now known. The urine in enteric fever is infected, and can convey the disease. Milk, water and foods are often infected by excretions, defects in the drains allowing the excretions to soak through and infect the waters of wells, or the water used in washing and cleaning conveys the infection to the utensils in which the milk is received and the food cooked. These articles of diet may also be infected by direct contact with the excretions of a carelessly treated patient, resulting in localized epidemics of infectious disease. Contamination of food often occurs through the medium of flies. (See INSECTS IN RELATION TO DISEASE.)

If the person is susceptible to the disease, a period elapses after the organism is received, known as the incubation period, during which no symptoms develop, but during which the organism multiplies and produces its poison. This period varies with each disease. (See INCUBATION; INFECTION.)

METHODS OF PREVENTION may embrace removal of cases to hospital or isolation at home; disinfection of clothing, bedding and premises; isolation, if necessary, of persons who have been in contact with certain diseases; closure of schools if the disease is being spread by the school connection (see INFECTION); stoppage of milk supplies if these be infected, and injection of protective sera, as in those exposed to diphtheria, and the performance of vaccination upon persons who have come in contact with cases of smallpox.

SMALLPOX – Smallpox was formerly an extremely common disease in this country, but is now relatively rare. The exhalations and purulent crusts are the chief means of conveying infection. (See SMALLPOX; VACCINATION.)

SCARLET FEVER – The greatest number of cases occurs in young children. It is generally endemic in the large towns of Britain, but from time to time assumes epidemic proportions. The fatality rate has been greatly reduced in recent years, the type of the disease being milder. The infection is chiefly spread by discharges from the throat and nose. Milk is occasionally infected and spreads the disease. (See SCARLET FEVER.)

DIPHTHERIA – Infection passes from case to case by the exhalations and discharges from the nose and throat. Milk epidemics occasionally occur where the milk has become infected by the discharges from some patient living at the dairy or from some case infecting the milk during the course of distribution. Schools aid in spreading the disease by the presence of some child suffering from a mild, unrecognized attack. The most important preventive measure is the inoculation of school children and the pre-school child with diphtheria prophylactic, as, for example, with alum-precipitated toxoid (APT). As a result of the increasing extent to which the child-population has been immunized in this way, there has been a dramatic fall both in the incidence and the severity of diphtheria. (See DIPHTHERIA.)

ENTERIC or TYPHOID FEVER – Its prevalence has been largely reduced by adequate water supplies and improved sanitary conditions. The excreta are highly infectious and must be carefully disinfected. Milk and water have been contaminated and have led to large epidemics. (See ENTERIC FEVER.)

TYPHUS FEVER – Poverty, with its consequences in privation, overcrowding and filth, is the chief predisposing cause of this disease. (See TYPHUS FEVER.)

MEASLES and WHOOPING-COUGH are largely diseases of childhood. With increase of years the liability to attack is reduced. The severity is greatest in the very young, who should therefore be protected from infection and not exposed. Convalescent serum and immune globulin are useful in preventing measles in the very young or frail, or in modifying the disease in the robust child, when known exposure to infection has occurred. A vaccine is now available for both diseases. (See MEASLES; WHOOPING-COUGH.)

PULMONARY TUBERCULOSIS is the most serious of all the infectious diseases. Preventive measures include mass miniature radiography, and the use of BCG vaccine (qv). (See TUBERCULOSIS.)

Disinfection and disinfectants – Disinfection consists in the destruction of the organisms or other agencies of disease. It is accomplished by means of disinfectants, of which sunlight, fresh air and fire are the most efficient and natural. During epidemics, milk or water, if suspected of being infected, should be boiled. All cloths and the like, used to clean up discharges from infectious cases should, if possible, be destroyed, whilst, if the bedding and clothing are totally worthless or in a wretched condition, they may also be burned. Many of the ordinary disinfectants, though containing disinfectant materials, are used in such strength as only to act as deodorants, and so, while removing the noxious odours, particularly of excreta, do not destroy the infecting material and consequently give only a false sense of security. For the varieties and uses of disinfectants see DISINFECTION.

Disposal of the dead – The chief object in the disposal of the dead is the speediest method by which the body can be dissolved into its simplest components. Two methods are in vogue in Britain: namely, burial and cremation.

BURIAL, from a sanitary point of view, should take place in a loamy or sandy porous soil, well drained, and so situated as not to contaminate any water supply, and preferably removed from the neighbourhood of houses. The body should be confined in a thin, easily disintegrated coffin. Oak and lead coffins and brick vaults all violate the first principles of burial. Coffins must be separated from each other by at least 1 foot (30 cm) of earth, and no coffin is permitted to be nearer the surface of the ground than 4 feet (120 cm).

The Burial Acts, 1853–1906, provide for the closing of overcrowded churchyards and the discontinuance of burials in them. Under this power many of the old overcrowded churchyards have been closed.

CREMATION is, perhaps, the best sanitary method of disposal, especially in cases of infectious disease, the germs of some of which can exist in the soil. The sanitary reason for it is powerful, but its adoption prevents the possibility of exhumation, and so might occasionally prevent the detection of crime. (For further details, see DEAD, DISPOSAL OF.)

SAPHENOUS is the name given to the two large superficial veins of the leg. The small saphenous vein which runs up the outside and back of the leg joins the deep veins at the bend of the knee; the great saphenous vein, the longest vein in the body, which has a long course from the inner ankle to the groin, is specially subject, with its branches, to become the seat of varicose veins.

SAPO is the Latin name for soap.

SAPRAEMIA is the name applied to a mild form of blood-poisoning. (See BLOOD-POISONING.)

SAPROPHYTE is the term applied to organisms which live usually upon decaying and dead matter and produce its decomposition.

SARCINA is a microscopic vegetable growth, which is found in the material vomited or drawn off by the stomach tube from a dilated stomach.

SARCO- is a prefix signifying flesh or fleshy.

SARCOIDOSIS is a chronic disease of unknown origin. In certain cases it is a manifestation of tuberculosis. It involves the skin, lymph nodes, eyes, salivary glands, lungs and bones of the hands and feet.

SARCOMA (see CANCER and illustration 98).

SARCOPTES SCABIEI is the mite which causes scabies (qv).

SARSAPARILLA is the root of various species of *Smilax*. It is largely used in domestic medicine as a 'blood-purifier', and is an ingredient of many patent medicines. Its main use today is as a flavouring agent.

SASSAFRAS is the name for a genus of laurel trees. The root bark of *Sassafras albidum* contains an oil, and its fluid extract was formerly much used in the treatment of various skin diseases. Mucilage derived from sassafras is also used in bronchial and gastric affections.

SATURNINE POISONING is another name for lead-poisoning. (See LEAD-POISONING.)

SAUNA is a hot-air, steam or smoke bath, combined with ice-cold water bathing or douching. An old Finnish practice, practically every house or block of flats there has its sauna. Originally, these log cabins were heated by wood-burning stoves made of rough stones, but the modern sauna has an electric oven surrounded by stones. The sauna cabin has a tightly fitting door and narrow vents in the walls, but no windows. The bathers sit or lie naked, according to their preferences, on wooden benches. Before entering the sauna, with its temperature of 110° C, a cold shower is taken. Periodically the bathers come out and plunge into a nearby ice-cold lake or have another cold shower. At some stage of the sauna mas-

sage is given, or alternatively the bathers beat each other with birch twigs. After this a further session is spent in the heat, and the course ends with a cold bath. The bather should rest for twenty minutes or until he has ceased to sweat before beginning to dress. The precise therapeutic value of saunas may not be clear, though the Finns claim that they are a well-proven means of maintaining health. There is some evidence that they may be good for the skin, the upper air passages, weight reduction, and for the relief of rheumatic pains.

SCAB is the name given to the crust which forms on superficial injured areas. It is composed of fibrin, which is exuded from the raw surface, together with blood corpuscles and epithelial cells entangled in its meshes. Healing takes place naturally under this protection, and the scab dries up and falls off when healing is complete. Scabs appearing on the face without any previous abrasion are often of infectious nature. (See IMPETIGO.)

SCABIES is a skin disease caused by the *Sarcoptes scabei* (illustration 354), which resembles the cheese mite in appearance. It is a minute oval-shaped mite possessing four pairs of legs. It is just visible to the naked eye, the female measuring about 250 to 350 micrometres in length; the male is smaller. The female burrows in the skin, particularly that on the front of the wrist, the web and sides of

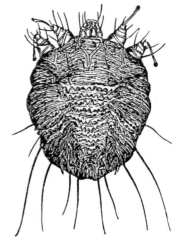

354 – The female sarcoptes, magnified about 80 times.

the fingers, the buttocks, the genitals, and the feet, forming small tunnels in which she lays her eggs (25 to 30). The sides and legs may also be affected in the same way, though rarely the upper parts of the body. The eggs hatch in the burrows in four to five days, and it is the movement of the larvae which causes the intense itching which gives scabies its popular name of itch. The scratching caused by this itching is responsible for much of the eruption of scabies. The larvae ultimately leave the burrows and develop in the skin, a female becoming mature in about two weeks.

Scabies is rife among the population of Great Britain. Personal contact is the most important factor in keeping this infestation going. This is why it is so important that all members of a household in which a case occurs should be carefully examined, and treated if found to be infected. Less stress is now laid on dissemination of the mite by infested clothes and blankets.

Symptoms – The person complains of great itchiness and heat, felt particularly soon after he goes to bed, and preventing sleep in the early part of the night. The spaces between the fingers, the backs of the hands, and the front of the wrists are red and scabbed as the result of scratching, or the surface in these localities may even be much inflamed.

Treatment – The patient is scrubbed with soft soap in a hot bath, to open up the burrows. Immediately after drying, the official *British Pharmacopoeia* 25 per cent preparation of benzyl benzoate, known as Benzyl Benzoate Application B P, is applied to the whole surface of the body below the chin. A second and a third application is made at twelve-hourly intervals. The patient then has a bath, puts on clean underclothes, and has his bed clothes changed. In infants and young children, in whom benzyl benzoate may cause unpleasant stinging, monosulfiram or gamma benzene hexachloride may be used as an alternative.

SCALD HEAD is the old name for favus. (See RINGWORM.)

SCALDS (see BURNS AND SCALDS).

SCALP is the soft covering of the skull on the top of the head. It consists of five layers, which from the surface inwards are as follows: the skin, thickly furnished with hair; next a subcutaneous layer of fat, rendered tough and stringy by many bands of fibrous tissue passing through it to bind the skin and the third layer together; thirdly, a tough membrane composed of fibrous tissue, known as the epicranium; fourthly, a loose layer of connective tissue attaching the epicranium to the deepest layer, and permitting the free movements of which the scalp is capable; and, finally, another fibrous layer clinging closely to the skull, and known as the pericranium.

SCALPEL is a small, straight, surgical knife.

SCAPULA is the technical name for the shoulder-blade. (See SHOULDER-BLADE.)

SCAR is the name applied to a healed wound, ulcer or breach of tissue. A scar consists essentially of fibrous tissue, covered by an imperfect formation of epidermis in the case of scars on the surface of the skin. The fibrous tissue is produced by the connective tissue corpuscles that wander into the wound in the course of its repair (see WOUNDS), and is at first delicate in texture and richly provided with blood-vessels. Accordingly a scar at first is soft, and has a redder tint than the surrounding skin. Gradually this fibrous tissue contracts, becomes more dense, and loses its blood-vessels, so that an old scar is hard and white.

The more specialized textures are not repaired when a scar forms: thus on the skin-surface the scar does not reproduce hairs and sweat-glands, only the general epithelium growing over the wounded surface. Similarly in the case of internal organs, such as the stomach, no glands form anew in the scar. When muscles or nerves are wounded, however, new muscle- or nerve-fibres grow into the scar. Bone is repaired by a formation of fibrous tissue, which is produced just as in the soft parts, and later lime salts are deposited in the scars. (See BONE.)

The contraction that takes place in a scar has already been mentioned. The more quickly the surfaces of a wound are brought into contact with one another, the less fibrous tissue is produced for the union. Consequently a wound whose edges are accurately brought together and in which healing is rapid shows far less contraction afterwards, and leaves a fainter scar, than one in which the wound is allowed to gape, and in which healing is slow. Burns are therefore followed by very marked scars and great contraction, which often produces marked deformity of the part concerned. Similarly, when inflammation takes place, as when an operation wound becomes infected, or when such a disease as lupus is present, causing great irritation of the wound, a wide, unsightly scar results and causes much puckering of the surrounding skin as it contracts. Such scars are also of low vitality, stretch easily, so as to become still more evident, and if irritated, as, for example, by the pressure of a boot or badly fitting artificial limb, readily give way and produce an ulcer which is slow to heal. Unsightly scars, on the face for example, can often be removed by the plastic surgeon.

Scars are sometimes extremely painful, especially those which are left after the amputation of part of a limb. This is caused in general by the involvement of a sensory nerve in the hard contracting tissue of the scar. (See also KELOID.)

SCARF-SKIN is another name for the epidermis, or outer layer of the skin. (See SKIN.)

SCARIFICATION means the making of shallow cuts in the skin for the purpose of drawing blood.

SCARLET FEVER, or SCARLATINA, is an acute infectious disease, characterized by high fever, sore throat and a diffuse red rash upon the skin, due to infection with a haemolytic streptococcus. This fever appears to have been first accurately described by Sydenham in 1676, before which period it had evidently been confounded with smallpox and measles.

Causes – Scarlet fever is highly contagious. The patient is infectious from the time of the first symptoms, and the infectivity is greatest at the height of the fever, thereafter gradually falling off as the disease declines. The period of isolation is until clinical recovery or not less than seven days from onset, provided that at the end of this time the patient has no infectious discharges, as from the nose. The disease may also be carried by milk, which has been contaminated by some infected person working on its distribution or in the dairy, or has come from a cow with mastitis. Scarlet fever is a disease especially of young children. Adults may also suffer if they have not had this fever in childhood, but one attack usually confers immunity from a second. Women in the puerperal state are particularly liable to contract the disease.

Surgical scarlatina is a name given to a mild condition of fever with red rash and sometimes enlargement of glands, which may accompany septic conditions such as

burns, empyema and other abscesses. It appears to be due to streptococcal infection.

Symptoms – The period of incubation (ie. the time elapsing between the reception of infection and the development of symptoms) varies somewhat. In most cases it lasts only two to three days, but in occasional cases the patient may take a week to develop his first symptoms. The invasion of fever is usually short and sharp, with rapid rise of temperature to 104° F (40° C) or thereabouts in the first few hours. There also occur shivering, vomiting, headache, sore throat and marked increase in the rate of the pulse. In young children convulsions or delirium may also usher in the fever. The rash usually appears within 24 hours of the onset of fever. It is first seen on the neck, chest, arms and hands, but quickly spreads all over the body and legs. The rash consists of minute, thickly set, red points which coalesce to form a general redness not unlike that produced by application of mustard to the skin. The rash tends to avoid the region of the nose and lips (circumoral pallor). Sometimes the redness is accompanied by small vesicles containing fluid. In ordinary cases the rash is at its height in about two days and then begins to fade, being gone at the end of a week from its first appearance. The tongue at first is covered by thick, white, creamy fur through which, on the second day, red papillae project, giving the appearance of a white strawberry tongue. The fur is then gradually denuded, and by the fourth or fifth day the tongue is red, bare and glazed – red strawberry tongue. The interior of the throat is red and swollen, especially the uvula, soft palate and tonsils, and a considerable amount of secretion is found on the inflamed surfaces. The glands under the jaw are slightly swollen and tender. In favourable cases the fever falls distinctly about the third day, the symptoms at the same time rapidly improve and the rash fades. The throat becomes more comfortable, and peeling of the skin shows itself first about the cheeks and neck, and later spreads all over the surface of the body. The amount of peeling varies widely, and to a certain extent it tends to be worst in the more severe cases. In the mild cases being encountered in Britain today it is very slight.

Complications – The most common and serious of these is *inflammation of the kidneys*, or *glomerulonephritis*, which may arise during any period in the course of the fever, but is specially apt to appear in convalescence, while desquamation is in progress. Its onset is sometimes announced by a return of feverish symptoms, accompanied with vomiting and pain in the loins; but in a large number of instances it occurs without these and comes on insidiously. One of the most prominent symptoms is slight swelling of the face, particularly of the eyelids, which is rarely absent in this complication. The urine is diminished in quantity and of dark smoky or red appearance, due to the presence of blood and contains albumin. Microscopic examination reveals the presence of tube casts containing blood and epithelium. In favourable cases these symptoms may soon disappear, but they may, on the other hand, prove extremely serious – the risks being the suppression of urine, leading to uraemic poisoning and causing convulsions which may terminate fatally, or the rapid development of general dropsy, and death from this cause. If this complication ensues, it commonly does so about the third or fourth week after the beginning of the illness. Occasionally this condition does not wholly pass off, and consequently lays the foundation for chronic Bright's disease. (See BRIGHT'S DISEASE.) Another complication of scarlet fever is *suppuration of the ears*, due to the extension of the inflammatory process from the throat along the Eustachian tube into the middle ear. (See EAR, DISEASES OF.) Other maladies affecting the heart and lungs occasionally arise in connection with scarlet fever, the chief of these being *endocarditis*, which may lay the foundation of valvular disease of the heart later in life. Arthritis or *scarlatinal rheumatism* is another complication of the disease, producing swelling and pain in the smaller rather than in the larger joints. This complication usually occurs in the second week of illness.

Treatment – In view of the mild type of scarlet fever at present prevailing there is a tendency in Great Britain not to admit such cases to hospital unless they are particularly severe, the home conditions are unsatisfactory, or there is some risk to the public: eg. a member of the household works in a dairy and may therefore be responsible for infecting milk. Children who have been in contact with cases of scarlet fever are allowed to go to school provided they are sent home at the first suggestion of fever or malaise.

When the patient is treated at home, the sick-room should contain only such furniture as may be required, and the atten-

dants should come as little as possible in contact with other members of the household. It is usual to keep the patient in bed for two weeks from the onset of the disease, and thereafter great care must be taken to avoid chills, owing to the danger of kidney complications. All body or bed linen when removed should be placed at once in boiling water, or in some disinfecting fluid. All books, toys, etc., used by the patient during the illness should be destroyed if of no value, or alternatively, carefully disinfected. The chief sources of contagion are the discharges of ear, nose, and throat. The desquamating skin is not infectious.

As scarlet fever is predominantly a streptococcal infection, the sulphonamide drugs or penicillin should be given. Preference is now generally shown for penicillin, and this should be given in every case. As to general management during the progress of the fever, in favourable cases little is required beyond careful nursing and feeding. The diet all through the fever and convalescence should be light but nourishing, consisting mainly of milk foods. During the febrile stage plenty fluid must be taken, which can be flavoured with fruit juices. A useful drink may be made from bitartrate of potassium (see CREAM OF TARTAR), of which the patient may partake freely.

The treatment of the kidney complication and its accompanying dropsy is similar to that for acute Bright's disease. The management of the sore throat, enlarged glands and joint affections, is conducted on general principles.

SCHISTOSOMIASIS, also known as BILHARZIASIS, is one of the most important diseases in the tropics. The responsible parasites, *schistosomes* or blood flukes, which are responsible for the disease, occur in Egypt, many parts of tropical Africa, and South America. The male is about 12 millimetres long. The female, which is about 24 millimetres in length, lies partly enclosed in a groove down the body of the male (illustration 355). The ova, or eggs, are provided with a sharp spike which is terminal in S. haematobium (illustration 356) and lateral in S. mansoni. The schistosomes live in the portal vein and its branches. The ova ultimately reach either the bladder (*S. haematobium*) or the rectum (*S. mansoni* and *S. japonicum*), whence they are voided in the urine or faeces. The next stage of development takes place in certain snails (illustration 357). Human infection occurs by wading or bathing in infected water, the infection occurring through the skin, whence the immature schistosome ultimately reaches the portal vein.

SCHISTOSOMA HAEMATOBIUM is widely distributed throughout North Africa, including Egypt, East Africa, and South Africa. It is also found in the Middle East, Portugal and Cyprus. As the ova are excreted through the bladder, the main symptoms are cystitis and haematuria (ie. the passage of blood in the urine). In chronic cases there may be formation of stones in the bladder, and sometimes cancer develops in the bladder.

SCHISTOSOMA MANSONI is found predominantly in the Nile valley, East Africa, and West Africa. It is also found in Israel, Yemen, Central and South America and the Caribbean Islands. As the ova are mainly excreted through the rectum, the first manifestation of the disease is usually diarrhoea, with the passage of much blood in the stools. As with S. haematobium

356 - Egg of Schistoma haematobium. From Blacklock and Southwell. Human Parasitology. H. K. Lewis & Co. Ltd.

infections, there is often irritation of the skin or dermatitis, and there is always some anaemia, which may become severe. The spleen usually becomes enlarged, sometimes to a very considerable extent.

SCHISTOSOMA JAPONICUM is confined to the Far East, particularly the Yangtse valley. Here again the ova are found in the rectum, and the main manifestations of the infection are chronic dysentery, enlargement of the liver and the spleen, and anaemia.

The treatment of schistosomiasis consists of the injection of various antimonial preparations, including stibocaptate, and two recently introduced drugs known as niridazole and lucanthone.

SCHISTOSOME DERMATITIS (see BATHER'S ITCH).

SCHIZO- is a prefix signifying splitting.

SCHIZOPHRENIA is a term applied to forms of psychosis in which there is a cleavage of the mental functions, associated with assumption by the affected person of a second personality. (See MENTAL ILLNESS.)

SCHOOL CHILDREN – With regard to the earliest period of life, the manage-

355 – Diagram showing cylindrical female schistosome (2) lying in the gynaecophoric canal of the male schistosome (1). From Blacklock and Southwell. Human Parasitology. H. K. Lewis & Co. Ltd.

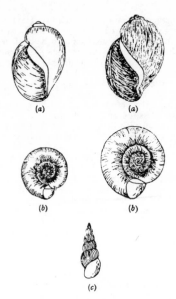

357 – Snails which act as intermediate hosts for schistosomes. (*a*) *Bulinus* and *Physopsis* genus, which are intermediate hosts for *S. haematobium*. (*b*) *Planorbis* genus, intermediate host for *S. mansoni*. (*c*) *Oricomelania* genus, intermediate host for *S. japonicum*. From Blacklock and Southwell, *Human Parasitology*. H. K. Lewis & Co. Ltd.

ment of children will be found under INFANT FEEDING and CHILDREN, PECULIARITIES OF. After infancy, there follows a period between the ages of 2 and 5, during which the child is more or less independent but requires a considerable amount of care, which at the present day is supervised by Child Welfare Clinics. Thereafter from about the age of 6 to 14 years the child comes under the discipline of school, and special arrangements for the welfare of children are then made through the educational agencies.

Schools are now built on a pavilion plan, and great care is taken in regard to their site, construction, ventilation, warming, etc. The appropriate temperature for teaching rooms and nursery playrooms, when the outside temperature is 32° F (0° C), is 62° F (16·5° C). For assembly halls, gymnasia, and dining-rooms a temperature of 57° F (14° C) is considered adequate. Some form of central heating is necessary, and also some system of artificial ventilation. When there is not more than 180 cubic feet (2·8 cubic metres) of space per child, six changes of air an hour

are necessary but if the available space is 500 cubic feet (8·5 cubic metres) per child, one and a half changes of air per hour is sufficient. The prescribed minimum of floor space depends upon the number of, and ages of, the children, varying in secondary schools from 38 to 52 square feet (3·53 to 4·83 sq. metres) per child.

Seats and desks are important both in regard to the comfort and, more particularly, in regard to the development of growing children, because if they are badly constructed or unsuitable in size the child is apt to assume unsuitable postures and undergo deformity in development. (See SPINE, DISEASES OF.) The seats and desks should be arranged in parallel rows at right angles with the windows, and, if possible, the chief illumination should be from the left. The desks should be from 15 to 18 inches (32 to 40 cm) wide and slightly sloped. The height of the seat from the ground should be equal to the length of the child's leg from the sole of the foot to the knee, and the front of the seat should be almost under the edge of the desk. The height of the edge of the desk above the seat should be one-sixth of the child's height. Seats and desks should be carefully adjusted to growing children twice yearly, and it must be remembered that the heights of children of the same age often vary as much as 10 inches (25 cm), whilst children often increase in height 4 to 6 inches (10 to 15 cm) in a year. Each pupil should have from 20 to 40 inches (0·5 to 1 metre) of seat room.

The provision of cloakrooms with pegs, of covered sheds for recreation, and of suitable lavatory and washing facilities is equally important.

Drinking-water is an important matter, because drinking-cups often form a means of communicating disease such as diphtheria. In the crystal stream drinking-fountains provided in American schools no cups are necessary, scholars drinking directly from a weak upward jet of water. Small folded paper cups are cheap and can be thrown away after use.

In Britain, education authorities are required to provide milk and meals for school children on days when the school meets, and they are empowered to provide such refreshment on other days. The **diet** for school children should be plain, generous, easily digested and varied, with ample eggs, butter, fish, meat and a liberal allowance of cooked and fresh fruit. Milk is a highly nutritious food, which is specially suitable for children. The craving for sweet things should be met by supplying these at the end of a meal after the appetite has been satisfied. Over 75 per cent of the elementary school children of Great Britain give evidence of **dental caries,** and an early investigation of the teeth is desirable, together with inculcation by the teacher of the use of the toothbrush as an essential act of cleanliness.

Under the Education Acts of Great Britain, children from 5 to 16 years of age must attend school, whilst mentally subnormal, blind and deaf children must receive education up to the age of 16 years. For the successful teaching of children it is important that they should not suffer from **mental fatigue.** This is brought about not so much by long hours of work as by a wrong system of teaching. No individual subject should be pursued for longer than three-quarters of an hour, and the succession of subjects taught should be suitably varied. There should be sufficient intervals for rest, play, physical exercise and food. In the classroom, quiet and fresh air are very important. (See FATIGUE.) For the amount of sleep requisite at different ages see CHILDREN, PECULIARITIES OF. The teaching of mentally subnormal children presents special problems, as these children make very slow progress. (See MENTAL SUBNORMALITY.) In any case, children up to the age of 5 years whose nervous system is rapidly developing and easily tired should be educated chiefly through their senses and physical activities. For the next five years, which is probably the chief period of character formation, the important object is the development of good habits; and after the age of 10 the child's reasoning powers and imagination can be most suitably developed.

The **eyesight** of about 20 per cent of schoolchildren is defective, and in 10 per cent seriously defective. Young children are specially handicapped by short sight; and at a later stage, when reading of books is a more essential part of study, those who suffer from long-sight are apt to develop symptoms of eye strain. (See VISION, DISORDERS OF; and SPECTACLES.)

Defective hearing due to ear disease is present in between 10 and 20 per cent of schoolchildren. The effect of this as regards lessons is that the child misses spoken words and shows seeming inattention or stupidity. Owing to the strain of his attention in class he is more readily exhausted by lessons. Physical symptoms are earache, headache, discharge from the ears and, if the condition is complicated by adenoids and enlarged tonsils, a habitually open mouth which gives him a still

further appearance of stupidity. The hearing should be carefully tested once a year, and if children are found to be deaf they should undergo the necessary treatment and should be given a suitable position in the class. (See DEAFNESS.)

Exercise (see EXERCISE) is a matter of great importance, partly because, when physical exercises are suitably interspersed with lessons, the circulation and general sense of well-being are increased so that more ready attention is given to teaching. Also physical exercises can be made to correct faulty and defective conditions in development and bad habits in regard to posture. Combined exercises, in which a large number take part, aid in school discipline and develop qualities of alertness, decision and activity. These exercises should, if possible, take place in the open air, should be carefully graded to suit the ages of the children, and should be designed to develop specially important muscles and movements such as those of deep breathing. Special attention should be given to children who develop faulty postures or have a tendency to deformities. These include children with the chest defectively formed as the result of rickets or early tuberculous disease, and particularly children with a tendency to lateral curvature of the spine or the development of round shoulders. Also at lessons the maintenance of a good posture is important, the child sitting squarely to his desk with the head erect, the shoulders squared, the back straight, and the elbows kept at the same level.

Among the **diseases** for which the teacher must be specially on the lookout are measles, diphtheria and scarlet fever among the infectious diseases (see INFECTION); discharges from the nose and from the ears which indicate inflammation in these cavities; the presence of bald patches indicating ringworm (see RINGWORM); and also the presence of scabies about the hands, and impetigo as shown by crusts about the face.

SCHOTT TREATMENT is a system of treatment devised by a German physician for persons suffering from disorders of the heart. The treatment is specially carried out at Nauheim in Germany, and consists in a combination of baths in spring-water containing brine or carbonic acid gas, with carefully graduated exercises, and suitable rules for the guidance of the daily life.

SCIATICA means pain in the distribution of the sciatic nerve. It is often accompanied by pain in the back, or lumbago. It may be due to a number of causes, such as a tumour in the spine or spinal column, tuberculosis of the spine, ankylosing spondylitis. (See SPINE, DISEASES AND INJURIES OF,) or a tumour in one of the organs in the pelvis such as the uterus. In the vast majority of cases, however, it is due to a prolapsed intervertebral disc (qv) pressing on one or more of the nerve roots issuing from the lower part of the spinal cord that make up the sciatic nerve. The precise distribution of the pain will thus depend on which of the nerve roots are affected. As a rule, the pain is felt in the buttock, the back of the thigh and the outside and front of the leg, sometimes extending on to the top of the foot. In other cases the pain is felt in the buttock, the back of the thigh and the calf, and then along the outer border of the foot towards the little toe. What probably happens is that degenerative changes take place in the annulus fibrosus. (See SPINAL COLUMN.) Ultimately this ruptures, either as a result of some special strain such as is induced by heavy lifting, or spontaneously. The cushioning disc between the two neighbouring vertebral bodies slips through the rent in the annulus fibrosus, and presses on the neighbouring roots, thus causing the pain.

The condition usually occurs in adults under the age of 60. The pain may come on suddenly when the person concerned is undertaking some unusual effort, such as heavy lifting, and may be so severe that the victim faints and, when he comes to, he may be locked in one position. More commonly it comes on gradually and keeps on recurring over long periods of time. In these cases the amount of pain varies tremendously: from little more than a recurrent nuisance to a pain of almost unbearable intensity.

Treatment consists essentially of rest in bed in the early stages until the acute phase is over. Boards should be placed underneath the mattress to ensure adequate support for the back. Alternatively, the mattress may be put on the floor for the patient to sleep on. Anodynes, such as aspirin and codeine, are given to relieve the pain. A few days' rest in bed at the beginning of the trouble probably reduces the risk of further trouble. Expert opinion varies as to the desirability of wearing a plaster of Paris jacket or a specially made corset. Some contend that such support is advisable. Others contend that it is seldom necessary. Certainly a corset of this type is uncomfortable to wear, and there is a tendency for some victims of the disease to become too dependent on it. Equally, opinion differs as to the desirability of manipulation of the spine and operation. By and large the tendency in recent years has been for a reduction in the number of operations performed for prolapsed intervertebral disc.

SCILLA is the Latin name for squills.

SCIRRHUS is the name applied to a hard form of cancer in which much fibrous tissue develops.

SCLERA, or SCLEROTIC COAT, is the outermost coat of the eyeball. (See EYE.)

SCLERITIS means inflammation of the sclerotic coat of the eye, usually of a rheumatic or gouty nature.

SCLERODERMA, or SCLERODERMIA, also known as 'hidebound disease', is a condition in which the skin becomes hard – like leather, causing stiffening of the joints, and leading to gradual wasting of the muscles.

SCLEROSIS means literally hardening, and is a term applied to conditions in which portions of organs become hard and useless as the result of an excessive production of connective tissue. The term is especially applied to a change of this type taking place in the nervous system. (See MULTIPLE SCLEROSIS.) When a change of this nature takes place in other organs it is generally known as cirrhosis or fibrosis. (See CIRRHOSIS.) These conditions are generally attributed to some form of chronic inflammation.

SCOLIOSIS is the name applied to curvature of the spine consisting partly of a bend to one side, partly of a rotary twist. It may result from disease of the spine, but in weakly children it may arise from so slight a cause as a bad habit in standing or in leaning one arm on the table at lessons. It also arises from disease affecting one side of the chest, such as chronic pleurisy or tuberculosis. (See SPINE, DISEASES OF.)

SCOPARIUM is the tops of *Cytisus scoparius*, the common broom. It has a diuretic action.

SCOPOLAMINE is an alkaloid identical with hyoscine and used in combination with morphine for an anaesthetic, or as a hypnotic in delirium or to produce twilight sleep.

SCOTOMA is the term applied to a blind or partly blind area in the visual field. It may affect either the outer part of the visual field (peripheral scotoma), or the blindness may affect the centre, vision being retained round about (central scotoma).

SCRIVENER'S PALSY is another name for writer's cramp. (See CRAMP.)

SCROFULA, or STRUMA, is a state of constitutional weakness, generally exhibiting itself in early life, and characterized mainly by defective nutrition of the tissues, which renders them a ready prey to tuberculosis. The condition, as it manifests itself in disease of the glands in the neck, was formerly known in England as 'king's evil', from the belief that the touch of the sovereign could effect a cure. This superstition can be traced back to the time of Edward the Confessor in England, and to a much earlier period in France. Samuel Johnson was touched by Queen Anne in 1712, and the same supposed prerogative of royalty was exercised by Prince Charles Edward in 1745.

SCROTUM is the name applied to the pouch of integument within which the testicles are suspended. It consists of a purse-like fold of skin, within which each testicle has a separate investment of muscle fibres, several layers of fibrous tissue, and a serous membrane known as the tunica vaginalis.

SCRUM-POX is a popular name for a contagious affection of the face and head affecting football players. (See IMPETIGO.)

SCURF, or DANDRUFF, is a popular name for the scaly condition that is often found on the scalp, and often precedes baldness. (See SEBORRHOEA.)

SCURVY, or SCORBUTUS, is a deficiency disease characterized by the occurrence of extravasations of blood in the tissues of the body, and due to an insufficiency of vitamin C, or ascorbic acid, in the diet.
Causes – In former times this disease was extremely common among sailors, and was responsible for a high mortality rate. It is now of rare occurrence at sea, its cause being well understood and its prevention readily secured by simple measures. Scurvy has also frequently broken out among soldiers on campaign, in beleaguered cities, as well as among communities in times of scarcity, and in prisons, workhouses and other public institutions. In all such instances it has been found to depend closely upon the character and amount of the food, the occurrence of serious illness, and a diet too limited, either in amount or variety. These conditions predispose to scurvy, but the essential cause lies in deprivation of fresh food and especially of fresh vegetables for a period of four to six months. The want of vitamin C, which is soluble in water and is found chiefly in citrus fruits, potatoes, green vegetables and black currants, is the essential deficient factor. Besides this essential defect, a diminution in the total amount of food, the large use of a salted meat or fish, and all causes of a depressing kind, such as exposure, anxiety, bad hygiene, will contribute to the development of the disease.

Infants, too, may suffer from scurvy as the result of insufficiency of vitamin C in the diet.

Symptoms – The symptoms of scurvy come on gradually, and its onset is not marked by any special indications beyond a certain failure of strength, most manifest on making efforts. Breathlessness and exhaustion are thus easily induced, and there exists a corresponding mental depression. The countenance acquires a sallow or dusky hue; the gums are tender and the breath offensive almost from the first. These preliminary symptoms may continue for weeks, and in isolated cases may readily escape notice, but can scarcely fail to attract attention where they affect large numbers of men. Later the gums are livid, spongy, ulcerating and bleeding; the teeth are loosened and drop out; and the breath is excessively foetid. Extravasations of blood now take place in the skin and elsewhere. These may be small, like the petechial spots of purpura (see PURPURA), but are often large, and cause swellings of the muscles in which they occur, having the appearance of extensive bruises, and tending to become hard and brawny. These extravasations are most common in the muscles of the lower limbs; but they may be formed anywhere, and may easily be produced by very slight pressure upon the skin or by injuries to it. Bleeding into joints is a troublesome symptom because it produces stiffness later. In addition, there are bleedings from mucous membranes, such as those of the nose, eyes and alimentary or respiratory tracts, whilst effusions of fluid take place into the pleural, pericardial or peritoneal cavity. Painful, extensive, and destructive ulcers are apt to break out on the limbs. There is also a considerable amount of anaemia. The further progress of the malady is marked by profound exhaustion, with a tendency to fainting, and with various complications, such as diarrhoea and lung or kidney troubles, any of which may bring about a fatal result. On the other hand, even in desperate cases, recovery may be hopefully anticipated when the appropriate remedy can be obtained.

Treatment – No disease is more amenable to treatment, both as regards prevention and cure, than scurvy. This consists of the administration of vitamin C in adequate amounts, either in the form of tablets of ascorbic acid or foodstuffs rich in this vitamin. Potatoes, cabbages, tomatoes, swede turnips, many fresh fruits, especially black currants, oranges and lemons, will be found of great service for this purpose. Orange-juice or lemon-juice is often employed, either fresh or canned. The use, in a fresh state, of lime-juice in the British Navy, which has been practised since 1795, had the effect of virtually extinguishing scurvy in the Service, whilst similar regulations introduced by the British Board of Trade in 1865 had a like beneficial result as regards the mercantile marine. It is only when these regulations have not been fully carried out, or when the supply of lime-juice has become exhausted, that scurvy among sailors has been noticed in recent times. The anaemia and debility are best overcome by the continued administration of iron, aided by fresh air and other measures calculated to promote the general health.

SCYBALA is the name applied to the extremely hard condition which the stools assume in aggravated constipation.

SEA-SICKNESS is a characteristic set of symptoms experienced by many persons when subjected to the pitching and rolling motion of a vessel at sea, of which depression, giddiness, nausea and vomiting are the most prominent.

Causes – Although the vast majority of people appear to be liable to this ailment at sea, they do not all suffer alike. Many endure distress of a most acute and even alarming kind, whilst others are simply conscious of transient feelings of nausea and discomfort. In long voyages, whilst many are affected with sea-sickness for the first few days only, others are tormented

with it during the entire period, especially on the occurrence of rough weather. In short voyages, such as across the English Channel, not a few, of those susceptible, escape, whilst others suffer in an extreme degree, the sickness persisting long after arrival on shore.

A great number of theories have been advanced to account for the connection between the motion of a ship and sea-sickness. The conditions concerned in the production of the malady are apparently of complex character, embracing more than one set of causes. In the first place, the rolling or heaving of the vessel disturbs that feeling of the relation of the body to surrounding objects upon which our sense of security rests. The nervous system being thus subjected to a succession of shocks or surprises fails to effect the necessary adjustments for equilibrium. Giddiness, nausea and vomiting follow. Much importance has been laid by some upon the effects of the displacement of the abdominal viscera, especially the stomach, by the rolling of the vessel; but, while this may possibly operate to some extent, it can only be as an accessory cause. The same may be said of the influence of the changing impressions made upon the vision – which has been regarded by some as so powerful in the matter – since attacks of sea-sickness occur also in the dark, and in the case of blind persons. Other contributory causes may be mentioned, such as the feeling that sickness is certain to come, which may bring on the attack in some persons even before the vessel has begun to move. The sense of the body being in a liquid or yielding medium as it descends with the vessel into the trough of the sea, the varied odours to be met with on board ship, and circumstances of a like nature, tend also to precipitate or aggravate an attack. In the few rare instances where sea-sickness has proved fatal, *post-mortem* appearances have been almost entirely negative, and only such as are met with in death from syncope.

Symptoms – The symptoms generally show themselves soon after the vessel has begun to roll, by the onset of giddiness and discomfort in the head, together with a sense of nausea and sinking at the stomach, which soon develops into intense sickness and vomiting. At first the contents of the stomach only are ejected; but thereafter bilious matter, and occasionally even blood, are brought up by the violence of the retching. The vomiting is liable to exacerbations according to the amount of oscillation of the ship; but seasons of rest, sometimes admitting of sleep, occasionally intervene. Along with the sickness there is great physical prostration, as shown in the pallor of the skin, cold sweats and feeble pulse, accompanied with mental depression and wretchedness. In almost all instances the attack has a favourable termination, and it is extremely rare that serious results arise, except in the case of persons weakened by other diseases, although occasionally the symptoms are for a time sufficiently alarming.

Treatment – Innumerable preventives and remedies have been proposed, but most of them fall far short of the success claimed for them. No means has yet been discovered which can altogether prevent the occurrence of sea-sickness, nor is it likely any will be found, since it is largely due to the pitching movements of the vessel, which cannot be averted. Swinging couches or chambers have not proved of any practical utility. No doubt there is less risk of sickness in a large and well-ballasted vessel than in a small one; but, even though the rolling may be considerably modified, the ascending and descending movements which so readily produce nausea continue. None of the medicinal agents proposed possesses infallible properties; a remedy which suits one person will often wholly fail with another. Experience gained during the 1939–45 War has shown that the most satisfactory remedy is hyoscine hydrobromide, grain $\frac{1}{100}$ to $\frac{1}{200}$ (0·6 to 0·3 mg). Other recently introduced drugs which are proving of value in the prevention of sea-sickness include avomine, dramamine and marzine.

When the vessel is in motion, or even before starting, the recumbent position with the head low and the eyes closed (so that the motion of the ship and sea cannot be seen) should be assumed by those at all likely to suffer, and, should the weather admit, on deck rather than below – the body, especially the extremities, being well covered. Many persons, however, find comfort and relief from lying down in their berths with a hot bottle to the feet, by which means sleep may be obtained, and with it a temporary abatement of the distressing giddiness and nausea. Individuals who tend to be constipated should ensure an adequate evacuation of the bowels before embarking. Should sickness supervene, small quantities of some light food, such as thin arrowroot, gruel or soup, ought to be swallowed if possible, in order to lessen the sense of exhaustion, which is often extreme, as well as to mitigate the

pain of retching by giving the stomach something upon which it can contract The vomiting may be mitigated by saline effervescing drinks, ice, chloroform (3 or 4 drops on a piece of sugar), or dilute hydrocyanic acid. Alcohol usually tends to aggravate the sickness, but brandy has long had a reputation as a useful means of treatment in the early stages.

SEASIDE, SEA-VOYAGES (see CLIMATE IN RELATION TO DISEASE).

SEAT-WORM is another name for threadworm. (See ENTEROBIASIS).

SEBACEOUS CYST is the term applied to a cyst in the skin formed as a result of blockage of the duct of a sebaceous gland.

SEBACEOUS GLANDS are the minute glands situated alongside of hairs and opening into the follicles of the latter a short distance below the point at which the hairs emerge on the surface (illustration 363). These glands secrete an oily material. and are especially large upon the nose, where their openings form pits that are easily visible. Some varieties of eczema, as well as acne, result from disorders of these glands. (See SKIN.)

SEBORRHOEA is the name given to a group of diseases of the skin in which the sebaceous or oil-forming glands are at fault. It manifests itself either by accumulation of dry scurf, or by the formation of an excessive oily deposit on an otherwise healthy skin.

Seborrhoeic dermatitis (or eczema), which is also known as SEBORRHOEA CAPITIS, is the form of seborrhoea which involves the scalp. In its mildest form it is little more than an exaggeration of the normal casting off of the superficial layers of the skin of the scalp (see SKIN), which manifests itself as the white scales popularly known as dandruff or scurf. In the more severe cases the amount of scaling is increased and is accompanied by redness of the scalp. This in turn may progress to such a stage that it is accompanied by a profuse discharge, sufficient to soak the victim's pillow at night. In these more severe cases the condition may spread to the forehead, eyebrows and back of the neck.

Treatment in the milder cases consists of washing the hair twice weekly with spirit soap or a soapless shampoo. The addition of 2 per cent cetrimide is sometimes beneficial. If there is no active eczema present, selenium sulphide (qv) may be used. In the more severe cases an antibiotic ointment, or lotion, which also contains a steroid, is often used.

SEBUM is the secretion of the sebaceous glands (qv). It acts as a natural lubricant of the hair and skin and protects the skin from the effects of moisture or excessive dryness. It may also have antibacterial action.

SECRETIN is the name given to a hormone secreted by the mucous membrane of the duodenum, the first part of the small intestine, when food comes in contact with it, which, on being carried by the blood to the pancreas, stimulates the secretion of pancreatic juice.

SECRETION is the term applied to the material formed by a gland as the result of its activity. For example, saliva is the secretion of the salivary glands, gastric juice that of the glands in the stomach wall, bile that of the liver. (See GLANDS.) Some secretions consist apparently of waste material which is of no further use in the chemistry of the body. These secretions are often spoken of as excretions: for example, the urine and the sweat. (For further details, see SALIVA; URINE; ENDOCRINE GLANDS, and also under the headings of the various organs.)

SECUNDINES is another name for the afterbirth, consisting of the placenta and membranes expelled in the final stage of labour.

SECUNDUM ARTEM is a Latin expression meaning in a skilful professional manner.

SEDATIVES are drugs and other measures which soothe over-excitement of the nervous system, whether the effect of this excitement be pain, sleeplessness, delirium or muscular spasm. Those sedatives that soothe pain are generally spoken of as anodynes; sedatives in sleeplessness or delirium are known as hypnotics; sedatives of spasm are called antispasmodics. (See ANODYNES; COLIC; HEADACHE; HYPNOTICS; NEURALGIA; PAIN.)

SEDIMENTATION RATE, or ERYTHROCYTE SEDIMENTATION RATE to give it its full title, is a test for measuring the activity and progress of certain diseases. If blood is drawn and put into a test-tube the red blood corpuscles sink and leave a clear layer above. In disease the rate of sinking is increased and can be measured. The more active the disease, the higher the rate of sinking of red blood corpuscles.

SEIDLITZ POWDER, or COMPOUND EFFERVESCENT POWDER, is a mild purgative composed of Rochelle salt and bicarbonate of soda, which are wrapped together in a blue paper, and tartaric acid, which is wrapped in a white paper. The contents of each paper are dissolved separately in half a tumblerful or less of water; the two solutions are mixed and swallowed while effervescing.

SEIGNETTE SALT is another name for Rochelle salt.

SELENIUM SULPHIDE is used as a shampoo in the treatment of dandruff (qv) and seborrhoeic eczema (or dermatitis) of the scalp. In view of its potential toxicity it should only be used under medical supervision. It must never be applied to inflamed areas of the scalp, and it must not be allowed to get into the eyes, as it may cause conjunctivitis or keratitis.

SELLA TURCICA is the name applied to the deep hollow on the upper surface of the sphenoid bone in which the pituitary gland is enclosed.

SEMEIOLOGY is the part of medical science dealing with the symptoms and signs of disease.

SEMEN is the richly albuminous fluid in which spermatozoa are suspended.

SEMILUNAR CARTILAGES are two crescentic layers of fibro-cartilage on the outer and inner edges of the knee-joint, which serve to form hollows on the upper surface of the tibia in which the condyles at the lower end of the femur rest. The inner cartilage is especially liable to be displaced by a sudden and violent movement at the knee. (See KNEE.)

SEMINAL VESICLE is one of the small paired sacs lying on either side of the male urethra (qv), the function of which is to collect and store spermatozoa. (See TESTICLE.)

SEMOLINA is a preparation of wheat. It is prepared by crushing wheat and removing the endosperm. It has the nutritive value of very low-extraction flour. Its main use is for the making of puddings. (See CEREALS.)

SENEGA is the root of *Polygala senega*, a small plant of the United States. It has an action as a stimulating expectorant, and its preparations are used in cough mixtures.

SENILITY (see AGE, NATURAL CHANGES IN).

SENNA is the leaves of various species of *Cassia senna*, being known as Tinnerelly senna and Alexandrian senna, according to its source. It is one of the most active of the simple laxative drugs, producing considerable griping if used alone. Senna is excreted in the urine, giving it a dark red or yellow colour. In the case of nursing mothers, some of the drug is excreted in the milk and may have a purgative effect upon the nursling. A standardized preparation of senna, Senokot, is now available which has none of the disadvantages of senna itself and is widely used for the management of constipation in old people.

SENSATION (see PAIN; TOUCH).

SENSITIZATION of a person means the production of anaphylaxis by a particular food, vaccine, or the like. (See ANAPHYLAXIS.)

SEPSIS means poisoning by the products of a putrefactive process. This process is set up by the growth of microorganisms in the body, and the general symptoms which accompany it are those of inflammation. (See INFLAMMATION.) It is prevented by the various procedures mentioned under ASEPSIS, and is neutralized, when it has occurred, by various substances. (See ANTISEPTICS.)

SEPTICAEMIA is a serious form of blood-poisoning due to the multiplication in the blood of bacteria – in fact, it is an infection of the blood. (See BLOOD-POISONING.)

SEQUELAE is the term applied to symptoms or effects which are liable to follow certain diseases. For example, bronchitis and other chest complaints may be sequelae of measles; heart disease is often a sequel of rheumatic fever; paralysis may follow diphtheria.

SEQUESTRUM is the name given to a fragment of dead bone cast off from the living bone in the process of necrosis. (See BONE DISEASES.) A sequestrum often remains in contact with, and partly enveloped by, newly formed bone, so that a sinus is produced, and a constant discharge goes on, till the dead bone is removed.

SEROUS MEMBRANES are smooth, transparent membranes that line certain large cavities of the body. The chief serous membranes are the peritoneum, lining the cavity of the abdomen; the pleurae, one of which lines each side of the chest, surrounding the corresponding lung; the pericardium, in which the heart lies; and the tunica vaginalis on each side, enclosing a testicle. The name of these membranes is derived from the fact that the surface is moistened by thin fluid derived from the serum of blood or lymph. Every serous membrane consists of a visceral portion, which closely envelops the organs concerned, and a parietal portion, which adheres to the wall of the cavity. These two portions are continuous with one another so as to form a closed sac, and the opposing surfaces are close together, separated only by a little fluid. This arrangement enables the organs in question to move freely within the cavities containing them. For further details see under PERITONEUM.

SERPENTARIA, or SNAKEROOT, is the root of various species of *Aristolochia* plants of the Southern United States. It has a stimulating action, and is used as a bitter in combination with other remedies in the treatment of indigestion.

SERPIGINOUS is a term used in connection with ulcers or eruptions that spread in a creeping manner.

SERUM is the fluid which separates from blood, lymph and other fluids of the body when clotting takes place in them. (See HAEMORRHAGE.) Blood plasma is the name given to the fluid of the blood circulating in the vessels, by which the corpuscles are carried along. As clotting takes place, fine threads of fibrin form from the fibrogen contained in the plasma. These threads produce a network of increasing density in which the corpuscles are entangled, and, as a result, the fluid (serum) which is left outside this clot is clear, unmixed with corpuscles, and of a pale yellow colour.

The relation of these substances is seen at a glance from the following table:

$$\text{Blood} = \begin{cases} \text{Plasma} = \begin{cases} \text{Serum} \\ \text{Fibrin} \end{cases} \\ \text{Corpuscles} \end{cases} = \text{Clot.}$$

Serum is a clear, yellowish fluid and contains, in addition to water, about 7 per cent of albumin and globulin, with smaller quantities of salts, fat, sugar, urea, uric acid and other extractives, as well as minute amounts of other albuminous bodies, which are of great importance in the prevention of disease. (See IMMUNITY.) The chief salt in the serum is common salt.

Serum is derived from the lymph also, and the fluid which is found in effusions into the pleura and other cavities of the body is very similar in composition.

The serum used for the administration of antitoxins in cases of diphtheria, tetanus, and other diseases, is generally derived from the blood drawn from horses which have been subjected to a long course of treatment. (See IMMUNITY; and SERUM THERAPY.)

SERUM THERAPY is the treatment of disease by the administration of serum (usually horse serum, sometimes human) containing antibodies against bacteria or viruses, or antitoxins against toxins, which are causing the symptoms of the disease. If bacteria are injected into an animal in gradually increasing doses – perhaps of dead bacteria first and of living bacteria later – antibodies to the bacteria appear in the blood serum of the animal injected. Similarly, if the toxins of bacteria are injected, antitoxins are produced. This reaction is the basis of immunity. The serum is then collected from the animal (usually a horse) for injection into a human being infected with the micro-organism against which the serum has been prepared. Serum therapy has proved highly successful in those infections in which the damage to the infected person is done by the toxins of the infecting micro-organism. For example, in diphtheria the diphtheria bacilli multiply in the throat, and the toxins there produced by the bacilli are absorbed into the blood, circulate round the body, and damage such structures as the heart and the nervous system. Here an antitoxic serum will provide the infected body with ready-made antitoxins which by uniting with the toxins will render them inert. Antitoxic serum is also of much value in the treatment of tetanus, botulism and gas gangrene. There is also a scorpion venom antiserum and a snake venon antiserum. (See also IMMUNOGLOBULIN.)

Dangers of serum – The serum which contains the antitoxic and other bodies is derived from the horse, and being different from human serum, it occasionally sets up serious symptoms when it is injected. The use of serum has even been known to cause death in very susceptible persons. (See ANAPHYLAXIS.)

SESAME OIL is the oil expressed from the seeds of *Sesamum indicum*. It is sometimes used to replace olive oil when the latter is in short supply.

SESAMOID BONES are rounded nodules of bone usually embedded in tendon. They are usually a few millimetres in diameter, but some are larger, such as the patella (qv), or knee-cap.

SETON is the name applied to a few strands of silk or thin strip of lint or gauze passed through the skin and underlying tissues by means of a large flattened needle, and left projecting at both ends.

SEWAGE AND SEWAGE DISPOSAL – Sewage consists of excreta (that is, urine and faeces), waste water from houses, effluent from factories, rain water and road washings. There are two major methods of disposing of it: the *conservancy method* and the *water carriage system.*

CONSERVANCY METHOD – This involves the retention of urine and faeces in or near the house, with removal as soon as possible. Waste waters are dealt with separately.

Privies are closets in which the excreta are deposited in a closed receptacle of such a size that weekly removal is necessary. They are an insanitary and unpleasant hangover from an age of slums, and are not now permitted in the planning of new buildings.

Earth Closets are based on the use of earth as a deodorizer, drier and disintegrator of excreta. The receptacle is made of galvanized iron and should have a capacity of not more than 2 cubic feet (57 cubic decimetres). At least half a pound (230 grams) of earth, which should be light loam, is needed for each user. Modern models are fitted with a simple method for the application of the earth. They must be built so that they can be entered only from the external air, and be so sited as not to render liable to pollution any well, spring or stream that is likely to be used for drinking or domestic purposes. The floor must be non-absorbent, 3 inches (7·5 cm) above the ground and must have a fall to the door. There must be no connection with any drain, and the receptacle must be protected from rain, easily accessible, watertight and non-absorbent.

Pail Closets are closets containing metal pails or tarred wooden tubs with a capacity not exceeding 2 cubic feet (57 cubic decimetres). Fine household ashes or sawdust may be used as covering.

None of these conservancy systems is satisfactory, and in all civilized communities they are steadily, if at times only gradually, being replaced by the water carriage system.

Chemical Closets are a more satisfactory means of conservancy disposal. In these the receptacle contains a disinfectant solution: either an alkaline emulsion of coal tar or some such product, or a strong solution of caustic soda. The contents are disposed of by burial or, if liquified, may be discharged into a soakaway approved of by the local authority. They are an acceptable form of closet for isolated houses, and, in portable form, are used for public gatherings and in boats, trains and aeroplanes.

'Multrum' is a method based on biological decomposition, or composting as it is known to gardeners. The 'multrum', converter (illustration 358) is a tight container with an air intake and a ventilation duct. It is equipped with a lavatory bowl and a garbage shute. Within the converter faeces, urine and paper are mixed with organic waste. Microbiological action turns the waste into an inodorous, inoffensive and stable product. This is a system that has been successfully used in Sweden for many years. In a more recent modification of it the converter is equipped with a thermostat regulated electric coil which

heats the compost to around 60° C. This cuts the cost by speeding up the process and thereby reducing the size of the converter.

Cesspools are used for houses which have a piped water supply but are too isolated to be linked to a water carriage system of drainage. They must be watertight, covered, effectively ventilated and provided with a means of access. They should never be less than 50 feet (15·25 metres) from a dwelling, or 100 feet (30·5 metres) from a well. To reduce the volume of sewage dealt with in them rain-water should be treated separately, and either taken away in a soakaway, disposed on the land, or run into a nearby stream. A cesspit has to be emptied at regular intervals.

WATER CARRIAGE SYSTEM – In this system all excreta and liquid wastes are removed by gravity to disposal works by a system of drains and sewers. *Drains* are pipes used for the draining of one building or 'any buildings or yards appurtenant to buildings within the same curtilage'. They are private property belonging to the owner of the premises drained who is responsible for their construction and maintenance. *Sewers* are either private or public property. A *private sewer* is 'a sewer constructed after 1937, and used for the purpose of draining a particular group or block of buildings'. It is private property, generally laid in the gardens or yards of the premises it serves, and is constructed and maintained by the person to whom it belongs. A similar sewer constructed before 1937 comes into the category of a public sewer, maintained by the local authority but at the expense of the premises it serves. A *public sewer* is one that belongs to, or is vested in, a local authority, which provides and maintains it. It is, for example, a sewer under a public road or street, into which the drains of neighbouring properties discharge.

Water Closets are closets which have a separate fixed receptacle connected to a drainage system and separate provision for flushing from a supply of clean water either by the operation of mechanism or by automatic action. They should have a smooth and easily cleaned non-absorbent surface. The flush of water should be 3 gallons (13·5 litres), delivered by a pipe at least $1\frac{1}{4}$ inches (3 cm) in diameter. The flushing cistern, with siphonic action, should have an overflow pipe discharging into the outer air. The room containing the water closet, the lavatory as it is often referred to, must have a window or similar

gases

358 – 'Multrum' sewage system.

means of ventilation opening directly into the external air, and the area capable of being opened should be not less than one-twentieth of the floor area, or there should be mechanical means of ventilation effecting not less than three changes of air per hour. It must not open directly into a habitable room (unless the room is used solely for sleeping or dressing), a kitchen or scullery or a room in which any person is habitually employed in any manufacture, trade or business.

Traps are contrivances which prevent air from the drainage system entering the house. The trap consists of a pipe bent on itself so as to retain a certain amount of water in the bend (illustrations 359, 360). This water is known as the 'seal', and should be about 2 inches (5 cm) in depth.

Sewers are underground channels used to carry off all household effluents, liquid trade wastes, water used for municipal purposes and surface or rain water.

SEWAGE DISPOSAL – Today, it is an offence to permit any noxious or polluting matter to enter a river, stream, watercourse or inland water.

Discharge into the sea – The sewage may be discharged directly into the sea, the outfall of the sewer being placed below the level of the lowest tide, and so situated that the sewage will be carried out at once into the sea by currents, and not cast up on the shore in front of the town. To prevent the sea water entering the sewer, a tidal valve should be placed over the end of the sewer, so that the opening may be closed by the force of the water dashing against it. If there is difficulty at low tides, the sewage can be stored in tanks, and then allowed to flow out at times when the tide is suitable. This is the most economical mode of disposal. It has, however, many objections and, whilst these are mainly aesthetic, an increasing number of seaside holiday resorts are treating the sewage before disposing of it in the sea. Disposal of crude sewage into tidal estuaries is even more undesirable than disposal into the sea, and is gradually being given up.

359 – Diagram showing a suitable form of trap for disconnecting the house drain from the sewer. The opening on the house side is for ventilation, that on the sewer side for cleansing.

360 – Diagram of a siphon trap attached to baths, wash-basins and sinks.

Treatment of water-carriage sewage – This is one of the major problems facing public health authorities today. The problem is that ultimately the final outcome of such treatment has to pass into the rivers of the country, and it is the waters of many of these rivers that provide the drinking water for many conurbations today. The method of treatment therefore must be such that it guarantees the final effluent cast into such rivers to be clean and safe in every sense of the term. The methods used have been classified as follows: (1) Separation of suspended solids from the liquid. (2) Coagulation of the colloidal and very finely divided solids by chemical precipitation and/or physical and bacteriological action. (3) Removal of the polluting properties of the solids in solution by biological oxidation. (4) Hygienic disposal of the separated solids.

After passing through a *screening plant* for the removal of large floating solids, and then through *grit collectors* to remove grit, the sewage is passed through a series of *settling tanks*. The next process is one of oxidation of the sewage. This can be done by means of *percolating filters*. These consist of a circular clinker bed, over which rotates a central pipe with four perforated arms extending out from it, and through these arms passes a fine spray of sewage. In this way the organic impurity in the sewage is broken down and oxidized. Effluent from the filter beds is led into a humus tank where solid matter settles. After two hours in this tank the treated sewage is ready for discharge into a stream. An alternative method is the *activated sludge process*, in which the sewage passes into a special tank with a layer of biologically active sludge, the aerobic micro-organisms in which utilize oxygen to oxidize impurities. Air pipes discharge large volumes of air into the tank, which mixes the sewage and the activated sludge and provides the necessary oxygen. A

Compressed air
Inlet
Sludge recycle
Outlet
Start-up air
Process air

361 – ICI's deep-shaft effluent sewage pit.

third method now being used is the *electrolytic method*, in which sewage passes through a disintegrator, is then mixed with sea water, and then enters an electrolytic cell for a few seconds where the chlorine released at the anode deodorizes and disinfects the sewage.

The most recent method of all is the *deep-shaft effluent treatment*. It employs a shaft around 400 feet (130 metres) deep in which sewage and what is known as biodegradable effluent are poured down an inner section by compressed air and progress back to the surface through the outer section (illustration 361). A culture of micro-organisms is maintained in the effluent to purify the waste. The compressed air, along with the micro-o:ganisms, promotes the biological digestion of the sewage, as well as circulating the effluent. The great advantage of this new system is that it cuts sewage works to half their normal size by doing away with the large settling tanks of conventional sewage works. It is also said to be cheaper and produce only half the sludge. This is apart from the amenity effect by reducing in size sewage farms, a recurring eyesore throughout the country, and their accompanying smell.

Sludge disposal – This is carried out in several ways. If there is direct access to the sea, as in London and Glasgow, it can be discharged into the sea. It can be ploughed into dry land, but this can create consider-

able nuisance in wet weather. It can be disposed of for agricultural purposes, either after being dried (but this again creates a local nuisance in wet weather), or digested, which produces a thick tarry mud (as well as methane gas which can be used for driving engines on the sewage farm), or mixed with 1 per cent lime and made into cakes for agricultural use.

SEX CHROMOSOMES – In the human being there are 23 pairs of chromosomes. Male and female differ in respect of one pair. In the nucleus of the female somatic cell the two members of the pair are identical and are called X-chromosomes. In the male nucleus there is one X-chromosome and another, unequal, dissimilar chromosome called the Y-chromosome. In the sex cells, after reduction division, all cells in the female will contain X-chromosomes. In the male, half will contain X-chromosomes and half Y-chromosomes. If, then, a sperm with an X-chromosome fertilizes an ovum (with, of course, an X-chromosome) the offspring will be female. If a sperm with a Y-chromosome fertilizes the ovum the offspring will be male. It is the sex chromosomes which determine the sex of an individual. (See also CHROMOSOMES; and HEREDITY.)

SHAKING PALSY is another name for Parkinsonism (qv).

SHELL-SHOCK was a form of war neurosis which presented one of the major medical problems in the 1914–18 War.

SHIGELLA is the name given to a group of rod-shaped, Gram-negative bacteria that are the cause of bacillary dysentery. (See DYSENTERY.)

SHINGLES is a popular name for herpes zoster, which forms more or less of a belt round the body. (See HERPES.)

SHIN SPLINTS is the term applied by athletes to a condition characterized by pain over the inner border of the shin, which occurs in most runners and sometimes in joggers. It is due to muscular swelling resulting in inadequate blood supply to the muscle; hence the pain. It usually disappears within a few weeks, responding to rest, physiotherapy, with or without injections. In some cases, however, it becomes chronic and so severe that it occurs even at rest. In such cases, relief is usually obtained by a simple operation to relieve the stress and strain in the affected muscles. Technically it is known as the medial tibial syndrome.

SHOCK is the name applied to a condition in which the vital activity is profoundly lowered, usually as a result of severe injury.

The problem of shock – to the fore in the two world wars of 1914–18 and 1939–45 – is still unsolved. Surgical shock may result from injury or haemorrhage, or from both. The modern view relates the shock of both injury and haemorrhage to the same underlying cause: diminution of the fluid element of the blood. The blood, in other words, becomes concentrated. In treatment therefore the aim is to restore the blood volume, and to this end plasma is often given as a transfusion fluid.

Symptoms – The person suffering from shock is in a state of great prostration, but can be roused to answer intelligently. The face and skin generally are pale, and copious perspiration breaks out. The lips and ears are pallid, and the voice whispering. The pulse is rapid and often almost imperceptible, the respiration irregular and sighing, and the temperature may be subnormal. The patient complains greatly of thirst.

Treatment – The immediate treatment of shock is to keep the patient flat and at complete rest, to keep him warm – but not too warm – with blankets and hot-water bottles, to relieve pain, and to give hot fluids to drink provided there is no abdominal injury. The foot of the bed is raised; the limbs are often bandaged.

SHORT-SIGHT is a condition in which objects near at hand are seen clearly, while objects at a distance are blurred. The condition is technically known as myopia. (See MYOPIA; SPECTACLES; and VISION.)

SHOULDER is the joint formed by the upper end of the humerus and the shoulder-blade or scapula. The acromion process of the scapula and the outer end of the collar-bone form a protective bony arch above the joint, and from this arch the wide and thick deltoid muscle passes downwards, protecting the outer surface of the joint, and giving to the shoulder its rounded character. The joint itself is of the ball-and-socket variety, the rounded head of the humerus being received into the hollow glenoid cavity of the scapula, which is further deepened by a rim of cartilage. One tendon of the biceps muscle passes through the joint, grooving the

humerus deeply, and being attached to the upper edge of the glenoid cavity. The joint is surrounded by a loose fibrous capsule, strengthened at certain places by ligamentous bands. The main strength of the joint comes from the powerful muscles that unite the upper arm with the scapula, clavicle and ribs.

SHOULDER-BLADE, or SCAPULA, is a flat bone, about as large as the flat hand and fingers, placed on the upper and back part of the thorax. Many of the large muscles that move the arm are attached to it. It is not in contact with the ribs, and its only attachemnt to the trunk of the body is through a joint between its acromion process and the clavicle on the tip of the shoulder and by the powerful muscles which suspend it from the backbone and ribs. With the arm hanging by the side the scapula extends from the second to the seventh rib, but, as the arm is raised and lowered, it slides freely over the back of the chest. From the hinder surface of the bone springs a strong process, the spine of the scapula, which arches upwards and forwards into the acromion process. The latter forms the bony prominence on the top of the shoulder, where it unites in a joint with the outer end of the clavicle.

SIALAGOGUES are substances which produce a copious flow of saliva.

SIAMESE TWINS, or CONJOINED TWINS, is the term applied to twins who are united bodily but are possessed of separate personalities. Their frequency is not known, but it has been estimated that throughout the world six or more conjoined twins are born every year who are capable of separation. The earliest case on record is that of the 'Biddendon Maids' who were born in England in AD 1100. The 'Scottish Brothers' lived for 28 years at the court of James III of Scotland. Perhaps the most famous, however, were Chang and Eng, who were born of Chinese parents in Siam in 1811. It was they who were responsible for the introduction of the term, 'Siamese twins', which still remains the popular name for 'conjoined twins'. They were joined together at the lower end of the chest bone, and achieved fame by being shown in Barnum's famous circus in the United States. They subsequently married English sisters and settled as farmers in North Carolina. They died in 1874.

The earliest attempt at surgical separation is said to have been made by Dr

Farius of Basle in 1689. The first successful separation in Great Britain was in 1912. Both twins survived the operation and one survived well into adult life. This is said to be the first occasion in which both twins survived the operation. The success of the operation is largely dependent upon the degree of union between the twins. Thus, if this is only skin, subcutaneous tissue and cartilage, the prospects of survival for both twins are good, but if some vital organ such as the liver is shared the operation is much more hazardous.

SIBBENS is an old name for a disease formerly prevalent in Scotland, which was probably syphilis.

SICK-HEADACHE (see HEADACHE).

SICKLE-CELL ANAEMIA is a form of anaemia in Negroes, which is so-called because of the sickle shape of the red blood cells. The fundamental abnormality is the presence of an abnormal form of haemoglobin. This leads to the sickle shape of the red blood cell. Such a cell is more fragile than the normal red blood cell, and it is this fragility of the cell which is responsible for the anaemia.

SICKNESS (see VOMITING; and SEA-SICKNESS).

SICK-NURSE (see NURSING).

SICK-ROOM (see NURSING).

SIDEROSIS is a name given to chronic fibrosis (qv) of the lungs occurring in iron-workers and due to the inhalation of fine iron particles. The term is also applied to the condition in which there is an excessive deposit of iron in the tissues of the body.

SIGHT (see VISION).

SILICA is a major constituent of the earth's crust. Its main danger to health arises from free silica, present mainly as quartz and flint and as an important constituent of granite, sandstone and slate. (See SILICOSIS.)

SILICONES are organic compounds of silicon, with a structure of alternate atoms of silicon and oxygen with organic groups, such as methyl and phenyl attached to the silicone atoms. As they produce a flexible and stable water-repellent film on the skin, they are used as barrier creams (qv).

SILICOSIS constitutes the most important industrial hazard in those industries in which silica is encountered: ie. the pottery industry, the sandstone industry, sand-blasting, metal grinding, the tin-mining industry, anthracite coal mines. It is a specific form of pneumoconiosis (qv) caused by the inhalation of free silica. Among pottery workers the condition has for long been known as potter's asthma, whilst in the cutlery industry it was known as grinder's rot. For the production of silicosis the particles of silica must measure 0·5 to 5 μ in diameter and they must be inhaled into the alveoli of the lungs, where they produce fibrosis. This diminishes the efficiency of the lungs, which manifests itself by slowly progressive shortness of breath. The main danger of silicosis, however, is that it is liable to be complicated by tuberculosis. The incidence of silicosis is steadily being reduced by various measures which diminish the risk of inhaling silica dust. These include adequate ventilation to draw off the dust; the suppression of dust by the use of water; the wearing of respirators where the risk is particularly great and it is not possible to reduce the amount of dust: eg. in sand-blasting; periodic medical examination of workpeople exposed to risk. In 1976, there were 171 notified cases.

SILK, OILED, consists of silk fabric made waterproof with drying oils or oil-modified synthetic resins. ·

SILVER is used in medicine externally in the form of three of its salts. *Silver nitrate*, also known as lunar caustic, is a caustic that is used to destroy warts. It is also bactericidal, ie. it kills bacteria, and in this rôle is used as a 0·2 to 0·6 per cent solution as eye-drops, particularly as a preventive of ophthalmia neonatorum, (see EYE DISEASES), but for this purpose it is largely being replaced by antibiotics and the sulphonamides. *Silver protein*, also known as Protargol, is prepared by the interaction of a silver compound and gelatine in the presence of an alkali. It has antibacterial properties and is used as eye-drops in the treatment of conjunctivitis. *Mild silver protein*, also known as Argyrol, contains a higher percentage of silver than silver protein, but is less irritating to the tissues. It is used as a 20 per cent solution in the treatment of conjunctivitis and for the prevention of ophthalmia neonatorum (though here it is largely being replaced by antibiotics and the sulphonamides). As a 50 per cent solution it is used in the treatment of corneal ulcers. (See EYE DISEASES.) All silver salts, if used for any length of time, are liable to produce discoloration of the skin; the condition known as argyria (qv).

SIMMONDS' DISEASE, or PITUITARY CACHEXIA, is a rare condition in which cachexia, wasting of the skin and the bones, impotence, loss of hair, and premature senility occur as a result of destruction of the pituitary gland.

SIMPLE is an old term applied to a herb with real or supposed medicinal virtues.

SINAPISM is an application containing mustard. (See MUSTARD.)

SINGER'S NODULE is the term applied to a minute warty excrescence on the vocal cords interfering greatly with the voice, which tends to develop in those who use their voice professionally: hence its name. (See LARYNGITIS.)

SINGULTUS is the Latin term for hiccup.

SINUS is a term applied to narrow cavities of various kinds, occurring naturally in the body, or resulting from disease. Thus it is applied to the air-containing cavities which are found in the frontal, ethmoidal, sphenoidal and maxillary bones, and which communicate with the nose. The function of these paranasal sinuses, as they are known, is doubtful, but they do lighten the skull and add resonance to the voice. They enlarge considerably around puberty and in this way are a factor in the alteration of the size and shape of the face. The term is also used in connection with the wide spaces through which the blood circulates in the membranes of the brain. Cavities which are produced when an abscess has burst but remains unhealed, are also known as sinuses. (See ABSCESS; FISTULA.)

SINUSITIS is inflammation of a sinus. It is usually applied to inflammation of the sinuses in the face. (See NOSE, DISEASES OF.)

SINUSOIDAL CURRENT (see ELECTRICITY IN MEDICINE).

SKATOL is a strongly smelling, crystalline substance contained in the stools, produced by decomposition of protein material.

SKELETON is the comprehensive term applied to the hard structures that support or protect the softer tissues of the body (illustration 83). Many animals are possessed of an exoskeleton, consisting of superficial plates of bone, horn, or the like; but in man the skeleton is entirely an endoskeleton, covered everywhere by soft parts, and consisting mainly of bones, but in places also of cartilages. The chief positions in which cartilage is found in place of bone are the larynx and the front of the chest. (For the details of the skeleton, see BONE.)

SKIAGRAM is the name applied to a photograph – strictly speaking, a 'shadowgraph', for this is what it is – made by X-rays.

SKIN is the membrane which everywhere envelops the outer surface of the body, meeting, at the various orifices of the body, with the mucous membrane which lines the internal cavities. The skin consists of two distinct layers (illustrations 362, 363), which differ entirely in structure and in origin. These are (a) the epidermis, also known as scarf-skin, cuticle, or epithelium, which is a cellular covering formed from the outer layer of the embryo; and (b) the corium, also known as the cutis vera, true skin, or dermis, which is a fibrous covering developed from the middle embryonic layer.

(a) **The epidermis** is the cellular layer which covers the outer surface of the body, varying in thickness from $\frac{1}{20}$ of an inch (1 mm) on the palms and soles to $\frac{1}{200}$ inch (0·1 mm) on the face. It is composed of four layers, which, from the surface inwards, are as follows:

(1) THE HORNY LAYER, or STRATUM CORNEUM, made up of several thicknesses of flat cells, forming an impervious covering pierced only by the openings of the sweat-glands and by the hairs. The flat cells are rubbed off the surface constantly as minute white scales, being replaced by growth from below.

(2) THE CLEAR LAYER, or STRATUM LUCIDUM, in which the cells are firmly fixed together into a kind of membrane.

(3) THE GRANULAR LAYER, or STRATUM GRANULOSUM, in which the cells are undergoing a change in form and substance from those of the fourth layer to those of the two on the surface.

(4) THE MALPIGHIAN LAYER, or GERMINATIVE ZONE, as it is sometimes known, which is made up of the STRATUM SPINOSUM (or PRICKLY CELL LAYER) and the STRATUM

785

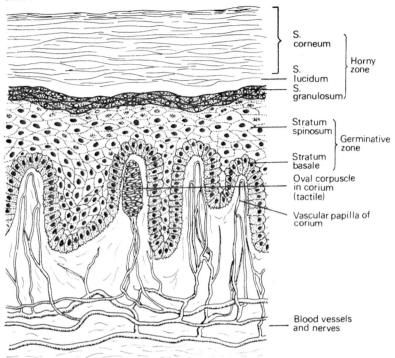

S.
corneum

S.
lucidum

S.
granulosum

Horny
zone

Stratum
spinosum

Stratum
basale

Germinative
zone

Oval corpuscle
in corium
(tactile)

Vascular papilla of
corium

Blood vessels
and nerves

362 – Vertical section of epidermis and corium. Cunningham's *Anatomy*, 11th edition. 1972. Oxford
University Press.

BASALE, in which the cells are soft, tender and living. These cells live in several rows, the deepest (the stratum basale) being set directly upon the uneven surface of the true skin, which is richly supplied with blood-vessels that nourish the cells. These cells divide continually and as they multiply they are pushed upwards to supply the constant wear and tear on the surface of the horny layer. There are no blood-vessels in the epidermis, but fine sensory nerves terminate between the cells of the Malpighian layer. These cells are joined together by cement substance and by minute processes that are continued from each cell into its neighbours. The cells in the stratum basale include the melanocytes which are responsible for the production of melanin, the pigment responsible for suntan. (See MELANIN; SUNBURN.)

NAILS (illustration 364) are analogous to the horny layer, but the cells of which they are composed are harder and more adherent. Beneath the nail is the nail bed, which is made up of the germinative zone

together with the corium. Underneath the greater part of the nail the corium has a very liberal blood supply, which gives the nail its pink colour. Towards the root of the nail, however, the nail becomes denser and the corium has a less liberal blood supply. As a result the nail is whiter. This is the part known as the lunule, which is most evident in the thumb, and gradually becomes covered by the nail fold towards the little finger where the lunule is usually hidden completely. The stratum corneum of the nail fold is prolonged over the nail as a thin fold known as the eponychium. All growth of the nail occurs at its root. Finger nails grow at an average rate of 0·5 mm a week. There is a gradual slowing of the rate with age, and a slight variation from finger to finger, the longer the finger the faster the rate of growth. Growth is quicker in summer than in winter. Toe nails grow more slowly than finger nails—at about a fourth of the rate of the latter.

A *blister* is a collection of fluid separating the Malpighian layer from the superficial ones.

(b) **The corium** is the fibrous layer which forms the chief part of the bodily covering. It varies greatly in thickness from about $\frac{1}{50}$ inch to $\frac{1}{8}$ inch (0·5 to 3 mm), being coarser on the back than on the front of the body, and thicker in men than in women. It contains many nerves, which play an important part in affording sensations of touch, pain and temperature, and blood-vessels which, in addition to nourishing the skin, are largely concerned in regulating the temperature of the body. The corium bears also the hairs which pierce the epidermis, and the sweat-glands, whose ducts also penetrate the epidermis to reach the surface. Beneath the corium lies a loose fibrous layer of

subcutaneous tissue which joins the skin to deeper parts and contains more or less fat, according to the stoutness of the person.

The fibrous tissue of the corium is composed of interlacing bundles of white fibrous tissue that form a dense feltwork. Here and there, elastic fibres are mixed with the others, and these serve to give the skin pliability, and at the same time to keep it always stretched. On the surface the network is very fine and close, and the skin is raised up into projections, known as papillae, which fit into corresponding depressions on the under-surface of the epidermis, and thus render the two inseparable. The corium is crossed everywhere by numerous folds, which are specially plentiful over joints and on the

363 – Section through the skin, showing the epidermis and corium, a hair in its follicle, the arrector pili muscle which raises the hair, and sebaceous glands opening into the hair-follicle. From *Gray's Anatomy*. Longman.

palms of the hands, and which are followed closely by the epidermis. There is a special arrangement on the palms and soles, where the papillae are so placed as to form continuous ridges with intervening grooves. These ridges remain permanent throughout life, and, as the formation by them of whorls and loops upon the finger-tips is distinctive and unchanging in each individual, an impression, or fingerprint, of these in ink is a most effective and reliable means of identifying a person. Hence their world-wide adoption as a means of identifying criminals. On the summit of each ridge the orifices of the sweat-glands can be seen, with the help of a magnifying glass, arranged in a row.

The endings of the sensory nerves in the skin have been described under NERVES.

HAIRS spring from the true skin, each having a root and a stem or shaft (illustration 363). The stem is generally rounded, and varies greatly in thickness, while in the case of curly hair it is oval or flattened in section. The surface is covered by scales, imbricated like the tiles on a roof, and it is in consequence of their projecting edges that felted or matted hair is so difficult to separate. The chief part of the stem is of a fibrous character, the fibres being composed also of elongated cells. Some hairs have, running up the centre, a pith composed of soft cells with air-spaces between them. The varying tint of hair is due to pigment scattered in varying amount throughout the hair, while a white hair is produced by the formation of very numerous air-spaces throughout the cells composing it. The root of the hair ends in a knob, and is set upon a fibrous papilla,

from which the hair appears to derive its principal nutriment. This root is set deep in the true skin, and is the growing part of the hair which pushes the older part of the hair out through the epidermis. In the scalp each hair grows steadily and continuously for three to five years at a rate of a little over 0·3 mm daily. Growth then ceases and after three to four months the hair is shed. In the latter half of this resting period the follicle forms a new hair which replaces the old one. The average daily moult varies from 50 to 100 hairs. The tube which contains the part of the hair embedded in the skin is known as the hair follicle and is lined by a fibrous coat derived from the true skin and a cellular coat developed from the cuticle, each of which consists of three layers (illustration 365). When a hair is roughly pulled out, the clear membrane that is often found surrounding it is part of the cellular root sheath. The follicle does not run straight down into the skin, but has a considerable obliquity, so that the part of the hair above the surface has a natural slope to one side. Attached to the underside of each sloping hair-follicle, near its deep end, is a small muscle, whose other end is attached to the surface of the true skin a little distance off. These muscles have the action of raising the hair, and also of producing goose-flesh, when stimulated to contract by the influence of cold or of fear.

GLANDS are found in immense numbers in the skin, and are of two kinds: *sebaceous glands*, which secrete a fatty substance, and *sweat glands*, which secrete a clear, watery fluid.

The *sebaceous glands* lie in the true skin,

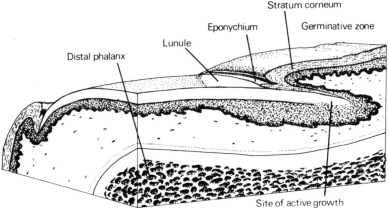

Stratum corneum

Eponychium   Germinative zone

Lunule

Distal phalanx

Site of active growth

364 – A longitudinal section through the root of a nail. From *Gray's Anatomy*, 35th edition, 1973. Longman.

Hyaline layer of dermic coat

Cortex of hair

Medulla of hair

Huxley's layer

Henle's layer

Outer layer of dermic coat

365 – Transverse section through one-half of a hair-follicle. From *Gray's Anatomy*. Longman.

and open into the follicles of the hairs a little way from the surface. Each consists of a bunch of small sacs, within which fatty material is produced. The secretion reaches the surface by the hair-follicle, and serves to lubricate the hair and give pliability to the surface of the skin (illustration 363).

Sweat glands, or sudoriparous glands, are very numerous (there are around 3 million of them), are found all over the surface of the body at a slightly deeper level than the sebaceous glands, and have no connection with the hairs. Each consists of a long tube, coiled up into a ball, from which a duct leads in a zigzag manner up towards the surface (illustration 366). The outlets of these ducts can just be seen with the naked eye as minute openings (pores), though with a magnifying glass they are readily visible. The number is said to vary from 400 in a square inch, on the lower limbs and back,

to 2800 in the same area on the palm of the hand. The structure of these glands is simple. Each is a coiled-up tube, which is lined by a layer of cells surrounded by muscle fibres, and these again by a thin membrane. In the fibrous tissue between the coils of the glands run many small blood-vessels, and from the blood in these the materials that form the sweat are extracted.

Functions of the skin – The main use of the skin is a *protective* one. It covers the underlying muscles, both protecting them from injury and, especially by virtue of the layer of fat immediately beneath the skin, warding off extremes of temperature. The epidermis forms a highly impenetrable surface, its horny character and elasticity being well calculated to resist wounds; whilst the sebaceous matter with which it is provided renders it almost waterproof. Thus poisons, drugs, and the like are not absorbed in any appreciable

789

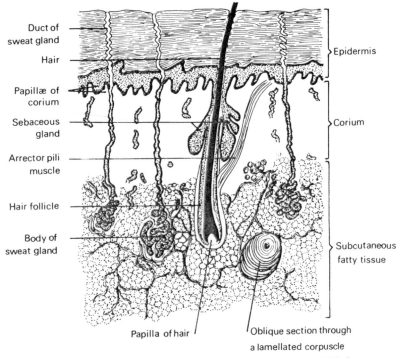

Duct of sweat gland

Hair

Papillæ of corium

Sebaceous gland

Arrector pili muscle

Hair follicle

Body of sweat gland

Epidermis

Corium

Subcutaneous fatty tissue

Papilla of hair

Oblique section through a lamellated corpuscle

366 – Schematic vertical section of skin. From *Gray's Anatomy*, 35th edition, 1973. Longman.

amount through the unbroken skin, unless combined with some fatty material, as in ointments, and diligently rubbed in.

Secretion is an important function of the skin, the two secretions being sebaceous material and perspiration. Of these, the former is a lubricant for the hair and skin, the latter is treated of under PERSPIRATION.

Heat regulation is one of the most important functions of the skin. Man is a warm-blooded animal, that is to say, his temperature remains constant in health between 98° and 99° F (36·7° and 37·2° C), no matter what the temperature of the surrounding medium may be. In order to maintain this constancy, it is evident that he must be provided with some means of quickly developing heat which will come into action when the body is cooled down by exposure to cold, and also some mechanism which can quickly get rid of heat when necessary. The main source of heat in the body lies in the muscular tissue, which develops heat every time a contraction takes place. The skin also plays a very prominent part in this

connection. When cold air or water come into contact with the surface, the skin blanches, the numerous blood-vessels of the the true skin contracting and thus preventing much blood from circulating through the skin, and being thereby unduly cooled. On the other hand, when the surface is exposed to a temperature approaching that of the body, say one of 80° or 90° F (26·7° or 32·2° C), or when an excessive amount of heat is produced by great muscular efforts, the blood-vessels of the surface dilate, the skin reddens as much blood comes to the surface, and there is a copious secretion of perspiration, which produces great cooling as it evaporates from the surface. These actions of narrowing and dilatation of vessels, and of sweat secretion, are brought about through reflex nerve influence. When the temperature rises so high that these processes are unable to take place, very serious results ensue. (See HEAT-STROKE.) It can be readily understood why the body tolerates high temperatures at a dry heat much better than continued moist heat, since evaporation of the perspiration takes place more readily the drier the surrounding air, and thus produces more rapid cooling. The serious effects of varnishing the skin or covering it with such an impervious material as gold-leaf, are due to interference with this process. The nerves of the blood-vessels appear to be thrown out of action, and delicate animals subjected to this process speedily die of cold.

Respiration is a function of the skin which in man is not of so great importance as in the lower animals. In the frog, the lungs and skin are of equal importance as breathing organs, although in man the amount of carbon dioxide given off by the skin is only about $\frac{1}{150}$ or $\frac{1}{200}$ of the amount given off by the lungs. It is probable however, that much of the organic matter which gives to impure air its disagreeable smell and contributes to its poisonous properties is given off by the skin.

SKIN CHAFING (see CHAFING OF THE SKIN).

SKIN DISEASES – These form a large and important class. In number they are very extensive, owing to the varied forms of change which the skin texture may undergo, and to the different structures in the skin which may be specially affected. Skin diseases are of great importance, not only from the fact that they have an influence on the general health, but also because these diseases are often the expression of constitutional conditions, inherited or acquired, the recognition of which is essential to their effectual treatment.

CANCER of the skin occurs in various forms. *Rodent ulcer* (qv), or basal cell epithelioma responds well to treatment. Cure is obtained in 98 per cent of cases if treated early. Anyone over the age of 50 with a persistent superficial crusted ulcer on the cheek or the side of the nose which has not healed over a period of months should seek medical advice in case it is a rodent ulcer. *Squamous cell carcinoma* which usually starts as a hard nodule, is usually the result of long excessive exposure to sunlight. *Malignant melanoma* (see MELANOMA) develops in a pigmented spot. Cancer of the skin may also be induced by exposure to tar, pitch, bitumen, the mineral oils, and X-rays. (See also ACNE; BOILS; BROMIDROSIS; DERMATITIS; ECTHYMA; ECZEMA; ERYSIPELAS; ERYTHEMA; ERYTHRASMA; HERPES SIMPLEX; HERPES ZOSTER; HYPERIDROSIS; ICHTHYOSIS; IMPETIGO; ITCHING; KERATOSIS; LEUCODERMA; LICHEN; LUPUS; MOLLUSCUM CONTAGIOSUM; NAPKIN RASH; NEURODERMATOSES; PEMPHIGUS; PITYRIASIS ROSEA; POMPHYLYX; PRURIGO; PRURITUS; PSORIASIS; RINGWORM; ROSACEA; SEBORRHOEA; URTICARIA; WENS.)

SKIN-GRAFTING is an operation in which large breaches of surface due to wounding or ulceration are closed by transplantation of skin from other parts. There are three methods by which this is done. Most frequently the epidermis only is transplanted, according to a method introduced by Reverdin and by Thiersch, and known by their names. For this purpose, a broad strip of epidermis some inches long is shaved off the thigh or upper arm, after the part has been carefully purified, and is transferred bodily to the raw or ulcerated surface, or is cut into smaller strips and laid upon it. By a second method, small pieces of the skin in its whole thickness are removed from the arm and thigh, or even from other people, and are implanted and bound upon the raw surface. This method has the disadvantage that the true skin must contract at the spot from which the graft is taken, leaving an unsightly scar. When very large areas require to be covered, a third method is sometimes adopted, as follows. A large flap of skin, amply sufficient to cover the gap, is raised from a neighbouring or distant part of the body, in such a way that it remains attached along one margin, so that blood-vessels can still enter and nourish it. It is then turned so as to cover the gap; or, if it be situated on a distant part, the two parts are brought together and fixed in this position till the flap grows firmly to its new bed. The old connection of the flap is then severed, leaving it growing in its new place.

SKULL is the collection of flat and irregularly shaped bones which protect the brain and form the face (illustrations 367, 368). These number in all twenty-two, and the names of the individual bones composing the skull are given under BONE.

Arrangement of the bones – In early life the brain and organs of special sense are enclosed in a case which is formed partly of cartilage, partly of fibrous membrane. At various parts of this investment, ossification begins early in life, and the bone gradually spreads outwards from each of these centres. Certain of the bones so formed fuse together in early childhood, thus constituting the twenty-two bones of the adult skull, which maintain their

791

independence throughout the greater part of life. In old age, however, the bones fuse so completely that the cranium comes to be a solid bony case. Even before this happens, the bones are fastened to one another by sutures so tightly that their separation without breaking is very difficult. The sutures are joints in which each edge is locked with the edges of neighbouring bones by exactly fitting projections and depressions, resembling a complicated mortise-work. Occasionally small bones develop in the sutures between the ordinary, named ones, these extra bones being known as sutural bones.

The growth of the bones spreads outwards, as already stated, from certain centres, and at the time of birth the growth of several bones has not been quite completed, so that an infant's head presents six soft spots or fontanelles where the brain is covered only by skin and membranes, and at some of which the pulsations of its blood-vessels can be seen. One of these spots, the anterior fontanelle, situated on the top of the head, does not completely close till the child is nearly 2 years old. Another change takes place as age advances, consisting in the development of an outer and inner hard table in each of the cranial bones, the tables being separated by a layer of cancellous bone (*diploë*), and in some positions by spaces containing air, which communicate with the respiratory passages. (See SINUS.) This change begins at the age of 10 years, and leads to great thickening and increased strength in the skull.

Parts of the skull – The skull consists of two distinct parts: the cranium, which encloses the brain and consists of eight bones; and the face, which forms a bony framework for the eyes, nose, and mouth, and is composed of fourteen bones (illustration 368). These two parts can be detached from one another. The lower jaw is connected with the base of the cranium by a movable joint on each side, and when the bones are bare of soft parts there is no union between them. The ear, which lies just behind and above this joint, is enclosed in the substance of the temporal bone, lying beneath the brain and separated from it in places only by a very thin shell of bone. The interior of the cranium is moulded so as to form a support for the brain (illustration 369). Its base is divided by bony ridges into three fossae, which from before back support the frontal lobes, the temporosphenoidal lobes, and the cerebellum. Further, the inner surface of the bone shows grooves and hollows corresponding to the convolutions and blood-vessels of the brain. The bones,

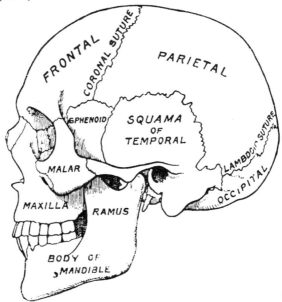

367 – Side view of skull. From Hill, *Manual of Human Physiology*. Edward Arnold & Co.

especially on the base of the skull, are pierced by many small canals (*foramina*) which transmit nerves, blood-vessels and the like. Of these, the largest is the foramen magnum, through which the medulla oblongata and the spinal cord are continuous with one another.

Shape of the skull – In the lower animals, the cranium is placed in the back part of the head, and the face looks upwards to a great extent as well as forwards. In man, as a consequence of the great development of the cerebral hemispheres of the brain, in connection with his mental activity, the cranium extends above, as well as behind, the face, which therefore looks straight forwards. A modified type of the lower class of skull is found in the more primitive races of mankind, in whom the forehead is low and sloping and the jaws prominent. This feature of the skull (prognathism) has been made, by the anatomist Camper and others, a basis for classification of the different races of mankind. The facial angle (ie. the angle between a line touching the most prominent points on the front of the face and the line on which the skull rests, when the lower jaw is removed) varies from an obtuse angle in the ancient Greeks, whose statues show an overhanging forehead, through a right angle in Romans and some of the higher Teuton types, to an acute angle in Negroes and Australian aborigines, and a still acuter angle in the man-like apes. Another method of classification is obtained by taking what is known as the cephalic index: ie. the percentage that the skull's breadth forms of its length. Long-headed peoples, like the Australian aborigines, are known as *dolichocephalic*; peoples with rounded heads, like most European races, are called *mesocephalic*; while races with broad heads, like some American Indians, are said to be *brachycephalic*.

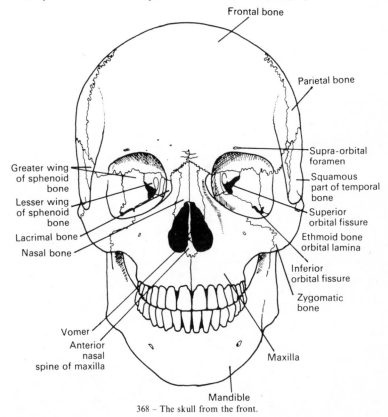

368 – The skull from the front.

369 – Skull divided in half to show cranial cavity. Names inside cavity indicate different parts of the brain. F. hole through which auditory nerve passes to ear. S. air sinus. From Hill, *Manual of Human Physiology.* Edward Arnold & Co.

Age makes considerable changes in the skull. The persistence of soft spots in the skull during the first two years of life, as well as the gradual obliteration of the sutures in later life, have been already mentioned. In children the size of the cranium is large compared with that of the face, which measures only one-eighth of the whole head, but increases till in adult life cranium and face are of almost equal proportions. In old age the face once more decreases, owing largely to loss of the teeth and consequent absorption of their bony sockets, which allows the cheeks to sink inwards and gives the appearance known as nut-cracker jaws. A similar result is produced earlier in life by premature extraction of the teeth. The child's head is gently rounded, and does not show the prominences above the eyebrows and behind the ears, due to the presence of air-cells at these localities in the full-grown skull. Further, the skull is thinner in childhood, does not show the heavy ridges for attachment of muscles displayed in later life, and is more vertical on the front and sides.

Sex also makes some differences, so that, as a rule, though not invariably, the skull of a woman can be told from that of a man. In the woman the characters resemble those of the child, the skull being lighter, smoother, and having less marked prominences. Further, the woman's skull has on an average only nine-tenths the capacity of the male skull.

Deformities result from various causes. The head is rarely symmetrical, one side almost always bulging more than the other. Premature closure of one of the sutures leads to increased growth at other sutures. Thus if the suture running from before backwards on the vertex of the head (sagittal suture) close too early, the result is a very long boat-shaped head. Some races, as, for example, the flat-head Indians of North America, show striking deformities of the head produced by applying boards and bandages in infant life. The natives in some parts of Southern France also show a curiously shaped head owing to the wearing in early life of a peculiar cap with tight strings.

SLAPPED CHEEK DISEASE (See ERYTHEMA.)

SLEEP is a periodic resting condition of the body, and especially of the nervous system. It helps children grow and it restores us all after a hard day's work. It is more than rest. It is a phase that ensures that the whole body, including the nervous system, can recuperate. It has been shown in animals that the formation of protein is more active during sleep, and the same presumably holds in man. It is the brain that controls sleep, and the benefit of sleep is most obvious for the brain. The highest rate of synthesis, or formation, of brain protein takes place during sleep. The nature and cause of sleep are a question that has excited discussion for many centuries, especially as to the part played by the mind in this resting condition.

Causes of sleep – There is a natural rotation of sleeping and waking every twenty-four hours, and sleep comes on commonly during the night when little work can be done. Sleep is not, however, a necessary consequence of darkness, as is proved by those persons who have to work in the night and sleep by day, and who speedily adapt themselves to this condition. Many persons, too, such as sailors, gain the power of sleeping as soon as they turn in, and for them short four-hourly periods of sleep and work become natural.

Many theories have been advanced as to the cause of sleep. One theory is that sleep is due to cerebral anaemia, or a poor blood supply to the brain. Against this is the fact that it has been shown that the total blood flow through the brain is not altered during sleep. On the other hand, this does not exclude the possibility that there may be local alterations in certain parts of the brain, such as the midbrain which is known to be concerned with the process of sleeping.

Another theory is the chemical one that sleep is due to want of oxygen in the nerve centres. It has been shown that, of the oxygen taken in during the twenty-four hours, 67 per cent is taken in during the twelve hours of day and 33 per cent during the twelve hours of night, while of the carbon dioxide given off, 58 per cent is the amount by day and 42 per cent by night. It is also well known that vitiated air containing an excess of carbon dioxide is capable, like many other substances, of causing drowsiness followed by unconsciousness. But these facts – while making it plain that want of oxygen or the presence of carbon dioxide and other products of activity in the tissues may cause sleep – do not explain why sleep comes on regularly in persons who are not exhausted by their day's work, nor why many people are able to compose themselves and fall asleep at any time they find convenient.

A third theory raises the question as to whether the mind remains active during the period of sleep. This theory brings forward the fact that all sensations, volitions, and other acts of consciousness are accompanied by chemical disturbances in the brain-cells that stimulate the mind to activity, just as bursting bubbles of gas escaping from the bottom of a pond agitate the surface of the water. When external impressions are cut off by closing the eyes and otherwise composing oneself for sleep, the mind ceases to be stimulated, and tranquil sleep ensues, just as the surface of the water becomes calm when the bubbles get few in number. What might be described as a slightly less fanciful variation of this theory is that during waking hours there is an accumulation in the brain of a sleep-inducing substance, and that after a period of time this ultimately induces sleep. None of these theories explains the direct cause of sleep, although each probably accounts for the main cause in different circumstances.

Sleep is not one steady process of gradually deepening sleep, as was at one time thought. It consists of several cycles of alternation between two stages: NREM or orthodox sleep, and REM or paradoxical sleep. On falling asleep we pass straight into the orthodox phase which lasts for about an hour or so. This is followed by the REM, so called because it is accompanied by Rapid Eye Movement (hence the abbreviation, REM) which lasts for two or fifteen minutes. This is the stage during which dreaming occurs. When it is over we pass back into the orthodox stage and so we alternate during the night, the orthodox stages tending to last longer in the earlier stages of sleep. By and large, however, orthodox sleep occupies about three-quarters of the sleep period in adults. In infants, however, it occupies only about half of the sleep period.

When sleep comes on, the eyes are closed as a rule, though in man, even when they are left open, the sense of sight is quickly lost as the sleep deepens. The pupils contract, also, during sleep, and dilate widely as the person awakes. Hearing is lost more slowly, and a person can be wakened even from deep sleep by a loud noise. In natural sleep, touch remains the least affected of the senses, and even the lightest touch will awaken many people from deep sleep. This does not hold good for sleep caused by drugs, many of which have a special effect in dulling general sensation, though much less effect upon the sense of hearing. With regard to the onset of sleep as it affects the mind, willpower is the first faculty to go and the last to appear in wakening. The association of ideas and power of reasoning next disappear, and people are often worried in light sleep by some simple idea which they cannot explain or understand. Memory and imagination remain longest, and, in dreams, the mind is presented with a series of bright, unconnected pictures, all jumbled together, which it does not attempt to explain. The part of the brain which regulates the power of movement is late in falling asleep, sleeps only lightly – since people may turn and make various other movements without waking – and usually wakens before the intellectual faculties and the special senses.

Other parts of the body, as well as the brain, rest during sleep. Thus the kidneys secrete less urine. the stomach secretes less gastric juice, and the liver secretes less bile, the heart beats less strongly, the blood pressure fall, and the respirations are slower and shallower than in the waking state. The skin becomes flushed with blood, so that it is specially necessary to keep the surface well covered during sleep in order to avoid chills. Some parts of the body never have a continued rest throughout life. Thus the heart, during the course of the two to three thousand million beats which it makes throughout an average life, never ceases longer than the fraction of a second that intervenes between each pair of beats, and, in each of these brief intervals, it recuperates itself for its next effort. Similarly the vital centres in the brain may be said never to sleep.

The amount of sleep suitable at different ages varies considerably as it also does from individual to individual. Some people keep going quite happily with five hours a night; others need eight hours or even more. Young people sleep easily but with increasing age sleep becomes more difficult. It becomes more broken and also less deep. At the same time there is a tendency for the elderly to require less sleep. (See also CHILDREN, PECULIARITIES OF.)

Dreams – The mind, like the vital centres, is probably never completely inactive during sleep, but is constantly receiving slight impressions which produce only a faint and quickly forgotten sensation. This is borne out by the fact that a sleeper may be awakened, not only by a loud sound or light touch, but by the ceasing of a continuous sound, as when machinery stops. A sleeper is also especially easily awakened by some sound or other sensation that he expects, and, in further proof of this constant wakefulness of the mind,

may be mentioned the fact that many people have the power of wakening after having slept for a period which they have previously determined. It has been already stated that the different parts of the brain and the different faculties of the mind go to sleep usually in a certain order. When the higher intellectual faculties of will and reason have become dulled, but deeper sleep does not at once come on, memory and imagination become increasingly vivid, so that brilliant pictures are presented to the mind. Often these are mingled with misinterpreted sensations from the surface of the body or from disordered internal organs, which serve to give them an unpleasant tinge. For example, dyspepsia following upon a late and heavy meal may give rise to sensations of falling over precipices, of vague depression, or of other unpleasant experiences which are in part memories of past events. Again, a wakeful memory and imagination may be associated with wakefulness of the motor portion of the brain, as when the person dreams that he is making desperate efforts to achieve some object or to escape pursuit, and his limbs go through movements associated with the ideas presented in his dream. Any sensation received from the surface of the body or from a disordered organ may suffice to produce the condition of partial sleep in which dreams occur, or it may become sufficiently strong to awaken the sleeper altogether. Again, the impression of the dream may produce so great an effect upon consciousness that the dream is remembered on waking, or it may fade so completely that only a sense of something forgotten is present, and a feeling that the slumber has been unrefreshing to the weary mind. Dreaming is really a form of partial insomnia, and is to be similarly treated. Much attention has been paid to dreams with the object of finding out repressed memories responsible for mental unrest in the person concerned. These often become more evident during sleep than in the waking hours, and, if the dreams are remembered, they give a guide to the identity of the disturbing memories. Appearances seen and things felt or heard in dreams often have a symbolic meaning; and the interpretation of this by those who practise psychotherapy often plays an important part in treatment.

Night terrors occur in nervous children and are allied to dreaming. The child goes to sleep after a day of unusual excitement or fatigue, or perhaps after partaking of some indigestible material, and in a short time, when sleep should be sound and dreamless, he awakens with a start and in a state of terror. Frequently the child screams with fear, cannot be pacified, and for several minutes does not seem to recognize those near him. When quieted, he can often give no reason for his fear, or he may attribute his behaviour to a dream. Children who suffer in this way should be guarded from excitement and fatigue, and, should the night terrors, or nightmares, persist, may well be taken to a child-guidance clinic or to a child psychologist.

Somnambulism, or habitual sleep-walking, is an imperfect form of sleep, in which the muscular apparatus, and the portion of brain controlling it, remain awake though the intellectual faculties are buried in slumber. In children it is not uncommon as an isolated phenomenon and is seldom of any significance, especially if it is ignored. Occasionally it may be associated with something that is worrying the child, either at home or at school. This is usually revealed by discreet enquiry, and relatively easily settled. In adults it may be a manifestation of a hysterical personality (see HYSTERIA) precipitated by some mental stress or strain though this may be difficult to ascertain in the hysteric. While the somnambulistic state persists the individual is unaware of his actions though he may see and avoid objects in his path, or may hear and answer questions, though seldom with coherence. It is almost unknown for somnambulists to injure themselves. On awakening they remember nothing of the episode.

Paralysed wakefulness is a condition of which people sometimes complain. This is the converse of somnambulism, the person waking from sleep to full consciousness and finding himself unable to make any movement for several seconds or minutes. In this condition the motor part of the brain seems to lag behind the intellectual and sensory part in waking up, but the condition is a transitory and unimportant one, though it can be quite terrifying for the victim.

Insomnia, or sleeplessness, is a condition that often causes annoyance, and by depriving the person of natural rest produces interference with the full activity during the day-time. When it becomes a habit, it may form a serious menace to health.

It may be due to a variety of causes, and these may act so effectively as to keep the person awake altogether, or they may serve, when present in a lesser degree, to produce one of the forms of dreaming and unrefreshing slumber already mentioned. In the first place, there are some persons of a nervous temperament whose sleep is much more liable to be interrupted by trivial causes than that of their more phlegmatic neighbours. In temporary cases of sleeplessness or dreaming, in which the affected person suffers from a disturbed night now and then, the cause is usually to be sought in some external source of irritation. A slight degree of pain, too light a bed-covering leading to general coldness, or even the presence of cold feet may be quite enough to prevent the brain from attaining the necessary degree of repose. Indigestion, due to eating a heavy meal shortly before retiring to rest, or some other internal disorder may act in a similar manner, even although there be no severe pain. In cases of habitual sleeplessness, a voluntary limitation of the hours of sleep, combined with overstudy, worry, or grief, is often instrumental in forming a bad habit which it is exceedingly hard to break. The brain in these cases remains fully active, despite the best endeavours of the sleepless person to compose himself for rest. A similar state of matters is often set up by poisonous materials circulating in the blood, as in fevers, malaria, gout, intemperance, and over-indulgence in tobacco. Another cause of sleeplessness or dreaming is found in persons suffering from depression, and these persons are often affected in such a way that they fall asleep on retiring to rest, enjoy only a light and partial slumber for an hour or two, and then lie wide awake till morning.

Treatment of disordered sleep – This varies greatly, depending indeed entirely upon the cause. A greater amount of exercise during the day, and care with regard to the diet may be sufficient in some of the slighter cases to remedy insomnia. In other cases a hot drink, eg. milk, just before retiring is an excellent sedative. In old people a hot whisky is often a most effective nightcap. As cold feet is a not uncommon cause of insomnia in old people, the wearing of bed-socks may ensure a good night's sleep. A comfortable warm bed can be better than any hypnotic. Where any known cause of pain or irritation exists, this must of course be remedied. Headache is not uncommonly a cause of sleeplessness, and the relief of this condition is then requisite and often sufficient to restore natural sleep. (See HEADACHE.) When a mental cause is at the root of the condition, the habit of overstudy, business worry, and the like which was originally responsible for the want of sleep, must be abandoned. Some change of occupation in the later part of the evening, such as reading some simple book or engaging in conversation, often helps to quiet the overworked brain. Cases which resist these simple means often yield to hypnotics. (See HYPNOTICS.) In cases in which the nervous system is thoroughly run down, treatment of a bracing nature is required. (See NEURASTHENIA.) Finally, any bad habits, like intemperance and excessive smoking, require appropriate treatment.

Coma is the name applied to a state of deep sleep from which the person cannot be roused. (See COMA.) The condition may be due to apoplexy, compression or concussion of the brain, poisoning by excess of alcohol or by narcotic poisons such as opium. (See OPIUM.)

is transmitted by various forms of the tsetse fly (illustration 371). The disease also occurs in cattle, when it is known as nagana. The most important species of trypanosomes are *Trypanosoma gambiense*, which only affects man, and *Trypanosoma rhodesiense*, and affects mainly man. *Trypanosoma brucei, Trypanosoma vivax,* and *Trypanosoma congolense* are all found in wild animals and are fatal to cattle and other domestic animals, but harmless to man. The tsetse flies responsible for the transmission of the disease are *Glossina morsitans* in the case of *Trypanosoma rhodesiense*, and *Glossina morsitans, Glossina swynnertoni,* and *Glossina pallidipes* in the case of *Trypanosoma gambiense*.

Other forms of the disease transmitted by other insects are also known, such as a disease occurring in Central and South

370 – *Trypanosoma gambiense.* 1, Long narrow form; 2, intermediate form; 3, thick, stumpy form; 4, posterior nuclear form; 5, red blood cell drawn to same scale to demonstrate size of trypanosome. From Blacklock and Southwell, *Human Parasitology.* H. K. Lewis & Co. Ltd.

Apparent death is a condition deeper than coma, in which persons are to all appearance dead. Cases have occurred of supposed death in which the person has been in a deep sleep or trance, from which some sudden shock has awakened him after several hours or even days. In all such cases, however, careful examination would reveal signs of life. (See CATALEPSY; and DEATH, SIGNS OF.)

SLEEPING SICKNESS, or AFRICAN TRYPANOSOMIASIS, is a disease occurring in West, East, Central and South Africa, between 14° N and 25° S latitude, and characterized by increasing weakness, lethargy, and a constant tendency to sleep, with gradual emaciation and finally death. It is one of the group of diseases caused by the presence in the blood of minute parasites known as *trypanosomes* (illustration 370). The discovery of these parasites in the blood in cases of sleeping sickness was first made in 1902. Later it was shown that this parasite

America called *American trypanosomiasis,* or Chagas' disease (qv).

The parasite, when introduced into the blood, produces its effects by developing in the small blood-vessels and in the lymphatic glands, around which its presence causes inflammation.

Symptoms – A few days after the person has been bitten by the fly, fever accompanied by a slight rash develops. This fever subsides but recurs at irregular intervals of

371 – Tsetse fly. The transmitter of sleeping sickness. From Manson's *Tropical Diseases.* Cassell & Co.

a few days or weeks. Gradually the fever becomes more pronounced, and in time the patient becomes weakened and anaemic. The glands of the neck and other parts of the body become enlarged and tender, and this state may last for months or even for years. Some cases appear to recover at this stage even after an illness of many months, and the parasite may disappear altogether from the blood. In most cases, however, the stage known as sleeping sickness gradually appears, although the lethargy may not set in for as long as seven years after the original infection. The patient now becomes disinclined for exertion, is slow mentally and weak physically, often complains of headache, and has an increasing tendency to sleep, although at first he is able to engage in conversation and to take his food. As time goes on, the weakness increases and the patient becomes more and more emaciated, bed sores form, and death finally takes place from weakness or from some intercurrent disease. The later symptoms appear to be due to the development of the parasites in the minute blood-vessels of the brain, around which, in consequence, inflammatory changes take place, with disorganization of the nervous tissues.

Treatment – For the prevention of sleeping sickness the chief essential is the avoidance of the flies which carry the disease. Fortunately, the occurrence of the flies is very definitely localized to certain regions, and, when such regions have to be traversed, the journey is made during the night-time when the flies do not feed. Those who live in fly-infested regions should have their houses and persons carefully protected against the fly. The wearing of long trousers and long-sleeved shirts gives some protection, as does the use of insect repellents such as dimethyl phthalate (qv). As the flies are mostly found close to streams, much has been done in certain localities by clearing the neighbourhood of streams in infested districts of all vegetation which would shelter the flies. The use of insecticides is proving more difficult than in the case of certain other insect-borne diseases, but promising results are being obtained from the hand-spraying of belts of vegetation bordering roads and tracks, and from aerial spraying of larger areas.

Suramin is the drug of choice in the treatment of *Trypanosoma rhodesiense* infections, and pentamidine in the treatment of *Trypanosoma gambiense* infections. Melarsoprol, a trivalent melaminyl arseni-

cal, has replaced tryparsamide in the treatment of advanced cases of the disease, but it is a drug which must be administered with great care on account of its toxicity.

SLEEPY SICKNESS is a popular name for encephalitis lethargica. (See ENCEPHALITIS.)

SLING means a hanging bandage for the support of injured or diseased parts. Slings are generally applied for support of the upper limb, in which case the limb is suspended from the neck. The lower limb is also frequently supported in a sling from an iron cage placed upon the bed on which the patient lies. In the latter case the object of slinging the limb is usually to aid the circulation, and so quicken the healing of ulcers on the leg.

372 – *a*, Sling for wrist; *b* sling for forearm.

373 – Sling for elbow; *a*, first stage; *b*, finished.

In the case of the upper limb, the sling is made from Esmarch's triangular handkerchief bandage, formed by cutting a yard of calico diagonally from corner to corner into two triangular pieces. There are four varieties of sling.

Sling for the wrist is made by folding the bandage up into a narrow cravat, laying the wrist upon the centre, and carrying one end up each side of the neck, behind which the two are tied (illustration 372).

Sling for the forearm is applied as follows (illustration 372b): the unfolded triangle is laid with one end over the shoulder of the sound side, the centre of the base at the wrist of the injured limb, and the point of the bandage at the elbow of the injured limb. The other end is

800

carried up in front of the injured limb, over the shoulder, and the two ends are tied behind the neck. The point is finally pinned neatly round the elbow.

Sling for the elbow is applied in much the same way, with this exception: that the point of the triangle is placed under the wrist, while the centre of the base supports the elbow (illustration 373a). The bandage is completed by turning the point up over the wrist and pinning it to the part of the bandage above (illustration 373b).

Sling for the shoulder is applied, as in the case of the sling for the elbow, with the centre of the base at the elbow, and the front end is carried over the opposite shoulder. The other end passes up behind the upper arm and across the back, the two ends being tied upon the sound shoulder. The object of this sling is to support, while avoiding pressure on the injured shoulder, as in fracture of the collar-bone. (See FRACTURES.)

SLIPPED DISC is the popular name for a prolapsed intervertebral disc (qv).

SLOUGH means a dead part separated by natural processes from the living body. The term is applied to hard external parts which the lower animals cast off naturally in the course of growth, like the skin of snakes or the shell of crabs. In man, however, the process is generally associated with disease, and is then known as gangrene. (See GANGRENE.) Sloughs may be of very small size, as in the case of the core of a boil, or they may include a whole limb, but in general a slough involves a limited area of skin or of the underlying tissues. The process of separation of a slough is described under gangrene.

SMALLPOX, or VARIOLA, is an acute infectious disease characterized by fever and by the appearance on the surface of the body of an eruption which, after passing through various stages, dries up, leaving more or less distinct scars. Few diseases have been so destructive to human life as smallpox, and it has ever been regarded with horror, alike from its fatality, its loathsome accompaniments and disfiguring effects, and from the fact that no age or condition of life is exempt from liability to its occurrence. In most civilized countries its ravages have greatly decreased, and there are now hopes that, as a result of the World Health Organization vaccination campaign, it may have been eradicated.

Much obscurity surrounds the early history of smallpox. It appears to have been imported into Europe from Asia, where it had been known and recognized from remote antiquity. The earliest accounts of its existence reach back to the sixth century, when it was described by Procopius and Gregory of Tours as occurring in epidemic form in Arabia, Egypt, and the south of Europe. The most reliable statements as to the early existence of the disease are found in Rhazes (c. AD 900), by whom its symptoms were clearly described, its pathology explained by a fermentation theory, and directions given for its treatment. During the period of the Crusades smallpox appears to have spread extensively through Europe, and hospitals for its treatment were erected in many countries. Smallpox was known in England as early as the thirteenth century, and had probably existed before. It appears to have been introduced into America shortly after the discovery of that continent, and there, as in Europe and throughout the known world, destructive epidemics were of frequent occurrence during succeeding centuries.

Causes – Smallpox is one of the most contagious of all diseases. It is due to infection with a virus. Its outbreak in epidemic form in a locality may often be traced to the introduction of a single case from a distance. By far the most common cause of conveyance of the disease is contact with the persons or the immediate surroundings of those already affected, but infection can also be carried by the clothes of third persons not themselves infected. The most infectious period extends from the appearance of the eruption till the drying up of the pustules. No age is exempt from susceptibility to smallpox. One attack of smallpox, as a rule, confers immunity from any recurrence. Overcrowding and all insanitary surroundings favour the spread of smallpox where it has broken out; but the most influential condition of all is the amount of protection afforded to a community by previous attacks and especially, in the present day, by vaccination. Such protection, although for a time most effectual, tends to become exhausted, unless renewed. Hence in a large population there is always likely to be an increasing number of individuals who have become susceptible to smallpox. This probably explains its occasional and even apparently periodic epidemic outbreaks in large centres, and the well-known fact that the most severe cases occur at the beginning of an epidemic – those least protected being necessarily more liable to be first and most seriously attacked.

Symptoms – The onset of the symptoms is preceded by a period of incubation, during which the patient may or may not complain. This period is from ten to sixteen (usually twelve) days. The invasion is sudden and severe, in the form of a rigor followed by fever (the *primary fever*), in which the temperature rises to 103° or 104° F (39·4° or 40° C) or higher (illustration 374). A quick pulse is present, together with thirst and constipation,

374 – Temperature chart of a case of smallpox, showing the primary and secondary fevers.

while intense headache, vomiting, and pain in the back are among the most characteristic of the initial symptoms. Occasionally the disease is ushered in by convulsions. These symptoms continue with greater or less intensity throughout two days, and during their course there may occasionally be noticed on various parts of the body, especially on the lower part of the abdomen and inner sides of the thighs, a diffuse redness accompanied by slight spots of extravasation (*petechiae*), the appearance somewhat resembling that of scarlet fever. On the third day the characteristic eruption begins to make its appearance. It is almost always first seen on the face, particularly about the forehead and roots of the hair, in the form of a general redness; but on this surface there may be felt by the finger numerous elevated points more or less thickly set together. The eruption, which is accompanied by heat and itching, spreads over the face, trunk, and extremities in the course of a few hours – continuing, however, to come out more abundantly for one or two days. It is always most marked on the exposed parts. The individual pocks are separated from each other (discrete). On the second or third day after its appearance the eruption undergoes a change – the pocks becoming vesicles filled with a clear fluid. These vesicles attain to about the size of a pea, and in their centre there is a slight depression, giving the characteristic umbilicated appearance to the pock. The clear contents of these vesicles gradually become turbid, and by the eighth or ninth day of the disease they are changed into pustules containing yellow matter, while at the same time they increase still further in size and lose the central depression. Accompanying this change, there are great surrounding inflammation and swelling of the skin, which, where the eruption is thickly set, produce much disfigurement and render the features unrecognizable, while the affected parts emit an offensive odour, particularly if, as often happens, the pustules break. The eruption is present not only on the skin but on mucous membranes, that of the mouth and throat being affected at an early period; the swelling produced here is not only a source of great discomfort but even of danger from the obstruction thus occasioned in the upper portion of the air passages. The mucous membrane of the nostrils is similarly affected, while that of the eyes may also be involved. The febrile symptoms, which ushered in the disease, undergo marked abatement on the appearance of

the eruption on the third day, but on the eighth or ninth day, when the vesicles become converted into pustules, there is a return of the fever (*secondary* or *suppurative fever*) (illustration 374), often to a severe extent, and frequently accompanied by nervous symptoms, such as great restlessness, delirium, or coma. On the eleventh or twelfth day the pustules show signs of drying up (desiccation), and along with this the fever abates. Great itching of the skin attends this stage. The scabs produced by the dried pustules gradually fall off and reddish-brown spots remain, which, according to the depth of skin involved in the disease, leave a permanent, white, depressed scar – this pitting, so characteristic of smallpox, being especially marked on the face.

In some outbreaks the type of the disease is much more severe than in others, and the mortality consequently greater. Smallpox is most fatal at the extremes of life. Numerous and often dangerous complications are apt to occur at or after the supervention of the secondary fever. The most important are inflammatory affections of the respiratory organs, such as bronchitis, pleurisy, pneumonia, suppurative conditions of the throat, and swelling of the mucous membrane of the larynx and windpipe. Involvement of the eyes is common and distressing, but serious permanent damage to the eyes is unusual. Persons of enfeebled health, and those whose constitution is impaired by intemperance, readily succumb to attacks of smallpox even of comparatively mild character. In the severe form of the disease in pregnancy death of the foetus and abortion practically always occur.

Varieties – *Confluent smallpox* shows much severer symptoms from the onset than those just described, and the eruption, instead of showing itself in isolated pocks, appears in large patches run together, giving a blistered appearance to the skin. This confluent condition is almost entirely confined to the face, and produces shocking disfigurement and deep scars. It is generally estimated that at least 50 per cent of the cases of confluent smallpox prove fatal, whilst in those who survive, convalescence is apt to be slow and interrupted. *Haemorrhagic smallpox* is a form in which bleeding takes place into the pocks after they are formed. This is apt to be accompanied by bleeding from various mucous surfaces (particularly in the case of females), occasionally to a dangerous degree. Many such cases also prove fatal. *Malignant smallpox* is a still more serious form, in which, as in the malignant forms of other infectious diseases (see MEASLES) the patient is from the outset overwhelmed with the poison and quickly succumbs, the rash scarcely appearing at all. Such cases are, however, rare. *Varioloid,* or *modified, smallpox* is the term applied to those cases which occur in people who are little susceptible to the disease, or in whom the protective influence of vaccination or of a previous attack of smallpox still exists to some extent.

Laboratory tests are now available to assist in diagnosis in difficult cases. The most reliable of these is the growing of the virus on the chorio-allantois of a fertile hen's egg. This is done by inoculating a sample of scrapings from the skin, or of fluid from a vesicle, into the egg.

Treatment – In the prevention of smallpox, with regard to the safety both of the individual and of the community, no measure has been so effective as vaccination. (See VACCINATION.) Promising results in the prevention of the disease have also been reported from the use of the drug known as methisazone.

The treatment of cases of smallpox is conducted upon the same general principles as that for the other infectious diseases. (See DIPHTHERIA; MEASLES; SCARLET FEVER.) The patient should lie on a soft bed in a well-ventilated but somewhat darkened room, and be fed with the lighter forms of nutriment, such as milk, soups, and the like. The skin should be sponged occasionally with tepid water, and the mouth and throat washed or sprayed with a solution of chlorate of potash, permanganate of potassium, or other safe disinfectant. In a severe case, with evidence of much prostration, stimulants are required. The patient should always be carefully watched, and special vigilance is called for when delirium exists.

Many applications have been proposed for preventing pitting, but probably the best are cold or tepid compresses of light weight kept constantly applied over the face and eyes. The fluid out of which these are wrung may be a weak lotion of boric acid, with which the eyes should also be frequently irrigated. When the pustules have dried up, the itching thus produced may be much relieved by the application of a dusting powder or lanolin or olive oil. Complications are to be dealt with as they arise, and the severer forms of the disease treated with reference to the special symptoms presented. Ventilation should be free, and all clothing, and the like should be afterwards burnt. The disease is con-

tagious from the appearance of the first symptoms to the disappearance of all scabs. The patient must therefore be kept in strict isolation until all the scabs have disappeared.

SMEGMA is a thick, cheesy secretion formed by the sebaceous glands of the glans penis. A bacillus, closely resembling the tubercle bacillus morphologically, develops readily in this secretion.

SMELL – The sense of smell is picked up in what is known as the olfactory areas of the nose. Each of these is about 3 square centimetres in area and contains 50 million olfactory, or smelling, cells. They lie, one on either side, at the highest part of each nasal cavity. This is why we have to sniff if we want to smell anything carefully, as in ordinary quiet breathing only a few eddies of the air we breathe in reaches an olfactory area. From these olfactory cells the olfactory nerves (one on each side) run up to the olfactory bulbs underneath the frontal lobe of the brain (qv), and here the impulse is translated into what we describe as smell.

SMELLING SALTS (see AMMONIA).

SMOKING (see TOBACCO).

SNAKE-BITE (see BITES).

SNAKE-ROOT is a popular term for several plants, including senega and serpentaria.

SNARE is a wire loop used by the ear, nose, and throat surgeon for removing polypi from the nose.

SNEEZING means a sudden expulsion of air through the nose, designed to expel irritating materials from the upper air passages. In sneezing, a powerful expiratory effort is made, the vocal cords are kept shut till the pressure in the chest has risen high, and air is then suddenly allowed to escape upward, being directed into the back of the nose by the soft palate.

Sneezing may be caused by the presence of irritating particles in the nose, such as snuff, the pollen of grasses and flowers. It is also an early symptom of colds, influenza, measles, and hay-fever, being then accompanied or followed by running at the nose.

SNORING is usually attributed to vibrations of the soft palate, but there is evidence that the main fault lies in the edge of the posterior pillars of the fauces (qv) which vibrate noisily. Mouth breathing is necessary for snoring, but not all mouth-breathers snore. The principal cause is blockage of the nose, such as occurs during the course of the common cold or chronic nasal catarrh. Such blockage also occurs in some cases of deviation of the nasal septum or nasal polypi. (See NOSE, DISEASES OF.) In children, mouth-breathing, with resulting snoring, is often due to enlarged tonsils and adenoids. A further cause of snoring is loss of tone in the soft palate and surrounding tissues due to smoking, overwork, fatigue, obesity, and general poor health.

Treatment therefore consists of the removal of any of these causes of mouth-breathing that may be present. Should these not succeed in preventing snoring, then measures should be taken to prevent the victim from sleeping lying on his back, as this is a habit which strongly conduces to snoring. Simple measures include sleeping with several pillows so that the head is raised quite considerably when asleep. Alternatively, a small pillow may be put under the nape of the neck. If all these measures fail, there is much to be said for the old traditional method of sewing a hair-brush, or some other hard object such as a stone, into the back of the snorer's pyjamas. This means that if he does turn on to his back while asleep, he is quickly awakened and therefore able to turn on his side again. (See also STERTOR.)

SNOW BLINDNESS, or ARC EYE, is the excruciatingly painful condition caused by excessive exposure to ultra-violet radiation. Treatment consists of the application of a local anaesthetic and of homatropine, and then bandaging the eyes for twenty-four hours.

SNUFFLES is the name applied to noisy breathing in children due to the constant presence of nasal discharge. (For treatment, see NOSE, DISEASES OF.)

SOAP is a substance made by boiling a fat or oil with an alkali. The most commonly used oil is olive oil, and the most frequent alkali is caustic soda. In the process of manufacture the fatty acids of the oil unite with the alkali, glycerin separating out. In soft soap or green soap, caustic potash is used in place of soda; marine soap is made with coconut oil; curd soap has tallow for its fat; while many toilet soaps have palm oil or

almond oil. Barilla soap is made from soda got by burning plants; in superfatted soaps care is taken that the fatty part is in excess, so that no crude alkali is left to irritate the skin; whilst glycerin soaps have a specially emollient action. Medicated soaps of various kinds are prepared, the chief drugs added to soap being of an antiseptic nature, such as carbolic acid, coal-tar, formalin, hexachlorophane, terebene.

Uses – The chief use of soap is, mixed with water, as a cleansing agent. Internally, hard soap is often used to make up the bulk of pills containing very active ingredients. As a purgative enema, soap is used made up into a strong solution in warm water. Soap liniment, better known as 'opodeldoc', is used as a popular remedy for stiffness or sprains.

SOCIAL CLASSES – As factors such as the cause of death and the incidence of diseases vary in different social strata, the Registrar-General evolved the following social classification, which has now been in official use for many years:

Class I   Professional occupations, such as lawyers, clergymen, and commissioned officers in the Armed Forces.
Class II   Intermediate occupations, such as teachers.
Class III   Skilled occupations, such as mine-workers, transport workers, and clerical workers.
Class IV   Partly skilled occupations, such as agricultural workers.
Class V   Unskilled occupations, such as building and dock labourers.

On the basis of the 1971 census families in Britain are divided into the different classes as follows:

Class I   762,000
Class II   3,145,000
Class III   7,745,000
Class IV   2,966,000
Class V   1,205,000

SODA (see ALKALI; SODIUM).

SODIUM is a metal, the salts of which are white, crystalline, and very soluble. The fluids of the body contain naturally a considerable quantity of sodium chloride, or common salt.

SODIUM CARBONATE, commonly known as SODA or WASHING SODA, has a powerful softening action upon the tissues.

SODIUM BICARBONATE, or BAKING SODA, is used as an antacid in relieving indigestion associated with increased acidity of the gastric secretion. It is taken in doses of 10 or 20 grains (600 or 1,200 mg), as a rule. (See ACIDITY.) The citrate and the acetate of sodium are used as diuretics and in the treatment of inflammatory conditions of the kidneys and bladder, although the corresponding potassium salts are more frequently employed.

SODIUM CALCIUMEDETATE is the name for the calcium complex of diamine tetra-acetic acid, which is proving of value in the treatment of lead poisoning and of chrome ulceration.

SODIUM CHLORIDE is the chemical name for common salt.

SODIUM CROMOGLYCATE is a drug used by inhalation in the preventive treatment of asthma.

SODIUM DIATRIZOATE is an organic iodine salt that is radio-opaque and is therefore used as a contrast medium to outline various organs in the body in X-ray films. It is given intravenously. Its main use is in pyelography (qv), that is in rendering the kidneys radio-opaque, but it is also used to outline the blood-vessels (angiography) and the gall-bladder and bile ducts (cholangiography).

SODIUM HYPOCHLORITE is a disinfectant by virtue of the fact that it gives off chlorine. For domestic use, as, for example, for sterilizing baby feeding bottles, it is available in a variety of proprietary preparations. (See also CHLORINATED LIME.)

SODIUM VALPROATE is a drug that is proving of value in the treatment of some cases of epilepsy which will not respond to any of the other drugs used for the treatment of this condition.

SOFTENING OF THE BRAIN (see APOPLEXY; BRAIN, DISEASES OF).

SOFT SORE, or CHANCROID, is an infective venereal ulceration due to the *Haemophilus ducreyi,* which is common in the tropics and subtropics. It is a local condition, not spreading beyond the glands in the neighbourhood of the original ulcer, although there is always a possibility that syphilis may be contracted along with this disease and may show itself later. The condition begins within a few hours after infection as a pimple which enlarges rapidly and ulcerates. The glands in the groin speedily become affected, and as these may soften and ulcerate, the condition sometimes results in a tedious illness.

Treatment consists in the administration of full doses of one of the sulphonamides by mouth. The affected glands are not drained, but if they become fluctuant the pus may be aspirated with a needle and syringe. In resistant cases, streptomycin or tetracycline may be tried.

SOLAPSONE is a sulphone derivative which is used in the treatment of leprosy. It can be given by mouth or by injection.

SOLARIUM is the term applied to a room enclosed by glass in which sun baths are taken while protection is afforded from the weather.

SOLDIER'S HEART, or DISORDERED ACTION OF THE HEART (DAH), or EFFORT SYNDROME, is a term applied to a set of symptoms arising under conditions of great anxiety and unusual physical strain, and consisting of palpitation, shortness of breath, speedy exhaustion, depression, and irritability. The condition received its name on account of the frequency with which it was noticed during the 1914–18 War. (See HEART DISEASES.)

SOLOMON'S SEAL is a popular name for *Polygonatum officinale.* The fluid extract has astringent properties and is used as an application to bruises.

SOLUTION (see LIQUOR).

SOMATIC means relating to the body, as opposed to the mind.

SOMNAMBULISM means sleep-walking. (See SLEEP.)

SOPORIFICS are measures which induce sleep. (See HYPNOTICS.)

SORDES is the name applied to the thick offensive material which gathers on the lips, teeth, and tongue of persons who are very weak from fever or other cause. In healthy people the constant movements of the tongue and lips serve to keep them free of growing bacteria, remnants of food, and cells cast off from the mucous membrane of the mouth, which in the enfeebled state collect and form a brown or black putrefying deposit.

Treatment – The lips, tongue, and teeth should be wiped occasionally with a rag

SORE

dipped in borax and honey, or glycerin of borax, and the rag then burned. Syringing out the mouth with bicarbonate of soda solution, one teaspoonful to a tumblerful of warm water, is also helpful in very weak persons. If the person be strong enough, he may rinse his mouth with weak solution of permanganate of potassium in water, diluted to a pale pink colour.

SORE is a popular term for ulcer (qv).

SORE THROAT (see THROAT, DISEASES OF; and TONSILLITIS).

SOUND is a rod with a curve at one end used mainly for passing into the bladder to determine whether a stone is present or not. (See BLADDER, DISEASES OF.)

SOUR MILK (see LACTIC ACID BACILLI).

SOUTHEY'S TUBES are long, fine tubes for drawing off fluid slowly from cases of dropsy. (See ASPIRATION.)

SOYA BEAN is the bean of *Glycine soja*, a leguminous plant related to peas and beans. The outstanding characteristic of the soya bean is its very high protein and fat content. There is an almost complete absence of starch, but a large amount of mineral matter. Soya flour contains 40 per cent of protein and 20 per cent of fat. It yields 470 Calories per 100 grams as compared with 370 Calories for white wheat flour. Soya flour contains 0·2 per cent of calcium (about ten times as much as in white flour). It also contains a variable but large amount of iron: 6·7 to 30 mg per 100 grams of soya flour compared with 1 mg in white flour and 3 mg in 100 grams of wholemeal flour. It is a good source of thiamine and riboflavine, and of vitamin A in the form of carotene. (See BEANS.)

SPAGHETTI (see MACARONI).

SPANISH FLY is a popular term for cantharides, which is used as a blistering agent. (See CANTHARIDES.)

SPASM means an involuntary, and, in severe cases, painful contraction of a muscle or of a hollow organ with a muscular wall. Spasm may be due to affections in the muscle where the spasm takes place, or it may originate in some disturbance of that part of the nervous system which controls the spasmodically acting muscles.

806

Spasms of a general nature are usually spoken of as convulsions; spasms of a painful nature are known as cramp when they affect the muscles of the limbs, and as colic when they are situated in the stomach, bowels, or other organs of the abdomen. Spasm of the heart receives the name of breast-pang or angina pectoris, and is both a serious and an agonizing condition. When the spasm is a prolonged firm contraction, it is spoken of as tonic spasm; when it consists of a series of twitches or quick alternate contractions and relaxations, it is known as clonic spasm. Spasm is a symptom of many diseases.

SPASMODIC TORTICOLLIS, or WRY-NECK, is the term applied to a condition in which there is continuous or interrupted spasm of the muscles of one side or of both sides of the neck, the head being held or jerked either backwards or to one side. It is a nervous disorder.

SPASMOLYTICS are remedies which diminish spasm. They may achieve this in one of three ways: (*a*) by interfering with the transmission of the nerve impulses that are causing the spasm; (*b*) by a direct action on the affected muscle; (*c*) by depressing the central nervous system.

Varieties – In the past many of the favourites in this field, such as oil of cinnamon, oil of cloves, oil of peppermint, and valerian, achieved their reputation by virtue of their depressing effect on the sensitivity of the nerve endings. Others, such as lobelia and stramonium, often in the form of cigarettes to be inhaled, achieved a wide reputation as asthma cures.

Today, a more scientific approach is maintained, though there is still much to be said for the use of preparations, such as oil of cinnamon or of peppermint for the relief of mild spasm of the gut, and not a few asthmatics have implicit faith in the relieving power of lobelia or stramonium. The most widely used spasmolytics today are atropine and its derivatives, or its many synthetic substitutes. These act by paralysing the action of the parasympathetic nerve fibres that induce contraction of smooth muscle. They are most widely used in relieving spasm in the alimentary and renal tracts. For the relief of the spasm of asthma adrenaline and ephedrine are still great standbys, though isoprenaline and other similarly acting drugs are being used to an increasing extent. All these act through the sympathetic nervous system.

Of the spasmolytics acting directly on muscle, the best known group is the nitrites – amyl nitrite and glyceryl trinitrate – which are the great standbys for the relief of the spasm that induces angina pectoris. Other drugs that act in this way are theophylline and aminophylline. If the spasm is really severe, and therefore painful enough, general depression of the brain may be necessary by means of general anaesthetics. In less severe cases, the lesser degrees of depression of the brain induced by hypnotics may have a spasmolytic action. and. though it should seldom be used for this purpose because of its habit-forming propensities, even alcohol could rank as a spasmolytic.

SPASMOPHILIA is a term applied to a condition affecting certain persons, especially in childhood, in which the motor nerves are unusually sensitive to irritation. Such patients show an abnormal tendency to convulsions and spasms on very slight cause.

SPASMUS NUTANS is the term for describing the rhythmic nodding of the head sometimes seen in infants during the first year of life.

SPASTIC is a term applied to any condition showing a tendency to spasm: eg. spastic gait. This is specially associated with some disease affecting the upper part of the nervous system connected with movement (upper neurone), so that its controlling influence is lost and the muscles are in a state of over-excitability.

SPATULA is the name of a flat, knife-like instrument used for spreading plasters and ointments, and also for depressing the tongue when the throat is being examined.

SPECIFIC is a term used in various ways. It is applied to remedies which appear to have a definitely curative effect in certain diseases, as, for example, to sodium salicylate. which is said to be specific in rheumatism, or to quinine, which is a specific for malaria. Again, it is applied to bacteria and other agents which form the chief cause of certain diseases, though there may be other minor contributing causes: for example, the comma bacillus is the specific cause of cholera, the sarcoptes parasite is the specific cause of scabies. The term is also used to designate diseases that have an identity of their own, have a definite cause, and do not consist merely of a group of symptoms: for example, scarlet fever, measles, typhoid fever are specific as compared with vague ailments such as enlargement of the glands in the neck, diarrhoea, or dyspepsia. The word specific is also sometimes used as a euphemism for venereal disease.

SPECTACLES are worn on account of some defect in the refractive (ie. focusing) power of the eye, or owing to the axis of the eye being misdirected (ie. squinting). or simply as a protection from bright light, wind, or dust.

Refractive errors consist of four types: (1) SHORT-SIGHT or MYOPIA, in which the refractive power of the eye is too strong or the globe of the eye too long from before backwards, so that rays of light from distant objects are brought to a focus in front of the retina, upon which blurred images are therefore formed. Spectacles containing concave lenses are used in order to correct this in viewing distant objects. Children with short-sight have difficulty in following their lessons, because they cannot see clearly maps, figures on blackboards, and other objects at a distance. They should therefore be early provided with appropriate glasses, since the error, if uncorrected, is liable to become more pronounced.

(2) LONG-SIGHT or HYPERMETROPIA, in which the globe of the eye is so short from before backwards, that rays of light from objects close at hand would come to a focus behind the retina and therefore produce blurred images, although the vision for distant objects may be perfect. In this case, convex spectacles are used for near work in order to increase the converging power of the lens of the eyes. Long-sighted eyes in school children and students are apt to be inflamed and productive of headache in consequence of the constant overstrain required to focus near objects, such as a printed page, upon the retina. The condition is very apt to pass unnoticed, since, except in extreme degrees of this malformation, the child or student has good vision for distant things. Constantly inflamed eyes, headache, and especially occasional blurring of the print after the eyes have been used for some hours in reading, should attract attention to this condition.

(3) ASTIGMATISM, in which the curvature of the cornea is not symmetrical. so that the rays of light in one plane cannot be focused upon the retina along with those in the plane at right angles to it. Such an eye, accordingly, sees objects, whether they be near at hand or far off, in a

distorted manner; a circle, for example, being seen as an ellipse and blurred at two points opposite one another. For the correction of this error extreme care is necessary. Spectacles have to be fitted in which the glasses, instead of being lens-shaped, consist of a slice from the side of a cylinder. That is to say, the glasses are flat in one direction, and curved in the axis at right angles to it. The axis of the cylinder must be set with great care in the spectacle frame at right angles to the axis of astigmatism. Astigmatism may occur in long-sighted or in short-sighted eyes, or the eye may be long-sighted in one meridian, short-sighted in the meridian at right angles to it (mixed astigmatism).

(4) PRESBYOPIA, or the condition which is a natural consequence of increasing age, in which the lens of the eye gradually hardens and so loses its power to become more convex and thus accommodate itself for the vision of near objects. This condition necessitates that reading, sewing, and the like shall be carried on, after the age of 40 or 45, at an inconvenient distance, if the details of the work are to be sharply focused on the retina. The condition is treated by wearing convex glasses for near work, although the eyes remain perfectly good for viewing objects at a distance. Thus it becomes possible for elderly people, aided by spectacles, whose strength is proportioned to their age, to read or sew, at the convenient distance of 12 or 14 inches (30 or 35 cm). One sometimes hears it said that a certain person has required no glasses for reading even in advanced old age, but this is simply equivalent to stating that the person has had short-sight all his days and has never had perfect vision for distant objects. In these persons the length of the eye is well adapted for focusing near objects, without artificial aid. Also in cases of commencing cataract in old people the vision for near objects improves a little at first. People of normal sight are usually benefited by spectacles for near work after passing the age of 45, and certainly after 50, since the effort to accommodate for near vision after this age fatigues the eyes and is productive of headache.

Squinting is usually caused by the excessive efforts made by long-sighted children to accommodate their eyes for near vision. In squints due to this cause the squint is remedied by convex glasses. Many other cases of squint (latent squint) are remedied by wearing prismatic glasses. (See SQUINTING.)

Protection of the eyes is afforded usually by glass, tinted grey, blue or black according to the degree of protection from light that is required. The disease in which protection is specially required is iritis.

The lenses of spectacles, then, are concave or convex lenses, cylinders, prisms, and plane glasses. In many cases a cylinder has to be combined with a lens, and then the lens shape is usually ground upon one side of the glass, the cylinder upon the other. The nature of the glass can be told by holding it close to the eye and moving from side to side. If the lens be convex, the objects seen through it appear to move in the opposite direction to that in which the glass travels. If it be concave, they move with the glass. If the glass contain a cylinder, the rate at which objects travel varies as the glass is moved up and down or from side to side. Often a person has to wear one pair of glasses for near, and another pair for distant work, and it is usual to combine these in what are known as bifocal lenses, by making the upper half of each glass the lens suitable for distant work, and adapting the lower half of each for near work. For the method of testing for spectacles see under VISION.

The frame in which lenses are set is important. It should be light, and, for persons who use glasses constantly, the spectacle form is best. For occasional use, some *pince-nez* form of frame is usually more convenient, but great care must be taken, especially if the lenses are strong, that the centre of each lens comes before the centre of the eye. For this reason the best form of eyeglasses is one in which the frame has a rigid bridge and is supported by springs that do not alter the position of the lenses.

SPECULUM is an instrument designed to aid the examination of the various openings on the surface of the body. Many specula are provided with small electric lamps so placed as to light up the cavity brilliantly.

SPEECH (see VOICE AND SPEECH).

SPERMATIC is the name applied to the blood-vessels and other structures associated with the testicle.

SPERMATORRHOEA is the name applied to the passage of semen without erection of the penis or orgasm.

SPERMATOZOON (plural: SPERMATOZOA) is the male sex or germ cell which unites with the ovum to form the embryo or foetus. It is a highly mobile cell approximately 0·1 mm in length. Each millilitre of semen (qv) contains on average about 100 million spermatozoa, and the average volume of semen discharged during ejaculation in sexual intercourse is between 2 and 4 ml. (See also FOETUS.)

SPES PHTHISICA is the term applied to the curious mental condition sometimes observed in a patient with advanced pulmonary tuberculosis, wherein he becomes hopeful of recovery and mildly exalted, and has a false sense of well-being. It appears to be a compensatory reaction to an inner knowledge of impending dissolution.

SPHACELUS is another name for gangrene. (See GANGRENE.)

SPHENOID is a bone lying in the centre of the base of the skull, and supporting the others like a wedge or keystone. (See SKULL.)

SPHINCTER means a circular muscle which surrounds the opening from an organ, and, by maintaining a constant state of moderate contraction, prevents the escape of the contents of the organ. Sphincters close the outlet from the bladder and rectum, and in certain nervous diseases their action is interfered with, so that the power to relax or to keep moderately contracted is lost, and retention or incontinence of the evacuation results.

SPHYGMOGRAPH is an instrument for recording the pulse. (See PULSE.)

SPHYGMOMANOMETER is the name of an instrument for measuring blood-pressure in the arteries. It usually consists of a pneumatic armlet, the interior of which communicates by a rubber tube with an air-pressure pump and a gauge. The armlet is bound about the upper arm and pumped up sufficiently to obliterate the pulse as felt at the wrist or as heard in the artery at the bend of the elbow. The pressure registered on the gauge at this point is regarded as the pressure of the blood at each heart-beat (systolic pressure). The pressure at which the sound heard in the artery suddenly changes its character marks the diastolic pressure.

SPICA BANDAGE is a method of applying the ordinary roller bandage in order to cover a joint. When it is finished the overlapping turns of bandage give it the appearance of a head of wheat. (See BANDAGES.)

SPINA BIFIDA is one of the commonest of the congenital malformations. In the British Isles the combined incidence of ancephaly (qv) and spina bifida at birth is around 4 to 5 per 1000, but there are marked regional variations. It takes two main forms. SPINA BIFIDA OCCULTA is much the commoner of the two and consists of a defect in the posterior wall of the spinal wall, usually in the lumbar region. As a rule it has no deleterious effects unless the underlying spinal cord is affected. It has been said that one in every ten individuals has such a defect.

SPINA BIFIDA CYSTICA, the other form, is a much more serious condition. Here the defect in the spinal canal is accompanied by protrusion of the spinal cord which, in turn, may take one of two forms. One is a *meningocele*, in which the meninges (qv), containing cerebrospinal fluid, protrude through the defect. The other is a *meningomyelocele*, in which the protruding sac contains spinal cord and nerves. This is much the more serious condition of the two and, unfortunately, much the commoner, accounting for 90 per cent of all cases. The over-all incidence of spina bifida cystica varies from one part of the country to another, but in England and Wales, in 1966, 1206 babies were born alive with this condition, representing a rate of 1·4 per 1000 births. This compares with a rate of 4·1 per 1000 births in rural areas of South Wales. The cause is not known but there is a strong genetic factor. Thus, a couple who have had one baby affected with spina bifida have a 5 to 8 per cent chance that any subsequent babies they have will have a major malformation of the central nervous system. If they have already had two or more affected infants, the risk of any further having a similar condition is about 1 in 4 to 1 in 8. Tests are now available, whereby severe cases of spina bifida (and anencephaly) can be recognized in the unborn child during pregnancy.

The usual site of the defect is in the lumbo-sacral, or lower, part of the spine. When the baby is born the protruding sac is quite soft but if it is a meningomyelocele, as it usually is, the baby's condition rapidly deteriorates, with the development of paralysis and incontinence, and a high risk of meningitis. This is why it is now recommended that the baby

should be operated on as soon as possible
– preferably in a special centre. Many of
these babies also have hydrocephalus (qv).
So successful are the results of operation
on carefully selected cases in special
centres that it is now claimed that 'the
majority of adequately treated children
with spina bifida associated with hydrocephalus will grow up with a normal intelligence, although the average intelligence
of the whole group falls below the 100 IQ
figure which applies to the general
population'. The emphasis here, however,
is on 'carefully selected cases', and 'adequately treated' and 'special centre'. Indeed, the decision as to how to deal with
a severe case of spina bifida can be one of
the most heart-rending and difficult in the
whole of medicine.

Parents of children with spina bifida or
hydrocephalus are recommended to join
the Association for Spina Bifida and
Hydrocephalus, Devonshire Street House,
30 Devonshire Street, London W1N 2EB,
which has branches in all parts of the
country. In this way they will receive continuing help, advice and encouragement in
coping with what is often a trying problem.

SPINAL COLUMN, also known as the
SPINE, CHINE, BACKBONE, and VERTEBRAL
COLUMN, forms an important part of the
skeleton, acting both as the rigid pillar
which supports the upper parts of the
body and as a protection to the spinal
cord and nerves arising from it. The spinal
column is built up of a number of bones
placed one upon another, which, in consequence of having a slight degree of
turning-movement, are known as the
vertebrae. The possession of a spinal cord
supported by a vertebral column distinguishes the higher animals from the lower
types, and gains for them the general name
of vertebrates. Of the vertebrates, man
alone stands absolutely erect, and this
erect carriage of the body gives to the skull
and vertebral column certain distinctive
characters.

The human backbone is about 28 inches
(70 cm) in length, and varies little in full-
grown persons; differences in height
depend mainly upon the length of the
lower limbs. The number of vertebrae is 33
in children, although in adult life 5 of these
fuse together to form the sacrum, and the
lowest 4 unite in the coccyx, so that the
number of separate bones is reduced to 26.
Of these there are 7 in the neck, known
therefore as *cervical vertebrae*; 12 with ribs
attached, in the region of the thorax, and
known as *thoracic* or *dorsal vertebrae*; 5 in

the loins, called *lumbar vertebrae*; 5 fused
to form the *sacrum*; and 4 joined in the
coccyx. These numbers are expressed in a
formula thus: C7, D12, L5, S5, Coc4 = 33
(illustration 375). The formula in different
animals varies considerably, but throughout the class of mammalia the number of
cervical vertebrae is almost constantly
seven, even in long-necked animals like
the giraffe and short-necked animals like
the whale. Although the vertebrae in each
of these regions have distinguishing features, all the vertebrae are constructed on
the same general plan (illustration 376).
Each has a thick, rounded, bony part in
front, known as the body, and these bodies
form the main thickness of the column.
Behind the body of each is a ring of bone,
the neural ring, these rings placed one
above another forming the canal bone

375 – The spinal column. *C7*, Cervical; *D12*,
dorsal; *L5*, lumbar vertebrae; *S5*, sacrum; *Coc4*,
coccyx; *C, C*, the twelve ribs; *Ps, Ms, Xs*, three
parts of the sternum; *V, V*, vertical axis of the
spine showing its four curves.

376 – Human dorsal vertebra seen from above. K, Body of vertebra: R, neural ring enclosing the spinal cord: B, B, notches by which the nerves emerge: D, spinous process: Qu, Qu, transverse process: G, G, articular processes for the vertebra above: Rg, Rg, those for the head of the corresponding ribs.

which lodges the spinal cord. From each side of the ring a short process of bone known as the transverse process stands out, and from the back of the ring a larger process, the spinous process, projects. These processes give attachment to the strong ligaments and muscles which unite, support, and bend the column. The spines can be seen or felt beneath the skin of the back lying in the centre of a groove between the muscular masses of the two sides, and they give to the column its name of the spinal column. One of these spines, that of the 7th cervical vertebra, is especially large and forms a distinct bony prominence, where the neck joins the back. Between the bodies of the vertebrae lies a series of thick discs of fibro-cartilage known as intervertebral discs. Each disc consists of an outer portion, known as the annulus fibrosus, and an inner core, known as the nucleus pulposus. To these 23 discs the upper part of the spine owes much of its pliability, as well as a great deal of its resiliency and power of diminishing the effect of jars and blows communicated through the feet or head. There is also a small joint at each side upon the ring of the vertebra so that each vertebra comes in contact with the one above and the one beneath in three places.

The first and second cervical vertebrae are modified in a very special manner. The first vertebra, known as the atlas, is devoid of a body, but has a specially large and strong ring with two hollows upon which

the skull rests, thus permitting of nodding movements. The second vertebra, known as the axis, has a pivot upon its body which fits into the first vertebra and thus permits of free rotation of the head from side to side.

An important feature of the spinal column, and one especially marked in human beings, is the presence of four curves from behind forwards (illustration 375). Thus the cervical vertebrae are arranged with a curve whose hollow looks backwards, the dorsal vertebrae have a marked curve with the hollow forwards; in the lumbar region the hollow is directed backwards, while the sacrum and coccyx form a marked hollow to the front. The effect of the dorsal and sacral curves is greatly to increase the size of the cavities of chest and pelvis, while the compensating curves of the neck and loins serve to keep the general axis of the spinal column in a vertical line. The curves have also an action very similar to that of the springs of a vehicle, in minimizing jolting and jarring of the internal organs. There is usually a very slight curve to one side in the upper dorsal region, resulting from the greater development and use of the right arm.

The neural rings placed one above another form a canal, which is wide in the neck, smaller and almost round in the dorsal region, and wide again in the lumbar vertebrae. This canal lodges the spinal cord, and the nerves that issue from the cord pass out from the canal by openings between the vertebrae which are produced by notches on the upper and lower margins of each ring. The intervertebral foramina formed by these notches are so large in comparison with the nerves passing through them that there is no chance of pressure upon the latter, except in very serious injuries which dislocate and fracture the spine.

SPINAL CORD is the lower portion of the central nervous system which is situated within the spinal column. Above, it forms the direct continuation of the medulla oblongata, this part of the brain changing its name to spinal cord at the *foramen magnum*, the large opening in the base of the skull through which it passes into the spinal canal. Below, the spinal cord extends to about the upper border of the second lumbar vertebra, where it tapers off into a fine thread, known as the filum terminale, that is attached to the coccyx at the lower end of the spine (illustration 377). The spinal cord is thus considerably shorter than the

SPINAL CORD

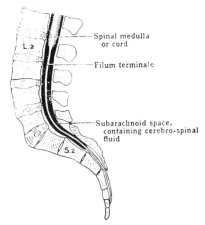

Spinal medulla
or cord

Filum terminale

Subarachnoid space,
containing cerebro-spinal
fluid

377 – Diagram of the lower end of the spinal
cord. L.2, 2nd lumbar vertebra, S.2, 2nd sacral
vertebra. From J. C. Boileau Grant, *An Atlas of
Anatomy.* E. & S. Livingstone.

spinal column, being only 15 to 18 inches
(37 to 45 cm) in length, and weighing around
30 grams. In its course from the base of the
skull to the lumbar region the cord gives off
thirty-one nerves on each side, each of
which arises by an anterior and a posterior
root that join before the nerve emerges from
the spinal canal. The openings for the nerves
formed by notches on the ring of each
vertebra have been mentioned under SPINAL
COLUMN. To reach these openings the upper
nerves pass almost directly outwards, whilst
lower in the series their obliquity increases, until below the point where the
cord terminates there is a sheaf of nerves,
known as the cauda equina, running
downwards to leave the spinal canal at
their appropriate openings. In shape the
cord is a cylinder, about the thickness of
the little finger, and slightly flattened from
before backwards. It has two slightly enlarged portions, one in the lower part of
the neck, the other at the last dorsal vertebra, and from these thickenings arise the
nerves that pass to the upper and lower
limbs. (See NERVES.) The spinal cord, like
the brain, is surrounded by three membranes, the dura mater, arachnoid mater,
and pia mater, from without inwards
(illustration 378). The arrangement of the
dura and arachnoid is much looser in
the case of the cord than their application
to the brain. The dura especially forms a
wide tube which is separated from the
cord by fluid and from the vertebral canal
by blood-vessels and fat, this arrangement

protecting the cord from pressure in any
ordinary movements of the spine.

IN SECTION, the spinal cord consists
partly of grey, but mainly of white, matter.
It differs from the upper parts of the brain
in that the white matter in the cord is arranged on the surface, surrounding a mass
of grey matter, while in the brain the grey
matter is superficial. The arrangement of
grey matter, as seen in a section across the
cord, resembles the letter H (illustration
379), each half of the cord possessing an
anterior and a posterior horn, and the
masses of the two sides being joined by a
wide posterior grey commissure. In the
middle of this commissure lies the central
canal of the cord, a small tube which is the
continuation of the ventricles in the brain.
The horns of grey matter reach almost to
the surface of the cord, and from their
ends arise the roots of the nerves that
leave the cord, but elsewhere the grey is
completely surrounded by white matter.
The white matter is divided almost completely into two halves by a posterior
septum and anterior fissure that project
inwards from the back and front surfaces,
the posterior septum reaching down to the
grey commissure, but the anterior fissure
being separated from it by a small anterior
white commissure that joins the white
matter of the two sides together. The white
matter is further divided into three columns, on each side, by the horns of grey
matter and the nerve roots passing from
them to the surface; these are known as
the anterior, lateral, and posterior
columns.

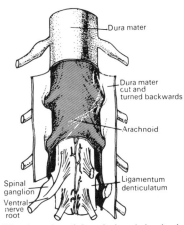

Dura mater

Dura mater
cut and
turned backwards

Arachnoid

Ligamentum
denticulatum

Spinal
ganglion

Ventral
nerve
root

378 – A portion of the spinal cord showing its
membranes.

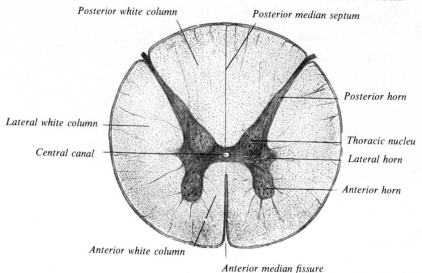

Posterior white column

Posterior median septum

Posterior horn

Lateral white column

Central canal

Thoracic nucleu

Lateral horn

Anterior horn

Anterior white column

Anterior median fissure

379 – Transverse section through the spinal cord in the thoracic region. Magnified eight times. From *Gray's Anatomy*. Longman.

Minute structure – The *grey matter* is found upon microscopic examination to consist largely of neuroglia, the connective tissue of the central nervous system, which is made up of small cells with long branching processes. This neuroglia forms a sort of felt-work, in the meshes of which lie numbers of multipolar nerve-cells (illustration 380) and the nerve-fibres that spring from them and unite one cell to another or pass out into the nerves. The *white matter* consists almost entirely of bundles of nerve-fibres provided in general with a medullary sheath, the white colour being due to the collective appearance of these sheaths. (See NERVES.) There is also in the white matter a small quantity of supporting connective tissue. Most of the nerve-fibres run vertically, so that a cross-section of the cord shows them as a collection of dots, each surrounded by a clear space. Blood-vessels are found in the cord both in grey and in white matter.

Functions – The cord is, in part, a receiver and originator of nerve impulses, and in part merely a conductor of such impulses along fibres which pass through it to and from the brain. The presence of centres in the cord, capable of receiving sensory impressions and originating motor impulses, is proved by several facts. Thus, it has been calculated that the number of nerve-fibres entering or leaving the cord

by the spinal nerves is twice as great as the number of fibres contained in the upper end of the cord, where it is continued into the brain. Again, if the cord be severed in the dorsal region, as by a fracture of the spine, the centres which govern the evacuation of the bladder and bowel do not lose their power of controlling these organs immediately upon being severed from the brain. Many of these centres are known to exist in the cord, such as centres for regulating the size of the blood-vessels, for altering the size of the pupil of the eye, for sweating, for breathing. Over most, if not all, of these centres, however, the brain exerts a controlling influence, and before any incoming sensation can produce an effect upon consciousness, it is in all probability necessary that it should obtain a clear passage up to the brain.

Many of these centres act in a rhythmical or *automatic* way. Other cells of the cord are capable of originating movements in response to impulses brought direct to them through sensory nerves, such activity being known as *reflex* action. (For a fuller description of the activities of the spinal cord, see NERVES.)

By observing the process of degeneration that takes place when nerve-fibres are cut off by disease or injury from the cells to which they belong, and by observing also the manner in which the fibres in dif-

813

Axon

Axon

Axon

380 – Three nerve cells from the anterior column of the spinal cord. From Cunningham's *Anatomy*. Oxford University Press.

ferent portions of the cord develop, it has been found possible to divide the three white columns of the cord into tracts, in each of which the fibres have a special function (illustration 381). Thus the posterior column consists of the *fasciculus gracilis* and the *fasciculus cuneatus* both conveying sensory impressions upwards. The lateral column contains the ventral and the dorsal spino-cerebellar tracts passing to the cerebellum, the crossed pyramidal tract of motor fibres carrying outgoing impulses downwards together with the rubro-spinal, the spino-thalamic, the spino-tectal, and the postero-lateral

tracts. And, finally, the anterior column contains the direct pyramidal tract of motor fibres and an anterior mixed zone. The pyramidal tracts have the best-known course (illustration 382). Starting from cells near the central sulcus on the brain (see BRAIN), the motor nerve-fibres run down through the internal capsule, pons, and medulla, in the lower part of which many of those coming from the right side of the brain cross to the left side of the spinal cord, and vice versa. Thence the fibres run down in the crossed pyramidal tract to end beside nerve-cells in the anterior horn of the cord. From these nerve-cells other fibres pass outwards to form the nerves that go direct to the muscles. Thus the motor nerve path from brain to muscle is divided into two sections of neurons, of which the upper exerts a controlling influence upon the lower, while the lower is concerned in maintaining the muscle in a state of health and good nutrition, and in directly calling it into action.

SPINE AND SPINAL CORD, DISEASES AND INJURIES OF – These

are considered together, because the chief danger of interference with the spinal column lies in the risk of injury to the spinal cord and nerves. Only some of the chief diseases will be dealt with.

LATERAL CURVATURE OF THE SPINE, or SCOLIOSIS, consists chiefly in bending of the spine over to one side, although, in consequence of the vertebrae being broader in front than behind, this is accompanied by a certain amount of twisting of the vertebrae round their vertical axis. The shape of the chest becomes, in consequence, markedly altered, the ribs on one side projecting behind at their angles, and causing the shoulder-blade to be very prominent, while on the other side the chest is flattened. (See CHEST DEFORMITIES.) The shoulder of the bulging side is usually considerably elevated. This condition may be started by slight injuries of the spine, by

rickets in early life, by diseases in the chest, such as pleurisy, which cause partial collapse of one side, or by weakness of the muscles, such as occurs in certain diseases of the nervous system: for example, cerebral paralysis (qv). *Idiopathic scoliosis*, so called because the cause is not known, occurs in babies, most commonly boys, and usually rights itself spontaneously within three years. Not uncommonly it develops in adolescents of feeble muscular power, especially in rapidly growing girls from about 12 to 16 years of age, who adopt some bad habit of posture. Such a habit may consist in always crossing one leg over the other in sitting, leaning constantly on the same elbow at lessons, standing habitually with the weight of the body on one foot, or carrying a heavy burden on one arm.

The consequences of this deformity are a bad carriage and awkward gait, while, if it be very marked, the lungs are more liable to be attacked by various diseases, although there is no tendency for the spinal cord to suffer any damage.

Treatment consists in avoiding the bad postures mentioned above, and in making sure that the general health is maintained as high as possible by fresh air and exercise. Above all, some special form of gymnastics, combined sometimes with massage, is advisable in order to strengthen

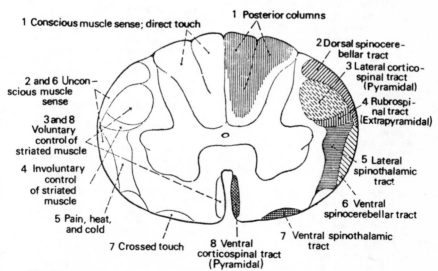

1 Conscious muscle sense; direct touch

1 Posterior columns

2 Dorsal spinocerebellar tract

3 Lateral corticospinal tract (Pyramidal)

4 Rubrospinal tract (Extrapyramidal)

2 and 6 Unconscious muscle sense

3 and 8 Voluntary control of striated muscle

4 Involuntary control of striated muscle

5 Pain, heat, and cold

7 Crossed touch

5 Lateral spinothalamic tract

6 Ventral spinocerebellar tract

7 Ventral spinothalamic tract

8 Ventral corticospinal tract (Pyramidal)

381 – Diagrammatic representation of cross section of spinal cord. The nerve tracts are shown on the right and their functions on the left. From Chaffee and Greisheim. *Basic Physiology in Anatomy.* Lippincott.

382 – Diagram showing the course of the motor tracts through the brain and spinal cord. The front half of the brain is supposed to have been removed, and the reader is looking at its interior. CH, Cerebral hemisphere: Cb, cerebellum: OT, optic thalamus: LN, lentiform nucleus: M, medulla oblongata: P, pons; SC, spinal cord. Note that the great majority of nerve-fibres cross over in the medulla from the right side to form the crossed pyramidal tract on the left side of the cord, while a smaller number continue straight down as the anterior pyramidal tract on the right side.

the feeble muscles of the back. In severe cases, which do not respond to such treatment, the wearing of a corset, known as the Milwaukee brace, or an operation may be necessary.

ANGULAR CURVATURE OF THE SPINE is a very much more serious condition. It not only produces more evident deformity, but many cases are accompanied by a certain degree of pressure upon the spinal cord. The condition was described by the famous surgeon. Percivall Pott (1714–88), after whom it is also called *Pott's disease.* This deformity is produced in the great majority of cases by caries of the vertebrae, the result of tuberculosis; the body of one or more vertebrae crumbles away, and the spinal column curves sharply forwards, so that the spinous processes stand out prominently at the site of the disease. A similar condition occasionally comes on after a fall in the case of a young child, or a severe blow upon the back of an older person. The symptoms are not at all well marked in the early stages. There is a general loss of health and strength, and the person becomes easily tired. The affected part of the spine is tender when pressure is made on the back, and the child holds himself stiffly. If the neck be diseased the head is not turned from side to side, and the child often supports the chin on his hand. If the back be the part concerned, the child holds himself very erect, and when he wishes to pick something off the floor, goes down upon his knees rather than bend the back. When the lumbar region of the spine is diseased a not uncommon result is a psoas abscess which burrows towards the back or into the groin.

Treatment is essentially that applicable to tuberculous disease affecting any other organ, consisting of chemotherapy combined with good food and fresh air. (See TUBERCULOSIS.) So effective is chemotherapy that, in the case of children anyhow, admission to hospital may not be necessary, and the child may often be treated as an outpatient. Even plaster-of-Paris jackets are seldom considered necessary nowadays, and surgical treatment is only required in a small majority of cases.

COMPRESSION OF THE CORD may arise from various causes. The seriousness of most diseases affecting the spine is, in fact, measured by their tendency to interfere with the spinal cord. This condition may be caused suddenly by a severe crush or blow upon the back, which produces a fracture of the spine with displacement of the fragments. Or it may come on slowly, and is then in the great majority of cases due to Pott's disease (see above). Compression of the cord in the neck is speedily fatal as a rule, owing to the involvement of important vital centres; but when it occurs in the region of the chest (illustration 383), the person may live a long time a more or less invalid life.

Symptoms comprise interference with sensation below the level of compression, and, in chronic cases, pain round the body at this level; more or less complete rigidity and paralysis of the lower limbs; interference with the functions of the bladder and rectum, and a special tendency to bed sores in the paralysed parts.

Treatment, in cases due to accident, is not as a rule hopeful, since the spinal cord is generally lacerated, as well as compressed, by the damage to the spine. But cases which come on slowly, for example, as the result of Pott's disease, often yield to treatment. This consists in the prolonged rest and support to the spine mentioned above; whilst brilliant results are often obtained, even after several months of complete paralysis, by an operation designed to remove the bone or inflammatory product which is pressing upon the cord. Apart from the question of recovery, these cases require special care and watchfulness in nursing because of the great tendency that is present to the formation of bed sores, and because the patient loses to a great extent the power of voluntary control over the bladder and bowels, so that septic inflammation of the bladder and kidneys is very apt to ensue and to terminate the patient's life. Modern methods of rehabilitation, however, have done much to ensure that, paralysed though they may be, many of the victims of severe damage to the spinal cord can return to a useful life in the community.

SPONDYLITIS, or inflammation of the vertebrae of the spine, may occur at any age, but the most important form is *ankylosing spondylitis,* also known as bamboo

383 – Fracture of of the spine with compression of the spinal cord. Outline of spinal cord shown by double dotted line. From Illingworth, *A Short Textbook of Surgery,* 9th edition. Churchill Livingstone.

spine and poker spine. This is a disease predominantly of young men between the ages of 20 and 40. Unless treated in the early stages, it tends to run an inexorable course, leading in the end to complete fixation of the spine as a result of bony ankylosis between the vertebrae.

Treatment consists of deep X-ray therapy and, if given early in the disease, the results are excellent. Even in the later stages it may give considerable relief and slow the progress of the disease. Promising results are also being obtained from the use of the drug known as phenylbutazone.

A National Association for Ankylosing Spondylitis has been formed which is open to those with the disease, their families, friends and doctors. Those interested should apply to the secretary, 4 Beaconsfield Road, Clifton, Bristol BS8 2TS.

SPONDYLOLISTHESIS is a congenital defect of the spine, usually the fifth lumbar vertebra. This results in slipping forward of the affected vertebra which induces backache. This usually responds to treatment with a spinal support, but in more severe cases an operation may be necessary.

MENINGITIS, or inflammation of the membranes surrounding the cord, is dealt with under MENINGITIS.

MYELITIS, or inflammation situated in the spinal cord itself, may be of an acute or chronic nature, and gives rise to symptoms much resembling those of compression though unaccompanied by pain. (See MYELITIS.) A special form of myelitis is poliomyelitis, affecting only the grey matter of the cord. (See POLIOMYELITIS.)

SCLEROSIS is a very chronic condition of the cord in which certain parts become increasingly hard in consequence of disappearance of the white nerve-fibres and their replacement by an overgrowth of the connective tissue of the cord. This change is due to various causes, and the symptoms which it produces depend mainly upon the particular tracts of fibres that are affected. Sclerosis in the posterior part of the cord, for example, produces the disease known as locomotor ataxia (see LOCOMOTOR ATAXIA); whilst another disease, known as multiple sclerosis, in which the degenerated patches are scattered through the nervous system, affects mainly the lateral portions of the cord. (See MULTIPLE SCLEROSIS.)

PROGRESSIVE MUSCULAR ATROPHY is the chief member of a group of diseases in which the main characteristic is loss of power and muscular wasting, due to a gradual degeneration in the grey matter of the spinal cord and brain. (See PARALYSIS.)

SYRINGOMYELIA is a disease in which fissures and cavities exist in the cord together with an overgrowth of the supporting neuroglia. (See SYRINGO-MYELIA.)

INJURIES TO THE SPINE AND CORD are of various grades of severity. *Sprains* of the back due to a twist and leading to tearing of muscles and ligaments, and to deep-seated effusion of blood, may be productive of long-continued pain and even of a considerable amount of paralysis. In most cases this is probably due to some injury of the spinal nerves, but the symptoms pass off in general with rest and time. *Fracture of the spine* has been mentioned under the heading of COMPRESSION. *Concussion of the cord* is a term which includes a number of possible injuries that may have been inflicted upon the cord by severe jarring or shaking of the body.

SPIRAMYCIN is an antibiotic isolated from *Streptomyces ambofaciens*, which is useful in the treatment of certain cases of staphylococcal infection.

SPIRILLUM is a form of micro-organism of wavy or spiral shape. (See BACTERIOLOGY.)

SPIRIT is a strong solution of alcohol in water. (See ALCOHOL.) Proof spirit is one containing 57 per cent of alcohol by volume or 49 per cent by weight, and is so named because it can stand the proof of just catching fire. Rectified spirit contains 90 per cent of alcohol by volume or over 85 per cent by weight. Proof spirit is generally used in the preparation of tinctures. Spirits of various drugs contain a solution of any given drug in rectified spirit. Among the most commonly used spirits are spirit of chloroform (also known as chloric ether), sweet spirit of nitre (spirit of nitrous ether), aromatic spirit of ammonia (sal volatile), spirit of ether, spirit of Cologne (eau-de-Cologne), spirit of camphor, and spirit of various volatile oils. Methylated spirit (also known as wood naphtha or wood spirit) is distilled from wood. When taken internally, it is a dangerous poison producing neuritis with great readiness, and especially neuritis of the optic nerves which may result in blindness. Mineralized or denatured methylated spirit is one to which crude pyridine and mineral naphtha have been added in small proportions, together with a minute quantity of methyl violet for colouring, to prevent its being drunk.

The term spirit is also used popularly in a loose application to various active substances: eg. spirit of turpentine (oil of turpentine), spirit of hartshorn (ammonia in water), spirit of nitre (nitric acid), Mindererus spirit (liquor ammonii acetatis), and spirit of salt (hydrochloric acid).

Uses (for internal uses, see ALCOHOL) – Externally, methylated spirit or eau-de-Cologne is used to sprinkle on the skin or to apply on lint, as an evaporating lotion for its cooling and soothing effect. (See LOTIONS.) Methylated spirit is also used to harden the skin for the prevention of bed sores and foot soreness. The spirits of the various oils form a convenient method of administering these oils as expectorants, or for colic, flatulence, etc. (See OILS.)

SPIROCHAETE is an order of bacteria which have a spiral form.

SPIROCHAETOSIS ICTEROHAE-MORRHAGICA, or WEIL'S DISEASE, is the term applied to an acute infection with the *Leptospira icterohaemorrhagiae* which is transmitted to man by rats, these animals excreting the organism in their urine; hence the liability of sewer workers to the disease. The condition is characterized by fever, jaundice, enlarged liver, nephritis, and bleeding from mucous membranes.

SPIRONOLACTONE belongs to the group of substances known as spirolactones. These are steroids similar to aldosterone (qv) in structure which competitively act as inhibitors of it. They can thus antagonize the action of aldosterone in the renal tubules. As there is evidence that there is an increased output of aldosterone in dropsical conditions, such as congestive heart failure, which accentuates the dropsy (or oedema), spironolactone is used, along with other diuretics, in resistant cases of oedema – to antagonize the fluid-retaining action of aldosterone.

SPLANCHNIC means anything belonging to the internal organs of the body as distinguished from its framework.

SPLEEN is an organ deeply placed in the abdomen.

Position and size – The spleen lies behind the stomach, high up on the left side of the abdomen, and corresponds to the position of the 9th, 10th, and 11th ribs, from which it is separated by the diaphragm. It is a soft, highly vascular, plum-

384 – Diagram of human spleen. A, artery and vein (V) in a trabecula (T) of the capsule (C); ZA, central artery of the corpuscle of Malpighi (MK); P, small arteries; HA, arteries with a sheath; AK, arterial capillaries which terminate in the sinuses (1) or in the meshes of the reticulum (2); MS, venous sinuses. From Best and Taylor, *The Physiological Basis of Medical Practice*. The Williams & Wilkins Co.

coloured organ, and has a smooth surface, being almost completely covered by peritoneum. There are two wide peritoneal ligaments that support the spleen, the one attaching it to the stomach, the other to the kidney. Through the latter ligament the large vessels that supply the spleen with blood make their way. The size of the spleen varies widely. It is usually about 5 to 6 inches (12·5 to 15 cm) in length, and weighs about 6 ounces (170 grams) or more, but these dimensions depend upon the amount of blood contained in it, for it contracts from time to time, and after meals is much smaller than at other times. In diseased conditions the organ may reach a weight of 18 to 20 pounds (8 to 9 kg).

Structure (illustration 384) – The spleen is enveloped by peritoneal membrane like the stomach and intestines, and this smooth coat greatly facilitates its movements. Beneath the peritoneum is a strong elastic tunic, composed partly of fibrous tissue containing many elastic fibres, and partly of unstriped muscle. This elastic coat allows of the free expansion and contraction of the organ according to the varying amount of blood present in it. From the inner surface of the membrane fibrous partitions known as trabeculae run down into the substance and form a network in which the dark spleen pulp is contained. If the spleen be cut open and the pulp washed away, these trabeculae stand out as shaggy projections on the cut surface. The pulp consists of delicate connective tissue fibres passing between the various trabeculae and of white and red

blood corpuscles lying in this meshwork. Round the smaller arteries there are condensed areas of this pulp formed of developing white blood corpuscles, and known as Malpighian bodies or corpuscles.

BLOOD-VESSELS pass to the spleen, and are so large compared with the size which would be necessary in order simply to carry nutritive material to the spleen as to render it clear that the organ has some important action connected with the maintenance of the blood. The arteries which enter the spleen at the hilum become smaller and smaller till they end in capillaries, which open freely into the pulp. The blood thus escapes readily into the substance of the spleen, and, after passing through its meshwork, is collected by veins that unite into larger trunks till they form the splenic vein, which leaves the organ and joins the portal vein. There are also numerous lymphatics in the organ, which run in the trabeculae or surround the veins.

Functions – These are at best only vaguely known. The organ certainly plays some part in the formation of the white corpuscles of the blood, because a great number of these is to be found in blood drawn from the splenic vein, and because, if the spleen be stimulated to contract by an application of electricity to the surface overlying it, the number of white corpuscles in the blood is found much increased. In some animals the spleen also forms red blood corpuscles, and it appears to do this in the human foetus, though not after birth. In human beings useless or worn-out red and white blood corpuscles and blood platelets are broken up by this organ. Nevertheless the spleen does not appear to be absolutely essential to life, since its removal is followed by increase in size of the lymphatic glands all over the body, and does not necessarily interfere with health.

SPLEEN, DISEASES OF – In certain diseases associated with marked changes in the blood, such as leukaemia, and malaria, the spleen becomes chronically enlarged. In some of the acute infectious diseases, it becomes congested and acutely enlarged: for example, in typhoid fever, anthrax, and infectious mononucleosis. Rupture of the spleen may occur, like rupture of other internal organs, in consequence of extreme violence, but in malarious countries, where many people have the spleen greatly enlarged and softened as the result of malaria, rupture of this organ occurs now and then as the result of some quite trivial blow upon the left side. The spleen, in consequence of its structure, bleeds excessively when torn, so that this accident is generally followed by collapse, signs of internal haemorrhage – and death if not dealt with promptly by operation.

SPLENECTOMY means removal of the spleen. This operation may be necessary if the spleen has been severely injured or in the treatment of the severe form of purpura known as purpura haemorrhagica. (See PURPURA.)

SPLENIC ANAEMIA (also known as BANTI'S DISEASE) is a chronic disease, of unknown cause, characterized by enlargement of the spleen and anaemia. In the later stages the liver becomes enlarged, and there may be severe haemorrhage from the stomach. The condition usually begins before the age of 30 years. There is no specific treatment, but some cases respond to removal of the spleen. In the majority of cases, however, all that can be done is to maintain, so far as possible, the general health of the patient and to treat the anaemia with full doses of iron. Blood transfusion is necessary if haemorrhage occurs.

SPLENOMEGALY means enlargement of the spleen beyond its normal size.

SPLINTS are supports for an injured or wounded part. They are most commonly employed in cases in which a bone is fractured, and consist then of some rigid substance designed to take the place of the broken bone in maintaining the shape of the limb, as well as to keep the broken ends at rest and in contact, and thus to ensure their union. Splints are most commonly made of wood either shaped to the limb or consisting merely of strips of wood about the width of the injured limb, and carefully padded with wool or similar soft material. Splints are also made of metal, poroplastic felt, leather, and cotton stiffened with plaster of Paris, as well as other materials. Splints may be improvised for first-aid out of walking-sticks, rifles, broom-handles, branches, folded-up newspapers, and in fact anything of suitable length and rigidity. (See FRACTURES.)

SPONDYLITIS is another name for arthritis of the spine. (See SPINE AND SPINAL CORD, DISEASES OF.)

SPONDYLOLISTHESIS (see SPINE AND SPINAL CORD, DISEASES OF).

SPONDYLOSIS is the condition characterized by ankylosis (qv) of the vertebrae.

CERVICAL SPONDYLOSIS is the form of spondylosis confined to the vertebrae of the cervical spine (the spine in the neck) and is characterized by degenerative changes in the intervertebral discs. These changes produce pain and stiffness in the neck, pain in the arms and, in the more advanced cases, weakness in the legs. Most men over 50 and women over 55 have X-ray evidence of cervical spondylosis, but it is only in a few that these changes cause trouble. Treatment consists of resting the muscles of neck, which may involve the wearing of a plastic collar, and physiotherapy. In the most severe cases a surgical operation may be necessary to reduce pressure on the spinal cord.

SPONGES are animals of lowly organization which develop on the bottom of shallow seas, and are gathered chiefly in the Levant and the West Indies. Small sponges which have been steeped in some antiseptic are still sometimes used by surgeons for wiping up blood at operations, but their place is generally taken by swabs of sterilized gauze. A domestic sponge should not be used to wash a wound, because the animal tissue it contains is likely to swarm with microbes. As a medicinal agent, burnt sponge was used for some time in treating goitre because of the iodine it contains. (See GOITRE.)

SPORADIC is the term applied to cases of disease occurring here and there, as opposed to epidemic outbreaks.

SPOTTED FEVER (see MENINGITIS, EPIDEMIC CEREBROSPINAL; and TYPHUS FEVER).

SPRAINS are injuries in the neighbourhood of joints, consisting usually in tearing of a ligament with effusion of blood. (See JOINTS, DISEASES OF.)

SPRAYS (see INHALATIONS).

SPRUE, or PSILOSIS, is a disease of uncertain origin, characterized by diarrhoea with the passage of large, fatty stools, anaemia, sore tongue, and loss of weight. The name was first given to the condition in 1879 by Sir Patrick Manson, and it was then considered to be a disease of tropical climates. Subsequent investigations have shown that a similar condition occurs in individuals who have never been in the tropics. To this latter condition the name of non-tropical sprue is usually given. The following description applies predominantly to the condition as it occurs in the tropics.

Causes – Many theories have been advanced concerning the cause of sprue, but the general consensus of opinion today is that it is due to an inborn error of metabolism characterized primarily by inability to absorb fats from the intestine. This explains the bulky, frothy stools due to excess of fat. Subsequently there is interference with the absorption of carbohydrate, vitamins, and minerals. The poor absorption of vitamins is responsible for the anaemia and sore tongue, whilst the decreased absorption of calcium is responsible for the low level of calcium in the blood. One advantage of this theory is that it correlates three somewhat similar conditions: (1) tropical sprue; (2) non-tropical sprue; (3) coeliac disease, which is a condition found in children. In all these the fundamental cause is the same. In children with coeliac disease the error of metabolism is so marked that the condition appears early in life. In adults the error is less marked and requires either some precipitating factor to provoke it, or else the normal ageing process. In the case of tropical sprue these precipitating factors are one or more of the following: an attack of dysentery; the strain of living in a hot, damp climate; dietetic indiscretions; the highly spiced diet so commonly eaten by Europeans in the tropics.

Tropical sprue is found chiefly in India, Burma, Malaysia, the East Indies, and China. It also occurs in the Southern States of USA, the West Indies, and South America. It is more common in Europeans than in natives, and is more common in women than in men. As a rule it occurs after long residence in the tropics, and the onset is usually after the rains. There is quite often a preceding history of dysentery.

Symptoms – The onset may be gradual or rapid. Initially there is weakness, soreness of the tongue, difficulty in swallowing, indigestion, and diarrhoea. The diarrhoea is usually worst in the morning, and the stools are pale, bulky, and frothy. The appetite is usually poor. There is a marked degree of anaemia, usually of the macrocytic type: ie. there is a high colour index. The tongue is smooth and red. Gastric acidity is low. Other characteristic findings are that the rise in the blood sugar level following the taking of sugar is less than normal, and there is an increase in the amount of fat in the stools. In untreated cases the patient steadily loses weight and becomes emaciated. Death is usually due to exhaustion and some intercurrent infection. The prognosis depends largely upon the stage at which treatment is begun.

Treatment – The essentials of treatment are rest in bed, a high-protein diet, and treatment of the anaemia and any other deficiency that may be present. It is usual to start the diet with skimmed milk and gradually add other items such as meat. Some authorities, on the other hand, recommend beginning with a diet consisting largely of beef. Whichever diet is used, the essential fact to be borne in mind is that the patient cannot tolerate fats, but that a high caloric intake is necessary to ensure that the patient is adequately nourished. This can best be done by a diet consisting predominantly of protein. For the anaemia folic acid and cyanocobalamin are required. Large doses of the vitamin B complex are also helpful: eg. Marmite. As the blood calcium level is also diminished, vitamins A and D should be given, and it is sometimes useful to supplement this by calcium lactate. As has already been pointed out, convalescence is often prolonged, resulting sometimes in marked depression on the part of the patient. Satisfactory results are seldom obtained unless the patient is sent home to a temperate climate. An individual who has had sprue should never return to residence in the tropics unless it is absolutely essential.

SPUTUM means material spat out of the mouth. It may consist of saliva from the mouth, of mucous secretions from the throat or back of the nose, but is generally expectorated by coughing from the lower air passages. (See EXPECTORATION.)

SQUILL is the sliced bulb of *Urginea maritima*, a plant from the shores of the Mediterranean. It contains several substances which exert an irritating, or, in small doses, a stimulating effect upon the kidneys and the mucous membrane of the stomach and bronchial tubes.

Uses – The tincture, syrup, and vinegar of squills are now used mainly as constituents of expectorant (or cough) mixtures. Squill is also a constituent of Guy's pill which is used in the treatment of dropsy due to heart failure.

SQUINTING is a condition in which the two eyes do not look in the same direction at one time. The movements of the eyeballs depend upon the action of six muscles, four being straight and two oblique. (See EYE.) Of these muscles the outer and inner straight (*recti*) muscles turn the eye from side to side and enable the two eyes to act together. The external rectus muscle and the internal rectus muscle are therefore the most important of the six, and defects connected with them produce inward or outward squint. Other squints upwards or downwards are occasionally, though only rarely, met with, and will not be further referred to.

Causes – A squint which appears in early childhood is often due to some optical error in the eye, generally in the direction of LONG-SIGHTEDNESS. Such a condition causes squinting inwards of one or both eyes, especially when the child looks at something close at hand. The reason for this is that the person with the long-sighted (hypermetropic) eye makes an excessive effort in accommodating his vision for near objects. The muscle of accommodation is supplied by the same nerve (third cranial) as the internal rectus muscle, and the excessive effort also affects the muscles which pull the eye inwards. The two eyes, when thus directed across one another, cannot act together, and the person therefore uses only one at a time, directing it straight forward and turning the other still farther inwards. If the eyes are equally good, the person adopts a habit of looking straight forward first with one eye, then with the other, and is said to have an alternating squint. If, however, the refractive error in one eye be much greater than that in the other, the better eye is always used, and the squint in the other becomes a permanent squint. The power of vision may be so little developed in the brain centre corresponding to a permanently squinting eye that even at an early age it may be almost lost, although the person is unaware of the fact till careful examination reveals it.

SHORT-SIGHT is also productive of a squint which is usually outwards in persons who are not provided with proper spectacles. In reading, writing and other near work such people bring their work much closer up to the eyes than is natural, and the internal recti muscles of the two eyes get a disproportionate amount of work in constantly making the eyes converge. These muscles increase in power therefore and produce the permanent degree of convergence which is occasionally seen in short-sighted students.

DEFECTIVE VISION in one eye is another, though much less frequent, cause of squinting. That is to say, quite apart from mere refractive errors which can be corrected by spectacles, there is some defect in power of seeing. In such a case the defective eye is not controlled by its muscles, as no attempt is made to use the eyes together, and it has a great tendency to roll outwards at times.

PARALYSIS, caused by some affection of the brain or of the nerves supplying the eye muscles, is the usual cause of a squint which suddenly appears after the person has passed the years of childhood. The sixth nerve, which has a long course over the base of the skull and supplies the external rectus muscle, is especially liable to suffer in this way. This produces a strong inward squint of one eye, when the glance is directed towards the side to which the eye belongs, since the eye cannot be turned outwards.

Treatment – In order to obtain the best results it is essential that treatment should be begun as soon as a squint is noticed in a child. Treatment may take one or more of four forms. When the squint is due to hypermetropia (ie. long-sightedness) all that may be necessary may be the wearing of suitable *spectacles*. In cases in which the hypermetropia has persisted for some time before treatment it may be necessary to supplement the wearing of spectacles by *occlusion* of the good eye. This is done so as to ensure that the child uses the bad eye, which otherwise he would not do. At a more advanced stage *orthoptic* supervision will be necessary. This consists of a carefully graduated series of exercises whereby the child is trained to use his eye muscles correctly and thereby overcome the squinting defect which is his untrained (and wrong) method of overcoming the defect. Finally, *operation* may be required, either to strengthen a poorly acting eye muscle or to weaken an over-acting one.

STABS (see WOUNDS).

STAMMERING is a condition in which a person hesitates in the act of speaking, being unable for a time to pronounce certain syllables or repeating the same syllable over and over. For example, in pronouncing such a word as 'Peter' the person may at the beginning of the word be unable to sound the 'P' for a time, remaining with the mouth open, or with the lips compressed, and often making vigorous movements with the hands or feet in the fruitless endeavour. Or he may repeat this sound, pronouncing 'Pe-pe-peter', and being unable for a time to pass off the 'P' to the rest of the word. The latter variety of stammering is generally called 'stuttering'.

Causes – Stammering is not due to any defect in the brain or in the speech organs, and may be described as a functional disease, or a bad habit, or a sign of diffidence. It begins usually in childhood, and is a practice which one child readily learns from another, just as any peculiarity of speech in one person is liable to be unconsciously mimicked by those around. It is more common in twins. The actual cause of the stammering is a want of coordination between the various parts concerned in speech. The speech mechanism consists of three parts, and may be roughly compared to an organ. The chest corresponds to the bellows of the organ, the larynx, where the voice sounds are produced, to the keyboard and pipes of the organ by which the different notes are sounded, and the changes in the mouth effected by the tongue, palate, and lips, resemble the stops of the organ which modulate the notes. Just as these three parts of the organ must be worked in unison for the production of perfect music, so the three parts of the speech apparatus must work together. In stammering there is some error; either the mouth does not shape itself at once to produce the necessary consonants when the stream of air is turned on and the larynx thrown into

action, or the mouth is rigidly held in the proper attitude but no laryngeal note is sounded.

Treatment – This consists of education in proper voice and speech production, and of psychological treatment. The importance of the psychological element is becoming more and more recognized. The stammerer, if a child, should in the first instance be removed from the others from whom he is learning to stammer. Later on, the cure depends upon the amount of care with which the person strives to regulate his vocal organs. (See VOICE AND SPEECH.) One of the most important points for the stammerer to recognize is the difference between those syllables and letters which are produced with full voice and those which have little voice. For example, in the words 'Peter' and 'Beater' the initial letter is hardly sounded in the first, the stress being thrown upon the *e*, while in 'Beater' the *B* receives its full sound. The stammerer's difficulty in many cases arises from a reversal of this process, and disappears when he learns to recognize this difference. Sometimes, before starting a course of treatment with a view to cure, the stammerer does well to remain absolutely silent for a week, with the view of losing his faulty method of speech.

STANNOSIS is the form of pneumoconiosis (qv) caused by the inhalation of stannous (tin) oxide, which occurs in tin ore mining.

STAPHYLOCOCCUS is the name given to a bacterium which under the microscope appears in small masses like bunches of grapes. It is one of the commonest infectious micro-organisms and is found, for example, in the pus discharged from boils.

STARCH is a substance belonging to that group of carbohydrates known as the amyloses. It is converted into sugar when treated with heat in presence of a dilute acid. It is changed largely into dextrin when exposed to a considerable degree of dry heat, as in toasting bread; and a similar change into dextrin and malt-sugar takes place under the action of various ferments such as the ptyalin of the saliva. Starch forms a chief constituent of the carbohydrate foods (see DIET), and in the process of digestion the above-mentioned change takes place in order to prepare it for absorption.

Starch is used externally to form a poultice for softening the skin in skin diseases.

(See POULTICES.) It is also used as a constituent of dusting powders for application to chafed or irritable areas of the skin. (See CHAFING.) Starch enema is administered in inflammatory conditions of the bowel, and is made by boiling two tablespoonfuls of starch in a pint (570 millilitres) of water and then adding hot water till the mixture is reduced to a syrupy consistency. This starch enema is used as the basis for several kinds of soothing enema. For example, a teaspoonful of laudanum may be added to the starch. (See ENEMA.)

STARVATION – Partial starvation, as a method of treatment, is used in certain diseases associated with previous excess of food, particularly obesity. (See CORPULENCE.) When a person is completely deprived of food for a time, not only is there great loss of weight but the chemical processes of the body are altered, and a poisoning effect is produced by the formation of acetone and other ketone bodies. In cases of slow starvation, the vitality of the tissues is reduced and they become more liable to tuberculosis and other diseases. (See also FASTING.)

STASIS is a term applied to stoppage of the flow of blood in the vessels or of the food materials down the intestinal canal. (For Blood Stasis, see CIRCULATION, DISORDERS OF.)

STATUS LYMPHATICUS is another name for lymphatism (qv).

STAVESACRE is the seeds of *Delphinum staphisagria*, which are crushed and made into an ointment for use as a parasiticide.

STEATORRHOEA is any condition characterized by the passing of stools containing an excess of fat. (See MALABSORPTION SYNDROME.)

STENOSIS is a term applied to a condition of unnatural narrowing in any passage or orifice of the body. The word is specially used in connection with the four openings of the heart at which the valves are situated. (See HEART DISEASES.)

STEPPAGE GAIT is the name given to the peculiar walk characteristic of neuritis affecting the muscles of the leg and causing drop-foot. The feet are lifted high so that the toes may clear the ground.

STEREOGNOSIS means the faculty of recognizing the solidity of objects, and thus their nature, by handling them.

STEREOTAXIS is the procedure whereby precise localization in space is achieved. It is applied to that branch of surgery known as *stereotactic neurosurgery*, in which the surgeon is able to localize precisely those areas of the brain on which he wishes to operate.

STERILIZATION means either (1) the process of rendering various objects, such as those which come in contact with wounds, and various foods, free from microbes, or (2) the process of rendering a person incapable of producing children.

The manner of sterilizing bedding, furniture, and the like, after contact with a case of infectious disease, is given under DISINFECTION, whilst the sterilization of instruments, dressings, and skin surfaces, necessary before surgical procedures, is mentioned in the same article and also under ANTISEPTICS, ASEPSIS, and WOUNDS. For general purposes, one of the cheapest and most effective agents is boiling water or steam.

Use of sterilization – Milk is the chief article of food that calls for special sterilization. With regard to other foods, ordinary cooking has this for one of its chief objects. Milk, even from healthy cows, is contaminated by the hands of milkers and by organisms that fall into it from the surrounding air, so that an ounce of milk may be found to contain as many as 2,800,000 bacteria within a short time after milking. Further, milk may be drawn from tuberculous cows. For healthy adults these impurities may not be of such great importance as they undoubtedly are in the case of children liable to tuberculosis, those suffering from gastroenteritis, and persons of weak digestive powers. The origin of epidemics, too, is often traced back to a dairy, especially in the case of typhoid fever. For all these reasons it is necessary to sterilize cow's milk, particularly before giving it to children.

Method of sterilization – One of the most effective modes is simply to boil the milk for a prolonged period in a covered pan; but this changes its taste considerably, and is therefore unsuitable for children and invalids, who tend to drink large amounts of milk.

Another method is to place the milk in a flask or bottle of which the neck is closed by a plug of cotton-wool, and set it in a pot of water, from the bottom of which it is separated by a triangle of wire or other means. The pot is placed upon the fire and the water boiled for three-quarters of an hour, by which time the milk is sufficiently sterilized without appreciably affecting its taste. Many forms of sterilizer are on the market, but all depend upon this principle of having an inner vessel or set of bottles suspended within an outer pot containing water, which is boiled for three-quarters of an hour to one hour. Care must be taken that the milk is not uncovered, after being sterilized, until just before it is to be used.

Pasteurization is a slightly different method of treatment, which is sufficient to destroy the microbes that cause gastro-enteritis, as well as those of many other diseases such as tuberculosis and typhoid fever, while preserving the natural state of the milk. (See PASTEURIZATION.)

Koch's method of sterilization is used in bacteriological investigation, where even the spores of bacteria must be destroyed. It is carried out by steaming the objects to be sterilized on three successive days. (See BACTERIOLOGY.)

BACTERIOLOGICAL STERILIZA-TION may be effected in many ways, and different methods are used in different cases, for it is evident that processes applicable to clothing or to a room may be quite unsuited for the sterilization of food.

SEXUAL STERILIZATION is being used to an increasing extent. In women it is performed by ligating, or cutting, and then tieing the Fallopian tubes (qv), the tubes that carry the ovum from the ovary to the uterus. It is usually performed through a small incision, or cut, in the lower abdominal wall. It has no effect on sexual or menstrual function, and, unlike the comparable operation in men, it is immediately effective. The sterilization is almost always permanent, but very occasionally, for some unknown reason, the two cut ends of the Fallopian tubes reunite, and pregnancy is then again possible. Removal of the uterus and/or the ovaries also causes sterilization, but such procedures are only used when there is some special reason, such as the presence of a tumour.

The operation for sterilizing men is known as vasectomy (qv).

STERNUM is another name for the breast-bone.

STERNUTATORIES are substances that provoke sneezing.

STEROID is the group name for compounds that resemble cholesterol chemically. The group includes the sex hormones, the hormones of the adrenal cortex, and bile acids.

STERTOR is a term applied to noisy breathing resembling snoring. It is due usually to flapping of the soft palate between a stream of air entering by the nose and one entering by the mouth. In ordinary snoring (qv) this results from the habit of sleeping with the mouth open, and in certain serious disorders it arises from paralysis of the soft palate. Some of these conditions affecting the nervous system and thus leading to paralysis of the soft palate are: apoplexy, suffocation, concussion of the brain, drunkenness, poisoning by opium or by chloroform. (For the means of distinguishing between these conditions see OPIUM POISONING.) In some of these paralytic conditions the snoring is very loud, and the noise is due then, not to flapping of the soft palate, but to lolling back of the tongue against the back of the throat as the patient lies on his back. In this case the breathing is at once relieved by pulling forward the lower jaw, by pulling the tongue out of the mouth, or by turning the patient upon one side, as is done, for example, in suffocation due to drowning.

Stertorous breathing is not to be confused with *sniffing* breathing produced by paralysis of the muscles that should hold the nostrils still and open; nor with *puffing* breathing due to paralysis of the muscles in the cheeks and lips; though all three conditions may be produced by the same causes. Nor must it be mistaken for *stridor*, or crowing breathing, due to spasmodic narrowing in the larynx (see LARYNGISMUS); nor for the prolonged, noisy, *wheezing* breathing of asthma produced by narrowing of the bronchial tubes.

STERULE is a term applied to a glass capsule containing a sterile solution for hypodermic administration.

385 – Binaural stethoscope.

STETHOSCOPE is an instrument used for listening to the sounds produced by the action of the lungs, heart, and other internal organs. (See AUSCULTATION.)

STHENIC is a term applied to certain

STIBOCAPTATE

diseases, especially fevers, to indicate that they are not associated with prostration.

STIBOCAPTATE is an organic antimony compound which is used in the treatment of schistosomiasis. (See SCHISTOSOMIASIS.)

STIFFNESS is a condition which may be due to a change in the joints, ligaments, tendons, or muscles, or to the influence of the nervous system over the muscles of the part affected. Stiffness is associated with various forms of rheumatism. Stiffness of the neck muscles resulting in bending backward the head, and of the hamstring muscles, causing difficulty in straightening the lower limbs, is a sign of meningitis. Stiffness or spasticity also occurs in certain diseases of the central nervous system.

STIGMA means any spot or impression upon the skin. The term, stigmas of degeneration, is applied to physical defects that are found in mentally defective persons. (See MENTAL SUBNORMALITY.)

STILBOESTROL is the name given to a synthetic oestrogen. Its physiological actions are closely similar to those of the natural ovarian hormone, and it has the great merit of being active when taken by mouth. An interesting property of stilboestrol is seen in the relief it affords when given to patients suffering from cancer of the prostate, inducing in some cases, it appears, regression of the primary tumour and of secondary deposits in bone. (See HEXOESTROL; and OESTROGEN.)

STILET, or STILETTE, means the delicate probe or the wire used to clear a catheter or hollow needle.

STILLBIRTH (see BIRTH).

STILL'S DISEASE is a disease of childhood first described by Sir Frederic Still (1868–1941). It is characterized by inflammation of several joints (similar to the changes found in rheumatoid arthritis), enlarged spleen and lymph glands, and fever.

STIMULANTS are drugs and other agents employed to call forth special powers of the body or of individual organs in order to effect some special purpose or to offer resistance to some acute attack of disease. The use of stimulants presupposes a certain amount of reserve power on the part of the body or of the organ

stimulated, which is lying dormant and requires an appropriate stimulus before it can be brought into action. In its broadest sense, the term stimulant includes all remedies which are not simply foods destined to supply the wear and tear of the body and to provide it with a store of energy-producing material. It also excludes remedies which have a sedative action upon the nervous system or other organs, and remedies which act directly upon the causes of disease without any reference to the body, such as antiseptics.

(For drugs which stimulate the intestines, see PURGATIVES; for those that stimulate the liver, see CHOLAGOGUES; for those that stimulate the kidneys, see DIURETICS; and for those that increase the activity of the skin secretion, see DIAPHORETICS.) Many substances, such as aromatics, spices, and bitters, stimulate the function of the stomach.

STINGS (see BITES, STINGS AND POISONED WOUNDS).

STITCH is a popular name for a sharp pain in the side. It is generally due to cramp following unusually hard exertion (see CRAMP), but care must be taken that this trivial condition is not taken for pleurisy or for a fractured rib.

(For the stitches used to unite the edges of wounds, see WOUNDS.)

STOKES-ADAMS SYNDROME is a term applied to a condition in which slowness of the pulse is associated with attacks of unconsciousness, and which is due to a state of heart-block.

STOMACH – The stomach is a dilated portion of the alimentary canal, which in man has a shape somewhat resembling that of a pear. The larger end, known as the fundus, lies in the hollow of the left side of the diaphragm, and at one side of this is the opening from the gullet. The greater part of the stomach, into which the gullet opens, is known as the cardiac part, whilst the lower and narrower portion is known as the pyloric part. The two openings into and out of the stomach are known as the cardia, or cardiac orifice, and the pylorus. The stomach is slightly flattened from before backwards, and the two edges are known as the lesser curvature, which runs from one opening to the other direct, and the greater curvature, which sweeps round the fundus from the cardia to the pylorus (illustration 386).

826

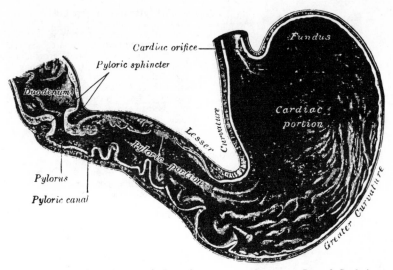

386 – The interior of the stomach. From *Gray's Anatomy*. Longmans, Green & Co. Ltd.

Size and position – The stomach hangs freely suspended in the upper and left part of the abdomen (illustration 387), so that changes in position and shape take place readily according to the amount of food it contains. On the surface, the stomach corresponds to the ribs on the left side from about the fifth to the ninth, and extends below their protecting margin about halfway down to the navel, while the person is recumbent, and slightly below the navel when he stands up. The fundus lies immediately below the heart and base of the left lung, separated from them only by the diaphragm and their enveloping membranes. This explains the embarrassment of the heart's action and of breathing sometimes experienced by dyspeptics. The stomach is attached at the cardiac opening to the gullet, and at this point it is further secured to the diaphragm by a ligament. A broad band of peritoneum (small omentum) attaches the lesser curvature to the under surface of the liver, and a similar peritoneal fold unites its hinder surface to the spleen. The pyloric end, like the cardiac opening, is to a great extent fixed in position, but the greater curvature is quite freely movable.

The greatest length of the stomach from the fundus to the greater curvature near the pylorus is about one foot (30 cm), and the greatest breadth does not exceed 4 to 5 inches (10 to 12·5 cm). The capacity varies greatly in different persons, but is usually

387 – A drawing of the abdominal contents, the anterior abdominal and thoracic walls having been removed. From J. Boileau Grant. *An Atlas of Anatomy*. E. & S. Livingstone.

about 1 to 1½ litres in adults. At birth its capacity is around 30 millilitres.

Structure – The stomach possesses four coats similar to those of the intestine, which are, from within outwards, a mucous membrane, submucous layer, muscular coat, and peritoneal coat (illustration 388).

388 – Diagram of section through wall of stomach. *M*, mucous membrane; *e*, epithelium; *d*, surface of gland duct; *m.m.*, muscularis mucosae; *sm*, submucosa; *c.m.*, circular muscular layer; *l.m.*, longitudinal muscle layer; *s*, serous, or peritoneal, coat. From Schafer's *Histology*. Longman.

MUCOUS MEMBRANE lines the interior of the stomach and is of smooth, soft texture, though raised up into ridges when the stomach is empty. The surface can be seen with the naked eye to be thickly covered by minute pits into each of which several tube-shaped glands are found, on microscopic section, to open. The mucous membrane in fact consists almost entirely of these glands placed side by side, and supported by a small quantity of connective tissue and by fibres of unstriped muscle. The surface of the mucous membrane is composed of a single layer of columnar cells, and these also line the pits referred

to. Each gland is composed of large cubical cells so arranged as to form a tube, open at the upper end where it meets the pit, and closed beneath. These cells secrete the gastric juice which exudes from all the minute tubes as digestion is proceeding. In the cardiac end of the stomach there are other larger cells in addition, mingled with those just described, and the large cells are supposed to secrete the acid of the gastric juice. Between the tubular glands lies some supporting connective tissue in which run numerous blood-capillaries and lymph-vessels.

SUBMUCOUS COAT is a loose connective tissue layer which joins the mucous coat to the muscular coat, and in which the large blood-vessels of the stomach run. The loose arrangement of its fibres allows the mucous membrane to glide freely over the muscular coat in the movements and variations in size of the stomach.

MUSCULAR COAT is of considerable thickness in the stomach, and is of great importance in varying the size of the organ according to the amount of food it contains, in making the peristaltic movements which mix the food with the digestive juice, and finally in expelling the softened food from the stomach into the small intestine. This coat consists of three layers: an outer one in which the fibres run lengthwise, a middle one where they are circular, and an inner layer in which they run obliquely across the stomach.

PERITONEAL COAT is similar to the peritoneum covering the other organs of the abdomen. (See PERITONEUM.)

VESSELS – The stomach is abundantly supplied with blood from the coeliac trunk, a short, wide artery which comes directly from the aorta and also gives branches to the liver, pancreas, and spleen. There is a large arterial arch round either curvature, and from these two arches smaller branches run into the wall of the stomach and reach the submucous coat, from which minute branches are distributed to the other coats. The blood is collected by veins which ultimately return it to the portal vein.

NERVES – The stomach is very richly supplied with nerves both from the brain and from the autonomic system. The tenth cranial nerve (vagus) of each side has a long course down the side of the gullet (hence its name: vagus or wanderer), and after giving branches to the larynx, heart, lungs, and other organs, terminates in the stomach, which has therefore important nervous connections with these vital organs. Other branches come from the solar (or coeliac) plexus of the sympathetic system. These nerves form a plexus in the submucous coat and another in the muscular coat, which exert a powerful influence over the secretions and movements of the organ, although these functions are, in the main, carried out automatically.

Functions of the stomach – The part played by the stomach in digestion consists in storing, warming, and softening the food, as well as partially digesting it, and then in passing it on in small quantities to the intestine, where the more important digestive processes that prepare it for absorption take place. The action of the gastric juice upon the food has been described under DIGESTION. The action of the muscular coat of the stomach is also very important. In birds, which have no teeth, the gizzard is a powerful muscular organ that grinds down the grain and other food into a pulp, but in man the muscular action is much gentler. This, together with other facts regarding the stomach, was first carefully observed between 1825 and 1833 by the American physician, William Beaumont, in the case of a man named Alexis St. Martin, whose stomach had been so exposed by a gunshot wound that a large opening existed through which its interior could be inspected. The movements, as seen by the aid of X-rays, consist of a series of waves, each of which takes about half a minute to pass along the stomach. These movements have also the effect of separating the more fluid parts from lumps still left in the later stages of digestion which are retained in the cardiac part of the stomach while the pylorus relaxes as each wave reaches it to allow some of the softened mass to pass through into the small intestine. This muscular movement takes place in health without causing any sensation, but in irritable conditions of the stomach, when digestion is not proceeding naturally, it may increase in force and give rise to irregular spasms which come and go, and which are attended by much pain. (See DYSPEPSIA.)

STOMACH, DISEASES OF – Only the more common and serious varieties of gastric disease can be considered here. The majority of them exhibit, as their most marked and sometimes their only feature, the symptoms of dyspepsia. (See DYSPEPSIA.)

ACUTE GASTRITIS: **Causes** – Of these, the most important are: (1) Dietetic indiscretions: eg. a large indigestible meal, or the excessive consumption of alcohol;

(2) food poisoning; (3) infections: eg. influenza, septicaemia; (4) toxins: eg. uraemia, gout; (5) the swallowing of poisons: eg. acids, alkalis.

Symptoms – The chief change the stomach undergoes affects its mucous membrane, which is in a state of congestion, either throughout or in parts. The symptoms are those well known as characterizing an acute 'bilious attack', consisting in loss of appetite, sickness or nausea, and headache, frontal or occipital, often accompanied with giddiness. The tongue is furred, the breath foetid, and there is pain or discomfort in the region of the stomach, with sour eructations, and often vomiting, first of food and then of bilious matter. An attack of this kind tends to subside in a few days, especially if the exciting cause be removed. Sometimes, however, the symptoms recur with such frequency as to lead to the more serious chronic form of the disease.

Treatment – The patient must be kept in bed. If the irritant causing the gastritis has not been got rid of by vomiting, vomiting should be induced by giving the patient half a pint (280 ml) of water, containing a teaspoonful of sodium bicarbonate, to drink. Hot applications, eg. a rubber hot-water bottle, to the abdomen are the best way of relieving pain and easing vomiting. If there is constipation a saline aperient should be given. Nothing but sips of water should be given by mouth until the vomiting has ceased. Subsequently warm milk diluted with water should be given in small amounts at frequent intervals, eg. hourly, and the diet gradually increased until the patient is again taking a normal diet.

CHRONIC GASTRITIS may arise after repeated attacks of the acute form or may come on independently. It is of several types. The result of the chronic irritation of the gastric mucous membrane may be an excessively acid gastric juice, which gives rise to an acid dyspepsia. After a long period of irritation an atrophy of the secreting structures of the stomach may be produced, and there is then little or no secretion of gastric juice. In addition to this failure to secrete a proper gastric juice, the interior of the stomach becomes constantly coated with tough mucus, which further prevents digestion from proceeding normally. The mucous membrane is permanently in a state of congestion, it becomes thickened and thrown into deep ridges and furrows, and frequent haemorrhages take place from its dilated veins. At a later stage, great thickening of the other coats may take place (cirrhosis), leading to still further impairment of digestion, since the stomach becomes small, its movements impeded, and the outlet often blocked by thickening in the region of the pylorus.

Causes – Chronic gastritis is more common in women than men, and its incidence increases with age. A high proportion of its victims have a long-standing iron-deficiency anaemia. (See ANAEMIA.) Overeating and alcoholic excess are two common causes. It may be the result of some other disease such as cirrhosis of the liver or heart failure.

Symptoms – The symptoms are those of dyspepsia in an aggravated form (see DYSPEPSIA), of which loss of appetite, discomfort and pain after food, with distension and frequent vomiting, are the chief.

Treatment – This consists essentially of ensuring that the affected individual is having a bland diet which is well cooked and that meals are taken regularly. Careful chewing of food must be insisted upon, and this is often facilitated by not drinking with meals. Alcohol and smoking should be avoided. Particular care must be taken not to eat coarse foods, fruit skins or pips, or pickles or sauces. Neither bitters nor alkaline mixtures should be taken until careful dieting has been given a full trial. Any underlying cause for the gastritis should be treated. Careful dental treatment is necessary if there is any evidence of dental sepsis or if there are not sufficient teeth to ensure adequate chewing of food.

ULCER OF THE STOMACH, GASTRIC ULCER, is of frequent occurrence, and may be a disease of much gravity. It occurs more often than is generally supposed, the result of necropsies showing that one person in every twenty or thereabout suffers from gastric ulcer at some period of life.

Causes – These are not fully understood, but the following points may be regarded as generally admitted: (1) gastric ulcer is more common in men than in women; (2) it becomes more frequent as age increases.

It is held that when any degenerative change takes place in the mucous membrane of the stomach the part is less able to resist the action of the gastric juice upon it, and is apt to undergo disintegration all the more readily. Hence an ulcer is formed. This ulcer is usually of small size ($\frac{1}{4}$ to 1 inch [5 to 25 mm] in diameter), of round or oval form, and tends to advance, not superficially, but to penetrate through

the coats of the stomach. Its most usual site is upon the posterior wall towards the upper or lesser curvature of the stomach and near to the pyloric orifice. This is the point at which the mucous membrane is subjected to most friction by the food as it leaves the stomach. The ulcer may undergo a healing process at any stage, in which case it may leave but little trace of its existence. On the other hand, its scar may produce such an amount of contraction as to lead to narrowing of the pylorus, and later dilatation of the stomach. Also, perforation may take place, which, if not quickly operated upon, may be rapidly fatal, unless previously the stomach has become, as it may, adherent to another organ, by which the dangerous effects of this occurrence may be averted. It may also lead to severe bleeding, the condition known as haematemesis (qv). Usually there is only one ulcer, but sometimes there are more.

Symptoms – The symptoms to which this disease gives rise are sometimes indefinite and obscure, and in some cases the diagnosis has been first made by the sudden occurrence of a perforation. First among the symptoms is *pain*, which is usually worse before food. This pain is situated either in front, at the lower end of the breast-bone, or behind, about the middle of the back. It is often severe, and is usually accompanied with much tenderness to touch, and also with a sense of oppression and inability to wear tight clothing. Accompanying the pain there may be vomiting, particularly in more advanced cases. This tends in some measure to relieve the pain and discomfort, and in many instances the patient rather encourages this act. *Vomiting of blood* (haematemesis) occurs in about 25 per cent of cases and is most important diagnostically. It may show itself either to a slight extent, and in the form of a brown or coffee-like mixture, or as a copious discharge of pure blood of dark colour and containing clots. The source of the blood is some vessel or vessels which the ulcerative process has ruptured. Vomiting of blood, however, does not always indicate the presence of a gastric ulcer. Blood is also found mixed with the discharges from the bowels, rendering them dark and tarry-looking. There is usually constipation of the bowels. X-ray examination gives little evidence of the presence of an acute ulcer, beyond showing that there is much irritation near the pyloric opening, with spasm in the rest of the stomach; but in chronic cases the deep ulcer often fills up with the barium that has been administered for the examination, and its outline can then be readily seen.

The course of a case of gastric ulcer is very variable. In some instances it is acute, making rapid progress to a favourable or unfavourable termination. In others, however, the disease is chronic, lasting for months or years, and in those cases where the ulcers are multiple or of extensive size, incomplete healing may take place and relapses of the symptoms occur from time to time. Ulcers are sometimes present and yet give rise to no marked symptoms, and one occasionally meets with cases where fatal perforation has suddenly taken place and where *post-mortem* examination reveals the existence of a long-standing ulcer which has furnished little or no evidence of its presence during life. Again, an unsuspected ulcer may run a favourable course, and the contraction of its scar may, at a later period of life, cause interference with the exit of food by the pylorus and consequent dilatation of the organ, and thus give the only evidence that an ulcer has at one time been present.

Although the majority of cases of gastric ulcer respond satisfactorily to a course of medical treatment, the relapse rate is high. This, however, has been reduced since the introduction of carbenoxolone in treatment. Further, as already noted, there is also the possibility of three serious complications developing: (i) haemorrhage; (ii) perforation; (iii) obstruction of the pylorus as a result of contraction of the wall of the stomach produced by the ulcer.

Duodenal ulcer, in which a condition similar to gastric ulcer is found just beyond the pyloric opening, has symptoms like those of gastric ulcer, but is six to twelve times more common in males than females, and tends to occur at an earlier age. (See DUODENAL ULCER.)

Treatment – The mainstay of treatment is a derivative of liquorice known as carbenoxolone. This has largely replaced all other drugs. So effective is it that in many cases admission to hospital is no longer necessary. Attention to the diet, however, is still advisable.

The essentials of an effective diet are small feeds every two hours, starting off with milk, or equal parts of milk and cream, and gradually working up to a diet which the individual can take while going about his daily work. In practice, this means breakfast, lunch and dinner (or supper) with a glass of milk in mid-morning, mid-afternoon, and at bedtime. Highly spiced foods should be avoided. Alcohol should be taken in strict moderation and only with food – preferably in the form of light wines. Smoking should be given up.

When haemorrhage occurs, it is treated by complete rest in bed, morphine, and small two-hourly feeds of diluted milk for the first twenty-four hours. When much blood has been lost a transfusion may be necessary. In the event of perforation, treatment is by an immediate operation in which the peritoneal cavity is cleansed and the opening in the stomach wall stitched together. Most surgeons consider that such an operation must be performed at the earliest possible moment in order to afford good hope of recovery.

Surgical treatment, usually in the form of removal of that part of the stomach containing the ulcer, is indicated: (i) in the presence of perforation of the ulcer; (ii) in the presence of severe pyloric obstruction; (iii) in the absence of satisfactory response to medical treatment.

CANCER OF THE STOMACH is the second most common form of cancer in men. In 1977, there were 10,570 deaths from cancer of the stomach in England. In all except the oldest age-groups its incidence has been falling in England and Wales over the last forty years. It occurs for the most part in persons at or after middle life, and is more common in men and in individuals belonging to blood group A. (See BLOOD GROUPS.)

The most common parts affected are at the outlet (or pylorus) and along the lesser curvature, but the disease may spread widely in the stomach wall. When it is situated in the neighbourhood of the pylorus, a stricture may be produced as the disease advances. The growth spreads in the submucous tissue, but as it progresses it tends to ulcerate through the mucous membrane, and in this process bleeding and vomiting of blood may occur. The early symptoms of this disease are in many instances so indefinite as to render the diagnosis for a long time conjectural. They are mostly those of dyspepsia, with more or less pain, discomfort, and vomiting, particularly after meals. The vomited material is often of coffee-ground appearance, due to admixture with blood, but copious haematemesis is less frequent than in cases of gastric ulcer. The patient loses flesh and strength, and soon comes to acquire the cachectic aspect commonly associated with cancer. (See CANCER.) The diagnosis is rendered all the more certain when, as is often the case, a tumour can be detected on examination over the region of the stomach; but where no such evidence is obtained, the nature of the disease is left to be made out by the age of the patient, by absence of free hydrochloric acid from the gastric juice, by progressive loss of weight, and by X-ray examination. Cases of cancer of the stomach advance with more or less rapidity to a fatal termination. Treatment can usually be only palliative, but much relief may be afforded by a careful attention to diet, by the treatment applicable to dilatation of the stomach, and by the use of morphine and other drugs which relieve pain. In early cases an operation can sometimes be performed by which the disease is completely removed, or, when this cannot be carried out, vomiting, pain, and other symptoms of obstruction are relieved by making a communication between the stomach and a loop in the small intestine (gastroenterostomy).

CONGENITAL PYLORIC STENOSIS is a congenital defect that occurs once in every 300 births. It is much more common in baby boys than baby girls, about 85 per cent of cases occurring in boys. It consists of marked hypertrophy, or enlargement of the muscles round the pylorus (qv): the opening from the stomach into the duodenum. The baby appears healthy at birth but within a fortnight he starts vomiting towards the end of his feed. The vomiting is described as projectile because the baby shoots the food out in one forceful volley. As the baby feeds, movements of the distended stomach can be seen moving across from left to right (*visible gastric peristalsis*), and the hypertrophied pylorus can be felt as a tumour or swelling. If surgical facilities are available operation is the recommended treatment. In mild cases, or if proper surgical facilities are not available, medical treatment with atropine methonitrate may be tried. If diagnosed and treated early, the results are excellent.

STOMACH TUBE is a soft rubber or plastic tube with rounded end, and usually about 30 inches (75 cm) in length (illustration 389), which is used for washing out the stomach when it contains some poisonous material, or when it is dilated and filled with fermenting food. (See WASHING OUT STOMACH.) A narrower rubber tube, about the thickness of a quill and of 36 or more inches (90 cm) in length (illustration 390), is used for the purpose of obtaining a sample of gastric juice for examination. (See also TEST MEAL.) Such a tube can also be allowed to pass out of the stomach into

389 – Stomach tube of india-rubber connected by glass junction with india-rubber tube and funnel.

the duodenum so that the contents of the upper part of the small intestine are similarly obtained for analysis.

STOMATITIS means inflammation of the mouth. (See MOUTH, DISEASES OF.)

-STOMY is a suffix signifying formation of an opening in an organ by operation: eg. gastrostomy (qv) and colostomy (qv).

STONE (see CONCRETIONS; BLADDER, DISEASES OF; GALL-STONES).

STOOLS consist of the remainder of the food after it has passed through the alimentary canal and been subjected to the action of the digestive juices, and after the nutritious parts have been absorbed by the intestinal mucous membrane. The stools also contain various other matters, such as pigment, derived from the bile, and large quantities of bacteria. The stools are passed once daily by most persons, but infants have several evacuations of the bowels in twenty-four hours. To some per-

390 – Ryle's stomach (or duodenal) tube. From Pye's *Surgical Handicraft*. John Wright & Sons Ltd.

sons the habit of opening the bowels only once or twice a week seems to be quite natural, though such cases are not common.

The *colour* of the stools is naturally of a dark brown, due to a pigment known as stercobilin, derived from the bile. This colour may be changed to green by the action of certain bacteria when decomposition is proceeding to a greater extent than usual in the bowels, and a deep green colour is also produced by some vegetables, such as spinach. White stools, having an appearance like that of clay or putty, are found in cases where the outlet of bile into the small intestine is stopped, and where jaundice is consequently present (acholic stools). When an excess of fat is taken in the food, as in the case of children fed on great quantities of cream, the digestive organs are unable to deal with it, and much of it is passed in the stools, giving the stools in these circumstances also a whitish colour. Black or slaty-grey stools are produced when certain drugs are taken, as, for example, iron and bismuth; and a tarry blackness known as melaena is sometimes imparted to them when bleeding takes place from the stomach, the iron in the blood being acted upon by the sulphuretted hydrogen always present in the stools to produce the black sulphide of iron. Bright yellow stools are produced in diarrhoea, when the bile is passed almost unchanged, and a similar colour is caused by rhubarb, senna, and some other drugs. Mucus in the stools, whether in strings, or mixed with the food remnants, or in the form of membranes coating the hardened stools, is almost always a sign of irritation or inflammation in the mucous membrane low down in the bowel (colitis). Red blood in the stools signifies some diseased condition situated near the lower end of the bowel, such as an ulcer or piles. When the blood proceeds from a point higher up, such as an ulcer of the stomach, it is changed by the action of the digestive juices as already described.

Incontinence of the bowels, or inability to retain the stools, is found in several diseases of a prostrating nature in which the sphincter muscles, that naturally keep the bowel closed, relax. It is also a symptom of disease in, or injury to, the spinal cord.

Pain at stool is a characteristic symptom of a fissure at the anus or of inflamed piles, and in such cases is of a very sharp nature. Pain of a duller character associated with the movements of the bowels is often caused by inflammation in the other pelvic organs.

CONSTIPATION and DIARRHOEA have been considered under separate headings.

STOUTNESS (see CORPULENCE).

STRABISMUS is another name for squinting (qv).

STRAMONIUM is the leaf of *Datura stramonium* (thorn-apple, devil's apple, Jimson weed). It contains an alkaloid named daturine, which is almost identical with atropine, and upon which its action depends. Certain preparations of stramonium are used similarly to those of atropine or of belladonna for various conditions. (See ATROPINE.)

STRANGULATION is the term applied to the stoppage of circulation which sometimes occurs in a hernia, owing to the pressure caused by the edges of the opening through which the affected organ protrudes. A strangulated hernia must be operated on immediately.

STRANGURY is the name given to a condition in which there is constant desire to pass water, accompanied by a straining sensation, though only a few drops can be voided. It is a symptom of inflammation situated in the kidneys, bladder or urinary passages.

STRAPPING means the application of strips of adhesive plaster, one overlapping the other, so as to cover a part and make pressure upon it. This method of treatment is used in cases of injury or disease when it is desired to keep a part at rest: for example, strapping may be applied to the chest in cases of pleurisy and fracture of the ribs. Also, it is often used to prevent the movement of joints which are sprained or otherwise injured.

STREPTOCOCCUS is the name given to a variety of bacterium which under the microscope has much the appearance of a string of beads. It is responsible for erysipelas and other virulent forms of inflammation. (See BACTERIOLOGY.)

STREPTOKINASE is a substance produced by certain streptococci, which has the property of removing blood clot and inflammatory material. It is now available on a commercial scale and is being used in the treatment of bruises and inflammatory conditions in order to facilitate the absorption of extravasated blood and inflammatory exudates. It is also being used to try and overcome the ill effects produced by the formation of clots (emboli or thrombi) in large blood-vessels.

STREPTOMYCIN is an anti-bacterial substance obtained from the soil mould, *Streptomyces griseus.* It was first isolated in 1944 by Dr Waksman in the United States of America. Its outstanding therapeutic advantages are twofold. In the first place, it is the most active known anti-tuberculous substance which can safely be used in the treatment of tuberculosis in man. Carefully controlled clinical trials have shown that it is of value in all acute forms of tuberculous infection.

Its second great advantage is that it is active against a range of Gram-negative bacteria which are relatively (or wholly) insensitive to penicillin. These particular organisms are responsible for certain chronic infections, particularly of the genito-urinary tract, which have hitherto proved resistant to all other known forms of treatment. Tularaemia (qv), an important disease in the United States of America, also responds to streptomycin, as do certain infections of the intestine.

Streptomycin, unfortunately, has also two big disadvantages. The most important of these is the tendency of organisms to become resistant to streptomycin. This means that the administration of this antibiotic must be carefully supervised to ensure that correct dosage is being used. This disadvantage can be overcome to a certain extent by combining it with the administration of para-aminosalicylic acid and/or isoniazid. The other disadvantage is that streptomycin produces toxic effects more easily than penicillin, especially disturbance of the vestibular and hearing apparatus. This may result in deafness, giddiness, and tinnitus (qv). Whilst in many cases these toxic manifestations disappear when the antibiotic is withdrawn, they may be permanent. For this reason therefore streptomycin must always be used with special care.

STRETCHERS (see INJURED, REMOVAL OF).

STRIAE ATROPHICAE is the term applied to atrophied strips of skin where this has been excessively stretched, as, for example, in pregnancy, when the greyish atrophied strips are known as STRIAE GRAVIDARUM.

STRICTURE means a narrowing in any of the natural passages of the body, such as the gullet, the bowel, or the urethra. It may be due to the development of some growth in the wall of the passage affected, or to pressure upon it by such a growth in some neighbouring organ, but in the majority of cases a stricture is the result of previous ulceration on the inner surface of the passage, followed by contraction of the scar. (See INTESTINE, DISEASES OF; THROAT, DISEASES OF; URETHRA, DISEASES OF.)

STRIDOR is crowing breathing due to spasmodic narrowing of the larynx. (See LARYNGISMUS.)

STROKE is a popular name for apoplexy (qv).

STROMA is the name applied to the tissue which forms the framework and covering of an organ.

STRONGYLOIDIASIS is the disease produced by *Strongyloides stercoralis*, a small nematode, which is found throughout the tropics, particularly in the Far East. It produces a characteristic itching skin rash, known as 'creeping eruption', as well as severe diarrhoea which, like hookworm, may lead to severe anaemia and prostration. The drug used in its treatment is thiabendazole.

STROPHANTHUS is the seed of an East African climbing plant, *Strophanthus kombé*, from which the natives made Kombé arrow-poison. From these seeds an active principle, strophanthin, can be separated, and upon this substance the activity of the drug depends. Its action upon the heart is almost identical with that of digitalis. (See DIGITALIS.) Strophanthin-K must be distinguished from ouabain (qv), which is strophanthin-G.

Uses – It is specially in cases of heart disease in which the heart is beating feebly and the pulse weak and irregular – ie. cases of atrial fibrillation – that strophanthus is used. The effects of this drug, like those of digitalis, are often remarkable in removing dropsy, breathlessness, dyspepsia, and various other symptoms due to some defect in the heart. (See also OUABAIN.)

STROPHULUS, or RED GUM, is a rash consisting of numerous small red pimples, which appears in young children usually about teething-time, and is associated with excessive sweating. It is relieved by light clothing, the exclusion of nylon and by frequent use of some astringent dusting powder.

STRUMA is an old term which was applied to swellings in the neck: either tuberculous glands or enlargement of the thyroid gland. In the former sense it is equivalent to scrofula. (See SCROFULA.) (For the second meaning, see GOITRE.) The term strumous is equivalent to tuberculous.

STRYCHNINE is an alkaloid derived from *Strychnos nux-vomca*, the seeds of an East Indian tree, as well as from the seeds of several other closely allied trees and shrubs. It is a white crystalline body possessed of an intensely bitter taste, more bitter perhaps than that of any other substance, and it is not very soluble in water. It stimulates all parts of the nervous system, and was at one time widely used for this purpose. Today, however, its use has largely been given up, though it is still found as a constituent of some so-called 'tonics'.

STRYCHNINE POISONING is fortunately of rare occurrence. When it does occur today in Britain, more often than not it is the result of a child helping himself to a generous dose of the family stock of one of the so-called 'tonic' tablets containing strychnine, such as Easton's tablets. It shows itself in convulsions, which come on very speedily after the person has taken the poison. These convulsions are brought on by slight causes, and the sufferer becomes quite flaccid between them. The mental faculties remain unaffected, and the symptoms end in death or recovery within a few hours. These symptoms serve to distinguish strychnine poisoning from tetanus or lock-jaw, the only malady which it resembles. (See TETANUS.)

Treatment – The patient should be kept quiet by himself in a darkened room, all noise and disturbance being reduced to a minimum. At the earliest moment a barbiturate is injected intravenously in a large enough dose to stop the convulsions and put the patient to sleep: sodium pentobarbitone or sodium amylobarbitone can be used for this purpose. If the patient is seen early enough after taking the poisonous dose, potassium permanganate, tannic acid, or charcoal may be given by mouth. To wash out the stomach or to induce vomiting in a patient with convulsions is not free from risk. If the muscles of respiration are fixed in spasm, artificial respiration is needed.

STUPE is the name applied to a hot fomentation with turpentine sprinkled on it. (See FOMENTATIONS.)

STUPOR (see UNCONSCIOUSNESS).

STUTTERING (see STAMMERING).

STYE (see EYE, DISEASES OF).

STYPTICS are applications which check bleeding, either by making the blood-vessels contract more firmly or by causing rapid clotting in the blood. Some possess both modes of action.

Varieties – Many substances have this action on account of their chemical or physical properties. Among them may be mentioned ice; hot water at 120° F (49° C) if brought directly in contact with the bleeding surface; perchloride of iron; acetate of lead and Goulard's water; nitrate of silver; sulphate of copper; sulphate of zinc; alum; tannin; hazeline; ergot; adrenaline; and Russell-viper venom.

Uses – The use of styptics is mentioned under HAEMORRHAGE.

SUB- is a prefix signifying under, near, or moderately.

SUBACUTE SCLEROSING PANENCEPHALITIS is a rare complication of measles due to infection of the brain with the measles virus. It develops two to eighteen years after the onset of the measles, and is characterized by mental deterioration leading on to convulsions, coma and death. The annual incidence in Britain is about 1 per million of the childhood population. The risk of its developing is five to twenty times greater after measles than after measles vaccination.

SUBARACHNOID HAEMORRHAGE is a haemorrhage into the subarachnoid space. It is usually the result of rupture of an aneurysm on the circle of Willis (qv).

SUBARACHNOID SPACE is the space between the arachnoid and the pia mater, two of the membranes covering the brain (qv).

SUBCLAVIAN is the name applied to a large artery and vein which pass to the upper arm between the collar bone and the first rib.

SUBCONSCIOUS is the term applied to a state of being partially conscious, or to the condition in which mental processes occur and outside objects and events are perceived with the mind nearly or quite unconscious of them. Such subconscious impressions or events may be forgotten at the time but may nevertheless exert a continued influence over the conscious mind, or may at a subsequent time come fully into consciousness. Much importance is attached to the influence of painful or unpleasant experiences which, though forgotten, continue to influence the mind, and these are held to be largely responsible for neurasthenic and similar states. This injurious influence is removed when the subconscious impressions come fully into consciousness and are then remembered and clearly seen in their relative importance.

SUBCUTANEOUS means anything pertaining to the loose cellular tissue beneath the skin: eg. a subcutaneous injection. (See HYPODERMIC INJECTION.)

SUBINVOLUTION is a term used to indicate that the womb has failed to undergo the usual involution, or decrease in size, which naturally takes place within one month after a child is born.

SUBJECTIVE is a term applied to symptoms, and sensations, perceived only by the affected individual. For example, numbness is a purely subjective sensation, whilst the jerk given by the leg on tapping the tendon of the knee is an objective sign.

SUBLIMATION is a term applied to the processes of converting a solid substance into a vapour and recondensing it. The term is also used in a mental sense for the process of converting instinctive sexual desires to new aims and objects of a higher type devoid of sexual significance.

SUBLUXATION means a partial dislocation, and is a term sometimes applied to a sprain.

SUBSTITUTION is a term used in pharmacy for the replacing of one substance by another, often in a fraudulent manner.

SUBSULTUS means the twitching of the muscles that sometimes occurs in weakening fevers.

SUCCINYLSULPHATHIAZOLE is a sulphonamide drug which is absorbed only slowly from the intestine, and on that account used in the treatment of intestinal infections.

SUCCUSSION is a method of examination by shaking the body of a patient in order to elicit splashing sounds, with a view to determining the presence of gas and fluid in a cavity such as the interior of the stomach or the pleural cavity.

SUCKLING (see INFANT FEEDING; BREASTS, DISEASES OF).

SUCROSE, or CANE SUGAR (see SUGAR).

SUDAMINA are small vesicles which appear underneath the surface layer of the skin during diseases associated with constant perspiration: e.g. rheumatic fever.

SUDORIFICS are drugs and other agents which produce copious perspiration. (See DIAPHORETICS.)

SUFFOCATION (see ASPHYXIA; and CHOKING).

SUGAR is a substance containing the elements, carbon, hydrogen, and oxygen, and belonging therefore to the chemical group of carbohydrates. This group includes three subdivisions as follows:

(1) Monosaccharides ($C_6H_{12}O_6$)
    eg. Glucose, or dextrose, or grape sugar.
       Fructose, or laevulose, or fruit sugar.
       Galactose.
(2) Disaccharides ($C_{12}H_{22}O_{11}$)
    eg. Sucrose, or cane sugar, or beet sugar.
       Lactose or milk sugar.
       Maltose or malt sugar.
(3) Polysaccharides ($C_6H_{10}O_5$)
    eg. Starch.
       Glycogen or animal starch.

Glucose, also known as grape sugar because it is found in various kinds of fruit. including grapes, is the form of sugar produced by the tissues and excreted in large amount by the kidneys in diabetes.

Sucrose is widely distributed through the vegetable kingdom, though it is specially plentiful in the juice of the sugarcane, beetroot, and maple. When taken as a food, it is converted by the digestive juices into glucose before it is absorbed, this process being known as inversion. It is a valuable food, being utilized in the production of heat and energy, although it is also to a certain extent a tissue-builder so far as fat is concerned. It is to be avoided by persons who tend to corpulence, as well as by diabetics.

Lactose is found in milk, and it is to the fermentation of this sugar and consequent production of lactic acid by certain bacteria that the souring of milk is due. The extent to which it is present in the milk of different animals is mentioned under INFANT FEEDING. It has little sweetening power compared with cane sugar, but it is used sometimes as a laxative.

Maltose is produced by the action of the ferment, diastase, upon the starch contained in barley, and also by the ferments of the saliva and pancreatic juice, and is still further changed by the intestinal ferments into glucose before it is absorbed.

Invert sugar is a natural mixture of dextrose and laevulose resulting from a chemical decomposition of cane sugar or of starch.

Starch is mentioned under a separate heading, and its use as a food under DIET and CEREALS.

The energy-producing value of sugars generally is taken as being, on the average, 4 Calories for each gram of sugar.

SUGAR OF LEAD (see LEAD).

SUGGESTION TREATMENT (see PSYCHOTHERAPY).

SUICIDE (see under MENTAL ILLNESS).

SULCUS is the term applied to any groove or furrow, but especially to a fissure of the brain.

SULFADOXINE is a long-acting sulphonamide (qv) with a range of action comparable to that of sulphamethoxypyridazine (qv). Along with pyrimethamine it is used in the prophylactic, or preventive, treatment of malaria. (See FANSIDAR.)

SULFAMETOPYRAZINE is a long-acting sulphonamide. Given in one weekly dose of 2 grams it is proving of value in preventing relapses during the winter in patients with chronic bronchitis.

SULINDAC is a recently introduced drug that is proving of value in the treatment of rheumatic conditions.

SULPHACETAMIDE is one of the sulphonamides. It is used in the treatment of infections of the urinary tract, as it is active against *E. coli*. Its main use today, however, is in the form of eye drops of the sodium salt used locally in the treatment of infections of the eye.

SULPHADIAZINE is one of the sulphonamides. It is a highly active drug and in moderate dosage produces a high and persistent blood concentration. It is relatively non-toxic and is particularly useful in the treatment of meningitis.

SULPHADIMETHOXINE is one of the long-acting sulphonamides, only one dose of which is required daily.

SULPHADIMIDINE is comparable in activity to sulphadiazine, and has the advantage of being even more non-toxic and of producing higher blood concentrations.

SULPHAFURAZOLE is one of the more recent additions to the range of sulphonamide drugs. It has a wide range of anti-bacterial action, but, in view of its high solubility, it is particularly useful in infections of the urinary tract.

SULPHAGUANIDINE is a sulphonamide which is not readily absorbed from the intestine, and is therefore of value in the treatment of bacillary dysentery.

SULPHAMERAZINE is a sulphonamide which is absorbed rapidly from the gut and is excreted slowly by the kidneys. The concentration of the drug in the blood therefore remains high for a long time, and so its action against bacterial infection is correspondingly maintained. Its therapeutic use is similar to that of sulphadiazine.

SULPHAMETHOXAZOLE is one of the long-acting sulphonamides. It is related to sulphafurazole, has a duration of action of 12 hours, and is said to be particularly effective against streptococci.

SULPHAMETHOXYPYRIDAZINE is one of the new long-acting sulphonamides, only one dose of which is required daily.

SULPHAMEZATHINE is another term for SULPHADIMIDINE (qv).

SULPHANILAMIDE, or *p*-aminobenzene-sulphonamide, is a drug the discovery of which is one of the most important in medicine in the twentieth century. It was the first of the sulphonamide drugs. In 1935 the German chemist,

SULPHAPHENAZOLE

Gerhard Domagk, announced the discovery of the effect of prontosil on streptococci. It was later found that this action was due to conversion in the body of prontosil into sulphanilamide, which acts by inhibiting the growth of various bacteria, especially the ubiquitous and dangerous *Streptococcus haemolyticus.* Although many other sulphonamides with various advantages have been subsequently introduced, sulphanilamide is still used to a certain extent. (See also SULPHONAMIDE.)

SULPHAPHENAZOLE is one of the long-acting sulphonamides.

SULPHASALAZINE is a sulphonamide which is proving of value in the treatment of ulcerative colitis.

SULPHASOMIZOLE is one of the long-acting sulphonamides.

SULPHATES are salts of sulphuric acid, and their action and uses vary much according to the metal with which the acid is combined. The sulphates of the heavy metals, which are soluble in water, viz. the sulphates of iron (green vitriol), zinc (white vitriol), and copper (blue vitriol), have a powerful astringent action; whilst sulphates of the alkalis, viz. the sulphates of sodium, potassium, and magnesium (Epsom salts), are used as saline purgatives.

SULPHATHIAZOLE, another drug related to sulphanilamide, is effective against a variety of germs. It is the only sulphonamide active against staphylococci. Its liability to produce toxic effects is steadily reducing its use.

SULPHETRONE is a sulphone, a group of drugs allied to the sulphonamides. It was originally introduced as an anti-tuberculous drug, but is now used in the treatment of leprosy.

SULPHINPYRAZONE is a derivative of phenylbutazone (qv) which is proving of value in the treatment of gout. It is also being used in the treatment of myocardial infarction. (See CORONARY THROMBOSIS.)

SULPHONAMIDE – A drug having the sulphonamide grouping – $SO_2 NH_2$. In 1935, Gerhard Domagk, a German chemist, announced the discovery of the effect of prontosil on streptococci. Subsequent work showed that this action was due to the conversion in the body of prontosil to sulphanilamide. The action of the sulphonamides is bacteriostatic and not bactericidal: ie. they do not directly kill the bacteria but so interfere with their growth that they are unable to multiply. This action of the sulphonamides is now believed to be due to the similarity of their chemical structure to that of *p*-aminobenzoic acid. This latter substance is essential for the growth of many bacteria. If the bacteria are surrounded by a sulphonamide in greater concentration than *p*-aminobenzoic acid, then the bacteria take up the sulphonamide. This interferes with their development and they therefore never mature; nor are they able to reproduce themselves. Although the sulphonamides are being replaced to an increasing extent by penicillin, which is active against many of the same organisms, they are still a useful addition to our ability to control diseases due to bacterial infection.

SULPHONES are a group of drugs allied to the sulphonamides. They are used in the treatment of leprosy. The members of this group include dapsone, solapsone (or sulphetrone), diasone, acedapsone, and promin.

SULPHONYLUREAS are sulphonamide derivatives which lower the blood-sugar, when they are given by mouth, by enhancing the production of insulin. They include acetohexamide (qv), chlorpropamide (qv), glymidine (qv), tolazamide (qv), and tolbutamide (qv). In around 10 per cent of patients a sulphonylurea, particularly chlorpropamide, causes undue sensitivity to even small amounts of alcohol, resulting in severe flushing of the face, throbbing headache and a feeling of intoxication. (See DIABETES MELLITUS.)

SULPHUR is a non-metallic element. Crude sulphur is obtained in volcanic districts, and from it sublimed sulphur is prepared by heating. This sublimed sulphur is either run into moulds as rolled sulphur, or allowed to deposit as flowers of sulphur, which consists of a fine gritty powder and is the most commonly used form. The sublimed sulphur may be boiled with slaked lime and treated with hydrochloric acid, when the sulphur settles down in the form of a fine greyish-yellow powder – precipitated sulphur.

Action – The action of sulphur depends partly upon the grittiness of the flowers of sulphur, and mainly upon the readiness with which sulphur enters into chemical combinations to form sulphides and sulphates. In consequence of this property, it is possessed of disinfectant and antiparasitic powers. When taken internally, the sulphides that are formed stimulate the action of the bowels, and, being excreted partly from the surface of the skin and mucous membranes of the air passages, they also stimulate these.

Uses – Sulphur is burned in order to produce sulphurous acid gas, which is used as a disinfectant. (See DISINFECTION.) Externally, sulphur ointment is an old remedy against the minute parasite that is responsible for the itch; and milk of sulphur is used in lotions for acne on the face. Sulphur is also used in baths for its stimulating action on the skin in cases of skin disease and rheumatism. For this purpose either plain sulphur or, more commonly, sulphurated potash is added in the amount of a quarter or half a pound (113 or 226 grams) to 30 gallons (135 litres) of hot water. Internally, sulphur is a time-honoured remedy for constipation, in doses of a teaspoonful or thereabout made into a paste with treacle. It may be used for the same purpose in the more palatable form of lozenges, several of these being taken at one time, and has a gentle laxative action. In old persons who suffer from rheumatism and who are liable to constipation and to bronchitis, sulphur has been long used in combination with various anti-rheumatic drugs in the confection known as Chelsea Pensioner. (See CONFECTIONS.)

SULPHURET OF POTASH, or SULPHURATED POTASH, also known on account of its appearance as liver of sulphur, is used in baths for the treatment of skin diseases. (See SULPHUR.)

SULPHURIC ACID, or OIL OF VITRIOL, is, in its undiluted state, one of the most powerful of the mineral acids. It is a heavy, colourless liquid of oily consistence and is largely used in various manufacturing operations, so that poisoning by sulphuric acid is not uncommon. It chars any organic substance with which it is brought in contact, and acts as a violent corrosive poison. The treatment of sulphuric acid poisoning is that for corrosive poisons generally: eg. to administer weak alkalis such as baking soda, whitening, magnesia, or soap in water, and to apply oil to the injured surfaces.

Uses – Dilute sulphuric acid, or aromatic sulphuric acid containing cinnamon and ginger, and commonly known as elixir of vitriol, is used in cases of diarrhoea for its astringent properties, in doses of 5 or 20 drops well diluted in water. A lemonade is also made, containing small quantities of sulphuric acid, for use by lead-workers; since it forms an insoluble sulphate with lead, and thus prevents absorption of any lead which may be accidentally swallowed at work.

SULPHURIC ETHER is a name sometimes applied to the ether used for cleansing purposes, because sulphuric acid is employed in its preparation. (See ETHER.)

SULPHUROUS ACID is a saturated solution of sulphur dioxide. It has an extremely pungent odour and strong disinfectant power. Dissolved in water mixed with glycerin it is used for application to the skin in various parasitic skin diseases.

SUMMER DIARRHOEA (see DIARRHOEA; and INFANT FEEDING).

SUNBURN includes the various effects produced on the skin by the sun's rays. Comparable effects may be produced by exposure to the heat of furnaces and by prolonged repeated exposure to electric arc lamps. The effects produced on the skin by sunlight are predominantly due to the ultra-violet rays. They are more marked in fair-skinned than in dark-skinned people, and consist predominantly of darkening, or tanning, of the skin as a result of the production in the skin of a dark pigment known as melanin (qv), which protects the skin against the deleterious effects of continued exposure to ultra-violet rays. In addition there is thickening of the superficial layer of the skin (qv). This production of melanin is preceded by reddening of the skin due to dilatation of the blood-vessels of the skin, and it is this action on the unprotected white skin that is responsible for the painful manifestations of sunburn, using this word in the strict sense of the term. In northern Europe the sensitivity of the skin to sunshine decreases during the late spring and early summer, to increase again in the autumn. This is probably a result of increasing exposure to the sun inducing thickening of the superficial layers of the skin and increasing their content of melanin.

The first manifestation of sunburn, the reddening of the skin, begins to develop in a few hours. This persists for about two days, when it is gradually replaced by tanning or darkening of the skin which gradually develops in extent and depth, depending on how long the body is exposed to the sun's rays and the intensity of the sunlight. The effect of the sun in this respect is much diminished by cloud, and increased by snow. This latter effect is the result of reflection of the ultra-violet rays by the snow, and explains why particular care must be exercised when exposing oneself to the sun in snowy conditions, as on a skiing holiday. There is probably little extra risk of sunburn from exposure to the sun at sea as the surface of the sea does not reflect ultraviolet rays to any appreciable extent.

Symptoms – If the body is over-exposed to the sun, the initial reddening of the skin increases. The skin begins to itch and tingle, becomes swollen, and then blisters begin to form, with peeling of the skin. The speed with which these changes occur, and their extent, depend upon the individual susceptibility of the skin and also the degree and extent of exposure to the sun, but in severe cases the effects may be extensive enough to cause a general upset accompanied by fever.

Prevention – All these unpleasant effects of sunburn can be avoided by gradual exposure of the body to the sun. How gradual this should be depends on the susceptibility of the individual's skin to sunlight, and the intensity of the sun's rays. For the first few days such exposure should not exceed an hour or so, and initially only part of the body should be exposed. Those who are proposing to indulge in sunbathing in warm climes, as around the Mediterranean, would be well advised to 'get into training' by preliminary sunbathing in the garden at home. It is the parts of the body that are normally not exposed to the sun that are most susceptible to sunburn.

Other preventive measures include the sensible use of 'beach umbrellas', and there is much to be said for the old-fashioned parasol of demure brown colour – or even veils for the ladies who are particularly sensitive. Straw hats also play a useful part in protecting the face. Oiling of the skin is an ancient practice that has stood up well to the test of time. There is now a wide range of sunscreen preparations on the market, the active constituents of which include titanium dioxide and zinc oxide. Care, however, must be exercised in the choice of these, as there is by no means invariably a direct correlation between price and efficacy. A basic formula which seems to be standing up to the test of time is 5 per cent

para-aminobenzoic acid in 70 per cent ethanol. A more complicated prescription for those who are particularly sensitive to sunlight is 5 per cent para-aminobenzoic acid, 2·5 per cent amyl dimethylaminobenzoate, and 70 per cent ethanol. The French swear by a preparation of horsechestnut known as Esculoside.

Treatment – Once sunburn, as opposed to suntan, has developed, the affected individual must keep in the shade. The itching and tingling of the skin may be relieved by applying calamine lotion, calamine lotion containing 1 per cent phenol, or 2·5 per cent solution of coal tar. In milder cases the dabbing on of an evaporating fluid such as eau-de-Cologne, elder-flower water, or rose water may be helpful, as may be sponging the affected skin with an astringent such as Goulard's water (qv) or hazeline (qv).

SUNLIGHT (see LIGHT TREATMENT).

SUPER- is a prefix signifying above or implying excess.

SUPERFOETATION is the term applied to the condition in which there is fertilization of a second ovum in a woman already pregnant.

SUPERINVOLUTION is a term applied to the process by which the womb decreases in size after childbirth, when, instead of stopping at the point when the womb reaches its usual size, more or less complete wasting away of this organ takes place.

SUPINATION means the turning of the forearm and hand so that the palm faces upwards.

SUPPOSITORY is a small conical mass made of oil of theobroma, to which white beeswax is sometimes added, or glycerin-jelly, and containing drugs intended for introduction into the rectum. This method of using drugs may be chosen for various reasons. For example, the suppository, as in the case of soap or glycerin suppositories, may be used to produce an aperient action. Other suppositories, such as those of morphine, are used to quiet pain and check the action of the bowels. Others are used for the sake of their influence on neighbouring organs.

There are five suppositories in the *British Pharmacopoeia* 1973: bisacodyl suppositories; glyceryl suppositories; indomethacin suppositories; phenylbutazone suppositories. In addition, the following suppositories are included in the *British Pharmaceutical Codex* 1973: bismuth subgallate suppositories; compound bismuth subgallate suppositories; chlorpromazine suppositories; cinchocaine suppositories; hamamelis suppositories; hamamelis and zinc oxide suppositories; hydrocortisone suppositories; morphine suppositories.

Method of use – The suppository is placed with its pointed end against the anus and with a firm but gentle screwing movement is pushed upwards. With the point of the forefinger, it must be pushed onwards for about 1 inch (25 mm), past the sphincter muscle, otherwise it will not be retained. It must be quickly introduced, as the material of which it is composed rapidly softens when brought into contact with the body.

SUPPRESSION is the name applied to a failure on the part of the kidneys to secrete urine. This is sometimes a complication of fevers or of acute nervous affections, such as meningitis, but it is chiefly found in acute Bright's disease, and leads then to the dangerous condition known as uraemia. (See URAEMIA.) Sometimes in children during a feverish attack the urine is almost completely suppressed for some days with little ill result.

SUPPURATION means the process of pus formation. When pus forms on a raw surface the process is called ulceration, whilst a deep-seated collection of pus is known as an abscess. (For more detailed information, see ABSCESS; INFLAMMATION; PHAGOCYTOSIS; ULCER; WOUNDS.)

SUPRA- is a prefix signifying above or upon.

SUPRAPUBIC operation is one in which the abdomen is opened in its lower part, immediately above the pubic bones. (See LITHOTOMY.)

SUPRARENAL GLANDS, also known as ADRENAL GLANDS, are two organs situated one upon the upper end of each kidney. Each measures about 2 inches (5 cm) in length from above downwards, rather less than that from side to side; and each is about a quarter of an inch (6 mm) thick. The two together weigh about a quarter of an ounce (7 grams).

Structure – Each suprarenal gland has an enveloping layer of fibrous tissue. Within this the gland shows two distinct parts: an outer, firm, deep-yellow, *cortical*

layer, and a central, soft, dark-brown, *medullary* portion. The cortical part consists of columns of cells running from the surface inwards, whilst in the medullary portion the cells are arranged irregularly and separated from one another by large capillary blood-vessels. Both the blood-vessels and the nerves of the suprarenal glands are large and numerous, considering the small size of the organ.

Functions – It has long been known that removal of the suprarenal glands in animals is speedily followed by great muscular prostration and death in a few days. In human beings, disease of the suprarenal glands is apt to bring on Addison's disease, in which the chief symptoms are increasing weakness and bronzing of the skin. The medulla of the glands produces a substance – adrenaline – the effects of which closely resemble those brought about by activity of the sympathetic nervous system: dilated pupils, hair standing on end, quickening and strengthening of the heart-beat, immobilization of the gut, increased output of sugar from the liver into the blood-stream. From the cortex of the gland are produced a series of hormones which play a vital, though as yet incompletely elucidated, rôle in the metabolism of the body. Some (such as aldosterone) control the electrolyte balance of the body, others are concerned in carbohydrate metabolism, whilst others again are concerned with sex physiology. Cortisone is another suprarenal cortical hormone which is now believed to be of value in the treatment of rheumatoid arthritis and certain other rheumatic diseases, as well as Addison's disease. (See ADRENALINE; ADDISON'S DISEASE; CORTISONE.)

SURAMIN is the *British Pharmacopoeia* name for a drug which has been much used, and with success, in the treatment of trypanosomiasis (qv).

SURFACTANT is a surface-active agent lining the alveoli of the lungs, which plays an essential part in respiration (qv) by preventing the alveoli collapsing at the end of the expiration. Absence, or lack, of surfactant is believed to be one of the factors responsible for hyaline membrane disease (qv).

SURMA is a fine powder which is applied to the inner surface of the eyelids in the same way as mascara is applied to the outer surface. Its name is derived from the Urdu for antimony, but in practice it may contain salts of antimony, zinc, and

SURROGATE

lead. Lead sulphide (galena) is the most common constituent, often combined with camphor or menthol to induce watering of the eyes. It is used by Asians, mainly as a cosmetic, but also to relieve eyestrain. It has been shown to induce lead poisoning in Asian children. Since January 1979 the use and sale of surma and other lead-containing cosmetics have been prohibited in Great Britain.

SURROGATE is a term applied in medicine to a substance used as a substitute for another.

SUSPENDED ANIMATION (see DEATH, SIGNS OF; and SLEEP).

SUSPENSORY means anything serving to hold up a part, and is a term specially applied to bandages for the breast, testicle, and other dependent parts.

SUTURE is the name given either to the close union between two neighbouring bones of the skull, or to the series of stitches by which a wound is closed. (See WOUNDS.)

SWAB is a term applied to a small piece of gauze, lint, or similar material used for wiping out the mouth of a helpless patient or for drying out a wound. The term is also applied to a tuft of sterilized cotton-wool wrapped round a wire and enclosed in a sterile glass tube used for obtaining matter or membrane from the throat, from wounds, or the like, in order that this may be subjected to bacteriological examination.

SWEAT (see PERSPIRATION).

SWEAT GLANDS (see SKIN).

SWEATING SICKNESS was the name given to a malady that appeared in Europe, and especially in England, during the fifteenth and sixteenth centuries. It was named after its most prominent symptom, appears to have been a disease of sudden onset which caused extreme prostration, and was very fatal. There were several epidemics during the centuries mentioned, and the disease seems to have been regarded with great dread, although it is difficult to identify it with any infectious malady at present known.

SWEETBREAD is a popular term applied to several glands used for food, including the thymus gland of young animals (neck sweetbread), the pancreas (stomach sweetbread), and the testis.

SWEET SPIRIT OF NITRE, also known as NITROUS ETHER SPIRIT, consists of a mixture of water, alcohol, acetaldehyde, and various nitrous bodies. Like other drugs containing nitrites, sweet spirit of nitre has an action in checking spasm of all sorts and in dilating the blood-vessels. (See GLYCERYL TRINITRATE.) In certain circumstances it is a diaphoretic, causing copious perspiration and thus reducing feverishness. In other circumstances it acts as a diuretic, increasing the action of the kidneys. When kept in unstoppered bottles, it rapidly loses strength and to be of any value, must be used fresh.

SYCOSIS is the name given to a skin disease in which the hair follicles, especially of the chin, are inflamed, forming pustules round the hairs, surrounded by a swollen and reddened area of skin. The disease is directly due to infection of the hair follicles with staphylococcus or ringworm. The infection is generally attributed to a barber's utensils, and the condition is sometimes known as barber's itch, foul shave, or ringworm of the beard. (For treatment, see IMPETIGO; and RINGWORM.)

SYMPATHETIC is a term applied to certain diseases or symptoms which arise in one part of the body in consequence of disease in some distant part. Inflammation may arise in one eye, in consequence of injury to the other, by the spread of organisms along the lymphatic channels connecting the two, and is then known as sympathetic inflammation. Pain also may be of a sympathetic nature. (See PAIN.)

SYMPATHETIC SYSTEM is part of the autonomic nervous system (qv). It consists of scattered collections of grey matter known as ganglia, united by an irregular network of nerve-fibres, those portions where the ganglia are placed most closely and the network of fibres is specially dense being known as plexuses. The chief part of the sympathetic system consists of two ganglionated cords that run through the neck, chest, and abdomen, lying close in front of the spine. (For further details, see NERVES.)

SYMPATHOMIMETIC DRUGS are those producing an effect comparable to those produced by stimulation of the sympathetic nervous system: eg. adrenaline (qv).

SYMPTOM is a term applied to any evidence of disease. The term, physical sign, is generally applied to symptoms of which the patient does not complain but which are elicited upon examination. For the symptoms indicative of the various diseases see under the headings of each disease.

SYN- is a prefix signifying union.

SYNAPSE is the term applied to the anatomical relation of one nerve-cell with another which is effected at various points by contact of their branching processes. The state of shrinkage or relaxation at these points (synapses) is supposed in some cases to determine the readiness with which a nervous impulse is transmitted from one part of the nervous system to another. Many drugs act upon the nervous system through their effect in closing or widening these junctions.

SYNCOPE is another name for fainting. (See FAINTING.)

SYNDACTYLY is the condition which a child is born with, in which two or more fingers or toes are fused together to a varying extent (illustration 391). The condition is popularly known as webbed fingers or toes (qv).

SYNDROME is a term applied to a group of symptoms occurring together regularly and thus constituting a disease to which some particular name is given: eg. *Stokes-Adams Syndrome*, of slow pulse and giddiness, forming a sign of degeneration of the heart-muscle causing heart-block; *Korsakoff's Syndrome*, of loss of appreciation of time and place combined with talkativeness, forming signs of alcoholic delirium.

SYNECHIA is the term applied to adhesions between the iris and the cornea or lens.

SYNOSTOSIS is the term applied to a union by bony material of adjacent bones normally separate.

SYNOVIAL MEMBRANE forms the lining of the soft parts that enclose the cavity of a joint. (See JOINTS.)

SYNOVITIS means inflammation of the membrane lining a joint. It is usually painful and accompanied by effusion of fluid within the synovial sac of the joint. It

391 – Syndactyly involving fusion of the second and third toes. *The Practitioner.*

is found in acute rheumatism, various injuries and inflammations of joints, and in chronic form in tuberculosis.

SYNTHETIC is a term applied to substances produced by chemical processes in the laboratory or by artificial building up.

SYPHILIS is a contagious disease of slow development, which, at its start, shows a characteristic sore at the site of infection, later brings on constitutional effects resembling those of other infectious diseases, and at a still later period produces certain changes in the central nervous system, the arteries and elsewhere. Because, in the majority of cases the disease is acquired as a result of sexual intercourse with an infected individual, it is classed as one of the *venereal* diseases, or sexually transmitted diseases as they are now known. Syphilis affects only human beings, though it has been experimentally produced in anthropoid apes.

The disease seems to have first attracted public attention about or soon after the year 1494 in consequence of a severe and widespread outbreak among the French soldiers then occupied in the siege of Naples. For long it was known as the Neapolitan disease, French Pox, or Great

Pox; and, in consequence probably of the licentiousness and the want of cleanliness that then prevailed in persons and dwellings, it spread in epidemic form. Later, it came to be called syphilis, the name being derived from that of the chief character in a Latin poem published by Fracastoro in 1530. It has been suggested that the disease existed in ancient times among the natives of America, and that the infection was brought to Europe by the followers of Columbus, but there are also grounds for supposing that the disease occurred among the Eastern races in ancient times, although it was most likely confounded with leprosy and tuberculosis.

Causes – The causative organism is the *Treponema pallidum*, a long, thread-like wavy organism with pointed tapering ends. It is found in large numbers in the sores in the primary stage of the disease and in the skin lesions in the secondary stage.

The number of cases of syphilis reported in England in the year ending June 30, 1977, was 5562 (4490 males, 1072 females). The number of cases of late syphilis was 681. The number of deaths from the disease in England in 1977 was 85.

Syphilis may be ACQUIRED from persons already suffering from the disease, or it may be CONGENITAL. The acquired form is usually got by sexual intercourse, but it may also result from kissing or from contact with a sore upon another person through some wound or abrasion. The epithelium covering the general surface of the skin seems to be an efficient protection, but the infective material apparently has the power of penetrating mucous membranes. Not only may the disease be spread as a venereal affection, but cups, spoons, towels, sponges, sheets, which have been used by the diseased, have been known to convey the contagion to others, although fortunately such inanimate articles appear to retain their infectiveness only for a short time. The acquired form of the disease is infectious from contact with sores, both in its primary and secondary stages; whilst infants suffering from the congenital form are also highly infectious. Accordingly any one frequently handling such an infant, runs great risk of infection, although the mother may handle the babe with impunity (Colles' Law).

Symptoms – The *acquired form* of the disease is commonly divided into three stages – PRIMARY, SECONDARY, and TERTIARY, although in many cases the tertiary stage is wanting, whilst in others there is no dividing line between the secondary and tertiary symptoms. To certain late affections, which may appear after the lapse of several years, such as locomotor ataxia and general paralysis, the terms parasyphilis and QUATERNARY syphilis are sometimes applied. The disease presents great variations of intensity, being occasionally of a 'malignant' type, in which widespread ulceration speedily comes on and even causes death; and in other cases showing little more than a slight skin eruption, although probably it exerts, even in such mild cases, a highly prejudicial effect upon the constitution. There are several laboratory tests for confirming the diagnosis.

The incubation period ranges from 10 to 90 days, though most frequently it occupies about four weeks. Then a small ulcer appears at the site of infection, which is accompanied by a typical cartilaginous hardness of the tissues immediately round and beneath it, and characterized by its resistance to all healing treatment. This, which is known as the PRIMARY SORE (or *chancre*), may be very much inflamed, or it may be so small and occasion so little trouble as to pass almost or quite unnoticed. A few days after this sore has appeared, the lymphatic glands in its neighbourhood, and later then all over the body, become swollen and hard. This condition lasts for several weeks as a rule, and then the sore slowly heals and the glands subside. After a variable period, which, however, may in most cases be placed at about two months from the date of infection, the SECONDARY SYMPTOMS appear and resemble the symptoms of an ordinary fever in so far as they include rise of temperature and feverishness, loss of appetite, vague pains through the body, and a faint red rash seen best upon the front of the chest. The rash may also show other characters. Other symptoms often present at this stage, including falling out of the hair, bloodlessness, the appearance of sores in the mouth and throat (mucous patches), fleshy-looking masses round the genitalia (*condylomatua lata*), headache with, occasionally, mental deterioration, and painful swellings on the bones due to periostitis. There is also general enlargement of the lymphatic glands. The duration of this stage is largely dependent upon the efficiency with which it is treated.

In untreated or inadequately treated cases manifestations of the TERTIARY STAGE develop after the lapse of some months or years. These consist in the growth, here and there throughout the body, of masses of granulation tissue known as gummas. These gummas may appear as hard nodules in the skin, or form tumour-like masses in the muscles, or cause great thickening of bones, or they may develop in the brain and spinal cord, where their presence causes very serious symptoms. Those which lie beneath the skin or a mucous membrane may break down and form deep ulcers with characteristic thickened, sharply cut edges. These often leave rounded brownish scars when they heal. Gummas yield readily, as a rule, to appropriate treatment, and generally disappear speedily when this is secured.

Still later effects are apt to follow, such as disease of the arteries, leading to aneurysm (see ARTERIES, DISEASES OF; and ANEURYSM), to apoplexy, and to early mental failure (see MENTAL ILLNESS); also certain nervous diseases, of which locomotor ataxia and general paralysis are the chief.

The *congenital form* of syphilis, or *congenital syphilis* as it is usually known, of which there were 141 cases in England in the year ending June 30, 1977, may affect the child before birth, leading then as a rule to miscarriage, or to a stillbirth if he (or she) be born at full time. Or he (or she) may show the first symptoms a few weeks after birth, the appearances then corresponding to the secondary manifestations of the acquired form. The child, apparently at first quite healthy, begins to waste, so that the skin appears loose and wrinkled. Eruptions develop and the breathing is of a snuffling character, in consequence of inflammation in the mucous membrane of the mouth and nose. Deafness is also a common result of inflammation in the delicate structures of the inner ear. On the other hand, no symptoms may appear till later in life, when the nose becomes sunken and broad at the bridge, and the eyes are dull as the result of the inflammation affecting the cornea (keratitis) or iris (iritis). These changes often appear about the age of 12 or 14, causing dimness of vision. When the permanent teeth appear, the central incisors are often notched at the edge (Hutchinson's teeth).

Treatment – Any person who suffers from this disease forms a source of infection to those around, and it is his duty to take precautions that he may not spread it. He should bear in mind the fact that, whilst the natural secretions of the body are harmless, the discharge from any sore or abraded surface is highly contagious. He should, if suffering from any sore about the lips or mouth, be most careful not to drink from any public drinking utensil, and he should never allow any one else to use his sponge or towel or to wear any of his clothes. He must remember, too, the fact that the disease is transmissible to his offspring so long as he shows any manifestation of its presence; and in this relation it is usual for physicians to advise a person suffering from syphilis not to marry till at least a year has elapsed since any sign of the disease has been present, and then only if an energetic course of treatment has been carried out.

For generations, salts of mercury were the traditional drugs for the treatment of syphilis, given by mouth or by inunction, and later by intramuscular injection. Following the discovery by Ehrlich, in 1910, of the anti-syphilitic action of organic arsenical preparations, these became the essential part of the treatment of the condition, supplemented by bismuth salts.

For nearly forty years the organic arsenical preparations, in one form or another, constituted the first line of attack on syphilis. During the last thirty years, however, they have been replaced by penicillin which, used in the correct dosage, is now accepted as the drug of choice in the treatment of syphilis in all its stages.

The successful introduction of penicillin, however, has not altered the three essential bases of successful treatment: (1) treatment must be instituted as soon as possible after infection is acquired; (2) a full course of treatment is essential in every case, no matter how mild the disease may appear to be; (3) periodic blood examinations or must be carried out on every patient for at least two years after he or she has been apparently cured.

SYRINGE is the name of an instrument for injecting liquids into the body. Syringes vary considerably in shape and size according to the purpose for which they are used. (For the method of using a hypodermic syringe, see HYPODERMIC.)

SYRINGOMYELIA is a rare disease affecting the spinal cord, in which are found irregular cavities surrounded by an excessive amount of the connective tissue of the central nervous system. These cavities encroach upon the nerve tracts in the cord, producing especially loss of the sense of pain or of that for heat and cold in parts of the limbs, although the sensation of touch is retained. Another symptom sometimes present is wasting of certain muscles in the limbs. Changes affecting outlying parts like the fingers are also found. On account of their insensitiveness to pain, the fingers, for example, are often burnt or wounded, and troublesome ulcers, or loss of parts of the fingers, result. The condition of the spinal cord is probably present at birth, though the symptoms do not usually appear till the period of youth is reached. The disease is slowly progressive, and the treatment consists simply in the maintenance of general good health.

SYRUP, formed of a mixture of sugar and water, is a fluid often used for the administration of drugs. It is employed partly on account of its pleasant taste, and largely also because it retards changes in drugs which deteriorate on exposure to the air. The dose of most syrups is about a teaspoonful. The *British Pharmaceutical Codex* 1973 contains the following syrups: black currant syrup; codeine phosphate syrup; compound figs syrup; ginger syrup; invert syrup; lemon syrup; orange syrup; raspberry syrup; squill syrup; tolu syrup; wild cherry syrup.

SYSTOLE means the contraction of the heart, and alternates with the resting phase, known as diastole. The two occupy, respectively, about one-third and two-thirds of the cycle of heart action.

T

TABES means, literally, a wasting disease, and is an old name applied to various diseases, such as locomotor ataxia, and tuberculosis accompanied by enlargement of glands. At present the name *tabes dorsalis* is used for locomotor ataxia (see LOCOMOTOR ATAXIA) and *tabes mesenterica* is used for tuberculosis affecting the glands in the abdomen: two diseases totally different in their nature and cause.

TABLET is the name given to a solid disc-like preparation made by compression and containing drugs mixed usually with sugar and other indifferent material. Tablets are widely used because of their convenience and accurate dosage. The word, 'tabloid', indicates a proprietary preparation.

TACHE CÉRÉBRALE is a sign often observed in meningitis. The sign consists in the production of a bright-red line of congestion when the finger-nail is drawn across the patient's skin – for example, across his abdomen.

TACHYCARDIA means a rapid pulse rate. (See HEART DISEASES.)

TACHYPNOEA means unusual quickness of breathing.

TAENIASIS is the disease caused by taeniae, or tapeworms. These parasites illustrate well the degeneration consequent upon a parasitic life. They exist solely to feed and to propagate their kind, discharging apparently no useful function in the economy of nature. Accordingly their shape is modified to present as large an absorbing surface as possible to the digested food passing down the intestine, so that they are flat, white and long (up to 12 metres [40 feet] in length), like a piece of tape, as their name implies. Each consists of a head (illustration 392), the size of a small pin's head, provided with suckers, and sometimes with hooklets, for adhesion to the bowel wall, and from this head segments are produced that gradually increase in size and develop ova the farther they recede from the head. The mature segments at the extremity of the worm are crammed full of ova, and are constantly splitting off to be discharged in the stools. When these mature segments, or proglottides, are discharged, they fall upon the ground, and the ova they contain are after-wards conveyed either by food or drink into the stomach of an intermediate host, which may be a pig, ox or cattle, in the case of different parasites. The geographical distribution of different tapeworm infestation depends largely upon the eating habits of the inhabitants. Thus *Taenia saginata*, or the beef tapeworm, is found in beef-eating areas, especially in Europe and Mohammedan countries. *Taenia solium*, the pork tapeworm, is found most commonly in Germany and the Slav countries. *Echinococcus granulosus* is found where dogs are widely used, as in Iceland or sheep-rearing countries such as Australia, New Zealand and Argentina. When the ova reach the stomach of the intermediate host their capsule is dissolved, the embryos escape and find their way through the wall of stomach or intestine into the blood-vessels, by which they are carried to distant

392 – Head of *Taenia solium*. Magnified by 20.

parts of the body. In the case of TAENIA SOLIUM the intermediate host is the pig, in the case of TAENIA SAGINATA it is cattle. In the muscles of these animals the embryos of the worm become encysted and remain so till they die, or till the animal's flesh happens to be eaten by the proper host, when they develop again into a new tapeworm in his intestine. The flesh of a pig thus infected shows plainly the encysted embryo (known as *Cysticercus cellulosae*), and is called measly pork. DIPHYLLO-BOTHRIUM LATUM is seldom met with, save in the north of Europe and Asia, and the intermediate hosts are several varieties of fish. In the case of the tapeworm known as *Echinococcus granulosus*, relations are reversed, and man plays the rôle of intermediate host, the host of the mature tapeworm being the dog, from which the human being derives the embryo worm by allowing the dog to lick his hands and face, or to contaminate his food. Although the worm in the dog is very small (having only three segments, as a rule), yet the encysted form in man, known as a hydatid cyst, may reach a large size, situated in the liver, lungs, kidney or brain.

In the case of infestation with *Taenia saginata* there may be no symptoms or signs at all, and the 'host' only becomes aware that he is infested, when he sees the tapeworm, or rather part of it, in the stools. In the case of *Taenia solium*, the outlook is more serious because the eggs, when swallowed, are liable to migrate into the tissues of the body, as they do in the pig, and cause cysts. If these occur in the muscles they may cause little trouble but, if they occur in the brain, they can prove very serious.

Hydatid cysts often grow to a great size, budding off in their interior smaller cysts, which may have still smaller ones within them, the final contents of the smallest cysts being a salt, watery fluid and numerous heads of echinococci, each provided with a circle of hooks, and each capable, under proper conditions, of forming a new worm. The symptoms produced by a hydatid cyst depend mainly upon the effects of its size and consequent pressure. Very small cysts in the brain may produce serious results, like those of a tumour, whilst in the liver a cyst may grow to the size of a man's head before causing much trouble.

Treatment of tapeworm infestation consists of the administration of mepacrine, niclosamide or dichlorophen, followed by a purgative. Castor oil must not be used for this purpose. During treatment the stools must be carefully examined for the head of the tapeworm. Unless the head is passed in the stools, the worm will grow again. The treatment of hydatid cyst is surgical: ie. the cyst must be removed by operation.

TAKA-DIASTASE (see DIASTASE).

TALAMPICILLIN (see PENICILLIN.)

TALC is a soft mineral consisting of magnesium silicate. It is much used as an ingredient of dusting powders.

TALIPES is the technical name for club-foot (qv).

TALUS is the name applied to the somewhat square-shaped bone which forms the lower part of the ankle-joint and unites the leg bones to the foot.

TAMARIND is the preserved pulp of the fruit of *Tamarindus indica*, a West Indian tree. It contains a large amount of vegetable acid, and has a laxative action.

TAMOXIFEN is a drug that is proving of value in the treatment of some cases of cancer of the breast.

TANNIN, or TANNIC ACID, is an uncrystallizable white or yellowish-white powder, which is soluble in water or glycerin. It is a complicated organic acid with the empirical formula of $C_{76}H_{52}O_{46}$. It is extracted from oak-galls in large amount, but it is also present in almost all vegetable infusions. Tannic acid, when brought in contact with any mucous membrane, acts as an astringent and diminishes its secretion. It coagulates albuminous substances and thus hardens animal food with which it is mixed, and also leads to rapid clotting of blood with which it is brought in contact.

Uses – Tannin is used as a styptic to apply directly to bleeding wounds or surfaces with which it can be brought in contact, as the mouth, interior of the stomach, or of the rectum, and since its action in coagulating albumin is powerful, it speedily causes a clot to form. It is applied to relaxed mucous membranes, employed, for instance, in lozenges when the throat is relaxed, or applied in ointment for piles. Glycerin of tannin is a convenient method of applying this substance as an astringent, by painting, to the throat. Tannin is used to check diarrhoea, administered either in the form of some vegetable astringent infusion, or in a chemical combination which is not destroyed in the stomach, such as acetannin or albumin tannate.

As tannin neutralizes many poisonous alkaloids, it is often administered as an antidote to vegetable poisons.

Many vegetable astringents owe their usefulness to the tannin they contain, as, for example, catechu, kino, and rhatany.

TAPEWORM (see TAENIASIS).

TAPPING is the popular name for the withdrawal of dropsical fluid from the cavities or the subcutaneous tissues of the body. (See ASPIRATION.)

TAR, or PIX LIQUIDA, is a thick, dark, oily substance obtained by the destructive distillation of several species of pine-tree. It is slightly soluble in water, more readily so in alcohol, oils, and strong alkaline solutions. Other tars of similar physical and medicinal properties are obtained from other woods, as well as from coal, shale, and peat: for example, birch-tar, well known for the aroma it imparts to Russian leather. Tar is a substance of complex chemical composition, varying not only according to the source from which it is derived, but still more with the temperature at which it has been distilled. Generally speaking, wood-tar contains resin, creosote, and turpentine in considerable quantities, also benzol, carbolic acid, acetic acid, wood-spirit or methyl alcohol, methyl acetate, acetone, and wood-naphtha. The aniline dyes, many antipyretic bodies, saccharin, and various other medicinal substances and disinfectants are obtained indirectly from coal-tar.

Action – In consequence of the numerous medicinally active bodies it contains, tar exerts many marked effects upon the body. By reason of the creosote, carbolic acid, and methyl alcohol that it contains, it possesses an antiseptic and preservative power. Certain of its ingredients are of an irritating nature, and tar therefore stimulates the action of any skin surface with which it is brought in contact, as well as the respiratory and other mucous membranes by which it is excreted after being taken internally.

Uses – Bishop Berkeley in 1744 published his *Siris*, a treatise upon the virtues of tar-water, in which he extolled this substance as an almost universal remedy.

Externally, tar is one of the most efficient preservatives of animal and vegetable tissues that we possess. For its germicidal action and stimulating properties it is used in chronic skin diseases, particularly psoriasis and dry eczema. To this end it is employed most commonly in the form of tar ointment. An alcoholic extract known as coal tar solution is also used to cleanse areas of skin affected by the disease.

Internally, it is sometimes used in chronic bronchitis as an expectorant. It both checks excessive expectoration and renders coughing easier. For this purpose it is most commonly used in the form of *tar-water*, made by shaking up one part of tar with ten of water, allowing to settle, and decanting the clear liquid. This tar-water may be taken in wine-glassful doses. Syrup of tar is tar-water sweetened with sugar.

TARAXACUM, or DANDELION, is a very old remedy for dyspepsia associated with torpidity of the liver. The fresh milky juice of the flower-stalks is also sometimes used as a remedy for warts.

TARSUS is the name applied to the region of the instep with its seven bones, the chief of which are the talus supporting the leg-bones and the calcaneus or heel-bone, the others being the navicular, cuboid, and three cuneiform bones.

TARTAR is a concretion that forms on the teeth near the margin of the gum, consisting chiefly of phosphate of lime deposited from the saliva. Mixed with this are food particles, and in it flourish numberless bacteria. It is important that it should be prevented from forming by regular brushing of the teeth, or removal after it has formed by regular visits to the dentist, because it gives rise to wasting of the gums and loosening of the teeth.

TARTAR EMETIC is another name for antimony potassium tartrate, a drug used in the treatment of schistosomiasis. (See SCHISTOSOMIASIS.)

TARTARIC ACID is almost indentical with citric acid in appearance, chemical properties, and medicinal uses. Tartaric acid is obtained from grapes, whilst citric acid is contained in many fruits like the lemon, lime, and orange. (See CITRIC ACID.)

TASTE (see TONGUE).

TATTOOING is performed by implanting particles of colour pigment into the deeper layer of the skin known as the dermis (see SKIN). This is done by means of a needle or needles. The pigments commonly used are carbon for black, cinnabar (red mercuric sulphide) or cadmium salts for red, chrome salts for greens and yellows, cobalt for blue, ferric (iron) salts for browns, pinks and yellows, and titanium for white. The main medical hazard of tattooing is infection, particularly of the liver, which may be fatal. The tattooed person may also become allergic to one of the pigments used, particularly cinnabar. Removal, which should only be done by a plastic surgeon, always leaves a residual scar. Removal is not allowed under the National Health Service unless there is some medical reason: for example, allergic reactions to it.

TAXIS is the name given to the method of pushing back, into the abdominal cavity, a loop of bowel which has passed through the wall in consequence of a rupture.

TEA (see COFFEE AND TEA).

TEARS (see EYE).

TEETH are hard organs developed in

849

connection with the mucous membrane of the mouth and implanted in the jawbones. In man they serve for biting and grinding the food, as well as aiding in speech, whilst in many animals they are adapted as weapons.

Structure – Each tooth is composed of four substances: dentine, enamel, cement or *crusta petrosa*, and pulp (illustrations 393, 394, 395).

394 – Diagram of vertical section through molar tooth. 1, enamel; 2, dentine; 3, pulp cavity; 4, cement; 5, dental periosteum; 6, bone of jaw. From *Hewer's Histology*.

393 – Diagram of vertical section through incisor tooth. 1, enamel; 2, dentine; 3, pulp cavity; 4, cement; 5, dental periosteum; 6, bone of jaw. From *Hewer's Histology*. Wm. Heinemann Ltd.

DENTINE, or IVORY, makes up the greater part of each tooth, both in the crown, where it is covered by a layer of enamel, and in the fang, where it is surrounded by cement; whilst in the centre of the tooth it is hollowed out to lodge the pulp. The dentine is composed of an intimate mixture of organic matter and inorganic salts, chiefly lime salts, in the proportion of 72 per cent of the latter, and 28 per cent of the former. When examined in thin slices, the dentine is found to con-

sist of a dense yellowish-white substance pierced by minute tubes that run in a wavy manner from the pulp cavity, giving off branches as they go, to end under the enamel and cement. At their widest part, these tubes are about $\frac{1}{4500}$ inch (5·5 micrometres) across, and each lodges a fine thread-like fibril that runs out through the tooth from the pulp. In some animals the dentine closely resembles bone in structure.

ENAMEL is a brilliant white layer forming a sort of cap to the tooth. It is thickest on the cutting or grinding surface and thins away towards the gum, disappearing at the neck of the tooth. It is the hardest tissue in the body and contains 96·5 per cent of earthy matter, mainly phosphate of

395 – Transverse section across the crown of a tooth. *p*, Pulp cavity; *d*, dentine; *e*, enamel. Magnified by 6.

lime. It is composed of long rods or prisms placed side by side, with one end resting on the dentine, the other forming part of the surface of the tooth. When the tooth appears, there is a thin, horny layer, known as Nasmyth's membrane, or the skin of the tooth, covering the enamel, but this is speedily worn away when the teeth come into use. Indeed, in persons who live on very hard food the upper surface of the tooth may, in advanced years, be worn quite flat and the dentine exposed.

CEMENT, *crusta petrosa*, or tooth bone, is simply a thin layer of bone covering the dentine in the fang where enamel is absent.

PULP is one of the most important parts of the tooth. In structure it is soft, consisting of connective tissue, the cells which form the dentine, the blood-vessels, and the nerve-fibres derived from the fifth cranial nerve. From its cells spring the fibrils that run into the tubes of the dentine, and upon this connection the sensitiveness of the tooth depends.

Arrangement and form – Teeth are present in most mammals and nearly all have two sets – temporary or milk teeth in early life, and permanent or adult teeth developed later. In some animals, like the toothed whales, all the teeth are similar, but in most mammals and in man there are four different shapes of teeth: incisors, canines or eye-teeth, premolars or bicuspids, and molars or grinders. Each tooth possesses a *crown* which projects into the cavity of the mouth and a root or *fang* which is embedded in a socket in the jaw-bone; at the point where crown and fang join, there is usually a constriction known as the *neck* (illustration 396).

The shape of the teeth is adapted very much to the habits and character of their owner. Thus in rodents the incisor teeth are long, chisel-shaped, and keep on growing all the animal's life at the same rate as they are worn away by gnawing. In some animals, such as the dog and boar, the canine teeth are elongated so as to be dangerous offensive weapons. In carnivorous animals generally, the back teeth are not flat-topped grinders, but have a jagged cutting edge, so that the upper and lower teeth tear the prey like a pair of shears. In herbivorous animals the teeth are flat-topped for crushing herbs and fruit. The elephant has peculiarly modified incisors in the upper jaw (tusks), and molars which appear one at a time: and in the narwhal, one of the canine teeth is developed into a long spear-like organ.

In man, the shape of the various teeth indicates that they are adapted for the

396 – The permanent teeth of the right side. From *Gray's Anatomy*.

397 – The permanent teeth of the lower jaw. From *Gray's Anatomy*.

mixed diet that custom has found most convenient. The adult set consists of two chisel-shaped incisors in each half jaw, one pointed canine tooth, two premolars, each with two cusps on the crown, and three flat-topped molars; thirty-two in all (illustrations 396, 397). In the child the molars have no predecessors, so that the teeth in a child are two incisors, one canine, and two premolars in each half-jaw, or twenty teeth in all.

Development – The first stage in the formation of the teeth consists of a groove produced in the soft connective tissue underlying the mucous membrane of the gum by the downgrowth of a ridge of cells derived from the epithelium on the surface of the mucous membrane. Here and there at the bottom of this groove, papillae of connective tissue appear, similar to those of the skin upon which hairs are developed. From each of these papillae, ten in number in the lower jaw, and ten in the upper jaw, the pulp, dentine, and

398 – The teeth of a 6-year-old child. The permanent teeth are coloured black. From *Gray's Anatomy*.

cement of a milk tooth are produced, while the caps of epithelial cells lying on the papillae form their enamel. The neck of epithelial cells which joins the enamel of each tooth to the surface is next cut off and each tooth becomes surrounded by a sac. Finally, when the child reaches a certain age, each tooth begins to develop a fang, which, as it grows. pushes the tooth out of its sac and through the mucous membrane of the gum. The permanent teeth are developed in a similar manner, and their formation begins before the milk teeth are completely formed (illustration 398). When the time approaches for the milk tooth to be shed, its fang is gradually absorbed and the growing permanent tooth pushes out the crown. If this process of absorption does not take place properly, the new teeth are apt to come through crooked.

Time of appearance – The teeth appear in a definite order and at definite periods, but there may be several months' delay without this being of any significance. The usual order for the milk teeth is:

Middle incisors	6–8 months
Lateral incisors	8–10 „
First molars	12–16 „
Canines (eye-teeth)	16–20 „
Second molars	20–30 „

The usual order for the permanent teeth is:

First molars	6–7 years
Middle incisors	6–8 „
Lateral incisors	7–9 „
Canines	9–12 „
First and second premolars	10–12 „
Second molars	11–13 „
Third molars (wisdom teeth)	17–21 „

TEETH, DISEASES OF – From the fact that the teeth are highly sensitive, that any interference with their use causes marked disturbance of digestion, and that good teeth form a highly aesthetic feature, disorders of these structures are of great importance. Only the most common disorders will be mentioned here; some conditions affecting the gums are mentioned under MOUTH, DISEASES OF (see also GUMBOIL; and NOSE, DISEASES OF).

TEETHING, or the process of eruption of the teeth, may be accompanied by certain symptoms due to the irritation produced by the erupting tooth as it pushes through the resistant gum. The most common symptoms are irritability and loss of sleep. The infant may also refuse feeds, and this may lead to loss of weight. The source of irritation is generally quite evident, as the child continually rubs the part of his gums beneath which the growing teeth are situated. Even adults possessed of a small lower jaw sometimes suffer great pain during the cutting of the lower wisdom teeth, the reason being that there is not enough space left for the new tooth in the corner between the second molar and the vertical portion of the jaw.

Treatment – In children, comfort is often obtained when the child is given some hard object, such as a bone or a rusk, against which it can press the gums. Should it not respond to this simple remedy, the local application to the affected gums of Choline Salicylate Dental Paste of the *Dental Practitioners' Formulary* will bring relief.

TOOTHACHE is a symptom of several affections of the teeth and neighbouring parts. The pain may vary from slight annoyance to great agony, and it often comes on at fairly regular intervals.

Causes – Much the commonest cause of toothache is caries or decay affecting one or more teeth, particularly when the cavity in a tooth reaches near to, or exposes, the pulp. A gumboil, consisting of an inflammatory condition connected with the root of the tooth, which often proceeds to the formation of an abscess, is another cause of dull, throbbing pain. (See GUMBOIL.) The want of effective cleansing of the mouth, leading to the presence of acid secretion on the gums and between the teeth, which eats gradually into the enamel, is another cause of annoying though less severe toothache. Certain general causes also, especially digestive disturbances, general debility, and pregnancy, render persons much more liable to suffer from toothache than when they are in ordinary health. Given some of these conditions, an attack of toothache is often started by exposure to cold, a hot drink, or some sweet or acid article of food.

Treatment – Expert dental advice should be sought at once. There is a tendency to avoid seeking such advice should the toothache settle quickly. Such delaying action is merely asking for trouble in the future. Toothache is a warning that something is wrong – and the sooner expert advice is sought the better. During an attack of toothache affecting a whole row of teeth relief can often be obtained by rinsing the mouth with warm bicarbonate of soda solution. If a tooth with a large cavity be affected, the pain can generally be eased by filling the hole with a small piece of cotton-wool dipped in an essential oil, such as oil of cloves, or in a mixture of chloral and menthol, or of zinc oxide and oil of cloves. In any case, pain can be temporarily abolished by an injection, with a hypodermic syringe, of procaine into the space between the root of the tooth and the jaw. If the tooth be so far decayed as to be useless for chewing, it should be extracted. (See also NEURALGIA.)

CARIES OF THE TEETH, or DENTAL CARIES, is an extremely common condition among civilized peoples, and is most common in childhood and early adult life. A high percentage of all children attending school have at least one carious tooth, while many show advanced dental disease. Thus, in Britain, only 50 per cent of children of 3 years of age are caries-free. By the age of 5 years this percentage has fallen to 20 per cent, whilst by the age of 12 years only 8 per cent of children are caries-free, and by the age of 15 the figure has fallen to 5 per cent. The sad tale is capped by the fact that 50 per cent of adults over the age of 35 have lost all their teeth. In Scotland, 44 per cent of all inhabitants aged 16 and over have lost all their natural teeth.

Causes – The precise cause of caries is still unknown, but the general consensus of expert opinion accepts what is known as the 'acidogenic theory'. In essence, this theory is that acids are produced at or near the surface of the tooth by bacterial fermentation of dietary carbohydrates, particularly sugar, and that these acids dissolve the calcium phosphate crystals which make up over 95 per cent of the mass of enamel in the tooth.

In areas where the fluorine content of drinking water is 0·75 to 1 part per million, the incidence of caries in young children is much less than in areas where the fluorine content of the water is lower. In some persons the teeth decay much more readily and more quickly than in others. This is in many cases due to bad quality of the teeth, in others due to overcrowding or a bad arrangement in the jaw which allows food particles to accumulate between the teeth and prevents opposing teeth from meeting one another properly in chewing. Decay rarely appears on free, smooth surfaces that are exposed to the rubbing of the lips and tongue and the scouring of the food; or among primitive peoples who subsist on coarse food that requires a great deal of chewing. It begins usually in some groove or pit in the enamel or between the teeth (illustration 399), and when the process has made a small opening through the enamel it may spread widely in the dentine, so that the first sign the person gets, apart from discoloration of the tooth, may be its sudden caving in during a meal. For this reason the teeth should be carefully inspected by a dentist once or twice every year.

Treatment – In early life the provision of suitable and sufficient food is of great importance in forming strong teeth. The prevention of caries, though not always successful, may be greatly assisted by constant care of the teeth. This consists mainly in cleaning the teeth after every meal and before retiring to bed at night.

right   left

399 – (Above) Natural crevices on healthy back teeth in which food collects and leads to decay and formation of cavities. (Below) Front teeth of the upper jaw showing places between teeth where food has collected and led to decay.

TEETH, DISEASES OF

Any simple tooth-powder or toothpaste should be used. Substances like charcoal, which impart a brilliant polish to the teeth, should not be often used, since they scratch the enamel and help to erode it. Persons taking medicines containing acids, like some of the iron preparations, should rinse the mouth out with water immediately after each dose.

The question of food is important, especially in children. The chewing of hard foods scours the teeth and stimulates the circulation in the jaw and gum. It is important also for the child, and for the pregnant mother, to have foods with calcium salts in them, such as milk, cheese, and green vegetables. For the calcium to be of use to the body, vitamin D is necessary, which is present in eggs, milk, butter, liver, and fish-liver oils. Equally important is the avoidance of too much confectionery. Children should never be allowed to eat sweets between meals or just before going to bed at night. They should be encouraged to eat as much fresh fruit as possible, especially apples. (See also NURSING-BOTTLE MOUTH.)

Promising results have been reported from many countries, including Britain, USA and New Zealand, from the adding of very small amounts of fluorine (up to 1 part per million) to drinking water, in the prevention of caries. Indeed, these reports are so overwhelmingly convincing that there are good grounds for recommending that fluoridation should be adopted on a national scale. (See FLUORINE.)

IRREGULARITY OF THE TEETH, when the permanent set appears, may be due to defective development of the jaw, to a highly arched palate, or to slowness in casting off the temporary set. Slight irregularities disappear as the jaw grows, but if the deformity be great, much may be done to remedy it by judicious extraction of some teeth and by wearing appliances in the mouth which maintain a steady pressure upon others.

LOOSENING OF THE TEETH may be due to accident, to wasting of the gums in consequence of the irritation set up by tartar on the teeth, or to the degenerative processes of advancing age. A tooth knocked out by injury may be washed and replaced in its socket, when it will usually again become firmly fixed, and the same is true of teeth which have been merely loosened. When the gums are receding and the teeth loosening in consequence of a deposit of tartar and inflamed gums, the tartar should be removed by a dentist and some antiseptic mouthwash used.

INFLAMMATION OF THE GUMS, or GINGIVITIS, may occur as an acute or as a chronic condition. The acute form, which is often part of a generalized infection of the mouth, ie. gingivo-stomatitis, occurs principally in children and young adults. The chronic form is more liable to occur at a later age, and is more common in women than in men. The gums are congested, often bleed either when food is chewed or when the teeth are brushed, and often show a certain amount of ulceration and purulent discharge at their edges. There is a considerable amount of tenderness leading to solid food being swallowed without proper chewing, and hence producing dyspepsia. Tartar, at the same time, collects on the teeth and the inflammation in severe cases spreads to the palate and the interior of the cheek. Various bacteria and spirochaetes are found on the inflamed parts. At a later stage, the gums waste and their margins shrink away from the teeth, leaving the necks of these exposed. The person whose teeth show either of these changes generally suffers from indigestion and often from diarrhoea and may have a considerable degree of anaemia. There is, however, no discharge of pus from the sockets of the teeth, a condition which distinguishes this disease from pyorrhoea. The tartar should be carefully scraped from the teeth and a mild antiseptic mouth-wash should be used daily. The gums should be regularly brushed with a soft tooth-brush and antiseptic aromatic tooth-paste, or, if too tender for this, should be wiped with tincture of myrrh on a pledget of cotton-wool. Daily massage of the gums with the fingers improves the circulation in the gums and their nutrition.

PYORRHOEA ALVEOLARIS, or RIGG'S DISEASE, now usually known as PARODONTAL DISEASE, is a condition characterized in the final stages by the promotion of pockets of purulent material around the teeth and loosening of the affected teeth. Although the precise cause is still a matter of debate, the general consensus of opinion is that the condition is the resultant of inadequate roughage in the diet and inadequate care of the teeth. These two factors lead to stagnation of food between the teeth and excessive formation of tartar. This in turn leads to proliferation of bacteria. The prolonged contact of tartar, food débris, and organisms with the surface of the gum results in ulceration of the gum and chronic inflammatory changes.

The effect of the condition upon the general health is variable, but there is no doubt that the condition tends to become worse if the individual develops some other illness. It is also liable to worsen during pregnancy. Pain is not a feature of parodontal disease, but it often gives rise to an unpleasant taste in the mouth and an unpleasant odour of the breath (halitosis). A characteristic feature in the later stages is a tendency for the gums to bleed easily. It is often accompanied by dyspepsia.

Treatment –. At one time, almost wholesale extraction of teeth was performed in an attempt to eradicate the disease. It is now realized that much can be done to cure the condition by careful hygiene of the mouth, including regular removal of tartar and attention to prevent food stagnating between the teeth by use of wooden points. In more advanced cases the free edge of the gum which forms the outer wall of the pocket, is removed.

INFLAMMATION OF THE TOOTH FANG is a condition which may be present in various degrees. There may be simple acute inflammation following a blow on the tooth; less acute inflammation due to the presence of an imperfect stopping; and in the severest form pyorrhoea.

Symptoms – There are pain and inflammation in a tooth or teeth without any obvious cause in the form of decay. Tenderness is present when the affected tooth is touched, and especially when the tooth is used for biting. The tooth usually appears to the individual to stand up a little higher than the other teeth and congestion is often visible in the neighbouring gum. Such a condition may come and go for a long time. If an X-ray photograph is taken of the teeth, a clear or rarefied area may be seen round the fang or as a small rounded area at its tip (*root abscess*). This condition may at times cure itself by the formation of an acute abscess, which distends the socket and bursts through the gum (see GUMBOIL), or it may remain for many years and ultimately develop into the condition of pyorrhoea.

Treatment – In the early stages, painting the gum with weak tincture of iodine or other counter-irritant is sufficient to abate inflammation, but the tooth may require to be extracted. In more advanced conditions a certain amount of extraction of the teeth is necessary. All decayed teeth which cannot be satisfactorily stopped, all roots which have lost their crown, and all teeth which are unopposed in the opposite jaw or which show a considerable amount of pyorrhoea should be extracted. The other

teeth should be treated by the application of antiseptic lotions night and morning. The mouth should be kept clean by the use of an aromatic mouth-wash. The general condition of the patient as regards dyspepsia and anaemia often requires considerable attention also.

PREVENTION OF DENTAL DISEASE – If parents would spend a little more on dental treatment and a little less on confectionery for their children, they would be providing their children with one of the greatest possible boons. At the moment so many parents are ruining the teeth of their children by allowing them to eat sweets morning, noon and night that they are piling up for these unfortunate children a dreadful account of unnecessary pain and unnecessary dental disease in the years to come. It is an indictment of which the nation should be ashamed.

TEETH GRINDING, or BRUXISM as it is technically known, is quite common in children during sleep, when it is of no significance unless really persistent. During the day it may be an attention-seeking device, often perpetuated by the anxiety which it elicits in the parents. There is no treatment for it and if ignored it will stop, though any genuine anxiety or worry on the part of the child should be dealt with. It is more common and persistent in mentally retarded children.

In adults it is usually associated with stress or anxiety, but may be due to some local condition in the mouth such as an unsatisfactory filling. It may also be caused by certain drugs, including fenfluramine and levodopa. More rarely it may be due to brain disease. Some families seem to be more prone to teeth grinding than others. If not controlled, it produces excessive wear of the enamel covering of the teeth. Treatment consists of alleviation of any condition in the mouth, and it may be useful to wear a splint covering the teeth of one jaw at night. Treatment should also be aimed at the alleviation of anxiety and stress.

TEETHING (see TEETH, DISEASES OF).

TELANGIECTASIS means an abnormal dilatation of arterioles and capillaries, forming sometimes a tumour or TELANGIOMA.

TEMAZEPAM is a relatively quick-acting hypnotic of short duration so that there is little or no 'hangover' the next morning. It is a derivative of diazepam (qv).

TEMPERAMENT is a term that includes those vague general peculiarities of mind and body that render some persons more liable than others to be affected by particular diseases. (See CONSTITUTION; IDIOSYNCRASY; IMMUNITY; and also ALCOHOLISM; HYSTERIA; MENTAL ILLNESS; NEURASTHENIA.)

TEMPERATURE of the body is a subject of great importance. For the proper temperature of rooms, baths and the like, see NURSING; BATHS; COLD, USES OF.

Animals are generally divided as regards their temperature into two classes: *cold-blooded animals*, including reptiles, amphibians, fishes, and invertebrates generally, whose temperature varies to a great extent according to that of the surrounding medium; and *warm-blooded animals*, including mammals and birds, whose temperature remains almost constant, no matter how the surrounding temperature falls or rises. In warm-blooded animals, this constancy of body temperature is effected by a perpetual balancing of the various forces which produce heat and give off heat. The chief heat producer in the body is the oxidizing action that takes place on muscular contraction, and the chief cooling agents are the skin and lungs, which act by the exposure of the blood circulating in them to the air, and by the evaporation of moisture from their surfaces. The temperature of different warm-blooded animals varies considerably, being high in birds, about 105° to 107° F (40·5° to 41·7° C), whilst in man it is somewhere between 98° and 99° F (36·7° and 37·2° C). It varies in different persons, but is generally stated to be about 98·4° F, or 37° C. Even in a given healthy individual the temperature is constantly changing, and may vary by 1° or 2° F in the day, being lowest in the early morning and highest in the evening. The chief reason for this change is to be found probably in the variations as regards activity at different periods of the day. The temperature also varies in different parts of the body, that of the skin being about half a degree lower than that taken within the hollow organs of the body; and in stout people this difference between the surface and the interior is still more marked. In parts exposed to cold or provided with a feeble blood supply, such as paralysed limbs, the temperature may sink very low.

Temperature in disease – The maintenance of a nearly steady temperature is the result of a constant process of balancing between heat-production and heat-loss, controlled probably by a special centre in the nervous system. In disease, one or other of these processes may be impaired or the controlling mechanism may be thrown completely out of gear. The general temperature may rise as high as 110° F (43·3° C), or sink to 90° (32·2° C) for a time; but the risk to life is great when it passes above 106° F (41° C) or below 95° F (35° C).

Fall of temperature may be due to many causes. Thus it generally accompanies great loss of blood, starvation, and the collapsed condition which sometimes results from severe attacks of fever, peritonitis, and other devitalizing acute diseases. Certain chronic diseases are generally accompanied by a subnormal temperature; of these, myxoedema is the most outstanding.

Rise of temperature is a characteristic of acute diseases, and of diseases due to micro-organisms, the poisonous products of which lead to increased waste of the tissues. Injuries to the nervous system, even unpleasant sensations in children and nervous people, may have a similar effect. In persons dying in a feverish condition, the temperature often rises very high immediately before death, owing probably to failure of the circulation and other conditions which diminish the body heat. Rapid rise of temperature in such a case is therefore an ominous sign.

Many diseases have a characteristic course of temperature, so that in hospital a glance at the temperature chart is often sufficient to acquaint a physician with the disease from which the patient is suffering. Thus pneumonia, enteric fever, measles, and malaria show, as a rule, quite recognizable temperature records.

High temperature in some diseases is a much less serious feature than in others. Thus in enteric fever or pneumonia 105° F (40·5° C) is an ordinary temperature, whilst in rheumatic fever and diphtheria the temperature generally ranges between 101° and 103° F (38·3° and 39·5° C), so that in these diseases a temperature of 104° F (40° C) gives cause for anxiety.

In most diseases the temperature gradually abates as the patient recovers, but others, for example pneumonia and typhus fever, end rapidly by a *crisis* in which the temperature falls, perspiration breaks out, the pulse becomes slower, and the breathing quieter. The reason for the sudden change lies probably in the fact that in favourable cases, after the disease has lasted a certain time, the resisting power of the body becomes able fully to neutralize the poisons produced by the organisms of the disease. This crisis is often preceded by an increase of all the symptoms, including an epicritical rise of temperature.

Record of temperature – Temperature is generally measured by a thermometer (illustrations 400, 401). Those intended for clinical use possess a long, narrow bulb, an index registering from 95° to 110° F (35° to 43·3° C), and are made so that the column of mercury does not fall back into the bulb till it is shaken down (illustration 400).

400 – Clinical thermometer.

There are two scales in common use: the Fahrenheit scale and the Centigrade or Celsius scale. Hitherto, in Britain the term Centigrade has been preferred, but under the new International System of Units (see WEIGHTS AND MEASURES) the term Celsius is recommended. The difference consists in this, that in the Centigrade scale the freezing-point of water is marked 0° and the boiling-point 100°, while in the Fahrenheit scale these are 32° and 212°, respectively. Accordingly 100 divisions on the Centigrade scale are equivalent to 180 divisions on the Fahrenheit scale, and 1 degree C equals 1·8 degrees F. To convert from degrees F to degrees C the following formula may be used:

$$n° \text{ Fahr} = \left[(n-32) \times \tfrac{5}{9}\right] C,$$

and to convert from degrees C to degrees F the following:

$$n° C = \left[(n \times \tfrac{9}{5}) + 32\right] \text{Fahr}$$

For examples:

$$98\cdot6° \text{ Fahr} = \left[(98\cdot6 - 32) \times \tfrac{5}{9}\right] = 66\cdot6 \times \tfrac{5}{9}$$
$$= 37° C$$
$$38° C = \left[(38 \times \tfrac{9}{5}) + 32\right] = 68\cdot4 + 32$$
$$= 100\cdot4° \text{ Fahr}$$

The Réaumur scale, in which the freezing-point is 0° and the boiling-point 80°, is also used in some countries, eg. France, though not for scientific purposes.

As to the part of the body where the temperature is taken, the mouth is preferable, the bulb of the thermometer being placed beneath the tongue. The instrument must be carefully washed with cold water before use, so that it does not convey infection,, and care taken to ensure that the mercury

is shaken down to below 96° F. The patient must be directed to keep the mouth shut but not to bite the thermometer with the teeth, and breathe through the nose. It is essential to ensure that the patient has not just had a hot drink. The thermometer must be kept in the mouth for at least three minutes. After use the thermometer must be thoroughly rinsed under running cold water and the mercury shaken down to below 96° F. When taken in the armpit the skin should be wiped dry, the bulb of the thermometer placed as high as possible, and the arm tightly folded across the chest. To obtain a correct reading, it is necessary to leave the thermometer in

401 – Thermometer scale ranging from room temperature to that of water used for douches, and the like and showing the corresponding points upon Fahrenheit and Centigrade scales.

Day of Dis.	1	2	3	4	5	6	7	Day of Dis.
Pulse	110	125	120	110	80	85	80	Pulse

402 – Temperature chart from a case of scarlet fever, showing the method of registering the temperature.

place for at least five minutes, because the skin surfaces do not at once represent the internal temperature of the body. Occasionally the temperature is taken by inserting the thermometer bulb about 2 inches (5 cm) into the rectum, a method which gives the most correct result of all, and is the most satisfactory in infants.

To keep a record, a piece of paper ruled with vertical lines to represent the periods at which the temperature is taken, and with horizontal lines corresponding to degrees, is used. A large dot is marked in the proper place each time the temperature is taken and the successive dots are afterwards joined by straight lines (illustration 402).

Treatment of high temperature is mentioned under ANTIPYRETICS; COLD, USES OF; and FEVER.

TEMPLE is the name given to the side of the head above the line between the eye and ear. The term, temporal, is applied to the muscles, nerves, and artery of this region. The hair usually begins to turn grey first at the temples.

TENDERNESS is the term usually applied in medical nomenclature to pain experienced when a diseased part is handled, the term, pain, being reserved for unpleasant sensations felt apart from any manipulation.

858

TENDON, SINEW, or LEADER, is the cord that attaches the end of a muscle to the bone or other structure upon which the muscle acts when it contracts. Tendons are composed of bundles of white fibrous tissue arranged in a very dense manner, and are of great strength. Some are rounded, some flattened bands, whilst others are very short, the muscle-fibres being attached almost directly to the bone. Most tendons are surrounded by sheaths lined with membrane similar to the synovial membrane lining joint-cavities. In this sheath the tendon glides smoothly over surrounding parts. The fibres of a tendon pass into the substance of the bone and blend with the fibres composing it. One of the largest tendons in the body is the tendo Achilles, which attaches the muscle of the calf to the calcaneus or heel-bone.

TENDOVAGINITIS means inflammation of a tendon and of the sheath enveloping it.

TENESMUS is a term applied to a symptom of disease affecting the lower part of the large intestine, such as dysentery, piles, or tumour. It consists of a constant sense of weight about the lower bowel and desire to go to stool, coupled with straining at stool and the passage of little but mucus and perhaps some blood.

TENNIS ELBOW (see ELBOW).

TENO- is a prefix denoting some relation to a tendon.

TENOSYNOVITIS, or TENOSITIS, means inflammation of a tendon.

TENOTOMY means an operation in which one or more tendons are divided, usually with the object of remedying some deformity. The operation is, in general, a slight one.

TENTORIUM is the name of a wide process of dura mater forming a partition between the cerebrum and cerebellum and supporting the former.

TENTS are instruments used for dilating narrow openings. The tent consists of some substance, like sea-tangle or sponge, which shrivels up when dried, and expands powerfully as it absorbs moisture. It is introduced dry into the opening it is to dilate, and expands in the course of some hours without producing pain.

TERATOGENESIS is the production of physical defects in the foetus. A teratogenic drug is a drug which, when administered to a pregnant mother, induces some physical defect in her unborn child. The term has come into common usage since the thalidomide disaster.

Thalidomide was a most effective non-barbiturate hypnotic which had passed most stringent tests before being released for general use. In spite of this it produced a large number of congenital defects, especially of the limbs, in children born to mothers who had taken the drug while pregnant. As soon as this was discovered the drug was withdrawn from use.

Subsequently the Government set up a Committee of Drug Safety to try and ensure that there was no recurrence of such a distressing episode with subsequent drugs. Even the most stringent precautions, however, cannot ensure the complete elimination of this risk. Fortunately the risk is a remote one, but it is now realized that no drug should be given to a pregnant woman, particularly during the first few months of pregnancy unless it is absolutely essential for her health or that of her unborn child.

TERATOMA is the term applied to a tumour that consists of partially developed embryonic tissues. The most common sites of this tumour are the ovary and the testicle.

TERBUTALINE is a drug that is proving of value in the treatment of asthma. It is given by injection under the skin or by inhalation.

TEREBENE is a clear, colourless fluid, with an odour like fresh pine sawdust, prepared by the action of sulphuric acid upon turpentine. It is used as an expectorant in bronchitis.

TEREBINTHINA is the Latin name for turpentine.

TERTIAN FEVER is the name applied to that type of malaria in which the ague-fit reappears every other day. (See MALARIA.)

TESTICLE – The testes, or testicles, are the two male sexual glands. Each is developed in the corresponding loin, but before birth they descend through openings in the lower part of the front of the abdomen into a fold or pouch of skin known as the scrotum. This fold is strengthened by a layer of muscle fibres and fibrous tissues, and within it each testicle possesses a separate covering known as the tunica vaginalis. This tunic is a double layer of serous membrane similar in structure to the peritoneum or pleura, and it is derived from the peritoneum while the testicle is still within the abdomen. Occasionally, as the result of defective development, a more or less open channel of communication is left between the peritoneum and tunica vaginalis, and down this channel a hernia is liable to form in childhood or later. Throughout life, the openings in the abdominal wall remain, but these inguinal canals should be just large enough to allow the passage of the two spermatic cords, each of which is composed of the vas (or ductus) deferens, together with the blood-vessels, nerves, and lymphatics proceeding to the gland. Within the tunica vaginalis lies a dense fibrous coat known as the tunica albuginea, which affords protection to the gland. On microscopic examination, each testicle is found to consist of a series of minute tubes, from eight hundred to one thousand in number, supported by fibrous tissue in which the nerves and blood-vessels run, and lined by cells from which the spermatozoa are formed. These tubes communicate with one another near the centre of the testicle, and are connected by a much convoluted tube, the epididymis, with the ductus, or vas, deferens, which enters the abdomen, and passes on to the base of the bladder (illustration 403). This duct, after joining a reservoir known as the seminal vesicle, opens, close to the duct from the other side of the body, into that part of the urethra which is surrounded by the prostate gland. Owing to the convolutions of these ducts leading from the testicles to the urethra, and their indirect route, the passage from testicle to urethra is over twenty feet (6 metres) in length. In addition to producing spermatozoa, the testicle also forms an internal secretion which is responsible for the development of male characteristics. This hormone has been isolated and is known as testosterone.

TESTICLE, DISEASES OF – The pouch of skin, or scrotum, in which the testicles lie is liable to various general skin diseases, but particularly to eczema, which in many cases is often difficult of cure. Cancer of the skin in this region is specially common among chimney-sweeps, shale workers and cotton spinners, the result of chronic irritation by a carcinogenic agent in soot and paraffin products. Hernia, which in some cases passes into the scrotum, is treated under a special heading. (See HERNIA.) Sometimes, owing to defective development, the testicles are retained within the abdomen.

HYDROCELE is a local dropsy affecting one tunica vaginalis, and distending that side of the scrotum with fluid. (See HYDROCELE.)

part, careful regulation of the bowels, and the support of a suspensory net bandage afford all the treatment that is necessary in many cases; but an operation may sometimes be advisable.

INFLAMMATION of an acute type (orchitis) may arise in persons suffering from cystitis, stone in the bladder, and various forms of inflammation in the urinary organs, the most common cause of all

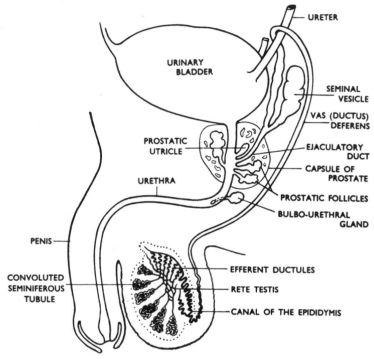

URETER

URINARY
BLADDER

SEMINAL
VESICLE

VAS (DUCTUS)
DEFERENS

PROSTATIC
UTRICLE

EJACULATORY
DUCT

CAPSULE OF
PROSTATE

URETHRA

PROSTATIC FOLLICLES

BULBO-URETHRAL
GLAND

PENIS

CONVOLUTED
SEMINIFEROUS
TUBULE

EFFERENT DUCTULES

RETE TESTIS

CANAL OF THE EPIDIDYMIS

403 – Diagram of the male sex organs. From Bell, Davidson and Elmslie-Smith, *Textbook of Physiology and Biochemistry*, 8th edition, 1972. Churchill Livingstone.

VARICOCELE is a condition in which the veins of the spermatic cord, especially on the left side, become unusually numerous and distended, the causes being much the same as those of varicose veins in other parts. The chief symptom is a dragging sensation in the testicle, which in some cases becomes at times very painful. This symptom is specially marked in warm weather and after exertion, the mass of veins at such a time becoming very distinct and resembling a 'bag of worms', though they empty quickly when the person lies down. Cold sponging of the

being gonorrhoea. It may follow also upon some cases of mumps. The symptoms are intense pain and swelling with redness of the skin over the affected testicle; and the usual treatment consists of rest in bed, support of the scrotum with a suspensory bandage or wads of cotton-wool, the administration of analgesics (in some cases the pain may be so severe that morphine may be necessary), and the administration of antibiotics if there is some definite causative micro-organism. In some cases the condition goes on to the formation of an abscess which bursts through the skin with immediate relief of pain. The condition is then treated as an abscess elsewhere.

TORSION of the testes, or, strictly speaking, of the spermatic cord, is a relatively common occurrence in adolescent and young adult males. It can occur during sleep, at rest, while playing games or doing hard physical work. About half the cases occur in the early hours of the morning during sleep. It makes itself felt by pain of varying severity – from slight to excruciating – either in the lower part of the abdomen or in the scrotum. In time the pain diminishes or disappears. The testes become hard and swollen. Treatment consists of immediate undoing of the torsion. If this is done within a few hours no harm ensues as a rule, but it should be followed within six hours by surgical operation to ensure that the torsion has been successfully undone and to fix the testes so that there should be no recurrence.

TUBERCULOSIS occurs in the testicle occasionally, especially when some other organ, such as the bladder, is already the seat of the disease. It causes practically no pain, and is therefore often far advanced before it attracts attention. It responds well to chemotherapy with streptomycin, para-aminosaliylic acid and/or isoniazid.

TUMOURS of the testes occur in around 600 males annually in Britain. They represent the second commonest form of malignant growth in young males. There are two types: seminomas and teratomas (qv). When adequately treated the survival rate for seminomas is 95 per cent, whilst that for teratomas is 50 per cent.

INJURIES of the testicles are relatively rare. A severe blow may lead to shock and symptoms of severe collapse for a time, and may cause an effusion of blood into the tunica vaginalis. These symptoms are usually relieved by rest in bed.

TEST MEAL is a term originally applied to a meal given for the purpose of testing the digestive powers. At the present day the original gruel meal has been replaced by the injection of histamine (qv), which is a powerful stimulator of gastric juice. In this *histamine test*, as it is known, samples of the fasting gastric juice are withdrawn through a Ryle's tube (see STOMACH TUBE) before and after a subcutaneous injection of histamine. A modification of this test is the *augmented histamine test*, in which a larger dose of histamine is injected preceded by a dose of an antihistamine drug. This allows a larger dose of histamine to be given because the

antihistamine counteracts its unpleasant effects, and the response to the larger dose provides a more accurate picture of the degree of acidity of the gastric juice. Other tests that have been introduced, and named, respectively, after the stimulating substance used are the *ametazole test*, the *pentagastrin test*, and the *insulin test*.

Tubeless test meals, so-called because they do not involve the passage of a stomach tube, have been evolved. These depend upon the dissociation of a cation-exchange resin (see ION EXCHANGE RESINS) by the hydrochloric acid in the gastric juice. The cation is then absorbed and the amount excreted in the urine is measured. The results, however, are not particularly reliable, and these tests are therefore only used when it is difficult or impossible to pass a stomach tube.

TESTOSTERONE is the name given to the male sex hormone secreted by the testes. It has also been prepared synthetically and has the formula $C_{19}H_{28}O_2$. In true eunuchoid conditions it has the power of restoring male sexual characteristics.

TEST-TUBE is a tube of thin glass closed at one end, which is used for observing chemical reactions or for bacterial culture.

TETANUS, or LOCKJAW, is a disorder of the nervous system, consisting in a greatly increased excitability of the spinal cord and manifesting itself by painful and lengthened spasm of the voluntary muscles throughout the body. The disease was well known in former wars, and Hippocrates (400 BC) refers to its rapidly fatal character.

Causes – The onset of the disease generally follows a wound, especially a deeply punctured, lacerated, or gunshot wound, usually appearing some 4 or 5 days after the wound has been inflicted, although it may be delayed for 3 or 4 weeks, by which time the wound is likely to be completely healed up. The presence in a wound of some foreign body, such as a splinter of wood or a portion of a bullet, seems to favour the onset of tetanus.

The direct cause of tetanus was discovered in 1889 by Kitasato, a Japanese observer, to be a bacillus: *Clostridium tetani*. This organism has a characteristic appearance, being long and bearing often at one end a large spore which gives to it a drumstick outline. It inhabits earth and dust, living especially a little distance below the surface in places where the manure of horses and cattle is collected. Hence it is found especially in the neighbourhood of stables, and is liable to infect wounds soiled with heavily manured earth. The bacillus develops a poison or toxin in the wound, and this, being absorbed, finds its way up the motor nerves to the spinal cord, which it renders excessively sensitive, so that its cells are excited by mild stimuli that under ordinary conditions would produce no reaction. After death, patients who have died of tetanus show very few lesions except congestion of the brain and spinal cord and degenerative changes in the cells of the latter.

In England, in 1974, there were 14 cases of tetanus, with 8 deaths.

Symptoms – The onset of tetanus usually occurs within two days to three weeks of the wound responsible for the introduction of the infection. This is not necessarily an incubation period in the strict sense of the term because the causative organism may be dormant in the tissues of the body before producing toxin. The importance of this is that, whilst generally speaking, it is a fact that the longer the period between the wound and the onset of tetanus, the better the outlook, there are occasions when a delayed onset of the disease is acute and dangerous because a hitherto dormant strain of the organism has suddenly started to produce large amounts of toxin. The first signs of the disease usually show themselves as stiffness in the muscles near the wound, followed later, no matter where the wound is situated, by stiffness about the muscles of the jaw, causing difficulty in opening the mouth, which soon increases to *lockjaw* or trismus. This is accompanied by spasm in neighbouring muscles, and the drawn features and exposed teeth give to the countenance the peculiar expression known as *risus sardonicus*. The rigidity extends to the muscles of the neck, back, chest, abdomen, and extremities, and the body may assume a bent attitude, either backward (*opisthotonos*), forward (*emprosthotonos*), or laterally (*pleurosthotonos*). This general muscular rigidity, which at first is not constant but occasionally undergoes relaxation, is accompanied by frequently recurring convulsive seizures, which are readily excited by the slightest irritation, such as from a draught of cool air, a bright light, the closing of a door. In such attacks there is great suffering and the expression of the face is indicative of agony. The function of respir-

ation may be seriously involved and asphyxia threaten or actually take place. The temperature sometimes rises to a high degree, and copious perspiration is also a constant symptom. These acute symptoms may subside after a few days and the patient gradually recover. On the other hand, the symptoms may increase in severity and death ensue either by asphyxia from prolonged spasm of the respiratory muscles, or exhaustion consequent on the violence of the symptoms, together with the absence of sleep. Throughout the whole course of the disease the mind is clear, and the patient waits with anxiety for the next convulsive attack. In milder cases the symptoms are less severe, the course more chronic, and recovery more common.

Tetanus sometimes occurs in new-born children, showing itself within a week of birth by obvious difficulty in the acts of sucking and swallowing, and, by the supervention of lockjaw, together with prolonged contraction of the muscles of the limbs and body, accompanied by convulsive seizures. *Local cases* of tetanus occur in which the muscles of a limb in the neighbourhood of the wound show spasms, but these do not become general, or they pass off after appearing to a slight extent. Such cases often show stiffness for several months.

The symptoms of strychnine poisoning bear a strong resemblance to those of tetanus, but in the former case they are more acute, less prolonged than the spasms of tetanus, come on after something has been swallowed, and end either in death or in recovery within a few hours. Hydrophobia, too, resembles tetanus in some respects.

The outcome depends upon various factors, including the virulence of the toxin, the age of the patient, his state of immunity and the availability of expert medical and nursing attention. The very young and the old do badly. The mortality is often said to be 40 per cent, but among the 59 cases treated in the Leeds Tetanus Unit in the decade, 1966–76, the mortality rate was only 13 per cent, all but one of the eight deaths occurring in patients over the age of 50. As an expert in this field has said, in the absence of the highest medical and nursing skill, tetanus is a highly fatal disease.

Prevention – The outlook in tetanus has been entirely altered by the introduction of tetanus antitoxin and of tetanus toxoid. The latter provides effective protection against the disease. Tetanus immunization is now an accepted part of the immunization programme for children in the United Kingdom. (See VACCINE.) Sportsmen using muddy playing fields are especially vulnerable and should have effective immunization, as should regular gardeners. Some authorities recommend booster injections of vaccine at intervals of ten years to maintain protection against the disease.

Whilst antitoxin is of primary value from the point of view of treatment, it is of prophylactic value if given immediately after an individual has received a wound which may be contaminated with the tetanus organism.

Treatment – Tetanus tends especially to follow wounds infected by stable refuse, by street dust, or by the deeper soil thrown up by shells on the battlefield. In all such cases, 1500 international units of antitoxin must be injected as soon as possible, unless it is definitely known that the individual has been completely immunized by a previous course of toxoid.

If the wound is only slight, all that may be required may be a dose of tetanus toxoid (0·5 ml) with or without an intramuscular injection of 1·2 mega units of benzathine penicillin. In addition careful cleaning of the wound is required. All these are preventive measures. In actual treatment expert opinion differs as to whether or not antibiotics and tetanus antitoxin should be given routinely. If the latter is given, particular care must be taken as to whether or not the patient suffers from asthma or any other allergic condition, as he may be allergic to the horse serum in which the antitoxin is contained, and react in a violent manner, which might even prove fatal. Tetanus immunoglobulin (See IMMUNOGLOBULIN) is now available and an injection of 250 units provides immunity for four weeks.

Various drugs, which diminish the reflex excitability of the spinal cord and relax spasm, help in relieving the patient's sufferings and in carrying him over the period during which the toxin of the disease is being excreted. These include thiopentone, barbiturates, paraldehyde, and one of the muscle-relaxant drugs. Quietness around the patient, a darkened room, and the absence of all noise and excitement are of great importance in preventing convulsions, and the patient must receive fluid nourishment of a stimulating character.

TETANY is a condition characterized by spasm of muscle usually caused by a fall in the ionic calcium of the blood. This fall in ionic calcium results in hyperexcitability of the muscles, which are thus liable to go into spasm on the slightest stimulus. This is well demonstrated in two of the classical signs of the disease: *Chvostek's sign*, in which the muscles of the face contract when the cheek is tapped over the facial nerve as it emerges on the cheek; *Erb's sign*, in which muscles go into spasm in response to an electrical stimulus which normally causes only a contraction of the muscle. Tetany is most common in infants, in whom it may arise as a result of rickets, excessive vomiting, or certain forms of nephritis. It may also be due to lack of the active principle of the parathyroid glands. Overbreathing may also cause it. Treatment consists of the administration of calcium salts, and in severe cases this is done by giving calcium gluconate intravenously or intramuscularly. The active principle of the parathyroid glands, is given in cases in which the tetany is due to deficiency of this principle.

TETRACYCLINES are a group of antibiotics which include chlortetracycline, oxytetracycline, tetracycline, demethylchlortetracycline, methacycline, lymecycline, minocycline, and clomocycline. Chlortetracycline, which is derived from *Streptomyces aureofaciens*, was the first to be discovered, followed by oxytetracycline which is derived from *Streptomyces rimosus*. Subsequently it was discovered that the active constituent of both these antibiotics was tetracycline, which can be prepared on a large scale by the catalytic hydrogenation of chlortetracycline. Methacycline, lymecycline, and clomocycline are subsequently discovered derivatives.

From the point of view of antibacterial activity, all the preparations are virtually identical, being active against both Gram-negative and Gram-positive bacteria, as well as certain rickettsiae (qv) and some of the larger viruses, including those causing Q fever, typhus, psittacosis, and lymphogranuloma inguinale.

It is this wide range of activity, which has given them the name of broad-spectrum antibiotics, combined with the fact that they are given by mouth, that has made them such a useful contribution to the treatment of infective diseases. They must be used with discrimination in young children as they are liable to produce permanent discoloration of the teeth.

TETRALOGY OF FALLOT is the most common form of cyanotic congenital heart disease. The tetralogy consists of: (*a*) stenosis of the pulmonary valve; (b) a defect in the septum separating the two ventricles; (c) the aorta over-rides both ventricles; (d) marked hypertrophy of the right ventricle.

TETRAMINE is a preparation which is of value in the treatment of certain forms of malignant disease, including Hodgkin's disease and chronic leukaemia.

TETTER is a vague name for skin diseases of the eczema type.

THALAMENCEPHALON, also known as the INTERBRAIN or TWEENBRAIN, is the part of the brain lying below the cerebrum, around the third ventricle and containing the optic tracts, the grey matter of the optic thalami, the infundibulum, pineal body, and other parts.

THALASSAEMIA, also known as Cooley's anaemia, is a condition characterized by severe anaemia, due to the individual having an abnormal form of haemoglobin in his blood. It is a genetically inherited disease which is widely spread across the Mediterranean through the Middle East and into the Far East. It has a particularly high incidence in Greece and in Italy. Thus in the Po valley 20 per cent of the population are said to have the disease.

THENAR EMINENCE is the name given to the projecting mass at the base of the thumb: what is popularly known as the ball of the thumb.

THEOBROMINE is the alkaloidal principle upon which the stimulating action of cocoa and chocolate depends. (See CHOCOLATE.)

THEOPHYLLINE is an alkaloid similar to theobromine and occurs in small amounts in tea. It is a diuretic, usually administered in the form of theophylline and sodium acetate or of theophylline with ethylenediamine (aminophylline).

THERAPEUTICS is the general name applied to the science and art of healing.

THERAPY means the treatment of disease.

THERIAC means an antidote or substance given to neutralize poison. The name was specially given to Venice treacle, a celebrated mixture of 64 drugs

prescribed in olden times as an antidote for poisons and a preventive of disease.

THERMISTOR is an instrument for determining temperature. It is essentially a mixture of cobalt, nickel and manganese oxides with finely divided copper, the resistance of which decreases or increases with changes in temperature.

THERMO- is a prefix implying some relation to heat.

THERMOGRAPHY is a method of detecting cancer of the breast. It is based on the fact that abnormally hot areas of skin occur in an area of cancer. The process records such changes in temperature in a record known as a thermogram. Unfortunately, such hot areas of skin are caused by a number of other conditions. It is therefore a diagnostic method that can be used only as a rough screening procedure, but to this extent it is proving of some value in the early detection of cancer of the breast.

THERMOMETER SCALES (see TEMPERATURE).

THERMOPHORE is the name applied to a box or rubber bag filled with a mixture of glue, acetate of soda, chloride of soda, and sulphate of calcium. When it is placed in hot water for some time it has the property of retaining its heat for several hours and is used as a warm application.

THIABENDAZOLE is a drug that is proving of value in the treatment of various parasitic infections, including those due to guinea-worm and certain nematodes, as well as strongyloidiasis (qv).

THIACETAZONE was introduced into medicine by Domagk, the discoverer of the original sulphonamide, for the treatment of tuberculosis. It is also proving of value in the treatment of leprosy. It is administered by mouth.

THIAMBUTOSINE is a diphenylthiourea that is proving of value in the treatment of patients with leprosy who are intolerant of, or hypersensitive to, dapsone.

THIAMINE is the *British Pharmacopoeia* name for vitamin B_1. Also known as ANEURINE, it is found in the husks of cereal grains. Its deficiency may be produced by too careful milling of rice in the East, or by a diet of white bread to the exclusion of brown bread and other cereal sources of this vitamin. The resulting disease is a form of neuritis with muscular weakness and heart failure, common in Japan and other parts of the East and known as beriberi (qv). Vitamin B$_1$ has been isolated in crystalline form, and a minute dose of this rapidly cures the symptoms of beriberi. The best sources of this vitamin are wholemeal flour, bacon, liver, egg-yolk, yeast and the pulses. The daily requirement is dependent, among other things, upon the total food intake, and has been estimated to be in the region of 0·5 mg of thiamine per 1000 Calories, increased during pregnancy to 2 mg daily as a minimum.

THIAZIDES (see BENZOTHIADIAZINES).

THIERSCH'S GRAFT is the term given to a method of skin grafting in which strips of skin are shaved from a normal area and placed on the abnormal area to be grafted.

THIGH is the portion of the lower limb above the knee. The thigh is supported by the femur or thigh-bone, the longest and strongest bone in the body. This fits by a rounded head at its upper end into the acetabulum, a hollow at the side of the pelvis, and at the lower end two large rounded condyles or knuckles rest upon the head of the tibia, and, along with the patella, or knee-cap, form the knee-joint. A large four-headed muscle, the quadriceps, forms most of the fleshy mass on the front and sides of the thigh and serves to straighten the leg in walking and to maintain the erect posture of the body in standing. At the back of the thigh, lie the hamstring muscles; and on the inner side the adductor muscles, attached above to the pelvis and below to the femur, pull the lower limb inwards. The large femoral vessels emerge from the abdomen in the middle of the groin, the vein lying to the inner side of the artery. These pass downwards with an inclination inwards deeply placed between the muscles, and at the knee they lie behind the joint. The great saphenous vein lies near the surface and can be seen towards the inner side of the thigh passing up to the groin, where it joins the femoral vein. The femoral nerve accompanies the large vessels and controls the muscles on the front and inner side of the thigh; while the sciatic nerve, about the thickness of a lead pencil, lies close to the back of the femur

and supplies the muscles at the back of the thigh and muscles below the knee.

Deep wounds on the inner side of the thigh are dangerous by reason of the risk of damage to the large vessels. Pain in the back of the thigh is often due to inflammation of the sciatic nerve. (See SCIATICA.) The veins on the inner side of the thigh are specially liable to become dilated. (See VARICOSE VEINS.)

THIOPENTONE SODIUM is the *British Pharmacopoeia* name for a commonly used intravenous anaesthetic. Its main use is for inducing anaesthesia, which it does rapidly and painlessly.

THIORIDAZINE is a tranquillizer that is proving of value as an anti-psychotic drug.

THIOSULPHATE OF SODIUM, or sodium hyposulphite, is much used in photography as a solvent of silver, and in medicine is used, in conjunction with sodium nitrite, in the treatment of cyanide, or prussic acid, poisoning. (See PRUSSIC ACID POISONING.)

THIOTEPA is one of the alkylating agents that is proving of value in the treatment of certain forms of malignant disease, including cancer of the breast and ovary.

THIOURACIL has the property of interfering with the synthesis of thyroxine in the thyroid gland. It was therefore introduced, with success, for the treatment of thyrotoxicosis, and is now widely used for this purpose, either as the methyl or the propyl salt. The use of thiouracil is not without its risks, but these are negligible provided the drug is only used under medical supervision. Thiouracil is used in one of two ways: (*a*) to control thyrotoxicosis, and for this purpose it usually needs to be taken for long periods; (*b*) as a preoperative measure in cases in which it has been decided that operation is necessary.

THIRST, like appetite, is an instinctive craving for something necessary to the continuance of bodily activity. The sensation of thirst is generally referred to the back of the throat, because, when there is a deficiency of water in the system, the throat and mouth especially become parched by evaporation of moisture from their surface. The mere swallowing of water, however, is not sufficient to abolish thirst, as appears in cases where a fistulous opening into the gullet exists, through which the water escapes. Thirst is increased by heat, and is a constant symptom of fever; it is also present in diseases which remove a considerable amount of fluid from the system, such as diarrhoea, diabetes, and after great loss of blood by haemorrhage. A desire for water is also a feature of many conditions associated with great exhaustion.

THORACIC DUCT is the large lymph-vessel which collects the contents of the lymphatics proceeding from the lower limbs, the abdomen, the left arm, and left side of the chest, neck, and head. It is about the size of a goose quill, is provided with numerous valves, and opens into the veins at the left side of the neck. (See GLANDS; LYMPHATICS.)

THORACOCENTESIS means the withdrawal of fluid from the pleural cavity. (See ASPIRATION.)

THORACOPLASTY is the operation of removing a varying number of ribs so that the underlying lung collapses.

THORAX is another name for the chest.

THORN-APPLE is a popular name for stramonium. (See STRAMONIUM.)

THREADWORM (see ENTEROBIASIS).

THREE-DAY FEVER, (see SANDFLY FEVER).

THRILL is a tremor or vibration felt on applying the hand to the surface of the body. It is felt particularly over the region of the heart in conditions in which the valve openings are narrowed or an aneurysm is present.

THROAT is, in popular language, a vague term applied indifferently to the region in front of the neck, to the larynx or organ of voice, and to the cavity at the back of the mouth. The last-mentioned use of the word, to denote the pharynx or cavity into which the nose, mouth, gullet, and larynx all open, is the correct one. (See PHARYNX. Information will also be found under NECK; LARYNX; TONSILS; NOSE.)

THROAT, DISEASES OF (see CHOK-ING; CLERGYMAN'S SORE THROAT; CROUP; CUT-THROAT; DIPHTHERIA; LARYNGISMUS; LARYNGITIS; MOUTH, DISEASES OF; NOSE, DISEASES OF; PHARYNGITIS; TONSILLITIS).

FOREIGN BODIES sometimes lodge in the throat, being either of the nature of food which has been swallowed in too large or too hard pieces, or of the nature of indigestible substances like coins which children are apt to place in the mouth. Bodies which lodge in the respiratory part of the throat, ie. at the entrance to, or in the cavity of, the larynx, set up immediate symptoms of choking (qv).

INJURIES OF THE THROAT from without have been briefly referred to under CUT-THROAT.

THROMBOANGIITIS OBLITER-ANS, also known as BUERGER'S DIS-EASE after the American surgeon who gave the first coordinated description of it in 1908, is an inflammatory disease involving the blood-vessels of the limbs, particularly the lower limbs. The cause is not known, but the use of tobacco is an important factor in its causation. It is almost entirely confined to men, and is more common in Jews than in Gentiles. Pain is the outstanding symptom, accompanied by pallor of the affected part. Sooner or later ulceration and gangrene tend to develop in the feet or hands. There is no specific treatment, but, if seen in the early stages, considerable relief may be given to the patient.

THROMBOCYTE (see PLATELETS).

THROMBOCYTOPENIA is the disease characterized by absence, or marked diminution, of platelets (or thrombocytes) in the blood. (See PLATELETS.)

THROMBOPHLEBITIS is the condition characterized by inflammation of the veins combined with clot formation. (See VEINS, DISEASES OF.)

THROMBOSIS means the formation of a blood-clot within the vessels or heart during life. The process of clotting within the body depends upon the same factors as in clotting of blood outside the body, involving the fibrinogen and lime salts circulating in the blood, as well as blood platelets. The indirect cause of thrombosis is usually some damage to the smooth lining of the blood-vessels brought about by inflammation, or the result of atheroma, a chronic disease of the vessel walls. The blood is also specially prone to clot in certain general conditions such as anaemia, the ill-health of wasting diseases like cancer, and in consequence of the feeble circulation of old age.

Thrombosis may occur in the heart and terminate some chronic wasting disease; it often takes place in the vessels of the brain and thus causes apoplexy in persons whose arteries are much diseased. It is sometimes a salutary thing, as in aneurysm, where the deposition of a clot within the sac forms the natural cure of this condition.

Thrombosis of a coronary artery of the heart is a very serious condition which affects, as a rule, middle-aged or elderly persons, appearing suddenly during rest and causing great pain in front of the chest or upper part of the abdomen, with pallor, feeble pulse, breathlessness, and sometimes vomiting. These symptoms may last for several hours or days, the pain being lessened by injections of morphine; but recovery takes place from about one-half of such attacks after a period of carefully supervised rehabilitation. (See also ARTERIES, DISEASES OF; CLOT; COAGULATION; CORONARY THROMBOSIS; and APOPLEXY.)

THRUSH is a type of inflammation affecting particularly the mouth of weakly children and causing a patchy white appearance on the lips, tongue, or palate. It is caused by the growth of a fungus on the surface of the mucous membrane. (See MOUTH, DISEASES OF.)

THUMB-SUCKING, or FINGER-SUCKING, is a universal habit in infancy. It is a harmless habit and nothing should be done to prevent it. After the age of 1 year it is usually indulged in on going to sleep. It is usually gradually given up during the pre-school period, but quite often persists after school age especially if the child is tired, lonely or unhappy. In these cases the remedy is to deal with the cause. On no account should threats be used to try and stop the habit. These only tend to make matters worse by inducing the child to persist in the habit in order to attract attention. On the other hand, if the habit is persistent and excessive after the age of 3 the child may be helped to stop it by being appealed to on the grounds that he is getting too old for such a baby habit. There is no evidence that in the vast majority of children it has any effect on the shape of the mouth. Indeed, there is evidence that children who suck their thumbs are more likely to be free of caries of the teeth than those who are not thumb-suckers.

THYMOL is a white, crystalline substance derived from oil of thyme and other volatile oils. It has an antiseptic action. It is also used, either alone or in combination with menthol, as a local application for the relief of pruritus (ie. itching of the skin).

THYMUS GLAND, so called by Galen in the second century A D because of its resemblance to a bunch of thyme flowers, has two lobes and lies in the lower part of the neck and the upper part of the chest. Each lobe is made up of a number of lobules divided into an outer portion, or cortex, and a central portion, or medulla. The cortex resembles lymphoid tissue and is made up of masses of small round cells (thymocytes), whilst the medulla contains small round masses known as Hassall's corpuscles. A striking feature of the gland is that it decreases in size after puberty. The main function of the thymus gland is the control of the production of lymphocytes (qv). In the neonatal period, that is, the first month of life, the thymus is essential for the normal development of the lymphatic tissues (see GLANDS). In this way it plays an important part in the immune processes of the body. (See IMMUNITY.) It also plays a part in the regulation of transmission of impulses from nerves to muscles. Enlargement occurs in disturbances of certain other endocrine glands, and has been reported in cases of acromegaly and eunuchoidism, and following castration. The observation that certain cases of myasthenia gravis (qv) are associated with enlargement of, or a tumour of, the thymus gland has led to the use of removal of the gland (ie. *thymectomy*) as a means of treatment of this condition.

THYROCALCITON is a hormone produced by the thyroid gland which helps to control the metabolism of calcium.

THYROID CARTILAGE is the largest cartilage in the larynx and forms the prominence of the Adam's apple in front of the neck. (See LARYNX.)

THYROID GLAND is a highly vascular organ situated in front of the neck. It consists of a narrow isthmus crossing the windpipe close to its upper end, and joining together two lateral lobes which run upwards, one on each side of the larynx. The gland is therefore shaped somewhat like a horseshoe, each lateral lobe being

404 – Section through thyroid gland of adult. Magnified 112 times. From *Hewer's Histology*. Wm. Heinemann Ltd.

about 2 inches (5 cm) long and the isthmus about ½ inch (12 mm) wide, and it is firmly bound to the larynx. The weight of the thyroid gland is about one ounce (28·5 grams), but it is larger in females than in males, undergoes in many women a periodic increase at each time of menstruation, and often reaches an enormous size in the condition known as goitre (qv).

Minute structure – The gland is enveloped in a layer of fibrous tissue and possesses a rich blood supply. It is composed of multitudes of closed vesicles (illustration 404), each formed by a layer of cubical cells and containing a thick yellow fluid (colloid). Round the vesicles there is a dense network of capillary blood-vessels, whilst the finest lymphatic vessels communicate with the interior of these vesicles.

Function – The chief function of the thyroid gland is to produce a hormone rich in iodine. The main active ingredient of this hormone is thyroxine, and its probable mode of manufacture is:

iodine + tyrosine = di-iodotyrosine
2 molecules of di-iodotyrosine = thyroxine.

This hormone, or secretion, which passes directly from the thyroid into the bloodstream, is de-iodinated in the body cells to triiodothyronine which exerts the physiological action of the thyroid hormone. This hormone is one of the most important in the body and controls the rate of metabolism. Thus, if it is deficient in children they fail to grow, a condition known as CRETINISM (qv). If the deficiency develops in adult life, the individual becomes obese, lethargic, and develops a coarse skin, a condition known as MYXOEDEMA (qv). Over-action of the thyroid, or HYPER-THYROIDISM, results in loss of weight, rapid heart action, and a highly strung nervous temperament. The condition known as EXOPHTHALMIC GOITRE, THYRO-TOXICOSIS, or GRAVES' DISEASE, is practically the same as hyperthyroidism, but, in certain cases at least, there is evidence to suggest that not only is the output of the secretion of the thyroid increased, in addition there is some abnormality in it.

The production of the thyroid hormone is controlled by a hormone of the pituitary gland – the thyrotrophic hormone.

THYROID GLAND, DISEASES OF (see CRETINISM; GOITRE; MYXOEDEMA).

THYROTOXICOSIS (see GOITRE).

THYROXINE is a crystalline substance, containing iodine, isolated from the thyroid gland and possessing the properties of thyroid extract. It has also been synthesized. It is used in cases of defective function of the thyroid, such as cretinism, and myxoedema.

TIBIA is the name of the larger of the two bones in the leg. One surface of the tibia lies immediately beneath the skin in front and towards the inner side of the leg, forming the shin. Fractures of this bone are accordingly very liable to wound the skin and become compound. The thigh-bone rests upon the larger upper end of the tibia at the knee-joint, whilst below, the tibia and fibula together enter into the ankle-joint, the two bosses or malleoli at the ankle belonging, the inner to the tibia, the outer to the fibula.

TIC is the term applied to the habit spasm which forms a personal peculiarity in neurotic subjects. (See CRAMP.)

TIC DOULOUREUX is another name for facial, or trigeminal, neuralgia due to some affection of the fifth cranial nerve, and characterized by pain, situated somewhere about the temple, forehead, face, or jaw, and sometimes by spasm in the muscles of the affected region. (See NEURALGIA.)

TICK is the general name given to a group of arachnid insects, some of which act as transmitters of diseases.

Ticks are blood-sucking arthropods which are responsible for transmitting a wide range of diseases to man, including Rocky Mountain spotted fever, African tick typhus and fièvre boutonneuse (see TYPHUS FEVER). Apart from being transmitters of disease, they cause intense itching and may cause quite severe lesions of the skin. The best repellents are dimethyl phthalate and diethyltoluamide. Once bitten, relief from the itching is obtained from the application of calamine lotion. Tick-bites are an occupational hazard of shepherds and gamekeepers. (See BITES AND STINGS.)

TINCTURE is an alcoholic solution, generally of some vegetable substance. *The British Pharmacopoeia* 1973 includes tinctures of hyoscyamus, belladonna, colchicum, ginger (weak and strong), hyoscyamus, iodine, ipecacuanha, nux vomica, opium, stramonium. In addition, there are compound tinctures of cardamom, and of rhubarb, and a camphorated opium tincture (paregoric). In addition, the *British Pharmaceutical Codex* 1973 contains tinctures of benzoin, capsicum, catechu, gelsemium, myrrh, orange. It also contains compound benzoin tincture (Friars' balsam); aromatic cardamom tincture (carminative tincture); chloroform and morphine tincture (chlorodyne); compound gentian tincture; ethereal lobelia tincture; concentrated compound opium tincture.

TINEA is the technical name for ringworm. (See RINGWORM.)

TINNITUS means a noise heard in the ear without any external cause. It is a frequent accompaniment of deafness. (See DEAFNESS; and EAR, DISEASES OF.)

TIN-POISONING from canned food seldom occurs at the present day. When it does occur, the tin comes from the solder used in sealing the tin in the hole and cap variety, and in modern canning the food has practically no contact with the solder. Tin has been found occasionally in cheese wrapped in tin-foil, due to the action of free lactic acid.

The strong soluble salts of tin used by dyers and calico-printers act as irritant poisons. (See POISONS.)

TIRED ARM SYNDROME is the condition occurring mainly in middle-aged women, in which during the night aching and throbbing pain occurs in the upper limbs, especially the forearm and sometimes with weakness of the hand. The right upper limb is usually affected in right-handed people, and the hand feels stiff when the affected individual wakens in the morning. No treatment is needed, as the condition clears in due course.

TISANE is a name sometimes given to barley-water. (See BARLEY-WATER.) The term is also applied to a variety of herbal tea.

TISSUES OF THE BODY are the simple elements from which the various parts and organs are found to be built. All the body originates from the union of a pair of cells but as growth proceeds the new cells produced from these form tissues of varying character and complexity. (See CELL.) It is customary to divide the tissues into five groups:

(1) Epithelial tissues, including the cells covering the skin, those lining the alimentary canal, those forming the secretions of internal organs. (See EPITHELIUM.)
(2) Connective tissues, including fibrous tissue, fat, bone, cartilage. (See these headings.)
(3) Muscular tissues (see MUSCLE).
(4) Nervous tissues (see NERVES).
(5) Wandering corpuscles of the blood and lymph (see BLOOD; LYMPH).

Many of the organs are formed of a single one of these tissues or of one with a very slight admixture of another, such as cartilage, or white fibrous tissue. Other parts of the body that are widely distributed are very simple in structure and consist of two or or more simple tissues in varying proportion. Such are blood-vessels (see ARTERIES; VEINS), lymphatic vessels (see LYMPHATICS), lymphatic glands (see GLANDS), serous membranes (see SEROUS MEMBRANE), synovial membranes (see JOINTS), mucous membranes (see MUCOUS MEMBRANE), secreting glands (see GLANDS; SALIVARY GLANDS; THYROID GLAND) and skin (see SKIN).

The structure of the more complex organs of the body is dealt with under the heading of each organ.

TITRATION is the term applied to a form of chemical analysis by means of standard solutions of known strength.

TITUBATION means a staggering or reeling condition, especially due to disease of the spinal cord or cerebellum.

TOAST is made by applying dry heat to bread, which drives off some of the moisture, produces changes in the starch grain, and renders machine-made British bread more palatable. Its brown colour is due to the formation of caramel.

TOAST WATER is a fluid for administration to invalids, containing a small amount of protein and carbohydrate nourishment. To prepare it, take two or three slices of bread, toast them thoroughly without burning, put them into a large jug, and pour over them a quart of boiling water. This is strained when cold, sweetened with sugar, and flavoured with lemon.

TOBACCO is the leaf of several species of Nicotiana, especially of the American plant *Nicotiana tabacum.*

The practice of smoking has probably been known for ages, but did not come into use in Europe till it was introduced from the West Indies by the followers of Columbus. The use of tobacco was popularized in England during the sixteenth century by Sir John Hawkins and Sir Walter Raleigh, and the plant was at that time successfully grown in England and Scotland. From the first, smoking was bitterly opposed by many who did not care for the practice. Popes issued edicts against it; in Turkey and Russia it was made a punishable offence, and in England James I was constrained to issue his *Counterblaste to Tobacco,* in which he described smoking as 'a custom loathsome to the eye, hateful to the nose, harmful to the brain, dangerous to the lungs, . . . resembling the horrible Stygian smoke of the pit that is bottomless'.

Composition – In addition to vegetable fibre, tobacco leaves contain a large quantity of ash, the nature of this depending largely upon the minerals present in the ground where the tobacco plant has been grown, but amounting to 12 or 20 per cent of the whole. Of the organic constituents the brown fluid alkaloid known as nicotine is the most important, as the special action of tobacco depends upon it. The nicotine content of tobacco ranges from 1·5 to 3 per cent of the dried leaf in Havana tobacco to 6 to 8 per cent in Virginian tobacco. Some Algerian tobaccos contain much larger amounts. The amount of nicotine entering the mouth of a smoker is 0·92 mg per cigarette, 3·6 to 7·9 mg per cigar, and 2·7 mg per gram of pipe tobacco. The amount of nicotine absorbed depends upon whether or not the smoker inhales. Most of the nicotine inhaled into the smaller air-passages of the lungs is absorbed, whereas without inhalation, much less per cigarette is absorbed. As a cigarette or cigar is smoked the stub becomes richer in nicotine. It has been estimated that if not more than two-thirds of a cigarette is smoked, some two-thirds of the nicotine is retained in the stub. The amount of nicotine that can be recovered from the mainstream smoke of one cigarette varies from 1 to 3 milligrams and smokers who inhale may absorb up to 90 per cent of this; those who do not inhale absorb as little as 10 per cent.

Tobacco smoke also contains some sixteen substances capable of inducing cancer in experimental animals. One of the most important of these is benzpyrene. Other constituents of tobacco smoke include pyridine, ammonia, and carbon monoxide. The last is the most abundant of these, but American workers have stated that an individual walking along a street with heavy motor traffic would absorb more carbon monoxide than he would from heavy smoking.

Action and use – The action of tobacco depends largely upon the constitution of the smoker, his habituation to the drug, and the circumstances under which he smokes.

A very small amount of nicotine, such as that derived from a single cigarette, has a stimulating effect upon the mental and bodily powers.

In larger amount, the action is a depressant and narcotic one, which in habitual smokers is modified to a sedative and quieting effect upon the nervous system, without much depression of the heart or other organs. The most suitable time for smoking is generally admitted to be after meals, and especially in the evening after the day's work is at an end, when the sedative action is most beneficial to the nervous system. Different people vary widely in their susceptibility to the influence of tobacco. In some, and particularly in young persons, very small quantities suffice to cause depression and irritability of the nervous system, the heart's action, and the digestive and other powers; whilst others, especially those who lead an open-air life, are not in the least affected by large amounts. Generally speaking, excessive smoking is a harmful thing, particularly for young people.

Among the evil effects of smoking may be mentioned the temporary nausea, depression, giddiness, and vomiting which affect the unaccustomed smoker. These effects, however, pass off quickly, and the tendency to their occurrence disappears as the person becomes habituated to tobacco. Of more importance is the group of symptoms produced by continued and excessive smoking, especially of cigarettes. These include palpitation and irregularity of the heart, giddiness, and a tendency to sudden attacks of faintness, symptoms often grouped together under the popular name of 'tobacco heart'. Other common symptoms are liability to fatigue on slight exertion, dyspepsia, and dimness of vision associated with impairment of power for seeing colours, especially green and red. These symptoms also pass off gradually when smoking is discontinued, or when the amount of tobacco consumed is reduced within suitable bounds; but, while they last, they may cause great impairment of the health.

The greatest hazard of smoking, however, is the correlation that has been shown to exist between excessive cigarette smoking and cancer of the lung. On the available evidence there seems to be little doubt that anyone who smokes 20 or more cigarettes a day is definitely increasing the risk that he or she will develop cancer of the lung. Hence the justification for the current campaign to persuade youngsters never to start smoking, and adult cigarette smokers to cut down their daily consumption.

Almost equally serious is the undoubted correlation between heavy cigarette smoking on the one hand, and chronic bronchitis and duodenal ulcer on the other, and there is a growing volume of evidence of a correlation between cigarette smoking and coronary heart disease.

Another set of symptoms frequently arising in those who smoke, and often attributed to a mistaken cause, consists of irritable cough and soreness of the throat. These symptoms pass off when smoking is discontinued.

The habit also has an adverse effect on the foetus, and is therefore contraindicated during pregnancy.

Acute nicotine-poisoning seldom occurs. It may be due to the accidental swallowing of nicotine insecticides, or to the inhaling of tobacco dust in industrial processes. Occasionally it may occur in children as a result of swallowing tobacco. Nicotine is one of the most rapidly fatal poisons. The fatal dose for man is about 40 mg. The fatal dose of tobacco is about 2 grams. The symptoms vary from those of smoking in the unaccustomed smoker to immediate prostration leading rapidly to collapse and death. Treatment consists of washing out the stomach, the administration of charcoal or potassium permanganate (1 in 5000 solution), and artificial respiration.

TOBRAMYCIN is an antibiotic related to gentamicin (qv) and with a similar range of activity. It is given by injection.

TOES (see CORNS; FOOT; NAILS).

TOLAZAMIDE is a sulphonylurea compound, like tolbutamide (qv), which is proving of value in the treatment of certain forms of diabetes mellitus when given by mouth. One of its practical advantages is that it only needs to be taken once a day.

TOLAZOLINE is a drug that antagonizes some of the effects of adrenaline, and is used in the treatment of peripheral vascular disorders due to arterial spasm or occlusion.

TOLBUTAMIDE is a sulphonamide derivative which lowers the level of the blood sugar in diabetes mellitus. As it is rapidly excreted from the body, it has to be taken twice daily. (See also DIABETES MELLITUS.)

TOLNAFTATE is a preparation which, in the form of a 1 per cent solution, is proving useful as a local application in the treatment of certain forms of ringworm, particularly ringworm of the foot. It may also be used as a powder or cream. It is also used in the treatment of tinea versicolor (see RINGWORM) and erythrasma (qv).

TOLU (see BALSAM).

TOLUENE, or METHYLBENZENE, is a product of the distillation of coal tar widely used as a solvent in the manufacture of paint and rubber and plastic cements.

-TOMY is a suffix indicating an operation by cutting.

TONGUE – The tongue is made up of several muscles, is richly supplied with blood-vessels and nerves, and is covered by highly specialized mucous membrane. It consists of a free part known as the tip, a body, and a hinder fixed part or root. The under surface lies upon the floor of the mouth, whilst the upper surface is curved from side to side, and still more from before backwards so as to adapt it to the roof of the mouth. At its root, the tongue is in contact with, and firmly united to, the upper edge of the larynx; so that in some persons who can depress the tongue readily the tip of the epiglottis may be seen projecting upwards at its hinder part.

Structure – The *substance* of the tongue consists almost entirely of muscles running in various directions. One runs along the upper surface and another along the lower surface from root to tip. Other fibres run vertically from the upper to the lower surface, whilst the chief bulk of the tongue is made up of muscle-fibres running from side to side. These various fibres are chiefly concerned in making changes in the shape of the tongue and moving it within the mouth. In addition to these, the tongue has numerous outside attachments; one muscle on each side unites it to the lower jaw-bone just behind the chin, and this muscle serves to protrude the tongue from the mouth; other muscles, which retract the tongue, attach it to the hyoid bone, the larynx, the palate, and the styloid process on the base of the skull.

The *mucous membrane* on the under surface of the tongue is very thin, so that the large blood-vessels on each side can easily be seen through it. In the middle line a fold of mucous membrane, the frenum, passes from the under surface to the floor of the mouth, and, when this frenum is attached too far forwards towards the tip of the tongue, the movements of the organ are impeded, and the condition is known as tongue-tie. On the upper surface or dorsum of the tongue the mucous membrane is thicker, and in its front two-thirds is studded with little projections of three kinds. The majority of these projections or *papillae* are of conical shape, and when the tongue becomes furred the appearance is due to an unhealthy collection of epithelium upon them. Some of them end in long filaments, and are then known as *filiform* papillae. The roughness of the tongue in cats and other carnivorous animals is due to large backwardly directed conical papillae, which assist in cleaning the flesh off bones. On the tip, and towards the edges of the tongue, small red rounded *fungiform* papillae are seen, which act in all probability as end-organs for the sense of taste. On a line dividing the front two-thirds from the hinder one-third, and set in the shape of a V, is a row of seven to twelve large flat-topped *circumvallate* papillae, each placed in a corresponding depression and just visible, in most mouths, when the tongue is pressed firmly down with some flat instrument. These also act as end-organs for the nerves of taste. Each circumvallate papilla is surrounded by a trench, and upon both sides of the trench open numerous *taste-buds* (illustration 405). A taste-bud is shaped somewhat like a barrel, with an outer covering of flattened stave-like cells, enclosing a bundle of spindle-shaped cells which end in hairlike processes at the mouth of the bud, and are connected at their deeply placed end with some filaments from the nerves of taste. These taste-buds are also found in the fungiform papillae, though in smaller numbers, and they are scattered over the throat, fauces, and palate; so that the popular expression 'a fine palate', as applied to the sense of taste, is quite correct.

Nerves – No fewer than five nerves supply branches to each side of the tongue. These are the *lingual* branch of the 5th nerve, which is the nerve of ordinary sensation, to the front two-thirds of the tongue; the *chorda tympani* branch from the 7th nerve, which is supposed to be the nerve of taste, for a similar extent; the *glossopharyngeal* or 9th nerve, which conveys sensations both of touch and taste from the hinder third; the *superior laryngeal* branch of the 10th nerve, also sensory; and the *hypoglossal* or 12th nerve, which supplies the muscles of the tongue.

Functions – The chief uses of the tongue are of three kinds: (*a*) to push the food

Gymnaema sylvesie, to do away with the power of tasting bitter and sweet substances, while the sensation for acids and salts remains, so that in all probability there are different nerve-fibres and end-organs for the different varieties of taste. Many tastes depend upon the ordinary sensations of the tongue, such as the constringent taste of tannin and the metallic taste of a weak galvanic current passed through the tongue.

Like other sensations, taste can be very highly educated for a time, as in tea-tasters and wine-tasters, but this special adaptation is lost after some years.

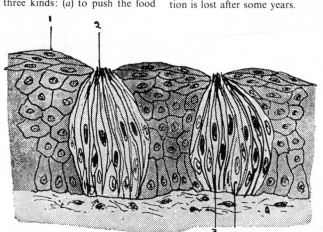

405 – Section showing taste-buds, magnified 420 times: 1, stratified epithelium; 2, gustatory pore; 3, gustatory cell with hairlet; 4, sustentacular cell. From *Hewer's Histology*. Wm. Heinemann Ltd.

between the teeth for mastication, and then mould it into a bolus preparatory to swallowing; (*b*) as the organ of the sense of taste, and as an organ provided with a delicate sense of touch; and (*c*) to play a part in the production of speech. (See VOICE AND SPEECH.)

As to taste, the Greeks recognized nine varieties, but it is usual to classify any taste as —

1. Sweet	3. Bitter
2. Salt	4. Acid

since finer distinctions are largely dependent upon the sense of smell. The loss of keenness in taste brought about by a cold in the head, or even by holding the nose while swallowing, is well known. Sweet tastes seem to be best appreciated by the tip of the tongue, acids on its edges, and bitters at the back. It is possible, too, by chewing the leaves of an Indian plant,

TONGUE, DISEASES OF (see MOUTH, DISEASES OF).

TONGUE, FURRING OF (see MOUTH, DISEASES OF).

TONICS are 'substances whose continued administration gives strength and vigour to the body, without producing sudden excitement or subsequent depression'. This is a 100-year old definition of a term which is gradually passing out of medical phraseology. In the old days, when knowledge of disease processes and of how to treat them was much less than it is to-day, there was a real place for remedies which would help to combat the weakness, lassitude, and loss of appetite which accompanied and followed most illnesses. At the present day it is so often possible to treat the underlying cause that tonics are seldom required. It is also recognized now that to treat symptoms of a disease, without discovering their cause, may do more harm than good. For instance, a middle-aged man's loss of appetite may be due to cancer of the stomach. To treat this by a bitter is obviously wrong, because the only hope of cure is an early operation. Similarly, the young woman's lassitude may be the first manifestation of pulmonary tuberculosis, the treatment of which is not a tonic but the appropriate chemotherapy. Or, to take one other example, an individual's lack of concentration may be due to diminished activity of the thyroid gland, ie. myxoedema, a condition which can be immediately and effectively controlled by the administration of thyroid extract.

Thus, the use of tonics is very much less than it was. But there are still occasions when they may be of value; for instance, in convalescence from a serious illness. Even in those cases in which they are still used, however, tonics are tending to be used with more discrimination and need not necessarily take the form of drugs. For the over-worked professional man or business executive who finds that he is unable to carry out his duties satisfactorily, is losing his appetite, and is not sleeping well, the best tonic is a holiday. To give such a man a bitter to stimulate his appetite, a nerve tonic to 'buck him up', a tranquillizer to take the edge off life for him, and a sedative to allow him to sleep, is simply equivalent to whipping a tired horse to make renewed efforts. There may well be a response, but merely a temporary one achieved at the risk of doing permanent harm.

For individuals who are run down, and in whom no disease or special cause can be found, the best tonics include a well-balanced diet, adequate sleep, ample fresh air and exercise. Cold baths or sprays are also of value in youngsters. During convalescence bitters such as nux vomica, quinine, quassia, and gentian may be useful adjuncts to re-stimulating an active interest in food, although this can usually be achieved much more satisfactorily by presenting the patient with a well-cooked variety of food served in an attractive manner.

An unbalanced diet is often a cause for debility, particularly in children and adolescents. Here the best tonic is a well-balanced diet, ensuring an adequate supply of all the vitamins, first-class protein, and essential salts and metals such as iron and calcium. Vitamin deficiency is no longer a major problem in

Great Britain, but this state of affairs can only be maintained if every individual up to the age of at least 18 years receives supplementary doses of vitamins A, D, and C during the winter months. Milk, eggs, and meat are the best sources of first-class protein.

Iron is often given as a tonic, but this is only of value when the individual is suffering from an iron-deficiency anaemia. Its use for this purpose is often indicated in adolescent girls in whom there is a heavy loss of blood during the menstrual period. Although there is not usually a marked degree of anaemia in these girls, there is often sufficient lack of iron in the diet to render beneficial the administration of additional iron. There is no justification for the use of liver extracts as a tonic.

The best heart tonic is rest. Digitalis is sometimes described as a heart tonic but this is not justified. Whilst digitalis is the sheet-anchor in the treatment of heart failure, it is always used in conjunction with rest. To give digitalis to an individual with a failing heart, and not restrict his activities, is merely putting an unnecessary strain on the heart muscle.

No account of tonics would be complete without at least a brief reference to three iron-containing tonics which are still widely used: Parrish's food (compound syrup of iron phosphate), Easton's syrup (syrup of iron phosphate with quinine and strychnine) and syrup of iron iodide. The first of these is still a favourite for use in children, whilst Easton's syrup is a useful bitter for adults. None of them contains sufficient iron to relieve an iron-deficiency anaemia. If such be present, iron must be given in much larger doses.

TONSILLITIS means inflammation of the tonsils and may be either acute or chronic.

ACUTE TONSILLITIS – It must never be forgotten that the infection is never entirely confined to the tonsils; there is always some involvement of the surrounding throat. Just as in many cases of 'sore throat' the tonsils are involved in the generalized inflammation of the throat.

Causes – The most common cause is the haemolytic streptococcus. Its highest incidence is between October and March. In children it is particularly important because it may be the precursor of rheumatic fever. When it occurs in hospitals or institutions it may be highly infectious, and, particularly in children's hospitals, care must be taken to prevent spread of the infection. In the early stages it may be difficult to differentiate from diphtheria, and should there be any doubt as to the diagnosis, a throat swab must be taken and sent immediately to the nearest laboratory so that the infecting organism can be determined. Occasionally the infection may spread to the surrounding tissues and cause abscess formation – a peritonsillar abscess or quinsy.

Symptoms – The onset is usually sudden, with pain in swallowing, a sensation of chilliness and fever. On examination, one or both tonsils are found to be enlarged, engorged and covered with a varying amount of whitish or grey material. This material, or exudate as it is known, consists of purulent discharge from the tonsil. It may occur as scattered areas over the surface of the tonsil, the condition known as follicular tonsillitis and usually due to the haemolytic streptococcus. In other areas there may be a more extensive exudate covering practically the whole of the tonsil; this is the type of tonsillitis which is most difficult to differentiate from diphtheria. The inflammatory process is seldom restricted to the tonsil (or tonsils), and the whole of the throat is reddened and inflamed. The tongue, particularly the posterior part, is covered with a thick fur, and the breath has often an unpleasant odour. On pressure on the tonsils further purulent material may be pressed out of them. The glands underneath the angle of the jaw are enlarged and tender; the enlargement may be marked. There is sometimes pain in the ear on the affected side; this may indicate spread of the infection to the Eustachian tube. Particular attention must be paid to this in children, as it may lead to infection of the ear – with serious consequences.

Occasionally an abscess develops around the affected tonsil – a peritonsillar abscess, or quinsy. This manifests itself by increased swelling in front of the tonsil, which is pushed backwards and also bulges farther into the throat. This is not a particularly serious complication provided it is treated properly. It may develop quite early in an attack of tonsillitis; in other cases it comes on as the tonsillitis is apparently settling.

Treatment – This consists of rest in bed so long as the temperature is raised. Except in mild cases, full doses of sulphonamides are given by mouth or penicillin is given intramuscularly or by mouth.

In view of the pain on swallowing, the diet must be bland and fluid: eg. milk, milk puddings, boiled or poached eggs. The patient should be encouraged to drink freely, and if he is taking plenty of milk (2 pints daily (1 litre)) and fruit drinks there is no need to worry about the amount he is eating during the acute phase. The sucking of pastilles helps to overcome the unpleasant dryness of the mouth which is so often complained of. Local applications to the throat or tonsils are of little value in acute tonsillitis, but hot menthol inhalations through the mouth are sometimes comforting. When the glands in the neck are enlarged, kaolin poultices to the neck are useful. To relieve the general discomfort and to ensure a good night's rest the best remedies are Dover's powder, aspirin, or a combination of aspirin, paracetamol and codeine.

Particular attention must be paid to tonsillitis in children because it may be the precursor of rheumatic fever or of acute nephritis (ie. Bright's disease). The best way of reducing the risk of such complications is to keep the child strictly confined to bed until the temperature has been settled for two days. Such complications are most likely to occur when the infecting organism is the haemolytic streptococcus. Some authorities recommend that full doses of penicillin should be given routinely to children with a haemolytic streptococcal tonsillitis in order to diminish the risk of rheumatic fever developing. Because of the risk of nephritis developing, the urine must be examined regularly in all cases. When a haemolytic streptococcal tonsillitis develops in an individual who has had rheumatic fever, the administration of penicillin is essential and the individual must be confined to bed for at least a week.

The treatment of quinsy is as for acute tonsillitis, except that the abscess is incised under a general anaesthetic when it is fully formed.

CHRONIC TONSILLITIS may occur either as a result of one attack of acute tonsillitis or, more commonly, as the result of recurrent attacks. In children there is usually also chronic inflammation of the adenoid tissue in the pharynx. (See NOSE, DISEASES OF.) Chronic tonsillitis is more likely to occur in debilitated children or in those who are living under unhygienic conditions: eg. overcrowded houses, inadequate exercise and fresh air, and poor diet.

The condition manifests itself by chronic enlargement of the tonsils, which tend to have a dull-red colour instead of the normal bright-red colour. On pressure on the tonsil, purulent material can often be exuded from it. If the adenoids are also enlarged, the child breathes through the mouth instead of the nose. Such individuals are liable to be susceptible to repeated 'colds', sore throats or infections of the sinuses.

Removal of the tonsils is indicated: (*a*) when the tonsils and adenoids are permanently so enlarged as to interfere with breathing – in such cases the adenoids are removed as well as the tonsils; (*b*) when the individual is subject to recurrent attacks of acute tonsillitis; (*c*) when there is definite evidence of persistent active inflammation of the tonsils which will not respond to medical treatment. Such treatment consists of local applications to the tonsils, e.g. Mandl's paint or an astringent paint, a nourishing diet, full doses of cod-liver oil and vitamin C, and iron if there be any anaemia. Steps must also be taken to ensure that the child is living under as satisfactory conditions as possible, and a holiday in the country or at the sea often works wonders. In dealing with suspected cases of chronic tonsillitis in children it must never be forgotten that an enlarged tonsil is not necessarily an inflamed or abnormal one.

TONSILS are two almond-shaped glands situated one on each side of the narrow fauces where the mouth joins the throat. Each has a structure resembling that of a lymphatic gland, and consists of an elevation of the mucous membrane presenting twelve to fifteen openings, which lead into pits or lacunae. The mucous covering is formed by the ordin-

ary mucous membrane of the mouth, which also lines the pits; and the main substance of the gland is composed of loose connective tissue containing lymph corpuscles in its meshes, and packed here and there into denser nodules or follicles. The tonsils play an important rôle in the protective mechanism of the body against infection.

TOOTHACHE (see TEETH, DISEASES OF).

TOPHUS is the name given to the concretions which form in connection with joints or tendon sheaths as the result of attacks of gout (illustration 406). At first the tophus is a soft mass, but later becomes quite hard. It is composed of biurate of soda. (See CONCRETIONS; GOUT.)

TORMINA is a technical name for griping pains felt round the navel, as the result of spasmodic action of the muscular coat in the small intestine. (See COLIC.)

TORPOR is a condition of bodily and mental inactivity, not amounting to sleep, but interfering greatly with the ordinary habits and pursuits. It is often found in persons suffering from fever, and is a common symptom in aged people whose arteries are diseased. It may annoy young persons after meals when they are the subjects of constipation or of dyspepsia, due to eating too much indigestible food.

TORSION means twisting. The term is applied to the process in which organs,

406 – Tophi on the hands in a case of gout. Professor E. G. L. Bywater.

or tumours, which are attached to the rest of the body by a narrow neck or pedicle, become twisted so as to narrow the blood-vessels or other structures in the pedicle. (See TESTICLES, DISEASES OF.)

Torsion is also the term applied to the twisting of the small arteries severed at an operation, by which bleeding from them is stopped.

TORTICOLLIS means wry-neck. (See CRAMP; SPASMODIC TORTICOLLIS; WRY-NECK.)

TORULA is a yeast, now known as cryptococcus, that causes an infection known as torulosis or cryptococcosis.

TORULOSIS is a disease due to a yeast, *Torula histolytica*, which is usually characterized by meningitis or meningo-encephalitis.

TOUCH, according to the popular idea, is the fifth sense diffused all over the body, by which we become conscious of our surroundings otherwise than by the four special senses of hearing, seeing, tasting and smelling. But when this diffused sensitiveness is examined it is found to consist of a group of senses, several of which have special end-organs situated in the skin, muscles and elsewhere and special nerve-paths to convey their impressions to the brain. It is convenient, however, to adopt the popular view, and to consider all these under one heading. The cutaneous sense, then, is made up of the following:

Touch sense proper, by which we perceive a touch or stroke and estimate the size and shape of bodies with which we come in contact, but which we do not see.

Pressure sense, by which we judge the heaviness of weights laid upon the skin, or appreciate the hardness of objects by pressing against them.

Heat sense, by which we perceive that a body is warmer than the skin.

Cold sense, by which we perceive that a body touching the skin is cold.

Pain sense, by which we appreciate pricks, pinches and other painful impressions.

To these we may for convenience add:

Muscular sensitiveness, by which the painfulness of a squeeze is perceived. It is produced probably by direct pressure upon the nerve-fibres in the muscles.

Muscular sense, by which we test the weight of an object held in the hand, or gauge the amount of energy expended on an effort.

Sense of locality, by which we can, without looking, tell the position and attitude of any part of the body.

Common sensation, which is a vague term used to mean composite sensations produced by several of the foregoing, like tickling, or creeping, and the vague sense of well-being or the reverse that the mind receives from internal organs. (See the article on PAIN.)

The structure of the end-organs situated in the skin, which receive impressions from the outer world, and of the nerve-fibres which conduct these impressions to the central nervous system, have been described under NERVES.

Touch affects the Meissner's or touch corpuscles (illustration 407) placed beneath the epidermis; as these differ in

407 – Tactile corpuscle of Meissner in a skin papilla. From *Hewer's Histology.* Wm. Heinemann Ltd.

closeness in different parts of the skin, the delicacy of the sense of touch varies greatly. Thus the points of a pair of compasses can be felt as two on the tip of the tongue when separated by only $\frac{1}{24}$ of an inch (1 mm), on the tips of the fingers they must be separated to twice that distance, whilst on the arm or leg they cannot be felt as two points unless separated by over an inch (25 mm), and on the back they must be separated by over two inches (50 mm). On the parts covered by hair, the nerves ending round the roots of the hairs also take up impressions of touch.

Pressure is estimated probably through the same nerve-endings and nerves that have to do with touch, but it depends upon a difference in the sensations of parts pressed on and those of surrounding parts. Heat-sense, cold-sense and pain-sense all depend upon different nerve-endings in the skin; and thus, with care and delicate instruments like needles, bristles in holders and metal pencils through which hot or cold water can be made to circulate, the skin may be mapped out into a mosaic of little areas where the different kinds of impressions are registered. Whilst the tongue and finger-tips are the parts most sensitive to touch, they are comparatively insensitive to heat, and can easily bear temperatures which the cheek or elbow could not tolerate. The muscular sense, in all probability, depends on the sensory organs known as muscle-spindles, which are scattered through the substance of the muscles, and the sense of locality is dependent partly upon these and partly upon the nerves which end in tendons, ligaments and joints.

Disorders of the sense of touch occur in various diseases.

HYPERAESTHESIA is a condition in which there is excessive sensitiveness to any stimulus, such as touch. When this reaches the stage when a mere touch or gentle handling causes acute pain it is known as HYPERALGESIA. It is found in various diseases of the spinal cord immediately above the level of the disease, combined often with loss of sensation below the diseased part. It is also present in neuralgia, the skin of the neuralgic area becoming excessively tender to touch, heat or cold. Heightened sensibility to pain is seen sometimes in drunkards, who wince at a mere touch when not under the influence of alcohol. Heightened sensibility to temperature is a common symptom of neuritis. (See PAIN.)

ANAESTHESIA, or diminution of the sense of touch, causing often a feeling of numbness, is present in many diseases affecting the nerves of sensation or their continuations up the posterior part of the spinal cord. The condition of *dissociated analgesia*, in which a touch is quite well felt, though there is complete insensibility to pain, is present in the disease of the spinal cord known as syringomyelia, and affords a proof that the nerve-fibres for pain and those for touch are quite separate. In locomotor ataxia there is sometimes loss of the sense of touch on feet or arms; but in other cases of this disease there is no loss of the sense of touch, although there is a complete loss of the sense of locality in the lower limbs, thus proving that these two senses are quite distinct.

PARAESTHESIAE are peculiar forms of perverted sensation such as creeping, tingling, pricking or hot flushes.

TOURNIQUET is an instrument used for the temporary stoppage of the circulation in a limb, to control bleeding. There are various forms of tourniquet, the simplest being a *tourniquet improvised* from a band such as that made by a handkerchief folded cravat-wise, tied round the limb, and then twisted up by means of a rigid object passed beneath it (illustrations 408, 409a). *Petit's tourniquet* has a linen strap passing over two pairs of brass rollers, which can be separated from one another by a screw, thus tightening

408 – Improvised tourniquet.

the strap after it has been buckled round the limb. *Esmarch's tourniquet* (illustration 409b) consists of an elastic band which is wrapped with moderate tightness round the limb, and then prevented from unwrapping by tapes. It is the form generally used. (See HAEMORRHAGE.) A rubber tube knotted, or fixed with a clip, round the limb (illustration 410) is also often used for arresting the blood-flow. In applying a tourniquet for bleeding, it must be rendered sufficiently tight to stop the circulation completely. Otherwise if the veins only are compressed and the arteries still open, the bleeding is made worse. A

409 – Two simple forms of tourniquet. *a*, An improvised tourniquet, the knot being over the femoral artery, and the lower band being intended simply to keep the handle of the tourniquet from unwinding; *b*, Esmarch's elastic band tourniquet.

410 – A tourniquet improvised from a rubber tube.

tourniquet must not be left in position longer than is absolutely necessary; otherwise gangrene of the limb may result. It must be loosened cautiously after not more than 15 minutes. If bleeding has not stopped, it is tightened again. This procedure must be repeated every 15 minutes.

TOW is a form of jute which is very hygroscopic, absorbing up to 25 per cent of moisture.

TOXAEMIA is a term applied to forms of blood-poisoning due to the absorption of bacterial products (toxins) formed at some local site of infection, such as abscesses. In other cases the toxaemia is due to defective action of some excretory organ, such as the kidney. As regards treatment, the most important consideration is to remove the source of infection.

Toxaemia of pregnancy is a term sometimes used to describe the two complications of pregnancy known as pre-eclampsia and eclampsia (qv).

TOXICOLOGY is the science dealing with poisons. (See POISONS.)

TOXINS are poisons produced by bacteria. (See BACTERIOLOGY; IMMUNITY; SERUM THERAPY.) Toxins are usually soluble, easily destroyed by heat, sometimes of the nature of crystalline substances, and sometimes albumins. When injected into animals in carefully graduated doses, they bring about the formation of substances called antitoxins which neutralize the action of the toxin. These antitoxins are generally produced in excessive amount, and the serum of the animal when withdrawn can be used for conferring antitoxic powers upon other animals or human beings to neutralize the disease in question. The best known of these antitoxins are those of diphtheria and tetanus. Toxins are also found in many plants and in snake venom.

Some toxins are not set free by bacteria, but remain in the substance of the latter and then are known as endotoxins and are not capable of producing antitoxins.

TOXOCARIASIS is a disease acquired by swallowing the ova of a roundworm which lives in the intestine of cats (*Toxocara cati*) or dogs (*Toxocara canis*). In man, the small larval worms produced by these ova migrate to various parts of the body, including the retina of the eye, where they then die, and produce a small granuloma (qv) which in turn may produce allergic reactions. In the eye it may cause choroidretinitis. It is said that 2 per cent of apparently healthy people in Britain have been infected in this way. A course of treatment with diethylcarbamazine is said to kill the worm.

TOXOID is toxin (qv) which has been rendered non-toxic by certain chemicals, or by heat, or by being partly neutralized by antitoxin. The best-known example is diphtheria toxoid. (See IMMUNITY.)

TOXOPLASMOSIS is a disease which is due to infection with protozoa of the genus *Toxoplasma*. The infection may be acquired from eating raw or undercooked meat, from cats, or from gardening or playing in contaminated soil. It occurs in two forms: an acquired form and a congenital form. The acquired form may run such a benign course that it is not recognized, the patient scarcely feeling ill. In the congenital form the unborn child is infected by the mother. The congenital form, in turn, may develop in one of two ways. The infant may either appear generally ill, or the brunt of the infection may fall on the nervous system causing hydrocephalus (qv), mental retardation, or loss of sight. In some cases the infection may be so severe that it kills the foetus, resulting in a miscarriage or stillbirth. In other cases the infection is so mild that it is missed until in later life the child begins to show signs of eye trouble. As the congenital form of the disease, which is most serious, seems to develop only if the mother acquires the infection during pregnancy, it would appear to be a wise precaution that pregnant women should avoid contact with cats and eating raw or undercooked meat foods.

TRACE ELEMENTS are chemical elements that are distributed throughout the tissues of the body in very small amounts and are essential for the nutrition of the body. Nine such elements are now recognized: cobalt, copper, fluorine, iodine, iron, manganese, molybdenum, selenium and zinc.

TRACHEA is another name for the windpipe (qv). (See also AIR PASSAGES.)

TRACHEITIS means inflammation of the trachea. It may occur along with bronchitis, or independently, due to similar causes.

TRACHEOTOMY, or TRACHEOSTOMY, is the operation in which the windpipe is opened from the front of the neck, so that air may obtain direct entrance into the lower air passages. The opening is made through the second and third rings of the trachea (qv).

Reasons for operation – Inflammatory conditions, which lead to narrowing of the opening into the larynx and threaten to prevent the entrance of air, such as diphtheria (qv), laryngo-tracheo-bronchitis (qv) and epiglottitis (qv), may require tracheotomy, in order to provide an opening lower down. Wounds of the larynx, followed by inflammation, as in cutthroat, require it sometimes for the same reason. Or the blockage of the larynx may be due to some foreign body which has gone down into the air passages, or to some tumour growing in the larynx, or tuberculous disease of the vocal cords. It may also be needed in comatose states, such as may accompany head injuries or barbiturate poisoning, to ensure that the lungs are being properly ventilated. Similarly, it may be needed in conditions, such as poliomyelitis or polyneuritis, in which normal breathing is difficult because of interference with the relevant nervous pathways. In young children the operation of *intubation* is sometimes preferred, and, as the tube in this case is pushed in through the mouth, no cutting operation is required. Although intubation of the larynx has several points of advantage, tracheotomy is generally more successful when an operation becomes absolutely necessary.

Tracheotomy tubes – When the trachea has been opened by a vertical slit on its front surface, after division of the skin and separation of the fatty tissue on the neck, it is necessary to introduce a tube in order to keep the opening from closing. The tubes are made either of hard rubber or more often of metal; and there is always an *outer tube* which is fixed in position by tapes passing round the neck, and an *inner tube* which slides freely out of and into the other, so that it may be removed at any time for cleansing, and is readily coughed out should it happen to become blocked by mucus.

A dressing of lint is generally applied between the edges of the outer tube and the wound, while the entrance to the inner tube is protected by a few layers of gauze wrung out of hot water and sprinkled with terebene, so as to form a filter for the air entering the trachea.

The inner tube must be removed and washed several times daily, and if at any time it gets blocked by coughed-up mucus, it must be instantly removed and wiped. The outer tube is not removed till one or two days have elapsed after the operation, and then it is replaced by a fresh tube carefully introduced.

After-treatment – When the operation has been performed for some permanent obstruction, the tube must be worn permanently; and the double metal tube is in such cases replaced after a short time by a soft rubber single one. When the operation has relieved some passing condition like diphtheria, the tube is left out now and then for a few hours, and finally, at the end a week or so, is removed altogether, after which the wound quickly heals up.

TRACHOMA is a chronic, persistent and severe form of conjunctivitis rampant amid the dirt and poverty of the tropics and subtropics, and also found in Eastern and Central Europe. It is the greatest single world cause of serious and progressive loss of sight. It is estimated that there are 400 million victims of the disease, 1 per cent of whom are blinded by the disease. Although one of the oldest known and most widespread of diseases, it was only a few years ago that the cause of it was discovered. Its name is *Chlamydia trachomatis*. Trachoma is characterized by the appearance of nodules, pale in colour, and often compared to boiled sago grains, situated on the conjunctiva lining the lids (illustration 411). Very often the cornea in its upper half becomes covered with a hazy

411 – Trachoma. From Parsons and Duke-Elder, *Diseases of the Eye.* J. & A. Churchill Ltd.

film containing a network of superficial blood-vessels. In the later stages of the disease there is much scarring and shrinking of the conjunctiva, and the lids are apt to be turned inwards, thereby causing the lashes to rub on the cornea. Loss of transparency of the cornea and consequent dimness of vision are therefore common results of this disease.

Treatment is by the local application to the eye of antibiotics, combined with the administration of sulphonamides by mouth. No final decision has yet, been reached as to the best combination of these drugs. The usual course of treatment is chlortetracycline, oxytetracycline or tetracycline, in the form of a 1 per cent ointment in oily suspensions applied to the eye three times or more daily for two months. In addition, the patient is given a triple sulphonamide mixture by mouth, 40 mg per kilogram of body weight daily in divided doses, for 20 successive days. This course of sulphonamides is repeated after a ten-day interval.

TRACTOTOMY (see CORDOTOMY).

TRAGACANTH is a gummy exudation obtained from *Astragalus gummifer*, which swells out and forms a mucilage when mixed with water. It is used as a demulcent, or in mixtures to suspend heavy particles, such as bismuth.

TRAINING (see DIET; EXERCISE).

TRANCE is the term applied to a profound sleep from which a person cannot for a time be aroused, but which is not due to organic disease. The power of voluntary movement is lost, though sensibility and even consciousness may remain. It is usually due to hysteria, and may be induced by hypnotism. (See CATALEPSY; ECSTASY; and SLEEP.)

TRANEXAMIC ACID is a drug used in the control of bleeding. Its mode of action is similar to that of aminocaproic acid (qv).

TRANQUILLIZER – A tranquillizer is a drug which induces a mental state free from agitation and anxiety, and renders the patient calm, serene and peaceful. Strictly speaking, tobacco, alcohol and the barbiturates might be included in this category, but the term 'tranquillizer' is usually restricted to certain new groups of drugs whose main action is the control of anxiety and psychomotor agitation without producing sleepiness, or clouding of consciousness. Among the more widely used drugs in this group are chlorpromazine, reserpine, diazepam and chlordiazepoxide.

TRANSFUSION OF BLOOD is an old method of restoring a person believed to be dying by passing blood from another person into his veins. The practice was in vogue during the seventeenth century, and was performed either by bleeding a healthy person into a basin, and, by means of a syringe, injecting the blood into a cannula previously tied in one of the sick person's veins; or by uniting a vein in the healthy person with one in the sick person by means of two cannulae and a connecting tube, so that the blood passed directly from one to the other. In spite of all speed, the blood introduced by either of these methods was apt to clot; and the practice was adopted of whipping the blood with fine twigs, or straining it through muslin so as to remove its fibrin, and thus introduce merely the serum and blood corpuscles.

TRANSILLUMINATION

Apart from the difficulty caused by the tendency to clot, the major drawback to transfusion is that the corpuscles are liable to break up in the new circulation into which they are introduced; and the person into whom the new blood is transfused may suffer to a dangerous degree from symptoms such as nettle-rash, difficulty of breathing, purging, and signs of shock, whilst the immediate destruction of the red blood corpuscles leads to the passage of blood pigment in the urine and jaundice in some cases. A fatal result may quickly supervene.

To avoid this, it is necessary to find out that the blood of the donor is compatible with the blood already in the circulation of the recipient. (See BLOOD GROUPS.) Whenever possible, this should be done by persons specially trained in the technique. In an emergency in a remote area, however, where such facilities are not available, compatibility of blood can be investigated by a relatively simple technique. A little blood is drawn from the recipient, and a drop of its serum mixed with a minute drop of blood from the donor, which has been allowed to drop into citrate of soda solution. If, in the course of a few minutes, the serum of the recipient causes clotting or breaking up of the donor's corpuscles, the two bloods are incompatible, and another donor of new blood must be chosen and similarly tested. Standard sera can also be obtained for testing the group to which the blood of the donor and that of the recipient belong.

Various methods of transfusion have been used at different times: such as by uniting a vessel in the donor with a vessel in the recipient by means of a short tube, while the two lie side by side; by withdrawing the blood into a syringe and then injecting it through a cannula into the recipient's vein; or, most commonly, by withdrawing the blood from the donor into a large glass vessel, which has been coated with paraffin, and which contains a small amount of citrate of soda solution intended to prevent clotting.

In Great Britain, however, all these methods have been largely given up since the inception, in 1946, of the National Blood Transfusion Service, which is responsible for the collection of blood from voluntary donors and for its storage in blood-banks throughout the country. A standard transfusion bottle has been evolved, with special apparatus for the taking and the giving of blood. When such a set is used with the proper technique, the blood can be safely stored at a temperature of 2° to 6° C for three weeks before use. In addition to whole blood, plasma or serum may be used for transfusion purposes. When stored in the dried form, human plasma and serum have proved to be valuable substitutes for whole blood. In the dried state human plasma is stable for five years provided it is stored at a moderate temperature (4·4° to 21·1° C) and is not exposed to direct sunlight. It is reconstituted by adding pyrogen-free distilled water.

EXCHANGE TRANSFUSION is the method of treatment in severe cases of haemolytic disease of the newborn (qv). It consists of replacing the whole of the baby's blood with Rh-negative blood of the correct blood group for the baby.

TRANSILLUMINATION means the inspection of the interior of a cavity, eg. of one of the sinuses connected with the nose, by means of a strong light passed through its walls, in a dark room. The condition of the cavity as regards the presence of pus or a tumour can thus be readily demonstrated.

TRANSPLANTATION of organs of the body has become a practical possibility within recent years. It is still in its infancy, however, and many problems have to be solved before it can be used on anything like a large scale. The major outstanding problem is how to prevent the recipient's body from rejecting and destroying the transplanted organ. Such rejection of a foreign body is part of the normal protective mechanism of the body and is essential for the maintenance of the integrity of the body.

If the transplant comes from another person it is known as an *allotransplant*. If it comes from the patient himself – for example, a skin graft – it is known as an *autotransplant*. If it comes from an animal it is known as a *xenotransplant*.

Hitherto the major success has been achieved with transplantation of the kidney, and this has been most successful when the transplanted kidney has come from an identical twin. Less successful have been live transplants from other blood relatives, while least successful have been transplants from other live donors and cadaver donors. Thus in its 12th report published in 1975 the Transplantation Registry showed that of 20,000 transplantations reported to it, the survival rate with a life-sustaining transplant at the end of one year was 90 per cent for identical twins, 75 per cent for blood-relative donors, and 55 per cent for cadaver donors. At the end of two years the comparable figures were 86, 70, and 48 per cent, respectively. The longest survival periods were 17 years when the donor was an identical twin, 14 years for a blood-relative donation, and 11 years for a cadaver donation. In the United Kingdom the number of kidney transplants was 706, but this is far short of the 2000 to 3000 patients who could benefit from one. This tragic discrepancy is largely due to the lack of kidneys, which in turn, is due to the failure of people to donate their kidneys for this purpose when they die. Donor cards for the purpose are now available in all general practitioners' surgeries and pharmacies. The tragedy is that of the 16 million cards distributed since 1972, so few have been used.

Drugs are now available that can temporarily depress the immune reactions of the recipient, which are responsible for the rejection of the transplanted organ. By means of these drugs it has proved possible to transplant kidneys, not only from near relatives, but also from cadavers. By these and other means, such as careful typing of the donor kidney, results are steadily improving. One of the more promising developments is the development of an anti-lymphocytic serum (ALS) which reduces the activity of the lymphocytes (qv), cells which play an important part in maintaining the integrity of the body against foreign bodies. Other organs that have been transplanted are the heart, the lungs, the liver, bone marrow, and the cornea of the eye. With the exception of the last two of these, the transplantation has never been more than temporarily successful but the results are improving. Thus, in one centre in U.S.A., of 150 heart transplantations done in a 10-year period (1968–78), the one-year survival rate was 70 per cent, and one patient is still alive eight years after the operation. The heart, however, seems to be more liable to rejection than the kidney. The liver seems to be less susceptible to rejection, and of the 200 patients who have had the operation, one is alive eight years after transplantation, and has given birth to a normal child. (See also DONORS.)

TRANS-SEXUALISM is the psychosexual abnormality characterized by feelings of belonging to the gender opposite to that of the genitalia and the secondary sex characteristics.

TRANSVESTITISM, or TRANSVESTISM, is the term given to a psycho-sexual abnormality in which there is a repetitive compulsion to dress in the clothes of the opposite sex to achieve orgasm.

TRAUMA is the term used to indicate disorders due to wounds or injuries.

TRAVEL MEDICINE – There are reciprocal health arrangements with the other European Economic Community (EEC) countries and with the following countries – Austria, Bulgaria, the Channel Islands, Czechoslovakia, German Democratic Republic (East Germany), Gibraltar, Malta, New Zealand, Norway, Poland, Romania, Sweden, USSR, and Yugoslavia – under which British visitors may receive emergency treatment free or at reduced cost. Information about these arrangements is available in leaflets SA28 (EEC countries) and SA30 (other countries), which may be obtained from Leaflets Unit, Department of Health and Social Security, Government Buildings, Honeypot Lane, Stanmore, Middlesex HA7 1AY, or from local offices of the Department. The Department also publishes a useful leaflet (SA 35), *Notice to Travellers: Health Protection,* which gives information about the health aspects of foreign travel, such as personal protection against various diseases and the like. This is available free of charge from International Relations Division, Room D312, Alexander Fleming House, Elephant and Castle, London SE1 6BY, or through travel agents.

TRAVEL SICKNESS is the sickness that is induced by any form of transport, whether by sea, air, motor-car or train. (See SEA-SICKNESS.)

TREATMENT – Special forms of treatment are considered under such headings as DIET; LIGHT TREATMENT; SERUM THERAPY. The treatment appropriate to each disease will be found under the headings of the various diseases.

TREMOR means a very fine kind of jerking spasm. Tremors may be seen in projecting parts like the hands, head and tongue, or they may involve muscles or even the individual fibres of a muscle here and there. They are of various grades of fineness. Very coarse tremors, which prevent a person from drinking a glass of water without spilling it, are found in multiple sclerosis and in chorea (see under these headings); somewhat finer tremors, which produce trembling of the hands or tongue when they are stretched out, are caused by alcoholism (see ALCOHOLISM,

CHRONIC), by poisoning with other substances like lead, by Parkinsonism (qv), and by the weakness which follows some acute disease or characterizes old age; a fine tremor of the outstretched fingers is a characteristic of thyrotoxicosis (see GOITRE); very fine tremors, visible in the muscles of face or limbs, and known as fibrillary tremors, are present in general paralysis of the insane, and in progressive muscular atrophy or wasting palsy.

TRENCH FEVER is an infectious disease caused by *Rickettsia quintana* which is transmitted by the body louse. Large epidemics occurred among troops on active service during the 1914–18 War. It recurred on a smaller scale in the 1939–1945 War, and is endemic in Mexico.

TREPHINING, or TREPANNING, is an operation in which a portion of the cranium is removed. Originally the operation was performed with an instrument resembling a carpenter's brace and known as the trephine or trepan, which removes a small circle of bone; but now this instrument is only used, as a rule, for making small openings, whilst, for wider operations, gouge forceps, circular saws driven by electric motor, or wire saws are employed in order to give greater ease and speed.

The operation is one requiring nicety of manipulation, but is neither difficult nor serious, and was one of the commonest major operations of antiquity. It is said, from the appearances presented by skulls found in old French burial mounds, to have been practised by prehistoric peoples; at all events Hippocrates describes fully the operation and the conditions that call for it, whilst Galen mentions two varieties of the instrument in common use. Both among the Greeks and Romans, and in the Middle Ages, resort seems to have been made to trephining on very slight provocation for conditions traceable to the head.

At the present time, the conditions under which it may be thought advisable to trephine the skull are chiefly as follows. In cases of fracture, with splintering of the skull, the operation is performed to remove the fragments of bone and any foreign bodies, like a bullet, which may have entered, in order that the wound may be thoroughly cleansed. In compression of the brain with unconsciousness following an injury, the skull is trephined and any blood-clots removed, or torn vessels ligatured. When an abscess is present within

the skull, the operation is called for in order to evacuate the pus. In certain forms of epilepsy, or in continued headache, when the symptoms point to a definite part of the brain being involved, the skull may be trephined over this area, so that any clot, scar, thickening of the bone or cyst, which is setting up the irritation, may be discovered and removed. For a cerebral tumour, trephining is often performed either with the view of removing the tumour, if that be possible, or at all events of relieving the great pressure within the skull caused by the growing mass.

TREPONEMA is the name of a genus of spirochaetal micro-organisms which consist of slender spirals and which progress by means of bending movements. *Treponema pallidum* (formerly called *Spirochaeta pallida*) is the causative organism of syphilis.

TRIAMCINOLONE is one of the newer corticosteroids, which has a potency equivalent to that of prednisone, but is less likely to cause retention of sodium.

TRIAMTERINE is a diuretic which is active when taken by mouth.

TRICHIASIS means a diseased condition of the eyelids, generally the result of old-standing inflammation, in which the eyelashes grow inwards towards the eye so as to cause great pain and irritation. (See EYE DISEASES.)

TRICHINIASIS (see TRICHINOSIS).

TRICHINOSIS, or TRICHINIASIS, is the name of a disease set up by eating diseased pork, in which the immature *Trichinella spiralis* is encysted. The full-grown female worm, which inhabits the intestine, is $\frac{1}{8}$ inch (3 mm) in length, and the larvae, to whose movements the disease is due, are much smaller (illustration 412). The disease is acquired by eating raw or underdone pork from pigs that have been infected with the worm. When such a piece of meat is eaten, the embryos contained in it are set free, develop into full-grown trichinellae, and from each pair of these 1000 or more new embryos may arise in a few weeks. So soon as this new generation of embryos is produced they bore their way into the wall of the bowel, setting up sometimes severe irritation and diarrhoea, and thence wander all over the body, finally depositing themselves between the fibres of

412 – *Trochinella spiralis*. A, adult female; B, larva; C, adult male. From Macfarlane, *A Short Synopsis of Human Protozoology and Helminthology*. E. & S. Livingstone.

the voluntary muscles. During this migration, which lasts four or five weeks, they set up fever and pain in the limbs and muscles, often mistaken for rheumatism. Death may even result, but if the person survives to the end of four or five weeks, the trichinellae, which are now encysted in the muscles (illustration 413), give no further trouble.

Prevention is based on thorough inspection of meat in slaughter-houses, for even cooking, unless the meat be in slices, is not an efficient protection. Pigs should not be fed on unboiled garbage. Rats may be a source of sporadic outbreaks, as infected rats have been found near piggeries. The disease is now a rare one, thanks to sanitary inspection though it still occurs in these parts of the country, such as the Midlands, where raw sausage meat is considered a delicacy. The encysted trichinellae are just visible as fine white specks.

Treatment – In the early stages, tetra-

413 – Larva of *Trichinella spiralis* in muscle. From Macfarlane, *A Short Synopsis of Human Protozoology and Helminthology*. E. & S. Livingstone.

chloroethylene, followed by a sharp purge, is of value. Recently, thiabendazole, which has proved of value in the treatment of affected pigs, has been used with promising results in human victims.

TRICHLOROETHYLENE, also known as TRILENE, is a volatile anaesthetic which has the advantages of being nonirritant and of inducing anaesthesia rapidly and pleasantly. It has been used mainly for inducing analgesia or light anaesthesia in obstetrics and dentistry. In an impure form it is used commercially in the dry-cleaning industry.

TRICHO- is a prefix denoting relation to hair.

TRICHOMONAS VAGINALIS is a protozoon normally present in the vagina of about 30 to 40 per cent of women. It sometimes becomes pathogenic and causes inflammation of the genital passages, with vaginal discharge. A man may become infected and have a urethral discharge as a result; it may also cause prostatitis. Excellent results are being obtained from the use of metronidazole in its treatment. To obtain a satisfactory result it may be necessary to treat the husband as well as the wife.

TRICHOPHYTON is the name of the vegetable parasite that causes ringworm. (See RINGWORM.)

TRICHORRHOEA is the term applied to the falling-out of hair. It is usually due to some general disease such as scarlet fever or typhoid fever. When there is no obvious cause, such as this, treatment consists of attention to the general hygiene of the scalp. Vigorous massage is to be avoided.

TRICHOTILLOMANIA is the term given to the condition in which a person has an obsessional impulse to pull out his own hair.

TRICHURIASIS is a worldwide infection, particularly common in the tropics. It is caused by *Trichuris trichiura*, or whipworm, so called because of its shape, the rear end being stout and the front end hairlike, resembling the lash of a whip. The male measures 2 inches (5 cm) and the female $1\frac{1}{2}$ inches (4 cm) in length. Infection results from eating vegetables, or drinking water, polluted with the ova (eggs). These

TRICRESOL

hatch out in the large intestine. The diagnosis is made by finding the eggs in the stools. The worms seldom cause any trouble unless they are present in large numbers when, especially in malnourished children, they may cause bleeding from the bowels, anaemia and prolapse of the rectum. The most effective drug at the moment is mebendazole: 100 mg twice daily for three days.

TRICRESOL is the name of a clear, colourless, strongly antiseptic mixture of the three forms of cresol. It may be mixed with water in any proportions. (For uses see CRESOL.)

TRICUSPID VALVE is the valve, with three cusps or flaps, that guards the opening from the right atrium into the right ventricle of the heart. (See HEART.)

TRIGEMINAL NERVE is the fifth cranial nerve. It consists of three divisions: (1) the ophthalmic nerve, which is purely sensory in function, being distributed mainly over the forehead and front part of the scalp; (2) the maxillary nerve, which is also sensory and distributed to the skin of the cheek, the mucous membrane of the mouth and throat, and the upper teeth; and (3) the mandibular nerve, which is the nerve of sensation to the lower part of the face, the tonngue and the lower teeth, as well as being the motor nerve to the muscles concerned in chewing. The trigeminal nerve is of special interest, owing to its liability to neuralgia (qv), trigeminal neuralgia (qv), or tic douloureux as it is also known, being the most painful form known of neuralgia.

TRIGEMINAL NEURALGIA, or TIC DOULOUREUX as it is also known, is one of the most severe forms of neuralgia. It affects the great nerve of sensation in the face (trigeminal nerve), and may occur in one or more of the three divisions in which the nerve is distributed. It is usually confined to one side. Women suffer, on the whole, more often than men, and they are usually over the age of 50. The attack is often precipitated by movements of the jaw, as in talking or eating, or by tactile stimuli such as a cold wind or washing the face. When the *first or upper division of the nerve* is involved, the pain is mostly felt in the forehead and side of the head. It is usually of an intensely sharp, cutting, or burning character, either constant or with exacerbations, and often periodic, returning at a certain hour each day while the attack

886

continues. Occasionally the paroxysms are of extreme violence, and are brought on by the slightest provocation, such as a draught of cool air. The skin over the affected part is often red and swollen, and, even after the attack has abated, feels stiff and tender to the touch. As in all forms of neuralgia, there are certain localities where the pain is more intense, these painful points, as they are called, being for the most part in those places where the branches of the nerves emerge from bony canals or pierce the fascia to ramify in the skin. Hence, in this form, the greater severity of the pain above the eyebrow and along the side of the nose. There is also pain in the eyelid, redness of the eye and increased flow of tears. When *the second division of the nerve* is affected, the pain is chiefly in the cheek and upper jaw, the painful points being immediately below the lower eyelid, over the cheekbone and about the upper lip. This form is accompanied by pain of similar character to that affecting the first division; the pain often appears suddenly on slight provocation such as by taking a mouthful of hot or cold fluid. When *the third division of the nerve* suffers, the pain affects the lower jaw, and the chief painful points are in front of the ear and above the chin. Attacks of tic douloureux, extremely distressing as they are, may recur for years; and although, by depriving the sufferer of sleep and interfering with the taking of food, they may in some measure impair the health, they rarely appear to lead to any serious results. Nevertheless, the pain may be so intolerable as to make life a burden.

Treatment – The outlook in trigeminal neuralgia has been radically altered by the introduction of the drug carbamazepine, which is proving of outstanding value in relieving the pain of what is one of the most devastating of all forms of neuralgia. In view of its potential side-effects, it must only be taken under medical supervision. The introduction of this drug has radically cut down the need for killing the ganglion of the nerve, or its branches, by the injection of alcohol, electrocoagulation, percutaneous or radio frequency gangliolysis, or rhizotomy (qv).

TRIGGER FINGER, or SNAPPING FINGER, is the condition in which when the fingers are straightened on unclenching the fist one finger, usually the ring or middle finger, remains bent. The cause is obscure. In severe cases treatment consists of opening up the sheath surrounding the tendon of the affected finger. When confined to the thumb it is known as TRIGGER THUMB.

TRIGGER THUMB (see TRIGGER FINGER).

TRIGONE is the base of the bladder between the openings of the two ureters and of the urethra.

TRIIODOTHYRONINE is the substance which exerts the physiological action of thyroid hormone. It is formed in the body cells by the de-iodination of thyroxine (tetra-iodothyronine) which is the active principle secreted by the thyroid gland. It has also been synthesized, and is now available for the treatment of myxoedema (qv). It is three times as potent as thyroxine. (See also THYROID GLAND.)

TRILENE (see TRICHLOROETHYLENE).

TRIMIPRAMINE is a relatively weak antidepressant drug which also acts as a sedative.

TRIMUSTINE is a nitrogen mustard derivative (qv) used in the treatment of certain forms of malignant disease. It is administered intravenously.

TRINITRIN (see GLYCERYL TRINITRATE).

TRIPLETS (see MULTIPLE BIRTHS).

TRISMUS is another name for lockjaw. (See TETANUS.)

TROCAR is an instrument provided with a sharp three-sided point fitted inside a tube or cannula, and used for puncturing cavities of the body in which fluid has collected.

TROCHANTER is the name given to two bony prominences at the upper end of the thigh-bone. The *greater trochanter* can be felt on the outer side of the thigh. The *lesser trochanter* is a small prominence on the inner side of this bone.

TROCHES is another name for lozenges. (See LOZENGES.)

TROCHLEAR NERVE is the name of the fourth cranial nerve, which acts upon the superior oblique muscle of the eye.

TROPHIC is a term applied to the influence that nerves exert with regard to the

healthiness and nourishment of the parts to which they run. When the nerves become diseased or injured, this influence is lost and the muscles waste, while the skin loses its healthy appearance and is liable to break down into ulcers. (See NERVOUS DISEASES; BED SORES.)

TROPHOBLAST is the outer layer of the fertilized ovum which attaches the ovum to the wall of the uterus (or womb) and supplies nutrition to the embryo.

TROPICAL DISEASES – This term includes some diseases that occur in temperate climates, but are more common or more severe in hot latitudes; as well as some that are found only in the tropics. (See ANCYLOSTOMIASIS; BERIBERI; BLACK-WATER FEVER; CHOLERA; CLIMATE; CLOTHING; DENGUE; DRACONTIASIS; DYSENTERY; ELEPHANTIASIS; FILARIASIS; FRAMBOESIA; HEAT-STROKE; HOOKWORM; LEISHMANIASIS; LEPROSY; LIVER, DISEASES OF; MALARIA; ORIENTAL SORE; PLAGUE; PRICKLY HEAT; SCHISTOSOMIASIS; SLEEPING SICKNESS; STRONGLYLOIDIASIS; SUNBURN; YELLOW FEVER.)

TROXIDONE is the *British Pharmacopoeia* name of one of the most effective drugs for the treatment of *petit mal.*

TRUSS is an instrument used to support a hernia, or to retain the protruding organ within the cavity from which it tends to pass.
Varieties of truss – The nature of trusses varies according to the situation of the opening which the truss has to cover; but every truss possesses a pad of some sort to cover the opening and a belt or spring to keep it in position.
VENTRAL TRUSSES intended for a hernia protruding through the wall of the abdomen, either at the navel or at some weak spot caused by a strain or by a wound, consist of a large flat pad kept in position by a belt passing round the waist. Sometimes a small pad made to fit the opening is adopted, but this is a mistake, as its pressure tends to enlarge the aperture.
INGUINAL TRUSSES are much more commonly required than any other, and though many forms are made by different makers, all possess an oval obliquely placed pad with a spring pressing upon it. In the *ordinary truss* (illustration 414), there is a spring firmly fixed at one end to the pad, from which it passes right round the waist, to be bound at the other end by

414 – Simple truss for right inguinal hernia.

415 – Truss for double inguinal hernia.

416 – Double truss with celluloid pads in position.

a short strap to the pad. Also there is a short strap passing down between the legs and fastened to the truss before and behind so as to keep the pad from slipping upwards as the person moves. This is one of the cheapest and most generally used forms. *Double trusses* (illustrations 415, 416) are fashioned like the ordinary truss. but have a pad for each side, and are advisable in the case of very stout people, in whom the retention of a hernia upon one side is sometimes apt to produce a hernia at the other side.

FEMORAL TRUSSES are made in various forms similar to those of inguinal trusses. The pad, which comes down on the thigh, is small and triangular, so as not to press upon the femoral vessels. Such a truss is difficult to keep in position, and this is sometimes effected by having attached to

the pad a thigh-piece which can be laced on the outer side of the thigh.

Before applying a truss the wearer must make certain that the hernia has been reduced. This may mean lying down before applying the truss. The skin should be washed twice daily with soap and water, then wiped gently with surgical spirit, and finally dusted with some benign dusting powder. In this way there is little risk of the underlying skin becoming sore and irritated. Saddle soap is used to keep the leather parts of the truss in good condition.

TRYPANOSOMA is the name of a genus of microscopic parasites, several of which are responsible for causing sleeping sickness and some allied diseases. (See SLEEPING SICKNESS.)

TRYPANOSOMIASIS (see SLEEPING SICKNESS).

TRYPSIN is the name applied to the chief protein ferment of the pancreatic secretion. It changes proteins into peptones and forms the main constituent of pancreatic extracts used for digestion of food. (See PANCREAS; and PEPTONIZED FOOD.)

TSETSE FLY is the name of an African fly of the genus *Glossina*. One or more of these is responsible for carrying the trypanosome which causes sleeping sickness and thus spreads the disease among cattle and from cattle to men. (Illustration 371.)

TSUTSUGAMUSHI, or JAPANESE RIVER FEVER, is a disease of the typhus group. (See TYPHUS.)

TUBERCLE is a term used in two distinct senses. As a descriptive term in anatomy, a *tubercle* means a small elevation or roughness upon a bone, such as the tubercles of the ribs. In the pathological sense, a *tubercle* is a small mass, barely visible to the naked eye, formed in some organ as the starting-point of tuberculosis (illustration 417). The name of *tubercle bacillus* was originally given to the microorganism that causes this disease but this has now been changed to *Mycobacterium tuberculosis*. The term tubercular should strictly be applied to anything connected with or resembling tubercles or nodules, and the term *tuberculous* to anything pertaining to the disease tuberculosis.

When *Mycobacteria tuberculosis* have

417 – Section of tubercle (highly magnified). The tubercle is surrounded by a zone of normal tissue. The ring of dark dots round the tubercle are leucocytes. Inside the tubercle five giant cells are seen.

gained entrance to an organ, no matter whether inhaled, or whether absorbed from food and circulated through the lymphatics or blood-vessels, the following results ensue. The individual bacilli multiply, and around each group forms a minute tubercle, or granule, which is of a size almost invisible to the naked eye, and greyish in colour. These tubercles fuse together, and, at the same time, soften to a cheesy substance, so as to form yellow bodies about the size of pin-heads. Each grey tubercle, under the microscope, shows the appearance of a group of cells of medium size (epithelioid cells), surrounded by many smaller cells (connective tissue cells and white blood corpuscles), attracted to the spot as a result of the inflammation set up. Scattered between these cells lie the mycobacteria. Near the centre of the older tubercles there are often seen one or more large cells with many nuclei (giant cells). The larger yellow tubercles form a more or less structureless mass in the centre, but show numbers of the small grey tubercles round their edge. Thus the process spreads, the healthy tissue being broken down and giving place to the soft, cheesy mass, which, in the case of the lungs, finally bursts into a bronchial tube, is coughed

up, and leaves a ragged cavity in its place. Another change, however, takes place at the same time, for, in consequence of the irritation set up by the tubercle, strands of fibrous tissue are built up round its edge, and, when the process is a very chronic one, these come to form a dense capsule for the tuberculous area, cutting it off from further advance on healthy tissue, and forming Nature's cure.

TUBERCULIDE is the term given to any skin lesion which is the result of infection with the tubercle bacillus, or *Mycobacterium tuberculosis* as it is now known.

TUBERCULIN is the name originally given by Koch in 1890 to a preparation derived from the tubercle bacillus, or *Mycobacterium tuberculosis* as it is now known, and intended for the diagnosis or treatment of tuberculosis.

Varieties – *Old Tuberculin* (OT) is the heat-concentrated filtrate from a fluid medium on which the human or bovine type of *Mycobacterium tuberculosis* has been grown for six weeks or more. It contains 100,000 Units per millilitre, and the final product is distributed in sterile glass containers which are sealed to exclude micro-organisms. The standardization, or biological assay as it is known, is done by comparison with the Standard Preparation. This consists of a concentrate of the culture filtrate of the human type of *Mycobacterium tuberculosis* in a 50 per cent w/v solution of glycerol. The unit of tuberculin is contained in 0·000011111 millilitre of the Standard Preparation of Old Tuberculin. Thus, 1 millilitre contains 90,000 Units. *Tuberculin Purified Protein Derivative* (Tuberculin PPD) is the active principle of Old Tuberculin, and is prepared from the fluid medium on which the *Mycobacterium tuberculosis* has been grown. It is supplied as a liquid, a powder, or as sterile tablets. The liquid contains 100,000 Units per millilitre, and the dry powder contains 30,000 Units per milligram. It is distributed in sterile containers sealed so as to exclude micro-organisms. It is more constant in composition and potency than Old Tuberculin.

Uses – The basis of the tuberculin reaction is that any person who has been infected with the *Mycobacterium tuberculosis* gives a reaction when a small amount of tuberculin is injected into the skin. This reaction consists of an inflammatory area, at least 5 mm in diameter, which develops at the site of the test within two to four days of the test being made. If the area is less than 5 mm in diameter the reaction is said to be negative. A negative reaction means that either the individual has never been infected with the tubercle bacillus, or that the infection has been too recent to have allowed of sensitivity developing. The only exceptions are that occasionally a negative reaction may be obtained in tuberculous subjects (*a*) in severe forms of the disease, (*b*) during pregnancy, (*c*) during an intercurrent infection.

To avoid serious reactions the test must be carried out in the first instance with a dilution of tuberculin of 1/10,000. If no reaction is obtained, the strength can be gradually increased: 1/1000; 1/100; 1/10. The amount used of any dilution is 0·1 millilitre.

There are various methods of carrying out the test, of which the following are the most commonly used. The *Mantoux Test* is the most satisfactory of all and has the advantage that the size of the reaction is a guide to the severity of the tuberculous infection. It is performed by injecting the tuberculin into the skin on the forearm. The *Heaf Multiple Puncture Test* is being used on an increasing scale because of its simplicity and reliability. It is carried out with the multiple puncture apparatus, or Heaf Gun, which enables six punctures to be made of equal depth: 2 mm for adults, 1 mm for children, depending upon which of the two detachable endpieces is used. The *Vollmer Patch Test* is particularly useful in children because of the ease with which it can be carried out. A piece of filter paper impregnated with tuberculin is fastened to the skin with adhesive plaster and left in position for forty-eight hours.

TUBERCULOSIS is the general name for the whole group of diseases associated with the presence of the *Mycobacterium tuberculosis*, of which pulmonary tuberculosis is the most important. (See BACTERIOLOGY.)

Tuberculosis not only affects the lungs, but may invade almost any organ, being seldom found, however, in the muscles or in tissues with few blood-vessels, like cartilage and sinews. The disease spreads usually by way of the lymphatic vessels. The severity of the disease varies considerably, according to the organ attacked – thus tuberculosis affecting the membranes of the brain and causing meningitis is a particularly dangerous disease, especially in infants and young children. Chronic inflammation of bones and white swelling of joints are manifestations of the disease, having less influence upon the general health. The enlargement of glands, most common in the neck, to which the name of scrofula was formerly given, because the swollen neck gives to the physiognomy a pig-like expression, is a well-known form of tuberculous disease. This form of the disease seems to have been much more widespread in former times, and was known also as 'king's evil', from the superstition that a touch of the royal hand conveyed a cure to the affected person. Many chronic abscesses are tuberculous in origin, arising from this affection in a bone, a gland, or the cellular tissue. The disfiguring skin disease known as lupus vulgaris is another of the manifestations of the disease. Other sites in which tuberculosis is apt to occur are the bowels and the genito-urinary tract: ie. the kidneys, bladder and epididymis.

Consumption, or phthisis, is the name given, in popular language, to tuberculosis. It dates from the days when there was no effective treatment for tuberculosis, and the disease tended to be characterized by a rapid or gradual wasting away of the body. The term, phthisis, was usually restricted to that form of the disease in which the infection was restricted to the lungs: ie. pulmonary tuberculosis.

The essential part of the disease, from which it receives its name of tuberculosis, is the formation in the substance of an organ of tubercles (illustration 417), fine granules of a size barely visible to the naked eye, these tubercles multiplying and changing in such a way as to lead finally to the destruction of the organ in which they are found.

Nature of the disease – Tuberculosis has been recognized as a disease from the earliest times. Hippocrates (460–375 BC) bestowed the name of phthisis upon the disease as it affects the lungs, and descriptions of the condition are found in the writings of classical authors. About AD 980 Haly Abbas of Baghdad, and again in 1779 Cullen, recognized the infectious nature of phthisis, but not till after the middle of the nineteenth century was it proved, by means of inoculating animals with tuberculous material from phthisical patients, that tuberculosis is really an infective disease, and that the tubercles result from an inflammatory process, due to some poison introduced with the diseased products. The nature of the poison was much disputed till 1882, when Koch announced the discovery of the tubercle bacillus, or *Mycobacterium tuberculosis* as it is known, and so answered this important question.

The manner in which these bacilli gain access to the body is important. There are three possible channels:

(*a*) BY INOCULATION – A person may prick himself with a knife contaminated by the sputum of a tuberculous patient, or may rub some of this material into a cut. Generally this results merely in a local skin disease, and it occurs only in doctors, nurses and others dealing with tuberculous patients.

(*b*) BY INHALATION – The sputum and other discharges from tuberculous persons swarm with bacilli. It has been calculated that a person suffering from a cavity in the lung may spit up 4,000,000,000 bacilli in the course of twenty-four hours, and each of these, when dried and blown about on dust, is potent for evil. Neither drying, nor freezing, nor putrefaction, nor the lapse of months destroys these bacilli, but direct sunlight is speedily fatal to them, so that dust which has lain for a short time in the open on a bright day becomes rapidly harmless. In rooms inhabited by tuberculous patients, and in hospital wards, the dust from the floor often contains *Mycobacterium tuberculosis*.

Probably almost all cases in which this disease primarily affects the lungs are due to inhalation of dust laden with the bacilli or inhalation of droplets coughed into the air by a tuberculous patient, whilst those cases in which the glands of the neck are first attacked arise by absorption of the bacilli through the tonsils.

That this manner of infection is of great importance is shown by the fact that, of all persons dying of tuberculous diseases generally in England and Wales over nine-tenths die from this disease as it affects the lungs.

(*c*) BY INGESTION – It has long been known that tuberculosis, like other infectious diseases, can be conveyed by means of milk and other articles of food, and, acting upon this belief, sanitary authorities have enforced regulations designed to protect the public from the effects of consuming diseased meat and milk. In the case of meat there is practically no danger, as the muscular tissues are exempt from the disease, and those parts which are diseased being, in the 'dressing' of the meat, carefully removed, any accidental contact with them is rendered harmless by the cooking of the meat.

The Royal Commission on Tuberculosis in its report issued in 1907, as well as various other observers, found that the bovine tubercle bacillus was present in a large proportion of diseased glands in children. It has also been found that in tuberculosis affecting the bones and joints of children from one-third to one-half are caused by the bovine bacillus, the rest by the human bacillus. We may therefore conclude that the tissues of healthy human adults are more capable of resisting the bacillus of bovine source than are those of children, but that bovine tuberculosis may be, and often is, communicated through milk to children.

Much progress has been made of recent years in eradicating tuberculosis from cattle in this country, and on October 1, 1960, the Ministry of Agriculture, Fisheries and Food declared the whole of Great Britain an attested area, thus marking the successful completion of the official scheme to eradicate bovine tuberculosis as a disease of cattle on a nation-wide scale. Even though milk from such attested cattle, as they are known, is safe to drink from the point of tuberculosis, it is still a wise precaution to allow children to drink only pasteurized milk.

Mortality – The figures in table 40 show the steady decline in the number of deaths due to tuberculosis in England and Wales. In England in 1977 there were 473 deaths from respiratory tuberculosis and 425

891

	Respiratory	Other forms	All forms
1851–1860	1336	1926	1438
1861–1870	1236	1872	1346
1871–1880	1063	1796	1190
1881–1890	863	1682	1004
1891–1900	675	1525	815
1901–1910	540	1232	649
1911–1920	479	898	541
1921–1930	336	524	362
1931–1939	223	336	245
1940–1944	209	309	221
1945–1949	169	204	174
1950–1954	85	82	85
1955–1959	37	31	36
1966	16	14	16

Table 40 – Tuberculosis Standardized Mortality Ratios for England and Wales.

deaths from other forms of the disease. In the same year, notifications of all forms of tuberculosis totalled 9051; of these, 6718 were respiratory tuberculosis.

A much larger number of the population suffer from early tuberculosis (it may be quite unsuspected) and recover. This is proved by the frequent presence on X-ray examination of old calcified tuberculous glands and by healed scars in the lungs found at post-mortem examination.

Causes – The direct cause of the disease is the tubercle bacillus, or *Mycobacterium tuberculosis*. (See BACTERIOLOGY.) But, in view of the fact that many people suffer from the disease in a mild degree and afterwards recover, and that many limited cases of tuberculosis in bones, skin and glands are successfully treated, it appears that there are other factors which determine whether a given case is serious or not, and whether it is likely to proceed towards recovery, if properly treated, or to end inevitably in death.

HEREDITY – There is probably a hereditary element in the predisposition to the disease. Over a long period those who are susceptible are gradually eliminated by the disease.

AGE is an important point. Young children are liable to tuberculosis affecting the bowels and the glands connected with them, and the meninges of the brain. At a slightly later age there is a greater tendency to that type of the disease formerly known as scrofula, the glands of the neck particularly being affected, and the greatest mortality from lung (or pulmonary) tuberculosis takes place after the age of 20 is reached. In recent years there has been an increasing incidence of respiratory, or pulmonary, tuberculosis in old folk. In England, in 1970, of the 819 deaths from respiratory tuberculosis, more than one-half, 445, occurred in people aged 65 years or over, and 169 of these occurred in people aged 75 and over.

ATMOSPHERE – The character of the atmosphere in which work is carried on has much to do with the onset of tuberculosis. Those who habitually live and work in ill-ventilated rooms are at a great disadvantage compared with those who lead an open-air life, or, at all events, keep their rooms well ventilated. Further, the amount and nature of the dust in the air are highly important.

OTHER DISEASES are of great importance in relation to tuberculosis. For example, a person who has long suffered from asthma or bronchitis may develop tuberculosis in the end, and diabetics not uncommonly contract this disease, but this has occurred less often since the introduction of insulin. It is not uncommon that a person suffers from tuberculosis and apparently recovers; then, when some business reverse or family trouble comes, the disease reappears.

Varieties – The forms of tuberculosis other than pulmonary tuberculosis, such as tuberculous disease of joints, bones and spine, meningitis, lupus, are considered under these headings. The lung disease has, however, itself several varieties, differing much from one another.

1. ACUTE MILIARY TUBERCULOSIS – In this form not only the lungs but the whole body becomes studded with the tubercles of the disease as a result of rupture of a tubercle or tuberculous gland into the blood stream, and the resultant dissemination of mycobacteria by the blood stream throughout the body. Untreated the sufferer dies, from fever and exhaustion, in two or three weeks. This is the most rapid form, and, with the second variety, constituted what was for long known as 'Galloping Consumption'.

2. ACUTE CASEOUS TUBERCULOSIS is a slightly slower form. The lungs only are affected, and, either in consequence of the bacilli inhaled into the lungs being specially virulent, or, more likely, owing to the person having acquired no immunity to the disease, or being in a particularly weak state, or of unhealthy constitution, tubercles form, undergo the caseous change, and break down to form cavities with great rapidity (illustration 418), the patient dying in two or three months.

3. FIBRO-CASEOUS TUBERCULOSIS is the usual form and may last for years. The change which occurs in the lungs is very much the same as in the last form, but, in addition, and in consequence of greater resisting power on the sufferer's part, there is

an attempt at nature's cure, and much fibrous tissue is formed. The lung becomes denser, cavities gradually form here and there, and the downward progress is slow or may be arrested.

4. FIBROID TUBERCULOSIS is a form in which areas of the lung are converted into fibrous masses, which are in reality scars of previous disease that has undergone nature's cure, and there are no cavities.

Symptoms – In the following brief account, the symptoms of an average case, in which fibrous formation and the caseous change leading to production of a cavity take place side by side, will be described. They fall conveniently into three stages of the disease:

(a) EARLY STAGE – In this stage the tubercles are being deposited in the lung, almost always near the apex; and this part of the lung becomes, in consequence, more solid. There is cough of an irritative nature, particularly in the morning, either without any expectoration or accompanied by a little clear mucus. Sometimes, the first sign of all is the spitting up of blood (haemoptysis), which is never copious at this stage, and is due to congestion caused by the irritation of the tubercles. (See HAEMORRHAGE.) There is generally, from the first, loss of appetite, colour and

418 – Lung showing acute caseous tuberculosis, with large masses of caseous material in the upper half, breaking down to form numerous large cavities. In the lower part are numerous scattered tubercles.

strength, followed soon by actual emaciation and loss of weight. Perspiration upon slight exertion is usual, and, very often, night sweats are a symptom. An important sign is a regular rise of temperature, either in the forenoon, or more often in the early afternoon, with a fall below normal in the early morning, but this is not an invariable symptom at this stage. The digestive functions are usually thrown out of gear, and there is apt to be sickness, diarrhoea or constipation. A slight attack of pleurisy, causing pain in the chest, is often a precursor of, or accompanies, these symptoms. This is the stage in which the disease is readily curable.

(b) STAGE OF ADVANCING DISEASE – By this time, the tubercles have fused to form caseous masses, and these are breaking down and being spat up, leaving a ragged cavity, while the disease is slowly advancing to new areas of the lung. The surface of the cavity becomes infected sooner or later with other inhaled organisms, and these keep up the ulcerative process on the surface of the cavity and prevent its healing. The symptoms are mainly an increase of those present in the first stage. The cough is more troublesome and the spit is thick and yellow, contains large numbers of bacilli, which can be stained and microscopically examined, and is occasionally streaked with blood. The sufferer is much weaker, and has greatly lost in weight. The temperature is of a swinging hectic type, rising to 100° or 101° F (37·8° or 38·3° C) in the late afternoon and falling, sometimes below normal, in the early part of the day. Drenching night sweats are apt to break out during sleep in the early hours of the morning, and attacks of vomiting or diarrhoea are not infrequent. The disease may at this stage be found in both lungs or in other organs, such as the throat or intestine, with which the sputum comes in contact. An important sign is that of falling in of the chest over the excavated area, so that a flat place or depression is found in its upper part.

(c) LATE STAGE – In this stage, large cavities have usually formed in the lung, or there has been a production of fibrous tissue, the lung being shrunken and consisting of a mass of matted fibrous tissue and smaller cavities. Accordingly, the whole side has usually fallen in considerably. The second lung is by this time extensively affected; the voice may be husky on account of disease in the larynx, or there may be troublesome diarrhoea, due to affection of the bowels. Haemorrhage is not uncommon in this stage, and death may be brought about by this means. The emaciation is now extreme, and bed-sores are apt to form. The swinging temperature and the excessive sweats continue, and the cough is often most troublesome. All through the disease, even to the very end, there is often a curious mental state known as the spes phthisica, the sufferer being buoyed up by the daily recurring belief that he is better, and is beginning to recover.

The duration of the illness is largely dependent upon four factors: the acuteness of the infection, the age of the patient, the stage at which efficient treatment is started, and the natural resistance of the patient to the disease. Acute miliary tuberculosis, for instance, is rapidly fatal unless treatment is initiated at an early stage, and the disease runs a more rapid course in children, adolescents and young adults than in the middle-aged.

Treatment – This falls very naturally into two classes: (a) preventive, and (b) remedial.

(a) PREVENTIVE TREATMENT – The problem of prevention is partly social and partly medical. Tuberculosis is commoner among the ill-fed and the badly housed. Abolition of overcrowding, provision of good homes, an adequate supply of protective foods and enough money to buy them have all gone a long way towards diminishing the incidence of tuberculosis. To a considerable extent, tuberculosis is a social disease. On the medical side, the problem is essentially to prevent uninfected susceptible people – especially children – from coming into contact with the infecting agent – the Mycobacterium tuberculosis. The great risk to the child is coming into contact with an adult who has the causative organism in his or her sputum. Every attempt must therefore be made (1) to detect all sufferers from tuberculosis, (2) to treat them and isolate them until they know how to safeguard other people, as, for instance, by the proper use of sputum pots, and (3) to examine and follow up all contact cases – especially children known to have been in close contact with adults suffering from tuberculosis.

Two of the most important preventive measures introduced of recent years have been BCG vaccination (qv) and mass miniature radiography (qv). By means of the former an immunity to the disease can be given to those who have not acquired a natural immunity. By means of mass miniature radiography the disease can often be detected at an early stage when it is most likely to respond to treatment.

(b) REMEDIAL TREATMENT – For all practical purposes this now consists of chemotherapy.

Chemotherapy – The outlook in tuberculosis has been revolutionized by the introduction of effective antituberculous drugs. Since the isolation, in 1944, of streptomycin, the first chemotherapeutic substance to be of any value in the treatment of tuberculosis, several other drugs have been introduced for this purpose, but the two important ones are para-aminosalicylic acid (PAS) and isoniazid. This triad – streptomycin, PAS, and isoniazid – now constitute the basis of treatment of all forms of tuberculosis. Each of these is discussed under its name, but there are two general aspects of the chemotherapy that should be mentioned here. The first is that the *Mycobacterium tuberculosis* has the unfortunate habit of becoming resistant to each of these drugs if it is given by itself. This can be prevented by giving two or more of them together. Thus, the routine treatment of tuberculosis now consists of the administration of (a) streptomycin combined with either PAS or isoniazid; or (b) PAS and isoniazid. The second is that whilst their introduction has marked a big advance in the treatment of tuberculosis, they are merely ancillary to the other well-established lines of treatment: eg. rest, fresh air and good food. It is when they are carefully integrated into a well-planned programme of treatment, under the supervision of a skilled physician, that they bring most benefit to the patient.

Eradication of Tuberculosis – Since the turn of the century there has been a marked fall in the incidence of tuberculosis, as is well shown in table 40, which gives the standardized mortality ratios for England and Wales from the decade, 1851–60, to 1966. This shows that the ratio for pulmonary tuberculosis fell from 1336 in 1851–60 to 16 in 1966. The figures for recent years are the most striking of all. Thus, in England and Wales the standardized mortality ratio for pulmonary tuberculosis fell from 85 in 1950–54 to 16 in 1966.

Apart from the treatment of individual cases, the general measures adopted for its eradication are:

1. PREVENTION OF BOVINE INFECTION, especially by obtaining a pure supply of milk, cream and butter from healthy cows; or if the milk be suspected, by sterilization of all milk to be consumed by children. (See MILK.)

2. BCG VACCINE, for the protection of infants born to tuberculous mothers, of senior schoolchildren and of young adults particularly exposed to risk of infection: eg. medical students and nurses.

3. MASS MINIATURE RADIOGRAPHY for the detection of cases at an early stage of the disease, when it is most amenable to treatment. This is also a valuable means of detecting the disease in individuals who, unbeknown to themselves and others, are suffering from the disease and spreading it to others with whom they live or work.

TUBEROSE SCLEROSIS, or EPILOIA, also sometimes known as TUBEROUS SCLEROSIS, is a hereditary disease due to a developmental abnormality of the brain. The incidence is 1 in 50,000 of the population. It is characterized by mental retardation (usually from birth), epilepsy which usually starts before 2 years of age and multiple small nodules or tumours in the face which usually appear around puberty. Relatives of those with this condition can obtain help and guidance from the British Tuberous Sclerosis Association, Church Farm House, Church Road, Northleigh, Oxfordshire OX8 6TX.

TULARAEMIA is a disease of rodents such as rabbits and rats, caused by the bacillus, *Francisella tularense*, and spread either by flies or by direct inoculation, for example, into the hands of a person engaged in skinning rabbits. In man the disease takes the form of a slow fever lasting several weeks, with much malaise and depression, followed by considerable emaciation. It was first described in the district of Tulare in California, and is found widely spread in North America and in Europe, but not in Great Britain. Streptomycin, the tetracyclines and chloramphenicol, have proved effective in treatment.

TUMOUR means literally any swelling, but, by common consent, the term is held not to include passing swellings caused by acute inflammation, whilst the collections of diseased material arising in the course of chronic inflammation, like tuberculosis, syphilis, leprosy and glanders, sometimes are and sometimes are not classed as tumours, according to their size and appearance.

Varieties – Some are of an infective nature, as already stated; some arise undoubtedly as the result of injury; several contributing factors are mentioned under the heading of CANCER, but for the rest, the causes of tumours are really still undiscovered.

An old idea divides tumours into two great classes. On the one hand, some are *simple* or *benign*, growing slowly at one spot, pressing neighbouring parts aside but not invading them, not recurring after removal, and having little tendency to ulcerate; whilst others are *malignant*, spreading quickly from point to point, invading and destroying surrounding tissues, tending to recur after apparently complete removal, and being liable to ulcerate. This distinction is as old as the days of Hippocrates, who gave to gnawing tumours the name of carcinoma. Although in the majority of cases it is easy to decide whether a given tumour is of simple or malignant character, there is no sharp dividing line between the two kinds. Thus an expert sometimes has difficulty in stating from the microscopic characters of an *adenoma* (glandular tumour) growing in the breast or in the bowel, whether its progress will show a simple or malignant course. Again, *rodent ulcer*, a small ulcerating tumour situated generally on the face, may remain restricted to a single spot for twenty or thirty years, although it has the microscopic characters of a malignant tumour and finally spreads like one. Another fact connecting the two groups is that some simple tumours, persisting as such through middle life, are liable to assume a malignant character when old age is reached.

Formerly tumours were named according to some peculiarity of shape, colour, or the like. Thus a fungoid tumour was one resembling a mushroom, a polypus one which seemed to have one stalk with many feet, a mole was a dark hairy growth resembling the animal of that name, and sarcoma was originally the name given by Galen to a tumour of fleshy appearance. The use of the microscope, however, has brought about a more precise grouping, and tumours are now classed according to the tissues of which they are built, somewhat as follows:

(1) Simple tumours of normal tissue.
(2) Hollow tumours or cysts, generally of simple nature.
(3) Malignant tumours: (*a*) of imperfect cellular structure, resembling the cells of skin, mucous membrane, or secreting glands; (*b*) of imperfect connective tissue.

(1) *SIMPLE TUMOURS* OF NORMAL TISSUE – ADENOMA is a tumour growing from a gland and composed of gland-like tissue. These tumours are specially common in the breasts of young women; there may be several together, but usually they are easily removed.

419 – Microscopic section of cancer of the breast, showing columns of cancer cells (1), surrounded by fibrous tissue (2). Kettle's *Pathology of Tumours*. H. K. Lewis & Co. Ltd.

420 – Small round-celled sarcoma of muscle. (1) Sarcoma cells, (2) muscle fibres. Kettle's *Pathology of Tumours*. H. K. Lewis & Co. Ltd.

ANGIOMA is a tumour formed by a mass of small blood-vessels or spaces in which blood circulates. These tumours may exist in internal organs, or on the skin, when they do not project much, and are known as naevi or 'mothers' marks'.

CHONDROMA is a tumour mainly formed of cartilage. These tumours develop especially on the fingers and toes.

FIBROMA is the name given to a tumour consisting mainly of fibrous tissue. Soft fibromas are often seen as wrinkled brownish tags upon the face or body.

LIPOMA means a tumour mainly composed of fat. Such tumours may be found in any part of the body, but they are especially common just beneath the skin. It is sometimes hard to distinguish such a tumour, which is very soft, from a chronic abscess; but the fatty tumour generally has a firm edge and can be seen to be attached at several points to the skin, which is puckered by these attachments.

MYOMA is a tumour composed largely of muscle fibres, usually unstriped muscle. These tumours are far more commonly found in the wall of the womb than in any other position, being known as fibroid tumours.

NEUROMA is a tumour growing upon a nerve, and therefore in many cases producing pain.

OSTEOMA is a tumour composed of bone. These are usually of small size and cause little trouble, except in so far as their position occasions discomfort.

PAPILLOMA is a tumour projecting from the surface of the skin or of a mucous membrane. It is composed of a core of fibrous tissue, which represents an over-development of the papillae naturally found in these situations, covered by masses of cells. Warts are examples of papillomas on the skin (see WARTS), whilst soft papillomas sometimes develop in the bladder or bowel and cause much bleeding.

(2) *HOLLOW TUMOURS* are described under a special heading. (See CYSTS.)

(3) *MALIGNANT TUMOURS* of imperfect cellular structure resembling the cells of skin, mucous membranes or secreting glands, are known generally as CANCERS. This group and the following group are treated together under the heading of CANCER AND SARCOMA (qv). Many names are applied to cancers of different parts and according to their appearance. The name, CARCINOMA, is generally reserved at the present day for malignant epithelial tumours. EPITHELIOMA is a cancer springing from the skin surface, and ADENOCARCINOMA means one originating in glandular tissue. SCIRRHUS is a hard cancer in which much fibrous tissue has been developed (illustration 419); MEDULLARY or SOFT cancer is one in which the softer cellular element forms large masses; and COLLOID cancer is one in which a characteristic glue-like transformation takes place.

Malignant tumours of imperfect connective tissue are known as SARCOMAS; and, according to the shape of the embryonic cells, or the nature of attempts at the formation of connective tissues, these are subdivided as ROUND-CELLED (illustration 420), SPINDLE-CELLED, MELANOTIC, MYELOID.

Symptoms – The symptoms of a simple tumour are, as a rule, nothing beyond the presence of a swelling, and such accidental symptoms as those set up by its pressure upon neighbouring important organs, by the inconvenience of its size, its position, and the like. (For special symptoms of malignant tumours see CANCER and SARCOMA.)

Treatment – The treatment of a tumour is, in general, its removal by operation. With regard to simple tumours, the advantage gained by removal may not be worth the inconvenience caused by an operation, and such tumours may be left alone. In particular cases the unsightliness of the tumour, the inconvenience of its size, or the tendency that some simple tumours have to become malignant may call for removal. If a tumour be malignant, or if there be any doubt as to its character, an operation should be performed at the earliest possible opportunity. For some surface tumours, and also for inoperable tumours in internal organs, the application of radiotherapy and X-rays has, in recent years, played a great part. (See RADIOTHERAPY; RADIUM; and X-RAYS.) Chemotherapy is also playing an increasingly important part in treatment. (See CANCER and SARCOMA.)

TUNNEL-WORM is another name for ancylostoma. (See ANCYLOSTOMIASIS.)

TURNING (see VERSION).

TURNER'S SYNDROME is a congenital malformation characterized by webbing of the neck, deformity of the forearm, dwarfism and persistent infantilism.

TURN OF LIFE is a term applied to the menopause. (See CLIMACTERIC.)

TURPENTINE is the oleo-resin which exudes from trees of the pine family when the bark is injured. The oil distilled from this is known as oil of turpentine, rectified turpentine or spirit of turpentine, the residue being the resin or rosin. The natural turpentine, containing resin, is not used in medicine, since it is highly irritating; and when the word turpentine is used, the distilled product is always understood. The turpentine obtained from the ordinary yellow pine is the common form, that obtained from the silver fir is known as Canada balsam or balm of Gilead and that got from the larch as Venice turpentine.

Action – Turpentine has an action similar to that of other essential oils. It is highly irritating to any surface with which it is brought in contact, is antispasmodic, and, especially when it has been exposed to the air, is powerfully antiseptic.

Uses – *Externally*, turpentine is used as a counter-irritant. It forms one of the most common ingredients of liniments and embrocations for application to sprains and bruises. It is used with hot fomentations when a specially strong action is desired, a fomentation sprinkled with turpentine being known as a stupe. (See FOMENTATIONS.) In chronic bronchitis, rubbing the chest with turpentine is an old favourite household remedy.

Internally, turpentine is seldom administered now. In lumbago and other forms of chronic rheumatism, 5 drops of turpentine taken upon a lump of sugar thrice daily over a long period is an old household remedy. As an enema, half-an-ounce (14 ml) of oil of turpentine may be mixed with 15 ounces (420 ml) of soapy water in order to relieve severe cases of flatulence.

TWILIGHT SLEEP is the name given to a method of anaesthesia at one time used in child-birth, but now practically discarded. The unconsciousness of pain was brought about by the hypodermic injection of morphine in full dose, with a small dose of scopolamine which was repeated about once an hour throughout the course of the labour or until the patient was unconscious.

TWINS (see MULTIPLE BIRTHS).

TYMPANIC MEMBRANE is the ear-drum.

TYMPANITES means distension of the abdomen due to the presence of gas or air in the intestine or in the peritoneal cavity. The abdomen, when struck with the fingers, gives under these conditions a drum-like (tympanitic) note.

TYMPANUM is another name for the middle ear. (See EAR.)

TYPHLITIS means inflammation of the caecum or first part of the large intestine, into which the small intestine and the appendix vermiformis open. As the associated condition of appendicitis is of far greater importance than typhlitis, the latter name is little used.

TYPHOID FEVER (see ENTERIC FEVER).

TYPHUS FEVER is an infective disease of world-wide distribution, the manifestations of which vary in different localities. The causative organisms of all forms of typhus fever belong to the genus Rickettsia. These are organisms which are intermediate between bacteria and viruses in their properties and measure 0·5 micrometre or less in diameter. The accompanying classification of the typhus fevers provides a practical basis for discussion of the subject (table 41).

LOUSE TYPHUS, in which the infecting Rickettsia is transmitted by the louse, is of world-wide distribution. It includes

Epidemic Typhus, Brill's Disease which is a recrudescent form of Epidemic Typhus, and Trench Fever (qv).

Epidemic Typhus Fever, also known as exanthematic typhus, classical typhus, and louse-borne typhus, is an acute infection of abrupt onset which, in the absence of treatment, persists for fourteen days. It is of world-wide distribution, but is largely confined today to parts of Africa. The causative organism is the *Rickettsia prowazeki,* so-called after Ricketts and Prowazek, two brilliant investigators of typhus, both of whom died of the disease. It is transmitted by the human louse, *Pediculus humanus.* The rickettsiae can survive in the dried faeces of lice for 60 days, and these infected faeces are probably the main source of infection of man.

Symptoms – The incubation period is usually 10 to 14 days. The onset is preceded by headache, pain in the back and limbs and rigors. On the third day the temperature rises suddenly, and the face and eyes become congested. At the same time the headache becomes more intense, and the patient is drowsy or delirious. Sometimes on this day, but more usually on the fifth or sixth day, the characteristic rash appears on the abdomen and inner aspect of the arms, to spread over the chest, back and trunk, but seldom involving the face except in severe cases. It has been described as a 'mulberry rash' and consists essentially of reddish spots on a dusky background. During the second week a low muttering delirium develops, the patient becomes restless, and great prostration develops: the so-called 'coma vigil'. In cases which are not going to recover, death usually occurs from heart failure about the fourteenth day. In those who recover, the temperature falls by crisis about this time (illustration 421). In severe cases, and in neglected cases, gangrene is liable to occur. In diagnosis the Weil-Felix reaction is helpful. The death-rate is variable, varying from nearly 100 per cent in epidemics among debilitated refugees to about 10 per cent.

FLEA TYPHUS, in which the infecting Rickettsia is transmitted by the flea, is represented by Murine Typhus.

Murine Typhus Fever, also known as flea typhus, is world-wide in its distribution and is found wherever individuals are crowded together in insanitary, rat-infested areas. Hence the old names of jail-fever and ship typhus. The causative organism, *Rickettsia mooseri,* which is closely related to *R. prowazeki,* is transmitted to man by the rat-flea, *Xenopsyalla*

Louse-borne	Flea-borne	Tick-borne	Mite-borne
Epidemic typhus	Murine (endemic) typhus	Rocky Mountain spotted fever	Tsutsugamushi fever
Brill's disease		African tick typhus (Tick-bite fever)	(Scrub typhus)
Trench fever		Fièvre boutonneuse	Rickettsialpox

Table 41 – Classification of the typhus fevers.

cheopis. The rat is the main reservoir of infection. Once man is infected, the human louse may act as a transmitter of the Rickettsia from man to man. This explains how the disease may become epidemic under insanitary, crowded conditions. As a rule, however, the disease is only acquired when man comes into close contact with infected rats.

Symptoms – These are similar to those of louse-borne typhus, but the disease usually runs a milder course, and the mortality rate is very low (about 1·5 per cent).

TICK TYPHUS, in which the infecting Rickettsia is transmitted by ticks, occurs in various parts of the world. The three best-known conditions in this group consist of Rocky Mountain Spotted Fever, Fièvre Boutonneuse and Tick-bite Fever.

Rocky Mountain Spotted Fever was reported originally in the mountainous western states of the USA, but it is now found in many of the eastern states. The causal organism is *Rickettsia rickettsii.* The usual transmitters are the wood tick (*Dermacentor andersoni*) and the dog tick (*Dermacentor variabilis*) but there is evidence that other ticks may occasionally

transmit the disease. The highest incidence of the disease is in the spring and early summer, when the ticks are most active.

Symptoms – The incubation period is three to twelve days. After a day or two of headache, backache and loss of appetite the onset is rapid, with intensification of the headache, rigors, sickness and congestion of the eyes. The temperature rises by steps to 103° to 106° F (39·4° to 41·1° C). The rash usually appears on the second to fourth day, first in the wrist and ankles, and then spreading over the whole body. It is usually more florid than the rash of louse typhus. The temperature settles slowly by lysis after two or three weeks. Convalescence is slow. The mortality rate varies, averaging about 20 per cent; it is low in children and high in adults and the elderly.

Fièvre boutonneuse, also known as Marseilles fever and African tick fever, is a mild form of tick typhus which occurs along the Medterranean littoral, throughout the African continent and and in India. The causative organism is *Rickettsia conori.* It is transmitted by a dog tick, *Rhipicephalus sanguineus,* in Europe. Elsewhere other ticks are involved and the

421 – Chart showing the ordinary course of the temperature in a case of typhus fever. The fall by sudden crisis differs markedly from the gradual subsidence in typhoid fever.

vectors are rodents and other small wild mammals. One of the distinctive features of the disease is the development of a small area of gangrene at the site of the tick bite – the *tâche noire*.

Tick-bite Fever occurs in South Africa, the Rhodesias and East Africa. The Rickettsia is conveyed by a number of ticks which are conveyed to man by dogs and cattle. The initial infection takes place through a bite in the skin or through the conjunctiva. The manifestations of the disease are similar to those of Rocky Mountain spotted fever, but usually runs a much milder course, with a death rate of less than 1 per cent. The fever persists for about a fortnight.

MITE TYPHUS, in which the infecting Rickettsia is transmitted by mites, includes scrub typhus. or tsutsugamushi disease, and rickettsialpox.

Scrub Typhus, also known as tsutsugamushi fever, Japanese river fever and tropical typhus, has been known in Japan for over a thousand years. Its distribution includes the area bounded by Japan, Pakistan and Australia. The causative organism is *Rickettsia tsutsugamushi*, which is transmitted by the larvae, or chiggers, of various mites which become infected from wild rodents. The disease is most common among farmers, field workers, hunters and surveyors. Whilst in Malaysia it occurs all the year round, in Japan it is most common between June and October.

Symptoms – The incubation period is 5 to 21 days. The onset is usually sudden, with headache, backache, rigors and congestion of the eyes, as in other forms of typhus. A small ulcer usually develops at the site of the mite-bite, and the lymph glands draining this area are often enlarged. The temperature rises rapidly to $101°$ to $102°$ F $(38·3°$ to $38·9°$ C), and then climbs to about $104°$ F $(40°$ C). The rash appears about the fourth or fifth day – on the chest and abdomen, then spreading to the limbs, and sometimes to the face. Nervous manifestations are usually marked: apathy during the day; insomnia and delirium at night. The temperature usually subsides during the third week.

Rickettsialpox is a mild disease caused by *Rickettsia akari*, which is transmitted to man from infected mice by the common mouse mite, *Allodermanyssus sanguineus*. It occurs in USA, West and South Africa and USSR.

TREATMENT – The general principles of treatment are the same in all forms of typhus, and can be divided into prophylactic and curative.

Prophylaxis consists of either avoidance of, or destruction of, the vector. In the case of louse typhus and flea typhus, the outlook has been revolutionized by the introduction of efficient insecticides such as DDT and Gammexane. The value of the former was well shown by its use during the post-1939–45-War period. This resulted in almost complete freedom from the epidemics of typhus which ravaged Eastern Europe after the 1914–18 War being responsible for 30 million cases with a mortality of 10 per cent. At the present day there are only 10,000 to 20,000 cases a year, with around a few hundred deaths. Efficient rat control is another measure which reduces the risk of typhus very considerably. In areas such as Malaysia, where the mites are infected from a wide variety of rodents scattered over large areas, the wearing of protective clothing is the most practicable method of prophylaxis.

Curative treatment has also been revolutionized by the introduction of chloramphenicol and the tetracyclines. These antibiotics have altered the prognosis in typhus fever very considerably. Currently the most widely used is the long-acting tetracycline, doxycycline, one single oral dose of which is said to be curative.

U

ULCER means a breach on the surface of the skin or on the surface of the membrane lining any cavity within the body, which does not tend to heal quickly. The process by which an ulcer spreads and which involves the death of minute portions of tissue round its edge is known as ulceration. The process of ulceration and that of abscess formation are the same, since both are inflammatory processes, although ulceration takes place along a surface from which its discharge escapes at once, whilst an abscess spreads in every direction from a centre and its products are for a time retained. The microscopic changes that take place when an ulcer forms will therefore not be described in

Varieties – Ulcers are sometimes classified as *local* when they are found at one spot only, such as the varicose ulcer found on the lower part of the leg; and *constitutional* when there are usually several ulcers on different parts of the body, produced chiefly by some constitutional defect. LOCAL ULCERS are further subdivided as follows, according to their symptoms or appearance.

SIMPLE or SLOWLY HEALING ULCER has been already described. The floor is moderately red and slightly sunk, the skin around is healthy up to the margin of the ulcer, and at the edge there is a blue line, which is of great importance as showing the progress of the healing. Such an ulcer

422 – Vertical section through the edge of a simple ulcer. On the left is the healthy surface, to the right is the bare ulcerated surface. *a*. Malpighian (growing) layer of the epidermis spreading over the edge of the ulcer at *e*; *b*, its horny layer; *c*, granulation tissue forming the floor of the ulcer; *d*, discharge on its surface. Magnified by 21.

detail, as the features of an inflammatory process have been already described under ABSCESS, ACUTE.

An ulcer consists of a floor or surface, which, in consequence of the loss of tissue, is usually depressed below the surrounding healthy surface, and an edge where the healthy tissues end (illustration 422). The floor of a healing ulcer is composed of granulations, which are small masses of cells engaged in forming connective tissue and richly supplied with capillary blood-vessels that give the ulcer a bright-red appearance; whilst the edge shows a blue line of growing epithelial cells, which are constantly spreading inwards. In the process of healing, the fibrous tissue formed by the granulations contracts and thus draws the edges of the ulcer together and gives a puckered appearance to the scar. If anything interferes with these natural processes, the ulcer is prevented from healing.

has a very slight white discharge and is quite free from smell.

INFLAMED ULCER is one which, as the result usually of the presence of bacteria, or in consequence of continued irritation, is still spreading. The floor of such an ulcer is very red and bleeds easily, the skin around is red and swollen, there is a thick discharge of pus from the surface, and portions of the reddened skin at its edge or in its neighbourhood tend to die and thus form new ulcers.

WEAK ULCER is an appearance which the ulcers of weakly people, especially those suffering from dropsy, tend to assume. The granulations are soft, project above the surface, forming what is popularly known as 'proud flesh', bleed easily, and prevent the healing edge of the ulcer from growing inwards.

CALLOUS ULCER is the type of chronic ulcer most often met. The edge is thick and hard, the colour pale, few granulations are present, and the discharge in consequence is thin and small in amount, though often very offensive in smell.

IRRITABLE ULCER is one which resembles in a mild degree the inflamed ulcer, and has the special character of being extremely painful to touch.

VARICOSE ULCER (illustration 423) may belong to any of the above types. It generally comes on as the result of scratching

CONSTITUTIONAL ULCERS are generally the result of some widespread disease such as syphilis or tuberculosis. SYPHILITIC ULCERS have the characters of possessing a very abrupt edge, as if punched out, and of leaving behind after healing a brownish discoloured scar. TUBERCULOUS ULCERS may arise from the bursting of a tuberculous abscess under the skin; whilst the skin disease known as lupus vulgaris is a variety of tuberculous disease.

423 – Varicose ulcer. From Borrie, *Roxburgh's Common Skin Diseases.* H. K. Lewis & Co. Ltd.

the skin of a leg which has been rendered eczematous by the bad circulation. It will not heal so long as the patient walks about, and has a great tendency to develop into a callous ulcer.

INTERNAL ULCERS develop sometimes in the mouth (see MOUTH, DISEASES OF); in the stomach (see STOMACH, DISEASES OF); in the duodenum (see DUODENAL ULCER) in the bowels (see INTESTINE, DISEASES OF); in the lining membrane of the heart (see HEART, DISEASES OF); and in other parts.

MALIGNANT ULCERS are developed when a cancer spreads so as to involve the skin. Such an ulcer has often a very offensive smell, requiring the use of deodorant substances.

TROPHIC ULCERS are apt to appear as the result of weakened nerve influence: eg. the deep perforating ulcer on the sole of the foot in locomotor ataxia, or bed sores in people sick of some lingering disease. (See BED SORES.)

Causes – An ulcer may be set up by any

cause which damages the surface of the body and prevents immediate healing. Naturally, any constitutional condition which diminishes the vitality or the healing power of the body acts in this way, and among these causes may be mentioned old age, general ill-health, scurvy, diabetes, gout, syphilis and tuberculosis, so that wounds produced in persons suffering from any of these conditions are apt to form ulcers. Defective circulation in the direction either of a poor blood supply or of the stagnation which takes place in varicose veins is another important cause. Constant movement of any part on which there is a wound is quite sufficient to delay its healing and produce an ulcer. Everyone knows, for example, how difficult it is to heal a small crack at the corner of the mouth. Irritation of the ulcer by pressure, or by discharges pent up under dressings that are too seldom changed, or even by the application of strong lotions to the ulcer, may prevent its healing.

Dangers – A person afflicted with a large ulcer is to a great extent incapacitated from active work, and the presence of any such septic condition has a prejudicial effect upon the general health. Further, the person always runs the risk of an attack of acute inflammation starting from the ulcer. A varicose ulcer has a danger of its own, consisting in the liability of the veins to become ulcerated and to burst, causing profuse bleeding. Even after a very chronic ulcer has healed, its scar contracts, and in doing so may cause disfigurement or may even interfere with the usefulness of a limb, if situated near a joint. Finally, ulcers which have lasted many years may become the seat of cancer.

Treatment – In treating an ulcer, three objects must be kept in view: (1) to remove the cause of ulceration; (2) to render the floor and edge of the ulcer healthy so that healing may begin; (3) to assist the healing process and ward off any source of irritation.

(1) REMOVAL OF THE CAUSE – Any constitutional condition underlying the development of the ulcer must first of all be treated; otherwise the tissues surrounding the ulcer are unable to exert their power of healing. Thus syphilis or tuberculosis, if present, requires the special remedies suited to these diseases, whilst old age, scurvy, diabetes, and other conditions demand appropriate treatment. Bodily rest is also of great importance for the healing of an ulcer; and especially is this the case in ulcers of the leg, where

constant movement combines with bad circulation to prevent healing. Accordingly, large varicose ulcers may refuse to heal till the person takes to bed, but when this is done, improvement is often rapid. This beneficial effect is still further aided, in the case of varicose ulcers, by raising the leg on a pillow or by elevating the foot of the bed on props so that the ulcer is brought above the level of the heart. When for any reason the person cannot lie in bed for several weeks, the evils of movement and the dependent position of the leg can be neutralized to some extent by wearing an elastic bandage over the dressing, which is applied every morning before the patient gets out of bed. Although this treatment will benefit any ulcer of the leg, it is not likely to cure a large one. (See VEINS, DISEASES OF.)

(2) RENDERING THE ULCER HEALTHY aims at converting any of the severer forms, eg. the inflamed, weak, irritable, or callous ulcer, into the simple type, which is the first step necessary in the healing process. When the ulcer is *inflamed*, it must be treated with active antiseptics such as eusol, acriflavine, or perchloride of mercury lotion, and the dressing covered by oil-silk or gutta-percha tissue. Penicillin is most effective when the causative organism is penicillin-sensitive. As soon as the ulcer has been purified, however, these strong antiseptics must be discontinued, since they retard the healing process. Sometimes the ulcer is purified quickly by the surgeon, who makes an application of undiluted carbolic acid to its surface, or scrapes away the diseased tissues thoroughly under an anaesthetic. Oxygen is sometimes used as a purifying agent. In mild cases of inflammation, charcoal, iodoform, and various weak antiseptics are sometimes used. *Weak ulcers* are treated with blue-stone, red lotion (qv), silver salts, or other substances which have an astringen effect upon the proud flesh and stimulate the edge and floor of the ulcer. *Callous ulcer* is by far the most common variety that needs special treatment. The reparative material, which has been accumulated in the edges and floor, and which obstructs the circulation near the ulcer, and prevents healing, must be absorbed. This is effected sometimes in slight cases by massage of the skin near the ulcer, in other cases by blistering the thick edge all round the ulcer. Generally, continued pressure is the method chosen. The more frequently used method is to wear during the day a special supporting bandage, which is applied to the leg from the ball of

the foot up to the knee, passing over the dressing upon the ulcer with a very slight degree of pressure. There is now a range of such bandages, and medical advice should be sought as to the best one to use. To be successful, this treatment must be combined with complete rest and elevation of the ulcerated part.

(3) ASSISTANCE OF THE HEALING PROCESS – When the ulcer has been purified and its floor and edges rendered healthy, a very simple dressing must be used. Care should be taken in dressing not to irritate the ulcer and make it bleed, and the greatest care must be taken of the blue line at the ulcer's margin, as this is the healing part. The frequency of dressing the ulcer is a point of great importance; for, if the dressing be too frequently renewed, the healing tissues are unnecessarily disturbed and damaged, whilst if the dressing be very seldom changed, pus is apt to collect, and by its decomposition to inflame the ulcer. The usual interval allowed to elapse between the successive dressings of a healing ulcer is two or three days, or less if there be much discharge. The ulcer must be washed with some mild fluid like weak boric lotion. The best dressing is a piece of clean lint or gauze, but this should be kept from actual contact with the ulcer by a piece of oil-silk perforated here and there and just large enough to cover the red granulations of the ulcer's floor without touching the edge. At each dressing, the lint, etc., must be thoroughly soaked before removal, not pulled away roughly; otherwise the healing tissues, especially the blue line at the edge, are damaged and torn. At each dressing, too, the piece of oil-silk is reduced in size. When an ulcer has become quite clean and is healing rapidly, one of the best forms of dressing consists of a weak boric ointment spread on lint.

The healing of a large ulcer, after it has been rendered clean, may often be hastened by grafting its surface with skin from another part. (See SKIN-GRAFTING.)

For the treatment of internal ulcers, see under the headings of the organs in which they occur.

ULITIS means inflammation of the gums.

ULNA is the name of the inner of the two bones in the forearm. It is wide at its upper end, and its olecranon process forms the point of the elbow. In its lower part it is more fragile and is liable to be broken by a fall upon the forearm while

something is grasped in the hand. Chipping off of the olecranon process is a not uncommon result of falls upon the elbow. (See FRACTURES.)

ULOGLOSSITIS means inflammation of the gums and of the tongue.

ULTRA- is a prefix denoting excess.

ULTRASONICS relate to sound in the frequency above 15 kilocycles per second: that is, well above the upper frequency limit of the human ear. These frequencies are now being used to an increasing extent in medicine. In diagnosis they are proving useful in obstetrics in assessing the stage of pregnancy, in the investigation of disease in the bladder, kidneys, liver, ovaries and pancreas, and also in the diagnosis of brain tumours. Their great advantage is that they are harmless and therefore their use for diagnostic purposes can be repeated without any harm to the patient. They are also being used in the treatment of Menière's disease (qv) and of bruises and strains.

ULTRA-VIOLET RAYS (see LIGHT).

UMBILICUS is the technical name for the navel.

UNCINARIA is another name for hookworm. (See ANCYLOSTOMIASIS).

UNCINATE FIT is the term applied to a state in which the patient has a hallucination of smell or of taste; it may be a manifestation of epilepsy, or the result of a tumour pressing on that part of the brain concerned with the appreciation of smell and taste.

UNCONSCIOUSNESS is a condition depending usually on some disorder of the brain, and may be of various degrees.

Varieties – Sleep is a natural form of unconsciousness due to a resting condition of the brain (see SLEEP). When the brain remains irregularly active various peculiar forms of unconsciousness or of disturbed consciousness are apt to ensue, such as delirium, somnambulism, hypnotism, catalepsy, ecstasy. (See under these headings.) In syncope, or fainting, the brain ceases to act for a time in consequence of a bloodless state, brought on by feebleness of the heart's action. In the lesser forms of epilepsy (petit mal), the epileptic sometimes becomes unconscious of his surroundings, though able to perform such a simple act as to take off his

424 – Undine, used for irrigating the eye with fluid.

clothing, or to run some distance, or even to attack ánother person.

STUPOR is the name given to a partial state of unconsciousness from which the person can be roused for a moment by some powerful stimulus such as a shout.

COMA means a condition of complete oblivion from which the individual cannot be aroused.

Causes – Fainting is due to deficient supply of blood to the brain. Among injuries to the brain, apoplexy, compression and concussion of the brain, and inflammation affecting the brain or its membranes are the chief causes of unconsciousness. Epilepsy is also a cause of passing unconsciousness, either accompanied by a fit, or, in the slighter forms, without any such seizure. Narcotic poisons also produce stupor. The poisons that accumulate in the blood during various diseases, such as Bright's disease and diabetes, may produce coma, that due to the latter disease being curable by insulin.

Treatment – The cause of unconsciousness must first of all be determined. Fainting brings with it its own cure, and little is necessary beyond leaving the unconscious person recumbent. (See FAINTING.) The means of distinguishing the effects of narcotic poisons from those of apoplexy are given under OPIUM, and this distinction is important, since in apoplexy the main requirement is absolute quiet, while in opium poisoning energetic treatment is necessary. Unconsciousness, due to compression of the brain resulting from severe injury to the head, may have to be treated by trephining the skull. The un-

consciousness of uraemia due to Bright's disease is perhaps the form most liable to be mistaken or overlooked, but doubts as to this are set at rest by examination of the urine. In this case also prompt treatment is essential if life is to be saved. For the treatment of unconsciousness due to other causes, the special symptoms present will in general indicate the cause, and the treatment is given under other headings.

UNDECYLENIC ACID is a long chain fatty acid which is of value in the treatment of tinea pedis. (See RINGWORM.)

UNDINE is the name given to a small glass flask with drawn-out neck and an opening which can be closed by the finger. It is used for irrigating the eye with fluid (illustration 424). (See EYE DISEASES AND INJURIES.)

UNDULANT FEVER is another name for Malta fever, but especially for a variety of this disorder which occurs in temperate climates and caused by the *Brucella abortus*. This organism produces contagious abortion in cattle, and is apt to be conveyed to man by contact with them or by their milk, when it gives rise to symptoms described under BRUCELLOSIS.

UNGUENTUM is the Latin name for ointment.

UNIT is the term applied to a quantity assumed as a standard for measurement. Thus, the *unit of insulin* is the specific activity contained in such an amount (in 1968 this was 0·04167 mg) of the standard preparation as the Medical Research Council may from time to time indicate as the quantity exactly equivalent to the unit accepted for international use. The standard preparation consists of pure, dry, crystalline insulin.

URACHUS is the name of a corded structure which extends from the bladder up to the navel, and represents the remains of the canal which in the foetus joins bladder with allantois.

URAEMIA is the condition which results from failure of renal function, as in Bright's disease (qv). Whilst it is generally accepted that it is due to retention in the body of substances that normally are excreted by the kidneys, there is no definite evidence as to which of these substances is responsible for the condition.

Symptoms – Uraemia is sometimes

905

classed as *acute*, ie. those cases in which the symptoms develop in a few hours or days, and *chronic*, including cases in which the symptoms are less marked and last over weeks, months, or years. There is, however, no dividing line between the two, for in the chronic variety, which may be said to consist of the symptoms of chronic Bright's disease, an acute attack is liable to come on at any time.

Headache in the front or back of the head, accompanied often by insomnia at night and drowsiness during the day, is one of the commonest symptoms, although it is apt to be attributed to some other cause. Unconsciousness of a profound type, which may be accompanied by convulsions resembling those of epilepsy, is the most outstanding feature of an acute attack and is a very dangerous condition.

Another group of symptoms is associated with the lungs and may consist of great difficulty in breathing when the patient attempts to lie down, repeated attacks resembling asthma, or the peculiar type of breathing known as Cheyne-Stokes breathing (qv).

Still another symptom, which often precedes an acute attack, is severe vomiting without apparent cause. The appetite is always poor, and the onset of diarrhoea is a serious sign.

Treatment – The treatment of the chronic type of uraemia includes all the measures which should be taken by a person suffering from chronic Bright's disease. Cheyne-Stokes breathing is relieved by the intravenous administration of aminophylline.

URAMUSTINE is a nitrogen mustard derivative (qv) used in the treatment of certain forms of malignant disease. It is given by mouth in capsule form.

URANORRHAPHY is the name applied to an operation for closure of a cleft palate.

URATES (see URIC ACID).

UREA, or CARBAMIDE, is a crystalline substance of the chemical formula, $CO(NH_2)_2$, which is very soluble in water or alcohol. It is the chief waste product discharged from the body in the urine, being formed in the liver and carried to the kidneys in the blood. The amount varies considerably with the quantity and nature of the food taken, rising greatly upon an animal (protein) dietary. It also rises during the continuance of a fever.

The average amount excreted daily, during health, on a mixed diet is about 33 to 35 grams, or slightly over one ounce.

Urea is administered for its diuretic action, and also as a test of kidney action, in doses of 5 to 15 grams. It is also used as a cream in the treatment of certain skin diseases, characterized by a dry skin, such as ichthyosis (qv).

Urea is rapidly changed, by a yeast-like micro-organism, into carbonate of ammonia; and to this chemical change the ammoniacal smell of badly kept latrines is due.

URETER is the tube, about the thickness of a goose-quill, which on each side leads from the corresponding kidney down to the bladder (illustration 426). Each ureter begins above at the pelvis of its kidney and after a course of 10 to 12 inches (25 to 30 cm) through the loins and pelvis it opens by a narrow slit into the base of the bladder. The lower end pierces the wall of the bladder so obliquely (lying embedded in the wall for about $\frac{3}{4}$ inch [21 mm]) that, though urine runs freely into the bladder, it is prevented from returning up the ureter as the bladder becomes distended.

URETHANE is the official *British Pharmacopoeia* name for ethyl carbamate. It is of value in the treatment of chronic leukaemia. Injection of quinine and urethane is used as a sclerosing agent.

URETHRA is the tube which leads from the bladder to the exterior, and by which the urine is voided. It is about 8 inches (20 cm) long in the male (illustration 426) and $1\frac{1}{2}$ inches (3·5 cm) long in the female.

URETHRA, DISEASES OF – The chief conditions which cause pain in the urethra, or interfere with the passage of urine, are urethritis or inflammation of the mucous lining, and stricture or narrowing of the tube.

URETHRITIS is often difficult to tell from inflammation of the bladder (cystitis), which, however, it may accompany and of which it is often the cause.

Causes – The most frequent cause of urethritis is gonorrhoea (qv), and this disease produces the most severe type of inflammation. Another common cause is the condition known as non-specific, urethritis (qv). Like gonorrhoea, it is a venereal disease. Gout is another cause, producing its effects either owing to the repeated passage of irritating gravel with the urine, or to a highly acid state of this excretion. The damage caused by the passage of a rough stone from the bladder or of a catheter unskilfully introduced may also occasion a severe urethritis; and various drugs or articles of diet, such as alcohol or arsenic, may bring on an attack in those who are liable to suffer from it.

Symptoms – The symptoms consist chiefly in the constant oozing out of a small quantity of pus from the orifice of the urethra, a sense of scalding pain whenever urine is passed, increased redness of the mucous membrane as seen at the orifice, and tenderness along the course of the urethra. Subsequently, inflammation in neighbouring organs, eg. the bladder, testicle, or even kidney, may be set up.

Treatment – This varies with the cause of the inflammation, but in all cases the drinking of milk, water, and other bland fluids in large quantities is of advantage in order to flush out the urethra. The sulphonamide drugs and penicillin are highly effective in the treatment of gonorrhoea. The disease causing the inflammation requires special treatment according to its nature. (See also NON-SPECIFIC URETHRITIS.)

STRICTURE is an abrupt narrowing of the tube at one or more places.

Varieties and causes – SPASMODIC or CONGESTIVE STRICTURE is a temporary condition which is not of much importance. It follows upon exposure to cold, excessive exercise like bicycling, alcoholic indulgence, and often upon operations near the urethra, such as that for piles. It prevents the passage of urine for a few hours or days. It is treated simply by a warm sitzbath or warm fomentations to the fork, and, if necessary, the urine is drawn off by means of a soft or flexible catheter passed along the urethra and through the stricture.

ORGANIC STRICTURE is a much more serious condition. It is a scar, due to previous injury or ulceration of the mucous membrane, which, by contracting after the manner of all scars, produces narrowing of the urethral tube. This scar is almost always due to one or other of two conditions: severe laceration of the urethra as the result of injury, or long-continued chronic inflammation.

A stricture almost always occurs at one of two points: either just within the orifice of the urethra or in the fork, or crotch, where the urethra turns upwards as it enters the pelvis.

Symptoms – An organic stricture is of very slow development, and gives rise at first to few symptoms beyond those of the urethritis, which causes it. As the stricture narrows, the stream of urine becomes smaller than natural, and there is straining and pain each time it is voided. Occasional attacks of spasmodic stricture are brought on by injudicious acts on the part of the person who already has an organic stricture; and this further narrowing of the tube causes complete stoppage of the urine for a time, accompanied by great pain, which results from distension of the bladder. After a stricture has lasted some years, unless it has been very carefully treated, and the person has led a well-ordered life, inflammation of the bladder almost certainly comes on, and the death of the patient may ultimately ensue from the spread of this inflammation upwards to the kidneys.

The existence, position, and calibre of a stricture are verified by the surgeon, who passes metal bougies of various sizes along the urethra.

Treatment – The person who is the subject of a stricture must above all things live a moderate, well-regulated life, free from excesses of every kind. Highly spiced food, alcoholic beverages, and some forms of exercise, such as cycling and horseback riding, should be avoided. The diet should be simple and constipation must be prevented. By these means unnecessary irritation of the stricture is avoided, and thus spasmodic attacks with retention of the urine are warded off.

To check the gradual narrowing of the stricture some operative procedure is necessary, and, according to the situation and nature of the stricture, it is either *dilated* by means of bougies passed along the urethra, or it is divided by a special instrument passed along the urethra (*internal urethrotomy*), or by an incision made through the fork (*external urethrotomy*). After-treatment, consisting in the passage of a bougie at regular intervals of some weeks or months, is necessary after any of these operations, in order to counteract the permanent tendency of the stricture to contract.

INJURIES TO THE URETHRA may follow a severe crush which has fractured the pelvis, or a fall astride of some object. The signs of this are the presence of blood in the urine, or inability to pass urine at all, after such an accident. The great risks are the occurrence of an abscess round the urethra, and the formation of a stricture at a later period.

URETHRITIS means inflammation of the urethra (qv).

URIC ACID is a crystalline substance, very slightly soluble in water, of chemical formula, $C_5 N_4 H_4 O_3$. It is white in the pure state, but when found as a urinary deposit it is reddish-brown, presenting a

the two kidneys placed in the loins, two ureters leading from them to the bladder which is situated in the front of the pelvis, and the urethra which leads from the floor of the bladder out beneath the pubic bones to the exterior (illustration 426). (See BLADDER; KIDNEYS; URETERS; URETHRA.)

425 – Urate crystals (magnified × 400) from a tophus. From Copeman. *Textbook of Rheumatic Diseases*. E. & S. Livingstone.

supposed resemblance to cayenne pepper. The bi-urate of sodium and urate of ammonium occur in considerable amount in the urine during a feverish state or after great exertion, and produce, as the urine cools, a dense pink or yellow sediment. The average daily quantity of uric acid passed by human beings is 0·5 to 1 gram. In the urine of birds and reptiles uric acid is the chief nitrogenous constituent, taking the place of the urea excreted by human beings. Uric acid is formed in the liver and removed by the kidneys from the blood. The amount is increased in the following conditions:

(a) Excessive consumption of meat, combined with sedentary habits.
(b) Gout (illustration 425) (see GOUT).
(c) Diseases in which the white corpuscles of the blood are increased: eg. leukaemia.

Owing to their insolubility, uric acid and the various urates often produce deposits in the urinary passages, which are known as urinary sand, gravel, or stones according to their size.

URINARY ORGANS form the system by which the urine is extracted from the blood, stored up, and from time to time discharged from the body. They comprise

URINE is the excretion produced by the kidneys, and consists chiefly of waste substances resulting from the activity of the body, dissolved in water. The function of the kidneys consists almost entirely in selecting these substances from the blood; their actual formation takes place in the liver, muscles, etc. The urine and the perspiration are to a great extent interdependent; thus, if the kidneys are acting vigorously, the skin becomes very dry, whilst if there has been much perspiration, as in fevers, the urine is small in amount and highly concentrated. The amount of water lost from the body daily by perspiration is, in health, about half the amount passed as urine, and, though the sweat contains little of the waste material present in the urine, the glands of the skin can be made to take up the function of the kidneys to some extent when the latter organs are diseased. (See BRIGHT'S DISEASE.) Many poisons taken into the body are excreted by way of the urine, eg. morphine and strychnine, and so also are the germs of many diseases, eg. those of typhoid fever.

Composition – About 96 per cent of the urine is water, the remaining 4 per cent being solids dissolved in it. Of the solids, far the most important is urea, of which

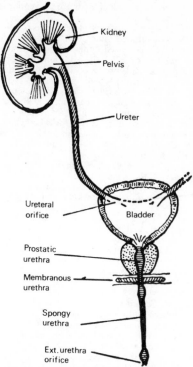

Kidney

Pelvis

Ureter

Ureteral orifice

Bladder

Prostatic urethra

Membranous urethra

Spongy urethra

Ext. urethra orifice

426 – Diagram of the male urinary system. From J. C. Boileau Grant, *An Atlas of Anatomy.* E. & S. Livingstone.

there is, on an average, 25 grams in 1 litre. Common salt stands next in quantity, the average amount in 1 litre of urine being 9 grams. Phosphates and sulphates are also important constituents combined with potassium, sodium, calcium, and magnesium, whilst there is less than 1 gram each of uric acid, and ammonia, and just over 1 gram of creatinine.

Pigments are also present in the urine, and to them its colour is due. These pigments, the chief of which is urochrome, are derived * indirectly from the colouring matter of the blood, and are produced also by the liver.

Amount – The amount of urine passed daily is about 50 ounces (1500 millilitres), subject to the variations mentioned above. A child, of course, passes much less than an adult; the average daily amount is: 15 ounces (430 ml) at two years; 20 ounces (570 ml) at four years; 30 ounces (850 ml) at seven years; and 40 ounces (1140 ml) at twelve years.

The amount of urine is *increased* in some diseases, of which diabetes and chronic Bright's disease of the cirrhotic type may be mentioned as the chief. In other conditions it is *diminished*, notably in acute Bright's disease, in fevers and feverish states generally, and in heart failure.

COMPLETE STOPPAGE of the urine may occur for a time in the feverish conditions of children, or it may be due to acute Bright's disease, when the condition is a very serious one. When the stoppage is due to failure of the kidneys to secrete any urine, the condition is known as *suppression* or *anuria*. When the stoppage is due to such a cause as blockage of the ureters by stones or of the urethra by a stricture, although secretion by the kidneys still goes on, it is known as *retention.* Stoppage of the urine, to whatever cause it be due, may often be relieved by placing the patient in a hot bath and administering to him sweet spirits of nitre or other diaphoretic.

Colour – The tint of normal urine is generally described as straw or amber coloured, but it may be considerably changed by various diseases or drugs.

PALLOR, giving the urine a watery appearance, is found in diabetes and in chronic Bright's disease, also in persons who drink large quantities of water.

ORANGE or RED COLOUR may appear when senna or rhubarb has been taken; when blood is present the colour may be pink or bright red; urates cause a turbid red or yellow appearance.

SMOKY TINT, depriving the urine of transparency, is caused by small quantities of blood.

GREEN or GREENISH-YELLOW urine is usually due to bile, or may be produced by taking santonin or quinine.

BLACK URINE may be due to absorption of carbolic acid from surgical dressings or from taking carbolic acid, lysol, or similar substances internally. It is often passed by those who are taking guaiacol or creosote. It may also be due to the presence of indican in cases of intestinal stasis, and is found in the form of sarcoma known as melanotic sarcoma when this involves the liver.

Odour – Healthy urine has a faint aromatic odour, but when it begins to decompose, an unpleasant ammoniacal smell is given off. Thus the presence of cystitis or of dribbling of the urine is betrayed by the odour of the patient's personal or bed clothes. When turpentine and some other aromatic drugs have been taken, the urine

909

acquires an odour of violets, and in diabetes it presents an aroma similar to that of new-mown hay.

Specific gravity of urine varies in health from 1015 to 1025 (distilled water being 1000). A urine of lower specific gravity suggests the presence of chronic Bright's disease, whilst a higher specific gravity may be due to diabetes, or to a feverish state.

Reaction – When the urine is tested with litmus paper it is found to be acid in general, and this is of importance, because the acid has an antiseptic action. This acidity is due, not to free acids, but to acid salts such as acid phosphate of sodium. In consequence of the secretion of acid from the blood into the gastric juice that is poured into the stomach shortly after meals, the urine may at such times become alkaline. In herbivorous animals and in vegetarians, owing to the great quantities of alkaline salts eaten in the diet, the urine is permanently alkaline.

Deposits – In healthy urine there is usually a fleecy deposit of mucus secreted by the mucous membrane of the urinary passages. A pink or yellow deposit, that settles as soon as the urine begins to cool, and that often leaves a stain upon the utensil in which the urine has stood, is due to urates. (See URIC ACID.) Uric acid is a rarer deposit, and, when present, falls in very scanty yellow or brownish, so-called 'cayenne-pepper' grains. A white deposit that collects upon the bottom of the utensil after the urine has stood undisturbed for some time may be due to phosphates, to pus, or to debris from diseased kidneys known as tube-casts.

Abnormal substances – Many unusual substances taken into or formed in the body are got rid of in the urine, sometimes just as they have entered the body, in other cases considerably changed, eg. drugs, and the poisons of various diseases. Further, various bacteria and parasites can be discovered in the urine in some diseases. Elaborate chemical or microscopical examination is necessary in order to reveal these, but there are six substances the detection of which is of great importance, and which are discovered with comparative ease. These substances are (1) albumin; (2) blood; (3) sugar; (4) pus and tube-casts; (5) bile; (6) acetone. Strip tests, which merely involve the placing in urine of small specially impregnated strips of paper, are now available for all of these, except pus and tube-casts. Whilst these are satisfactory and time-saving for routine purposes, they still require to be checked sometimes by the older, more conventional, methods.

(1) ALBUMIN is present in various conditions mentioned under ALBUMINURIA, and may be recognized by the following tests:

(a) *Boiling*, after the addition of a few drops of acid, produces a copious white cloud of coagulated albumin.

(b) *Salicylsulphonic acid* – Drop 25 per cent solution of salicylsulphonic acid into a test-tube containing urine. If albumin is present, each drop carries down a white cloud of coagulated albumin.

(2) BLOOD is present in acute Bright's disease, in congestion of the kidneys, or when a stone, ulcer, or tumour is present in any of the urinary organs. A drop of the urine must be examined under the microscope to find if blood-cells are actually present.

(3) SUGAR is a sign of diabetes mellitus (qv) when it is present constantly in the urine. It may also be found following upon a diet that contains a great deal of sugar – a harmless condition known as alimentary glycosuria. In some cases the difficulty lies in the kidneys – renal diabetes, which is also of little importance.

(a) *Fehling's test* – A special blue-coloured solution composed of copper sulphate, Rochelle salt, and caustic potash is placed in a test-tube and heated almost to boiling point. While it is hot, an equal volume of the suspected urine, which has also been heated in a separate test-tube, is added, and, if sugar is present, red and yellow cuprous salts are formed.

(b) *Benedict's test* – Benedict's reagent contains copper sulphate, sodium carbonate, potassium citrate, potassium thiocyanate, and potassium ferrocyanide, dissolved in distilled water. When urine containing sugar is boiled along with this pale-blue solution, the colour disappears. This reagent can be used for estimating approximately the amount of sugar present, the calculation being based upon the fact that 25 ml of the reagent are completely reduced by 50 mg of glucose, and rendered colourless.

(c) *Fermentation test* – A little yeast is shaken up with some of the urine, placed in a special glass which is closed at the upper end, and allowed to stand in a warm place overnight. If the urine contains sugar it will ferment and bubbles of carbon dioxide collect at the upper end of the glass.

(4) PUS AND TUBE-CASTS are the sign of inflammation or of ulceration somewhere in the urinary passages. Pus alone is generally a sign that the bladder is affected;

tube-casts always point to involvement of the kidneys. For the detection of pus or tube-casts in small amounts a drop of urine must be placed on a glass slide and examined with the microscope.

(5) BILE in the urine is a sign that the bile ducts are obstructed, and that bile is being absorbed into the blood. Sometimes the jaundice that accompanies this condition is so slight as to escape notice, so that the detection of bile in the urine is an important sign. Place some of the urine in a large conical glass, dilute it with water till quite transparent, and pour impure nitric acid down the side of the glass. If bile is present in the urine, a brilliant play of colours – yellow, red, violet, and green – takes place where the urine and acid meet. It is the green colour that is characteristic of bile.

(6) ACETONE may appear in the urine in cases of diabetes, general acidosis, and some other conditions.

Rothera's test – Place in a test-tube crystals of ammonium sulphate to a depth of about an inch (25 mm). Then add a few grains of sodium nitroprusside. Add sufficient urine to produce a saturated solution of the ammonium sulphate. This requires vigorous shaking of the test-tube, and, if the solution is saturated, there will be some undissolved crystals in the solution. A solution of strong ammonia is then added, and, if a purple colour develops, this denotes the presence of acetone bodies.

DIACETIC ACID, which is often also present with acetone, may be tested by adding to $1\frac{1}{2}$ inches (3·5 cm) of urine in a test-tube, solution of 10 per cent ferric chloride, drop by drop. A precipitate of iron phosphate first forms, which is filtered off. If diacetic acid be present, a dark-red colour next develops, which disappears on boiling the urine. This is known as *Gerhardt's test*.

URINE, EXCESS OF – The amount of urine passed in 24 hours is often markedly increased in diabetes, a fact which sometimes, without any other symptom, attracts the patient's attention. The bladder also requires to be emptied more than usual in the chronic forms of Bright's disease, but this is due rather to greater frequency than to increased quantity of urine. The increase in this case is noticed especially during the night. Any source of irritation or inflammation in the kidneys or bladder may also produce frequency, such as the formation of gravel or of a stone, tuberculosis of the kidney, inflammation of the bladder (cystitis), or enlargement of the prostate gland. The

bladder, however, varies greatly in size in different individuals, and the necessity to pass water frequently may simply be a lifelong personal peculiarity due to smallness of its capacity.

An annoying form of increase in the urine at night leads to wetting of the bed by children. (See NOCTURNAL ENURESIS.)

Treatment – Any increase in the amount of urine or the frequency with which it is passed calls for testing as to the presence of sugar, albumin, gravel, pus, and the like. The treatment consists in that suited to any disease that may be discovered.

URINE, RETENTION OF – The term, retention, is applied to cases in which urine is duly secreted by the kidneys, but for some reason is retained in the bladder; while the more serious condition, in which the kidneys fail to produce urine, is known as suppression or anuria. (See URINE, AMOUNT.)

Causes – The urine may be retained either because the bladder is too weak to expel it, or because of some obstruction to the passage by which it should be voided. Weakness is a rare condition and is generally the result of some damage to the nervous system, this being one of the troublesome symptoms that follow an injury to the spinal cord; it is accompanied by dribbling away of the urine when the bladder becomes fully distended. A similar condition results from long-continued distension produced by some obstruction to the outflow.

Among the cases due to obstruction, some are acute and merely temporary, such as the difficulty of passing water that follows upon any operation near the bladder, eg. one for piles, or that is apt to follow child-birth. In these cases the difficulty commonly is due to spasm, and does not persist more than a day or two. Among the more chronic cases of retention the commonest are those caused by enlargement of the prostate gland and consequent blockage of the outlet from the bladder; this condition is common in old men. In these the retention usually comes on gradually, and it is a common experience to find that the bladder never empties completely as it ought to do, but forms a sort of reservoir from which an overflow is discharged every few hours. The condition that leads to the most complete form of retention is a stricture or narrowing of the urethra due to the scar of previous injury or ulceration. (See URETHRA, DISEASES OF.) Similar blockage results also, in rare instances, from the pressure of some tumour upon the urethra, or the displacement of a neighbouring organ such as the womb in women.

Treatment – Cases in which retention is due to weakness of the bladder, in a chronic invalid, are treated by the regular use of a soft rubber catheter, and this forms one of the most important duties in the nursing of such a case.

In any case of retention where the urine accumulates in and causes painful distension of the bladder, the condition may often be relieved by the sufferer placing himself in a warm bath. This produces so much relaxation that the bladder often succeeds in emptying itself, a result which is still further assisted by the use of soothing draughts or the giving of an enema.

If relief is not gained by these means, the medical attendant withdraws the urine by means of a catheter passed along the urethra. (See CATHETERS.) The instrument chosen varies according to the cause of the retention; thus, in cases due to weakness of the bladder or to moderate spasm at the outlet, a soft rubber catheter only is necessary. In cases of severer spasm, and in cases where the prostate gland is enlarged, a flexible instrument or a hard rubber catheter with a bend upon the point (known as a *coudé* catheter) is generally chosen; while, in cases of very narrow stricture, the surgeon may require to pass a rigid metal instrument. As a rule, great difficulty is experienced only in the last-named class of cases; and in them it may occasionally be necessary to tap the bladder above the pubis by means of a hollow needle. After its contents have escaped, the patient gains immediate relief.

URINOMETER, or DENSIMETER, is an instrument designed for estimating the specific gravity of urine. It consists of a graduated stem supported upon a large glass bulb containing air which floats partly submerged, and which is kept upright by a smaller bulb containing mercury placed at its lower end. The urine is poured into a tall glass vessel, the urinometer placed in it, and, when it is floating motionless, the point on the scale which is at the surface of the urine registers the specific gravity.

UROGASTRONE is a depressant of gastric acidity which has been isolated from urine. Its precise function in the body and its constitution are not known.

UROLOGY is that branch of medicine which treats of disorders and diseases of the kidneys, ureters, bladder, prostate, and urethra.

URTICARIA is another name for nettle-rash (qv).

UTERUS or WOMB, is a hollow organ suspended in the cavity of the pelvis. In shape, it is triangular from side to side, and flattened from before backwards. The lower angle is prolonged into a rounded neck (*cervix*), about 1 inch (2·5 cm) long, which communicates through a narrow opening or mouth (*os uteri*) with the vagina, the passage leading to the exterior of the body. In size, the normal uterus is only about 3 inches (7·5 cm) long, 2 inches (5 cm) in its greatest width, and 1 inch (2·5 cm) in thickness from front to back, while the walls are so thick that the cavity consists of a mere slit. It weighs 30 to 40 grams. During pregnancy, however, it enlarges to an enormous extent, and the walls increase still further in thickness. (See MUSCLE.) The cavity is lined by a thick, soft, mucous membrane, and the wall is chiefly composed of muscle fibres arranged in three layers. The outer surface, like that of other abdominal organs, is covered by a layer of peritoneum. The uterus has a copious supply of blood derived from the uterine and ovarian arteries. It has also many lymphatic vessels, and its nerves establish wide connections with other organs. (See PAIN.) The position of the uterus is in the centre of the pelvis, where it is suspended by several ligaments between the bladder in front and the rectum behind. On each side of the uterus are the broad ligaments passing outwards to the side of the pelvis, the utero-sacral ligament passing back to the sacral bone, the utero-vesical ligament passing forwards to the bladder, and the round ligament uniting the uterus to the front of the abdomen.

UTERUS, DISEASES OF – Among the most common symptoms are pain or irregularity in the menstrual functions, the presence of a white discharge (*leucorrhoea*), constant pain or sense of weakness in the back, and often the inability to bear children.

MALFORMATIONS sometimes occur and give rise to trouble in child-birth: for example, the uterus may be double, having a partition down the middle. The cervix may be long and furnished with a very narrow mouth, which is sometimes a cause of pain in menstruation.

DISPLACEMENTS are more common. The uterus is slung in the centre of the pelvic cavity, and has great freedom of movement up and down and from before backwards. It lies naturally with its long axis directed upwards and forwards between the bladder and rectum, but its position at any time varies considerably according to the state of distension of one or other of these organs. A flabby state of the muscular wall of the uterus, or a contraction of some of the ligaments that suspend it, may produce a bend upon the organ itself, or may permanently tilt it forwards or backwards. Bending forwards is known as *anteflexion*, tilting forwards is called *anteversion*, and the corresponding conditions towards the back are known as *retroflexion* and *retroversion*. In the treatment of these conditions, two objects are kept in view, the one being to diminish the inflammation that is apt to accompany them, and the other consisting in the support of the uterus in its proper position by a suitably shaped instrument known as a pessary; or by an operation, when the displacement is very marked.

Downward displacement is known as *prolapse*, and in this condition the uterus slips bodily downwards in the space between the bladder and bowel, till, in bad cases, it may actually protrude from the vagina. The condition comes on in older women, usually those who are becoming stout, have a considerable amount of work to do, and have in child-birth suffered laceration of the parts that should support the uterus. When the condition is slight it may be relieved by wearing a suitably shaped pessary, and in cases which are not relieved by this simple measure an operation (colporrhaphy), designed to repair the injury previously done, will often remedy the displacement.

INFLAMMATION is, perhaps, the commonest type of uterine disorder. It is of several forms, but the general term *endometritis* is applied to inflammation affecting the mucous membrane, *metritis* to the rarer condition in which the muscular substance is involved. This condition is often due to child-birth which has not passed off quite successfully; and it is still more often due to miscarriage. Inflammation spreading upwards from the vagina, and displacements of the uterus are other, though less common, causes. The usual treatment consists in rest, the employment of hot, antiseptic douches and other applications to the vagina, and remedies to improve the general health. The sulphonamides or penicillin are given in severe cases. The interior of the uterus can often be brought quickly to a healthy condition by the operation of curetting, which consists in scraping away the unhealthy mucous membrane with a special instrument, the curette. After this operation the patient must observe the greatest caution till the next menstrual period shall have passed.

TUMOURS of the uterus are by no means uncommon. The two most important ones are fibroids and cancer.

Fibroid tumours, or fibromyomas, are the most common form of tumour in any part of the body. They consist of masses of muscle fibres, similar to those of the uterus, and white fibrous tissue. They vary in size from that of a small seed to a mass weighing several pounds. The cause is not known, but they are much more common in women who have never borne children than in those with children. Whilst they may occur any time between puberty and the change of life, they are usually first recognized between the ages of 35 and 45. The symptoms depend upon the size and site of the tumour, and many fibroids give rise to no symptoms at all. Speaking generally, the larger the tumour, and the more it involves the inner aspect of the uterus, the more likely is it to produce signs of its presence. The more important symptoms and signs are menstrual irregularity consisting of excessive loss of blood or excessive length of the period, sterility, frequency of micturition, and retention of urine. Pain is seldom a marked feature. Only those fibroids causing symptoms require treatment. If the symptoms are at all severe, operation is the treatment of choice. In some cases this involves removal of part, or the whole, of the uterus; in others it is possible to remove the tumour itself and leave the rest of the uterus intact. In cases with only mild symptoms, or in women approaching the menopause, when the tumour may decrease in size, medical treatment is sometimes used. This consists of rest in bed during menstruation, the administration of ergot to control the excessive bleeding, and full doses of iron to combat the anaemia usually present. In more severe cases, or in those in which such treatment fails, radiotherapy is sometimes used with benefit.

Cancer of the uterus is one of the most common forms of cancer in women. It may occur in either the neck (or cervix) of the uterus or in the body of the uterus. Cancer of the cervix of the uterus is more common than cancer of the body of the uterus, and 95 per cent of cases occur in women who have borne children. Cancer of the body of the uterus, on the other hand, is more common in unmarried women or women who have never borne children. Both forms occur most commonly between the ages of 40 and 55. Cancer of the body of the uterus is rare before the menopause. The first sign is usually a blood-stained discharge. Treatment consists of radiotherapy or surgery or a combination of both. By and large the earlier the cancer is detected and treated, the better the results. This is why it is so important that any woman over the age of 40 who has either excessive loss at the period, or irregular bleeding, should report at once to her doctor. In most cases there will be nothing serious to worry about, but if the bleeding should be due to cancer, then early diagnosis will permit of treatment being carried out at a stage when the expectation of cure is high. It is in the early diagnosis of cancer of the cervix that cervical cytology, as it is known, is so important. This consists of the perfectly simple procedure, which the woman can do herself, of taking a 'smear' of the cervix for examination in the laboratory. Such examination may reveal the presence of cancer long before it has produced any symptoms and signs, and treatment at this stage produces excellent results. The recommendation of the British Society for Clinical Cytology is that a woman should have this procedure carried out every five years from the age of 30 to that of 70. In 1977, in England there were 3417 deaths from cancer of the uterus.

UTICILLIN (see PENCILLIN).

UVEA is a term applied to the middle coat of the eye, including the iris, ciliary body and choroid.

UVEITIS is inflammation of the uvea. It is responsible for 2 to 3 per cent of the blind population in England. It is rare in childhood and old age.

UVULA is the small mass of muscle covered by mucous membrane that hangs down from the middle of the soft palate. It may be elongated in relaxed conditions of the throat, but should not be cut, since it recovers its proper size as the condition of the throat improves. Its elongation, when sufficient to make it reach the tongue, may set up a constant irritative cough and a tendency to retch.

V

VACCINATION means inoculation with the material of cowpox, performed for the purpose of affording protection to the inoculated person against an attack of smallpox, or at all events with the view of diminishing the seriousness of, and averting a fatal result from, any such attack. This is the strict sense of the term, and the sense in which it will be used here, but it is also used nowadays to describe the process of inoculating with any vaccine to obtain immunity, or protection, against the corresponding disease. The vaccine contains the living virus of smallpox, and is made from the lesions produced by the inoculation of vaccinia in the skin of healthy animals, usually calves or sheep. It may also be prepared by inoculating chick embryos with the virus. Glycerin is added to destroy any other disease-producing micro-organisms that may be present.

History – Among Eastern nations there existed a very ancient practice of inoculating healthy persons with the material from mild cases of smallpox, in the expectation of producing in them a mild attack which rendered them immune from accidental infection that might produce a serious attack at a later period. This practice was introduced into England from Turkey by Lady Mary Wortley Montagu about 1717, and the necessity for some such measure may be judged when it is stated that one in every twelve of the deaths in London during the eighteenth century was due to smallpox. This practice, however, involved a considerable element of danger, and after the introduction of vaccination it was abolished in Britain by Act of Parliament in 1840.

There had long been a tradition among the country people in the west of England that an attack of cowpox – an eruption upon the udders of cows liable to be communicated to the hands of milkers – afforded protection against a subsequent attack of smallpox. In 1796, Edward Jenner, a surgeon of Berkeley, performed his first experiment in this matter by inoculating James Phipps, a boy of eight, with cowpox material from the hand of Sarah Nelmes, a dairymaid. Six weeks later the boy was inoculated with smallpox material, but no disease followed. Subsequently, the experiment was successfully repeated both by Jenner and by other persons, and by 1801 Jenner claimed that over 100,000 persons had been vaccinated in England alone. With regard to the nature of cowpox, opinions have varied as to whether it is simply a modified smallpox or is a different disease. At the present day the general opinion agrees with that held by Jenner, that cowpox is simply smallpox much modified by passage through the cow. So important did vaccination appear to the governments of foreign countries, that its practice was in a few years made compulsory by several, although in England it was not enforced till 1853. Its efficacy was shown by the fact that, the smallpox death-rate for London in the eighteenth century, just before the introduction of vaccination, was 4000 per million living in every year, and in the beginning of the twentieth century, the death-rate from smallpox for England and Wales was only about 75 in every million living. That is to say, during the century in which vaccination was practised, smallpox decreased to one-fortieth of its previous importance as a cause of death.

A Royal Commission on vaccination was appointed by the British Government in 1889, and after exhaustive and careful examination of all the objections to vaccination, this Commission issued its report in 1896. The conclusions as to the value of vaccination in relation to smallpox arrived at by the Commission were as follows: 'We think –

'1. That it diminishes the liability to be attacked by the disease.

'2. That it modifies the character of the disease, and renders it (a) less fatal, and (b) of a milder or less severe type.

'3. That the protection it affords against attacks of the disease is greatest during the years immediately succeeding the operation of vaccination. It is impossible to fix with precision the length of this period of highest protection. Although not in all cases the same, if a period is to be fixed, it might, we think, fairly be said to cover in general a period of nine or ten years.

'4. That after the lapse of the period of highest protective potency the efficacy of vaccination to protect against attack rapidly diminishes, but that it is still considerable in the next quinquennium, and possibly never altogether ceases.

'5. That its power to modify the character of the disease is also greatest in the period in which its power to protect from attack is greatest, but that its power thus to modify the disease does not diminish as rapidly as its protective influence against attacks, and its efficacy during the later periods of life to modify the disease is still very considerable.

'6. That revaccination restores the protection which lapse of time has diminished, but the evidence shows that this protection again diminishes, and that to ensure the highest protection which vaccination can give the operation should be at intervals repeated.'

Dangers of vaccination – There are certain complications of vaccination. One is the development of the condition known as vaccinia which, for all practical purposes, is a mild attack of smallpox. In England and Wales, in 1970, there were 17 cases of vaccinia among the 417,803 people vaccinated, and three among the 114,452 people who were revaccinated. Another is the development of certain skin rashes but these are seldom severe except in eczematous subjects, and the general rule is not to vaccinate such individuals unless there is some special reason such as the occurrence of a local outbreak of smallpox, or the individual requiring an International Certificate of Vaccination for essential travel abroad. In England and Wales, in 1970, there were two cases of vaccination eczema (or eczema vaccinatum as it is known) both were in coloured children who had a history of eczema; both recovered. On the other hand, two eczematous children who came in contact with recently vaccinated relations, developed eczema vaccinatum and died. This is a reminder that recently vaccinated people must avoid all contact with eczematous children until the vaccination process is completed. A third complication, and most important of all, is the development of encephalitis (qv) or encephalomyelitis (qv). This is not common. In 1970 in England and Wales there were two cases, one of which proved fatal.

In the United Kingdom the recommended time for primary (or first) smallpox vaccination is the second year of life. In 1971, however, the Secretary of State for Health and Social Security decreed that vaccination against smallpox need no longer be recommended as a routine procedure in early childhood.

Method of vaccination – If the child suffers from any skin disorder, or from diarrhoea, or if there is any severe epidemic in the neighbourhood by which the child is likely to be infected, vaccination should be delayed till the child is better. If, however, there be smallpox in the child's vicinity, nothing should interfere with his vaccination.

The two main methods of vaccination

are the multiple pressure method and the scratch method. The former is the technique used in the United States of America, and is preferred by many experts in Great Britain. The advantages claimed for it are that it produces less severe reactions and smaller scars, and a larger number of 'takes'. Many, however, still prefer the scratch method which is officially recognized as an alternative procedure in Great Britain.

The part is either covered by a simple dry dressing or is left exposed, care being taken not to wet it. No change is noticed till about the third day, when a slight elevation appears at the vaccinated spots. By the fifth or sixth day this has developed into a distinct vesicle, with a central depression, and the vesicle has attained its full development and become of a pearl colour one week from the day on which the lymph was inserted. There is often a red ring of inflammation round each vesicle, and both this and the vesicle increase in extent for the next day or two, the arm at the same time becoming slightly swollen and the glands in the armpit enlarged. After this the inflammation subsides, the vesicle at the end of a fortnight dries up and forms a hard brown scab, which falls off about the end of the third week, leaving a permanent, depressed scar.

As a result of the World Health Organization (W H O) smallpox eradication campaign the disease has for all practical purposes been wiped out, only sporadic cases occurring in the Horn of Africa: three between October 1977 and August 1978. Vaccination, however, is still required by seventy countries, all outside Europe and North America, for all travellers from abroad. Anyone therefore travelling overseas who is not carrying a valid International Certificate of Vaccination, which is valid for three years, may find himself refused entry to another country or alternatively have to submit to immediate vaccination at the point of entry to the country in question – with all the disadvantages, practical, medical and financial that this may involve. In these circumstances anyone who has already been vaccinated, and is proceeding overseas, would probably be well advised to have himself vaccinated every three years until the International Certificate of Vaccination is withdrawn from official use. What line parents should take with their children is another matter, and one that should be discussed with their family doctor.

VACCINE is the name applied generally to a substance of the nature of dead or attenuated living infectious material introduced into the body with the object of increasing its power to resist or to get rid of a disease. (See also IMMUNITY.)

In cases where healthy people are inoculated with vaccine as a protection against a particular disease, this is done with the object of producing antibodies which will confer immunity against a subsequent attack of the disease.

Vaccines may be divided into two classes: stock vaccines, prepared from micro-organisms known to cause a particular disease and kept in readiness for use against that disease; and autogenous vaccines, prepared from micro-organisms which are already in the patient's body and to which the disease is due. Vaccines intended to protect against the onset of disease are necessarily of the stock variety.

Autogenous vaccines are prepared from the cultivation of bacteria found in the expectoration, the urine, the faeces, and in areas of inflammation such as boils. This type of vaccine was introduced by Wright about 1903. (See OPSONINS.)

Anthrax vaccine was introduced by Pasteur about 1882 for the protection of sheep and cattle against this disease. A safe and effective vaccine for use in human beings has now been evolved.

BCG vaccine is used to provide protection against tuberculosis. (See BCG VACCINE.)

Cholera vaccine was introduced by Haffkine in India about 1894. Two injections are given at an interval of at least a week; this gives a varying degree of immunity for six months.

Diphtheria vaccine is available in several forms. (See DIPHTHERIA.) It is usually given along with tetanus and pertussis vaccine in what is known as Triple Vaccine. This is given in three doses: the first at the age of 3 or 6 months, the second six to eight weeks later, and the third six months later, with a booster dose at the age of 5 years.

Hay fever vaccine – A vaccine prepared from the pollen of various grasses is used in gradually increasing doses for prevention of hay fever in persons susceptible to this disease.

Influenza vaccine – A vaccine is now available for protection against influenza due to the influenza viruses A and B.

Measles vaccine is now available in two forms: an inactivated vaccine and a live attenuated vaccine. One injection of the live attenuated vaccine is recommended officially in Britain early in the second year of life.

Plague vaccine was introduced by Haffkine, and appears to give useful protection, but the duration of protection is relatively short – from two to twenty months. Two injections are given at an interval of 4 weeks. A reinforcing dose should be given annually to persons exposed to the disease.

Poliomyelitis vaccine is now available which gives a high degree of protection against the disease. The Salk-type of vaccine, in which the virus is killed by formaldehyde, contains all three known types of poliomyelitis virus. Three intramuscular injections are required, with an interval of four to six weeks between the first and second, and seven to twelve months between the second and third. There is a growing volume of evidence that a fourth injection prolongs the duration of the protection provided by the vaccine.

The Salk vaccine has now been largely replaced by the live attenuated vaccine which is taken by mouth – a few drops on a lump of sugar.

Rabies vaccine was introduced by Pasteur in 1885 for administration, during the long incubation period, to persons bitten by a rabid dog, in order to prevent the disease from developing.

Rubella vaccine is now available to provide protection against German measles. The value of such a vaccine lies in the fact that it will allow immunity to be given to adolescent girls who have not had the disease in childhood and so ensure that they will not acquire the disease during any subsequent pregnancy. In this way it should prove possible to reduce the number of congenitally abnormal children whose abnormality is the result of their being infected with German measles before they were born, the infection being acquired through their mother having the disease. The recommendation is that it should be given to all girls at the age of 12 to 13 years who have not had the disease.

Smallpox vaccine was the first introduced. (See VACCINATION.)

Tetanus vaccine is given in two forms: (a) In the so-called Triple Vaccine, combined with diphtheria and pertussis (whooping-cough) vaccine. This is used for the routine immunization of children, the first dose being given at the age of 3 to 6 months, a second dose six to eight weeks later, and a third dose six months later. (b) By itself to adults who have not been immunized in childhood and who are particularly exposed to the risk of tetanus, such as soldiers and agricultural workers.

917

Typhoid vaccine was introduced by Wright and Semple for the protection of troops in the South African War and in India. The commonly used TAB vaccine contains 1000 million *Salmonella typhi* (the causative organism of typhoid fever) and 500 or 750 million *Salmonella paratyphi* A and 500 or 750 million *Salmonella paratyphi* B (the causative organisms of paratyphoid fever) in 1 millilitre. Two doses are given by subcutaneous injection at an interval of four to six weeks, and give protection for one to three years. There may be some reddening and discomfort at the site of injection accompanied sometimes by general malaise for 12 hours. There is also a vaccine available now, either with, or without, *S. paratyphi*, which is given intracutaneously (ie. into the skin).

Whooping-cough vaccine is prepared from the bacillus of Bordet and Gengou, or *Bordetella pertussis*, and is proving of value in prophylaxis against whooping-cough.

Yellow fever vaccine is prepared from chick embryos injected with the living, attenuated strain (17D) of pantropic virus. Only one injection is required, and immunity persists for many years. Reinoculation, however, is desirable every ten years.

The hazards of vaccination, or immunization are minimal, compared with its benefits. Complications, however, do occur. A Vaccine Damage Payments Scheme has therefore been introduced. This provides for the payment of £10,000 tax free in respect of persons who, since July 5, 1948, have suffered severe damage as a result of the following vaccinations which have taken place under routine public policy programmes: diphtheria, tetanus, whooping-cough, poliomyelitis, measles, German measles, tuberculosis (BCG), and smallpox (up to July 31, 1971).

VACCINIA is another term for cowpox, a disease in which vesicles form on the udders and teats, due to the same virus as is responsible for smallpox in man. It is also the term used to describe the reaction to smallpox vaccination.

VAGINA is the name given to the front passage leading from the exterior to the womb.

VAGINISMUS is the term applied to spasmodic contraction of the orifice of the vagina on attempted coitus. It is usually psychological in origin, due, for instance, to a neurotic temperament or to frigidity, but it may also be due to some local inflammatory condition.

VAGINITIS is inflammation of the vagina. (See WHITES.)

VAGITUS UTERINUS is the term applied to the crying of a child just before birth and while still in the uterus.

VAGOTOMY is the operation of cutting the fibres of the vagus nerve to the stomach. It is sometimes performed as part of the surgical treatment of duodenal ulcer, the aim being to reduce the flow or acidity of the gastric juice.

VAGUS, or PNEUMOGASTRIC, nerve is the tenth cranial nerve. Unlike the other cranial nerves, which are concerned with the special senses, or distributed to the skin and muscles of the head and neck, this nerve, as its names imply, strays downwards into the chest and abdomen, supplying branches to the throat, lungs, heart, stomach, and other abdominal organs. It contains motor, secretory, sensory, and vasodilator fibres.

VALERIAN is the root of *Valeriana officinalis,* a European plant. Its action, which is a sedative one upon the nervous system, depends mainly upon a volatile oil that it contains, and also to some extent upon valerianic acid.

Uses – Valerian was at one time widely used, chiefly in the form of the tincture of valerian, to quiet nervousness, insomnia, and hysterical attacks, being taken in doses of a teaspoonful. The oil of valerian, in doses of two or three drops on sugar, is an old remedy for the relief of dyspepsia associated with spasm of the stomach.

VALETUDINARIAN is a term applied to an invalid; also to a person who is constantly thinking about his own state of health.

VALGUS means literally knock-kneed, and is a bending inward at the knees (*genu valgum*), or at the ankle, as occurs in flatfoot (*pes valgus*).

VALVES are found in the heart, veins, and lymphatic vessels, for the purpose of maintaining the circulation of the blood and lymph always in one direction. (See HEART; LYMPH; VEINS.)

VALVULAR DISEASE (see HEART DISEASES).

VANCOMYCIN is an antibiotic derived from a streptomyces, which is active against a wide range of Gram-positive organisms, including the staphylococcus.

VAN DEN BERGH TEST is one performed on a specimen of serum of the blood in cases of jaundice, to decide whether this is due to ordinary bile (immediate reaction) or incompletely formed bile pigment (delayed reaction).

VAPOUR BATHS (see BATHS).

VARICELLA is another name for chickenpox (qv).

VARICOCELE means a condition in which the veins of the testicle are distended. (See TESTICLE, DISEASES OF.)

VARICOSE VEINS are veins that have become stretched and dilated. (See VEINS, DISEASES OF.)

VARIOLA is another name for smallpox (qv).

VARIOLOID is the name applied to a mild type of smallpox.

VARIX means an enlarged and tortuous vein.

VARUS, meaning bow-legged, is the term applied to a bulging condition at the hip (*coxa vara*), at the knee (*genu varum*), or at the ankle (*talipes varus*).

VAS is the Latin term for a vessel, especially a blood-vessel.

VASECTOMY is the surgical operation performed to render men sterile, or infertile. It consists of ligating, or tying, and then cutting the ductus, or vas, deferens (see TESTICLE). It is quite a simple operation carried out under local anaesthesia, through a small incision, or cut (or sometimes two) in the upper part of the scrotum. It has no effect on sexual drive or ejaculation, and does not cause impotency. It is not immediately effective, and several tests, spread over several months, must be carried out before it is safe to assume that sterility has been achieved. Although, in those who desire it, fertility can sometimes be restored by a further operation, to restore the continuity of the vas, this cannot be guaranteed, and only seems to occur in about one-fifth of those so operated on.

In 1976, 16,884 vasectomies were performed in National Health Service family planning clinics in England.

VASODILATORS are substances that cause dilatation of the blood-vessels. They may be drugs, such as amyl nitrite (qv), or natural substances in the body, such as kinins (qv).

VASOMOTOR NERVES are the small nerve fibres that lie upon the walls of blood-vessels and connect the muscle fibres of their middle coat with the nervous system. Through these nerves are retained in a state of moderate contraction. There are vasodilator nerves, through which are transmitted impulses that dilate the vessels, and, in the case of the skin-vessels, produce the condition of blushing. There are also vasoconstrictor nerves which transmit impulses that constrict, or narrow, the blood-vessels, as occurs on exposure to cold. (See HYPOTHERMIA.) Various drugs produce dilatation or contraction of the blood-vessels and several of the substances produced by ductless glands in the body have these effects: eg. adrenaline (qv).

VASOPRESSIN is the fraction isolated from extract of the posterior pituitary lobe which stimulates intestinal activity, constricts blood-vessels, and inhibits the secretion of urine. It is also known as the antidiuretic hormone because of this last effect, and its only use in medicine is, on account of this effect, in the treatment of diabetes insipidus (qv). (See also PITUITARY BODY.)

VEGANISM is a strict form of vegetarianism.

VEGETARIANISM means the principle of subsisting on a diet of vegetables which contains no meat. Such a diet may include milk, cheese and eggs, but there is a strict form of vegetarianism, known as veganism, the adherents of which will eat only vegetables and fruit. (See Quality of Food under DIET.)

VEGETATIONS is the term applied to roughenings that appear upon the valves of the heart, usually as the result of acute rheumatism, and that lead in time to narrowing of the openings from the cavities of the heart, or to incompetence of the valves that close these openings. (See HEART DISEASES.)

VEGETATIVE SYSTEM is a term applied to that part of the nervous system which acts in an involuntary manner, to a large extent independently of the brain and spinal cord, and which regulates and connects movements and secretions of internal organs. It is also known as the autonomic nervous system. The term includes the sympathetic and parasympathetic nervous systems (qv).

VEINS are the vessels which carry blood to the heart after it has circulated through the tissues of the body. In general the veins lie alongside corresponding arteries that carry outwards to the tissues the blood which afterwards returns by the veins. The veins are, however, both more numerous and more capacious than the arteries, and, as a rule, there are two accompanying veins for each artery of moderate size. In addition to these deeply placed veins, there are superficial veins in the limbs, which can be readily seen in their distended state lying immediately beneath the skin.

Structure – A vein is of similar structure to an artery, consisting of three coats: outer of fibrous, middle of muscular and elastic fibres, and inner composed of elastic membrane and flattened cells. Any vein has, however, a much thinner wall than its corresponding artery, especially as regards the middle coat. Most veins are provided with valves (illustration 427) similar in structure to the aortic and pulmonary valves of the heart, and consisting each of two segments or pouches, which lie flat against the wall of the vein as the blood passes in the proper direction, or which meet and close the passage whenever the blood tends to run backwards. The position of these valves can easily be seen upon the arm or leg by running the finger backwards along a large vein, when the distended vein shows a little swelling at each valve. The valves are most numerous in the veins of the lower limb, those in the arm stand next in point of

427 – A vein slit open to show the two pockets of a valve on its inner surface.

numbers, whilst there are few valves in the veins of internal organs.

Chief veins – Four *pulmonary veins* open into the left atrium of the heart, two coming from each lung. Into the right atrium there open some small veins from the walls of the heart, and two great vessels, superior vena cava and inferior vena cava, that bring back blood from the body generally. The *superior vena cava* brings the blood from the head, neck, and upper limbs. It is formed by the union of two *innominate veins*, each of which results from the junction, at the root of the neck, of the internal jugular vein, from the neck, and the subclavian vein, from the upper limb. The *internal jugular vein* receives the blood from within the skull and collects branches from the face and neck as it runs downwards alongside the carotid artery under cover of the thick sternocleidomastoid muscle. One of its most important branches is the *external jugular vein*, which runs beneath the skin from the angle of the jaw straight downwards to the middle of the collar-bone. This vessel can be readily seen when the veins of the neck are distended, and is liable to be opened in wounds of this region. The *subclavian vein* is the last section of the system of veins that accompany the arteries in the arm, each vein being named after its corresponding artery. The superficial veins of the arm are of special interest, because the large *basilic vein* that runs up the inner side of the upper arm is the vein usually opened in blood-letting. Its tributary, the median cubital vein, is used for punctures to get blood for various tests or in order to give intravenous injections. (See BLOOD-LETTING.)

The *inferior vena cava*, which lies to the right side and in front of the spinal column, starting at the junction of the two common iliac veins about the level of the navel, collects the blood from the lower limbs and abdomen. In the lower limbs and in the pelvis, the deeply placed veins correspond in name and in position to the arteries, while the surface veins of the lower limb empty their contents into the *small saphenous vein* on the back of the leg, and the *great saphenous vein* that runs from the instep up the inner side of the leg, knee, and thigh. These veins, and especially the great saphenous vein, are of special interest because of their liability to become distended or varicose. Within the abdomen, the inferior vena cava receives branches corresponding to several branches of the aorta, its largest branches being the *hepatic veins*, which return not only the blood that has reached the liver in the hepatic arteries, but also blood which comes from the digestive organs in the *portal vein* to undergo a second capillary circulation in the liver. (See PORTAL VEIN.)

It appears from what has been said that the blood circulating in the uppermost parts of the body is returned to the heart by the superior vena cava, that from below the diaphragm by the inferior vena cava. There are, however, several connections between these two great vessels, the most important being three *azygos veins* that lie upon the sides of the spinal column, the veins on the front of the abdomen, and some veins that emerge from the abdomen at the navel and connect the portal system with those of the inferior and superior vena cava. By these means the circulation is maintained even when one of these large vessels has been blocked by some disease within the chest or the abdomen.

VEINS, DISEASES OF – These vessels are subject to degenerative and inflammatory changes.

INFLAMMATION of a vein is a condition which is serious mainly on account of the clotting of blood that usually takes place within the inflamed part (thrombosis), and the risk that such a clot may break up and portions be swept away by the circulation to lodge in other vessels (embolism). *Phlebitis*, or *thrombophlebitis*, is the name commonly applied to general inflammation of a vein, while the term *peri-phlebitis* is used when the inflammation is limited to the loose connective tissue immediately surrounding the vessel. Occasionally the inflammation is of a very acute character, the vein becoming filled with a clot containing bacteria, which are carried to distant parts of the body and there produce abscesses. This condition, known as pyaemia, is an extremely grave one. (See BLOOD-POISONING.) As a rule, however, phlebitis is of a more chronic type, running a course of three or four weeks and then improving under careful treatment.

Causes – Thrombophlebitis may occur as a result of local injury to the affected part, eg. a bruise or a fracture, or it may be due to involvement of the vein from a neighbouring inflammatory or suppurative process. It not infrequently occurs in varicose veins. Most of the cases, however, occur following child-birth or an operation, and in these cases the main factor responsible for the condition is stagnation of the blood-flow through the veins. (See also WHITE LEG.) It may also occur in certain infectious diseases, particularly typhoid fever, and in certain non-infectious diseases, including gout. In all these conditions the actual cause is probably one or more of three factors: (1) injury or inflammation of the lining endothelium of the vein; (2) slowing of the blood-stream in the vein; (3) some alteration in the blood which makes it more liable to clot.

Symptoms – In a typical case, the skin near the inflamed vein becomes red; the affected part becomes hot, and indeed the general temperature of the body may sometimes be raised; there is swelling both around the vein and of the part beyond it, so that, if a vein in the leg be inflamed, the foot is swollen; finally, considerable pain and tenderness to touch are experienced along the vein. When a clot forms in the vein, as it commonly does, the vessel can be felt as a hard line, and this blocked condition may persist for the rest of life, the vein being converted into a firm, fibrous cord; or a passage may be tunnelled through the clot after the inflammation has subsided in the course of three or four weeks.

Treatment – When the veins of the lower limbs are involved, the patient should rest in bed with the affected limb elevated and resting on pillows. Hot wet packs are applied to relieve the pain and to help to maintain an adequate circulation. If the pain is severe, sedatives may be required. Anticoagulants such as dicoumarol (qv) and heparin (qv) are also given to prevent the clot increasing in size and to reduce the risk of pulmonary embolism (qv). Within three days of going to bed, the patient should be encouraged to move the affected limb and foot, as this speeds the process of recovery. It is now recognized that prolonged rest in bed tends to delay recovery.

VARICOSE VEINS are veins that have become stretched and dilated out of proportion to the amount of blood they have to carry. There are three positions in which the veins have a special tendency to become varicose. These are the veins about the lower end of the bowel, producing the condition known as haemorrhoids or piles (see PILES); the veins of the testicle. producing varicocele (see TESTICLE, DISEASES OF); and the great saphenous vein, with its branches on the inner side of the leg, knee, and thigh. Further, small veins are apt to become varicose here and there on a mucous membrane that is the seat of chronic catarrh and congestion;

these minute varicose veins are found especially on the mucous membranes of the throat and stomach, and may give rise, now and then, to haemorrhage, particularly in the case of persons addicted to alcoholism. Only the varicose veins of the limbs are considered here, the others having been dealt with elsewhere.

Causes – Undoubtedly some persons are more liable to the formation of varicose veins than others. The veins vary greatly in thickness in different persons and at different portions of the same vein, so that the formation of the vessel wall and the condition of surrounding parts have much to do with its dilatation. Thus the tendency to varicose veins is often hereditary. Employments that necessitate long-continued standing, with little vigorous muscular exertion, not only throw a great strain upon the veins of the leg, but fail to provide the pumping action that muscular contractions exert in emptying the veins. Thus barmaids, shop assistants and waitresses often suffer from varicose veins. The evil effects of prolonged standing are increased by tight garters. Pregnancy is another common cause of varicose veins, though the condition tends to disappear after the child is born.

An important consideration is that, after a vein has begun to dilate, its walls become weaker and its valves useless. Thus the weight of the column of blood in the limb presses down with increasing force, the condition tends to grow worse and worse, and to spread into neighbouring veins.

Symptoms – At first the only symptoms are a feeling of weight and aching in the limbs, accompanied sometimes by cramps. This is experienced either at night, after a long day's standing, or in the morning when the feet are first put to the ground. After the condition becomes marked, there is often swelling of the feet, especially above the ankles, that quickly disappears when the patient lies down. Varicose veins that have lasted many years are liable to become inflamed, and to produce eczema and ulceration of the skin (illustration 428). (See ULCERS.) Another risk attached to untreated varicose veins, particularly in older individuals, is that a blow on them may lead to severe haemorrhage.

Treatment – Varicose veins, as already noted, tend, when untreated, to become worse and worse. Treatment which is directed merely towards checking their increase and towards preventing ulceration is known as palliative treatment, whilst the entire removal of the distended veins is known as radical treatment.

PALLIATIVE TREATMENT – In slight cases, it is often sufficient to avoid the use of garters, to remedy constipation, to avoid standing as much as possible, and, after the day's work is done, to sit with the feet elevated on a couch or chair. In more marked cases, some mechanical support for the superficial veins is necessary, in order to counteract the downward pressure of the blood in the great saphenous vein, whose valves have become useless. For this purpose one may use an elastic or crêpe bandage, or elastic stockings. Elastic bandages are probably the most satisfactory method of support. They can be cleaned with soap and water, and, if carefully handled, will last for a year. There are two main types of elastic bandages: the two-way stretch bandage and the one-way stretch bandage. The former is rather more difficult to apply, but is the bandage of choice in severe cases. For many cases the one-way stretch bandage is eminently satisfactory. Elastic bandages must be removed at night before retiring to bed and reapplied before getting out of bed in the morning. Crêpe bandages are used in a similar manner. Some persons find elastic stockings more comfortable than bandages. There must be no tight band at the top of the stocking, but slipping down may be prevented by suspenders; of the various kinds, the spiral silk elastic stocking is generally regarded as the best. For the treatment of varicose ulcers see ULCERS.

Successful results are sometimes obtained from the injection, here and there into the veins, of some irritating substance, such as sodium tetradecyl sulphate or sodium morrhuate. A clot forms at once in the vein, which later becomes solid. This treatment is practically painless and devoide of later discomfort.

RADICAL TREATMENT is adopted when the veins are excessively dilated, when they cause much annoyance, or when the person suffering from them wishes to enter one of the public services. The most successful method consists in turning up a flap of skin on the inner side of the thigh or knee, ligaturing the vein in two places and removing the intervening dilated portions *en masse*. The wound heals quickly, and, in most cases, the cure is complete.

WOUNDS IN VEINS are not in general serious; for, although a considerable amount of dark blood flows steadily from that end of the vein more distant from the heart, it can be stopped by gentle pressure, and soon ceases of itself. When a varicose

428 – Varicose ulcer. From Borrie,
Roxburgh's Common Skin Diseases.
H. K. Lewis & Co. Ltd.

vein ruptures, as it may do if an ulcer be present, the condition is more serious. Blood, in this case, flows copiously from the end next the heart in consequence of the defects in the vein's valves, as well as from the other end; and the loss of blood may be great unless pressure be speedily applied. This also can be checked easily by pressure above and below the wound, and by raising the limb. Another danger, attaching to wounds of the veins in the neck, is that air may be drawn into them by the act of breathing, and great interference with the circulation may ensue which may well prove fatal.

VENA CAVA is the name applied to either of the two large vessels that open into the right atrium of the heart. (See VEINS.)

VENEPUNCTURE is the name applied to inserting a needle into a vein, usually for the purpose of injecting a drug.

VENEREAL DISEASES, SEXUALLY TRANSMITTED DISEASES, as they are now officially known, are certain contagious maladies which are, as a rule, communicated from one person to another by sexual intercourse. The two important diseases are: syphilis and gonorrhoea. (See articles under these headings.)

The number of patients with early syphilis attending venereal disease clinics in England for the first time in 1977 was 2593. The comparable figure for gonorrhoea was 58,978, 594 of whom were under the age of 16. In 1977, in England the number of deaths directly attributable to syphilitic disease was 85. These figures, however, do not by any means represent the amount of serious invalidism caused to the persons who have suffered from one of these diseases and to their children. The direct results of the diseases are mentioned under the headings GONORRHOEA and SYPHILIS. The results of congenital syphilis include deafness, various forms of skin and bone diseases, and mental defectiveness.

923

At one time a large proportion of cases of blindness in young persons were due to gonorrhoeal ophthalmia contracted at birth, but efficient treatment has now made this one of the rarer causes of blindness.

Among the means which have been proposed for reducing the amount of these diseases are: general instruction of the public in regard to their disastrous effects; provision of means for immediate self-disinfection; early treatment; and compulsory treatment of all persons found to be affected, the last measure almost necessarily implying notification of these diseases in the same manner as one of the ordinary infectious diseases. Such compulsory notification has never been favoured in Great Britain, though it is in force in certain European countries. For purposes of efficient treatment, clinics, where treatment is obtained free of charge, have been established in all the large towns in Great Britain.

VENESECTION means the withdrawal of blood by opening a vein. (See BLOOD-LETTING.)

VENOGRAPHY is the study of the veins, particularly by means of X-rays after the veins have been injected with a radio-opaque substance.

VENOMOUS BITES (see BITES).

VENTER is the Latin term for the belly.

VENTILATION – Ventilation consists in the continuous dilution or removal, by pure fresh air, of the vitiated products from respiration, combustion, putrefaction of animal and vegetable material, and from industrial processes and trades. It includes the ventilation of houses, factories, buildings of every description, as well as of streets, alleys, courts, and sewers. Different methods must be adopted for each variety of case. In streets and courts, reliance must be placed on the influence of winds, the height of the buildings, and the width of the street or space. In the confined areas of houses, means must be adopted for the ingress and exit of the air. Similar provision must be made in the case of sewers, the exit for which, however, must be placed where there is least chance of danger.

It is now recognized that lack of oxygen or excess of carbon dioxide plays little part in producing the discomfort of badly ventilated rooms. Nor is there any evidence that there is any organic poison in exhaled air. The main factor responsible is heat stagnation due to excess of moisture and lack of air movement. In other words, ventilation and warming must be considered together. A desirable atmosphere has been defined as 'cool rather than hot; dry rather than damp; and moving rather than still'. Various methods have been evolved for correlating these different factors, the most important of which include: The *kata-thermometer* (qv) which indicates the cooling power of the air. The *eupatheoscope*, an instrument which corresponds approximately to the human body in its sensitivity to air currents, and is read on a scale of equivalent temperature. The *globe thermometer*, which gives an index of the combined influence of air temperature and radiant heat. Another standard, used in the USA, is the *effective temperature*, which is defined as 'that temperature of saturated motionless air which would produce the same sensation of coolness as that produced by the combination of temperature, humidity, and air motion under observation'. In Great Britain the optimum conditions for sedentary work are a dry kata-thermometer cooling power of 6; an equivalent temperature of 62° F (16·7° C); a globe thermometer reading of 65° F (18·3° C); an effective temperature of 61° F (16·1° C).

Room	Air Supply per Hour
Living-room (4 persons)	2400 cubic feet (68 cubic metres)
Bedroom (2 persons)	1200 cubic feet (34 cubic metres)
Bedroom (1 person)	600 cubic feet (17 cubic metres)
Kitchen	1000 cubic feet (28 cubic metres)
Halls and passages	1 air-change
Bathroom and W.C.s	2 „ „ (or more)

Table 42 – Minimum standards of ventilation.

In the provision of ventilation, the amount of cubic space (table 42) and the superficial area allotted to each individual are important, the amount of floor space per person being a better standard than the amount of cubic space. With a greater cubic space the air can more readily be supplied without the production of a draught. Thus, other things being equal, a wide, low room is better ventilated than a high, narrow one. Some idea of the standards at present being observed may be obtained from the fact that the size of house officially recommended for five persons is 800 to 900 square feet. One of the official criteria of overcrowding is where more than one person is sleeping in a room with a floor area of 70 square feet or more, but less than 90 square feet.

In ventilation, we are either dependent on processes of Nature or on artificial interference, and ventilation may therefore be described as natural or artificial (mechanical).

Natural ventilation depends on the use of certain physical processes. The prevalence of winds by which volumes of air are driven ahead into spaces, or masses of air are aspirated as the wind passes horizontally over chimneys; the law of the diffusion of gases; and the fact that air, when heated, expands, and so becoming lighter bulk for bulk, rises, allowing colder air to rush in to take its place, all play their part in natural ventilation.

In the ordinary dwelling-house, no special provision is usually made for the inlet of fresh air. The windows, doors, and spaces between the skirting-boards and sashes act as inlets. The chimney provides the exit or exhaust. The chief objections, where there are no special inlets, are that one cannot control the source of the supply or ensure thorough mixture of the fresh and vitiated air.

Building regulations lay it down that, unless ventilated by mechanical means, every room for human habitation must be provided with at least one window or other means of ventilation opening directly into the external air. The area of the ventilation opening must equal at least one-twentieth of the floor area, and some part of the opening must be not less than $5\frac{3}{4}$ feet (1·75 metres) above the floor. Every habitable room, not situated in the roof, must be at least 7 feet (2·1 metres) in height. If the room is in the roof, it must be $7\frac{1}{2}$ feet (2·3 metres) in height over not less than one-half the area of the room measured at a height 5 feet (1·5 metres) above the floor.

Inlets, if the air can be warmed, should be placed preferably at the floor level. In cold climates like that of Britain, however, if the air is not specially warmed, the inlet should be placed above the occupants, with the stream directed upwards so that it may at once be well mixed with the general air of the room. A convenient special form of inlet is provided by double windows, the lower sash of the outer window being raised, and the upper sash of the inner window lowered. The air then enters between the windows.

Hinckes Bird's method of raising the lower sash about four inches (10 cm) by an accurately fitting wooden board, gives an

429 – Hinckes Bird's ventilator from inside room.

430 – Vertical section of a window, showing the board introduced beneath the lower sash.

inlet between the two sashes of a window (illustrations 429, 430). Louvres, preferably on the lowest plane of the upper sash, and revolving glass discs covering or exposing holes in the window when required, are largely used. Windows with the upper portion hinged to fall inwards and thus directing the current upwards, are commonly employed. Sheringham's valves, in which the air passes through a perforated plate and impinges on a hinged valve, serve the same end (illustration 431). Tobin's tubes have the air entering through a perforated plate at the floor level, from which it is

Sheringham's valve

Tobin's tube

431 – Vertical section of a house wall with a grating on the outer side and the valve on the inside.

432 – Vertical section showing the wall, grating, and flanges to direct the air over a tray of water on the floor and Tobin's tube running upwards about 6 feet.

conducted by a tube of about 6 feet (1·8 metres) in height through the wall and up its inner side (illustration 432). Ellison's bricks are bricks pierced with conical holes which have a small opening to the outside and a wide opening to the inside of the building. The air in this way is diffused as it enters.

Outlets should be placed at the highest parts of the room, or, if they can be heated, at any part. They should be protected by cowls to aid aspiration by wind, and to prevent their being closed or acting as channels for rain. They should be straight and smooth to lessen the retardation of the air by friction. The chimney with an open fire is still a not uncommon outlet in rooms, or the heat of the fire may be utilized by shafts round the smoke-flue opening from the upper parts of the room, or again a valve may open directly into the chimney, but so arranged as to prevent the reflux of smoke.

Artificial ventilation consists in the propulsion into a building of the required fresh air, or the extraction of foul air, by mechanical means. Various forms of air-conditioning plants are now in use which purify, heat, and moisten the air, and automatically change the air in a room so many times an hour.

The advantages of artificial ventilation are: the greater certainty that the source of fresh air is pure; the ease with which the supply can be regulated, filtered, warmed, or cooled; the more effective distribution of the air, and its independence of the weather conditions.

Air sterilization – In order to reduce the risk of cross-infection, particularly in schools, dormitories, and offices, much attention has been devoted in recent years to the problem of killing pathogenic organisms in the air of a room. Ultra-violet light has been used, but its use for this purpose is restricted. It has been used mainly in operating theatres and the like (illustration 288). By and large, the most practical way of ensuring as clean air as possible is to maintain adequate circulation of the air to keep it as free as possible from dust, and the wearing of masks on special occasions. (See also HUMIDIFICATION.)

VENTOUSE, or VACUUM EXTRACTOR, is used in obstetrics. It is based upon a suction-cup technique, whereby the baby is sucked out of the uterus instead of being drawn out by forceps.

VENTRAL means belonging to the belly.

VENTRICLE is the term applied to the two lower cavities of the heart (see HEART), and also to the cavities within the brain.

VENTRICULOGRAPHY is the term applied to the process of taking an X-ray photograph of the brain after the fluid in the lateral ventricles of the brain has been replaced by air; in this way any alteration in the outline of the ventricles (eg. from pressure by a tumour) can be detected.

VERAPAMIL is a drug that is used in the treatment of disordered rhythms of the heart and angina pectoris (qv). It is given by intravenous injection.

VERATRINE is a mixture of alkaloids, derived from the seeds of *Schoenocaulon officinale*, which has a paralysing effect upon nerves. The ointment of veratrine is used for the relief of pain in cases of rheumatism or of neuralgia.

VERATRUM, also known as green hellebore, Indian poke, and poke root, is the root of *Veratrum viride*, a plant of the United States. It acts as a sedative and depressant of the heart and nervous system by virtue of veratrine and other alkaloids that it contains. Alkaloids obtained from it are used in the treatment of high blood-pressure. (See ESSENTIAL HYPERTENSION.)

VERBIGERATION means the insane repetition of meaningless words and sentences.

VERDIGRIS is a basic acetate of copper. It may be formed by the action of fruit juice on copper saucepans or dishes which are not kept clean, and is said to have given rise to poisoning. (See COPPER POISONING.)

VERMICELLI (see MACARONI).

VERMICIDES, or VERMIFUGES, are substances that kill, or expel, parasitic worms from the intenstines.

VERMIN is a term applied in medicine to parasites on the surface of the body. (See INSECTS IN RELATION TO DISEASE.)

VERRUCA is the Latin term for a wart.

VERRUCOSE means covered with warts.

VERSION, or TURNING, is the name given to an operation in obstetrics which consists in turning the child in cases in which the lie of the child is abnormal.

VERTEBRA is one of the irregularly shaped bones that together form the vertebral column. (See SPINAL COLUMN.)

VERTIGO, or giddiness, is a condition in which the affected person loses the power of balancing himself, and has a false sensation as to his own movements or as to those of surrounding objects. The power of balancing depends upon sensations derived partly through the sense of touch, partly from the eyes, but mainly from the semicircular canals of the internal ear, and vertigo is in general due to some interference with this mechanism or with the centres in the cerebellum and cerebrum with which it is connected. Giddiness is very apt to be associated with headache, nausea, and vomiting.

Causes – The simplest cause of vertigo is some mechanical disturbance of the body affecting the fluid in the internal ear; such as that produced by moving in a swing with the eyes shut, the motion of a boat causing sea-sickness, or a sudden fall. (See SEA-SICKNESS.) The cause which produces the most severe and sudden giddiness is Menière's disease (qv), a condition in which there is loss of function of the labyrinth of the inner ear. The most serious form is that in which sudden haemorrhage takes place into the semicircular canals, producing an apoplectic-like fall, often of great violence. A condition of similar nature, though less violent and less permanent in its effects, is sometimes produced by the removal of wax from the ear, or even by syringing out the ear. (See EAR, DISEASES OF.) A third group of causes for vertigo is found in disorders of the stomach. Refractive errors in the eyes which have not received appropriate treatment by glasses, an overstrained nervous system, an attack of migraine, a mild attack of epilepsy, and gross diseases of the brain, such as tumours, form another set of causes acting more directly upon the central nervous system. Finally, giddiness may be due to some disorder of the circulation, eg. bloodlessness of the brain produced by fainting, or by disease of the heart.

Treatment, while the attack lasts, consists in maintaining a recumbent posture, in a darkened, quiet room. Sedatives are the drugs which have most influence in diminishing giddiness when it is distressing. After the attack is over, careful examination is necessary in order to determine the cause, for upon this depends the appropriateness of treatment.

VESICAL is the term applied to structures connected with, or diseases of, the bladder. (See BLADDER.)

VESICANTS are blistering agents. (See BLISTERS.)

VESICLE means a small collection of fluid in the epidermis. The fluid in some cases consists of a drop of sweat collected at the mouth of a sweat-gland, but in general it is serum from the blood. The skin disease specially associated with the formation of vesicles is herpes; in this disease the vesicles usually burst and then scab over. Some infectious diseases show an eruption composed of vesicles: eg. smallpox and chickenpox. When a large number of white corpuscles from the blood find their way into a vesicle, it becomes a pustule.

The term vesicle is also applied to minute sacs of normal structure, such as the air-vesicles in which the finest bronchial tubes end in the lungs.

VESTIBULOCOCHLEAR NERVE is the eighth cranial nerve. It consists of two sets of fibres, which constitute two separate nerves. One is known as the vestibular nerve, which is the nerve of equilibration or balance. The other is known as the cochlear nerve, which is the nerve of hearing. Disturbance of the former causes giddiness, whilst disturbance of the latter causes deafness.

VIABLE is a term applied to a newly born child to signify that he or she is capable of living separately from the mother. (See BIRTH.)

VIBRATOR is the name of an instrument used for vibratory massage in the mechanical treatment of disease. For its use see MASSAGE.

VIBRIO is the name applied to a bacterium of curved shape, such as the vibrio of cholera.

VIBURNUM, or BLACK HAW, is the bark of *Viburnum prunifolium* or of *Viburnum lentago*, of which the liquid extract is used in doses of 60 to 120 minims (4 to 8 ml) for treating painful menstruation.

VICARIOUS is a term applied to the temporary discharge by one organ of the functions of another. The word is chiefly used in connection with vicarious menstruation, when the blood that should be got rid of from the uterus runs from, for example, the nose, bowels or stomach.

VICHY WATER is an alkaline mineral water from springs at Vichy in France.

VILLUS is the name given to one of the minute processes which are thickly planted upon the inner surface of the small intestine, giving it, to the naked eye, a velvety appearance, and greatly assisting absorption. (See DIGESTION; INTESTINE.)

VINBLASTINE is an alkaloid (qv) derived from the periwinkle plant (*Vinca rosea* Linn.) which is of value in the treatment of certain forms of malignant disease, particularly choriocarcinoma and Hodgkin's disease.

VINCENT'S ANGINA is an ulcerative inflammation of the throat, often foul smelling, and caused by large, spindle-shaped bacilli and spirilla.

VINCRISTINE is an alkaloid derived from the common periwinkle which is proving of value in the palliative treatment of certain forms of malignant disease.

VINEGAR (see ACETIC ACID).

VINUM is the Latin name for wine. The wines used as medicinal remedies include wines of colchicum, antimony, ipecacuanha, citrate of iron, quinine and orange. They are seldom used now.

VINYL ETHER is an inhalational anaesthetic used in minor surgical procedures of short duration, and for the induction of anaesthesia.

VIOMYCIN is an antibiotic which is active against the *Mycobacterium tuberculosis*, but less active than streptomycin or isoniazid.

VIRGINIAN PRUNE BARK, or WILD CHERRY BARK, is the bark of *Prunus serotina*, which yields an oil containing hydrocyanic acid. It possesses tonic and sedative properties and in the form of tincture and syrup is used as a remedy for cough.

VIRAL HAEMORRHAIC FEVER or EBOLA VIRUS FEVER, is a highly fatal disease due to a virus related to that of Marburg disease (qv). Two outbreaks of it have been recorded, with a mortality, respectively, of 50 and 80 per cent. After an incubation period of 7 to 14 days, the onset is with headache of increasing severity and fever. This is followed by diarrhoea, extensive internal bleeding and vomiting. Death usually occurs on the eighth to ninth day. Infection is by person-to-person contact. Serum from patients convalescent from the disease is a useful source of antibodies to the virus.

VIRILISM is the term applied to the condition in which masculine characteristics develop in the female, and is commonly the result of an overactive suprarenal gland, or of a tumour of its cortex.

433 – Model showing the structure of influenza virus, by J. J. Skehel. (Medical Research Council)

VIRUS is the term applied to a group of infective agents which are so small that they are able to pass through the pores of collodion filters. They are responsible for some of the most important diseases affecting man: eg. influenza, poliomyelitis, smallpox, and yellow fever. Some idea of their size may be obtained from the fact that the virus of influenza (Illustration 433) measures 80 micrometres, whereas the staphylococcus measures 1000 micrometres. (1 micrometre = 0·000001 millimetre.)

VISCERA is the general name given to the larger organs lying within the cavities of the chest and abdomen. The term 'viscus' is also applied individually to these organs.

VISCEROPTOSIS, also known as splanchnoptosis, means a falling down of the viscera, especially those of the abdomen. In elderly women it may be associated with prolapse of the womb. (See PROLAPSE.)

VISION – The functions of the eye as an optical instrument which brings rays of light to the endings of the optic nerve, have been already considered (see EYE); in this article, vision will be dealt with as a sensation.

Rays of light pass, in the first place, through the cornea, then through the aqueous humour that fills the anterior chamber of the eye (illustration 434). The light then enters the hinder part of the eye through the pupil, a round hole in the iris which is automatically narrowed according to the strength of the entering light. Next it passes through the lens, which, by a similar automatic action, brings the rays to a correct focus upon the retina, where they finally arrive after passing through the vitreous humour (or body), a jelly-like substance that fills out the eyeball. (See ACCOMMODATION.)

In the retina, the sensory endings are the rods and cones, minute structures placed closely side by side (illustration 435). The number of cones in the human retina has been estimated at 6,500,000, whilst the number of rods is estimated at 110 to 125 million. At the *fovea centralis* or point of clearest vision, situated near the centre of the back of the eye, there are no rods, but only cones.

Light perception – The retina is extremely delicate in its power of perceiving

435 – Diagrammatic section of the retina showing its various layers. A, pigment cells; B, cones; C, rods; D,F, felt-work of dendrites; E. axon of one of the cells which lie between the rods and cones and G, the ganglion cells; H, axons passing from ganglion cells to optic nerve. From Hill, *Manual of Human Physiology.* Edward Arnold & Co.

a faint amount of light and very short flashes of light. Thus a flash from a rapidly revolving mirror lasting only one eight-millionth of a second is perceived. According to Weber's law, however, if the eye be subjected to a constant light, the light must be increased in strength by $\frac{1}{100}$ before any difference can be observed: for example, if a room be lighted by 1000 candles and the light be increased, no difference in brightness will be noticed if fewer than ten more candles be brought in at one time. The intensity of a sensation of light bears no relation to the time during which the light falls upon the eye, but a very important fact is that any image formed in the eye takes an appreciable time to fade away, lasting about $\frac{1}{8}$ of a second. Thus, if an appearance be repeated more frequently than eight times in a second it produces an impression of permanence, and, for this reason, the spokes of a quickly revolving wheel produce an appearance as if the wheel were solid.

Acuteness of vision – As in the case of the sense of touch, a sharp contrast between any object and its surroundings

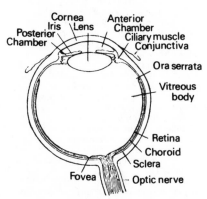

434 – A diagram of the eye. From *Hewer's Textbook of Histology for Medical Students.* Heinemann.

929

renders it more perceptible, whilst movement renders anything more easily seen, just as it makes a touch more easily felt. In order that an object may be distinguished, it must be of a certain size. Two points will not be seen as two unless they are at least so far apart that the lines joining them to the centre of the eye enclose between them an angle of about one-sixtieth of a degree. This distance enables the images of the two points to fall upon two cones, the centres of the cones, which are closely placed at the *fovea centralis*, being about $\frac{1}{7000}$ of an inch (3·5 micrometres) apart. In order that a complex object, such as a letter or figure, may be recognized, it must subtend an angle of about five times this size: that is, one-twelfth of a degree. On this principle Snellen's types for testing the acuteness of vision are constructed (illustration 436). The largest letters are of such

E V O

436 – Three test types of Snellen's scale (D = 6). These letters should be clearly visible to normal eyes at a distance of 6 metres.

a size that at 60 metres distance they occupy an angle of one-twelfth degree, and should therefore be clearly seen; whilst the smallest are of such a size that they occupy this angle at 6 metres distance, and should there be correctly read. The vision of a normal-sighted person, who can read these last types at 6 metres distance, is represented by the fraction $\frac{6}{6}$, whilst that of a person who can read only the largest type at the same distance is $\frac{6}{60}$, and intermediate degrees of faulty vision are $\frac{6}{12}$, $\frac{6}{18}$, $\frac{6}{24}$, etc. Still smaller types are used for testing the acuteness of near vision. It must be noted that efficiency of vision is not proportional to acuity of vision. Thus a man with vision = $\frac{6}{12}$ has half the visual acuity of a man with vision = $\frac{6}{6}$ but he has very little less efficiency. Indeed, for ordinary manual work, vision of $\frac{6}{12}$ gives practically full efficiency. This point is important in connection with accidents to the eye.

Colour sense is one of the most difficult to understand of the visual powers. It corresponds, broadly speaking, to the perception of the pitch of notes by the ear, depending upon the difference in rapidity of vibration of various rays of light. White light is compounded of a mixture in certain proportions of the other colours, into which it may be split by refraction through the prism. This band of colours,

or spectrum, may be again compounded into white light by passage through a second prism; or the same effect may be got by rotating rapidly before the eyes a disc with segments variously coloured. White light may also be formed by a disc of two colours, which are therefore known as complementary colours. These are red with bluish-green, orange with blue, or violet with yellow. Again, any colour may be produced by mixtures in varying proportions of red, green, and violet, these three being therefore known as cardinal or fundamental colours. Three theories have been suggested as to the manner in which various colours are produced.

(1) YOUNG-HELMHOLTZ THEORY is the one that finds most acceptance. It teaches that there are in the retina separate elements, probably cones, capable of being stimulated by the rays in different parts of the spectrum. Some of these react to red but not to green or violet, others to green but not to red or violet, and a third set to violet though not to red or green; whilst an appearance of white results when all are fairly equally stimulated.

(2) HERING'S THEORY demands the existence of chemical substances in the retina, three in number, which are constantly being either formed or broken down under the action of light. Each substance is supposed to correspond with a pair of colours, one with black or white sensations, one with red or green, and the third with yellow or blue. Destruction of each substance by light produces one colour of a pair, construction produces the other. Intermediate colours of the spectrum, such as orange, result from light affecting two of these substances.

(3) TELEPHONE THEORY is one that has been suggested, but has not found much favour. By it the rays of all wave-lengths are supposed to be received on the retina, where they set up differing nerve vibrations that are conveyed to the brain, where for the first time they are analysed into different sensations of colour, just as a telephone ear-piece reproduces the voice with all its original pitch and modulations.

Field of vision – When one looks straight forwards with one eye at a time, one sees with special clearness the object towards which the eye is directed and more vaguely objects for some distance around. The extent that can be seen without moving the eye is known as the field of vision (illustration 437). It is oval in shape and extends much farther outwards than in other directions. Towards the temple, indeed, the eye of a sharp-sighted person

437 – Diagram of the fields of vision. The outer circle represents the half of space lying in front of the observer. As he looks directly forwards, the figure 0 is straight above his head, 180 straight beneath his feet, and 90 straight out on either side. The two smaller circles rise 30° and 60° above the horizon. The two shaded areas represent the field visible to either eye, *LE* to the left eye, and *RE* to the right eye. The darker area, where the two overlap, is the part seen by both eyes.

looking straight forwards can see white objects about ten degrees behind the person. The fields of vision of the two eyes overlap to a great extent, so that objects around the centre and to the inner side of each field are viewed by both eyes. Accordingly there are corresponding points in the two retinae, an object to the right of the observer producing an image on the inner side of his right eye, but on the outer side of his left eye.

The optic nerves are arranged in correspondence with this, the nerve fibres from the left half of each retina passing to the left hemisphere of the brain, and those fibres from the two right halves going to the right hemisphere. Thus half of each optic nerve crosses from one eye to the other side of the brain at the optic chiasma.

It is interesting to note that the field of vision forms an inverted image on the retina (illustration 438), objects to the right falling upon the left side of each retina, those above upon its lower part, and vice versa. The mind, however, as the result of experience, analyses these images and so this inversion is not perceived.

The field of vision varies for different colours, that for white being largest, yellow next, then blue, and red, while green is only seen for a short distance round the centre of the field when the coloured areas are of equal size.

The existence of a blind spot is mentioned and the proof of its presence detailed under EYE.

Visual judgments – The sensations of sight imply a great amount of judgment, for whilst the other senses are influenced by direct physical impressions, in sight we have to examine an inverted image of microscopic size produced by ether waves upon each retina. We are, however, conscious neither of the minuteness of the visual image, nor of its inversion; nor are we aware of the blind spot in each field of vision, unless we search for it in the manner described under EYE.

The manner in which we estimate size and distance was inquired into by Bishop Berkeley in his *Essay towards a New Theory of Vision*, published in 1709, and his conclusions still in the main hold the field. He concluded that our idea of near distances was derived from three arbitrary signs: (*a*) the sense of muscular effort in converging the eyes when they are directed to something very close at hand, and of relaxation when they diverge to view some object farther off; (*b*) the blurred appearance presented by nearer objects, when we are looking at an object situated farther off, or vice versa; (*c*) the muscular effort of accommodating the eye for near or for distant vision. (See ACCOMMODATION.) In distant vision, too, he held that we are mainly dependent on the three signs: (*a*) evidence derived from experience mainly of the sense of touch, a certain combination of colours and form, for example, being associated with the idea of a man felt at close quarters, the same colours and form of smaller size suggesting a man some distance off; (*b*) the sense of blurring of distant objects, already mentioned, when we look at objects close at hand; (*c*) faintness in appearance of an object suggests distance, clearness suggests that the object is near at hand. When objects are seen under unusual conditions

438 – Diagram showing the inverted image on the retina produced by the lens.

of faintness or clearness it becomes very difficult to estimate their size and distance. Thus the moon low down near the horizon and partly obscured by mists rising from the earth, or figures of men on a foggy day, loom much larger than natural, because we over-estimate their distance, owing to their faintness.

Berkeley, however, took little note of the value of binocular vision and of the partial overlapping of the two fields already mentioned. He based his theory largely upon the axiom that 'distance being a line directed endwise to the eye, it projects only one point to the fundus of the eye – which point remains invariably the same, whether the distance be longer or shorter'. This, however, applies only to a one-eyed man, and, in binocular vision, each eye corrects this deficiency of the other, seeing as it were across the other eye's line of vision. Thus we can see in some degree behind or round the corners of nearer objects, and so obtain to a great extent our idea of depth, or solidity.

VISION, DISORDERS OF – Many disorders which indirectly affect the power of vision owing to inflammation or to a painful condition of the eye have been mentioned under EYE, DISEASES OF, and RETINA, DISEASES OF. Here we shall consider more permanent and direct disturbances of sight under the heads of: (a) Dimness of vision; (b) Colour blindness; (c) Decreased visual field; (d) Night-blindness. (See also BLINDNESS.)

Dimness of vision – The most frequent cause of dim vision, or even of total blindness, is some obstruction to the entrance of light through the parts that ought to be transparent.

CORNEAL OPACITIES may produce a ground-glass-like condition of the naturally transparent cornea, so that light may be prevented from gaining access to the eye at all. Thus a dark shadow is cast upon the vision, or complete blindness is produced, according to the breadth and density of the opacity. The most common diseases leading to this condition are keratitis and corneal ulcers. (See under EYE, DISEASES OF.)

REFRACTIVE ERRORS produced by malformations of the cornea, the lens, or the globe of the eye, are by far the commonest causes of defective vision. They are also the most important, both because they cause great interference with the ordinary pursuits of life and because the recognition and appropriate treatment of these errors are easily effected by the expert. The

symptoms due to refractive errors are sometimes grouped as the result of *eyestrain*, and include in the first place headache, inflammation of the eyes (*conjunctivitis* and *iritis*), and inability to use the eyes for long at one time. Children, especially, who have uncorrected errors of refraction have difficulty in keeping up with their fellows at school because of blurring of the page in reading (long-sight) or inability to see clearly maps, blackboards, and other objects at a distance (short-sight). The strain produced may even lead, in some children, to headaches or more serious nervous disorders, or to impairment of the general health. Further, children with such defects are apt to adopt a crouching position at lessons, and to evince a distaste for outdoor sports. This leads to curvature of the spine, defective chest development, and liability to lung diseases. The varieties and treatment of refractive errors are dealt with under SPECTACLES. (See also MYOPIA.)

CATARACT is an opaque condition of the lens coming on slowly, as a rule, in elderly people. (See CATARACT.)

VITREOUS HUMOUR OPACITIES are apt to be seen by anyone who looks steadily at a bright surface, particularly when the general health is not perfect. These may be due to the remains of former inflammation in the choroid coat, but as a rule they are simply the shadows of unimportant cells and fibres floating in the vitreous humour, and need not cause any worry.

DISEASE IN THE FUNDUS of the eye, consisting of chronic inflammation in the retina or choroid coat, or in both, is often a reason of diminishing vision, characterized especially by inability to see in a dim light. (See EYE, DISEASES OF; RETINA, DISEASES OF; CHOROIDITIS.)

DISEASES OF THE BRAIN OR OF THE OPTIC NERVE may lead to temporary dimness of vision, and sometimes blindness.

Colour blindness is a much more common disorder than is generally supposed, being present to an appreciable extent in about one person out of every fifty, and much more common in men than in women. It is usually congenital, being inherited through the female, who is usually unaffected. It is thought to be due to the absence of one of the photopigments normally found in the foveal cones. It persists through life, although it may be acquired as the result of poisoning by various substances, notably by excessive tobacco smoking.

Red-green blindness is the most common form, and is present in all grades of completeness, from that of a person for whom red simply loses its brilliance at a distance, to that of a person for whom vivid green and brilliant scarlet appear as one and the same colour. In one variety of red-green blindness the red, orange, yellow, and green of the spectrum appear all of one colour, green; while the blue and violet both appear as blue, with a gap in the spectrum where the normal eye sees a bluish-green colour.

One test for colour blindness consists in giving the person a skein of green or red wool, and asking him to select from many other skeins the colours which appear to him to match the one he holds. The colour-blind person confuses red with brown, greenish-brown, and yellowish-brown; and he confuses green with bluish-green, rose, and grey. This test, however, has been largely replaced by the Ishihara test (qv).

The importance in testing for colour-blindness any one who is to be a navigator at sea, an air pilot, an automobile driver, signalman or engine-driver is evident.

Decreased visual field is another form of visual defect. Complete blindness in one eye which has lasted since birth is often discovered only by accident in middle life, because the healthy eye has always had an unrestricted field. Another and rarer condition, which is more noticeable to the patient, consists in loss of one-half of the visual field, so that the person can see objects only at one side and must turn his head in order to appreciate his surroundings. This is due to some defect in one-half of the brain or in the optic tract. In this defect a corresponding part of each retina is thrown out of action. Local causes of decrease in the visual field of each eye are found in atrophy of the optic nerve and certain forms of inflammation of the retina. Some general conditions also produce a temporary narrowing of the field, notably great bloodlessness, and over-dosage with quinine.

These defects can be mapped out accurately by the help of an instrument called the perimeter.

Night-blindness, or NYCTALOPIA, an abnormal inability to see things in the night, is thought to be due in many cases to vitamin A deficiency; sometimes the condition is hereditary.

Yellow vision may appear from taking santonin or excessive doses of digitalis, or in jaundice.

VIS MEDICATRIX NATURAE is a Latin term meaning the healing power of Nature, and is often used to indicate the tendency of wounds to heal and of the bodily powers to subdue disease, when left to the operation of time and rest.

VITAMIN is a term applied to a group of substances which exist in minute quantities in natural foods, and which are necessary to normal nutrition, especially in connection with growth and development. Several of them have now been synthesized. When they are absent from the food, defective growth takes place in young animals and children, and in adults various diseases arise; whilst short of the production of actual disease, persistent deprivation of one or other vitamin is apt to lead to a state of lowered general health. Certain deficiencies in diet have long been known to be the cause of scurvy, beriberi, and rickets, but the so-called vitamin hypothesis was not introduced until the twentieth century.

Vitamin A is usually taken in more than ample quantity in the food, and is stored in the liver. It is developed originally by plants as a yellow colouring matter, carotene, for example in carrots, and it is also found in egg yolk, liver, milk, butter, and most green vegetables. When stored in the liver it is colourless and has a slight chemical difference from carotene. The two richest sources of this vitamin are halibut-liver oil and cod-liver oil. The daily requirement of vitamin A is in the region of 4000 international units. Children and pregnant women require relatively more than adults. Deficiency of vitamin A is responsible for serious inflammation of the eyes known as xerophthalmia, which is one of the chief causes of blindness in the developing world; also for night blindness, various skin eruptions, defective development of the teeth, and particularly for want of vitality in the tissues, which leads to localized inflammations.

Vitamin B₁ (see THIAMINE).
Vitamin B₂ (see RIBOFLAVINE).
Vitamin B₃ (see PANTOTHENIC ACID).
Vitamin B₆ (see PYRIDOXINE).
Vitamin B₁₂ (see CYANOCOBALAMIN).
Vitamin C is especially found in fresh fruits such as the orange, and also in fresh green vegetables, and to a smaller extent in milk, meat, and other fresh foods. Canned vegetables such as tomatoes also retain it if their reaction is acid. It is quickly destroyed by high temperature, by excess baking soda and other alkalis, and gradually by oxidation in process of keep-

ing. Its deficiency leads to symptoms of scurvy (qv), including muscular weakness, haemorrhages under the skin, swelling and inflammation of the gums with loss of teeth, and serious damage to joints by haemorrhage; it occurs in sailors and other persons long deprived of fresh foods, and also in babies fed persistently on artificial foods. This vitamin has not only been obtained in a pure state, but has been manufactured in a crystalline form as ascorbic acid. The daily requirement of vitamin C (in terms of ascorbic acid) is 30 mg for adults and 60 mg for children.

Vitamin D is of special importance for the growth of children, and its deficiency produces rickets (qv) with softening and irregular growth of bones, so that swollen joints, distorted limbs, deformities of the chest and similar malformations arise. It was formerly common in the dark and narrow streets of large manufacturing towns and is still found when children are kept too much indoors. Osteomalacia (qv), a similar disease affecting the bones of adult women, results from the same causes when lime salts are absorbed from the bones during pregnancy. Rickets is also common among young dogs and other animals. It has long been known that cod-liver oil was the chief remedy for rickets, and for a time it was supposed that its anti-rachitic action depended upon vitamin A, but it is now known to be vitamin D. There are two forms of vitamin D. Vitamin D_2, also known as calciferol or ergocalciferol, is obtained from ergosterol, a waxy constituent of plants, by ultra-violet irradiation. Vitamin D_3 or cholecalciferol, is the natural form of the vitamin. It is produced by the ultra-violet radiation of a sterol widely distributed in animal fats. This substance is also formed naturally in the fatty tissues of the body when the skin is exposed to the action of sunlight, or, when this is not available, to ultra-violet rays from an arc lamp. It can also be formed in food such as milk when this is similarly exposed to light. Only a few foods contain vitamin D naturally, including cod-liver oil and other fish liver oils (especially that from halibut liver), whilst egg yolk contains a smaller quantity; other fats and milk contain very small quantities. The mode of action of vitamin D is to aid the absorption of phosphorus and calcium from the food, increase their amount in the blood, and thus in the bones. In the case of this vitamin bad effects may follow overdosage, or hypervitaminosis, because if too much calcium and phosphorus are maintained in the blood the bones and teeth become over-calcified, the arteries may become unduly hardened and calculi may be formed in the kidneys and other organs. The daily requirement for infants and nursing mothers is 400 to 800 international units, whilst for adults it is probably about 400 units.

Vitamin E has been known since 1922, when it was found that its absence in the case of rats caused failure to produce young. It is derived especially from the oil contained in seeds and in green leaves, and also is present in smaller amounts in other fresh fats. It is readily stored, like vitamin A, in the body, and thus is unlikely to be found wanting in human beings except in cases of very severe under-nutrition. It is possible, however, that miscarriages may occasionally be due to its deficiency.

Vitamin K, also known as PHYTOMENA-DIONE, the anti-haemorrhagic vitamin, is essential for the proper clotting of blood. It has been given successfully in cases of bleeding in infants, and to patients with jaundice, who have a special tendency to bleeding. Bleeding in these conditions is thought to be due to deficiency of vitamin K. Synthetic chemical products with an identical physiological action have now been made. In the natural form it is widespread in nature, the main sources being spinach, leafy vegetables, tomatoes, and liver. The daily requirement of man is not known.

Vitamin P, CITRIN, or HESPERIDIN, present in citrus fruits, appears to be responsible for the resistance of the capillaries to pressure. If there is a deficiency of vitamin P in the diet the capillaries rupture easily, resulting, for example, in purpura.

It should be said in conclusion, with regard to the supply of vitamins, that any person using a diet containing the protective foods, such as milk, eggs, butter, cheese, fat, fish, wholemeal bread, fresh vegetables and fruit, should obtain an ample supply of vitamins. Infants should have a teaspoonful daily of cod-liver oil and two teaspoonfuls of orange juice or of tomato juice.

VITELLUS, or VITELLUM, is the Latin name for yolk of egg.

VITILIGO is the term given to a skin disease in which smooth light-coloured patches appear either on the skin or in the hair.

VITRELLA is a small, crushable, glass capsule enclosed in an absorptive and protective fabric, used for the dispensing of medicines such as amyl nitrite which are to be inhaled.

VITREOUS BODY is a semi-fluid transparent substance which fills most of the globe of the eye behind the lens.

VITRIOL, OIL OF, is an old name for sulphuric acid.

VOCAL CORDS (see LARYNGOSCOPE; and VOICE AND SPEECH).

VOCAL RESONANCE is the term applied to the buzzing sound that is heard when the ear is applied to the chest as the patient speaks.

VOICE AND SPEECH are two terms applied to the system of sounds which are produced in the upper air passages and in the mouth, and which form one of the means of communication between human beings.

Voice means the set of fundamental notes and tones produced by the larynx (illustration 439), which are modified in various ways during their passage through the mouth so as to form speech or song. Speech differs from song in being less sustained and of smaller compass with regard to pitch, and in presenting sounds which have not a musical character.

Voice is produced in the larynx of most animals, although birds have a special organ known as the syrinx in which their song takes origin. The question was formerly much debated as to what musical instrument most closely resembles the larynx. Ferrein held that the violin formed the nearest artificial approach, and hence the name of vocal cords. Other observers have, in a somewhat fanciful way, compared the air which the chest drives upwards to the bow, the larynx to the violin, and the tongue and lips, which modify the laryngeal notes, to the string-hand of the violinist. It is generally admitted, however, that the larynx more nearly resembles a wind instrument with a pair of vibrating reeds. Many persons have made a careful study of voice production by the aid of the laryngoscope (see LARYNX), an instrument which enables the changes that take place in the larynx, when different notes are sounded, to be clearly seen (illustration 440).

Musical notes vary in three characters: loudness, pitch, and quality or timbre. The *loudness* of the voice depends upon the volume of air which is available for agitating the vocal cords, and therefore upon the size of the chest and the vigour with which its muscles can be made to act.

The *pitch* of the voice is determined by several things, the chief points being the size of the larynx; the degree of tenseness at which the vocal cords are, for the time being, maintained by the laryngeal muscles; the fact as to whether the cords vibrate as a whole or merely at their

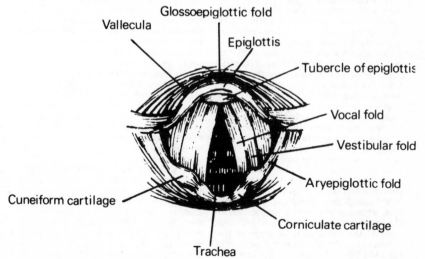

439 – A laryngoscopic view of the interior of the larynx. From *Gray's Anatomy*, Longman.

935

edges; and the shape which is given to the cavity of the larynx by movements of the arytenoid and epiglottic cartilages. In any given voice, the range of pitch seldom exceeds two and a half octaves, although the particular part of the musical scale that can be produced varies according as the voice is bass, tenor, contralto or soprano. Generally speaking, a large larynx with long vocal cords produces low notes, and hence men have a deeper voice than women. For the same reason the small larynx of childhood produces a shrill voice, whilst the rapid growth of the larynx at the time of puberty, and consequent uncertainty of muscular control over the vocal cords, produces the breaking of the voice that occurs in boys at this time. The manner in which the muscles of

the bad voice-production which leads to great straining of the throat, and is largely responsible for the throat affections of many of those who use the voice much. (See CLERGYMAN'S SORE THROAT.)

There are certain peculiar forms of voice production. The *falsetto voice* has been already mentioned. *Whispering* is a form of speech in which voice is completely absent, the larynx being wide open (illustration 440), and the sound produced entirely in the mouth. *Ventriloquism* is a form of speech in which the voice is produced by the indrawing of air, instead of in the usual way of expiration. Since it is always difficult to localize the source of sound, the ventriloquist can easily suggest to his audience a false place of origin for the unusual voice.

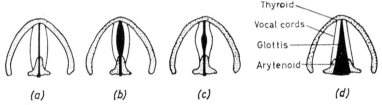

440 – Diagram of shape of glottis during phonation: (*a*) closed phase of phonation; (*b*) low voice; (*c*) falsetto voice; (*d*) whispering. From Scott Brown, Ballantyne and Groves, *Diseases of the Ear, Nose and Throat*. Butterworth.

the larynx act upon the cords allows the pitch to change at will. Thus if the thick part of each cord be held rigid and only the sharp free edge be allowed to vibrate, a high note is the result, and a still higher note is reached in men when only the front part of this free edge is allowed to move, as in the falsetto voice (illustration 440). On the other hand, by allowing a greater thickness of the cord to vibrate, the person loads the vibrating edge, and thus produces a much deeper note.

The *timbre* of the voice is partly due to these differences in the larynx, but chiefly to peculiarities and to voluntary changes in shape of the mouth and other cavities associated with the air passages. These changes in shape are chiefly concerned with the alterations of the fundamental notes which produce speech, and they are considered in detail below.

It should be remembered, however, that, while the muscular arrangements of the larynx are chiefly concerned with the pitch of the voice, and the shape of the mouth with its modulation, the *loudness* is varied by the movements of the chest. The neglect of this fact is often responsible for

Speech consists of a series of rapid modifications of the voice, produced by changes in position of the palate, tongue, and lips. EACH VOWEL has an appropriate pitch as ordinarily spoken, although it is possible to pronounce any of the vowels in any note within the compass of the voice. The appropriate pitch of *u* (pronounced *oo*) is lowest, and the vowels rise through *o*, *a* (pronounced *ah*), *e* (pronounced *eh*), to *i* (pronounced *ee*). Apart from this slight difference in pitch, the distinguishing character of each vowel is gained by alterations in the shape of the mouth cavity through which the stream of air passes. Anyone can at once prove this fact by opening his mouth widely and sounding musical notes of various pitch. All of these will have the character of *a*, nor can the vowel be changed till the mouth is shut somewhat and certain changes made in the position of the tongue and lips. These changes in the shape of the mouth have the effect of intensifying certain of the overtones in the fundamental laryngeal note, and thus the vowels are produced. The shape of the mouth in speaking the different vowels is somewhat as follows. In pronouncing a (ah) the mouth is something like a funnel open to the front, the lips and teeth being held wide apart. For sounding e (eh) the shape is slightly modified, the mouth being more closed. When u (oo) is pronounced the cavity of the mouth is shaped like a wide flask with a very narrow neck at the lips, which are protruded as far as possible. For o the flask shape is modified slightly, the neck being made shorter and wider by bringing the lips nearer the teeth and opening them a little. In pronouncing i (ee) the tongue is brought up to the teeth, so that the air passes through a long narrow cavity, and obtains free exit, the lips being drawn well back. Although the English language is usually said to include only five vowels, many others can be formed by slight variations in the shape of the mouth, as, for example, in the case of the modified ö and ü, and other vowels of Continental languages. Diphthongs, like ai, oi, ae, are produced simply by a rapid change from one mouth-shape to another while air is issuing through the larynx.

CONSONANTS are sudden sounds produced by cutting off the stream of air either wholly or partially, or by suddenly beginning it. Of necessity, a consonant forms either the beginning or end of a vowel sound, and the particular consonant produced depends upon the point at which the stream of air is checked. According to Brücke, there are four stop-positions:

(1) Between the lips.
(2) Between tip of tongue and roof of mouth.
(3) Between root of tongue and palate.
(4) In the larynx.

The character of the consonant varies also according as the stoppage of air is complete or its commencement sudden (*explosive consonants*); as the stoppage is only partial or the commencement gradual (*aspirate consonants*); or as the margins of the opening are thrown into vibration (*vibrative consonants*). Again, in the case of some consonants, the mouth is closed at different stop positions, and the air stream is allowed to pass out by the nose (*resonant consonants*). On this principle, consonants are classified as follows:

	Explosives	Aspirates	Vibratives	Resonants
1st Stop Position	P, B	F, V, W		M
2nd Stop Position	T, D	S, Z, L Sch, Th	R	N
3rd Stop Position	K, G	Ch, J	Palatal R	Ng
4th Stop Position		H	Saxon R	

Table 43 – Classification of consonants.

Another distinction, which is of great importance in the treatment of stammering, consists in the amount of force which is necessary to open the stop and sound the consonant, and the amount of voice which therefore accompanies it at the beginning of a syllable (table 44).

	Explosives	Aspirates
Voiceless	P, T, K	F, S, Sch, Th (as in *throw*), Ch
Voiced	B, D, G	V, Z, L, Th (as in *then*), J, H

The vibratives and resonants are all voiced.

Table 44 – Classification of explosives and aspirates.

One can test this by comparing, for example, the words 'Peter' and 'Beater'. In 'Peter' the P has little sound, the voice becoming full only on the E, while in 'Beater' the full volume of sound comes out at once on the B and dies away on the E. One cause of stammering is the attempt to pronounce, with full voice, the consonants at the commencement of words which should be voiceless, instead of touching off the consonant lightly and passing on at once to emphasize the vowel.

Defects of speech – The apparatus for speech being so complicated, and the changes which must take place constantly in its different parts so varied, it follows that the act of speech has a very elaborate controlling mechanism in the nervous system. Further, the power of speech is gained in early life by children hearing the sounds made by others and mimicking them, so that the centres for speech in the brain are intimately connected with those concerned in the sense of hearing.

MUTISM, or the entire absence of the power to speak, may be due to various causes, the most effectual being some mental deficiency which denies to the child sufficient intelligence to mimic the actions of those around him. In other cases the child seems to be quite intelligent, but, owing apparently to some defect in the nervous control of the voice and speech organs, or in these organs themselves, he is unable to make any sounds. A common cause of mutism is complete deafness present at birth, or caused by some ear diseases in early childhood. The child in this case cannot learn to speak, simply because he cannot hear, but, if properly educated, he can be taught to speak fluently and to understand what is said by watching the lips and throat of others. (See DUMBNESS.)

STAMMERING is a bad habit of speech due to want of co-ordination between the different parts of the speech mechanism. (See STAMMERING.)

TWANGS of various kinds are assumed very easily, and, indeed, often unconsciously, from those around. The ease with which the exact pronunciation of a foreign tongue is picked up by a person living in the country in question is well known. Many differences between different languages are to be explained by slight differences in shape between the speech organs of different races. Other differences are to be explained by different habits of opening the lips and mouth in various tribes of the same stock, due perhaps to external conditions, such as climate. Such minor peculiarities in speech as burrs and lisps are due to peculiarities in the action of the tongue or palate, whilst the deformities of tongue-tie and cleft-palate are accompanied by still greater defects of speech. When the nose is blocked by any condition, such as a cold in the head or polypus, the pronunciation of the resonants *m, n,* and *ng* is interfered with, these being heard as *b, d,* and *g,* respectively, for a reason which can be seen on consulting table 44.

APHASIA is a condition in which various forms of inability to speak, or to understand speech, come on, usually late in life, as the result of brain disease. (See APHASIA.)

APHONIA, or loss of voice, causes speaking to be carried on in a whisper. It is usually either due to some disorder of the vocal cords, as in the laryngitis which may form part of a cold (see THROAT DISEASES), or is a symptom of hysteria. It is generally of short duration.

VOLAR means something pertaining to the palm or sole.

VOLKMANN'S CONTRACTURE is the term applied to the condition in which, as a result of too great a pressure from splint or bandage in the treatment of a broken arm, the flexor muscles of the forearm contract and thus obstruct free flow of blood in the veins; the muscles then swell and ultimately become fibrosed.

VOLSELLA is a Latin term for a forceps with hooked blades.

VOLVULUS means an obstruction of the bowels produced by the twisting of a loop of bowel round itself. (See INTESTINE, DISEASES OF.)

VOMICA means a cavity in the lung produced by ulceration, which is usually a sign of tuberculosis.

VOMITING means the expulsion of the stomach contents through the mouth. When the effort of vomiting is made, but nothing is brought up, the process is known as retching. When vomiting occurs, the chief effort is made by the muscles of the abdominal wall and by the diaphragm contracting together and squeezing the stomach. The contraction of the stomach wall is no doubt also a factor, and an important step in the act consists in the opening at the right moment of the cardiac or upper orifice of the stomach. This concerted action of various muscles is brought about by a vomiting centre situated on the floor of the fourth ventricle in the brain.

Causes – Vomiting is brought about by some irritation of this nervous centre, but in the great majority of cases this is effected through sensations derived from the stomach itself. Thus, of the drugs which cause vomiting some act only after being absorbed into the blood and carried to the brain, although most are irritants to the mucous membrane of the stomach (see EMETICS); dyspepsia also acts thus, and lies at the root of most sick headaches; various diseases of the stomach, such as cancer, and ulcer, and food poisoning, act in a similar way. Irritation, not only of the nerves of the stomach, but also of those proceeding from other abdominal organs, produces vomiting; thus in obstruction of the bowels, peritonitis, gall-stone colic, renal colic, and even during pregnancy, vomiting is a prominent symptom.

Strong impressions of an unpleasant nature made upon the nerves of sense are apt to produce vomiting. Thus an offensive smell, a disagreeable sight, any interference with the balancing sense as in sea-sickness, irritation or even tickling of the throat, and the pain of an injury or operation are all likely to be attended by vomiting.

Direct disturbance of the brain itself is a cause: for example, a blow on the head, a cerebral tumour, a cerebral abscess, meningitis. Many cases of hysteria also show attacks of vomiting as one of their prominent symptoms.

Finally, the vomiting centre may be brought into action by various poisons introduced into the blood, like tartar emetic and apomorphine; or by the poisons of various acute and chronic diseases: eg. Bright's disease, smallpox, scarlet fever, typhus, and cholera. Vomiting, indeed, forms an important early symptom of these diseases.

Characters of the vomit – FOOD, more or

less softened and made sour and bitter by digestion, constitutes the vomit in the simpler cases, such as those due, for example, to emetics and sea-sickness. It should be remembered that when milk is vomited up curdled, this indicates simply that the first step in its digestion has taken place, and it is a mistake to conclude, as is often done, that the curdling indicates some intolerance of the stomach for milk.

WATERY FLUID, brought up irrespective of meals, forms the vomitus in conditions where the vomiting is due to disturbances of the brain: eg. brain tumours, and in certain other conditions such as the vomiting in the early months of pregnancy. When the vomiting continues long, it tends to bring up mucus and bile also.

MUCUS, when vomited in considerable amount in strings, and especially when sour in taste and brought up in the morning, is a sign of catarrh of the stomach, particularly that form associated with constant indulgence in alcohol.

BILE may be brought up by any long-continued attack of vomiting, after the contents of the stomach have been expelled and retching still continues: for example, in sea-sickness, or in migraine. Usually the bile is golden-yellow in colour; but sometimes it is grass-green.

FROTHY MATERIAL, with a yeasty smell, which divides into three distinct layers, froth on the surface, and a sediment of undigested food, with a layer of clearer fluid between, is characteristic of the vomit from a dilated stomach in which fermentative dyspepsia is taking place.

BLOOD may be red in colour, and brought up mixed with the food or in clots; but, much more often, it is vomited as a brown granular material, very much resembling 'coffee-grounds'. As a general rule, the vomiting of blood indicates some ulceration in the interior of the stomach, but the amount of blood is no guide to the size of the ulcer, because serious bleeding sometimes occurs from hardly perceptible erosions of the mucous membrane. Large quantities of blood are also occasionally brought up in chronic catarrh of the stomach (especially the alcoholic variety) which is accompanied by congestion.

Treatment must have two objects in view: (1) to relieve the source of the irritation, and (2) to soothe the nervous centre.

In the first place, the cause of the vomiting must be sought for, and in general this will be found to be some disorder of the stomach. If an indigestible meal has been taken some time previously, and its remnants be still loading the stomach, an emetic or a copious draught of warm water has the effect of getting rid of the indigestible material and allowing the irritation to subside. Various substances which have a soothing action upon the stomach may also be taken when the sickness continues, such as cream of magnesia, or a powder composed of rhubarb (2 parts), soda (2 parts), and bismuth (4 parts), in teaspoonful doses, or a tablespoonful of chloroform water.

The application of heat, such as a rubber hot water bottle, over the pit of the stomach, has often a marked sedative effect. In irritable stomach conditions, posture is an important matter: the sufferer lying quietly in bed in whichever position he finds most comfortable, with the head on a low pillow.

The vomiting due to such serious conditions as peritonitis subsides under the treatment appropriate to these conditions.

The special measures applicable to sea-sickness are given under SEA-SICKNESS.

Vomiting due to inflammation or some other source of irritation in the throat is greatly relieved by soothing gargles, or by sucking lozenges containing ammonium chloride or chlorate of potash.

Fresh air is of great importance, and the drawing of deep breaths has a distinct effect in checking the tendency to vomit. Mental quiet and a darkened room also assist in soothing the nervous system.

VULVA is the general term applied to the external female genitals.

VULVO-VAGINITIS is inflammation of the vulva and the vagina. It is more common in young girls than in adult women. It may be a manifestation of infection elsewhere in the body, or may indicate the presence of some infection in the vagina. (See WHITES.)

W

WAFER PAPERS are thin circular discs made of flour and water, which become pliable when wetted, and form a convenient wrapper for swallowing nauseous drugs without tasting them. (For the method of use, see POWDERS.)

WALK (see GAIT).

WARFARIN is an anticoagulant which is active whether given by mouth, intramuscularly, intravenously or rectally. It is usually given by mouth, when its maximum effect occurs within about 36 hours. Its action passes off within 48 hours of cessation of treatment.

WARMING (see HEATING).

WARTS, or VERRUCAE, are small, solid growths, arising from the surface of the skin. They are due to a papova virus infection of the skin. They are highly infectious, and it is estimated that 10 per cent of the population suffer from them. The infection is most likely to be spread in schools by hand-holding games, and among adolescents by walking barefoot on gymnasium floors and in swimming baths.

COMMON WARTS develop on the skin of children and young persons on the knuckles, on the backs of the hands and on the knees. Occasionally such warts come out in a crop. In structure, these warts consist of a bundle of fibres produced by overgrowth of the papillae in the true skin, each bundle enveloped by a cap of the horny cells that cover the surface of the epidermis, and the whole mass being surrounded by a ring of thickened epidermis. These fibres can easily be seen when the surface of the wart becomes worn away, and especially if the top of the wart be accidentally cut or knocked off, so that it bleeds. The dirty-brown colour of warts is due to dirt becoming lodged between these fibres. PLANE WARTS, which are flat-topped, are commonest on the face and the back of the hands. PLANTAR WARTS occur on the soles of the feet. They are found most commonly in older children and adolescents. Epidemics are not uncommon in schools, the infection being spread by the children walking with bare feet. They are usually painful. SENILE WARTS are usually hard, wrinkled, and slightly raised areas of skin found in old people. SOFT WARTS, consisting of little tags of skin, are found especially upon the neck, chest, ears, or eyelids of persons whose skin has been subjected for long to some irritation, such as that of working among paraffin. HORNS are formed sometimes upon the face or hands, as the result of the drying up of the sebaceous material exuding from the skin that covers a wart, and, as the secretion goes on, these horns occasionally reach a length of some inches. TUBERCULOUS WARTS are developed sometimes as the result of a wound in the skin of the hands, especially of those who have come in contact with persons or animals suffering from some form of tuberculosis: eg. pathologists and butchers.

Treatment – Quite often they disappear spontaneously. One-fifth of plantar warts disappear spontaneously in six months, and it is said that two-thirds of all warts disappear in two years. This explains the large range of vaunted 'cures'. All too often all that has happened is that the use of the 'cure' in question has coincided with the natural disappearance of the wart. As a rule, warts are removed painlessly by the application of some substance which dissolves the horny surface and cauterizes the parts beneath, such as 10 per cent salicylic acid in soft paraffin, or a combination of salicylic acid and lactic acid. The local application of carbon dioxide snow is a most effective form of treatment provided there are not too many warts. In some cases large warts on the fingers may need to be cut out under a local anaesthetic. The most effective treatment for plantar warts is to soak them in 3 per cent formalin. This is done by filling an old tin lid or saucer with the solution and soaking the part of the sole containing the wart in it for twenty minutes each night. Care must be taken not to soak more of the part than is absolutely necessary in the formalin solution. Each night, before soaking, the surface of the wart is rubbed with a nail file. The soaking may need to be repeated nightly for several weeks. Warts that hang by a pedicle are best removed by snipping off with scissors, the bleeding being easily checked by some astringent. (See also CONDYLOMA.)

WASHING (see BATHS; DISINFECTION).

WASHING OUT BLADDER (see BLADDER, DISEASES OF; and DOUCHES).

WASHING OUT STOMACH is performed for various reasons, particularly in order to remove poison that has been recently swallowed, before it shall have had time to act. Expert opinion today differs as to the value and safety of washing out the stomach in cases of poisoning. If it is done for this purpose, it should only be done by a doctor, nurse or experienced first-aider. The elementary rules are as follows:

(1) Place the head of the patient over the side of the bed so that the mouth and throat are at a lower level than the larynx and trachea.

(2) Use a wide-bore stomach tube (Jaques gauge 30) and lubricate it well with glycerin or some similar lubricant. In the adult 50 cm (20 inches) will reach the stomach. Make sure the tube is in the gullet (oesophagus) and not the trachea.

(3) For the first wash use 300 ml water, or olive oil if a tar oil derivative has been taken. Repeat this process, using 300–600 ml at a time, at least three or four times, saving all washings for analysis.

(4) If the patient is conscious, leave in the stomach 600 ml water containing 20 ml sodium or magnesium sulphate. If the patient is comatose, leave the stomach empty, and leave a nasogastric tube in place to keep the stomach empty.

Washing out is also employed to cleanse the stomach in cases in which the food tends to collect in the organ and to ferment. (See STOMACH TUBE.)

WASP STINGS (see BITES).

WASSERMANN REACTION is a test introduced for the diagnosis of syphilis by examination of the blood. It has now been largely supplanted by other more specific tests.

WASTING (see ATROPHY).

WASTING PALSY is a popular name for the disease more commonly known as progressive muscular atrophy. (See PARALYSIS.)

WATER-BEDS are flat, closed sacks of heavy india-rubber material, with a funnel-shaped orifice at one corner through which water can be poured, and which can be closed by a screw-stopper. They are made in various sizes, some being sufficiently large to cover a whole bedstead, though more often, for convenience in handling, they are of smaller size, and occasionally are made as small cushions, as rings with a hollow in the centre, or in horseshoe shape. Those of the largest size possess a special outlet at one corner through which air escapes as water enters at the opposite corner.

Water-beds have been replaced to a great extent by air-beds (qv).

WATERBRASH, or PYROSIS, is a condition in which, during the course of digestion, the mouth fills with tasteless or sour fluid, which is generally saliva, but sometimes seems to be brought up from the stomach. At the same time, a burning pain is often felt at the pit of the stomach or in the chest. The condition is a symptom of excessive acidity of the stomach contents, due sometimes to an irritating diet, and often characteristic of a duodenal ulcer.

WATER CANKER is another name for cancrum oris. (See CANCRUM ORIS.)

WATER-CLOSETS, DRAINS, and SEWERS (see SEWAGE AND SEWAGE DISPOSAL).

WATER-HAMMER PULSE is a name given to the peculiarly sudden pulse that is associated with incompetence of the aortic valve of the heart, and suggests the philosophical toy after which it is named. (See PULSE.)

WATERING-PLACES suited for the treatment of various diseases are mentioned under these headings, and the general principles underlying the choice of a watering-place are described under CLIMATE IN RELATION TO DISEASE.

WATER ON THE BRAIN is a popular name for hydrocephalus and for meningitis. (See HYDROCEPHALUS; MENINGITIS.)

WATER SUPPLY: Sources – RAINFALL forms the primary source of all water supplies. If collected under careful conditions, the vessels in which it is received being free from contamination and filth, it constitutes the purest and softest of waters, containing only such impurities as it has washed down or dissolved in its course through the atmosphere. In its passage through the air it becomes highly aerated and, except in the neighbourhood of towns and densely populated districts, where factories abound and the pollution of the atmosphere with impurities may be considerable, it is practically pure. The rainfall is usually collected from the roofs of houses and buildings by the gutters and rain-pipes, which should be regularly cleaned. These conduct the water to specially prepared underground cisterns or receptacles, preferably formed of slates, bricks set in cement, or good cement concrete. Sometimes special collecting surfaces are provided, portions of land being set aside, the surface of which is rendered impermeable with a layer of slates, and the water being conducted into a tank by a pipe to which the surface of the impermeable layer has been sloped. The first rain that falls should be rejected, as it will contain most of the impurities washed from the atmosphere and the collecting surface.

Rain-water, on account of its softness, is invaluable for washing. This quality of softness, however, renders it especially organic matter with which the water came in contact in the upper regions of the soil.

Springs are due to the water percolating through the soil and being prevented from going deeper by some impermeable stratum, above which the water accumulates as if in a reservoir. The point of issue of the spring is determined by the position where this impermeable layer crops out upon the surface of the soil. Where the collection of underground water is due to an impervious layer of clay just under a thin surface of gravel or sand, the springs are poor in their yield, subject to variations with the nature of the season, intermittent in their supply, and are therefore termed *land springs*. These intermittent springs are often found along the course of rivers in

441 – Diagram of a section across the bottom of a little valley, showing a water supply by wells. *a*, surface well polluted by *d*, a neighbouring cesspool; *b*, surface well at a safe distance; *c*, deep well (safe) lined with masonry down to the first impervious stratum, and protected above ground; *e* and *g*, permeable strata; *f* and *h*, impervious strata.

liable to dissolve lead, and consequently lead should not be used in any of the piping or other fittings. Its great disadvantage, as a sole source of supply, arises from the variability in the rainfall, and therefore it is advisable to have some other means of supply.

SPRINGS – The portion of the rainfall which percolates through the soil absorbs from the ground-air carbonic acid, which aids it in dissolving many of the mineral constituents with which it comes in contact, thus rendering it in many instances unsuitable for drinking purposes. On the other hand spring water is often rendered clear and bright by the purification it undergoes in moving through the strata of the earth before it reaches its point of issue, this natural filtration, if the water has penetrated far enough, being sufficient to remove completely the valleys bounded by hills, where the level of the underground water varies considerably with the seasons.

Main springs are deep-seated, where the water has percolated through thick masses of porous geological formations, such as chalk, overlying impermeable layers. Where the demand is not great, they usually yield throughout the whole year a sufficient supply of water which is clear, sparkling, well aerated, and cool, due to the natural purification it has undergone. It may be impregnated with various mineral salts, which render it hard and so interfere with its value for washing and cooking, although it may still be extremely palatable for drinking.

As the water from springs may be contaminated at the point of issue, the spring should be walled in and provided with a discharging pipe that passes some distance below the surface, thus conducting the water to the surface.

WELLS consist of two main forms, shallow and deep, a special form of the latter being known as artesian. The shallow wells (illustration 441 *a*) reach the same kind of water as was described in the case of land springs, and are liable to pollution by soakings through the soil from leaking cesspools and drains, from surface washings and manure, from animal and vegetable debris spread on the fields, the depth of such a well not being usually sufficient to allow of natural purification. Deep wells (illustration 441 *c*), in which the water is usually brought to the surface by pumping, tap the same kind of water as main springs, yielding usually an excellent, palatable supply, and, in order to protect them from pollution by surface and subsoil waters, they should be lined with bricks embedded in cement down to the depth of the impermeable layer, and built up and closed in above the ground to prevent them further from being contaminated at the surface.

Artesian wells pass through an upper impermeable layer to reach a store of water in a water-bearing stratum lying upon a second impermeable formation. This water-bearing permeable stratum has its outcrop at a higher level than where the well has been sunk, and consequently the water in its endeavour to find its own level rises up the well and issues at the top.

Tube wells are made by driving tubes, one section of which is screwed on to the next, down into the soil, the first one being provided with a steel point and perforated at the bottom for about 2 feet. These can be used to provide a small temporary supply of water, the water entering the tube through the perforations and being pumped up if the pressure is not sufficient to raise the water to the surface.

RIVER WATER – The quality of the water derived from rivers differs greatly according to the nature of the source from which it is obtained. Where the supply is drawn from a river high up near its origin among granite-bound hills, the water may be perfectly potable and pure, but if it is obtained from a river after it has received the washings and drainage of manured fields, the soakage from cesspools, and the sewage of hamlets and towns, it may be highly contaminated and unfit for drinking purposes. Every river in its course tends naturally to purify its water. The bulk of water dilutes any sewage entering the river, the grosser impurities are broken up against the stones of the river's bed or

destroyed by fish, and the oxygen which the moving water absorbs in large quantity from the air decomposes the organic matter into harmless substances. This natural purification is considerable where there is abundance of pure fresh water in the stream to mix with the sewage; but where there is extensive contamination from sewage, rivers and streams form a supply in which the process of natural purification will not have been sufficient to render the water free from danger.

UPLAND SURFACE WATER – The supply of water from such a source is usually good alike for domestic purposes and trade requirements. The water taken from streams near their source or from upland lakes resembles closely rain-water in composition, because it contains little dissolved solid matter, whilst the organic matter present is mainly of vegetable, not of animal, origin. These waters are usually highly palatable and pure, with the additional advantage of softness, which renders them suitable for trade purposes. Peaty matter is often found in such upland waters, giving the water a slight yellow discoloration and imparting a peaty taste, but this does not interfere with its potability, and the peaty matter may be removed, if desired, by filtration through filters of sand.

These upland waters form such good sources of supply, being removed largely from danger of contamination by human excretions, that many of the principal towns in Great Britain now obtain their supplies in this manner. Glasgow, Manchester, and Liverpool, to mention three examples, have all tapped such sources of supply many miles from their boundaries, and the water thus obtained for the inhabitants has contributed in no small degree to the health of the cities.

Quality – Apart from actual contamination, or the tendency to convey diseases (see below), water may be either soft or hard (illustration 442). The hardness is usually described as either temporary or permanent. Temporary hardness is due to the presence of the bicarbonates of calcium and magnesium held in solution by carbon dioxide, which may be driven off by boiling the water. This carbon dioxide may also be got rid of by adding slaked lime to the water, which causes the production of still more carbonate of lime. This, however, settles, with the carbonate originally present, in a sediment; and thus the temporary hardness is removed. Permanent hardness is due to the presence of the sulphates of calcium and magnesium, as well as iron

HARDNESS OF WATER
in parts per million (p.p.m.)

Very hard, 300 p.p.m. and over

Hard, 200 to 300 p.p.m.

Undifferentiated

Moderately soft, 50 to 100 p.p.m.

Soft, 0 to 50 p.p.m.

0   50 Miles
0   80 Kilometres

442 – Degree of hardness of waters supplied by direct supply water undertakings in Britain in 1968 (based on data in *Water Engineer's Handbook*, 1968). From Howe, *Man, Environment and Disease in Britain*. David & Charles.

and alumina, which cannot be got rid of by boiling.

Rain-water is the softest of all waters. Soft water is invaluable for washing and cooking, since hard water forms a precipitate with the fats of the soap, and thus prevents it from lathering till all the hardness has been neutralized. Hard water therefore entails a great waste of soap, and it is said that each degree of hardness means the waste of a pound of soap in every 1000 gallons of water used. In cooking, too, hard water deposits a layer on kettles and pots, and even on the food, thus preventing the boiling water from penetrating it. On the other hand there is some evidence indicating that soft water is associated with a higher death rate from ischaemic heart disease, or coronary thrombosis (qv).

Storage – In obtaining a supply of water for a town from gathering-grounds, it is customary to store the water in a reservoir so placed as to allow the water to pass into the distributing pipes by gravitation, and be so conveyed through the district supplied. The usual arrangement consists in carefully selecting the site for the impounding reservoir so that no leakage will occur, a dam being constructed across the valley to which the waters naturally flow, at such a place as will store up sufficient water for four to six months' supply, and where the construction of this barrier will entail as little expense as possible. Provision is also made to regulate the admission of water into the reservoir, since compensation water must be allowed to flow on in the streams, while an arrangement may be made to allow turbid storm water to pass on without entering the reservoir. Sluices and valves must be placed on the outlet culvert to regulate the discharge of the water to the town, and special service reservoirs for each district of the town may be formed at suitable places, so that the supply to each portion of the town may be known and regulated.

Filtration – The water supplied to a district should be selected from a source as little liable to pollution as can be obtained, but if there is the slightest chance that it is contaminated in any form, filtration and purification should be carried out before distribution. The main objects of filtration consist in the removal of deleterious ingredients such as mineral matters, eg. the salts of magnesia and lime leading to hardness, suspended materials, dissolved organic matters, and micro-organisms.

PUBLIC FILTRATION on a large scale is usually carried out in sand filter-beds, which consist of layers of fine sand about 3 feet (1 metre) in thickness, resting on layers of fine gravel, gradually increasing in size from above downwards till the last layer of coarse gravel and pebbles is reached, in which are found the mouths of the outlet pipes. The water is conducted on to the surface of the filter-beds to a suitable depth (usually not more than 2 feet [600 cm]), and allowed slowly to percolate downwards.

By this system of filtration, water is rendered pure and potable, the suspended matter being removed by the superficial layers of sand, mineral particles being detained in the same manner, whilst the organic matter present is aerated in the deeper portions of the filter, and rendered innocuous to a certain extent. Such filters remove micro-organisms from the water in a large degree. This is accomplished by a gelatinous film which forms on the surface of the sand and consists of the suspended materials and masses of bacteria. If proper precautions as to aeration, rate of filtration, and cleansing of the sand are carried out, such sand filters remove bacteria from the water in satisfactory proportions.

Sterilization – Filtration is usually followed by sterilization. This is usually carried out by chlorination or by the addition of *excess lime. Chlorination* is dependent upon the powerful bactericidal properties of chlorine which is added to the water either in the form of bleaching powder or of chlorine gas. The latter is used when large quantities of water have to be dealt with.

Domestic purification may be carried out, where required, in various ways. *Distillation* provides an excellent, pure water, which is, however, insipid because deficient as to aeration, and which acts easily on certain metals, such as copper. The water may be aerated by passing it in a finely divided spray through the air. *Boiling* renders the water softer and destroys micro-organisms, but leaves the water insipid, and therefore the water should be aerated again before use.

Domestic filters, as commonly employed, are often worse than useless, giving an idea of false security and rendering the water after so-called filtration more impure than it was before. When a domestic filter is employed therefore expert advice must be sought as to its choice. Once installed it must be regularly and systematically cleansed, for in certain forms the organic matter, if not removed, accumulates and constitutes an excellent nidus for the growth of bacteria, which still further pollute the water that is being filtered.

Diseases spread by water – In spite of the fact that there are 320 million cubic miles of sea water and that 35,000 cubic miles of rain fall annually, only around 3 per cent of this is fresh water and much of this is locked in the polar ice-caps. It has been estimated that only some 0·3 per cent of this apparently vast reserve is available as fresh water which could be used as drinking water. As each of us now uses 500 litres of water a day, and demand is rising by around 3 per cent annually so that it is estimated that it will be doubled by 2000 A.D., the problem of ensuring an adequate supply of safe water is assuming alarming proportions. The problem is not made any easier by the increasing pollution of water by industry and pesticides and the like.

A wide variety of illnesses and disease may be produced by impure water. Thus, excessive sulphates may induce diarrhoea, excess nitrates may induce cyanosis (qv) in infants, excessive lead may produce lead poisoning, lack of fluoride may enhance the incidence of dental caries, and lack of iodine may induce goitre (qv). There is also some evidence suggesting a correlation between the softness of the water and heart disease. Contamination with micro-organisms may be responsible for outbreaks of enteric fever, dysentery, infective hepatitis, Weil's disease and cholera. Parasites transmitted by water include those responsible for amoebic dysentery, hookworm, schistosomiasis, and filariasis.

Poisoning by various metals may arise from trade-washings that pass into a stream, or by the solution of the metallic constituents of the water-pipes. Lead-poisoning may arise from the latter cause, especially where the water contains a free acid, as in the case of peaty waters; but, if the water contains carbonate of lime, an insoluble protective coating is formed on the interior of the pipes. Many moorland waters have been found to act on lead, but this may be effectually prevented by treating the water with filters composed of sand and limestone. It is also possible to avoid the use of lead pipes where the water is known to act on the lead. The 1976 Brussels Directive on Water, to which member states of the EEC are supposed to adopt their laws within two years, and enforce within ten years, lays down the permitted quantity of lead as 0·05 mg per litre. It also decrees that bottled or other water used for baby feeds should not contain more than 25 mg of nitrate per litre.

WATER TREATMENT (see BATHS; COLD, USES OF; DOUCHES; WET PACK).

WAX is used in medicine as an ingredient of ointments, plasters, and suppositories. It is used either as yellow wax derived directly from honeycomb, or as white wax, which is the same substance bleached. It is also used in the form of paraffin wax to apply heat in the relief of rheumatic pains. (See BATHS.)

For wax in the ear, see EAR, DISEASES OF.

WEAKNESS (see ATROPHY; CACHEXIA; PARALYSIS; TONICS).

WEALS, or WHEALS, are raised white areas on the skin with reddened margins, which may result from sharp blows, or may be a symptom of nettle-rash.

WEANING (see INFANT FEEDING).

WEBBED FINGERS or TOES (illustration 443), or SYNDACTYLY, constitute a deformity sometimes present at birth, and liable to run in families. The web may be quite a thin structure, or the fingers may

443 – Syndactyly involving fusion of the second and third toes. *The Practitioner.*

be closely united by solid tissue. In any case, separation is a matter of considerable difficulty, because, if the web be simply divided, it heals up as before. A special operation is necessary, consisting in turning back a flap of the web upon each of the united fingers, or some other device to produce healing in the new position.

WEIGHT and HEIGHT – The weight of a child at birth is about 7 to 8 pounds (3·2 to 3·6 kg) and the height 20 inches (50 cm). During the first six months the infant puts on weight at the rate of about 5 ounces (140 G) per week if no illness occurs, and during the second six months of life about 1 pound (0·5 kg) per month. At the age of one year he weighs from 18 to 24 pounds (8·2 to 10·9 kg). In the first year he increases in height about 10 inches (25 cm), and measures almost 30 inches (75 cm) at one year old.

In both boys and girls the growth in height amounts to 3 inches (7·5 cm) per year from the second to the fifth years. Boys continue to grow at the rate of 2 inches (5 cm) per year from the sixth to the fifteenth years, whilst girls continue to grow at this rate from the sixth to the eleventh years. In general, it may be said that the height is doubled at the end of five years, and trebled in the thirteenth or fourteenth year. After adolescence growth is more vigorous in boys, but girls attain their full height earlier than boys. Increase in height is greatest in the late spring and early summer, and least in the winter.

As a rule increase in height and increase in weight run parallel. At 2½ years the birth-weight has usually been increased fourfold, whilst at 5 years it has been increased fivefold. The general tendency of weight increase can be summarized as follows: (1) rapid increase in infancy and early childhood; (2) slow but constant increase from 3 to 12 years; (3) marked acceleration during puberty; (4) very slow increase to age of 25 or 30 years.

The following tables (45–46) give a

| Age | Boys | | Girls | |
	Inches	Centi-metres	Inches	Centi-metres
Birth	20·0	50·9	19·5	49·5
2 weeks	20·3	51·7	20·1	51·0
3 months	23·7	60·2	23·2	58·8
6 months	26·2	66·7	25·6	65·0
9 months	28·0	71·2	27·4	69·6
1 year	29·6	75·1	29·1	73·9
2 years	34·0	86·4	33·7	85·5
3 years	37·8	95·9	36·9	93·8
4 years	40·6	103·0	40·0	101·6
5 years	43·1	109·5	42·9	108·9

Table 45 – Mean height of infants and young children. Thomson.

| Age | Boys | | Girls | |
	Pounds	Kilo-grams	Pounds	Kilo-grams
Birth	7·5	3·4	7·3	3·3
2 weeks	7·5	3·4	7·3	3·3
3 months	12·9	5·8	12·0	5·5
6 months	17·4	7·9	16·4	7·4
9 months	20·4	9·2	19·2	8·7
1 year	22·8	10·3	21·7	9·8
2 years	27·0	12·2	25·7	11·6
3 years	31·5	14·3	30·4	13·8
4 years	35·6	16·2	34·5	15·7
5 years	40·2	18·3	39·4	17·9

Table 46 – Mean weight of infants and young children. Thomson.

Weight in pounds

Height in inches	5 years	6 years	7 years	8 years	9 years	10 years	11 years	12 years	13 years	14 years
38	34	34								
39	35	35								
40	36	36								
41	38	38	38							
42	39	39	39	39						
43	41	41	41	41						
44	44	44	44	44						
45	46	46	46	46	46					
46	47	48	48	48	48					
47	49	50	50	50	50	50				
48		52	53	53	53	53				
49		55	55	55	55	55	55			
50		57	58	58	58	58	58	58		
51			61	61	61	61	61	61		
52			63	64	64	64	64	64	64	
53			66	67	67	67	67	68	68	
54				70	70	70	70	71	71	72
55				72	72	73	73	74	74	74
56				75	76	77	77	77	78	78
57					79	80	81	81	82	83
58					83	84	84	85	85	86
59						87	88	89	89	90
60						91	92	92	93	94
61							95	96	97	99
62							100	101	102	103
63							105	106	107	108
64								109	111	113
65								114	117	118
66									119	122
67									124	128
68										134
69										137
70										143
71										148

Table 47 – Correlation of height, weight, and age in boys.
Bird T. Baldwin and Thomas D. Wood, from Bridges' *Dietetics for the Clinician*.
Courtesy of Lea & Febiger and Henry Kimpton.

guide to the expected height and weight of children, but their interpretation in any one particular case must be made with care and discretion. Height, particularly, is a variable factor, and, if a child is under the average height for his age, this need not necessarily be of serious import. Family variations must be taken into consideration, as well as weight and the child's general health. Failure to gain weight is of more significance. Whilst this may be due to some underlying disease, the commonest cause is a diet containing inadequate calories. Over the last six decades or so there has been quite a striking increase in the heights and weights of European children. Thus, the average 13-year-old Glasgow boy was 13 cm taller and 21 kg heavier in 1966 than in 1910. Manufacturers of children's clothing, shoes and furniture have had to increase the size of their products. Growth is now completed at 20–21 years, compared with 25 at the turn of the century. This increase, and earlier maturation, it has been suggested, have been due to a com-

Weight in pounds

Height in inches	5 years	6 years	7 years	8 years	9 years	10 years	11 years	12 years	13 years	14 years
38	33	33								
39	34	34								
40	36	36	36							
41	37	37	37							
42	39	39	39							
43	41	41	41	41						
44	42	42	42	42						
45	45	45	45	45	45					
46	47	47	47	48	48					
47	49	50	50	50	50	50				
48		52	52	52	52	53	53			
49		54	54	55	55	56	56			
50		56	56	57	58	59	61	62		
51			59	60	61	61	63	65		
52			63	64	64	64	65	67		
53			66	67	67	68	68	69	71	
54				69	70	70	71	71	73	
55				72	74	74	74	75	77	78
56					76	78	78	79	81	83
57					80	82	82	82	84	88
58						84	86	86	88	93
59						87	90	90	92	96
60						91	95	95	97	101
61							99	100	101	105
62							104	105	106	109
63								110	110	112
64								114	115	117
65								118	120	121
66									124	124
67									128	130
68									131	133
69										135
70										136
71										138

Table 48 – Correlation of height, weight, and age in girls.
Bird T. Baldwin and Thomas D. Wood, from Bridges' *Dietetics for the Clinician*.
Courtesy of Lea & Febiger and Henry Kimpton.

bination of genetic mixing as a result of population movements, combined with the whole range of improvement in environmental hygiene, and not merely to better nutrition.

In the case of adults (tables 49–52), views have changed of recent years concerning 'ideal' weight. Life insurance statistics have shown that maximal life expectancy is obtained if the average weight at ages 25 to 30 years is maintained throughout the rest of life. These insurance statistics also suggest that it is of advantage to be slightly over average weight before the age of 30 years, to be of average weight from ages 30 to 40, and to be under-weight after the age of 40. In the past it has been usual, in assessing the significance of an adult's weight, to allow a 10 per cent range on either side of normal for variations in body build. A closer correlation has been found between thoracic and abdominal measurements and weight. As average weights are still often referred to, the tables of these in men and women have been retained in this edition, but two further tables have been added showing ideal weights in men and women.

Height		Small Frame	Medium Frame	Large Frame
Feet	*Inches*	*Pounds*	*Pounds*	*Pounds*
5	2	116–125	124–133	131–142
5	3	119–128	127–136	133–144
5	4	122–132	130–140	137–149
5	5	126–136	134–144	141–153
5	6	129–139	137–147	145–157
5	7	133–143	141–151	149–162
5	8	136–147	145–156	153–166
5	9	140–151	149–160	157–170
5	10	144–155	153–164	161–175
5	11	148–159	157–168	165–180
6	0	152–164	161–173	169–185
6	1	157–169	166–178	174–190
6	2	163–175	171–184	179–196
6	3	168–180	176–189	184–202

Table 49 – Ideal weights for men

Weight in pounds with clothes. Height in feet and inches, with shoes on.
From Metropolitan Life Insurance Company, as noted by Rynearson and Gastineau.

Height		Small Frame	Medium Frame	Large Frame
Feet	*Inches*	*Pounds*	*Pounds*	*Pounds*
4	11	104–111	110–118	117–127
5	0	105–113	112–120	119–129
5	1	107–115	114–122	121–131
5	2	110–118	117–125	124–135
5	3	113–121	120–128	127–138
5	4	116–125	124–132	131–142
5	5	119–128	127–135	133–145
5	6	123–132	130–140	138–150
5	7	126–136	134–144	142–154
5	8	129–139	137–147	145–158
5	9	133–143	141–151	149–162
5	10	136–147	145–155	152–166
5	11	139–150	148–158	155–169

Table 50 – Ideal weights for women

Weight in pounds with clothes. Height in feet and inches, with shoes on.
From Metropolitan Life Insurance Company, as noted by Rynearson and Gastineau.

Feet and Inches of Height with Shoes

Age	5-0	5-1	5-2	5-3	5-4	5-5	5-6	5-7	5-8	5-9	5-10	5-11	6-0	6-1	6-2	6-3	6-4	6-5
16	109	111	114	117	120	124	128	132	136	140	144	149	154	159	164	169	174	179
18	113	115	118	121	124	128	132	136	140	144	148	153	158	163	168	173	178	183
20	117	119	122	125	128	132	136	140	144	148	152	156	161	166	171	176	181	186
22	119	121	124	127	131	135	139	142	146	150	154	158	163	168	173	178	183	188
24	121	123	126	129	133	137	141	144	148	152	156	160	165	171	177	182	187	192
26	123	125	127	130	134	138	142	146	150	154	158	163	168	174	180	186	191	196
28	125	127	129	132	135	139	143	147	151	155	159	164	170	176	182	188	193	198
30	126	128	130	133	136	140	144	148	152	156	161	166	172	178	184	190	196	201
32	127	129	131	134	137	141	145	149	154	158	163	168	174	180	186	192	198	203
34	128	130	132	135	138	142	146	150	155	160	165	170	176	182	188	194	200	206
36	129	131	133	136	139	143	147	151	156	161	166	171	177	183	190	196	202	208
38	130	132	134	137	140	144	148	152	157	162	167	173	179	185	192	198	204	210
40	131	133	135	138	141	145	149	153	158	163	168	174	180	186	193	200	206	212
42	132	134	136	139	142	146	150	154	159	164	169	175	181	187	194	201	208	214
44	133	135	137	140	143	147	151	155	160	165	170	176	182	188	195	202	209	215
46	134	136	138	141	144	148	152	156	161	166	171	177	183	189	196	203	210	216
48	134	136	138	141	144	148	152	156	161	166	171	177	183	190	197	204	211	217
50	134	136	138	141	144	148	152	156	161	166	171	177	183	190	197	204	211	217
52	135	137	139	142	145	149	153	157	162	167	172	178	184	191	198	205	212	218
54	135	137	139	142	145	149	153	158	163	168	173	178	184	191	198	205	212	219

Table 51 – Average weight of men in pounds with clothes

Feet and Inches of Height with Shoes

Age	4-8	4-9	4-10	4-11	5-0	5-1	5-2	5-3	5-4	5-5	5-6	5-7	5-8	5-9	5-10	5-11	6-0
16	102	104	106	108	109	111	114	117	120	124	128	132	136	139	143	148	153
18	104	106	108	110	112	114	117	120	123	126	130	134	138	141	145	150	155
20	106	108	110	112	114	116	119	122	125	128	132	136	140	143	147	151	156
22	107	109	111	113	115	117	120	123	126	129	133	137	141	145	149	153	157
24	109	111	113	115	117	119	121	124	127	130	134	138	142	146	150	154	158
26	110	112	114	116	118	120	122	125	128	131	135	139	143	147	151	155	159
28	111	113	115	117	119	121	123	126	130	133	137	141	145	149	153	156	160
30	112	114	116	118	120	122	124	127	131	134	138	142	146	150	154	157	161
32	113	115	117	119	121	123	125	128	132	136	140	144	148	152	155	158	162
34	115	117	119	121	123	125	127	130	134	138	142	146	150	154	157	160	163
36	116	118	120	122	124	126	128	131	135	139	143	147	151	155	158	161	164
38	117	119	121	123	125	127	130	133	137	141	145	149	153	157	160	163	166
40	119	121	123	125	127	129	132	135	138	142	146	150	154	158	161	164	167
42	120	122	124	126	128	130	133	136	139	143	147	151	155	159	162	166	169
44	122	124	126	128	130	132	135	138	141	145	149	153	157	161	164	168	171
46	123	125	127	129	131	133	136	139	142	146	150	154	158	162	165	169	172
48	124	126	128	130	132	134	137	140	143	147	152	156	160	164	167	171	174
50	125	127	129	131	133	135	138	141	144	148	152	156	161	165	169	173	176
52	125	127	129	131	133	135	138	141	144	148	152	157	162	166	170	174	177
54	125	127	129	131	133	135	138	141	144	148	153	158	163	167	171	174	177

Table 52 – Average weight of women in pounds with clothes

WEIGHTS AND MEASURES

WEIGHTS AND MEASURES – As every British schoolboy (and schoolgirl), past and present, knows to his (or her) cost the British system of weights and measures is just about as archaic as it could be. As with so many other national customs and institutions, this is because it is based on history and tradition. A short review of this historical background is therefore called for.

The sixteen-ounce (avoirdupois) pound was introduced into Britain by the Romans, but the history of weights and measures in Britain dates essentially from 1266, with the passing of an Act, in the reign of Henry III, which declared that 'an English penny called the sterling, round and without clipping, shall weigh thirty-two grains of wheat, well dried and gathered out of the middle of the ear; and twenty pence (pennyweights) do make an ounce and twelve ounces a pound, and eight pounds do make a gallon of wine, which is the eighth of a quarter'. The next step was in 1304, when a statute of Edward I declared that 'every pound of money or of medicines is of twenty shillings weight, but the pound of all other things is twenty-five shillings weight'. Further, it declared, 'the ounce of medicines consists of twenty pence, and the pound contains twelve ounces (the Troy Pound), but in other things the pound contains fifteen ounces, in both cases the ounce weighing twenty pence'.

The troy pound is named after the French city of Troyes, which was one of the French cities in which, in the 8th and 9th centuries, fairs were held which provided a meeting place for traders from all over the then known world. In due course, Troyes came to be looked upon as the most important of these international fairs. In these days coins were sold by weight, mainly because they became so mutilated. As a consequence the standard weight of Troyes (duly abbreviated to Troy in this context) for selling coins was adopted throughout Europe for weighing of medicines and precious stones. Although originally the troy ounce and the avoirdupois ounce were meant to have the same weight, the enactment of Edward I meant that, even in those days, there was a difference between the troy and avoirdupois pound. Incidentally, it is to be noted that the weights in use today are one-sixteenth heavier than those decreed in the statute of 1304. This was by subsequent decree that also abolished the penny-weight standard. The responsibility for the adoption of troy weight for prescribing purposes in Britain lies at the door of Sir Theodore Turquet de la Mayerne who compiled the first *Pharmacopoeia* produced by the Royal College of Physicians of London in 1618.

The rest of the story can be briefly summarized. On January 1, 1826, what is known as the Imperial measures and standards were legalized in Britain. According to these, the pound Troy (containing 5760 grains) was standardized on the basis that a cubic inch of distilled water weighed with brass weights in air at 62° F, the barometer standing at 30 inches, weighed 252·458 grains. The standard for capacity was the imperial gallon, which contains 10 pounds avoirdupois (a pound avoirdupois being 7000 grains) of distilled water weighed in air at 62° F and 30 inches barometric pressure. The bushel was equivalent to 8 gallons. Just to complicate the issue, in 1836, after much heart searching, the United States of America adopted the imperial standards for the troy and the avoirdupois pounds and the yard, but defined the gallon as the old wine gallon of 231 cubic inches containing 58,372·2 grains of distilled water at its maximum density weighed in air at a temperature of 62° F and a barometric pressure of 30 inches, whilst the bushel contained 77·274 pounds of water at the same temperature and pressure.

	Name of Unit	Unit Symbol
Length	Metre	m
Mass	Kilogram	kg
Time	Second	s
Electric current	Ampere	A
Thermodynamic temperature	Kelvin	°K
Luminous intensity	Candela	cd
Amount of substance	Mole	mol

Table 53 – Basic units of the International System of Units (SI).

At long last it looks as if this traditional chaos were going to be overcome by the introduction of the metric system. This, however, has been a long time coming. It is over a hundred years (1864 to be precise) since the metric system was legalized in Britain (two years later in the United States of America). In medicine it has encountered a hard core of conservative resistance. Over fifty years ago it was being taught in progressive medical schools, such as that in the University of Edinburgh, but it was not until March 3, 1969, that it became illegal to use any system of weights and measures other than the metric system for dispensing prescriptions. This edict, however, applies only to dispensers. For some curious reason there is as yet no compulsion on doctors to use the metric system in prescribing.

To round off the picture, it should be noted that in recent years a rationalization of the metric system has been introduced, known as the International System of Units (SI). This has been described as 'a coherent system with seven basic units from which all other units are derived'. These are shown in table 53. Among these derived units is that for force – the newton, the symbol for which is N. The new unit of pressure is the pascal, the symbol for which is Pa, while the universal unit for energy is the joule, symbolized by J. Even in this scientifically perfect scheme, exceptions have had to be made for practical purposes. From the medical aspect, the most important of these is that the derived basic unit for volume, the metre cubed (m^3), is admitted to be too clumsy for medical purposes. The litre (l) is

APOTHECARIES' WEIGHT

					Metric Equivalent in Grams
Troy grains	20		=	1 scruple =	1·29
„ „	60 =	3 scruples =		1 drachm =	3·88
„ „	480 =	8 drachms =	-	1 ounce =	31·1
„ „	5760 =	12 ounces =		1 pound (lb) =	373

AVOIRDUPOIS WEIGHT

		Metric Equivalent in Grams
Troy grains 437·5 =	1 ounce (oz) =	28·35
„ „ 7000 =	1 pound (lb) =	453·60

IMPERIAL FLUID MEASURE

					Metric Equivalent in Millilitres
Minims	60	=	1 fluid drachm	=	3·55
„	480 = 8 fluid drachms	=	1 fluid ounce	=	28·41
„	9,600 = 20 fluid ounces	=	1 Imperial pint	=	568·25
„	19,200 = 2 Imperial pints	=	1 Imperial quart	=	1136·5
„	76,800 = 4 Imperial quarts	=	1 Imperial gallon	=	4546·0

N.B. – 1 Imperial pint = 1 pint 4 fluid ounces Apothecaries' Measure.

METRIC WEIGHT AND MEASURE UNITS

1 metre or unit of length	= 39·37 inches (approx 40 inches)
1 litre	= 35·196 fluid ounces (approx 35 fluid ounces)
1 gram	= 15·43 troy grains (approx $15\frac{1}{2}$ grains)
1 millilitre	= 16·89 minims (approx 17 minims)

METRIC MEASURES OF LENGTH

1 kilometre (km)	=	1000·0 metres	=	0·621 mile
1 hectometre	=	100·0 metres	=	109·30 yards
1 dekametre	=	10·0 metres	=	32·81 feet
1 metre (m)	=	1·0 metre	=	39·37 inches
1 decimetre (dm)	=	0·1 metre	=	3·94 inches
1 centimetre (cm)	=	0·01 metre	=	0·394 inch
1 millimetre (mm)	=	0·001 metre	=	0·039 inch
1 micrometre (μm)	=	0·000001 metre	=	0·000039 inch
1 nanometre (nm)	=	0·000000001 metre	=	0·000000039 inch

WEIGHTS AND MEASURES

METRIC MEASURES OF WEIGHT

1 Kilogram (kg)	=	1000·0 G	=	2·20 pounds (avoirdupois)
1 Hectogram	=	100·0 G	=	3·53 ounces (avoirdupois)
1 Dekagram	=	10·0 G	=	154·32 grains
	=	1·0 G	=	15·43 grains
1 Decigram	=	0·1 G	=	1·54 grains
1 Centigram (cg)	=	0·01 G	=	0·15 grain
1 Milligram (mg)	=	0·001 G	=	0·015 grain
1 Microgram (μg or mcg)	=	0·000001 G	=	0·00001 grain

METRIC MEASURES OF CAPACITY

1 Litre (L) = 1000 millilitres = 35·196 Imperial fluid ounces
1 millilitre (ml) = 0·001 litre = 16·89 minims

N.B. – 1 millilitre is approximately equivalent to 1 cubic centimetre (cc).

FACTORS FOR CONVERTING FROM ONE SCALE TO THE OTHER

To convert grams into grains	× 15·432
grams into avoirdupois ounces	× 0·0353
.. kilograms into pounds	× 2·205
„ grains into grams	× 0·065
„ avoirdupois ounces into grams	× 28·35
„ troy ounces into grams	× 31·104
„ mililitres into Imperial fluid ounces	× 0·0352
„ litres into Imperial fluid ounces	× 35·2
„ fluid ounces into millilitres	× 28·42
„ pints into litres	× 0·568
„ metres into inches	× 39·37
„ inches into metres	× 0·0254

APPROXIMATE VALUE OF DOMESTIC MEASURES

Tumbler = 10 fluid ounces	Table-spoon (small) = $\frac{1}{2}$ fluid ounce
Breakfast-cup = 8 „ „	Dessert-spoon = 120 minims
Tea-cup = 5 „ „	Tea-spoon = 60 minims
Wine-glass (large) = $2\frac{1}{2}$ „ „	Drop (of water) = 1 minim

Note – When medicine is measured this should be done by means of a standardized measure, because domestic utensils vary greatly in size.

IMPERIAL – METRIC CONVERSION TABLES

Minims	Milli-litres	Minims	Milli-litres	Grains	Milli-grams	Grains	Milli grans
1	0·06	47–55	3	1/600	0·1	1/10	6
2	0·12	56–64	3·5	1/500	0·125	1/8	7·5
3	0·18	65–74	4	1/300	0·2	1/6	10
4	0·25	75–84	4·5	1/240	0·25	1/5	12·5
5	0·3	85–93	5	1/200	0·3	1/4	15
6–7	0·4	94–110	6	1/150	0·4	1/3	20
8–9	0·5	111–130	7	1/120	0·5	1/2	30
10–11	0·6	131–149	8	1/100	0·6	3/4	50
12–13	0·7	150–167	9	1/75	0·8	1	60
14–16	0·9	168–185	10	1/60	1	2	125
17–18	1	186–200	11	1/50	1·25	3	200
19–22	1·2	201–220	12	1/40	1·5	4	250
23–27	1·5	221–250	14	1/30	2	5	300
28–32	1·8	251–275	15	1/20	3	$7\frac{1}{2}$	450
	2	276–300	17	1/15	4	10	600
	2·5	301–330	18	1/12	5	12	800

Grains	Grams	Grains	Grams
15	1	75	5
20	1·2	90	6
25	1·5	120	8
30	2	150	10
40	2·5	225	15
45	3	300	20
60	4	375	25

therefore to be retained as an alternative, with its various submultiples such as millilitre (ml). To avoid the possible confusion arising from the use of the comma, and not a full stop, for the decimal point in continental Europe, it is recommended that in writing large numbers, groups of three

greater care is necessary, and the thin skin over the wen, to which the lining membrane is adherent, is also removed. The little operation is usually performed under a local anaesthetic, and is accompanied by very little pain.

Multiple	Prefix	Symbol		Submultiple	Prefix	Symbol
10^1	deca	da		10^{-1}	deci	d
10^2	hecto	h		10^{-2}	centi	c
10^3	kilo	k		10^{-3}	milli	m
10^6	mega	M		10^{-6}	micro	u
10^9	giga	G		10^{-9}	nano	n
10^{12}	tera	T		10^{-12}	pico	p

Table 54 – Prefixes for decimal multiples and submultiples in the International System of Units.

figures be separated by a space, and not by a comma. Thus one-million-five-hundred-thousand is 1 500 000, or 2.5×10^6, or $2,5 \times 10^6$. Decimal multiples and submultiples will be as shown in table 53.

For yet another edition at least, however, details are given of both the imperial and metric systems (pages 953–954).

WEIL'S DISEASE is a form of jaundice due to infection with a leptospira (qv), also known as infectious jaundice and as SPIROCHAETOSIS ICTEROHAEMORRHAGICA (qv).

WEIR MITCHELL TREATMENT is a form of treatment which consists in absolute rest of body and mind, administration of highly nutritious and easily digestible food in large quantities, and massage to take the place of muscular exercise. (See NEURASTHENIA.)

WELLS (see WATER SUPPLY).

WENS are small cystic tumours in the skin, consisting of a collection of sebaceous material, due to blockage of the outlet from a sebaceous gland. They occur most commonly about the face and scalp, where they form smooth, rounded, elastic tumours, often of a considerable size, but give rise to no trouble save that occasioned by their position, by their unsightliness, and by the fact that they are liable to become inflamed from the pressure, for example, of the hat.

Treatment consists in opening the cyst, squeezing out its fatty contents, and carefully removing the lining membrane. If any part of the membrane lining the interior be left behind, the wound heals in such a way that the wen is apt to refill. On the scalp this membrane is tough and can generally be pulled out entire, but on the face

WET BRAIN is a term applied to an oedematous state of the brain caused by chronic alcoholism and associated with mental failure and delusions.

WET CUP is a form of cupping in which the cupping glass is applied after scarification of the skin. (See CUPPING.)

WET PACK is a method of treatment much in vogue in some countries for the purpose of applying a moderate degree of cold or of heat, for some time, to a patient's skin.

Uses – The conditions in which cold is beneficial are detailed under COLD, USES OF. The wet pack is a specially convenient method of applying cold when it is desired to exert a gentle cooling influence over a prolonged period, one hour or more, and at the same time to maintain the patient in a condition of absolute quiet and rest. It is used, for example, in such conditions as exhaustion due to heat. When a more rapid degree of cooling is desired, the patient is changed from one wet pack to another every quarter of an hour or thereabout, two beds being placed near one another for this purpose. Very rapid cooling may be achieved by wrapping the patient in a wet pack and rubbing down the sheet in which he is enveloped with pieces of ice.

Hot wet packs are also applied.

Method of application: (1) COLD PACK – A mackintosh sheet covered by a large blanket is spread upon the bed, and, when the patient is ready, a sheet is dipped in cold water, wrung out fairly dry, and laid over the blanket. The patient, stripped, is laid upon the sheet, which is quickly turned over him from both sides, and pushed between his legs and between each arm and the chest, so that skin does not touch skin anywhere. This must be done quickly, and the sheet being neatly tucked in round the neck and folded beneath the feet, every part of the body is covered saving the head and face. The head may also be wrapped in a wet towel. Finally the sides of the blanket are turned over the patient, and wrapped round him so as to lie smoothly everywhere. The patient, enveloped in this pack, lies absolutely helpless and should on no account be left by the attendant till the pack is removed, when he is put back into bed.

(2) HOT PACK (illustration 444) – A mackintosh sheet is spread on the bed as for a cold pack. Upon this is laid a dry blanket. A second blanket (which retains heat better than a sheet) is placed in a pail and boiling water is poured over it (illustration 445). The blanket is then taken out of the pail, wrung, shaken, and rolled up (illustration 446). It is next applied to the patient in the same way as the sheet in the case of the cold pack (illustration 447) The dry blanket is then also wrapped round the patient outside the wet blanket; a second mackintosh sheet is spread over him (illustration 448); and hot-water bottles, if desired, are placed alongside him; and several more blankets are laid on top of the mackintosh sheet. The patient may lie enveloped in the hot pack for twenty minutes; he is then quickly dried with warm towels, a warm flannel nightdress is put on and he is put back in bed. The patient must on no account be left alone while he is in the hot pack.

(3) WHISKY PACK – (See ALCOHOL.)

(4) MUSTARD PACK – A pack containing mustard is sometimes used as a last resort in cases of collapse or of failure of breathing in young children.

WHEEZING is a popular name applied to the various sounds produced in the chest when the bronchial tubes are inflamed. It is applied particularly to the long-drawn breathing of asthma, and to the whistling or purring noises that accompany breathing in cases of bronchitis. (See ASTHMA; BRONCHITIS.)

WHELK is a term applied to a weal, and also to a red protuberance on the face or nose seen in the case of a hard drinker. (See ROSACEA.)

WHEY (see JUNKET).

WHIPWORM is a popular name for *Trichuris trichiura*. (See TRICHURIASIS.)

WHISKY (see ALCOHOL).

956

444 – Requisites for hot pack

445 – Hot pack, first stage. Pail containing sheet for wringer and blanket for pack.

446 – Hot pack, second stage. Wringing out the blanket inside the sheet.

447 – Hot pack, third stage. Applying the hot wet blanket.

448 – Hot pack, fourth stage. Blanket tucked round patient, and upper mackintosh being laid over.

WHITE LEG is a fairly common and well-known condition in which a limb, usually one of the lower limbs, becomes enlarged, white, and painful.

Causes – Most commonly the condition occurs after child-birth; sometimes it occurs during convalescence from an acute febrile disease, especially typhoid fever or pneumonia. It is usually due to inflammation in, and blocking of, the veins of the limb, or may be caused by the spread of infection into the lymphatics of the limb from those within the pelvis, or to some morbid change in the blood causing it to clot.

Symptoms – The disease comes on during convalescence from one of the conditions mentioned above, beginning with slight feverishness and pain down the leg which is to be affected. The limb gradually swells, and in a few days may be greatly enlarged, hard, glossy, and of a strikingly white colour. The veins can generally be felt as solid lines down the inner side of the thigh, and the affected parts may be very tender to the touch. These symptoms persist for a week or so, but generally begin to subside within a fortnight from the onset, and about three-fourths of all cases recover completely in a few weeks. In other cases, some degree of muscular weakness, swelling, or aching of the limb remains permanently, but the condition, though a serious one demanding most careful treatment, is seldom fatal.

Treatment consists chiefly of rest in bed with the affected limb supported on a pillow. Pain is relieved by laudanum fomentations or simply by wrapping the limb in cotton-wool. Anticoagulants such as heparin and dicoumarol are given to prevent the process spreading.

This is one of the conditions, however, in which it is now recognized that preventive measures can be most effective. These consist principally of not allowing patients to stay in bed longer than necessary, or of giving massage to the legs in cases which are confined to bed for long periods. (See also VEINS, DISEASES OF.)

WHITE PRECIPITATE is the popular name for Ammoniated Mercury, B P, a substance used in the form of an ointment for application to various skin diseases. (See MERCURY.)

WHITES, or LEUCORRHOEA, is a symptom of many diseases peculiar to women, and may be of an acute nature, when the discharge is thick and white, consisting mainly of pus; or is more often chronic and catarrhal, when the discharge is usually thinner, sometimes of a clear mucous nature; in other cases acrid and offensive. In slighter cases, the discharge precedes or follows the menstrual flow; in severer cases it continues throughout the whole intervening periods. Persons affected in this manner are generally unhealthy in appearance, the face is pale and sallow, weariness is felt easily upon exertion, and a dull gnawing pain is often experienced in the lower part of the back.

Causes – Leucorrhoea may arise as a result of infection anywhere in the genital tract in women: ie. in the uterus, cervix, or vagina. The commonest cause is some chronic inflammation of the womb following on childbirth, and associated with some laceration of its neck. Another important cause is gonorrhoea. In other cases it is due to infection of the vagina with the *Trichomonas vaginalis* (qv). The condition may occur as a symptom of general debility accompanied by congestion of the uterus. It may also be due to a tumour in the uterus or the cervix. An occasional cause of very offensive discharge is found in the irritation set up by the presence of a foreign body, such as a pessary that has been introduced for the support of a displaced womb, and then forgotten. In young children the condition is not common, but may arise from the irritation set up by threadworms, as the result of general debility combined with want of cleanliness, or following upon some acute infective disease.

Treatment – This depends upon the cause of the discharge. Thus, if it is due to infection with *Trichomonas vaginalis* (qv) metronidazole should be given. If it is due to gonorrhoea it is this that must be treated. (See GONORRHOEA.) If it is due to an erosion of the cervix, or neck of the womb, this must be treated. In women past the menopause, or the change of life, the most effective treatment may be administration of an oestrogen (qv). (See also UTERUS, DISEASES OF.)

WHITE SWELLING is a popular name applied to tuberculous disease of joints. (See JOINTS, DISEASES OF.)

WHITLOW is a popular term applied to all acute inflammations of the deep-seated tissues in the fingers, whether the structure affected be the root of the nail, the pulp of the finger-tip, the sheaths of the tendons that run along the back and front of the fingers, or the bone. Acute inflammation of the bones in the finger is rare, and in general a whitlow begins in the last part of one finger, being, when situated towards the back, a small abscess at the root of the nail, and, when starting in front, an abscess in the fat and fibrous tissue that compose the pulp of the finger. Suppuration may also begin in the sheath of the tendon, generally in front of the finger.

WHOOPING-COUGH, also known as HOOPING-COUGH, PERTUSSIS, and CHIN-COUGH, is an infectious disease of the mucous membrane lining the air passages, which manifests itself by frequently recurring attacks of convulsive coughing, followed by a peculiar, loud indrawing of the breath, and often by vomiting. It occurs for the most part in children, and seldom more than once in a lifetime.

Causes – The cause of whooping-cough is a bacillus discovered by Bordet and Gengou in 1906 and found in the sputum. It is known as *Bordetella pertussis*. Although specially a disease of childhood, whooping-cough is by no means limited to that period, but may occur at any time of life, even to old age, should there have been no previous attack. It is most prevalent between the ages of 1 and 4, and is uncommon after 10. Whooping-cough can be a dangerous disease in infants, but is a much less serious malady in older children. It has been occasionally observed in newly born infants, and is more common in girls than in boys. Whooping-cough is infectious during any stage of its progress, but chiefly at its commencement. It prevails mostly in the winter months, doubtless owing to the increasing predisposition to affections of the respiratory passages. In recent years the disease has tended to occur in cycles, with periods of increased prevalence occurring every three to four years. The incubation period is usually 7 to 10 days.

In 1977, there were 17,470 cases of whooping-cough in England, with 7 deaths. This was the biggest outbreak since 1960 and its size was partly attributed to the fall in vaccination acceptance rates.

Symptoms – Three stages of the disease are recognized: (1) the catarrhal, (2) the spasmodic, (3) the stage of decline.

The *first stage* is characterized by the usual symptoms of a catarrh, with sneezing, watering of the eyes, irritation of the throat, feverishness, and cough, but in general there is nothing in the symptoms to indicate that they are to develop into whooping-cough. There may be a slight rise of temperature to 99° to 100° F (37·2° to 37·7° C) in the first few days. The catarrhal stage usually lasts from ten to fourteen days.

The *second stage* is marked by the abatement of the catarrhal symptoms, but at the same time by increase in the cough, which now occurs in irregular paroxysms both by day and by night. Each paroxysm consists in a series of violent and rapid expiratory coughs, succeeded by a loud sonorous or crowing inspiration – the 'whoop'. During the coughing efforts the air is driven with great force out of the lungs, and, as none can enter the chest, the symptoms of impending asphyxia appear. The patient grows deep-red or livid in the face, the eyes appear as if they would burst from their sockets, and suffocation seems imminent till relief is brought by the whoop. Occasionally blood runs from the nose or mouth, or is extravasated into the conjunctiva of the eyes. A single fit rarely lasts beyond from half to three-quarters of a minute, but after the whoop another recurs, and of these a number may come and go for several minutes. The paroxysm ends by the coughing or vomiting up of a viscid tenacious secretion, and usually after this the patient seems comparatively well, or, it may be, somewhat wearied and fretful. The frequency of the paroxysms varies according to the severity of the case, being in some instances only to the extent of one or two in the whole day, whilst in others there may be several in the course of a single hour. Slight causes serve to bring on the fits of coughing, such as the acts of swallowing, talking, laughing, crying, or they may occur without any apparent exciting cause. In general, children come to recognize an impending attack by a feeling of tickling in the throat, and they cling with dread to their mother or nurse, or take hold of some object near them for support during the paroxysm; but, although exhausted by the severe fit of coughing, they soon resume their play, apparently little the worse. The attacks are on the whole most severe at night. This stage of the disease usually continues during two to four weeks, but it may be shorter or longer. It is during this time that complications are apt to arise which may become a source of danger greater even than the malady itself. The chief of these are inflammatory affections of the bronchial tubes and lungs, and convulsions, any of which may prove fatal. A milder complication is the formation of a small ulcer under the tongue from rubbing against the teeth in coughing. Hernia and prolapse of the rectum sometimes are produced by the strain of violent coughing.

When, however, the disease progresses favourably, as it usually does, it passes into the *third* or *terminal stage*, in which the cough becomes less frequent and generally loses in great measure its whooping character. The patient's general condition undergoes improvement, and the symptoms disappear in from one to three weeks. It is to be observed, however, that for a long period afterwards in any simple catarrh from which the patient suffers the cough often assumes a spasmodic character, which may suggest the erroneous notion that a relapse of the whooping-cough has occurred.

In severe cases it sometimes happens that the disease leaves behind it such structural changes in the lungs (eg. emphysema) as entail permanent shortness of breathing, or a liability to attacks of asthma. Occasionally the violence of the cough may rupture a blood-vessel in the eye, or in the brain with hemiplegia as a result.

Treatment – As regards the treatment of whooping-cough in mild cases, little is necessary beyond keeping the patient warm and carefully attending to the general health. The remedies applicable in the case of catarrh or the milder forms of bronchitis are of service here. In mild weather the patient may be in the open air. In the more severe forms, efforts have to be employed to modify the severity of the paroxysms. Numerous remedies are recommended, the chief of which are phenobarbitone, camphorated tincture of opium, and atropine methonitrate. During convalescence, when the cough still continues to be troublesome, a change of air will often effect its removal.

Antibiotics, including tetracyclines, chloramphenicol, cephaloridine, erythromycin, and co-trimoxazole are of value, but it is not recommended that they should be used routinely. The main indications for their use are in young children and when there are complications.

A vaccine has been prepared which is effective as a prophylactic. This is given in the form of Triple Vaccine (Diphtheria, Tetanus, and Pertussis Vaccine) at age of 3 or 6 months. A second dose is given six to eight weeks later, and a third dose six months later. It should not be given to a child with any disease or disorder of the central nervous system, to a child with a history of convulsions or to a child with a family history of convulsions. Administration should also be postponed in the case of a temporarily unwell child until he is well again. A hyper-immune serum is also available but appears to be of doubtful value.

WIDAL REACTION (see AGGLUTINATION).

WILMS' TUMOUR, or NEPHROBLASTOMA, is the commonest kidney tumour in infancy. It is a malignant tumour, which occurs in around 1 per 10,000 live births. The survival rate with modern treatment (removal of the kidney followed by radiotherapy and chemotherapy) is now around 80 per cent.

WILSON'S DISEASE, or HEPATOLENTICULAR DEGENERATION, is a familial disease in which there is an increased accumulation of copper in the liver, brain, and other tissues including the kidneys. Its main manifestation is the development of tremor and rigidity, with difficulty in speech. In some cases there is improvement following the administration of dimercaprol or penicillamine; these two substances cause an increased excretion of copper.

WINDPIPE is the popular name for the trachea, which extends from the larynx above to the point in the upper part of the chest where it divides into the two large bronchial tubes, one to each lung. It thus extends through the lower part of the neck and upper part of the chest, and is about four inches (10 cm) in length. It consists of a fibrous tube kept permanently open by about twenty strong horizontally placed hoops of cartilage, each of which forms about two-thirds of a circle, but is defective behind where the two ends are united by muscle-fibres. This fibro-cartilaginous tube is lined by a smooth mucous membrane, richly supplied with mucous glands and covered by a single layer of ciliated epithelium. (See also AIR PASSAGES.)

WIND SUCKING (see AEROPHAGY).

WINE (see VINUM and ALCOHOL).

WINTER COUGH is a name sometimes given to chronic bronchitis which affects old people specially. The cough passes off during the summer and returns with the damp weather each winter. (See BRONCHITIS.)

WINTERGREEN (see GAULTHERIA).

WISDOM TOOTH is a popular name for the last molar tooth on either side of each jaw. These teeth are the last to appear and should develop in early adult life, but often they do not cut the gum till the age of twenty or twenty-five, or indeed they may sometimes remain permanently impacted in the jaw-bone. This occurs in up to 25 per cent of individuals. The lower third molar is often impacted against the second because of the direction in which it erupts. (See TEETH.)

WITCH-HAZEL is a preparation of the bark, twigs, and dried leaves from *Hamamelis virginiana*, a plant of the United States possessed of strong astringent properties. It is used to check haemorrhages and excessive mucous discharges, and also for piles. The most commonly used preparation is the liquid extract, which is sometimes given internally and more often used in the strength of 60 minims (4 ml) to 3 ounces (85 ml) of cold water, either as a lotion for bruises or as an enema for bleeding piles. Extract of hamamelis is employed as an application for varicose veins and ulcers; and ointments, known as hazeline snow and hazeline cream, are used as applications for irritable states of the skin.

WOLFSBANE is another name for aconite (qv).

WOMB (see UTERUS).

WOOD ALCOHOL is another name for methyl alcohol. (See SPIRIT.)

WOOD WOOL is the name of a fabric prepared from wood fibre, and much used for padding splints and other surgical purposes where the more expensive and softer cotton-wool is not necessary.

WOOLSORTERS' DISEASE is another name for anthrax. (See ANTHRAX.)

WORD BLINDNESS is the term applied to a condition in which, as the result of disease in the brain, a person becomes unable to associate their proper meanings with words, although he may be quite able to spell the letters. WORD DEAFNESS is an associated condition in which, though hearing remains perfect, the patient has lost the power of referring the names he hears to the articles they denote. (See APHASIA.)

WORMWOOD (see ABSINTHISM).

WOUNDS – A wound is any breach suddenly produced in the tissues of the body by direct violence. An extensive injury of the deeper parts without corresponding injury of the surface is known as a bruise or contusion.

Varieties – Classified according to the immediate effect produced, four varieties are usually described as *incised, punctured, lacerated,* and *contused.*

INCISED WOUNDS are usually inflicted with some sharp instrument, and are clean cuts, in which the tissues are simply divided without any damage to parts around. The bleeding from such a wound is apt to be very free, but it can be readily controlled.

PUNCTURED WOUNDS, or stabs, are inflicted with a pointed instrument. These wounds are the most dangerous, partly because their depth involves the danger of wounding vital organs, partly because bleeding from a stab is hard to control, and largely on account of the difficulty of purification. The wound produced by the nickel-nosed bullet is a puncture, much less severe than the ugly lacerated wound caused by an expanding bullet, or by a ricochet, and, if no clothing has been carried in by the bullet, the wound is clean and usually heals at once.

LACERATED WOUNDS are those in which great tearing takes place, such as injuries caused by machinery. The blood-vessels being torn and twisted, little bleeding is apt to result, and a limb may be torn completely away without great loss of blood. Such wounds are, however, specially liable to the danger of suppuration.

CONTUSED WOUNDS are those accompanied by much bruising of surrounding parts, as in the case of a blow from a cudgel or poker. In these wounds also there is little bleeding, but healing is slow on account of damage to the edges of the wound.

Any of these varieties may become infected by pus-forming germs and develop into a POISONED WOUND.

First-aid treatment – The first duty of a bystander who renders help to a wounded person is to check any bleeding. This may be done by pressure upon the edges of the wound with a clean handkerchief, or, if the bleeding is serious, by putting the finger in the wound and pressing it upon the spot from which the blood is coming. If necessary, the person may then at his leisure apply other methods described under HAEMORRHAGE and TOURNIQUET.

If a medical man is to see a wound within a few hours, it should not be interfered with further than is necessary to stop the bleeding and to cover the wound with a clean dry handkerchief or piece of lint. In cases in which expert assistance is not soon obtainable, one of the following procedures may be adopted. The bleeding being checked, the next step is to cleanse the wound and surrounding skin.

(*a*) *By painting freely with acriflavine cetrimide, chlorhexidine, or Dettol* the wound and the surrounding skin, and covering with a piece of clean dry lint; this answers well in the case of small wounds and abrasions. A small piece of sterilized lint attached to a strip of sticking plaster may be purchased ready for use and forms a convenient and quickly applied dressing.

(*b*) *By washing with clean water* (ie. boiled). For this purpose, one requires two *clean* bowls scalded out quickly with boiling water, and filled with *clean* warm water; also several *clean* cloths, which may be handkerchiefs, squares of lint (preferably boric lint), or newly washed rags.

(1) First, it is essential that the person who is to dress the wound should wash his own hands, and especially the nails, thoroughly with soap and water.

(2) Press a clean cloth upon the wound to prevent the entrance into it of dirty water, and carefully wash the skin around the wound with water, from one of the bowls, using soap if necessary.

(3) Wring out a fresh cloth from the clean water in the second bowl, and with it gently dab the wound. Remove, replace by another clean cloth similarly wrung out, and fix it on the wound with a folded handkerchief. (See BANDAGES.)

(4) The injured part is finally fixed so that movement is prevented or minimized. A wounded hand or arm is fixed with a sling (see SLINGS), a wounded leg with a splint (see SPLINTS).

(5) If the injury has caused severe shock, stimulants may be necessary. (See SHOCK.)

Healing of wounds – The reaction of the tissues to an injury is similar to that produced by any other irritation. If the wound has been accompanied by loss of tissue which has to be made good, or by death of a piece of tissue which has to be cast off as a slough, or by infection with bacteria which has to be overcome, the process of repair is tedious and in some cases permanent damage is produced. The new tissue formed in the wound is mainly fibrous tissue, like that composing the supporting framework of the body.

HEALING BY FIRST INTENTION – In a clean, incised wound of moderate severity, the immediate effect is bleeding from the ends of the vessels which have been cut. This, however, is soon arrested by the contraction and retraction of the coats of the divided vessels, and by the formation of blood-clots in their open ends. A small quantity of blood remains in the wound and clots. The blood-vessels round the injured part dilate, the blood flow becomes slowed, and there passes out from the blood a fluid known as lymph, which coagulates upon the surface of the wound, forming a sticky layer of fibrin which, if the injured surfaces are in contact, causes them to adhere to one another. This forms the temporary scaffolding within which the tissues of repair will be built, and possesses the other valuable property of being strongly germicidal to any organisms which may come in contact with it. White corpuscles also migrate through the walls of the dilated blood-vessels and pass into this exudate in the wound. This fact is of the greatest importance, since the white corpuscles eat up and destroy any foreign or dead substance which has to be removed in the process of repair. (See PHAGOCYTOSIS.) They remove the minute portions of tissue which have been killed by the injury, and the small quantity of blood which has accumulated in the wound. Following the entrance of the white blood corpuscles, within twenty-four hours after the infliction of the wound, there comes a host of cells produced by the rapid multiplication of the cells in the tissues around the wound. Some of these also have the power of phagocytosis, and others, called fibroblasts, become transformed into delicate fibrous tissue. Next, minute buds shoot in from the walls of the smallest blood-vessels and form minute blood channels, which pass from side to side of the wound, or form loops if a gap has been left. The tissue so formed is known as granulation tissue, because, when its surface is closely examined, it has a red, granular appearance due to these loops of vessels covered by masses of the cells mentioned above. The same form of tissue is readily seen on a healing ulcer. Epithelial cells from the surface of the skin now grow over and cover the wound, the whole process being completed usually in less than a week. The delicately formed tissue of the healed wound is gradually replaced by firm fibrous tissue containing fewer blood-vessels, and in a matter of·months, depending partly on where the scar has occurred, the angry, red scar of the recently healed wound is replaced by a white scar. As a rule wounds on the face heal very rapidly. With minor modifications, this process of repair takes place in all healing wounds.

HEALING BY SECOND INTENTION occurs in wounds which have broken down owing to suppuration, or where there is an ulcer, and the edges are gradually drawn together by the contraction of the newly formed fibrous tissue. This results in a wider, weaker, and more noticeable scar.

HEALING BY SCAB FORMATION occurs where the lymph dries up, and union is continued under the dry cake so formed.

HEALING OF POISONED WOUNDS – Where a wound becomes poisoned, or septic, the multiplication of the germs in it dissolves the fibrin and destroys many of the cells engaged in repair. The reaction of the tissues becomes intense, and the inflammation is so evident that the wound is popularly said to be inflamed. As a result of the destruction, many of the cells are discharged as pus. Granulation tissue is gradually formed around the site of infection, the bacteria are cast off in the pus, and healing by second intention takes place. A certain amount of the poison produced by the bacteria, however, escapes into the circulation and causes the symptoms of general ill-health which are present with a poisoned wound.

Dangers of wounds – BLOOD-POISONING usually means that the germs themselves have entered the circulation, which is a grave occurrence and may be fatal. (See BLOOD-POISONING.)

ERYSIPELAS, TETANUS and GAS GANGRENE are conditions in which the germs, (or their toxins) responsible for these diseases enter the lymphatics and bloodstream and produce widespread effects. (See ERYSIPELAS; TETANUS; GANGRENE.)

HAEMORRHAGE – *Primary haemorrhage* means bleeding which occurs at the time of the injury. A large vein or artery may have been divided and may require to be tied. (See HAEMORRHAGE.) A wound of a large vessel like the femoral or the popliteal artery may cause death in a few minutes if untreated. *Reactionary haemorrhage* takes place sometimes from wounds which do not bleed much when they are first inflicted. The explanation is that the shock caused by the injury enfeebles the action of the heart, and, when the wounded person recovers from the shock in a few hours, the increased force of the heart's beating causes bleeding to recommence in the wound. *Secondary haemorrhage* occurs only in the case of poisoned wounds. The spread of the infection breaks down the blood-clot which has formed in the open end of a blood-vessel

and allows the escape of blood. It is usually preceded by a slight oozing of blood, which serves to forewarn the medical attendant. This form of bleeding seldom occurs earlier than a week from the date of the injury.

PARALYSIS – In a wound of a limb, one of the nerves may be divided. When this has happened, a definite area of skin is found to have lost the sense of touch and pain, and the muscles supplied by the divided nerve have completely lost their power. The tendons, which attach the muscles to the bones, may also be divided, as, for example, by a wound behind or in front of the wrist, causing loss of power in the injured part. If either or both of these complications be present, it is of the greatest importance that the divided ends should be stitched together as early as possible, or a permanent loss of power may result.

SCALP WOUNDS usually heal well, but in deep scalp wounds there is a danger that suppuration may result and may pass within the skull. Again, a severe blow producing a scalp wound may cause fracture of the skull and concussion or compression of the brain. (See BRAIN, DISEASES AND INJURIES OF.)

CHEST WOUNDS – Stabs of the chest are serious chiefly because of the fatal bleeding likely to follow any wound of the heart or large vessels; a less serious danger attends wounds of the pleural cavity causing collapse of the lung or empyema.

ABDOMINAL WOUNDS – A penetrating wound of the abdomen, particularly when the bowel has been cut, is often fatal from the acute general peritonitis which it causes.

General treatment of wounds – The first-aid treatment, already described, has for its chief objects the arrest of bleeding and the covering of the wound by a clean dressing, so as to prevent the entrance of germs and to get rid of those which have gained entrance from the skin, or upon the object that inflicted the wound.

To prevent infection of a wound at an operation or in applying a permanent dressing, everything which comes in contact with it must be sterilized or rendered germ-free. To destroy the germs, the best and most easily obtained material is boiling water or steam. If subjected to the action of boiling water for one hour, all known germs are killed, whilst five minutes' boiling is found sufficient for practical purposes. Chemical agents, such as carbolic acid or perchloride of mercury, when used in solutions of given strength, are antiseptics or germicides, and are employed where heat is not applicable. The antiseptic method of treatment for a wound, as originally laid down by Lord Lister, was carried out by using, in addition to the preliminary sterilization of everything which could possibly contaminate the wound, antiseptic lotions with which to douche it. The disadvantage of this form of treatment is that an antiseptic powerful enough to kill any germs in the wound, will also kill the tissue cells. The aseptic method of treatment, on the other hand, is carried out when everything that can possibly convey infection to the wound is rendered free from germs, but none of the fluids or dressings which come in contact with the wound contains antiseptics. In hospitals it is usual to employ the aseptic method, and all gauze, lint, wool, and bandages are treated in a steam sterilizer before use, and kept covered till required.

CHANGING THE DRESSING – If the wounded surfaces are in contact, the dressing should not be changed unless pain is felt in the wound, discharge from the wound soaks through the dressing, a rise of temperature occurs, or the part feels uncomfortable, until the eighth to tenth day, when the dressing is removed.

DRESSINGS AND LOTIONS – The most satisfactory dressing is sterilized gauze but should this not be available, then either boric lint or cyanide gauze may be used. Cyanide gauze is gauze impregnated with the double cyanide of mercury and zinc.

Among the local applications the *flavines* are still among the most useful: acriflavine and proflavine are the most widely used. *Eusol* (qv) is also of value, particularly in wounds known to be infected; its major practical disadvantage is that it only retains its antiseptic properties for two or three weeks, and must therefore be made up fresh at regular intervals. *Iodine*, in 2 to 5 per cent alcoholic solutions, is a useful antiseptic if used with discrimination. *Biniodide of mercury* (1 in 500 solution in 75 per cent methylated spirit) is a potent antiseptic. *Perchloride of mercury* (1 in 2000 parts of water) is less potent but correspondingly safer. *Carbolic acid* (qv), 1 part in 20 parts of water, is less widely used than at one time, but is still a useful application to small, infected wounds. It must not be used for large wounds, nor must it be used with dressings impermeable to the air, because of the risk of excessive absorption leading to carbolic acid poisoning. *Saponaceous solution of cresol, B P* (perhaps better known as lysol), 1 part in 100 to 200 parts of water, is also used. Three widely used antiseptics at the moment are *cetrimide, chlorhexidine,* and *Dettol.*

STITCHES – If the wound be of the incised variety, with wide separation of the edges, it may require to be stitched. Horsehair, silkworm gut, silver wire, silk, or catgut may be employed for this purpose. One of the first three is used in cases in which there is a risk that the wound may become poisoned. Catgut, which is prepared from the intestine of the sheep, possesses the advantage over all the others that it is absorbed by the tissues, and thus does not require to be removed. Where stitches of any of the others have been used, they are generally removed about the tenth day. Sometimes a continuous suture is used for a long wound, but more commonly each stitch is put in and tied singly.

DRAINAGE TUBES – Sterilized indiarubber tubing is inserted down to the bottom of the wound in all cases in which suppuration is likely to occur in a deep wound, when there is much bruising of the tissues, or when blood is liable to accumulate in the wound. If the wound remains clean, the drainage tube will be removed on the third day. If suppuration occurs, it will be replaced and kept in until the discharge ceases or the deep wound closes up so far as to become a healing ulcer. For small wounds, a strip of gauze or a few strands of worsted or a folded strip of thin rubber tissue is often used as a drain instead of a tube.

Treatment of discharging wounds – If a wound should suppurate, it must receive treatment which will enable the pus to escape freely while the wound slowly closes. This is provided by inserting a drainage tube into the wound. To prevent the pus drying up and retaining the discharge, and to draw the pus out of the wound, a moist dressing is applied. A piece of lint soaked in sterilized water, or boric lotion (1 in 60), or perchloride of mercury lotion (1 in 3000), is applied to the wound. The lint is covered with a larger piece of waterproof material, such as gutta-percha tissue, oil-silk, or tin-foil; over this a still larger piece of cotton-wool is applied, and the whole is fixed by a bandage. This dressing is changed daily until the discharge ceases. If the pus is abundant and not escaping freely, the wound is, in addition, washed out with sterilized water or with lotion at each dressing. When improvement is very slow, a hot boric fomentation, changed every four hours, is to be recommended. Should blood-poisoning develop, special treatment is required, directed against the infection which is present throughout the blood. This includes the administration of penicillin or one of the sulphonamides.

WRIST is the joint situated between the arm above and the hand below. The

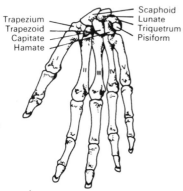

Trapezium
Trapezoid
Capitate
Hamate

Scaphoid
Lunate
Triquetrum
Pisiform

449 – The bones of the hand and wrist, anterior (or palmar) view.

region of the wrist contains eight small carpal bones, arranged in two rows, each containing four bones (illustration 449). Those in the proximal row, that is the row nearest the forearm, are from the outside inwards when looking at the palm of the hand, the scaphoid, lunate, triquetrum, and pisiform. Those in the distal row, that is the row nearest the hand, are the trapezium, trapezoid, capitate and hamate. These intervene between the arm bones and the five metacarpal bones in the hand, and have the effect of diminishing jars communicated to the hand in virtue of a certain amount of sliding movement over one another, of which they are capable. These small bones are closely bound to one another by short, strong ligaments, and the wrist-joint is the union of the composite mass thus formed with the radius and ulna in the forearm. The wrist and the radius and ulna are united by strong outer and inner lateral ligaments, and by weaker ligaments before and behind, whilst the powerful tendons passing to the hand and fingers give it a great measure of strength.

The joint is capable of movement in all directions, and, on account of its shape and its numerous ligaments, is very little liable to dislocation, although stretching or tearing of some of these ligaments is a common accident, constituting a sprain. (See JOINTS, DISEASES AND INJURIES OF.) Inflammation of the tendon-sheaths before and behind the wrist, causing the presence of fluid, also results occasionally from an injury, and produces a sense of weakness in the wrist. A fairly common condition is that known as a ganglion, in which an elastic swelling full of fluid develops on the back or front of the wrist in connection with the sheaths of the tendons. (See GANGLION.)

WRIST-DROP (see DROP-WRIST).

WRITER'S CRAMP (see CRAMP).

WRY-NECK is a condition in which the head is twisted to one side. It may be caused by the contraction of a scar, such as that resulting from a burn or by paralysis of some of the muscles, but in the great majority of cases it is a spasmodic condition due to excessive tendency of certain muscles to contract. (See CRAMP; and SPASMODIC TORTICOLLIS.)

X

X-RAYS, or RÖNTGEN RAYS – The discovery of these was recorded in January 1896 by Professor Röntgen, at that time professor of physics at Würzburg. This epoch-making discovery had been preceded by a series of experiments carried out by Crookes and Lenard. Crookes, employing vacuum tubes with residual air at $\frac{1}{1000000}$ of an atmosphere, produced cathodal rays from the negative pole on the passage of a high-potential electric current. Lenard passed these rays into the air through an aluminium window in the tube, and found that they could produce fluorescence of certain bodies, would pass through certain substances opaque to ordinary light, and would act on a photographic plate. Röntgen, using a still higher vacuum, succeeded in producing X-rays from the walls of the tube, these rays being unaffected by a magnet, and possessing greater power of penetration.

From these simple beginnings the science of Radiography and Radiotherapy has been slowly developed, until at the present day countless sets of apparatus are in daily use in X-ray departments of hospitals throughout the world. The uses of X-rays are, however, manifold. Hardly any scientific laboratory of the present day is complete without an X-ray installation. In industry X-rays are used for investigational purposes: thus, for example, with high-tension apparatus giving up to 300,000 volts, steel is examined for faults.

Röntgen named these new rays, or radiations, X-rays, because their character and quality were unknown. The name, however, has stuck, though they are often now referred to as Röntgen rays. It is now known that they are electromagnetic vibrations of short wave-lengths (illustration 450). They are produced by accelerating electrons in an electron field between two electrodes. In practice, this process is carried out in a glass vacuum bulb containing two electrodes. This is known as an X-ray tube. The X-ray tube used today is of a type (illustrations 451, 452), in which the cathode consists of a spiral filament of incandescent tungsten, and the anode consists of massive tungsten. The essence of what happens in such a tube is that the electrons come by thermionic emission from the electrically heated filament of tungsten (the cathode) and are halted by the mass of tungsten in the anode. The X-rays are produced by the interaction of the electrons from the filament, known as the cathode stream, with the material of the 'target' or anode.

FLUORESCENT SCREEN – Fluorescence is produced in various substances by the action of X-rays, but the two most used are barium platinocyanide and calcium tungstate, one of which, sprinkled on cardboard, forms the fluorescent screen in common use. In a darkened room, if a hand be placed close against the screen, between it and the tube which is emitting the rays, the screen will appear brightly illuminated, except in the region where, owing to the obstruction of the rays, there is a faint shadow of the flesh, a denser shadow of the bones, and, if there be a ring on the finger, a still darker shadow from the ring.

Radiography – X-rays act on a sensitized photographic plate in the same manner as ordinary light, but, as they penetrate paper, the exposure can be made in daylight by enclosing the plate in a black paper envelope, through which the daylight cannot pass. It must be remembered that the X-ray photograph differs from a photograph taken by ordinary light in that it is really a shadow-picture or skiagram. A skiagram differs from an ordinary photograph in that no lens is used; the X-rays pass in parallel lines from the focus spot in the X-ray tube. For this reason X-rays cannot be focused upon the object as in ordinary photography. Briefly, in order to obtain a skiagram, the method is as follows. The plate – a rapid one – is placed first in a yellow envelope, this again in a black one, the whole being placed close beneath the part to be photographed. The tube is situated directly opposite, with the limb or other object to be photographed a little distance off, but between the tube and the plate. The tube must be arranged so that the rays fall as perpendicularly as possible on to the part. The distance of the tube from the object and the duration of exposure are matters of experience; but the farther apart they are, the less chance there is of distortion. At two metres or more the amount of distortion is practically negligible: so that when working at that distance between the anode of the tube and the surface of the film or plate, the actual size of an organ within the body can be measured. This is taken advantage of in cardiac examinations, when measurements of the size of the heart can be obtained.

450 – Spectrum of electromagnetic radiations.

451 – Diagram of a modern X-ray tube. (a) anode; (b) cathode.

In order to show the position, shape, etc., of the stomach and intestine, some radio-opaque but harmless material, such as barium sulphate is administered by mouth. This throws a dense shadow, corresponding to the interior of the organ examined, upon the screen or photographic plate. For examination of the lungs, gall-bladder, and kidneys, other opaque substances, such as harmless compounds of iodine, are injected so as to pass into their interior.

For examination of other organs, such as the brain and abdominal organs,

oxygen is sometimes injected into the cavities in the brain or the peritoneal cavity, so as to render the outlines sharper when an X-ray photograph is taken.

THE EXPOSURE IN RADIOGRAPHY – The nearer we can get to an instantaneous exposure, the clearer is the outline, especially when dealing with the abdomen or thorax. In the early days, very long exposures were required because of the very low currents available and the imperfect development of the X-ray tube. At the present time it is possible to get exposures in as short a time as $\frac{1}{100}$ of a second through the thickness of the body of an average patient.

Amongst other uses for X-rays in diagnosis attention must be called to the localization of foreign bodies in various parts of the body. For this purpose localizers of various patterns and arrangements for taking stereoscopic photographs have been devised. These are of great importance in surgery for the purpose of fixing the position of foreign bodies, like steel

452 – Dynamax rotating anode X-ray tube. GEC Medical Equipment Ltd.

chips in the eye or bullets in the body, and also give valuable aid in determining the nature and position of fractures and other injuries of the bones.

Accelerating screens made of cardboard covered with fluorescent material are sometimes used. This screen is placed in contact with the photographic plate. Being caused to glow where the light falls upon it, the screen still affects the plate after the exposure is over. When the apparatus is not powerful enough to give very short exposures, accelerating screens are used. In this way an instantaneous photograph can be made in $\frac{1}{50}$ second or less from a distance of several feet. Thus the beating heart or the contractions of the stomach in digestion can be taken in a series of flashes and demonstrated on a cinematograph film.

In view of the increasing recognition of the hazards to health from irradiation in this nuclear-energy-oriented age the X-raying of patients is being reduced to a minimum. Particularly is this so during pregnancy and in children and adolescents.

Radiotherapy, or Treatment by X-rays – The two chief sources of the ionizing radiations used in radiotherapy are the gamma rays of radium (qv) and the pene-trating X-rays generated by apparatus working at various voltages. For superficial lesions energies of around 40 kilovolts are used, but for deep-seated conditions, such as cancer of the internal organs, much higher voltages are required. X-ray machines are now in use which work at two million volts. Even higher voltages are now available through the development of the linear accelerator (illustration 453), which makes use of the frequency magnetron which is the basis of radar. The linear accelerator receives its name from the fact that it accelerates a beam of electrons down a straight tube, 3 metres in length, and in this process a voltage of eight million is attained. The use of these very high voltages has led to the development of a highly specialized technique which has been devised for the treatment of cancer and like diseases.

Like the photographic effect, the therapeutic effects were discovered almost accidentally. It was observed that prolonged exposures to the rays caused inflammation, and even ulceration of the skin, and further, that they caused loss of hair, and that they improved various diseased conditions. Repeated exposures, for example, of the hands of physicians using this method of treatment, have been observed

453 – The Dynaray 4 clinical linear accelerator. Radiation Dynamics Ltd.

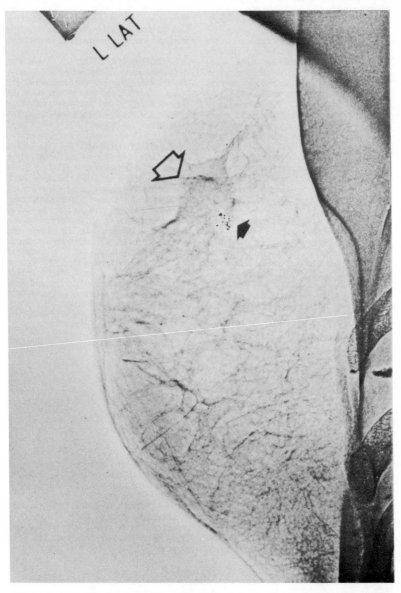

454 – Lateral xerogram of the breast. The outlined arrow shows the tumour with its strand-like extension into normal breast tissue. The solid arrow indicates calcification in the tumour. (*Understanding Cancer*, Ian Burn and Roger Meyrick, DHSS. By permission of the Controller of HMSO)

to produce pigmentation of the skin, excessive growth of its horny layer, and even epithelioma. X-rays are particularly hurtful to the testes and ovaries of young persons; and when these are exposed to the rays repeatedly, the genital glands must be covered by sheet-lead or some such protection, lest sterility result. Too severe a reaction to the irritating effect of the rays upon the patient's skin at a single sitting must also be avoided. It is important to protect the surrounding areas, and this is done by the use of masks of sheet-lead, with a hole cut out over the affected area, and by enclosing the tube in a metal-lined box, with an opening opposite the affected spot. By these means, as well as by wearing lead-lined gloves, and by frequently anointing the skin with some simple ointment, persons constantly applying the rays are effectually protected.

The greatest value of radiotherapy is in the treatment of malignant disease. In many cases it can be used for the treatment of malignant growths which are not accessible to surgery, whilst in others it is used in conjunction with surgery.

Leukaemia and other conditions, in which the spleen is enlarged, are often greatly benefited by exposure of the spleen or long bones to X-rays or radium. (See RADIOTHERAPY.)

In simple conditions, particularly superficial ones, X-rays have been used very successfully, but are being used less and less, in view of the increasing necessity to reduce to the absolute minimum the amount of irradiation to which the citizen of today is exposed.

XANTHOMA, also known as XANTHELASMA and VITILIGOIDEA, is a relatively rare skin disease in which yellow plates form in the surface of the skin, especially on the eyelids.

XENOGRAFT is a transplant from one animal to another of a different species. It is also known as a heterograft.

XERODERMA is the name applied to a rough, dry condition of the skin accompanied by the copious formation of scales.

XERODERMA PIGMENTOSUM is a rare hereditary affection of the skin appearing first in early childhood. It is characterized by a dry skin which is heavily freckled and hypersensitive to sunlight.

XEROPHTHALMIA is a dry, thickened state of the conjunctiva associated with chronic conjunctivitis, the result of deficiency of vitamin A in the diet. It is one of the four main causes of blindness in the developing world. (See EYE DISEASES AND INJURIES.)

XERORADIOGRAPHY is a method of radiography, originally used for X-raying the breast (illustration 454). It is now being used also in investigating the skull, neck and larynx. A xeroradiograph is made on an electrically charged selenium-coated aluminium plate. Exposure to an X-ray beam produces positive and negative changes in a pattern that differentiates the varying densities of anatomical structures being examined, according to the amount of absorbed radiation. When the plate is then dusted with a cloud of negatively charged blue plastic powder, an image is formed producing a vertical electrical field component with enhanced edges, which is then transferred to paper electrostatically.

XEROSIS means abnormal dryness, especially of the eye.

XEROSTOMIA is the condition of dryness of the mouth due to lack of saliva.

XIPHISTERNUM, or XIPHOID CARTILAGE, is the lowest part of the breast-bone, or sternum.

XYLITOL, or BIRCH SUGAR, is a sugar alcohol and therefore not strictly a carbohydrate. It has a very sweet taste, and occurs in fruits and mushrooms, but the commercial source is birch wood chips (hence its alternative name). There is some evidence that both it and fructose are less likely to cause caries of the teeth than sucrose.

Y

YAWNING consists of an involuntary opening of the mouth, which is accompanied by marked dilatation of the pharynx, a characteristic distortion of the face and usually stretching of the limbs. The cause and function of yawning are quite obscure. It is classically regarded as a sign of drowsiness or boredom, but it not infrequently occurs following a severe haemorrhage, and it is also sometimes associated with indigestion. An interesting feature of it is that it occurs in both birds and animals.

YAWS, known also as FRAMBOESIA and PIAN, is a disease of the tropics, especially of Africa and the West Indies, affecting both white and black races. It consists in the appearance of small tumours covered with yellow crusts, scattered over the surface of the body.

Cause – The disease is directly contagious from person to person, and the infection is probably also carried by flies, and certainly by clothing and by the unclean huts of the natives. The direct cause is a spirochaete known as *Treponema pertenue*, and the occurrence of the disease in a person of unhealthy constitution, or one who is suffering from another disease, such as syphilis or tuberculosis, renders the attack much more serious.

Symptoms – The disease does not appear for a fortnight or more after infection, and during this time fever, malaise, pains, and itching of the skin may come on. It begins as a scaly eruption about the body and legs, in which small lumps form, and grow till they reach a size even of several inches in diameter. The surface of these is covered by a yellow crust of dried-up secretion, and in unhealthy people the tumours may break down and produce deep ulcers. After a duration of weeks or months the tumours gradually shrink and disappear.

Treatment – The outlook in yaws has been transformed by the introduction of penicillin, the effects of which are dramatic in this disease.

YEAST consists of the cells and spores of unicellular fungi belonging to the family of Saccharomycetaceae. The main species of yeast used in medicine is *Saccharomyces cerevisiae*, which is used in the fermentation industries, such as brewing. It is a rich source of the vitamin B complex (see VITA-MIN), but its use has largely been given up since the various components of the vitamin B complex became available as separate entities.

YELLOW FEVER, also known as YELLOW JACK and VOMITO AMARILLI, is an acute disease of certain tropical localities, characterized by fever and jaundice.

Distribution – It is endemic in Africa from coast to coast south of the Sahara to Northern Rhodesia. It also occurs in the northern part of South America and to a less extent today in Central America. In 1793 a very serious epidemic spread over the Northern United States, and, in Philadelphia alone, over 10 per cent of the population were swept off in the course of four months. Numerous other epidemics invaded the States in the end of the eighteenth and during the course of the nineteenth centuries, the last severe one taking place in 1878. In Europe the disease has from time to time invaded some of the Portuguese and Spanish ports, but it has never gained any permanent hold. When cases of yellow fever arrive at British or other northern European ports, no spread of the disease takes place. It is also unknown in the Far East.

Causes – The disease is due to a virus which is transmitted to man by the *Aedes aegypti* mosquito (illustration 455). Monkeys are an important reservoir of infection in areas where the disease is endemic. The virus is found in the blood of infected individuals during the first three

455 – *Aedes aegypti* (female). The transmitter of yellow fever and dengue. From Manson's *Tropical Diseases*.

or four days of the disease. The blood of a patient is directly infectious, and the deaths of three of the great investigators of the disease, Stokes, Noguchi, and Young, all of whom died of yellow fever, were probably due to direct contact with infected blood.

One attack gives more or less protection for life. Many adult natives in yellow fever areas therefore are protected against reinfection by having had the disease in childhood. In affected areas babies born to immune mothers are protected against the disease for several months.

Symptoms – Different cases vary greatly in severity, but the disease is apt to be especially serious during the prevalence of an epidemic, or when it affects persons newly arrived from healthier parts. The incubation period is usually 3 to 5 days, but may be up to 10 days.

Three stages are usually described in a severe case. The *first stage* begins suddenly with headache, chill, pains in the back and limbs, and rise of temperature. The eyes are bloodshot. Vomiting also occurs, the tongue is furred, and the bowels are constipated. An important point is that the urine decreases in amount, and, if tested, is found to contain albumin, the result of inflammation of the kidneys. The degree in which these signs are present forms a valuable indication of the severity of the case and of the need for special treatment.

These symptoms last for about three days and then sometimes abate to some extent for a day and the patient appears better. This constitutes the *second stage*.

The *third stage* begins usually about the fourth day. The patient now becomes very weak and the black vomit comes on. This consists in bringing up constantly from the stomach a clear fluid containing black flakes formed of blood that has been acted upon by the gastric juice. Although this black vomit is regarded as an alarming sign, it is by no means an index that the patient is sure to die. Jaundice also appears with the third stage, and is the symptom to which the disease owes its name. Usually it amounts only to a pale yellow discoloration of the skin, but it may become mahogany brown in hue, and small haemorrhages under the skin and mucous membranes are also common. In fatal cases examined after death, the principal changes found are fatty degeneration of the liver, acute inflammation of the kidneys, and an inflamed and congested state of the stomach, which contains some of the black fluid mentioned above.

Treatment – PREVENTIVE TREATMENT is important, and consists of vaccination of everyone travelling to and from those parts of the world where the disease occurs. Such vaccination is compulsory, not only for the inhabitants of endemic zones and for travellers going to these areas, but, in addition, many countries outside endemic areas require that travellers who have come from, or have passed through, yellow fever areas shall have been vaccinated. The protection it gives comes on within ten days and is long-lasting, but it is wise for residents in yellow-fever areas to have it repeated every ten years. The sick must be kept for the first three days of illness in rooms protected by mosquito-netting, so that they may not infect mosquitoes which would pass on the disease to healthy persons. The same general measures as in the case of malaria should be taken against mosquitoes.

CURATIVE TREATMENT must be directed towards checking symptoms as they arise. Vomiting is allayed by sucking ice or sipping iced water, and by the administration of dilute hydrocyanic acid in doses of two drops in water. Food should be, to a great extent, withheld in the early stage, but the patient must have plenty of water in small draughts, containing glucose, and flavoured with lime, orange, or grapefruit juice. Later on, the only food should be milk, thin soups, and similar liquid nourishment. When the patient is greatly prostrated, alcohol may be given, and, of this, champagne is the most approved form. The high temperature, which sometimes shows itself, is relieved by sponging or by the wet pack. One of the most important symptoms to treat is stoppage of the urine, and for this hot-air baths are employed, as in acute Bright's disease.

YERSINIA is a genus of bacteria which includes the causative organism of plague, *Yersinia pestis.*

YOGHURT is the name applied to sour milk curdled with one of the lactic-acid producing bacilli, such as *Lactobacillus acidophilus* or *Lactobacillus bulgaricus*. It contains all the protein, fat, calcium, and vitamins of the original milk, and is therefore a nutritious food, but there is no evidence that it has any unique beneficial properties of its own. In countries where standards of hygiene are low it has the advantage of having been sterilized by boiling and is therefore unlikely to be contaminated with dangerous micro-organisms.

Z

ZANDER APPARATUS is a collection of machines devised by J. G. W. Zander, a Swedish physician, for permitting within the limits of a gymnasium various active forms of exercise usually attainable only out of doors. It includes devices for exercising the muscles employed in rowing, those used in bicycling and horseback riding, as well as apparatus for moving individual joints and so increasing their suppleness after injury or disease.

ZINC is a metal, several salts of which are used in medicine for external application. It is essential for growth and development in animals and plants. The average human body contains a total of 1 to 2 grams, and most human diets contain 10 to 15 mg. Oysters are reputed to be a rich source. In human beings, deficiency of zinc results in lack of growth, slow sexual development and anaemia. Such a condition has been reported in Iran and the Middle East. In pigs zinc deficiency produces the condition known as parakeratosis, characterized by dermatitis, diarrhoea and vomiting.

Uses – Zinc chloride is a powerful caustic and astringent which, combined with zinc sulphate, is used as an astringent mouth-wash. Zinc sulphate is also used in the form of eye-drops in the treatment of certain forms of conjunctivitis. (See EYE DISEASES AND INJURIES.) At one time widely used as an emetic it is seldom used for this purpose now.

Zinc oxide, zinc stearate, and zinc carbonate are made up in dusting powders, in ointments, or suspended in water as lotions for the astringent action they exert upon abraded surfaces of the skin. Zinc and castor oil ointment of the *British Pharmacopoeia* is a well-tried treatment for napkin rash.

Zinc undecenoate is used as an ointment and as a dusting-powder in the treatment of ringworm (qv).

ZONA and ZOSTER are two names for the eruption popularly known as shingles. (See HERPES.)

ZONULOLYSIS is the process whereby the ciliary zonule, which is the suspensory ligament of the lens of the eye, is lysed, or digested, by chymotrypsin, which is an enzyme obtained from mammalian pancreas. Zonulolysis is now being used as an aid in cataract surgery.

ZOONOSES are animal diseases which can be transmitted to man. There are over 150 infections of domestic and wild vertebrates which can be transmitted in this way, including bovine tuberculosis, brucellosis, hydatid cysts, ringworm, toxocariasis, toxoplasmosis, leptospirosis, listeriasis, and rabies. (See separate entries for details of these diseases.)

ZYGOMA is the name given to a bridge of bone formed by the union of a process from the temporal bone with one from the malar bone. It lies in the region of the temple, gives attachment to the powerful masseter muscle which moves the lower jaw, and forms a protection to the side of the head.

ZYMOTIC DISEASES is an old term for the acute infectious maladies. As originally employed by Dr. Farr of the Registrar-General's department, the term included the diseases which were 'epidemic, endemic, and contagious', and owed their origin to the presence of some morbific principle in the system acting in a manner analogous to, although not identical with, the process of fermentation. A very large number of diseases were accordingly included under this designation. The term, however, came to be restricted to the chief fevers and contagious diseases (eg. typhus and typhoid fevers, smallpox, scarlet fever, measles, erysipelas, cholera, whooping-cough, diphtheria), but is seldom used nowadays, on account of the theory which it suggests.